D1759117

BRITISH MEDICAL ASSOCIATION
1003541

Complications in Neurosurgery

"asato mā sadgamaya
tamasomā jyotir gamaya
mrityormāamritam gamaya
"From ignorance, lead me to truth;
From darkness, lead me to light;
From death, lead me to immortality

Brihadaranyaka Upanishad. [700 BC]

To my wife, Laura, my children, Alexander, Christopher and Mary Catherine.
and to my mother, Uma Nanda and late father Dr. K.G.S.Nanda

Complications in Neurosurgery

Anil Nanda, MD, MPH, FACS

Professor and Chairman, Department of Neurosurgery
Rutgers-Robert Wood Johnson Medical School
Professor and Chairman, Department of Neurosurgery
Rutgers-New Jersey Medical School
Senior Vice President of Neurosurgical Services
RWJBarnabas Health

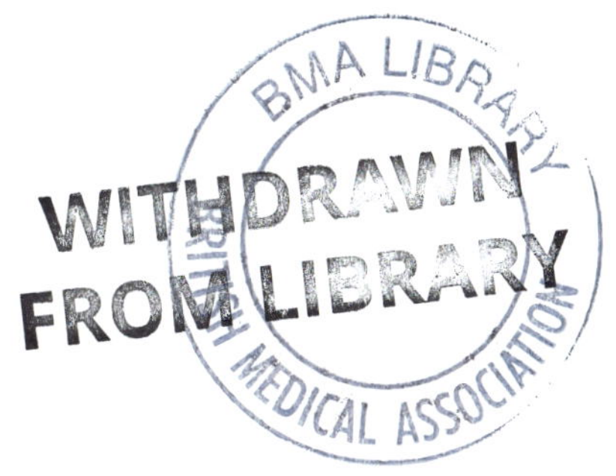

For additional online content visit ExpertConsult.com

ELSEVIER

Edinburgh London New York Oxford Philadelphia St Louis Sydney 2019

ELSEVIER

Notices

Practitioners and researchers must always rely on their own experience and knowledge in evaluating and using any information, methods, compounds or experiments described herein. Because of rapid advances in the medical sciences, in particular, independent verification of diagnoses and drug dosages should be made. To the fullest extent of the law, no responsibility is assumed by Elsevier, authors, editors or contributors for any injury and/or damage to persons or property as a matter of products liability, negligence or otherwise, or from any use or operation of any methods, products, instructions, or ideas contained in the material herein.

Although all advertising material is expected to conform to ethical (medical) standards, inclusion in this publication does not constitute a guarantee or endorsement of the quality or the value of such product or the claims made of it by its manufacturer.

ISBN: 978-0-323-50961-9

Content Strategist: Belinda Kuhn
Content Development Specialist: Trinity Hutton
Project Manager: Joanna Souch
Design: Brian Salisbury
Illustration Manager: Amy Naylor
Marketing Manager: Melissa Fogarty

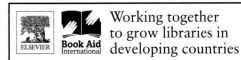

Printed in China

Last digit is the print number: 9 8 7 6 5 4 3 2 1

Contents

Section 3: Spinal and Peripheral Nerve Surgery Complications

General and Degenerative Spinal Disease Surgery Complications

Spinal Neoplastic and Vascular Lesion Surgery Complications

Spinal Trauma and Peripheral Nerve Surgery Complications

Foreword

I am truly honored to be asked by Dr. Nanda to write the foreword for this important comprehensive text on neurosurgical complications. Dr. Nanda is in a particularly advantageous position to edit this book because he is one of the few neurosurgeons of his generation that, while achieving true technical mastership in some of the most difficult neurosurgical specialties such as skull base and neurovascular surgery, continues to accumulate vast experience in practically all areas of neurosurgery. It is also appropriate that he edits and personally writes a good portion of this book because of his well-earned reputation for honest assessment and discussion of his complications. To watch a master surgeon like Anil operating on a difficult petroclival meningioma or basilar aneurysm and to hear of his excellent results leaves us in awe of his virtuosity and with admiration and not infrequently envy of his results. However, to hear an honest and thoughtful discussion of his complications and possible ways to avoid them educates us and makes us better and safer neurosurgeons to the advantage of our future patients.

I am not sure if Dr. Nanda asked me to write this foreword because of the quantity and variety of complications that I have encountered in my career or because he may have heard me say that of the papers and chapters I have written in neurosurgery the ones that have given me the most pride and satisfaction have been those I have written about my own complications. These writings have certainly not been frequently quoted and have not significantly contributed to my "quotation index" but, much more importantly, have not infrequently led to a colleague stopping me in a meeting to thank me for having written about that personal complication and how I could have avoided it. This led him to prevent this complication and result in a good outcome on a patient he recently encountered. I am sure that any of us would rather hear that comment than hear somebody telling us "Wow, I was so impressed by those wonderful results you reported in that recent paper."

I teach my residents that there are three levels where complications should be discussed. The first level is at the time when they occur, which in our case is usually at surgery. When we make the wrong move, which results in massive rupture of the aneurysm, there is no point in telling our assisting resident, hopefully after the situation was controlled, that the rupture resulted from "bad luck" or "abnormal anatomy". Much better is to discuss exactly what was the mistake made and how it could have been avoided; this the resident will not forget. The next level to discuss complications is at morbidity and mortality conference. I have always advocated for a brutally open and honest discussion of complications which has frequently not been popular with my colleagues. By giving our colleagues the opportunity to hear about our complications it offers them the opportunity to learn from them and avoid them in their own future practice. It would be a sad thing if the only complications that we could learn from were our own. Much safer for our patients is that we learn not only from our complications but also from those of others. The third level to discuss complications is to talk about them in formal lectures and write about them in papers, chapters or in a comprehensive text of which I am sure this one will be a model.

This foreword is just that and it is not a book review so I will not make it insufferably long by describing the contents of the book in detail. Suffice it to say that the list of senior authors of each chapter compiled by the editor reads like a "who is who" of American neurosurgery and, for good measure, Dr. Nanda has also included contributions from several international neurosurgical eminences. Of the chapters that Dr. Nanda has contributed himself, I particularly enjoyed reading the proofs of his first chapter "Historical Perspective". In his uniquely elegant and scholarly fashion Anil begins the chapter by telling us that the first punishment for surgical complications was spelled out in the Code of Hammurabi, a Babylonian king of the 17th century BC. Fortunately, the punishment he decreed for surgical complications was not as severe as that for stealing which was death! What a lovely historical pearl!

I know that this book will make us better neurosurgeons. I could not imagine that the library of any conscientious colleague would be complete without it. Congratulations Anil!

Roberto C. Heros

Preface

"This above all: to thine own self be true.
And it must follow, as the night the day,
Thou canst not be false to any man."
William Shakespeare
Hamlet: Act 1, Scene 3

The great Roman, Seneca, has contributed richly to the world's aphorisms. Shakespeare provided an English translation of one of Seneca's most quoted guidelines for professional conduct. This aphorism about not being false to any man extends to our surgical sphere and is the Magna Carta of our art, our profession, and our oath.

I am delighted to welcome you to a book solely focused on complications. One might ask, why? As someone put it best, "Victory has a thousand fathers and defeat is an orphan." Too often in our specialty, we inflate our bravado to talk about triumphs and too little of the klieg light is focused on our failures. I remember as a young attending going to a major meeting where a prominent surgeon said that all his patients went home after an acoustic neuroma on post-op day two. I felt incomplete and inadequate, since most of my patients were still in the ICU. But I think it is important to talk about this. We have taken an entire textbook and devoted it to the different facets of complications.

On a theological note, talking about your worst-case disaster can be almost like a religious experience. In the Jewish faith, they talk about *cheshbon hanefesh*, a personal accounting about what has gone wrong. As my Catholic wife would remind me, *mea maxima culpa* is one of the cornerstones of Catholicism. So, to improve your surgical karma, it is most important to look at complications with complete dispassion and honesty, learn what went wrong, and most importantly, share what happened with others so if they go down that path they are guided and may perhaps find their way out of these dark corners.

Much like Odysseus on his perilous journey home to Ithaca, we take you through a veritable odyssey of complications. We begin with section one, the history of complications, all the way from the Code of Hammurabi almost 4000 years ago, where you would lose your hand if you had a mortality – something most of us would dread since we all confront surgical mortalities – through the Renaissance and Victorian times, where Robert Liston had a 300 percent mortality when the patient, his assistant, and an observer died in the same operation! In the general chapters, we have looked at wrong level disc-surgery, wrong-side craniotomies, post-op hematomas (both in the back and spine), the medical legal aspects, and how, in fact, surgical consent has been framed by certain landmark neurosurgical cases. Section two is mainly cranial complications, which are divided into vascular and endovascular, as well as skull base, primary brain tumors, and functional neurosurgery. Section three is focused on spine and peripheral nerve complications, including adjacent level disc disease, graft related complications, neurological deteriorations, as well as vascular injuries during approaches to the spine. The contributing authors have done a great job providing us with surgical pearls and a neurosurgical "selfie" moment with their worst-case disasters

As a resident and young attending, Dr. Charles Drake's brutal honesty, in terms of complications, was inspirational and the gold standard for all of us. In this generation, I think that mantle has been carried by Dr. Roberto Heros, with his unabashed honesty while talking about his complications with AVMs, aneurysms, and other topics. I feel privileged that he agreed to write the foreword to this book. He has been an incredible mentor and a blessing to so many of us. I am deeply grateful to him.

An offering of this sort is never an individual work, but it has been an amazing team effort. I am deeply indebted to the fellows in my department who have richly contributed to this book, including Dr. Amey Savardekar, Dr. Devi Patra, Dr. Vinayak Narayan, Dr. Bhavani Kura, and Dr. Mohammed Nasser. I am also grateful to my PA, Alice Edwards, and editorial assistant, Cody Hanna, as well as Belinda Kuhn and Trinity Hutton from Elsevier, who were a pleasure to work with. Lastly, I am deeply indebted to my wife, Laura, and my children, Alexander, Christopher, and Mary Catherine, who have always inspired me and reminded me about what is truly important in life. Their love and affection have always sustained me.

In the end, as American poet John Berryman wrote in "Dream Song," "I am obliged to perform in complete darkness operations of great delicacy on myself." This offering is a book about mistakes and how to avoid them, with the hope that it benefits all of us and makes the profession stronger, deeper, and richer.

Anil Nanda, MD, MPH, FACS
Professor and Chairman, Department of Neurosurgery
Rutgers-Robert Wood Johnson Medical School
Professor and Chairman, Department of Neurosurgery
Rutgers-New Jersey Medical School
Senior Vice President of Neurosurgical Services
RWJBarnabas Health

List of Contributors

Muhammad M. Abd-El-Barr, MD, PhD
Assistant Professor
Department of Neurosurgery
Duke University School of Medicine
Durham, NC, USA
53. Vascular Complications in Cervical Spine Surgery (Anterior and Posterior Approach)

Vijay Agarwal, MD
Assistant Professor
Neurosurgery
Mayo Clinic
Rochester, MN, USA
20. Primary Brain Lesion Resection Complications: An Overview and Malignant Brain Swelling After Resection of Superior Sagittal Sinus Meningioma

Felipe C. Albuquerque, MD
Director, Endovascular Surgery
Professor of Neurosurgery
Department of Neurosurgery
Barrow Neurological Institute
St. Joseph's Hospital and Medical Center
Phoenix, AZ, USA
40. Procedure-Related Complications of Aneurysm Treatment: Intraprocedural Rupture, Thromboembolic Events, Coil Migration or Prolapse Into Parent Artery, and Recurrent Aneurysm Management

Hamidreza Aliabadi, MD, FAANS
Clinical Associate Faculty
Department of Neurological Surgery
University of California, San Francisco
San Francisco, CA, USA
Assistant Clinical Professor
California Northstate University College of Medicine
Elk Grove, CA, USA
Spine and Neurosurgery Associates
Roseville, CA, USA
30. Complications Associated With Cerebrospinal Fluid Diversion

Yasir Al-Khalili, MD
Chief Resident
Department of Neurology
Drexel Neurosciences Institute
Philadelphia, PA, USA
42. Procedure-Related Complications: Stroke

Rami O. Almefty, MD
Neurosurgery Resident
Barrow Neurological Institute
St. Joseph's Hospital and Medical Center
Phoenix, AZ, USA
59. Complications of Surgery for Spinal Vascular Malformations

Sepideh Amin-Hanjani, MD, FAANS, FACS, FAHA
Professor & Program Director
Co-Director, Neurovascular Surgery
Department of Neurosurgery
University of Illinois at Chicago
Chicago, IL, USA
12. Complications of Cerebral Bypass Surgery

Filippo F. Angileri, MD, PhD
Associate Professor of Neurosurgery
Department of Biomedical and Dental Sciences and Morphofunctional Imaging
University of Messina
AOU Policlinico "G. Martino"
Messina, Italy
16. Complications in Anterior Cranial Fossa Surgery

Cinta Arraez, MD
Department of Neurosurgery
Carlos Haya University Hospital
Malaga, Spain
13. Complications of the Surgery for Cavernomas

Miguel A. Arraez, Sr., MD, PhD
Professor and Chairman
Department of Neurosurgery
Carlos Haya University Hospital
Malaga, Spain
13. Complications of the Surgery for Cavernomas

Jacob F. Baranoski, MD
Neurosurgery Resident
Barrow Neurological Institute
St. Joseph's Hospital and Medical Center
Phoenix, AZ, USA
40. Procedure-Related Complications of Aneurysm Treatment: Intraprocedural Rupture, Thromboembolic Events, Coil Migration or Prolapse Into Parent Artery, and Recurrent Aneurysm Management

Daniel L. Barrow, MD
Pamela R. Rollins Professor and Chairman
Director, Emory MBNA Stroke Center
Department of Neurosurgery
Emory University School of Medicine
Atlanta, GA, USA
9. Intraoperative Rupture and Parent Artery Injury During Aneurysm Surgery

Bernard R. Bendok, MD
Professor and Chair
Department of Neurosurgery
Mayo Clinic
Rochester, MN, USA
39. Access-Related Complications in Endovascular Neurosurgery

Edward C. Benzel, MD
Emeritus Chair of Neurosurgery
Cleveland Clinic
Cleveland, OH, USA
48. Complications in Neurosurgery—Graft-Related Complications (Autograft, BMP, Synthetic)

Mitchel S. Berger, MD
Professor and Chairman
Berthold and Belle N. Guggenhime Endowed Chair
Department of Neurological Surgery
University of California, San Francisco
San Francisco, CA, USA
23. Thalamic and Insular Tumors: Minimizing Deficits

Indira Devi Bhagavatula, MS, MCh
Professor
Department of Neurosurgery
NIMHANS
Bangalore, India
25. Complications Associated With Surgery for Intracranial Infectious Lesions: Brain Abscess, Tuberculosis, Hydatid Disease, Neurocysticercosis

Dhananjaya I. Bhat, MCh
Professor
Department of Neurosurgery
NIMHANS
Bangalore, India
25. Complications Associated With Surgery for Intracranial Infectious Lesions: Brain Abscess, Tuberculosis, Hydatid Disease, Neurocysticercosis

Mark Bilsky, MD
Attending Neurosurgeon
Department of Neurosurgery
Memorial Sloan Kettering Cancer Center
Professor
Department of Neurosurgery
Weill Medical College of Cornell University
New York, NY, USA
60. Complications of Surgery and Radiosurgery in Spinal Metastasis

Mandy J. Binning, MD
Assistant Professor
Department of Neurosurgery
Drexel Neurosciences Institute
Philadelphia, PA, USA
42. Procedure-Related Complications: Stroke

Frederick A. Boop, MD
Professor and Chairman
Department of Neurosurgery
University of Tennessee Health Sciences Center
Memphis, TN, USA
28. Complications of Posterior Fossa Tumors: Ependymoma/Medulloblastoma/Pilocytic Astrocytoma

Alexa N. Bramall, MD, PhD
Neurosurgery Resident
Department of Neurosurgery
Duke University
Durham, NC, USA
21. Complications After Glioma Surgery

Jeffrey N. Bruce, MD
Edgar M. Housepian Professor of Neurological Surgery
Vice Chairman of Academic Affairs
Neurological Surgery
New York-Presbyterian Columbia University Medical Center
New York, NY, USA
24. Complications of Surgery for Pineal Region Tumors

Avery L. Buchholz, MD, MPH
Fellow
Neurological Surgery
University of Virginia
Charlottesville, VA, USA
55. Postoperative Spinal Deformities: Kyphosis, Nonunion, and Loss of Motion Segment

Kim J. Burchiel, MD
Professor and Head
Division of Functional Neurosurgery
Oregon Health and Science University
Portland, OR, USA
33. Complications of Deep Brain Stimulation (DBS)
34. Complications After Epilepsy Surgery

Jan-Karl Burkhardt, MD
Fellow
Department of Neurological Surgery
University of California, San Francisco
San Francisco, CA, USA
11. Complications of AVM Microsurgery; Steal Phenomenon and Management of Residual AVM

Salvatore M. Cardali, MD, PhD
Associate Professor of Neurosurgery
Department of Biomedical and Dental Sciences and Morphofunctional Imaging
University of Messina
AOU Policlinico "G. Martino"
Messina, Italy
16. Complications in Anterior Cranial Fossa Surgery

Hsuan-Kan Chang, MD
University of Miami
Miller School of Medicine
Miami, FL, USA
School of Medicine
National Yang-Ming University
Taipei, Taiwan
56. Complications of Minimally Invasive Spinal Surgery

Fady T. Charbel, MD, FAANS, FACS
Head, Department of Neurosurgery
Richard L. and Gertrude W. Fruin Professor
University of Illinois at Chicago
Chicago, IL, USA
12. Complications of Cerebral Bypass Surgery

Yi-Ren Chen, MD, MPH
Clinical Instructor and Fellow in Spine Surgery
Department of Neurosurgery
Stanford University School of Medicine
Stanford, CA, USA
62. Posttraumatic Syringomyelia

Jimmy Ming-Jung Chuang, MD
Assistant Professor
Department of Neurosurgery
Kaohsiung Chang Gang Memorial Hospital
Kaohsiung City, Taiwan
28. Complications of Posterior Fossa Tumors: Ependymoma/Medulloblastoma/Pilocytic Astrocytoma

Alan R. Cohen, MD
Chief of Pediatric Neurosurgery
Professor of Neurosurgery, Oncology and Pediatrics
Carson-Spiro Professor of Pediatric Neurosurgery
Johns Hopkins University School of Medicine
Baltimore, MA, USA
38. Complications of Ventricular Endoscopy

Alfredo Conti, MD, PhD
Associate Professor of Neurosurgery
Department of Biomedical and Dental Sciences and Morphofunctional Imaging
University of Messina
AOU Policlinico "G. Martino"
Messina, Italy
16. Complications in Anterior Cranial Fossa Surgery

Brian M. Corliss, MD
Fellow - Neuro-Endovascular Surgery
Department of Neurological Surgery
University of Florida
Gainesville, FL, USA
41. Procedure-Related Complications: AVMs

Randy S. D'Amico, MD
Neurological Surgery
New York-Presbyterian Columbia University Medical Center
New York, NY, USA
24. Complications of Surgery for Pineal Region Tumors

Roy Thomas Daniel, MCh
Professor
Neurosurgery
Lausanne University Hospital
Lausanne, Switzerland
45. Complications After Surgery for Chronic Subdural Hematomas

Stephanie A. DeCarvalho, BS
Department of Neurosurgery
Brigham and Women's Hospital
Boston, MA, USA
53. Vascular Complications in Cervical Spine Surgery (Anterior and Posterior Approach)

Anthony M. Digiorgio, DO, MHA
Resident
Department of Neurological Surgery
Louisiana State University Health Sciences Center
New Orleans, LA, USA
47. Adjacent Level Disc Degeneration and Pseudarthrosis

Kyle M. Fargen, MD, MPH
Assistant Professor
Department of Neurological Surgery
Wake Forest University
Winston-Salem, NC, USA
14. Complication of Carotid Endarterectomy

Michael G. Fehlings, MD, PhD, FRCSC, FACS
Professor of Neurosurgery
Vice Chair Research
Department of Surgery
University of Toronto
Head, Spinal Program
Toronto Western Hospital
University Health Network
Toronto, ON, Canada
50. Complications of Surgery at the Craniocervical Junction

Juan C. Fernandez-Miranda, MD
Associate Professor
Department of Neurological Surgery
University of Pittsburgh School of Medicine
Pittsburgh, PA, USA
36. Complications of Endoscopic Endonasal Skull Base Surgery

Bruno C. Flores, MD
Neurosurgery Fellow, Endovascular
Barrow Neurological Institute
St. Joseph's Hospital and Medical Center
Phoenix, AZ, USA
40. Procedure-Related Complications of Aneurysm Treatment: Intraprocedural Rupture, Thromboembolic Events, Coil Migration or Prolapse Into Parent Artery, and Recurrent Aneurysm Management

Jared Fridley, MD
Assistant Professor
Department of Neurosurgery
Rhode Island Hospital
Providence, RI, USA
58. Complications of Surgery for Vertebral Body Tumors

Allan Friedman, MD
Guy Odom Professor
Department of Neurosurgery
Duke University
Durham, NC, USA
21. Complications After Glioma Surgery

Michael A. Galgano, MD
Department of Neurosurgery
Brown University
Providence, RI, USA
58. Complications of Surgery for Vertebral Body Tumors

Mario Ganau, MD, PhD, FEBNS, FACS
Fellow in Complex Spine Surgery
University of Toronto
Toronto, ON, Canada
50. Complications of Surgery at the Craniocervical Junction

Paul A. Gardner, MD
Associate Professor
Department of Neurological Surgery
University of Pittsburgh School of Medicine
Pittsburgh, PA, USA
36. Complications of Endoscopic Endonasal Skull Base Surgery

Antonino F. Germanò, MD
Professor and Chairman of Neurosurgery
Department of Biomedical and Dental Sciences and Morphofunctional Imaging
University of Messina
AOU Policlinico "G. Martino"
Messina, Italy
16. Complications in Anterior Cranial Fossa Surgery

George M. Ghobrial, MD
Neurosurgeon
Novant Health Brain and Spine Surgery
Winston Salem, NC, USA
56. Complications of Minimally Invasive Spinal Surgery

Siraj Gibani, MD
Clinical Instructor, Spine Surgery
Department of Neurosurgery
Stanford University
Stanford, CA, USA
62. Posttraumatic Syringomyelia

John L. Gillick, MD
Assistant Professor
Department of Neurological Surgery
Rutgers-New Jersey Medical School
Newark, NJ, USA
54. Instrumentation-Related Complications

Ziya L. Gokaslan, MD, FAANS, FACS
Gus Stoll, MD Professor and Chair, Department of Neurosurgery
The Warren Alpert Medical School of Brown University
Neurosurgeon-in-Chief, Rhode Island Hospital and The Miriam Hospital
Clinical Director, Norman Prince Neurosciences Institute
President, Brown Neurosurgery Foundation
Rhode Island Hospital
Department of Neurosurgery
Norman Prince Neurosciences Institute
Providence, RI, USA
58. Complications of Surgery for Vertebral Body Tumors

M. Reid Gooch, MD
Assistant Professor
Department of Neurological Surgery
Thomas Jefferson University
Philadelphia, PA, USA
43. Complications in Endovascular Management of Carotid-Cavernous and Dural Arteriovenous Fistulas

Gerald A. Grant, MD
Associate Professor
Department of Neurosurgery
Stanford University School of Medicine
Stanford, CA, USA
30. Complications Associated With Cerebrospinal Fluid Diversion

Fabio Grassia, MD
Neurosurgery Resident
Department of Neurosurgery
University of Milan
San Gerardo Hospital
Monza, Italy
34. Complications After Epilepsy Surgery

Michael W. Groff, MD
Vice-Chairman
Department of Neurosurgery
Brigham and Women's Hospital
Harvard Medical School
Boston, MA, USA
53. Vascular Complications in Cervical Spine Surgery (Anterior and Posterior Approach)

Andrew J. Grossbach, MD
Assistant Professor
Department of Neurosurgery
The Ohio State University
Columbus, OH, USA
51. Neurologic Deterioration After Spinal Surgery

James S. Harrop, MD
Professor, Departments of Neurological and Orthopedic Surgery
Director, Division of Spine and Peripheral Nerve Surgery
Neurosurgery Director of Delaware Valley SCI Center
Thomas Jefferson University
Philadelphia, PA, USA
54. Instrumentation-Related Complications

Robert F. Heary, MD
Professor
Department of Neurological Surgery
Rutgers-New Jersey Medical School
Newark, NJ, USA
61. Spinal Fracture Complications

Hirad S. Hedayat, MD
Assistant Professor
Department of Neurosurgery
Drexel Neurosciences Institute
Philadelphia, PA, USA
42. Procedure-Related Complications: Stroke

Carl B. Heilman, MD
Chairman and Professor
Tufts University School of Medicine
Boston, MA, USA
18. Complications in Posterior Cranial Fossa Surgery

Robert S. Heller, MD
Resident
Department of Neurosurgery
Tufts University School of Medicine
Boston, MA, USA
18. Complications in Posterior Cranial Fossa Surgery

Vernard S. Fennell, MD, MSc
Endovascular Neurosurgery Fellow
Department of Neurosurgery
Jacobs School of Medicine and Biomedical Sciences University at Buffalo
Department of Neurosurgery
Gates Vascular Institute at Kaleida Health
Buffalo, NY, USA
10. Cerebral Vasospasm: Complications and Avoidance

Shawn L. Hervey-Jumper, MD
Associate Professor
Department of Neurological Surgery
University of California, San Francisco
San Francisco, CA, USA
23. Thalamic and Insular Tumors: Minimizing Deficits

Brian L. Hoh, MD
James and Brigitte Marino Family Professor
Department of Neurosurgery
University of Florida
Gainesville, FL, USA
41. Procedure-Related Complications: AVMs

Brian M. Howard, MD
Cerebrovascular Fellow
Department of Neurosurgery
Emory University School of Medicine
Atlanta, GA, USA
9. Intraoperative Rupture and Parent Artery Injury During Aneurysm Surgery

Joshua D. Hughes, MD
Chief Resident Associate
Neurologic Surgery
Mayo Clinic
Rochester, MN, USA
26. Management of Facial Nerve Injury in Vestibular Schwannoma

Ibrahim Hussain, MD
Resident
Department of Neurological Surgery
Weill Cornell Medical Center—New York Presbyterian Hospital
New York, NY, USA
60. Complications of Surgery and Radiosurgery in Spinal Metastasis

Corrado Iaccarino, MD
Neurosurgery-Neurotraumatology
University Hospital of Parma
Parma, Italy
45. Complications After Surgery for Chronic Subdural Hematomas

M. Omar Iqbal, MD
Resident Physician
Department of Neurological Surgery
Rutgers University
Newark, NJ, USA
61. Spinal Fracture Complications

Rashad Jabarkheel, MD
Medical Student
Stanford University School of Medicine
Stanford, CA, USA
62. Posttraumatic Syringomyelia

Darnell T. Josiah, MD, MS
Assistant Professor
Department of Neurosurgery
University of Wisconsin Hospitals and Clinics
Madison, WI, USA
49. Procedure-Related Complications (Inadvertent Dural Tear, CSF Leak)

Piyush Kalakoti, MD
Spine Research Fellow
University of Iowa Hospitals & Clinics
Iowa City, IA, USA
4. Medical Complications in Neurosurgery
34. Complications After Epilepsy Surgery

Joseph R. Keen, DO
Clinical Professor
Department of Neurosurgery
Ochsner Medical Center
New Orleans, LA, USA
22. Complications of Surgery for Pituitary Tumors

William J. Kemp, MD
Resident
Department of Neurosurgery
Cleveland Clinic Foundation
Cleveland, OH, USA
48. Complications in Neurosurgery—Graft-Related Complications (Autograft, BMP, Synthetic)

Irene Kim, MD
Assistant Professor
Department of Neurosurgery
Medical College of Wisconsin
Milwaukee, WI, USA
31. Complications After Myelomeningocele Repair: CSF Leak and Retethering

Bhavani Kura, MD
Fellow
Department of Neurosurgery
LSUHSC
Shreveport, LA, USA
1. Historical Perspective
19. Complications of Chiari Malformation Surgery

Domenico La Torre, MD, PhD
Associate Professor of Neurosurgery
Department of Biomedical and Dental Sciences and Morphofunctional Imaging
University of Messina
AOU Policlinico "G. Martino"
Messina, Italy
16. Complications in Anterior Cranial Fossa Surgery

Michael J. Lang, MD
Cerebrovascular Fellow
Department of Neurosurgery
Thomas Jefferson University
Philadelphia, PA, USA
43. Complications in Endovascular Management of Carotid-Cavernous and Dural Arteriovenous Fistulas

Ilya Laufer, MD
Associate Attending
Department of Neurosurgery
Memorial Sloan Kettering Cancer Center
Associate Professor
Weill Cornell Medical College
New York, NY, USA
60. Complications of Surgery and Radiosurgery in Spinal Metastasis

Michael T. Lawton, MD
Professor & Chairman, Department of Neurosurgery
President & CEO, Barrow Neurological Institute
Chief of Vascular & Skull Base Neurosurgery
Robert F. Spetzler Endowed Chair in Neurosciences
Barrow Neurological Institute
Phoenix, AZ, USA
11. Complications of AVM Microsurgery; Steal Phenomenon and Management of Residual AVM

Elad I. Levy, MD, MBA
Professor and L. Nelson Hopkins II MD Chair of Neurosurgery and Professor of Radiology
Jacobs School of Medicine and Biomedical Sciences University at Buffalo
Medical Director, Neuroendovascular Services
Gates Vascular Institute at Kaleida Health
Buffalo, NY, USA
10. Cerebral Vasospasm: Complications and Avoidance

Michael J. Link, MD
Professor
Neurologic Surgery
Mayo Clinic
Rochester, MN, USA
20. Primary Brain Lesion Resection Complications: An Overview and Malignant Brain Swelling After Resection of Superior Sagittal Sinus Meningioma
26. Management of Facial Nerve Injury in Vestibular Schwannoma

William B. Lo, MBBChir, FRCS(SN), FEBNS
Fellow in Pediatric Neurosurgery
Division of Neurosurgery
Hospital for Sick Children
Toronto, ON, Canada
29. Craniopharyngioma: Complications After Microsurgery

L. Dade Lunsford, MD
Lars Leksell Professor of Neurological Surgery
Distinguished Professor of Neurological Surgery
University of Pittsburgh
Director, Center for Image Guided Neurosurgery & Neurosurgery Residency Program
UPMC Presbyterian
Pittsburgh, PA, USA
27. Complications in Vestibular Schwannoma Patients

Rodolfo Maduri, MD
Medical Doctor
Department of Clinical Neurosciences, Service of Neurosurgery
Lausanne University Hospital (CHUV)
Lausanne, Switzerland
45. Complications After Surgery for Chronic Subdural Hematomas

Philippe Magown, MD
Department of Neurological Surgery
Oregon Health and Science University
Portland, OR, USA
33. Complications of Deep Brain Stimulation (DBS)

Tanmoy Kumar Maiti, MD
Clinical Fellow
Stereotactic and Functional Neurosurgery
Cleveland Clinic
Cleveland, OH, USA
8. Complications in Vascular Neurosurgery—Overview
37. Vascular Injuries During Transsphenoidal Surgery
52. Vascular Injury During Approach to Lumbar Spine

Kevin Mansfield, MD
Clinical Fellow in Stereotactic and Functional Neurosurgery
Oregon Health and Science University
Portland, OR, USA
34. Complications After Epilepsy Surgery

Mohammed Nasser, MD, MCh
Fellow
Department of Neurosurgery
LSUHSC
Shreveport, LA, USA
2. Informed Consent and Medicolegal Aspects of Neurosurgery
46. Overview of General and Degenerative Spine Surgery Complications

Edward Monaco III, MD, PhD
Assistant Professor
Department of Neurological Surgery
University of Pittsburgh
Pittsburgh, PA, USA
27. Complications in Vestibular Schwannoma Patients

Praveen V. Mummaneni, MD
Joan O'Reilly Endowed Professor and Vice Chairman
Department of Neurological Surgery
University of California, San Francisco
San Francisco, CA, USA
47. Adjacent Level Disc Degeneration and Pseudarthrosis

Vinayak Narayan, MD, MCh, DNB
Fellow
Department of Neurosurgery
LSUHSC
Shreveport, LA, USA
4. Medical Complications in Neurosurgery
15. Skull Base Surgery Complications: An Overview
17. Complications in Middle Cranial Fossa Surgery
20. Primary Brain Lesion Resection Complications: An Overview and Malignant Brain Swelling After Resection of Superior Sagittal Sinus Meningioma
57. Complications of Surgery for Intrinsic Spinal Cord Tumors

Ajay Niranjan, MD, MBA
Professor, Department of Neurological Surgery
Associate Director, Center of Image-Guided Neurosurgery
University of Pittsburgh
Pittsburgh, PA, USA
27. Complications in Vestibular Schwannoma Patients

W. Jerry Oakes, MD
Professor of Neurosurgery and Pediatrics
Department of Neurosurgery
University of Alabama-Birmingham
Birmingham, AL, USA
31. Complications After Myelomeningocele Repair: CSF Leak and Retethering

Jeff Ojemann, MD
Professor
Department of Neurosurgery
University of Washington
Seattle, WA, USA
34. Complications After Epilepsy Surgery

Nelson M. Oyesiku, MD, PhD, FACS
Professor and Vice-Chairman
Department of Neurosurgery
Emory University
Atlanta, GA, USA
22. Complications of Surgery for Pituitary Tumors

Aqueel Pabaney, MD
Fellow
Department of Neurosurgery
LSUHSC
Shreveport, LA, USA
17. Complications in Middle Cranial Fossa Surgery
57. Complications of Surgery for Intrinsic Spinal Cord Tumors

Devi Prasad Patra, MD, MCh
Fellow
Department of Neurosurgery
LSUHSC
Shreveport, LA, USA
5. Surgical Complications in Neurosurgery
32. Complications of Various Treatment Options for Trigeminal Neuralgia
37. Vascular Injuries During Transsphenoidal Surgery
52. Vascular Injury During Approach to Lumbar Spine

Bruce E. Pollock, MD
Professor
Departments of Neurological Surgery and Radiation Oncology
Mayo Clinic College of Medicine and Science
Rochester, MN, USA
35. Complications After Stereotactic Radiosurgery

John C. Quinn, MD
Spine Fellow
Department of Neurological Surgery
University of Virginia
Charlottesville, VA, USA
55. Postoperative Spinal Deformities: Kyphosis, Nonunion, and Loss of Motion Segment

John K. Ratliff, MD
Professor of Neurosurgery
Vice Chair for Operations and Development
Department of Neurosurgery
Stanford University
Stanford, CA, USA
62. Posttraumatic Syringomyelia

Roberta Rehder, MD, PhD
Research Associate
Division of Pediatric Neurosurgery
Johns Hopkins Hospital
Baltimore, MD, USA
38. Complications of Ventricular Endoscopy

Andy Rekito, MS
Department of Neurosurgery
Oregon Health and Science University
Portland, OR, USA
34. Complications After Epilepsy Surgery

Daniel K. Resnick, MD, MS
Professor and Vice Chairman
Department of Neurosurgery
University of Wisconsin School of Medicine and Public Health
Madison, WI, USA
49. Procedure-Related Complications (Inadvertent Dural Tear, CSF Leak)

Bienvenido Ros, MD
Associate Professor
Chief, Pediatric Division
Department of Neurosurgery
Carlos Haya University Hospital
Malaga, Spain
13. Complications of the Surgery for Cavernomas

Jeffrey V. Rosenfeld, MD, MS, FRACS, FRCS(Edin), FACS, IFAANS
Senior Neurosurgeon
Department of Neurosurgery
The Alfred Hospital
Melbourne, VIC, Australia
Professor
Department of Surgery
Monash University
Clayton, VIC, Australia
Adjunct Professor
Department of Surgery
F. Edward Hébert School of Medicine Uniformed Services University
Bethesda, MD, USA
44. Complications After Decompressive Craniectomy and Cranioplasty

Robert H. Rosenwasser, MD
Professor and Chair
Department of Neurological Surgery
Thomas Jefferson University and Hospitals
Philadelphia, PA, USA
43. Complications in Endovascular Management of Carotid-Cavernous and Dural Arteriovenous Fistulas

James T. Rutka, MD, PhD
Professor and R.S. McLaughlin Chair
Department of Surgery
University of Toronto Faculty of Medicine
Director of the Arthur and Sonia Labatt Brain Tumour Research Centre
Division of Paediatric Neurosurgery
Hospital for Sick Children
Toronto, ON, Canada
29. Craniopharyngioma: Complications After Microsurgery

Victor Sabourin, MD
Resident Physician
Department of Neurological Surgery
Thomas Jefferson University
Philadelphia, PA, USA
54. Instrumentation-Related Complications

John H. Sampson, MD, PhD, MHSc, MBA
Robert H. and Gloria Wilkins Professor of Neurosurgery
Chair, Department of Neurosurgery
Duke University Medical Center
Durham, NC, USA
21. Complications After Glioma Surgery

Mithun G. Sattur, MD, MBBS, MCh, FEBNS
Clinical Fellow
Department of Neurosurgery
Mayo Clinic
Phoenix, AZ, USA
39. Access-Related Complications in Endovascular Neurosurgery

Amey R. Savardekar, MD, MCh
Fellow
Department of Neurosurgery
LSUHSC
Shreveport, LA, USA
3. Wrong Side Craniotomy and Wrong Level Spine Surgery. "Res Ipsa Loquitor"
6. Venous Injuries and Cerebral Edema in Cranial Surgery
7. Postoperative Hematoma in Cranial and Spinal Surgery
8. Complications in Vascular Neurosurgery—Overview
25. Complications Associated With Surgery for Intracranial Infectious Lesions: Brain Abscess, Tuberculosis, Hydatid Disease, Neurocysticercosis

Franco Servadei, MD
Professor
Humanitas University and Research Hospital
Milan, Italy
45. Complications After Surgery for Chronic Subdural Hematomas

Christopher I. Shaffrey, Sr., MD
John A. Jane Professor
Departments of Neurological and Orthopaedic Surgery
University of Virginia Health System
Charlottesville, VA, USA
55. Postoperative Spinal Deformities: Kyphosis, Nonunion, and Loss of Motion Segment

Sophia F. Shakur, MD
Neurosurgeon
Peninsula Regional Medical Center
Salisbury, MD, USA
12. Complications of Cerebral Bypass Surgery

Carl H. Snyderman, MD, MBA
Professor
Department of Otolaryngology
University of Pittsburgh School of Medicine
Pittsburgh, PA, USA
36. Complications of Endoscopic Endonasal Skull Base Surgery

Hesham Soliman, MD
Assistant Professor
Director of Spinal Oncology
Department of Neurosurgery
Medical College of Wisconsin
Milwaukee, WI, USA
58. Complications of Surgery for Vertebral Body Tumors

Robert F. Spetzler, MD
Director and J.N. Harber Chair of Neurological Surgery
Barrow Neurological Institute
St. Joseph's Hospital and Medical Center
Phoenix, AZ, USA
Professor of Neurosurgery
Department of Surgery
University of Arizona College of Medicine
Tucson, AZ, USA
59. Complications of Surgery for Spinal Vascular Malformations

Robert J. Spinner, MD
Chair
Department of Neurological Surgery
Burton M. Onofrio Professor of Neurosurgery
Professor of Orthopedics and Anatomy
Mayo Clinic College of Medicine
Rochester, MN, USA
63. Complications of Surgery for Peripheral Nerve Injuries and Tumors

James A. Stadler III, MD
Assistant Professor—Pediatric Neurosurgery
Department of Neurological Surgery
University of Wisconsin-Madison
Madison, WI, USA
30. Complications Associated With Cerebrospinal Fluid Diversion

Hai Sun, MD, PhD
Assistant Professor and Director of Epilepsy Surgery, Department of Neurosurgery
Adjunct Assistant Professor, Department of Physiology
Adjunct Assistant Professor, Department of Pharmacology, Toxicology and Neuroscience
LSUHSC
Shreveport, LA, USA
Adjunct Faculty
Department of Biomedical Engineering
Center for Biomedical Engineering & Rehabilitation Science (CBERS) Louisiana Tech University
Rustom, LA, USA
34. Complications Following Epilepsy Surgery

Jin W. Tee, MD
Neurosurgeon
The Alfred Hospital
Melbourne, VIC, Australia
Senior Lecturer
Department of Surgery
Monash University
Clayton, VIC Australia
44. Complications After Decompressive Craniectomy and Cranioplasty

Alexander Tenorio, BA
Medical Student
School of Medicine
University of California, San Francisco
San Francisco, CA, USA
47. Adjacent Level Disc Degeneration and Pseudarthrosis

Francesco Tomasello, MD
Professor of Neurosurgery
University of Messina
Honorary President of World Federation of Neurosurgical Societies (WFNS)
President Network Innovation Technology in Neurosurgery/Neuroscience (NITns)
Messina, Italy
16. Complications in Anterior Cranial Fossa Surgery

Vincent C. Traynelis, MD
Professor and Vice Chair
Department of Neurosurgery
Rush University Medical Center
Chicago, IL, USA
51. Neurologic Deterioration After Spinal Surgery

Erol Veznedaroglu, MD
Professor and Robert A. Groff Chair
Department of Neurosurgery
Director, Drexel Neurosciences Institute
Philadelphia, PA, USA
42. Procedure-Related Complications: Stroke

Edoardo Viaroli, MD
Département de Neurosciences Cliniques
Service de Neurochirurgie
Centre Hospitalier Universitaire Vaudois (CHUV)
Lausanne, Switzerland
45. Complications After Surgery for Chronic Subdural Hematomas

Michael S. Virk, MD, PhD
Complex Spine Fellow
Department of Neurological Surgery
University of California, San Francisco
San Francisco, CA, USA
47. Adjacent Level Disc Degeneration and Pseudarthrosis

Eric W. Wang, MD
Associate Professor
Department of Otolaryngology
University of Pittsburgh School of Medicine
Pittsburgh, PA, USA
36. Complications of Endoscopic Endonasal Skull Base Surgery

Michael Y. Wang, MD
Professor
Departments of Neurosurgery and Rehab Medicine
University of Miami School of Medicine
Miami, FL, USA
56. Complications of Minimally Invasive Spinal Surgery

Matthew E. Welz, MD
Neurosurgery Research Fellow
Mayo Clinic
Phoenix, AZ, USA
39. Access-Related Complications in Endovascular Neurosurgery

James L. West, MD
Neurosurgery Resident
Department of Neurosurgery
Wake Forest Baptist Health
Winston-Salem, NC, USA
14. Complication of Carotid Endarterectomy

John A. Wilson, MD, FAANS, FACS
David L. and Sally Kelly Professor and Vice Chair
Department of Neurosurgery
Codirector, Neuroscience Service Line
Wake Forest Baptist Health
Winston-Salem, NC, USA
14. Complication of Carotid Endarterectomy

Thomas J. Wilson, MD
Clinical Assistant Professor
Co-Director, Center for Peripheral Nerve Surgery
Department of Neurosurgery
Stanford University
Stanford, CA, USA
63. Complications of Surgery for Peripheral Nerve Injuries and Tumors

Ethan A. Winkler, MD, PhD
Resident
Department of Neurological Surgery
University of California, San Francisco
San Francisco, CA, USA
11. Complications of AVM Microsurgery; Steal Phenomenon and Management Of Residual AVM

Stacey Quintero Wolfe, MD, FAANS
Associate Professor and Residency Program Director
Neurological Surgery
Wake Forest School of Medicine
Winston-Salem, NC, USA
14. Complication of Carotid Endarterectomy

Video Contents

1

Historical Perspective

BHAVANI KURA, ANIL NANDA

If a physician make[s] a large incision with the operating knife, and kill[s] him, or open[s] a tumor with the operating knife, and cut[s] out the eye, his hands shall be cut off.[1]

This is one of the 282 laws that constitute the Code of Hammurabi, a Babylonian king who ruled from 1792 to 1750 BC (Fig. 1.1). His decrees were inscribed on a stone pillar after his rule, and several of his rulings pertained to the practice of medicine, including the enacting of a heavy penalty for a surgical complication. It is a wonder that anyone would choose to perform surgery with such a possibility at a time when morbidity and mortality likely were very high. This punishment was still less severe than that of being caught committing theft, for which the penalty was death.[1]

The earliest evidence of surgical procedures is from trephinations performed approximately 12,000 years ago in the Mesolithic era.[2] The actual reason for these surgeries is unknown and may have been for ritualistic purposes, but there have been examples found from ancient civilizations throughout the world (Fig. 1.2). From ancient Egypt, the Edwin Smith papyrus, which dates back to approximately 1700 to 1600 BC, is the oldest known medical text and detailed 48 cases of surgical pathologies and their management, including those of injuries of the cranium and spine. These treatments largely involved stabilization to allow healing with time. The Ebers papyrus (circa 1550 BC) was more encouraging of surgical intervention and included descriptions of procedures for the removal of tumors and abscesses.[3]

The earliest documentation of trephination comes from Greece. Hippocrates (460–370 BC) is known as the "father of medicine" due to his incredible contribution to the advancement, analysis, and documentation of the practice of medicine (Fig. 1.3A). The Hippocratic Corpus, a large collection of medical works attributed to Hippocrates and others in the Hippocratic School, included the book *On Injuries of the Head*, which detailed several types of skull fractures and their recommended management.[4] In the most famous of the writings within the Corpus, the Hippocratic Oath (Fig. 1.3B), the responsibilities of the physician are outlined, including:

I will follow that system of regimen which, according to my ability and judgment, I consider for the benefit of my patients, and abstain from whatever is deleterious and mischievous.[5]

Similarly, in *Of the Epidemics*, the author notes:

The physician must ... have two special objects in view with regard to disease, namely, to do good or to do no harm.[5]

As in the texts from ancient Egypt, and unlike the code from ancient Mesopotamia, there is no indication of any penalties for complications, but in *On the Articulations,* Hippocrates does show disdain for those physicians lacking proper "judgment," to whom he attributes certain complications. He describes the inappropriate treatment of a nasal fracture leading to unsatisfactory healing[6]:

... those who, without judgment, delight in fine bandagings, do much mischief, most especially in injuries about the nose ... those who practice manipulation without judgment are fond of meeting with a case of fractured nose, that they may apply the bandage ... the physician glories in his performance ... and the physician is satisfied, because he has had an opportunity of showing his skill in applying a complex bandage to the nose. Such a bandaging does everything the very reverse of what is proper ... will evidently derive no benefit from bandaging above it, but will rather be injured...[5]

He also provides advice for the prevention of complications in *On Injuries of the Head.* The readers are advised to avoid incising the brain to prevent convulsions on the contralateral side and to make the operative wounds clean and dry to prevent gangrene.

Several centuries later, Galen of Pergamon (129–200 AD) followed and expanded on the teachings of Hippocrates. He used his surgical experiences and anatomic dissections of animals to provide detailed descriptions of anatomy, which remained the standard for a millennia, despite some errors.[7] He emphasized the importance of the knowledge of anatomy in surgery:

If a man is ignorant of the position of a vital nerve, muscle, artery or important vein, he is more likely to maim his patients or to destroy rather than save life.[2]

The first recorded medical malpractice case was *Stratton vs. Swanlond* in 1374 in London. The surgeon had attempted to repair the plaintiff's hand, which had been severely disfigured by trauma. The patient claimed that the surgeon had promised a cure, but her hand remained significantly deformed after the operation, and she filed a lawsuit for breach of contract. Although the case was actually thrown out on a technicality, the judge asserted that a physician would be held liable if harm came to the patient as a result of negligence, but not if he was unable to obtain a cure despite making every effort.[8] This decision became a part of English common law, or judge-made law. It countered people's expectation that only a complete cure could be a good outcome and not a complication. The term "malpractice" came about much later; it was coined from the Latin term *mala praxis* by Sir William

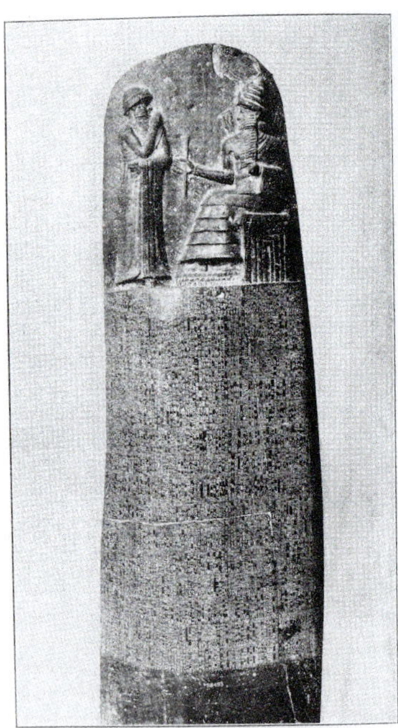

• **Fig. 1.1** The Code of Hammurabi inscribed on a stela. (Photo copyright Wellcome Library, London, supplied by Wellcome Collection, licensed under CC-BY.)

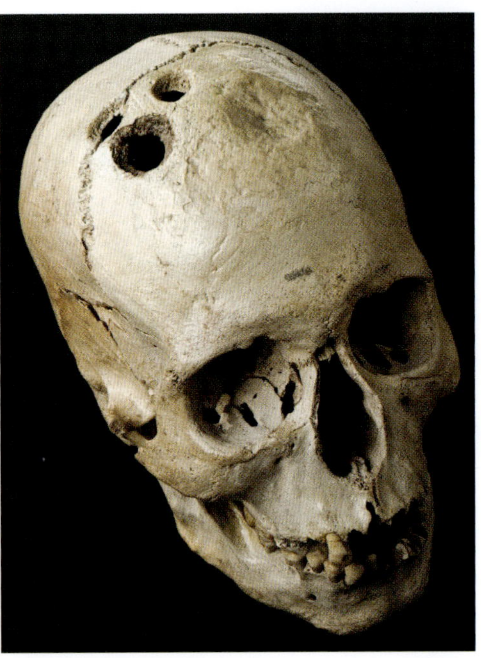

• **Fig. 1.2** A skull that had undergone several trephinations and shows evidence of healing, from 2200 to 2000 BC. (Photo copyright Science Museum, London, supplied by Wellcome Collection, licensed under CC-BY.)

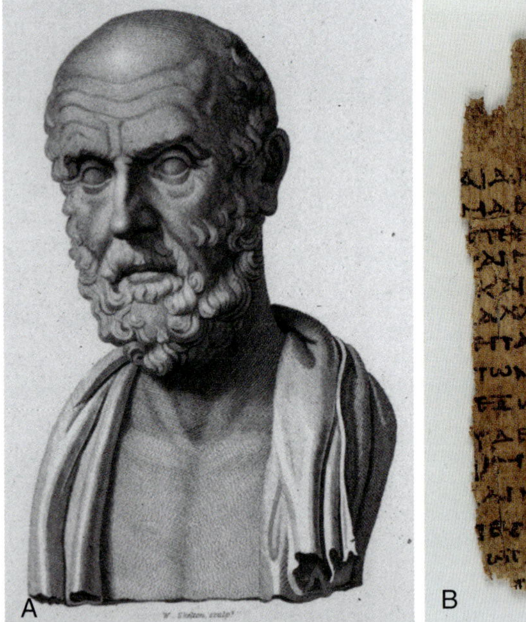

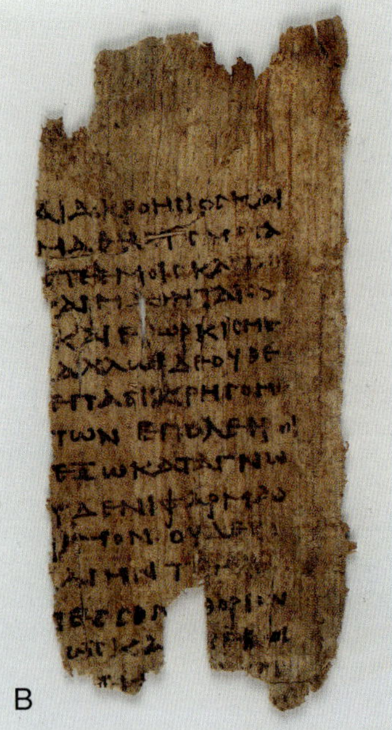

• **Fig. 1.3** (A) A bust of Hippocrates (from the National Library of Medicine). (B) A fragment of the Hippocratic Oath, from the 3rd century BC (from Wellcome Library, London).

Blackstone's *Commentaries on the Laws of England* in 1768. He described malpractice as injuries "by the neglect or unskillful management of his physician … breaks the trust which the party had placed in his physician, and tends to the patient's destruction."[9] The first malpractice case in the United States occurred in 1794, but the overall number of malpractice cases remained low until the mid-1800s.

Infection was a major cause of surgical morbidity and mortality during the long history of surgery before the introduction of antisepsis. Because there was limited understanding of the origin of infections, which were thought to arise by spontaneous generation, hospitals and operating rooms remained decidedly unsterile.[10] Many physicians made varied attempts to improve wound healing. Some physicians, such as Paul of Aegina (625–690 AD), used wine-soaked dressings, unknowingly applying antisepsis, but this was not the norm.[7] The theory of "laudable pus," that inducing pus formation encouraged wound healing, has been attributed to Galen as well as Roger of Salerno (fl. 1170) and remained the guideline for wound care until the 19th century.[4] Theodoric Borgognoni of Cervia (1205–1298 AD), among others, advocated against the idea of laudable pus. He recommended careful hemostasis, debridement of foreign and necrotic tissue, closure of dead space, and wine-soaked dressings, but his ideas were met with skepticism. Others attempted to explain the transmission of infection but were ignored or rebuked by the medical community. In the 19th century, 80% of patients undergoing surgical procedures developed "hospital gangrene," and they carried a 50% mortality rate.[10] The mortality rate of women giving birth actually increased at this time as physicians took over the job of delivering babies from midwives. Ignaz Semmelweis reported in 1847 that handwashing significantly reduced maternal mortality from puerperal fever, but it still took decades for the practice to become routine.[11]

Louis Pasteur's (1822–1895) discovery of the fermentation process supported the germ theory of disease rather than spontaneous generation. Joseph Lister (1827–1912) expanded on these findings to develop the concept of antisepsis, which he delineated in a landmark report in *Lancet* in 1867. He recommended using carbolic acid for sterilization of instruments, washing of hands, and dressing of wounds (Fig. 1.4).[12] Although many physicians were slow to accept Lister's conclusions, the use of antiseptic technique in operating rooms and for wound care reduced the mortality rate after amputations by 30%.[13] Even with the incredible reduction in complications that occurred with the introduction of antisepsis, surgeons continued attempting to reduce their rates of infection. Harvey Cushing, often referred to as the father of neurosurgery, noted:

> *Even to the painstaking final approximation of the scalp wound, every detail of the operation and the local after-treatment must be followed with the greatest care, if one wishes to avoid that most distressing of all complications, a fungus cerebri, which I am happy to say has occurred to me only twice.*[14]

The emergence of anesthesia in the 19th century was a significant breakthrough in the advancement of surgery. Surgeons had previously been limited by patients' tolerance for pain, requiring them to work as rapidly as possible. The British surgeon Robert Liston was known to be a very good, exceedingly fast surgeon and in fact operated with such speed that he reportedly once amputated his assistant's fingers in addition to his patient's leg (Fig. 1.5). Both the patient and assistant subsequently died from sepsis, and an observer died of shock, resulting in "the only operation

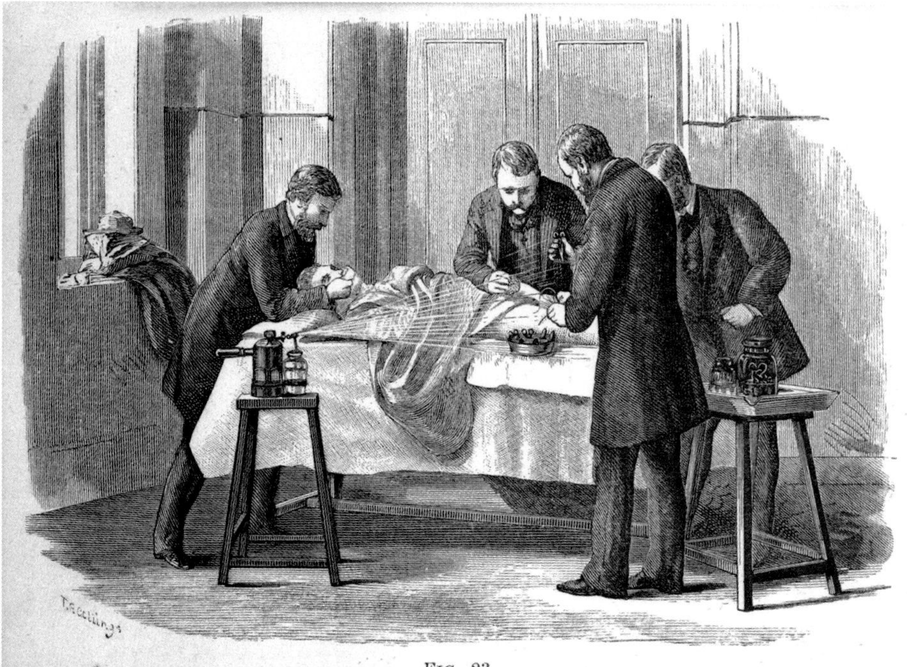
FIG. 23.
This figure represents the general arrangement of surgeon, assistants, towels, spray, &c., in an operation performed with complete aseptic precautions. The distance of the spray from the wound, the arrangement of the wet towels, the position of the trough containing the instruments, the position of the small dish with the lotion, the position of the house surgeon and dresser, so that the former always has his hands in the cloud of the spray, and the latter hands the instruments into the spray and various other points, are shown.

• **Fig. 1.4** Antiseptic surgery with the use of carbolic acid spray. The drawing is from a book by William Watson Cheyne published in 1882. (Photo copyright Wellcome Library, London, supplied by Wellcome Collection, licensed under CC-BY.)

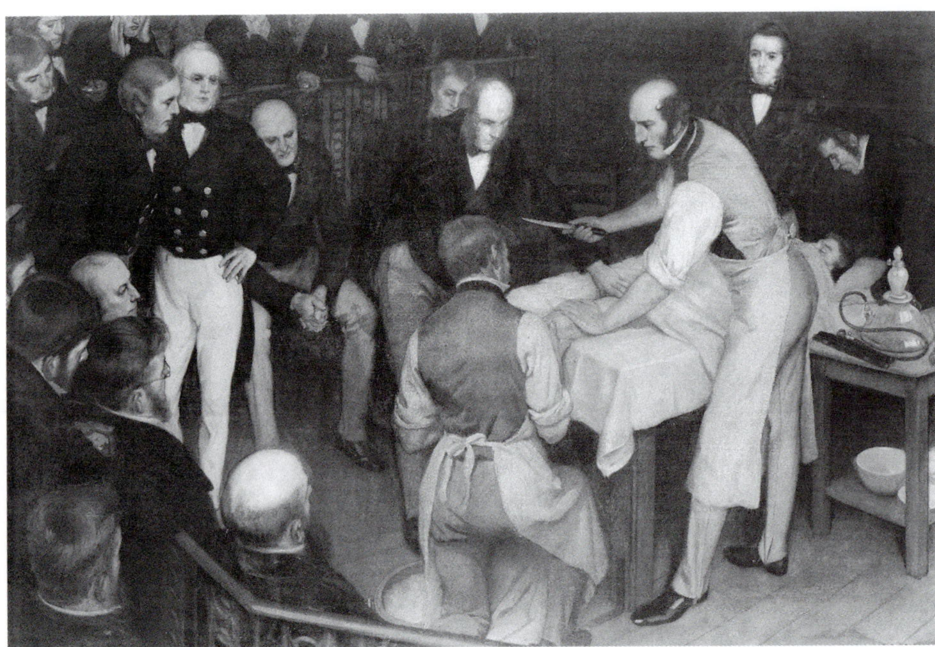

• **Fig. 1.5** A painting by Ernest Board of Bristol depicting Robert Liston in the operating theater. (Photo copyright Wellcome Library, London, supplied by Wellcome Collection, licensed under CC-BY.)

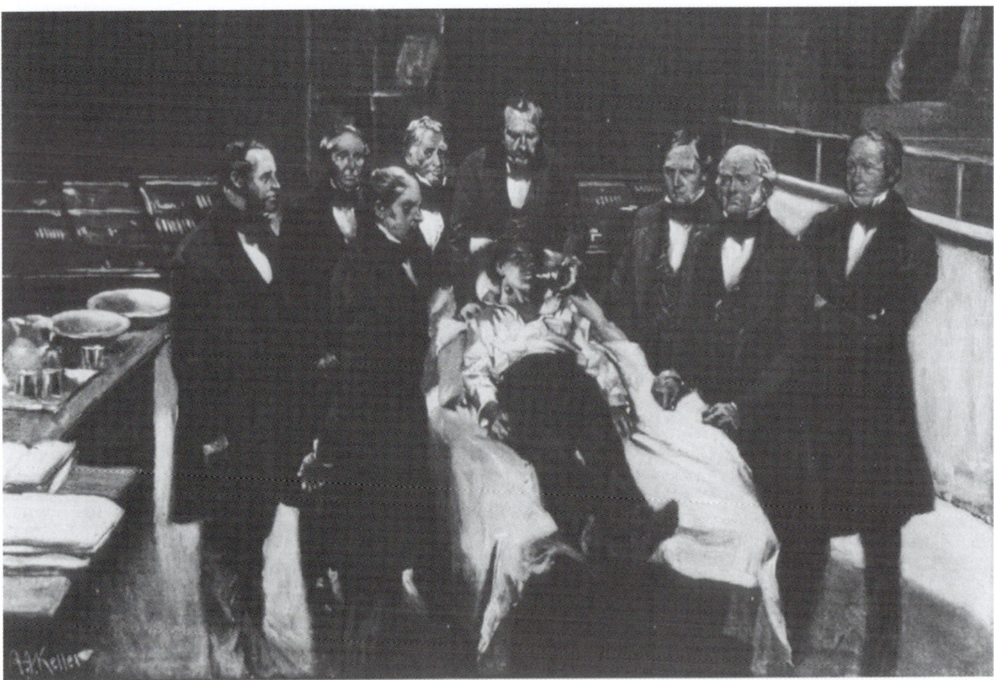

• **Fig. 1.6** The first public demonstration of surgical anesthesia, at Massachusetts General Hospital on October 16, 1846 (from the National Library of Medicine).

in history with a 300 percent mortality rate"[15] and giving new meaning to the word complication. In 1846, Dr. William Morton (1819–1868), a dentist, provided a public demonstration of the use of ether vapor for anesthesia at Massachusetts General Hospital as Dr. John C. Warren (1778–1856) resected a submaxillary vascular tumor (Fig. 1.6).[16] The introduction of anesthetics in the operating room gave surgeons time to be more precise in their technique.

With the innovations in anesthesia and antiseptic technique, surgeons could perform longer and more complex procedures with increased precision and decreased infection-related complications, leading to the flourishing of surgery as a whole as well as the subspecialty of neurosurgery. Of course, this meant that the proportions of other complications increased, requiring further investigation to prevent and manage them, while malpractice cases increased exponentially from the late 19th century and beyond.

References

1. The Code of Hammurabi. In: *The Avalon Project*; n.d. Retrieved from avalon.law.yale.edu/ancient/hameframe.asp.
2. Missios S. Hippocrates, Galen, and the uses of trepanation in the ancient classical world. *Neurosurg Focus*. 2007;23(1):E11.
3. Goodrich JT. History of spine surgery in the ancient and medieval worlds. *Neurosurg Focus*. 2004;16(1):1–5.
4. Goodrich JT, Flamm ES. Historical overview of neurosurgery. In: Youmans JR, Winn HR, eds. *Youmans Neurological Surgery*. Philadelphia, PA: Saunders/Elsevier; 2011:8–48.
5. Stevenson DC. Works by Hippocrates. In *The Internet Classics Archive*; 2009. Retrieved from http://classics.mit.edu/Hippocrates/artic.html.
6. Chapman A. A history of surgical complications. In: Hakim NS, Papalois VE, eds. *Surgical Complications: Diagnosis and Treatment*. London: Imperial College Press; 2007.
7. Goodrich JT. Landmarks in the history of neurosurgery. In: Ellenbogen RG, Abdulrauf SI, Sekhar LN, eds. *Principles of Neurological Surgery*. 3rd ed. Philadelphia, PA: Elsevier/Saunders; 2012:3–36.
8. Field R. The malpractice crisis turns 175: what lessons does history hold for reform? *Drexel Law Rev*. 2011;4(1):7–39.
9. Mohr JC. American medical malpractice litigation in historical perspective. *JAMA*. 2000;283(13):1731–1737.
10. Miller JT, Rahimi SY, Lee M. History of infection control and its contributions to the development and success of brain tumor operations. *Neurosurg Focus*. 2005;18(4):1–5.
11. Gawande A. Two hundred years of surgery. *N Engl J Med*. 2012;366:1716–1723.
12. Lister J. On a new method of treating compound fracture, abscess, etc., with observations on the conditions of suppuration. *Lancet*. 1867;89:326–329, 357–359, 507–509; 90:95–96.
13. Alexander JW. The contributions of infection control to a century of surgical progress. *Ann Surg*. 1985;201:423–428.
14. Voorhees JR, Cohen-Gadol AA, Spencer DD. Early evolution of neurological surgery: conquering increased intracranial pressure, infection, and blood loss. *Neurosurg Focus*. 2005;18(4):1–5.
15. Hollingham R. *Blood and Guts: A History of Surgery*. New York, NY: Thomas Dunne Books; 2008.
16. Chivukula S, Grandhi R, Friedlander RM. A brief history of neuroanesthesia. *Neurosurg Focus*. 2014;36(4):1–5.

2

Informed Consent and Medicolegal Aspects of Neurosurgery

ANIL NANDA, MOHAMMED NASSER

The theory of informed consent has its origins in a multitude of dimensions ranging from law, medical practice, ethics, political policies, social sciences, philosophy, and behavioral sciences. It cannot be viewed purely from the perspective of law or from that of medical science. To understand the doctrine, one needs to understand this multifaceted dimension of informed consent. Throughout history, it has been viewed as rather unethical to inform the patient about the risks involved in the treatment process. Today the medical science has far advanced beyond its own fears, and disclosures of the risks involved in the treatment process have become the norm. Informed consent refers to a set of legal principles that has been set up to define the physician-patient interaction occurring in clinical treatment scenarios. It is a theory based on ethical principles but given effect by legal rulings and put into practice by clinicians. Informed consent is a process of *active shared decision-making* based on mutual respect and participation and not a ritual of reciting from a piece of paper the possible complications of the intended treatment. Hence, in its essence, informed consent is an ethical principle.

Moral reasoning dictates that an action that leads to well-being is the right action. Beneficence is the core value on which medical practice is based. In beneficence, medical therapy aims at treating patients in ways that are likely to be beneficial to them. Autonomous action is an action that is self-propagated and legislated. Autonomy is a fundamental human right. Beneficence and autonomy are the two sides of the doctrine of informed consent.[1] Beneficence may not always uphold the principles of autonomy (i.e., a conflict between free choice and the patient's best interests). Autonomous action ceases to be autonomous when the person involved lacks the necessary cognition, or when the volition is impaired.[1] It is in this context that the concept of therapeutic privilege must be understood. *Therapeutic privilege* is the situation where the physician may at his or her discretion withhold information from the patient for the reason that disclosing certain information may likely result in serious physical or psychological harm and be detrimental to the patient's recovery; thereby the physician may be excused from divulging the information.[2] The information that can be withheld may be related to either the diagnosis or the treatment. Such therapeutic nondisclosure is especially important in a patient where psychiatric illness is diagnosed. Therapeutic privilege can be a defense against negligence to take informed consent only when the risks of full disclosure exceeds the risks of treatment. *Paternalistic deception* is a deception that is deliberately performed for the individual's own good. Patients may make an informed choice that may actually be medically improper. Paternalism may curb autonomy but may not always be wrong if it might result in the patient's well-being. The concept of paternalism does not imply that the action is justifiable or unjustifiable but rather that it is an act of beneficence similar to parental beneficence. Paternalism can be weak or strong. The philosophical debate between the paternalism and antipaternalism faces off with the new age concept of autonomy. For the patient to give informed consent, he should be competent enough to understand and make a decision, should receive adequate disclosure of the relevant information, and should make the decision voluntarily.

The History of Informed Consent

To understand the present-day theory of informed consent, it is important to understand the evolution of the theory of informed consent from the historical perspective. The historical incidents where physicians have been subjected to compensation, either in physical or financial form, are not rare. Four thousand years ago, medical malpractice was recognized and was punishable as a crime. The sixth Babylonian king, Hammurabi (1792–1750 BC), who lived in modern-day Iraq and eastern Syria, is best known for his testimony of legal codes, engraved on a 2.25-meter-high diorite stone stela that is on exhibit at the Louvre in Paris. The code has 282 laws pertaining to various civil and criminal matters with a description of their punishments. Code 218 says, "If a physician operate on a man for a severe wound with a bronze lancet and cause the man's death, or open an abscess in the eye of a man with a bronze lancet and destroy the man's eye, they shall cut off his hands" (Code No. 218 of Hammurabi).[3,4] Although the punishment of cutting the fingers of erring physicians is not comparable to present-day medical malpractice, the financial payment does have resemblance to modern-day medical litigation settlements. Codes 219 and 220 say that "if a physician makes a wound and cures a freeman, he shall receive ten pieces of silver, but only five if the patient is the son of a plebeian or two if he is a slave." *Sushruta Samhita*, a treatise on surgery from India written in the 3rd century BC, describes the need for obtaining the consent of the king in certain treatment scenarios like, "If surgical intervention is not done then the patient will die and after surgery it is not certain if surgery will be beneficial."[5]

In ancient Greece, the patient's participation in decision-making on medical treatment was considered undesirable.[6] It was thought that any discussion regarding the possible complications would decrease the patient's trust and confidence in the treatment. In the era of enlightenment, the medical community still felt that "deception" was required to facilitate the treatment. There were dichotomous views as to whether to disclose the prognosis to the patient or to hide it.[6] To effect a treatment cure, it was widely felt that authority must be coupled with obedience. The doctrine of assault versus battery evolved in early English common law. Gradually informed consent has emerged to be more patient oriented, and it has been established that a well-informed patient is a master of his or her own body. Since the 1930s, the courts have largely moved away from the *battery* theory of informed consent and have adopted the concept of *negligence* in its place. The negligence theory puts more emphasis on professional standards and expertise than the *battery* concept. During the 20th century, the courts extended the English common law tort doctrine of negligence to the field of surgery by equating negligence with breach of duty, and breach of duty with incomplete patient consent. The present concept of informed consent has evolved with several landmark judgements in the last century. It is essential that these cases be analyzed to understand the evolution of the present-day theory of informed consent. The first recorded case of medical litigation was *Stratton vs. Swanlond* in 1374. The case pertained to a surgery on the hand of a patient, which was injured in trauma. The surgery did not result in eradicating the problem. The patient contended that the promised cure was not achieved. The judge held that the physician could be held responsible if harm came to the patient as a result of surgery, and that he could not be held responsible if the intended cure was not achieved despite his best efforts.

In the aftermath of World War II, several trials were held against Nazi Party members for war crimes, under the orders of President Harry Truman. The trials began on December 9, 1946, in Nuremberg, Germany, and came to be known as the Nuremberg trials. One of the trials, the so-called "doctors trial" focused on the inhuman medical experiments that were carried out by the Nazi physicians. The trial promulgated six ethical principles of medical experiments, which later came to be known as the Nuremberg Code.[7] The first principle of the code states the absolute need for voluntary consent in medical experiments. The Nuremberg Code has not been officially accepted as a law by any nation or medical association, but it has formed the basis of many guidelines worldwide.

There are well-known cases involving neurosurgery that have shaped the legal doctrine of informed consent in the United States. The case of *Canterbury vs. Spence* is a landmark case that defined many issues of informed consent in present-day practice. Jerry Watson Canterbury was an FBI clerk who developed a prolapsed intervertebral disc in 1958 at the age of 19 years. He consulted a well-known neurosurgeon, Dr. William Spence. He was diagnosed to have a prolapsed disc at the T4 level as confirmed by a myelogram. Spence recommended that the patient have a laminectomy. After the surgery, Canterbury had a fall from his bed while still being hospitalized and developed paralysis from the waist down with urinary incontinence. Canterbury underwent a second operation due to the neurologic deterioration. He made some recovery in his motor function but continued to have issues with urinary incontinence. The court held that Spence was negligent in obtaining complete consent. On March 15, 2017, Canterbury passed away, and an obituary was posted in *The New York Times* about him.[8] This case was a landmark case in the medicolegal context. Before this judgement, the onus of soliciting information about treatment resided with the patient. Describing the risks involved in the proposed treatment was at the doctor's discretion. He was held negligent only when the treatment was carried out against the wishes of the patient. The 1972 ruling in this case made it mandatory for the doctor to disclose all pertinent information relating to the risks of treatment, and to inform the patient of any alternative forms of treatment available. According to professor Alan Meisel, "The opinion is the cornerstone of the law of informed consent not only in the United States, but in other English-speaking countries, too."[8] The case shifted the perceptions from "professional practice standard" to a "reasonable person standard." The *Johnson vs. Kokemoor* case has opened a new dimension to informed consent. Donna Johnson was diagnosed during an evaluation of her headaches to have a basilar aneurysm. She consulted Dr. Richard Kokemoor, who advised surgery for the aneurysm. Kokemoor informed the patient that he had performed the procedure "dozens of times"[9] and compared the risks involved with those of a tonsillectomy or gallbladder surgery. Kokemoor estimated the risk of death due to surgery at 2%, when in fact it was close to 30% when performed by inexperienced surgeons. Johnson underwent the surgical procedure but developed quadriparesis, incontinence with speech, vision problems, and swallowing disturbances. Johnson filed a suit against Kokemoor, and the jury deliberated in favor of Johnson. The court held that the actual risks involved in the surgery were not conveyed to the patient. Kokemoor had not disclosed the difference in results between experienced and inexperienced surgeons, and he had not disclosed that the mortality rate in the hands of inexperienced surgeons was much higher than what had been disclosed to the patient. It was brought to evidence that Kokemoor had performed the aneurysm clipping in six patients after his residency and had operated on a basilar aneurysm only twice. The plaintiff contested that the doctor should have referred her to a more experienced tertiary care center like Mayo Clinic, which was only 90 miles away. The court held that the defendant failed to do the following: divulge the extent of his experience in performing the specific operation, compare the mortality and morbidity between experienced and inexperienced surgeons, and refer the plaintiff to a more experienced treatment center.[10] The Wisconsin Supreme Court stated that "physicians must provide comparative risk in statistical terms to obtain informed consent."[10]

The Legal Doctrine of Informed Consent

Fig. 2.1 depicts the diverse areas that have an influence on the formation of the theory of informed consent. Tort law is an important basis for the current legal doctrine of informed consent. The word is derived from old French as a modification of the Latin "tortus," meaning crooked or twisted. In modern French, the word "tort" means "wrong."[11] A tort consists of four Ds: Duty, Dereliction, Direct causation, and Damage. A tort is a civil injury to one's person or property that is intentionally or negligently caused by another and which is measured in terms of, and compensated by, money damages.[12] In the parlance of common law, failure to obtain informed consent is a tort. American law is divided into common law, which is derived from the English medieval period, judge-made laws, and the law derived from the Constitution. Tort law is originally derived from the civil wing of common law. Informed consent is essentially a concept derived and developed from common law. The theory of liability that is applied in the context of informed consent has changed from that of "battery" to negligence. The debate between battery and negligence pertaining to the theory of informed consent has raised difficult legal issues. In the *battery*

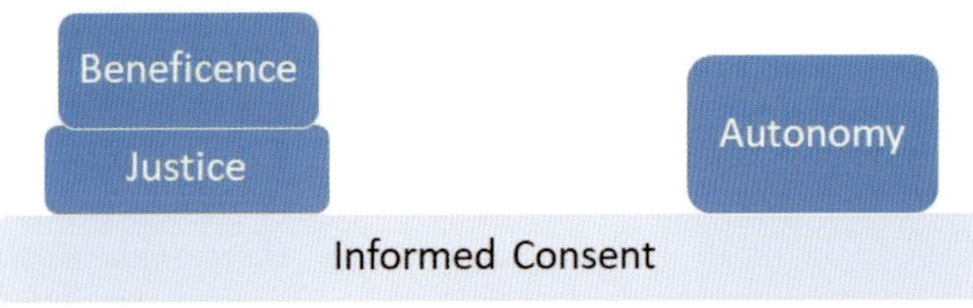

• **Fig. 2.1** Figure depicting the diverse areas that have an influence on the formation of the theory of informed consent.

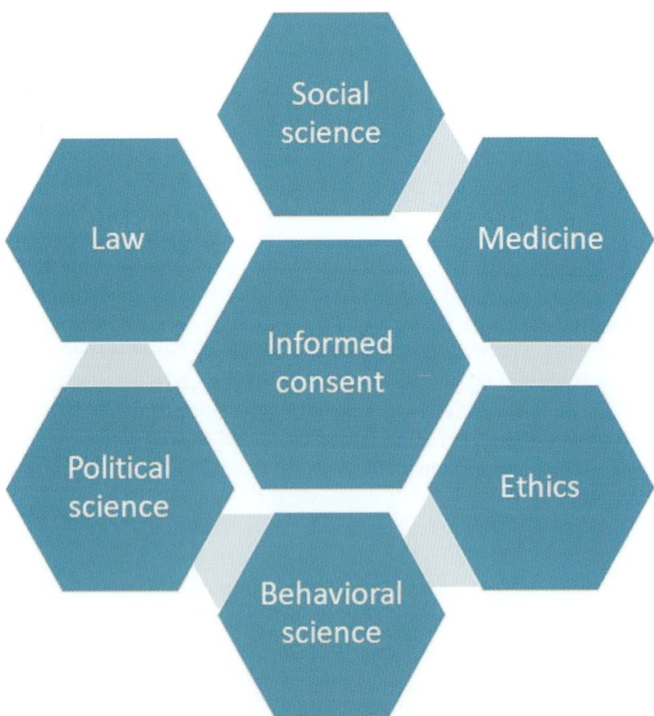

• **Fig. 2.2** Beneficence and autonomy are the two sides of the doctrine of informed consent. A balance needs to be achieved when there is a conflict between the free choice of the patient and the patient's best interests.

theory, the defendant can be held accountable for an intentional act that results in a physical contact for which no permission is given by the plaintiff. There is no requirement of an evil intent or injury to occur for applying the charge of battery. Just the unpermitted contact will suffice to bring the charge of battery. In the negligence theory, the careless act of commission or omission is considered. Negligence is a tort of unintended harmful action or omission.[12]

The Ethical Basis of Informed Consent

Fig. 2.2 shows the ethical basis of the informed consent. Ethics is a set of principles that determine right and acceptable conduct. The Hippocratic Oath is essentially an oath of ethics. The ethical foundation of informed consent is based upon personal well-being and autonomy. Clinicians often find themselves in the crossroads between the legal perspectives and the ethical theorists in deciding the complex clinical scenarios. Informed consent has both a legal and moral perspective. The legal perspective is codified and more focused on financial compensation, and the moral angle has more to do with the autonomy of choices and the ethical issues of medicine. The theory of informed consent is based on three principles: respect for autonomy, beneficence, and justice. Beneficence is the concept of doing good and has to be distinguished from mere avoidance of harm. It must be remembered that in clinical practice the risks of harm due to treatment must be constantly balanced with the possible benefits that the patient receives. The concept of "first do no harm" does not mean that there should never be any harm caused; it means that one should strive to have more benefits than harms, which is more often the case in clinical practice.

The costs involved in medical litigation are substantial. A study by Studdert et al.[13] retrospectively reviewed 1452 closed claims from 33,000 physicians, 61 acute care hospitals, and 428 outpatient facilities. The study found that 60% of the plaintiffs were females. Obstetricians were the most frequently sued physicians (19%), followed by general surgeons (17%) and primary care physicians (16%). In 3% of the claims, no adverse event was evident. Nine percent had allegations pertaining to the breaches of informed consent. Eight percent of the claims concerned significant or major physical injury. Fifty-six percent of the claims received compensation at an average of $485,348 per claim. It is estimated that 44,000 to 98,000 people die every year from medical errors in hospitals.[14] The famous Institute of Medicine report *To Err Is Human* draws attention to the burden of medical error–related deaths.[14] Classen et al. concluded that one-third of all hospital admissions suffer some form of adverse event.[15] Chassin and Loeb stated that "hospitals house patients who are vulnerable to harm due to medical negligence and the complexity of medical treatment system increases the likelihood of those errors."[16] Medical litigation is a direct result of the advancement of medical science and is not a by-product of lawmakers' intrusive policies. The threshold of treating difficult clinical scenarios has been ever-expanding. For instance, today surgeries on an elderly population are being done that previously were not done, more preterm babies are being supported to survive now than before, and more difficult cancer cases are being treated than before. This, coupled with ever-increasing costs of medical treatment, has propelled medical litigation to increase its reach and capacity. The political changes that are now bringing the Affordable Care Act into the limelight will only make the scrutiny on hospitals more stringent.

Conclusions

Medicine is not an exact science. A great responsibility lies in the judicial system to define the laws pertaining to medical practice so as not to hamper the innovations and developments. In conclusion, the evolution of informed consent— from battery to negligence to informing patients of the risks as well as professional competence—has seen several neurosurgical procedures, including brachial plexus injury, paraplegia after laminectomy, and aneurysm clipping. There are many unresolved moral issues pertaining to informed consent. There is a conflict between the right of autonomy that the patient may impose and the act of beneficence, which may take a course against autonomy in cases when the patient refuses treatment. It is important for neurosurgeons to be aware of the history of informed consent and to be vigilant in obtaining detailed consent in our current medicolegal atmosphere.

References

1. O'Neill O. Paternalism and partial autonomy. *J Med Ethics.* 1984;10:173–178.
2. van den Heever P. Pleading the defence of therapeutic privilege. *S Afr Med J.* 2005;95:420–421.
3. *Johns: Oldest Code of Laws in the World the Code of Laws Promulgated by Hammurabi, King of Babylon B.C. 2285-2242*, 1903.
4. Violato C. Doctor-patient relationships, laws, clinical guidelines, best practices, evidence-based medicine, medical errors and patient safety. *Can Med Educ J.* 2013;4:e1–e6.
5. Kumar NK. Informed consent: Past and present. *Perspectives in Clinical Research.* 2013;4:21–25.
6. Murray PM. The history of informed consent. *Iowa Orthop J.* 1990;10:104–109.
7. Shuster E. Fifty years later: the significance of the Nuremberg Code. *N Engl J Med.* 1997;337:1436–1440.
8. Roberts S. *Jerry Canterbury, Whose Paralysis Led to Informed Consent Laws, Is Dead at 78, in* The New York Times, 2017.
9. Menikoff J. *Law and Bioethics: An Introduction.* Washington, DC: Georgetown University Press; 2001.
10. Clarke S. *Informed Consent and Clinician Accountability: the Ethics of Report Cards on Surgeon Performance.* Cambridge: Cambridge University Press; 2007.
11. Shindell S. Survey of the law of medical practice: III. civil wrongs in the practice of medicine. *JAMA.* 1965;193:1108–1114.
12. Faden R, Beauchamp TL. *A History and Theory of Informed Consent.* New York, NY: Oxford University Press; 2010.
13. Studdert DM, Mello MM, Gawande AA, et al. Claims, errors, and compensation payments in medical malpractice litigation. *NEJM.* 2006;354:2024–2033.
14. Institute of Medicine Committee on Quality of Health Care in A. Kohn LT, Corrigan JM, Donaldson MS, eds. *To Err is Human: Building a Safer Health System.* Washington, DC: National Academies Press; 2000.
15. David C, Classen RR, Frances G, Frank F, Terri F, Nancy K. 'Global trigger tool' shows that adverse events in hospitals may be ten times greater than previously measured. *Health Aff.* 2011;30: 581–589.
16. Chassin MR, Loeb JM. The ongoing quality improvement journey: next stop, high reliability. *Health Aff (Millwood).* 2011;30: 559–568.

3

Wrong Side Craniotomy and Wrong Level Spine Surgery

"Res Ipsa Loquitor"

ANIL NANDA, AMEY R. SAVARDEKAR

HIGHLIGHTS

- Wrong-site surgery is a rare occurrence that can lead to significant clinical morbidity, increased healthcare costs, and medicolegal consequences.
- Wrong-site procedures occur in roughly one out of every 100,000 neurosurgical operations and have an average payout of $127,159 per occurrence.
- Although wrong-site surgery may never be completely eliminated, "zero tolerance" or "one hundred percent accuracy" should be the end goal of the neurosurgical community when dealing with this specific error.
- Emerging data suggest that preventing such errors will require the neurosurgeons and their allied specialties to recognize the importance of checklists and to increase the use of intraoperative imaging during neurosurgical procedures.

Background

Medical errors are essentially acts of commission (doing something wrong) or omission (failing to do the right thing) that can lead to an undesirable outcome for the patient or that have the potential for such an outcome.[1] They encompass a wide spectrum, but none is as hazardous to the patient or as detrimental to the psyche of the surgeon as a "wrong-site surgery." Surgeries carried out on the wrong side or on the wrong person are amongst the most serious of surgical errors.[2] These "surgical never events" have become a focus of media concern and attention, not to mention a source of negative publicity for the medical profession and surgical specialties.[3] Neurosurgery is as vulnerable to the occurrence of these errors as any other branch of surgery, if not more.[1]

Neurosurgery is the third most likely specialty to perform a wrong-site or wrong-level surgery, after orthopedic and general surgery.[1] Wrong-side or wrong-patient procedures occur in roughly 1 case out of every 100,000 operations and in 2.2 cases of every 10,000 craniotomies.[2] Surveys of neurosurgeons show that 25% of physicians have made an incision on the wrong side of the head, and 35% admitted to wrong-level lumbar surgery in their careers.[1] In a survey of members of the American Academy of Neurological Surgeons performed by Mody et al., 50% of responding surgeons reported that they had performed at least one wrong-level surgery during their career. Of 418 wrong-level surgeries, 17% resulted in litigation or monetary settlement.[4]

Is an Explanation Plausible?

Despite substantial efforts, including surgical checklists and other protective measures, the healthcare industry has not been able to eliminate the menace of wrong-site surgery.[5] Most of the adverse events related to wrong-side or wrong-patient surgery appear to arise from breakdowns in communication. In an anonymous survey, neurosurgeons recognized fatigue, unusual time pressure, and emergent operations as factors contributing to wrong-site surgery.[2]

It has to be recognized that for these fundamental errors, it is inappropriate to focus the responsibility entirely on the "end-of-the-line operator"—in this case the neurosurgeon.[6] The neurosurgery operating room is a complex adaptive network in which a mix of professionals must cooperate while performing demanding technical tasks and using complex technologies and techniques. Hence the complex network of systemic factors that surround the neurosurgeon (in addition to the neurosurgeon) should be considered while offering a plausible explanation for wrong-site neurosurgery. The Swiss cheese model effectively elucidates how the complexity of our systems, when combined with human factors, can synergistically promote errors like wrong-site surgery (Fig. 3.1).[6] In the context of the systems approach, it has been suggested that when an error occurs, it is more useful to correct the system that failed than to assign blame to the individual who committed the last act in the chain of events leading to the error.

Lessons From the Aviation Industry

Safety management in aviation and in the surgical suite is often comparable. This emulation is in the context of major achievements in the field of aviation: Despite the number of worldwide flight hours doubling over the past 20 years (from approximately 25 million in 1993 to 54 million in 2013), the number of fatalities has fallen from approximately 450 to 250 per year.[7] This stands in comparison to health care, where in the United States alone there are an estimated 200,000 preventable medical deaths every year, which amounts to the equivalent of almost three fatal airline crashes per day.[7]

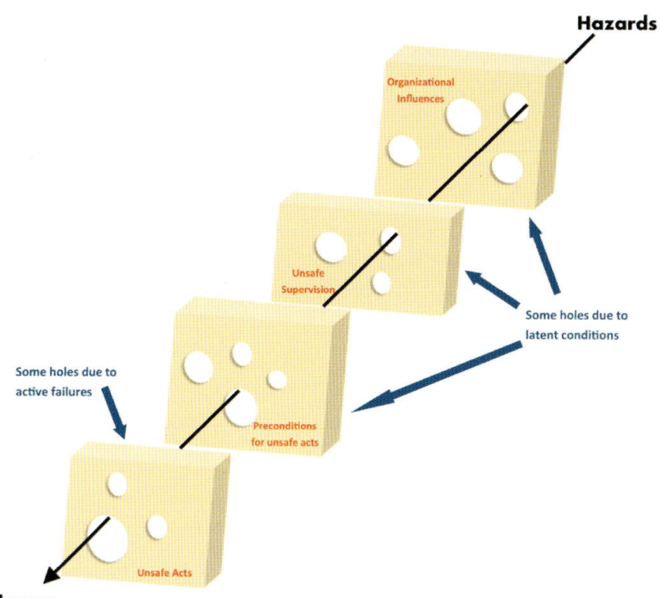

• **Fig. 3.1** The Swiss cheese model of accident causation. Despite the presence of multiple layers of defenses, barriers, and safeguards, an error can still occur if the "holes" are all aligned.

The aviation industry functions as a high-reliability organization that has used a variety of practices to maintain an enviable safety record, despite the inherent risks of flying. The inherent risks associated with air transport, the team structure of its air crews, and the importance of a methodic approach in completing critical tasks make it in many ways similar to the perioperative setting. The safety record of the surgical setup as a whole has failed to emulate the strides taken by the aviation sector. Over the past few decades, there has been a gradual but steady move toward attempting to integrate aviation safety principles to improve perioperative patient safety. Crew resource management (CRM), incident reporting, checklists, and readbacks have been some of the most prominent principles that are slowly being adopted in the surgical suite with the intention of preventing the "surgical never events."

Utilizing the long-term effectiveness of aviation strategies to improve perioperative safety is a work in progress, given some significant differences between aviation and the surgical suite.[8] At least three safety-related cultural attributes appear to distinguish aviation from health care.[7] Aviation has much more of a "blame-free culture" in the case of reporting and owning up to safety incidents. Secondly, there appear to be competing demands between economic factors and safety, with financial pressures and considerations constantly making news headlines. Thirdly, safety permeates all levels of aviation, whereas in health care it is still regarded as the priority of some, not the obligation of all. Empowering all participants in the surgical suite would be a significant step toward avoiding complications like wrong-site surgery.

Strategies to Avoid Wrong-Side Craniotomy

The Joint Commission—Universal Protocol for Preventing Wrong Site, Wrong Procedure and Wrong Person Surgery—has developed guidelines designed to encourage better communication among the surgical team, the anesthesiologist, the nursing staff, and the patient.[9] The Commission suggests that all members of the clinical staff, as well as the patient, should be involved in marking the site of surgery. Involvement of the patient helps ensure that everyone understands the surgery to be performed, and it allows the clinical team to confirm that the intended surgery coincides with the patient's symptomatology.[9] One disadvantage that may be inherent in the neurosurgical setting is that the patient may not always be conscious or cooperative in the preoperative period to be involved in marking the surgical site. In this context, extra precautions are mandated, and barcode-enabled patient identification systems may reduce the chance of errors.

The Joint Commission guidelines recommend that a formal "time out" process be performed immediately before making the incision.[9] In the neurosurgical setting, a systematic review of the patient's history, neurologic examination, radiologic studies, and allied specialty consults should be conducted to verify the correct diagnosis and the correct procedure for the patient.

As rightly suggested by Ladak et al., neurosurgeons must embark on creating an open forum in which team members feel safe to question the diagnosis, localization, and surgical plan preoperatively without reprimand.[3] This is best accomplished through a surgical "team huddle" in which the diagnosis, imaging/testing, and surgical plan are reviewed, including patient identifiers, surgical site, and planned surgical procedure. Another aspect of preventing such complications is the familiarity and comfort level of interaction between the team members of the surgical suite.[10] If everyone knows and is comfortable communicating with each other, it is more likely that at the first hint of trouble the issue will be addressed promptly. If people don't communicate (say the nurse is intimidated by a surgeon he or she has not met before, or the surgeon incorrectly presumes the anesthesiologist is doing something that the usual anesthesiologist does), problems may not be articulated or fixed quickly.

Technologic advances can be incorporated in an effort to eliminate the chance of such errors. An example is the introduction of image-guided neurosurgery such as frameless stereotactic navigation system. In addition to providing easier localization of intracranial lesions and avoiding critical structures like venous sinuses during craniotomy, this technology can help nearly eliminate the chance of wrong-sided surgery.[1]

Strategies to Avoid Wrong-Level Spine Surgery

Vigilance against wrong-site surgery should be particularly high for spine surgeons because there are several factors inherent to spine surgery that increase the risk of wrong-site surgery compared with other types of surgery. These include morbid obesity, thoracic location, presence of multiple lesions, transitional anatomy, and diminished mineralization of the bone (resulting in difficult intraoperative localization). Not only can a surgeon potentially operate on the wrong side of the spine or at the wrong level, but unique issues related to spinal localization also can be challenging for even the most experienced clinicians.

Almost 50% of reporting surgeons have performed wrong-level lumbar spine surgery at least once, and >10% have performed wrong-side lumbar spine surgery at least once.[5] Nearly 20% of responding surgeons have been the subject of at least one malpractice case relating to these errors. Only 40% of respondents believed that the site marking/"time out" protocol of the Joint Commission—Accreditation of Healthcare Organizations—has led to a reduction in these errors.[5] It is important to acknowledge that even a strict adherence to such organizational guidelines will not prevent all instances of wrong-site surgery during spinal procedures. It is clear that preoperative checklists should be only one component of an overall strategy to prevent wrong-site surgery in spinal procedures.[9]

Intraoperative localization of spinal lesions with accuracy and specificity is paramount in avoiding wrong-site spinal surgery. This task is especially challenging in certain clinical situations, including operations in morbidly obese patients, those with pathologic entities in the thoracic spine, and patients with variations in spinal anatomy. Preoperative anticipation of this difficulty and implementation of certain localizing maneuvers can facilitate the surgical outcome. Radiopaque skin markers can be placed before a magnetic resonance imaging study or computed tomography scan to localize spinal lesions intraoperatively. However, skin markers may be subject to significant localization errors because the skin and underlying subcutaneous tissues of patients may undergo dramatic shifting and/or folding during positioning, particularly in obese patients. In patients undergoing operative procedures in the high thoracic spine, the use of methylene blue dye has been described to mark the spinous process of interest. Although potentially useful for posterior approaches to the thoracic spine, it is not feasible for anterior surgical techniques. In addition, neurotoxicity of the dye and lack of specificity (due to the tendency of the dye to spread) are disadvantages. Oblique fluoroscopic view avoids much of the chest and shoulder mass and may assist in difficult situations during lower cervical or high thoracic spinal surgeries. Preoperative vertebroplasty can be used for thoracic spine localization; it is very specific but has a significant complication rate associated with the procedure. Radiopaque coils have been described for the purpose of thoracic spine localization and are specific with low complication rates. In extremely difficult cases, 3-dimensional intraoperative imaging for the spine can be utilized with the sole aim of accurate localization of the correct spinal level.

Future Directions

Zero tolerance, or 100% accuracy, is the professional end goal for all neurosurgeons and the expectation by patients and society from the neurosurgical specialty. Excellence can be achieved only by surpassing the expectation, and in this context, technologic innovations and change of the current safety practices (surgical pause and checklist) are required. Existing safety protocols may not be mitigating wrong-site surgery to the extent previously thought, and this is especially true in the field of spine surgery. Application of an aviation model of incident reporting, redefining the neurosurgical checklists, inclusion of technologic advances like intraoperative imaging/navigation, application of the systems approach, and strong commitment from the neurosurgical community will be the way to move forward.

References

1. Rolston JD, Bernstein M. Errors in neurosurgery. *Neurosurg Clin N Am*. 2015;26:149–155, vii.
2. Jhawar BS, Mitsis D, Duggal N. Wrong-sided and wrong-level neurosurgery: a national survey. *J Neurosurg Spine*. 2007;7:467–472.
3. Ladak A, Spinner RJ. Redefining "wrong site surgery" and refining the surgical pause and checklist: taking surgical safety to another level. *World Neurosurg*. 2014;81:e33–e35.
4. Mody MG, Nourbakhsh A, Stahl DL, Gibbs M, Alfawareh M, Garges KJ. The prevalence of wrong level surgery among spine surgeons. *Spine*. 2008;33:194–198.
5. Groff MW, Heller JE, Potts EA, Mummaneni PV, Shaffrey CI, Smith JS. A survey-based study of wrong-level lumbar spine surgery: the scope of the problem and current practices in place to help avoid these errors. *World Neurosurg*. 2013;79:585–592.
6. Ferroli P, Caldiroli D, Acerbi F, et al. Application of an aviation model of incident reporting and investigation to the neurosurgical scenario: method and preliminary data. *Neurosurg Focus*. 2012;33:E7.
7. Kapur N, Parand A, Soukup T, Reader T, Sevdalis N. Aviation and healthcare: a comparative review with implications for patient safety. *JRSM Open*. 2016;7:2054270415616548.
8. Ricci M, Panos AL, Lincoln J, Salerno TA, Warshauer L. Is aviation a good model to study human errors in health care? *Am J Surg*. 2012;203:798–801.
9. Hsu W, Kretzer RM, Dorsi MJ, Gokaslan ZL. Strategies to avoid wrong-site surgery during spinal procedures. *Neurosurg Focus*. 2011;31:E5.
10. McDonnell PJ. The lesson of flight 214, in *Ophthalmology Times*, 2013.

4 Medical Complications in Neurosurgery

VINAYAK NARAYAN, PIYUSH KALAKOTI, ANIL NANDA

HIGHLIGHTS

- Medical complication after a neurosurgical procedure is defined as an unanticipated adverse event that is not directly related to the neurosurgical technique or procedure.
- It includes venous thromboembolism; cardiorespiratory complications; acute renal failure; and infectious, gastrointestinal, metabolic, and hemorrhage or transfusion-related complications.
- The incidence of medical complications adversely influences the neurosurgical outcome.
- A multidisciplinary team approach, strict perioperative vigilance, early detection of the medical complication, and immediate intervention are the effective strategies for tackling medical complications.

Introduction

Medical complications after neurosurgical procedures are common and contribute substantially to morbidity and mortality. They can adversely impact the surgical outcome and are also implicated in increasing resource utilization by prolonging the hospital stay. Whereas most neurosurgical literature on outcome-based prediction has laid emphasis on surgery-related complications, the literature on medical complications based on current evidence is scarce. Considering the deleterious impact of medical complications on overall surgical outcome, it is pertinent to reiterate commonly occurring medical complications associated with neurosurgical care to optimize patient-oriented outcome and minimize resource utilization as well as cost of care. In this chapter, we provide a comprehensive overview of common medical complications that are likely to occur after a cranial or spinal procedure, their catastrophic impact on patient management, and the prophylactic/preventive strategies to reduce their incidence.

Definition and Classification Scheme

Medical complication after a neurosurgical procedure is defined as an unanticipated adverse event that is not directly related to the neurosurgical technique or procedure.[1] The timing of its occurrence can range from any time during initial hospitalization to later on as a part of routine care. These complications comprise a myriad of conditions such as venous thromboembolism, cardiorespiratory complications, acute renal failure (ARF), and infectious gastrointestinal (GI) and metabolic complications.[2–4] A recent proposition by Landriel Ibañez et al. aggregated 167 potential complications into a four-point scale grading system, of which 38 complications were classified as medical (grade IV) events not directly related to surgery or surgical technique; however, little information was provided on the specifics of the complications.[4] In the context of pediatric patients with spinal deformity, Smith et al. proposed a complication grading system that incorporated disease-related inpatient medical complications as a subset, emphasizing the impact of medical complications on outcomes.[5] Although disease- or procedure-specific grading systems are useful, most complications overlap several procedures. In the current chapter, we focus on medical complications that are limited to those occurring post–cranial or spinal interventions, rather than preoperatively occurring comorbidities or events. Based upon current literature, medical complications are broadly categorized based on the organ system involved; they are summarized in Table 4.1.

Thromboembolic Complications: Deep Venous Thrombosis and Pulmonary Embolism

Thromboembolic events are life threatening and can often lead to rapid clinical deterioration including mortality. Deep venous thrombosis (DVT) and pulmonary embolism are major contributors to this morbidity and mortality in postoperative neurosurgical patients. The incidence of thromboembolic events is estimated to be 0% to 50%, of which DVT, as measured by the labeled fibrinogen technique, accounts for around 29% to 43%.[6–11] Major events usually occur within the first week after a neurosurgical procedure. Most DVT patients are asymptomatic, and 15% of silent DVTs can lead to pulmonary embolism. Significant thrombi are thought to arise from the popliteal and iliofemoral veins. Risk factors include prolonged surgery and immobilization, previous DVT, malignancy, ischemic stroke, direct lower-extremity trauma, limb weakness, seizure disorder, chronic smoking, use of oral contraceptives, pregnancy and the puerperium, obesity, gram-negative sepsis, advanced age, pregnancy, and congestive heart failure.[7,9–12] Patients with deficiencies in antithrombin III, protein C, or protein S and with various genetic clotting factor abnormalities, such as factor V Leiden, are also at risk for venous thromboembolism. Specific to neurosurgical procedure, patients undergoing brain surgery for intracranial tumors—especially meningioma, traumatic brain injury, and spinal cord injury—are the high-risk groups for developing a thromboembolic event.[13]

Even though the clinical signs can give a clue regarding DVT, Doppler ultrasonography and impedance plethysmography are the preferred investigation modalities. When Doppler results are

TABLE 4.1 Common Medical Complications Following Neurosurgical Procedures

Thromboembolic complications	• Deep venous thrombosis • Pulmonary embolism • Phlebitis
Respiratory complications	• Pneumonia • Acute respiratory distress syndrome • Acute lung injury • Transfusion-related acute lung injury • Atelectasis • Pleural effusion • Pneumothorax (rare)
Nosocomial infections	• Meningitis • Urinary tract infections • Catheter-associated urinary tract infections • Systemic inflammatory response syndrome/ multiorgan dysfunction syndrome
Cardiac complications	• Acute myocardial ischemia • Arrhythmias • Hyper- or hypotension • Sudden cardiac death
Renal complications	• Acute renal failure • Urinary retention • Acute tubular necrosis
Gastrointestinal complications	• Gastric ulcers or hemorrhage • Pseudomembranous colitis • Cholecystitis • Pancreatitis • Noninfectious diarrhea • Necrotizing pancreatitis
Other complications	• Venous air embolism • Hemorrhagic and transfusion-related complications • Wound complications • Psychologic disturbances • Decubitus ulcer • Metabolic complications (hyponatremia, diabetes insipidus, hyperglycemia) • Anemia • Sepsis and shock

equivocal, extremity venography can be used to diagnose distal and proximal DVTs. Similarly, a postoperative patient developing acute-onset chest pain, hemoptysis, and breathlessness should be evaluated for pulmonary embolism, and computed tomography (CT) angiogram or pulmonary angiogram are considered the investigation methods of choice.

Because DVT can very often lead to pulmonary embolism, the prophylactic measures to prevent these complications are very important. Many studies have confirmed the utility of sequential pneumatic leg compression devices in preventing DVT.[7,8] These devices are placed on the patient preoperatively and should be continued until the patient is ambulatory. The prophylactic use of low-dose (minidose) subcutaneous heparin (e.g., 5000 IU twice daily) has been well studied over the past several years and has been demonstrated to be efficacious in preventing DVT. Several meta-analyses have been conducted, but it remains unclear whether unfractionated heparin or low-molecular-weight heparin is superior for DVT prophylaxis in neurosurgical patients, or whether increased efficacy correlates with increased hemorrhagic complications.[14–17]

Many neurosurgeons believe that in the immediate and early postoperative period, neurosurgical patients with documented DVT should undergo transvenous Greenfield filter placement. Anticoagulation using heparin followed by warfarin may be continued for 6 weeks to 3 months in uncomplicated cases.[14,15] The treatment guidelines followed for DVT are applicable for pulmonary embolism also. Pulmonary embolectomy may be performed as the last lifesaving measure when all other treatment options fail.

Pulmonary Complications

Pulmonary complications are common after neurosurgical procedures. They have been reported to cause almost 50% of deaths from medical causes. The major respiratory complications include hypoxemia, pneumonia, pulmonary edema, pulmonary embolism, respiratory infections, and acute respiratory distress syndrome. The major risk factors for respiratory complication after a neurosurgical procedure are older age, chronic obstructive pulmonary disease (COPD), history of ischemic stroke or transient ischemic attack (TIA), coagulopathy, and chronic smoking.[18,19] Irrespective of the etiology, whether cardiogenic or noncardiogenic, the treatment of pulmonary edema includes immediate intubation and ventilation, adequate oxygenation, positive end-expiratory pressure, furosemide, and measures to reduce increased intra-cranial pressure (ICP).

Ventilator-associated pneumonia (VAP) is a common complication in those patients who require prolonged postoperative mechanical ventilation. The high incidence of pneumonia (27.2%) and its association with increased mortality rate (9.7%) have been reported previously.[20] Prevention of pneumonia in these cases should include removal of nasogastric and endotracheal tubes as soon as indicated, avoidance of unanticipated extubation and gastric overdistention, strict handwashing, semirecumbent positioning of the patient, maintenance of adequate nutrition, oral intubation, proper ventilator care, optimum antibiotic coverage, chest physiotherapy, and early mobilization. Tracheostomy should be considered in a patient who has been intubated for 10 to 14 days and for whom extubation is not imminent.

Nosocomial Infections

Nosocomial infections, especially meningitis, in postoperative neurosurgical patients constitute the major cause of morbidity and mortality worldwide. The risk factors for meningitis include elderly age group, male gender, diabetes mellitus, tracheal intubation, presence of lumbar drain, enteral nutrition (percutaneous endoscopic gastrostomy [PEG] tubes), repeat surgery, Glasgow coma scale (GCS <12), and those undergoing emergent procedure.[21] Urinary tract infections (UTI) and respiratory and wound infections are the other common nosocomial infections seen in neurosurgical patients. *Staphylococcus aureus, Staphylococcus epidermidis,* and *Pseudomonas aeruginosa* are the common pathogens involved in hospital-acquired infections. The judicious use of antibiotics based on sensitivity pattern, careful use of steroid medications to avoid immunosuppression, strict glycemic control in diabetic patients, aseptic precautions during surgical procedures, and implementation of infection control protocol in the hospital are the primary measures to prevent nosocomial infection–related morbidity and mortality.[22]

Cardiac Complications

Cardiac complications after neurosurgical procedures are well described in the literature. The common cardiac issues usually encountered in neurosurgical setup include arrhythmias (atrial and ventricular fibrillation), blood pressure derangements (hyper- or hypotension), bradycardia, myocardial infarction, infective endocarditis, sudden cardiac death, and asystole.[23–25] The complications are commonly seen after tumor/vascular surgery. For brain tumor surgery, the incidence of inpatient cardiac complication is estimated to be 0.7% after glioma resection and 1.1% after a benign tumor resection.[18,19] In the context of cerebrovascular interventions, rates of cardiac complication are likely to be higher after microsurgical clipping compared with endovascular coiling for both ruptured (1.69% vs 0.95%) and unruptured aneurysms (1.28% vs 0.48%).[12,26] The general risk factors include advancing age, prior history of stroke, active smoking, cocaine abuse, cardiac comorbidities (coronary artery disease, congestive heart failure), altered mental sensorium, renal dysfunction, hyperlipidemia, coagulopathy, cardiac prosthesis, and peripheral vascular disease.[12,18,19,26] Neurogenic stunned myocardium, a severe cardiac injury, is a reversible pathology often found in patients who die after subarachnoid hemorrhage (SAH).

Electrocardiogram (ECG) and echocardiography are the standard investigation modalities to rule out cardiac disease. Strict intensive care management is essential to diagnose and treat cardiac complications in a postoperative neurosurgical unit. Medications such as beta-blockers and calcium channel blockers for hypertension, digoxin for cardiac failure, antiarrhythmic medications, vasodilators such as nitrates, and ionotropic agents like dopamine/dobutamine, as well as defibrillation/cardioversion, play a crucial role in the postoperative management of neurosurgical patients.[26–28]

Renal Complications

The incidence of renal complications such as ARF or acute tubular necrosis (ATN) in a neurosurgical setup can be due to nephrotoxic medication administration, dehydration, rhabdomyolysis, and radiocontrast injections. Major risk factors include advancing age, chronic renal dysfunction, history of ischemic stroke, coagulopathies, diabetes mellitus, congestive heart failure, peripheral vascular disease, and hypertension.[12,18,19,23,26]

Analysis of data from nonfederal U.S. hospitals demonstrated the estimated risk of postsurgical ARF of 1.3% and 1.5% after intracranial glioma and meningioma surgeries, respectively.[18,19] Lower rates were observed for patients undergoing microsurgical clipping or endovascular coiling of aneurysms (ruptured 0.8%; unruptured 0.1%).[12,26] On the contrary, a higher rate of over 4% was noted in patients undergoing fusion surgery for axis fracture.[29] Incidence of ARF was higher in patients undergoing secondary fusion (revision) surgery for lumbar degenerative disc disease than in patients undergoing primary fusion (1.2% vs 1.0%).[30] The use of imaging such as cerebral arteriogram or contrast-enhanced CT/MR (magnetic resonance), which requires injecting nephrotoxic contrast materials, should be judiciously used in patients with renal dysfunction. Removing the offending drug; avoiding radiocontrast injections; monitoring blood electrolytes, urea, and creatinine; maintaining adequate hydration; and monitoring blood pressure and urinary output help patients avoid complications due to renal dysfunction. Severe cases of ARF may require hemodialysis to prevent further renal damage.

Gastrointestinal Complications

The myriad of GI complications after neurosurgical interventions include postsurgical paralytic ileus, gastric or duodenal ulcers, GI bleeding, colitis, and noninfectious (antibiotic-associated or pseudomembranous colitis) diarrhea. The incidence of paralytic ileus ranges from 5% to 12% in patients undergoing spine procedures.[31] In selected patients implanted with a PEG tube for feeding, medical complications such as infection (methicillin-resistant *Staphylococcus aureus* [MRSA]) or sepsis, peristomal wound leakage, necrotizing fasciitis, tube dislodgement, and pneumoperitoneum may complicate the hospital stay.[32] The administration of appropriate antibiotics, stool softeners, and proton pump inhibitors; adequate hydration; strict asepsis; electrolyte monitoring; and judicious use of analgesics in the postoperative period are the basic prerequisites to avoid such complications. Surgery may be required in certain emergency situations such as gastric or intestinal perforation, mesenteric ischemia, or intestinal gangrene.

Other Complications

Venous air embolism (VAE) is also a catastrophic medical complication most commonly encountered in patients undergoing posterior cranial fossa surgery in seated position, even though other positions are also described in the literature.[33] Apart from sitting position, dehydration, and congenital heart diseases such as patent foramen ovale, right to left shunts are also major risk factors for VAE. It is caused by the entry of air through noncollapsible veins, venous sinuses, or diploic veins.[33] Its incidence varies from 1% to 60%, with a morbidity/mortality rate of less than 3% in most series. Early detection of this complication is the most important step in management, and the ideal diagnostic modalities are transesophageal echocardiography and Doppler. The treatment comprises hemodynamic stabilization, aspiration of air through right atrial catheter, discontinuation of nitrous oxide, and administration of pure oxygen in addition to the surgical sealing of the portal of air entry.

Two significant hemorrhage-related complications are disseminated intravascular coagulation and transfusion reactions. Even though both are related to excessive bleeding and transfusions, the former results in consumptive coagulopathy, while the latter results in shock. The transfusion-related disorders also include metabolic disorders and associated electrolyte disturbances. The methods to minimize allogenic transfusion and avoidance of aspirin in the perioperative period help prevent transfusion- and hemorrhage-related complications.

Similarly, wound-related complications at the operative site also contribute to poor surgical outcome; the major risk factors are malnutrition, obesity, smoking, prior radiotherapy or chemotherapy, prolonged steroid use, and reoperations. Off-midline incision in spine surgeries, avoidance of the incision in the impaired area, and maintenance of a clean and dry sterile wound area are the basic requirements to maintain wound integrity.

Endocrinologic disturbances such as diabetes insipidus, hyperglycemia, and fluid and electrolyte abnormalities (e.g., hyponatremia in syndrome of inappropriate antidiuretic hormone secretion [SIADH] or cerebral salt wasting [CSW]) after aneurysmal SAH or pituitary tumor surgeries are common in routine practice.[34] The basic management principle is to make an accurate diagnosis. Tight glucose control is the basis of hyperglycemia management. The key differentiating feature between SIADH and salt wasting is volume status. The primary treatment for salt wasting is adequate water and sodium replacement to maintain at least normovolemia and normal serum sodium, whereas in patients with SIADH, fluid restriction is the mainstay of treatment. Treatment of diabetes insipidus consists of replacement of fluid losses with hypotonic solutions such as 5% dextrose in water or 0.45% sodium chloride.

In the chronic phase, exogenous replacement of antidiuretic hormone may be required.[35]

Psychologic complications include mental health disturbances such as postoperative delirium or excessive anxiety, which can be managed with antipsychotic medications such as haloperidol and selective serotonergic reuptake inhibitor (SSRI) medications, respectively.[23] Anemia, decubitus ulcer, sepsis, and multiorgan dysfunction syndrome (MODS) are the other medical complications that are usually encountered in neurosurgical practice.

Conclusions

The surgical outcome of neurosurgical interventions can be improved with proper understanding of the complications that are likely to arise. The incidence of medical complications adversely affects postoperative recovery and prolongs the hospital stay of the patient. A strict perioperative vigilance, early detection of the medical complication, and immediate intervention are the effective strategies involved in ideal postoperative neurosurgical care. A multidisciplinary team approach involving neurosurgeons, intensivists, occupational therapists, and allied health professionals is required to reduce the incidence of such life-threatening complications and to improve the neurosurgical outcome.

References

1. Lebude B, Yadla S, Albert T, et al. Defining "complications" in spine surgery: neurosurgery and orthopedic spine surgeons survey. *J Spinal Disord Tech*. 2010;23(8):493–500.
2. Bonsanto MM, Hamer J, Tronnier V, Kunze S. A complication conference for internal quality control at the Neurosurgical Department of the University of Heidelberg. *Acta Neurochir Suppl*. 2001;78:139–145.
3. Houkin K, Baba T, Minamida Y, Nonaka T, Koyanagi I, Iiboshi S. Quantitative analysis of adverse events in neurosurgery. *Neurosurgery*. 2009;65(3):587–594.
4. Landriel Ibañez FA, Hem S, Ajler P, et al. A new classification of complications in neurosurgery. *World Neurosurg*. 2011;75(5–6):709–715.
5. Smith JT, Johnston C, Skaggs D, Flynn J, Vitale M. A new classification system to report complications in growing spine surgery: a multicenter consensus study. *J Pediatr Orthop*. 2015;35(8):798–803.
6. Khaldi A, Helo N, Schneck MJ, Origitano TC. Venous thromboembolism: deep venous thrombosis and pulmonary embolism in a neurosurgical population. *J Neurosurg*. 2011;114(1):40–46.
7. Bucek RA, Koca N, Reiter M, Haumer M, Zontsich T, Minar E. Algorithms for the diagnosis of deep-vein thrombosis in patients with low clinical pretest probability. *Thromb Res*. 2002;105(1):43–47.
8. Dearborn JT, Hu SS, Tribus CB, Bradford DS. Thromboembolic complications after major thoracolumbar spine surgery. *Spine*. 1999;24(14):1471–1476.
9. Ferree BA, Stern PJ, Jolson RS, Roberts JM, Kahn A. Deep venous thrombosis after spinal surgery. *Spine*. 1993;18(3):315–319.
10. Levi AD, Wallace MC, Bernstein M, Walters BC. Venous thromboembolism after brain tumor surgery: a retrospective review. *Neurosurgery*. 1991;28(6):859–863.
11. Marras LC, Geerts WH, Perry JR. The risk of venous thromboembolism is increased throughout the course of malignant glioma: an evidence-based review. *Cancer*. 2000;89(3):640–646.
12. Bekelis K, Missios S, Mackenzie TA, Fischer A, Labropoulos N, Eskey C. A predictive model of outcomes during cerebral aneurysm coiling. *J Neurointerv Surg*. 2014;6(5):342–348.
13. Eisenring CV, Neidert MC, Sabanés Bové D, Held L, Sarnthein J, Krayenbühl N. Reduction of thromboembolic events in meningioma surgery: a cohort study of 724 consecutive patients. *PLoS ONE*. 2013;8(11):e79170.
14. Melamed AJ, Suarez J. Detection and prevention of deep venous thrombosis. *Drug Intell Clin Pharm*. 1988;22(2):107–114.
15. Wen DY, Hall WA. Complications of subcutaneous low-dose heparin therapy in neurosurgical patients. *Surg Neurol*. 1998;50(6): 521–525.
16. Dickinson LD, Miller LD, Patel CP, Gupta SK. Enoxaparin increases the incidence of postoperative intracranial hemorrhage when initiated preoperatively for deep venous thrombosis prophylaxis in patients with brain tumors. *Neurosurgery*. 1998;43(5):1074–1081.
17. Mätzsch T. Thromboprophylaxis with low-molecular-weight heparin: economic considerations. *Haemostasis*. 2000;30 Suppl 2:141–145-9.
18. Bekelis K, Kalakoti P, Nanda A, Missios S. A predictive model of unfavorable outcomes after benign intracranial tumor resection. *World Neurosurg*. 2015;84(1):82–89.
19. Missios S, Kalakoti P, Nanda A, Bekelis K. Craniotomy for glioma resection: A predictive model. *World Neurosurg*. 2015;83(6):957–964.
20. Savardekar A, Gyurmey T, Agarwal R, et al. Incidence, risk factors, and outcome of postoperative pneumonia after microsurgical clipping of ruptured intracranial aneurysms. *Surg Neurol Int*. 2013;4(1):24.
21. Chen C, Zhang B, Yu S, et al. The incidence and risk factors of meningitis after major craniotomy in China: a retrospective cohort study. *PLoS ONE*. 2014;9(7):e101961.
22. Yamamoto M, Jimbo M, Ide M, Tanaka N, Umebara Y, Hagiwara S. Postoperative neurosurgical infection and antibiotic prophylaxis. *Neurol Med Chir (Tokyo)*. 1992;32(2):72–79.
23. Baron EM, Albert TJ. Medical complications of surgical treatment of adult spinal deformity and how to avoid them. *Spine*. 2006;31: S106–S118.
24. Chowdhury T, Petropolis A, Cappellani RB. Cardiac emergencies in neurosurgical patients. *Biomed Res Int*. 2015;2015:751320.
25. Tyler DS, Bacon D, Mahendru V, Lema MJ. Asystole as a neurologic sign. *J Neurosurg Anesthesiol*. 1997;9(1):29–30.
26. Bekelis K, Missios S, MacKenzie TA, et al. Predicting inpatient complications from cerebral aneurysm clipping: the Nationwide Inpatient Sample 2005-2009. *J Neurosurg*. 2014;120(3):591–598.
27. Hottinger DG, Beebe DS, Kozhimannil T, Prielipp RC, Belani KG. Sodium nitroprusside in 2014: a clinical concepts review. *J Anaesthesiol Clin Pharmacol*. 2014;30(4):462–471.
28. Varon J, Marik PE. Perioperative hypertension management. *Vasc Health Risk Manag*. 2008;4(3):615–627.
29. Kalakoti P, Missios S, Kukreja S, Storey C, Sun H, Nanda A. Impact of associated injuries in conjunction with fracture of the axis vertebra on inpatient outcomes and postoperative complications: a Nationwide Inpatient Sample analysis from 2002 to 2011. *Spine J*. 2016;16(4): 491–503.
30. Kalakoti P, Missios S, Maiti T, et al. Inpatient outcomes and postoperative complications after primary versus revision lumbar spinal fusion surgeries for degenerative lumbar disc disease: a nationwide inpatient sample analysis, 2002–2011. *World Neurosurg*. 2016;85: 114–124.
31. Althausen PL, Gupta MC, Benson DR, Jones DA. The use of neostigmine to treat postoperative ileus in orthopedic spinal patients. *J Spinal Disord*. 2001;14(6):541–545.
32. Koc D, Gercek A, Gencosmanoglu R, Tozun N. Percutaneous endoscopic gastrostomy in the neurosurgical intensive care unit: complications and outcome. *JPEN J Parenter Enteral Nutr*. 2007;31(6): 517–520.
33. Türe H, Harput MV, Bekiroglu N, Keskin O, Koner O, Türe U. Effect of the degree of head elevation on the incidence and severity of venous air embolism in cranial neurosurgical procedures with patients in the semisitting position. *J Neurosurg*. 2017;1–10.
34. Sherlock M, O'Sullivan E, Agha A, et al. The incidence and pathophysiology of hyponatraemia after subarachnoid haemorrhage. *Clin Endocrinol*. 2006;64(3):250–254.
35. Takaku A, Shindo K, Tanaka S, Mori T, Suzuki J. Fluid and electrolyte disturbances in patients with intracranial aneurysms. *Surg Neurol*. 1979;11(5):349–356.

5 Surgical Complications in Neurosurgery

ANIL NANDA, DEVI PRASAD PATRA

HIGHLIGHTS

- Avoidance of surgical complications is an important step in achieving a profitable health care system and therefore needs a judicious reporting system in defining the incidence of complications.
- Important complications after cranial surgery include cerebral edema, hemorrhage, infarction, wound infection etc. Important complications after spinal surgery include neurological deficits, dural tear and CSF fistula, vascular injury and instrumentation failure etc.
- Infectious complications are the most common cause of morbidity after neurosurgical procedures whereas intracranial hemorrhage is the most common cause requiring reoperation.
- Meticulous dissection, gentle handling of neural tissues, good hemostasis and appropriate use of intraoperative adjuncts are few amongst the invaluable tools in prevention of surgical complications.

Introduction

With the current economic reform in health care, the focus is on high-quality care and the pressing need for better performance by healthcare providers. The accountability of healthcare professionals has increased multifold with the current "value-based healthcare system," which is defined as the health outcome achieved per dollar spent.[1] An initiative by the Centers for Medicare and Medicaid Services (CMS) to compare and evaluate individual hospitals based on different outcome measures gives insight into the competitive market and the need for value-based care.[2] When the emphasis is on amalgamating cost containment and profitable care, surgical complications are considered most undesirable, both for the patient and the healthcare system. In this context, complications after neurologic surgery are fairly common and contribute significantly to overall postoperative morbidity and to health expenditure.

A common hindrance in addressing any surgical complication is its irregular reporting.[3,4] Many cases go unnoticed because of inherent avoidance of documentation by the surgeon himself. However, there has been improved reporting of adverse events and complications with the introduction of electronic data recording systems and with mandatory checklists that are maintained by independent treatment teams. In the past decade, many of the national databases in the United States have been committed to collecting data on complications based on objective criteria; these databases include the National Surgical Quality Improvement Program (NSQIP),[5] the Cleveland Clinic's cardiovascular information registry,[6] and the Agency for Healthcare Research and Quality.[7,8] In particular, NSQIP has well-defined criteria for documentation of surgical complications, with regular auditing of the reporting system to make it honest and reproducible.[4] Neurosurgical procedures are more prone to complications compared with nonneurosurgical procedures because of factors such as the increased number of inpatient procedures, longer operative time, and increased hospitalization days.[4]

A NSQIP database review of 38,000 neurosurgical cases during 2006 to 2011 reveals that the overall complication rate after neurosurgical procedures is 14.3%; the complication rate after cranial procedures was 23.6%, which was 2.6 times the rate with spinal procedures (11.2%).[4] The most common complication in this study was bleeding requiring transfusion, which occurred in 4.5% of patients. A recent analysis of an individual hospital–based patient registry of 2880 patients undergoing cranial surgery estimates the overall complication rate to be 24%.[9] However, another study of 5361 patients, from 19 physicians with a predominantly spinal procedure practice, reported a complication rate as low as 4.9%. The major complication in the series was cerebrospinal fluid (CSF) leakage (0.89%) and infection (0.61%).[10] Another study, based on the NSQIP database, compared the complication trend in neurosurgery and reported a decrease in complication rate from 11.0% in 2006 to 7.5% in 2013.[3]

Surgical complications are usually specific to a particular neurosurgical procedure, and these specific complications will be dealt with in the individual sections. This current overview focuses on the general complications that are common to all neurosurgical procedures.

Complications in Cranial Surgery

Cerebral Edema

Postoperative edema of the neural tissue is almost inevitable after any degree of surgical manipulation, but in most cases, this is not clinically significant. Subtle cerebral edema may lead to delayed return of normal neurologic function, but in severe cases may manifest as worsening level of sensorium, seizures, and neurologic deficits. In severe cases, it is referred to as malignant cerebral edema, which may lead to cerebral herniation and also death. The pathogenesis of cerebral edema involves both the macro- and microcirculation. Hemodynamic changes after damage or thrombosis of draining veins, accompanied by cytotoxic changes of brain parenchyma due to direct damage or ischemia from prolonged retraction, form a vicious cycle that produce macroscopic cerebral edema. Multiple factors have been correlated with the development of cerebral edema, including excessive brain manipulation, prolonged retraction, and excessive bipolar coagulation with resultant venous edema.[11]

Incorrect positioning or excessive head rotation that leads to impaired venous return may also result in brain edema that itself may become obvious during surgery. Some of the anesthetic agents can also cause cerebral edema by various mechanisms; for example, isoflurane and nitrous oxide may increase cerebral blood volume, and enflurane and halothane may reduce CSF absorption.[12] Cerebral venous thrombosis can also occur after an uneventful surgery because of dehydration and intraoperative hypotension. Patients with inherited coagulopathy are more prone to this complication. Cerebral edema is usually diagnosed in computed tomography (CT) scans as areas of hypodensity surrounding the surgical cavity with or without mass effect. Large areas of edema may be seen as loss of demarcation at gray-white matter interface. In magnetic resonance imaging (MRI), edema is more evident in T2 and fluid attenuation inversion recovery (FLAIR) sequences, where it appears as areas of hyperintensity due to increased water content. In most cases, postoperative edema is self-limiting and requires only careful observation and strict intake and output monitoring with maintenance of euvolemia and normotension. Resolution of edema becomes clinically evident with improvement in the sensorium and in neurologic deficits. In moderate cases, osmotic agents like mannitol and hypertonic saline as well as diuretics like furosemide are used to decrease the brain's hydrostatic pressure. Mechanical ventilation in obtunded patients is usually helpful in reducing edema by improving brain oxygenation and cerebral vasoconstriction. In cases of severe malignant edema with impending herniation, surgical intervention may be required in the form of decompressive craniectomy or lobectomy. Surgical strategies that are suggested to prevent significant postoperative edema include proper positioning to decrease venous compression, avoidance of excessive brain retraction, adequate intraoperative hydration, minimal manipulation of the normal brain parenchyma, judicious use of bipolar coagulation, and avoidance of coagulation of draining veins.

Cerebral Hemorrhage

Postoperative hematoma is one of the most common and catastrophic complications after intracranial surgery and is an important cause of postoperative morbidity and mortality. The reported rates of postoperative hemorrhage vary in the literature depending on the practice patterns and definitions of postoperative hemorrhage. Many patients have a small amount of blood in the operative cavity, and such radiologic incidence of hemorrhage ranges from 10% to 50%.[13–15] However, the incidence of hemorrhage having clinical implications that require some form of intervention is reportedly low, ranging from 0.8% to 6.9%.[16,17] Many factors have been correlated with the formation of postoperative hemorrhage. The most important are perioperative factors, which include the inability to achieve hemostasis, and intraoperative factors such as hypertension and intraoperative severe bleeding causing disseminated intra-vascular coagulation (DIC). Important preoperative factors include older age, hypertension, and hematologic abnormalities such as thrombocytopenia and coagulation abnormality. Some of the intracranial lesions have a greater propensity for developing postoperative hemorrhage, notably vascular tumors like meningioma, glomus tumor, and hemangiopericytoma; arteriovenous malformations; and high-grade gliomas, especially after subtotal resection. Conditions such as chronic subdural hematomas also have a propensity for recurrence, though this is not evident in the immediate postoperative periods. Similarly, patients with traumatic hemorrhage or contusion tend to have increased incidence of postoperative hematoma because of trauma-induced coagulopathy.[15,18]

Unless immediate postoperative CT scan is a norm, most postoperative hemorrhages are suspected based on clinical grounds, including lack of recovery from anaesthesia, deterioration of the sensorium, or development of focal neurologic deficits. Postoperative hemorrhages can be tumor bed hematomas or subdural or epidural hematomas. Although almost all postoperative hemorrhages are located in the primary surgical area, remote-site hemorrhages can occur in intraparenchymal, subdural, subarachnoid, and epidural locations and in different compartments as well. The incidence of remote-site hemorrhage is rare and has been estimated to be an average of 1 in 300 craniotomies.[19] Important causes of remote-site hemorrhage include coagulation disorders, older patients with an atrophic brain, rapid decompression of the brain after ventricular shunts or evacuation of hematomas, brain shrinkage due to excessive mannitol use, sitting or remaining in a prone position for a prolonged period, and inappropriate placement of head holders with injury of epidural or subdural vessels.[14,19] One study analyzing the NSQIP database reported that 1.5% of craniotomies required reoperation for hemorrhage.[20] The most common site of hemorrhage was subdural or epidural, comprising 88.5% of cases, whereas only 11.5% of cases had intraparenchymal hemorrhage. Although repeat surgery decreases the mortality rate, the neurologic deficits are less likely to improve completely, giving rise to a significant morbidity. Therefore a preventive strategy is considered wiser; this includes meticulous hemostasis using bipolar coagulation and various commercially available topical hemostats. Maintaining perioperative and postoperative normotension and preventing and managing coagulation disorders are among the few general measures that help reduce the incidence of postoperative hematoma.

Cerebral Infarction

The incidence of postoperative stroke and coma after neurosurgical procedures is 0.73% as estimated by one study using the NSQIP database.[21] Postoperative cerebral infarction can be arterial or venous. Arterial infarctions may occur due to intraoperative injury and sacrifice of major arteries, which are usually well delineated. Although sacrifice of a major artery almost definitely leads to the development of an infarction, in most cases the size of the infarction is limited due to the presence of collateral circulation. For this reason, watershed areas are more prone to the development of an infarction due to direct injury or even in the event of prolonged hypotension. Most of the arterial injuries are evident during surgery; however, in a few cases, injury of the perforating vessels may go unnoticed intraoperatively but give rise to significant postoperative deficits due to lacunar infarcts in the deep nuclear structures. Arterial injuries are dependent solely on the experience of the surgeons and on the type and extent of the lesions. Tumors with vascular encasements like meningiomas, chordomas, and hemangiomas are prone to arterial injury during dissection. Similarly, vascular lesions like aneurysms and arteriovenous malformations have an inherent tendency to induce vasospasm during/after surgery. Surgical experience has also been correlated with incidence of arterial injury. Inadequate knowledge of vascular anatomy, poor skills in microsurgery, inappropriate dissection techniques, and lack of expertise in vascular repairs are obvious surgeon-related factors associated with a higher incidence of vascular injuries. Arterial infarcts may develop in a delayed fashion due to vasospasm, most notably after subarachnoid hemorrhage due to aneurysm rupture. Some forms of vasospasm may be noted after resection of tumors from encased vessels and are related to prolonged dissection and manipulation of the vessel. In such cases arterial infarcts may not develop in all cases, but cerebral hypoperfusion can lead to altered sensorium and short-term neurologic deficits. Acute development of infarct is associated with some form of edema, which may give rise to mass effect and is therefore life-threatening. In such cases, intracranial pressure (ICP) reduction measures or even decompressive craniectomy may be required. The mortality risk decreases gradually once the infarct becomes well delineated; however, it carries a significant risk of permanent morbidity.

Venous infarcts develop after sacrifice of major cortical draining veins or venous sinuses but are rarely permanent. Apart from direct venous injury, other significant causes for the development of venous infarcts include venous thrombosis or sinus thrombosis. Important factors responsible for this include prolonged cortical exposure without saline irrigation, intraoperative hypotension, and inappropriate use of pressure or hemostats for bleeding control or ligation of proximal veins. The venous thrombosis may manifest acutely or develop in a delayed fashion. Venous infarctions mostly manifest as the development of cerebral edema with or without venous hemorrhage. The edema and mass effect are more significant than with arterial infarcts and therefore need anti-ICP measures or surgery in almost all cases. The edema tends to be progressive, which requires prolonged clinical and radiologic monitoring. However, once the edema subsides, neurologic recovery is usually more complete as compared with arterial infarcts.

Seizures

Postoperative seizures can occur in the immediate postoperative period or late in the recovery course. Early postoperative seizures can occur in 10% to 20% of supratentorial surgeries due to cortical irritation after manipulation of brain tumors like gliomas and meningiomas or of vascular lesions like arteriovenous malformations or pneumocephalus.[11,22] However, seizures can be the early manifestation of underlying severe complications like postoperative hematomas, venous edema, or infarction. Therefore all early postoperative seizures should be evaluated with brain imaging to rule out life-threatening events. Other causes of seizures during the postoperative period include recurrence in patients with previous seizures, electrolyte imbalance, hypoxia, and anaesthetic medication. Seizures may also occur during the late postoperative period due to cortical scarring or regrowth of the lesion. Postoperative seizures are usually managed conservatively with antiepileptic drugs, unless they are induced by life-threatening hematoma or edema. However, various systematic reviews as well as clinical trials have not proven any benefit of prophylactic use of antiepileptics for intracranial surgery.[22,23] Intraoperative precautions that are helpful in reducing the incidence of seizures include minimization of retraction, avoidance of excessive coagulation, frequent irrigation, and maintenance of proper hemostasis.

Neurologic Deficits

Neurologic deficits are among the most feared complications. Many of the neurologic deficits especially affecting the higher mental functions go unnoticed unless checked specifically. Significant neurologic deficits causing limb weakness, numbness, or speech difficulties pose significant morbidity in the postoperative period. Most patients recover to a great extent in the long term; however, complete recovery is rare. Neurologic deficits are usually predictable because they are specific to the site of surgery. In the initial postoperative period, the deficits are denser and more widespread because of the involvement of surrounding neurons, called "neural stunning," a condition that is usually transient. Once the neurons recover from the operative stress, the deficits gradually improve and become limited to the structures that were directly damaged. On the other hand, the deficits may appear in a delayed fashion with worsening of initial deficits; this is mostly due to damage to vascular structures, leading to gradual ischemia. The extent of damage required to produce a deficit greatly varies with the site involved. Sites with a great degree of plasticity like cerebral and cerebellar lobes require severe damage to produce deficits; however, deeper structures like the thalamus, internal capsule, and brainstem are less compliant, and small lesions may produce dense deficits. Cranial nerve deficits are not uncommon after posterior fossa surgery, especially around the cerebellopontine angle cistern. Sensory nerves are more prone to produce deficits as compared with motor nerves. Unfortunately, no specific therapy is available to treat neurologic deficits that have already occurred. However, physiotherapy and speech therapy are some interventions available to greatly improve the final outcome. The few intraoperative adjuncts available to decrease the incidence of postoperative deficits include cortical mapping, neuromonitoring, and intraoperative EEG. Other technical points that are important to prevent inadvertent injury include intratumoral dissection in lobar tumors, intraarachnoidal dissection in lesions around cisterns, and gentle manipulation of neural structures.

Hydrocephalus

Postoperative hydrocephalus is an important complication after surgeries around the third or fourth ventricles. Intraventricular surgeries for colloid cysts, central neurocytoma, ependymoma, thalamic tumors, medulloblastomas, and hemangioblastomas are a few examples where postoperative obstruction of the ventricular pathway can give rise to obstructive hydrocephalus. The cause of such obstruction may include intraoperative bleeding, debris, or postoperative edema of the surrounding tissues. Another important cause of postoperative hydrocephalus is subarachnoid hemorrhage, which impedes CSF absorption at the level of the arachnoid villi. Acute hydrocephalus in previously normal ventricles gives rise to a life-threatening increase in ICP and can be fatal unless addressed emergently. Patients with previously dilated ventricles may compensate to an extent before becoming symptomatic. Most patients with postoperative hydrocephalus are usually managed with an external ventricular drain (EVD), which may help in CSF diversion until the ventricular system clears up. A few patients may ultimately require permanent CSF diversion with insertion of shunts.

Cerebrospinal Fluid Fistula

CSF leak from the cranial wounds may complicate a significant number of craniotomies, but chronic fistula is rare. CSF leak in most cases is the result of faulty closure techniques including improper dural closure, dural tear due to stretching, and improper soft tissue and skin closure. In a few cases, increased CSF pressure due to hydrocephalus may give rise to wound dehiscence producing a leak. Similarly, wound breakdown due to ischemia after tight closure, closure of previously irradiated skin, or wound infection may produce CSF leakage. Posterior fossa craniotomies are especially prone to producing a CSF leak because of the thin and tight dura, which makes dural closure difficult. A CSF leak is manifested as clear discharge from the wound or wound bulge, which should be differentiated from benign wound seromas. Although CSF leaks are asymptomatic for the patient, persistent leakage may give rise to infectious complications like meningitis, empyema, or brain abscess. In few cases, CSF leak can manifest as CSF otorrhea or rhinorrhea instead of wound discharge. Notable examples include retromastoid craniotomies that produce CSF otorrhea or rhinorrhea due to CSF leakage through mastoid air cells into the middle ear cavity. Similarly, surgeries around the sella, especially endonasal approaches, can give rise to CSF rhinorrhea. Most postoperative CSF leaks are managed conservatively with revision of wound closure with or without CSF diversion. CSF rhinorrhea or otorrheas are managed with CSF diversion. Revision of dural closure with placement of dural substitutes that produce a watertight closure may be required for persistent leaks. Endonasal approaches are more prone to persistent leaks or delayed leaks, which may require reconstruction of the sellar floor using bone or fat-grafts along with dural substitutes. Most CSF leaks are due to technical failures and therefore are preventable. Meticulous watertight dural closure, adequate waxing of exposed air cells during the retromastoid or middle fossa approach, and proper reconstruction of the sellar floor are among the few important surgical steps that help in preventing CSF leak.

Infectious Complications

Postoperative infections are an important cause of postoperative morbidity and can complicate 0.7% to 1.1% of cranial procedures and 1.1% to 1.5% of spinal procedures.[4] One of the retrospective longitudinal studies from the Statewide Planning and Research Cooperative System (SPARCS) database found postoperative infection to be the most common cause of unplanned readmission after neurologic surgery.[24] Postoperative infections can be superficial surgical site infections, deeper infections like cranial osteomyelitis, meningitis, subdural empyema, or brain abscess. Another important site of infection is the hardware infection such as at the EVD, ventriculo-peritoneal shunt, bolts, or cranial or spinal implants. Surgical site infections manifest as erythema or edema around the incision site with or without purulent discharge. Postoperative meningitis can occur after 0.5% to 0.7% of neurosurgical procedures and is most commonly due to breach in antisepsis during surgery. Other causes include postoperative CSF leak and wound dehiscence with secondary contamination. Deeper infections are usually serious and can be life-threatening. Subdural empyema or abscess present as focal neurologic deficits with or without features of raised ICP. On imaging they present with enhancing walls with edema out of proportion to the size of the lesion. In some cases, necrosis of the residual tumor may simulate an abscess, which can be differentiated by diffusion-weighted MRI. The mainstay of postoperative infection is antibiotic therapy, so broad-spectrum antibiotics should be started in patients with clinical suspicion of infection. The surgical site of infection and meningitis can be treated with antibiotic therapy alone, although some cases may need surgical debridement of the wound or repair to treat CSF fistula. All deep infections like empyema or abscess are managed surgically, along with antibiotic therapy. Surgical drainage of the cavity is usually performed during a neurosurgical emergency both to decrease the raised ICP and to aid in isolating the organism for antibiotic sensitivity.

Complications in Spine Surgery

Neurologic Deficits

Postoperative neurologic deficits are frequently encountered complications after spine surgery and can occur due to a multitude of reasons. Although the reported incidence of major neurologic deficits after spinal surgery is small at around 0% to 2%, the consequences are often devastating.[25,26] The neurologic complications can occur due to direct injury to the nerve elements from laceration or traction or due to indirect pressure on the spinal cord or nerve roots from hematoma, hemostatic plugs, and spinal instrumentation. Other forms of injury can be due to edema and ischemia secondary to devascularization. In most cases, the neurologic deficits are evident immediately after the surgery and improve with time. Most cases are managed conservatively with short-term steroids and physiotherapy. However, early identification of reversible causes like postoperative hematoma and nerve root impingement by instrumentation is critical to prevent long-term morbidity. Neuromonitoring, avoidance of excess distraction, and minimal retraction of nerve roots or the spinal cord are among the few intraoperative adjuncts that help in reducing the incidence of neurologic complications.

Vascular Injury and Hemorrhage

Vascular injury or hemorrhage in spine surgery is a rare but devastating complication.[27] Cervical and lumbar spine surgeries are more prone to vascular injuries. Posterior approaches for cervical spine surgery have a risk of vertebral artery injury, especially in the upper cervical region, where the course of the vertebral artery is more complex and is exposed during surgery. Similarly, anterior approaches to subaxial cervical spine surgery require retraction of the carotid artery and therefore are susceptible to injury. In the lumbar spine, anterior approaches carry a risk of injury directly to the aorta or inferior vena cava or iliac arteries during exposure of L5–S1 region. Vascular injuries from posterior approaches to the lumbar spine are rare but are possible when there is a breach in the anterior annular ligament and the instrument is passed deeper beyond this limit. Compared with vascular injury, postoperative hemorrhages like epidural hematoma are more common and are usually the result of inappropriate hemostasis. Epidural hematomas that produce deficits usually present as a surgical emergency requiring urgent evacuation. Similarly, spinal cord contusions can produce significant neurologic deficits; however, these are managed expectantly.

Dural Tears and Cerebrospinal Fluid Fistula

Dural tear is a well-known and common complication of spine surgery. The incidence of dural tear has been variably reported and can range up to 16% to 20%.[28–30] Dural tears are common in lumbar spine surgery because the dura is thin and because the surgery is more frequent in older patients, who may have adherent dura and calcified ligamentum flavum. Khan et al., in their retrospective review of 3183 lumbar spine cases, found that the incidence of dural tear is almost double (15.9% vs 7.6%) in revision surgeries as compared with primary surgeries.[31] The usual mode of injury is during removal of the ligamentum flavum with a Kerrison punch. Similarly, dural tears can occur during removal of an extruded disk, or retraction of the thecal sac or nerve root. Most dural tears are evident during surgery and require prompt watertight closure using sutures or fibrin glue. However, in undetected cases, CSF leak may have significant consequences: it may begin as a wound discharge and become a pseudomeningocele, meningitis, or empyema. Postoperative CSF leaks are usually managed with bed rest and epidural blood patches. Some cases may require re-exploration and closure of the defect with CSF diversion by placement of a lumbar drain. Given the ominous consequences of a simple dural tear, the value of controlled bony work and meticulous dissection cannot be overemphasized.

Hardware Failure in Spinal Instrumentation

The true incidence of implant failure is unknown, and rates are infrequently reported. The implant failure can manifest as breakage of the implants, fracture of the body or pedicle, extrusion of the screws, or progressive kyphosis or lordosis without bony fusion.[32] The majority of the implant failures are due to improper planning and fusion techniques with persistent instability of the spinal column even after instrumentation. Hence, implant failure rates vary depending on the indication for spinal fusion. Broad classifications are degenerative spine, traumatic spine, and deformity spine surgery. The incidence of implant failure is more common in patients with spinal deformity where the complexity of the spinal orientation makes fusion techniques challenging. Smith et al. in their prospective multicenter study on adult spinal deformity patients found a 9.0% incidence of rod fractures, which increased to 22% in patients who received pedicle subtraction osteotomy.[33] Apart from fracture, implant migration can cause pain, progressive deformity and, in some cases, neural compression requiring immediate implant removal. Implant failures pose a great degree of morbidity that requires reoperation and long-term rehabilitation. A good understanding of the spinal biomechanics and good fusion techniques are essential to prevent such devastating complications.

Conclusion

Avoidance of surgical complications is an important step in achieving a profitable healthcare system. A judicious reporting system aids in defining the incidence of complications and helps in understanding their management issues. In spite of diligent efforts from the entire team, complications are an integral part of neurosurgery, so the best measure is to limit the consequences by prompt identification and early management. The majority of the complications are benign and do not lead to long-term consequences if promptly identified and treated. Infectious complications are the most common cause of morbidity after neurosurgical procedures, whereas intracranial hemorrhage is the most common cause requiring reoperation. Given the lower recovery potential of neural tissues, neurologic injuries are less likely to recover completely. Meticulous dissection, gentle handling of neural tissues, good hemostasis, and appropriate use of intraoperative adjuncts are the best tools for preventing surgical complications.

References

1. Porter ME. What is value in health care? *N Engl J Med.* 2010; 363(26):2477–2481.
2. https://www.medicare.gov/hospitalcompare/search.html.
3. Cote DJ, Karhade AV, Larsen AM, Burke WT, Castlen JP, Smith TR. United States neurosurgery annual case type and complication trends between 2006 and 2013: An American College of Surgeons National Surgical Quality Improvement Program analysis. *J Clin Neurosci.* 2016;31:106–111.
4. Rolston JD, Han SJ, Lau CY, Berger MS, Parsa AT. Frequency and predictors of complications in neurological surgery: national trends from 2006 to 2011. *J Neurosurg.* 2014;120(3):736–745.
5. Ingraham AM, Richards KE, Hall BL, Ko CY. Quality improvement in surgery: the American College of Surgeons National Surgical Quality Improvement Program approach. *Adv Surg.* 2010;44: 251–267.
6. Koch CG, Li L, Hixson E, Tang A, Phillips S, Henderson JM. What are the real rates of postoperative complications: elucidating inconsistencies between administrative and clinical data sources. *J Am Coll Surg.* 2012;214(5):798–805.
7. Kaafarani HM, Borzecki AM, Itani KM, et al. Validity of selected patient safety indicators: opportunities and concerns. *J Am Coll Surg.* 2011;212(6):924–934.
8. Romano PS, Geppert JJ, Davies S, Miller MR, Elixhauser A, McDonald KM. A national profile of patient safety in U.S. hospitals. *Health Aff (Millwood).* 2003;22(2):154–166.
9. Sarnthein J, Stieglitz L, Clavien PA, Regli L. A patient registry to improve patient safety: recording general neurosurgery complications. *PLoS ONE.* 2016;11(9):e0163154.
10. Theodosopoulos PV, Ringer AJ, McPherson CM, et al. Measuring surgical outcomes in neurosurgery: implementation, analysis, and auditing a prospective series of more than 5000 procedures. *J Neurosurg.* 2012;117(5):947–954.
11. Weiss N, P KD. Avoidance of complications in neurosurgery. In: Winn H, ed. *Youmans Neurological Surgery.* Philadelphia, PA: Elsevier; 2011:408–423.
12. Fugate JE. Complications of neurosurgery. *Continuum (Minneap Minn).* 2015;21(5 Neurocritical Care):1425–1444.
13. Fukamachi A, Koizumi H, Nukui H. Postoperative intracerebral hemorrhages: a survey of computed tomographic findings after 1074 intracranial operations. *Surg Neurol.* 1985;23(6):575–580.
14. Seifman MA, Lewis PM, Rosenfeld JV, Hwang PY. Postoperative intracranial haemorrhage: a review. *Neurosurg Rev.* 2011;34(4):393–407.
15. Touho H, Hirakawa K, Hino A, Karasawa J, Ohno Y. Relationship between abnormalities of coagulation and fibrinolysis and postoperative intracranial hemorrhage in head injury. *Neurosurgery.* 1986;19(4):523–531.
16. Kalfas IH, Little JR. Postoperative hemorrhage: a survey of 4992 intracranial procedures. *Neurosurgery.* 1988;23(3):343–347.
17. Taylor WA, Thomas NW, Wellings JA, Bell BA. Timing of postoperative intracranial hematoma development and implications for the best use of neurosurgical intensive care. *J Neurosurg.* 1995;82(1):48–50.
18. Kaufman HH, Moake JL, Olson JD, et al. Delayed and recurrent intracranial hematomas related to disseminated intravascular clotting and fibrinolysis in head injury. *Neurosurgery.* 1980;7(5):445–449.
19. Wijdicks E. Complications of craniotomy and biopsy. In: *The Practice of Emergency and Critical Care Neurology.* New York, NY: Oxford University Press; 2010:629–641.
20. Algattas H, Kimmell KT, Vates GE. Risk of reoperation for hemorrhage in patients after craniotomy. *World Neurosurg.* 2016;87:531–539.
21. Larsen AM, Cote DJ, Karhade AV, Smith TR. Predictors of stroke and coma after neurosurgery: an ACS-NSQIP analysis. *World Neurosurg.* 2016;93:299–305.
22. Pulman J, Greenhalgh J, Marson AG. Antiepileptic drugs as prophylaxis for post-craniotomy seizures. *Cochrane Database Syst Rev.* 2013;(2):CD007286.
23. Wu AS, Trinh VT, Suki D, et al. A prospective randomized trial of perioperative seizure prophylaxis in patients with intraparenchymal brain tumors. *J Neurosurg.* 2013;118(4):873–883.
24. Taylor BE, Youngerman BE, Goldstein H, et al. Causes and timing of unplanned early readmission after neurosurgery. *Neurosurgery.* 2016;79(3):356–369.
25. Cramer DE, Maher PC, Pettigrew DB, Kuntz CT. Major neurologic deficit immediately after adult spinal surgery: incidence and etiology over 10 years at a single training institution. *J Spinal Disord Tech.* 2009;22(8):565–570.
26. Papadakis M, Aggeliki L, Papadopoulos EC, Girardi FP. Common surgical complications in degenerative spinal surgery. *World J Orthop.* 2013;4(2):62–66.
27. Inamasu J, Guiot BH. Vascular injury and complication in neurosurgical spine surgery. *Acta Neurochir (Wien).* 2006;148(4):375–387.
28. Bosacco SJ, Gardner MJ, Guille JT. Evaluation and treatment of dural tears in lumbar spine surgery: a review. *Clin Orthop Relat Res.* 2001;389:238–247.

29. Epstein NE. The frequency and etiology of intraoperative dural tears in 110 predominantly geriatric patients undergoing multilevel laminectomy with noninstrumented fusions. *J Spinal Disord Tech*. 2007;20(5):380–386.
30. Luszczyk MJ, Blaisdell GY, Wiater BP, et al. Traumatic dural tears: what do we know and are they a problem? *Spine J*. 2014;14(1): 49–56.
31. Khan MH, Rihn J, Steele G, et al. Postoperative management protocol for incidental dural tears during degenerative lumbar spine surgery: a review of 3,183 consecutive degenerative lumbar cases. *Spine*. 2006;31(22):2609–2613.
32. Sodhi HBS, Savardekar A, Chauhan RB, Patra DP, Singla N, Salunke P. Factors predicting long-term outcome after short segment posterior fixation for traumatic thoracolumbar fractures. *Surg Neurol Int*. 2017;8:233.
33. Smith JS, Shaffrey E, Klineberg E, et al. Prospective multicenter assessment of risk factors for rod fracture following surgery for adult spinal deformity. *J Neurosurg Spine*. 2014;21(6):994–1003.

6

Venous Injuries and Cerebral Edema in Cranial Surgery

AMEY R. SAVARDEKAR, ANIL NANDA

HIGHLIGHTS

- The exact consequences of "venous injury," inadvertently caused during the course of routine neurosurgical operations, find scant mention in neurosurgical literature.
- Numerous so-called "unpredictable" postoperative complications in neurosurgery are related to the lack of prevention or nonrecognition of venous injury.
- The factors responsible for devastating postoperative venous complications are a combination of intraoperative venous compromise, iatrogenic brain injury, and prolonged lobe retraction.
- The frequency of postoperative venous infarction after manipulation/sacrifice of venous structures during cranial surgery is reportedly higher in older patients than in younger patients.
- There is no intraoperative test available to determine whether postoperative venous infarction will occur if we injure or sacrifice a particular vein during surgery.
- The unpredictable response of the brain to venous injury causes catastrophic complications in a few patients; to avoid these, meticulous venous preservation should be an aim in all neurosurgical procedures.

Background

Complications related to the intracranial venous system, especially the cerebral venous drainage, have received comparatively less attention in the neurosurgical literature. Consequently, venous complications are not given due recognition, even though most practicing neurosurgeons would agree that they are not uncommon.[1] Numerous so-called "unpredictable" postoperative complications in neurosurgery are most likely related to the lack of prevention or to the nonrecognition of venous problems, especially damage to the dangerous venous structures—namely the major dural sinuses, the deep cerebral veins, and some of the dominant superficial veins like the vein of Labbé, vein of Trolard, or the superior petrosal vein.

Frequent variations exist in the size and connections of the intracranial veins, and this has made it difficult to define their normal pattern. Hence, there is ambiguity in reporting the damage to the venous anatomy that usually occurs during the course of an intracranial surgery. Apart from the treatise on the neurosurgical perspective of the intracranial venous system published by Hakuba and the extensive reviews published by Sindou and Auque, the neurologic literature on venous injury and its consequences is scant.[2–4]

Incidence of Venous Injury and Its Sequelae

Kageyama et al. reported postoperative venous infarction (POVI) in 13% of the 120 cases operated on by them.[5,6] Saito et al. reported POVI in 2.6% of cases after the frontotemporal bridging vein was cut during the pterional approach, and Al-Mefty and Krisht showed that brain edema occurred in 10% of cases after sacrifice of the superficial sylvian vein.[6–8] Kubota reported that 4 of 10 patients with vein sacrifice during an interhemispheric approach suffered from brain damage.[6] Roberson et al. reported that the complication rate of venous insufficiency was 1.5 per 1000 cases of neurologic–skull base surgery.[9] Agrawal and Naik studied a total of 376 patients undergoing elective major cranial surgeries over a period of 8 months. In their study, 26 (7%) patients developed POVI, out of which 16 (61%) patients developed hemorrhagic POVI and 10 (39%) patients developed nonhemorrhagic POVI.[1]

The exact consequences of "venous injury," inadvertently caused during the course of routine neurosurgical operations, find scant mention in neurosurgical literature; some publications even suggest that veins could be sacrificed without any significant neurologic damage.[10] The reasons can be manifold. When we consider the postoperative computed tomography (CT) or magnetic resonance imaging (MRI) scan and visualize an area of cerebral contusion or hypodensity, adjacent to the operative site or in the trajectory of the neurosurgical approach, we tend to attribute it to several factors—namely retraction injury, retraction edema, pial transgression by the surgeon, arterial injury, presence of preoperative tumor edema, and after-effects of tumor manipulation. The extent of brain damage from venous cause is rarely quantifiable, and this may be due to the interplay of the above-mentioned confounding factors.

Consequences of Venous Injury

The incidence of intraoperative venous injury and subsequent POVI is difficult to determine due to an unclear definition, myriad postoperative neurologic presentations, and the inclusion of other factors during the operation itself (for example, brain retraction).[6]

Roberson et al. divided venous infarction into two types: the acute form and the chronic form.[9] The acute form manifests itself in the immediate postoperative period and can, at times, be life-threatening. The chronic form manifests itself months or years postoperatively with headaches, disequilibrium, and visual changes due to papilledema. In this setting, venous thrombosis from intraoperative venous injury progresses to the dural sinuses, thus influencing cerebrospinal fluid (CSF) absorption and eventually presenting as communicating hydrocephalus.

Nakase et al. further described two types of perioperative (acute) venous infarction in their study: severe and mild types.[6] The severe type requires extensive treatment like internal decompression and barbiturate therapy immediately after the operation. The mild type has a slow clinical deterioration by gradual thrombus evolution and can be treated conservatively. In all the severe cases documented in their series, the sacrificed cortical vein was the petrosal vein.

The variability of the intracranial venous system makes it difficult to predict the exact course and amount of flow in a particular draining vein during surgical approaches. The absence of valves in the veins and the presence of collateral drainage systems make it possible for the venous drainage to adapt to an intraoperative venous injury and limit the amount of brain damage. This is often used as an excuse by neurosurgeons to sacrifice veins during the surgical approach. However, it should be borne in mind that it is very difficult to predict the dominant venous drainage from a particular cerebral region intraoperatively and that sacrificing this dominant drainage can have disastrous consequences for the brain.

The fact that sacrifice of the individual cortical veins only infrequently leads to venous infarction, hemorrhage, swelling, and neurologic deficits is attributed to the diffuse anastomoses between the veins.[11] The intraoperative sacrifice of the anastomotic or bridging vein usually does not lead to venous infarction due to the absence of cerebral valves. The recruitment of collateral pathways occurs during the early phase of venous occlusion. The severity depends on the availability of individual venous collaterals. Only when the collateral venous flow is compromised by additional compression or under extraordinary physiologic conditions—for example, intraoperative brain retraction, excessive changes of systemic blood pressure, and an elderly patient—does venous infarction occur.[6,11] Although the brain may tolerate occlusion of the nondominant channels to a large extent, the occlusion of a dominant venous channel carries significant risk of POVI.

Types of Postoperative Venous Complications

Based on the published literature on this subject and on our current understanding of the venous system, the postoperative venous complications can be classified into the following categories.

Acute Decompensated Venous Injury

This injury is analogous to the severe acute venous infarction described by Nakase et al. and manifests immediately postoperatively as a hemorrhagic cerebral infarction in the territory of the injured draining vein. This usually presents with severe cerebral edema with consequent midline shift and may require extensive measures like decompressive surgery or barbiturate coma to manage the raised intra-cranial pressure (ICP).

Acute Compensated Venous Injury

When the venous injury results in the occlusion of the nondominant venous channels or in the occlusion of the dominant venous channel in a favorable setting (without the added insult of brain retraction or preexisting cerebral edema), the recruitment of venous collaterals may compensate for the venous injury and thus limit the damage to the brain. This usually manifests as mild to moderate cerebral edema and may resolve with cerebral protection strategies and antiedema measures.

Chronic Venous Insufficiency

In this entity, the intraoperative venous injury may go unnoticed or may manifest as mild cerebral edema. However, venous thrombosis due to intraoperative venous injury may progress to the dural sinuses, causing chronic dural venous thrombosis. Over time, this influences CSF absorption and may eventually present as a form of communicating hydrocephalus.

Factors Influencing the Outcome of a Venous Injury

During surgery, impaired venous outflow, along with prolonged brain retraction, might cause cerebral venous circulatory disturbances resulting in venous infarction.[12] The factors responsible for devastating postoperative venous complications are intraoperative venous compromise, iatrogenic brain injury, and prolonged lobe retraction.[13] Nakamura and Samii suggested four mechanisms for venous complication during surgery: lacerations of venous sinuses, obliteration of veins or venous sinuses, brain retraction interfering with venous flow, and hemodynamic changes in the venous system due to removal of extensive lesions.[14]

Age

Mild cerebral venous injury in aged patients is known to frequently cause unexpectedly severe postoperative complications in neurosurgical practice.[6] The frequency of POVI after venous injury/manipulation is reportedly higher in older patients than in younger patients.[6] Therefore venous infarction is an increasingly recognized cause of postoperative complications in older patients.

Extent of Anastomotic Channels

The severity of POVI depends on the availability of individual venous collaterals. When a cerebral venous outflow is sacrificed, either the venous drainage may redirect through available collaterals (due to absence of valves), or a severe POVI may develop.[11] The recruitment of collateral pathways occurs during the early phase of venous occlusion. Only when the collateral venous flow is compromised by additional compression or under extraordinary physiologic conditions—for example, intraoperative brain retraction, excessive changes of blood pressure, and an elderly patient—does venous infarction occur.[6,11]

Brain Retraction

Brain retraction induces local congestion by compressing the cortical venous network, reducing the venous flow by stretching bridging veins, and if compression is prolonged, thrombosis of veins.[3] Nakase et al. have proved with animal studies that, compared with vein occlusion or brain compression alone, the accumulated effects of brain retraction cause severe ischemia and increased vulnerability to brain damage.[6] Therefore it is advisable to retract the brain with the least force necessary and for the shortest time possible. Savardekar et al. note that intraoperative venous compromise and prolonged lobe retraction are synergistic mechanisms leading to devastating postoperative venous complications.[11] In the setting of a dominant venous drainage sacrifice planned during a skull base approach, they recommend ligating the bridging vein at first sitting, allowing the venous drainage to accommodate, and then removing the tumor at the second sitting. In such a setting, Sindou and Auque,[3] Auque and Civit,[15] and Auque and Huot[16] also recommend stopping the surgical procedure and postponing the removal of the tumor for some weeks, allowing the veins to reestablish an adequate blood supply. Thus brain retraction is a known contributory factor in the development of POVI and should be avoided in cases of intraoperative venous injury.

Perioperative Blood Pressure Changes

Ischemia mechanisms play an important role in the pathophysiologic consequences of venous injury: The supply of blood may fall below a critical threshold in circumscribed brain areas drained by the occluded veins.[6] Previous studies by Nakase et al. have shown that venous occlusion is followed by regional cerebral blood flow (rCBF) decreases in the adjacent cortical area and that 90% of histologically analyzed rat brains showed evidence of brain damage upon occlusion of two cortical veins.[17–19] Additional experiments in a similar setting proved the lower autoregulation limit to be shifted upward even after a single cortical vein occlusion in the rat.[20] With these results in mind, one may consider the brain of a patient to be at a particular risk for the development of neural damage during early postoperative periods. Along with an upward shift in the lower limit of autoregulation, these findings may have implications for perioperative hemodynamic regulation in patients with intraoperative coagulation of large cortical veins. This may be the pathophysiologic basis for subsequent hemorrhagic POVI. The fact that a brain with venous injury is very fragile has been underestimated so far. Extreme care to avoid significant hemodynamic changes should be taken in such an ailing brain because evidence suggests that autoregulation may be impaired.

Anatomic Considerations for the Venous System

The Dural Venous Sinuses

The concept that ligation or acute blockade of the middle and posterior third of the superior sagittal sinus (SSS) is associated with bilateral venous infarcts has been proven in both experimental and clinical settings. It is considered that ligation of the anterior third of the SSS is well tolerated by the brain.

In fact, the literature recommends ligation and division of the anterior third of the SSS to improve the surgical approach for parasagittal and anterior skull base lesions. It has definite advantages, because the working distance is reduced significantly, the retraction of frontal lobes is minimized, and larger anterior skull base tumors can be approached with relative ease, resulting in better resection. Despite these advantages, there are some disadvantages that simply cannot be overlooked and can occasionally prove fatal.

Nakamura et al. in their series of 82 olfactory groove meningiomas reported mortality in four cases (4.9%) operated via the bifrontal approach with ligation of the anterior third of the SSS.[21] They attribute the mortality to the venous edema and complications secondary to the ligation of the SSS and recommend the unilateral subfrontal approach over the bifrontal approach for olfactory groove meningiomas. This experience reiterates the sentiment that venous sacrifice is tolerated in many, but not all; to prevent complications in these few patients, it is appropriate to try to preserve venous structures in all.

The ligation of the anterior third of the SSS was considered safe, especially in anterior third parasagittal meningiomas from Cushing's time. However, ligation of the unoccluded anterior third of the SSS may produce severe blood flow disturbances in some cases, leading to cerebral edema and POVI.[22,23] Parasagittal meningiomas either infiltrate the sinus or compress the adjacent cortical veins, resulting in the opening up of collateral venous circulation; therefore ligation of the anterior third of the SSS may be safer in such cases. Recent literature has shown that ligation of the anterior third of the SSS may not be completely safe even for these tumors due to the extension of the thrombus in the occluded sinus posteriorly.[23]

The Bridging Veins

When analyzing the pterional approach, Kageyama et al. found that postoperative brain damage occurred in 13% of their 120 cases and was located mostly in the inferior frontal lobe. The two causative factors were duration of surgery and "sylvian" type of venous drainage pattern. They concluded that POVI during the pterional approach is the most important factor in postoperative brain injury.

Sindou and Auque state that when venous sacrifice is unavoidable, the safest approach is to divide a bridging vein. This is because the intraoperative sacrifice of the anastomotic or bridging vein usually does not lead to venous infarction due to the absence of cerebral venous valves, because redirection of venous outflow occurs.[3] Al-Mefty and Krisht also concur with ligating the vein as close to the dura as possible to preserve the anastomotic channels, if sacrifice is contemplated.[24] Savardekar et al. have proposed the idea of tackling the venous drainage redistribution through bridging vein ligation at one stage, followed by tumor resection through the preferred route in the second stage.[11] The rationale behind "bridging vein ligation" and protection of the cortical venous system stems from experimental studies stating that bridging vein or sinus occlusion results in only hydrostatic edema, and blood-brain barrier mostly remains intact.[11]

The Cortical Veins

Obliteration of the cortical veins during surgery does not always result in clinical damage because collateral pathways of the cerebral venous system vary greatly among individuals.[14] The injury to cortical veins can occur during resection of cortical lesions (which involve or are adhered to the veins) or during approach to deep parenchymal lesions (as a result of vein sacrifice during corticectomy or bystander injury to the vein due to retraction). In the first setting, the cortical lesions may have already caused collateral venous channels to develop, and hence cortical venous injury is mostly well tolerated. A few reports of venous complications arising in this setting have been described.[14] In the second setting, if the dominant venous channels are damaged, catastrophic consequences may occur.[25] Hence it is important to evaluate the venous drainage of the brain with preoperative venogram to understand the dominant venous drainage pathways and to follow the dictum of minimal venous sacrifice.

Surgical Strategy: Make Venous Preservation an Aim

There is no intraoperative test available to determine whether venous infarction will occur postoperatively if we injure or sacrifice a particular vein during surgery. Also uncertain are whether venous or tissue pressure recording could allow assessment of tolerance or intolerance, whether barbiturates or hypothermia could limit the deleterious effect of venous compromise, and whether heparin is useful in the setting of postoperative cerebral venous thrombosis. Obliteration of the superficial and deep bridging veins—including the great, basal, and internal cerebral veins—is inescapable in some operative approaches. However, the number of these veins and their branches to be sacrificed should be kept to a minimum because of the possible undesirable sequelae, which, although usually transient, can be permanent in a small percentage of cases. Before sacrificing any veins, the surgeon should try to work around them, displacing them out of the operative route or placing them under moderate or even severe stretch, accepting the fact that they may be torn, if this will yield some possibility of their being saved.

References

1. Agrawal D, Naik V. Postoperative cerebral venous infarction. *J Pediatr Neurosci*. 2015;10(1):5–8.
2. Hakuba A, ed. *Surgery of the Intracranial Venous System*. Berlin: Springer; 1996.
3. Sindou M, Auque J. The intracranial venous system as a neurosurgeon's perspective. *Adv Tech Stand Neurosurg*. 2000;26:131–216.
4. Rhoton AL Jr. The cerebral veins. *Neurosurgery*. 2002;51(4 suppl): S159–S205.
5. Kageyama Y, Watanabe K, Kobayashi S, et al. Postoperative brain damage due to cerebral vein disorders resulting from the pterional approach. In: Hakuba A, ed. *Surgery of the Intracranial Venous System*. Berlin: Springer; 1996:311–315.
6. Nakase H, Shin Y, Nakagawa I, Kimura R, Sakaki T. Clinical features of postoperative cerebral venous infarction. *Acta Neurochir (Wien)*. 2005;147(6):621–626; discussion 26.
7. Saito F, Haraoka J, Ito H, Nishioka H, Inaba I, Yamada Y. Venous complications in pterional approach; About frontotemporal bridging veins. *Surg Cereb Stroke*. 1998;26:237–241.
8. Kubota M, Ono J, Saeki N, Yamaura A. Postoperative brain damage due to sacrifice of bridging veins during the anterior inter-hemispheric approach. In: Hakuba A, ed. *Surgery of the Intracranial Venous System*. Berlin: Springer; 1996:291–294.
9. Roberson JB Jr, Brackmann DE, Fayad JN. Complications of venous insufficiency after neurotologic-skull base surgery. *Am J Otol*. 2000;21(5):701–705.
10. McLaughlin MR, Jannetta PJ, Clyde BL, et al. Microvascular decompression of cranial nerves: lessons learned after 4400 operations. *J Neurosurg*. 1999;90(1):1–8.
11. Savardekar AR, Goto T, Nagata T, et al. Staged 'intentional' bridging vein ligation: a safe strategy in gaining wide access to skull base tumors. *Acta Neurochir (Wien)*. 2014;156(4):671–679.
12. Ohata K, Haque M, Morino M, et al. Occlusion of the sigmoid sinus after surgery via the presigmoidal-transpetrosal approach. *J Neurosurg*. 1998;89(4):575–584.
13. Sakata K, Al-Mefty O, Yamamoto I. Venous consideration in petrosal approach: microsurgical anatomy of the temporal bridging vein. *Neurosurgery*. 2000;47(1):153–160; discussion 60-1.
14. Kiya K, Satoh H, Mizoue T, Kinoshita Y. Postoperative cortical venous infarction in tumours firmly adherent to the cortex. *J Clin Neurosci*. 2001;8(suppl 1):109–113.
15. Auque J, Civit T. [Superficial veins of the brain]. *Neurochirurgie*. 1996;42(suppl 1):88–108.
16. Auque J, Huot JC. [Deep venous system of the brain]. *Neurochirurgie*. 1996;42(suppl 1):109–126.
17. Nakase H, Heimann A, Kempski O. Alterations of regional cerebral blood flow and oxygen saturation in a rat sinus-vein thrombosis model. *Stroke*. 1996;27(4):720–727; discussion 28.
18. Nakase H, Heimann A, Kempski O. Local cerebral blood flow in a rat cortical vein occlusion model. *J Cereb Blood Flow Metab*. 1996;16(4):720–728.
19. Nakase H, Kempski OS, Heimann A, Takeshima T, Tintera J. Microcirculation after cerebral venous occlusions as assessed by laser Doppler scanning. *J Neurosurg*. 1997;87(2):307–314.
20. Nakase H, Nagata K, Otsuka H, Sakaki T, Kempski O. Local cerebral blood flow autoregulation following "asymptomatic" cerebral venous occlusion in the rat. *J Neurosurg*. 1998;89(1):118–124.
21. Nakamura M, Struck M, Roser F, Vorkapic P, Samii M. Olfactory groove meningiomas: clinical outcome and recurrence rates after tumor removal through the frontolateral and bifrontal approach. *Neurosurgery*. 2008;62(6 suppl 3):1224–1232.
22. Sahoo SK, Ghuman MS, Salunke P, et al. Evaluation of anterior third of superior sagittal sinus in normal population: identifying the subgroup with dominant drainage. *J Neurosci Rural Pract*. 2016;7(2):257–261.
23. Salunke P, Sodhi HB, Aggarwal A, et al. Is ligation and division of anterior third of superior sagittal sinus really safe? *Clin Neurol Neurosurg*. 2013;115(10):1998–2002.
24. Al-Mefty O, Krisht A. The dangerous veins. In: Hakuba A, ed. *Surgery of the intracranial venous system*. Berlin: Springer; 1996:338–345.
25. Koerbel A, Gharabaghi A, Safavi-Abbasi S, et al. Venous complications following petrosal vein sectioning in surgery of petrous apex meningiomas. *Eur J Surg Oncol*. 2009;35(7):773–779.

7

Postoperative Hematoma in Cranial and Spinal Surgery

ANIL NANDA, AMEY R. SAVARDEKAR

HIGHLIGHTS

- The cranial perspective
  - Postoperative hemorrhage is one of the most serious complications of any cranial neurosurgical procedure.
  - The incidence figures for clinically significant postoperative hemorrhage for cranial surgery ranges from 0.8% to 6.9%.
  - Hemostatic disturbances including coagulopathy and thrombocytopenia, as well as administration of antiplatelet agents, have been identified as general risk factors for postoperative hematomas after neurosurgical procedures.
  - Many of the best recommendation practices for preventing, detecting, and treating postoperative hemorrhage seem intuitive and are likely to be in practice in most neurosurgery units; however, dealing with this iatrogenic disaster just comes down to "doing the simple things right, each and every time."
- The spinal perspective
  - Symptomatic postoperative spinal epidural hematoma is a rare, yet well-recognized, complication of spinal surgery with the potential for leaving patients with devastating consequences.
  - The reported incidence of symptomatic postoperative spinal epidural hematoma in the literature varies significantly from 0.1% up to 1%.
  - Most clinically significant postoperative spinal epidural hematomas occur in the first few hours after surgery, highlighting the importance of close neurologic monitoring of patients during this period.
  - It usually requires emergent surgical evacuation, and early intervention is likely to result in better neurologic recovery.
  - Larger studies are needed to accurately identify those at high risk of developing spinal epidural hematoma after spinal surgery.

"The practice of neurosurgery, inherently, is more sensitive to any deficit in hemostasis than many of the other surgical disciplines."

MERRIMAN ET AL. (1970)

Introduction

Postoperative hemorrhage (POH) can develop after any neurosurgical operation and tends to have a devastating effect on the outcome, if not detected at an early stage. Thus avoidance of such a complication is of vital interest. Merriman et al. accurately noted "the practice of neurosurgery, inherently, is more sensitive to any deficit in hemostasis than many of the other surgical disciplines."[1] This puts the impetus squarely on the operating neurosurgeon to prevent this postoperative complication and, in the event of its occurrence, to detect and treat it early before the patient develops a lasting neurologic deficit. Due to the variation in the presentation, detection, and management of this complication in cranial vis-à-vis spinal surgery, we have dealt with these in two separate sections.

The Cranial Perspective

POH is one of the most serious complications of any cranial neurosurgical procedure. A number of studies have demonstrated the significant morbidity and mortality associated with intracranial bleeding after neurosurgery.[2] The rates of POH after intracranial procedures reported in the literature vary greatly, ranging from 0.8% to 50.0%.[3] However, meaningful comparison is difficult due to the variance in the definition of POH. It is generally defined as bleeding at the operative site after surgery; however, it may be argued that in most operative beds, some residual blood is to be expected. Also, it is clinico-radiologically difficult to acutely differentiate between expected residual blood and small de novo hemorrhages that are benign.[4] Incidence figures thus vary depending on definition, with rates of 0.8% to 6.9% reported for postoperative clinical deterioration and rates of 10.8% to 50.0% based on routine radiologic monitoring.[3] Postoperative clinical deterioration is the most consistent sign directing clinicians to suspect significant intracranial hematoma.[5] Hence, as per existing literature, the best definition for a postoperative intracranial hemorrhage is a hematoma, which is clinically significant and requires surgical evacuation.[3,4]

Location of Postoperative Hemorrhage

POH after a cranial surgery can occur at any of the following locations: epidural, subdural, intraparenchymal, remote, or mixed. Many studies have found that the majority of postoperative hematomas were epidural or intraparenchymal.[2] Kalfas and Little analyzed a series of 4992 intracranial procedures performed over an 11-year period for the occurrence of POH.[5] Forty patients (0.8%) experienced POH, out of which 24 (60%) were intracerebral, 11 (28%) were epidural, 3 (7.5%) were subdural, and 2 (5%) were intrasellar. POH in 33 patients occurred at the operative site, and in 7 it occurred remote from the operative site. Palmer et al., in a review of 6668 operations performed over 5 years, reported 71 surgically evacuated POH, accounting for an incidence of 1.1%.[6] POHs were intraparenchymal in 43% of cases, subdural in 5%, extradural in 33%, mixed in 8%, and confined to the superficial wound in 11%. In a study by Gerlach et al., 21 out of 296 patients operated for intracranial meningiomas developed a POH and needed resurgery.[7] Out of those 21, 9 patients had extradural hematoma (EDH), 3 patients had intraparenchymal hematoma (IPH), and the remaining 9 patients had mixed [EDH/subdural hematoma(SDH)/IPH] hematomas. In 2305 cranial neurosurgical procedures reviewed by Taylor et al., 50 (2.2%) developed a hematoma.[8] The hematomas were extradural in 26 patients (52%), intracerebral in 22 (44%) patients, and subdural in two (4%) patients.

Remote intracerebral hemorrhage is a rare complication of craniotomy with significant morbidity and mortality.[3,9] Brisman et al. reviewed 37 cases of remote POH occurring after cranial neurosurgery and concluded that such hemorrhages likely develop at or soon after surgery, tend to occur preferentially in certain locations, and can be related to the craniotomy site, operative positioning, and nonspecific mechanical factors.[9] They are not related to hypertension, coagulopathy, cerebrospinal fluid drainage, or underlying pathologic abnormalities.

Analysis of Causative Factors

A postoperative hematoma after elective surgery can have a devastating effect on the patient's outcome. However, in most of the patients with POH, no obvious cause for the hematoma can be found; it is related neither to the surgical technique nor to hemostatic parameters. Various predisposing risk factors have been analyzed: Hypertension was generally found to be significant in most studies, whereas diabetes mellitus, cerebral amyloid angiopathy, and atherosclerosis were generally not significant.[3,5] Basali et al. noted that patients with postoperative intracranial hemorrhage had a significantly greater rate of intraoperative and postoperative/prehemorrhage hypertension.[10] Intraoperative hypertension occurs during brain manipulation, head pin application, use of epinephrine containing anesthetics, periosteal dissection, and emergence. Basali et al. also found a significantly high odds ratio for intracranial hemorrhage when patients had blood pressure <160/90 intraoperatively but then had elevated blood pressure postoperatively.[10] This suggests that some vessels may not have been adequately tested intraoperatively for the possibility of leaking when blood pressure rises.[10]

Age is a significant risk factor for hematoma development—sixfold more likely at age over 70 and 12-fold over 75.[7,11] It remains speculative why the risk of bleeding increases with age. It can be speculated that POH in the elderly is attributed to changes in the blood vessels themselves and to the function of platelets. It was found that elderly patients have more thrombin activation/generation and fibrinolytic activity before surgery than younger patients.[7] Other risk factors include antiplatelet use, including aspirin and nonsteroidal antiinflammatory drugs, preoperative mannitol administration, excessive alcohol use, coagulopathies, disseminated intravascular coagulation, thrombocytopenia, acute decreases in platelet counts postoperatively, excessive intraoperative blood loss, poor response to preoperative platelet transfusions, factor XIII deficiencies, and decreased fibrinogen levels.[1–4,7]

One might expect that surgeons with greater levels of experience should encounter fewer postoperative hematomas. However, in the study by Taylor et al., there was no correlation between the rank of the surgeon and the occurrence of postoperative hematoma, with 27 hematomas (54%) occurring after operations by consultants and 23 (46%) after operations by registrars or senior registrars.[8]

Kim et al. conclude that large intraoperative blood loss and wide craniotomy area are risk factors for postoperative EDH after intracranial surgery.[12] However, this study had significant limitations because it did not examine the role of established risk factors for POH. In another series of patients, who underwent surgery to remove brain tumors, the highest rate of postoperative hematomas was found after meningioma surgery.[7] POH remains a major cause of poor outcome after meningioma surgery.

Timing of Occurrence of Postoperative Hemorrhage and Overall Outcome

Gerlach et al. found that the majority of their hematomas were discovered within 3 days of the initial operation.[7] Kalfas and Little found that 35% of their ICH cases were discovered within 12 hours.[5] Taylor et al., in their review of 2305 patients in which 50 developed postoperative hematomas, noted that 44 out of the 50 developed within 6 hours.[8] What has emerged through the literature review is that there are two distinct time periods in which neurologic deterioration secondary to a hematoma occurs, the first being within 6 hours of surgery and the second being 24 hours or more from the time of surgery. The first group likely represents continued active bleeding at the operative site, and the second group represents patients in whom active bleeding is likely to have come to a halt; their clinical deterioration may represent secondary swelling and edema formation around the hematoma. Desai et al., in their review of 3109 cranial operations, noted that when the initial operation was for evacuation of intraparenchymal hematoma, the return to the operating room for evacuation of a postoperative hematoma occurred sooner than for any other type of operation.[2]

Generally, outcome is poor with a range of mortality from 13% to 41% depending on the type of initial operation (tumor vs traumatic ICH, etc.). Good recovery, defined as Glasgow Outcome Scale (GOS) 4 or 5, has been reported in the range of 39% to 71% of the cases in which POH developed.[4–7]

Strategies—Preventive and Treatment

Close clinical and neurologic observations in the immediate postoperative period are the usual means of POH detection.[3] Failure to adequately awaken from general anesthesia or deterioration of observation parameters would prompt for an urgent scan to check for and treat POH.

Thus, our recommendations for clinical practice based on the literature reviewed would include:

1. Preoperative: Cease any antiplatelet and anticoagulant therapy for an adequate period; stop alcohol consumption; ensure platelet count, function, and coagulation parameters are normal; consider factor XIII screening; and optimize medical management of preexisting conditions, particularly hypertension.
2. Intraoperative: Avoid hypertension and excessive blood loss; replace blood losses promptly and sufficiently; aim for gross total resection of tumor wherever possible; meticulous technique and hemostasis including dural tenting, appropriate use of electrocoagulation and topical hemostats; Valsalva maneuver at the end of surgery; and a slow, gentle wean from general anesthesia.
3. Postoperative: Avoid hypertension; replace blood losses adequately; avoid upright patient positioning in the initial phase; close clinical monitoring in the first 6 h postsurgery; consider ICP monitoring or early postoperative imaging. ICP monitoring may be useful if there have been significant problems with hemostasis during surgery, if the lesion has been very vascular,

if blood loss has been great during surgery, or if the patient needs to remain sedated and/or ventilated after surgery.

The Spinal Perspective

Symptomatic postoperative spinal epidural hematoma (SEH) is a rare, yet well-recognized, complication of spinal surgery with potentially devastating consequences.[13] Some common complications, such as an incidental durotomy, have little long-term clinical impact; conversely, some rare complications, such as a clinically significant SEH, can lead to permanent neurologic deficits.[14] Most patients after spinal surgery demonstrate a varying degree of epidural hematoma on imaging; however, most remain asymptomatic.[13] It is therefore impractical and unnecessary to perform a postoperative MRI scan on all patients.[13,14] However, prompt attention should be paid to patients who develop either new or deteriorating neurologic signs and symptoms postoperatively.[15] In this section, we discuss the incidence, associated risk factors, diagnosis, and management strategies for this rare but important complication of spinal surgery.

Incidence of Postoperative Symptomatic Spinal Epidural Hematoma

The actual incidence of clinically silent epidural hematoma is reported to be much higher than that found for symptomatic hematomas. Postoperative SEH is a common radiologic finding identified in 33% to 100% of surgical cases by computed tomography (CT) scan or magnetic resonance imaging (MRI).[16] For example, in patients undergoing lumbar surgery, Sokolowski et al. identified a 58% incidence of asymptomatic postoperative epidural hematoma (diagnosed by MRI) compressing the thecal sac beyond its preoperative state at one or more levels.[17] The majority of radiologically diagnosed SEHs are clinically silent. As per literature review, most authors define a postoperative SEH as one that is clinically symptomatic rather than one that is asymptomatic and diagnosed by radiology alone.

Kao et al. reviewed over 15,500 lumbar spine surgeries and identified 25 patients with a symptomatic postoperative SEH for an incidence of 0.16%.[18] Awad et al. reviewed almost 15,000 consecutive spine cases at a single institution and identified 32 cases (0.2%) of symptomatic postoperative SEH.[19] In a study by Kou et al., out of approximately 12,000 spinal procedures performed over a 10-year period, 12 patients (0.1%) were identified who developed a new postoperative neurologic deficit that was surgically confirmed to be caused by a postoperative SEH.[20] All cases involved lumbar laminectomies. Aono et al. reported on 6356 spinal surgeries and identified 26 (0.41%) patients with symptomatic postoperative SEH.[21] The authors also identified the incidence by procedure. Zero hematomas were seen in 1568 lumbar discectomies; eight were identified in 1614 patients undergoing a lumbar laminectomy (0.5%), and eight were identified in 1191 patients undergoing a posterior lumbar interbody fusion (0.67%). As per the above-mentioned articles and a detailed review of literature, the risk of a clinically significant postoperative SEH appears to be low, the range being between 0% and 1%.[13,15]

Risk Factors for Postoperative Spinal Epidural Hematoma

The ensuing morbidity of postoperative SEH is substantial, and therefore it is a feared complication of spinal surgery.[21] Identification of potentially modifiable risk factors or preventive measures is of value to help decrease the risk of hematoma development in this patient population.[16] The rarity of this complication makes it difficult to study or draw conclusions on regarding potential predisposing risk factors. Although multiple large studies have been performed attempting to identify risk factors for this complication, there is still significant debate about the effect of subfascial drains, postoperative anticoagulation, and antiplatelet medication on the incidence of postoperative hematoma. Although there is no evidence that use of prophylactic doses of anticoagulation increases the risk of a symptomatic postoperative epidural hematoma, there is insufficient data available in the literature to define the safety profile of postoperative prophylactic anticoagulation.

Kao et al. performed a case-control analysis to identify risk factors.[18] Despite looking at over 20 possible risk factors including age, the use of anticoagulants, platelet count, and blood loss, the only significant risk factors for the development of a symptomatic SEH identified by the authors were an elevated preoperative diastolic blood pressure, the intraoperative use of Gelfoam for dura coverage, and high postoperative drain output. Awad et al. found the following risk factors associated with postoperative SEH: Preoperative risk factors included the use of nonsteroidal antiinflammatories, Rh-positive blood, and age above 60 years; intraoperative risk factors included surgeries involving >5 levels, significant blood loss of >1 L, and a hemoglobin of <10 g/dL; postoperative risk factors included Coumadin use only if the international normalized ratio (INR) was >2.0 in the first 48 hours.[19] They also found that well-controlled anticoagulation and the use of drains were not associated with an increased risk of postoperative SEH. Kou et al. conclude that patients who require multilevel lumbar procedures and/or have a preoperative coagulopathy are at a significantly higher risk for developing a postoperative epidural hematoma. They suggest that extra precautions for meticulous hemostasis during the surgical procedure should be considered in such patients and that postoperative neurologic examinations be done routinely for them.[20] Amiri et al., in their review of 4568 open spinal operations, found alcohol consumption greater than 10 units a week, multilevel procedure, and previous spinal surgery as risk factors for developing SEH.[13]

Studies specifically evaluating whether the presence of a postoperative subfascial drain affected the risk of symptomatic epidural hematoma have not found a significant protective effect from the use of a drain.[13,19,20] Similarly, a metaanalysis looking at the effect of drain use after all orthopedic procedures found that there was no decrease in the rate of a postoperative hematoma with the use of a closed suction surgical drain.[22] However, the use of a drain did lead to an increase in the need for blood transfusions. Despite the lack of evidence that subfascial drains decrease the risk of a symptomatic postoperative epidural hematoma, drains are still commonly used in lumbar spine surgery because they have been shown to decrease the risk of an asymptomatic postoperative epidural hematoma.[23,24] In a prospective study in which a lumbar spine MRI was obtained on postoperative day 1 in 50 patients who underwent lumbar spine surgery, Mirzai et al. reported that the use of a drain significantly decreased the incidence of an asymptomatic epidural hematoma from 89% to 36%.[24] Importantly, none of the patients in either of these studies had evidence of neurologic deficit related to the epidural hematomas.

Diagnosis and Management of Symptomatic Postoperative Spinal Epidural Hematoma

Once SEH has occurred, it is important to act rapidly to minimize any lasting disability. Delay in surgical evacuation has previously resulted in a successful litigation case.[13] Almost all patients who develop a symptomatic postoperative epidural hematoma have some evidence of neurologic compromise.[14] The symptoms of SEH usually occur within 24 hours after the initial surgery.[18,21] Kao et al. reported that 80% of patients with a lumbar epidural hematoma presented with progressive loss of postoperative muscle strength, 76% presented with some amount of saddle anesthesia, and 56% presented with a sudden severe increase in pain.[18] When any of these symptoms are present, the patient should undergo an emergent MRI to evaluate for a possible epidural hematoma. It is preferred to obtain an MRI on all patients with new neurologic findings postoperatively to ensure that the diagnosis of a postoperative SEH is not missed or delayed. Most authors agree that emergent surgical evacuation should be performed as soon as possible when neurologic deterioration is detected and postoperative SEH is suspected.[14,15,25] Delamarter et al. have demonstrated, in a model of dogs, that recovery from spinal cord compression is inversely associated with duration of compression, and that demyelination after compression occurs in direct proportion to the duration of compression.[26] Kebaish and Awad concluded that if patients undergo evacuation operation within 6 hours of symptom onset of postoperative deficit, the neurologic outcomes are usually better.[27] In a study of 30 cases of epidural hematoma with neurologic deficit due to various causes such as spinal surgery and anticoagulation medications, Lawton et al. revealed that the rapidity of taking patients to re-operation correlated with better neurological outcomes.[25] Hence, symptomatic postoperative SEH should be suspected in any patient with a new-onset neurologic deterioration in the postoperative period; the patient should be diagnosed with an MRI or CT (if urgent neuroimaging is possible), and an emergent decompression surgery should be performed as early as possible.

Conclusion

"A stitch in time saves nine."

POH in neurosurgery is a harbinger of poor neurologic outcome and hence should be given due importance. It is imperative to check hemodynamic and coagulation factors before taking up a patient for any neurosurgical procedure. However, the truth of the matter is that even after doing everything right both preoperatively and intraoperatively, POH can occur even in the absence of any risk factors. The neurosurgeon always has to be vigilant toward this dreaded complication. An examination/imaging study in time saves the patient valuable neurons and significantly improves the overall outcome.

References

1. Merriman E, Bell W, Long DM. Surgical postoperative bleeding associated with aspirin ingestion. Report of two cases. *J Neurosurg*. 1979;50(5):682–684.
2. Desai VR, Grossman R, Sparrow H. Incidence of intracranial hemorrhage after a cranial operation. *Cureus*. 2016;8:e616.
3. Seifman MA, Lewis PM, Rosenfeld JV, Hwang PY. Postoperative intracranial haemorrhage: a review. *Neurosurg Rev*. 2011;34:393–407.
4. Bullock R, Hanemann CO, Murray L, Teasdale GM. Recurrent hematomas following craniotomy for traumatic intracranial mass. *J Neurosurg*. 1990;72:9–14.
5. Kalfas IH, Little JR. Postoperative hemorrhage: a survey of 4992 intracranial procedures. *Neurosurgery*. 1988;23:343–347.
6. Palmer JD, Sparrow OC, Iannotti F. Postoperative hematoma: a 5-year survey and identification of avoidable risk factors. *Neurosurgery*. 1994;35:1061–1064, discussion 1064–1065.
7. Gerlach R, Raabe A, Scharrer I, Meixensberger J, Seifert V. Post-operative hematoma after surgery for intracranial meningiomas: causes, avoidable risk factors and clinical outcome. *Neurol Res*. 2004;26:61–66.
8. Taylor WA, Thomas NW, Wellings JA, Bell BA. Timing of postoperative intracranial hematoma development and implications for the best use of neurosurgical intensive care. *J Neurosurg*. 1995;82:48–50.
9. Brisman MH, Bederson JB, Sen CN, Germano IM, Moore F, Post KD. Intracerebral hemorrhage occurring remote from the craniotomy site. *Neurosurgery*. 1996;39:1114–1121, discussion 1121-1112.
10. Basali A, Mascha EJ, Kalfas I, Schubert A. Relation between perioperative hypertension and intracranial hemorrhage after craniotomy. *Anesthesiology*. 2000;93:48–54.
11. Gerlach R, Tolle F, Raabe A, Zimmermann M, Siegemund A, Seifert V. Increased risk for postoperative hemorrhage after intracranial surgery in patients with decreased factor XIII activity: implications of a prospective study. *Stroke*. 2002;33:1618–1623.
12. Kim SH, Lee JH, Joo W, et al. Analysis of the risk factors for development of post-operative extradural hematoma after intracranial surgery. *Br J Neurosurg*. 2015;29:243–248.
13. Amiri AR, Fouyas IP, Cro S, Casey AT. Postoperative spinal epidural hematoma (SEH): incidence, risk factors, onset, and management. *Spine J*. 2013;13:134–140.
14. Schroeder GD, Kurd MF, Kepler CK, Arnold PM, Vaccaro AR. Postoperative epidural hematomas in the lumbar spine. *J Spinal Disord Tech*. 2015;28:313–318.
15. Glotzbecker MP, Bono CM, Wood KB, Harris MB. Postoperative spinal epidural hematoma: a systematic review. *Spine*. 2010;35:E413–E420.
16. Goldstein CL, Bains I, Hurlbert RJ. Symptomatic spinal epidural hematoma after posterior cervical surgery: incidence and risk factors. *Spine J*. 2015;15:1179–1187.
17. Sokolowski MJ, Garvey TA, Perl J 2nd, et al. Prospective study of postoperative lumbar epidural hematoma: incidence and risk factors. *Spine*. 2008;33:108–113.
18. Kao FC, Tsai TT, Chen LH, et al. Symptomatic epidural hematoma after lumbar decompression surgery. *Eur Spine J*. 2015;24:348–357.
19. Awad JN, Kebaish KM, Donigan J, Cohen DB, Kostuik JP. Analysis of the risk factors for the development of post-operative spinal epidural haematoma. *J Bone Joint Surg Br*. 2005;87:1248–1252.
20. Kou J, Fischgrund J, Biddinger A, Herkowitz H. Risk factors for spinal epidural hematoma after spinal surgery. *Spine*. 2002;27:1670–1673.
21. Aono H, Ohwada T, Hosono N, et al. Incidence of postoperative symptomatic epidural hematoma in spinal decompression surgery. *J Neurosurg Spine*. 2011;15:202–205.
22. Parker MJ, Livingstone V, Clifton R, McKee A. Closed suction surgical wound drainage after orthopaedic surgery. *Cochrane Database Syst Rev*. 2007;(3):CD001825.
23. Leonardi MA, Zanetti M, Saupe N, Min K. Early postoperative MRI in detecting hematoma and dural compression after lumbar spinal decompression: prospective study of asymptomatic patients in comparison to patients requiring surgical revision. *Eur Spine J*. 2010;19:2216–2222.
24. Mirzai H, Eminoglu M, Orguc S. Are drains useful for lumbar disc surgery? A prospective, randomized clinical study. *J Spinal Disord Tech*. 2006;19:171–177.
25. Lawton MT, Porter RW, Heiserman JE, Jacobowitz R, Sonntag VK, Dickman CA. Surgical management of spinal epidural hematoma: relationship between surgical timing and neurological outcome. *J Neurosurg*. 1995;83:1–7.
26. Delamarter RB, Sherman J, Carr JB. Pathophysiology of spinal cord injury. Recovery after immediate and delayed decompression. *J Bone Joint Surg Am*. 1995;77:1042–1049.
27. Kebaish KM, Awad JN. Spinal epidural hematoma causing acute cauda equina syndrome. *Neurosurg Focus*. 2004;16:e1.

8

Complications in Vascular Neurosurgery—Overview

ANIL NANDA, TANMOY KUMAR MAITI, AMEY R. SAVARDEKAR

HIGHLIGHTS

- Cerebrovascular surgery is associated with relatively higher mortality and morbidity in comparison to other sub-specialties of neurosurgery.
- Advances in surgical technology, technical expertise, neuro-anesthesia and neuro-intensive care have improved the overall outcome in recent years for vascular neurosurgery.
- Understanding the common complications and the nuances to avoid them will guide neurosurgeons towards appropriate prognostication and formulation of treatment protocols.
- We present a brief overview of common complications encountered in the practice of vascular neurosurgery.

Introduction

Cerebrovascular surgery is a dual-edged sword. On one hand, this neurosurgical branch is highly rewarding, offering lifesaving treatments for potentially lethal intracranial vascular pathologies; on the other hand, it carries relatively higher rates of morbidity and mortality among neurosurgical specialties.[1,2] The latter can be very well gauged from the fact that the 30-day postsurgical mortality rates for clipping of unruptured aneurysms (1.0% to 5.5%) and for clipping of ruptured aneurysms (7.4% to 13.4%) are significantly higher than those for brain tumor surgery (2.3%) and epilepsy surgery (0%). Based on various single- and multi-institutional studies, the overall complication rate for cerebrovascular surgery ranges from 2% to 17%. However, a recent study analyzing the complication and mortality in cerebrovascular surgery based on the National Surgical Quality Improvement Program (NSQIP) database has revealed a complication rate of 30.9%, and patients who had at least one complication were found to have significantly increased odds for 30-day postoperative mortality.[3] Thus, complication avoidance in vascular neurosurgery is a vital component of achieving good patient outcomes and preventing postoperative mortality. A significant proportion of complications in cerebrovascular neurosurgery may be avoidable through specific technical practices, teamwork, and specialization. This overview and the ensuing section on complications in cerebrovascular neurosurgery represent a step toward recognizing and addressing these complications.

Neurosurgery for Intracranial Aneurysms

The single most important factor to improve the outcome can be ensured by individualizing the treatment of each patient. Since the publication of the International Subarachnoid Aneurysm Trial (ISAT) in 2002, there has been plenty of comparison between outcomes of endovascular coiling versus surgical clipping. A total of 2143 (endovascular = 1073 and surgical clipping = 1070) patients were randomized. About 23.7% of patients who underwent endovascular coiling were dependent or dead at 1 year compared with 30.6% of patients who had their aneurysm surgically clipped (P <0.002). This led to a relative/absolute risk reduction of dependency or death at 1 year of 22.6% versus 6.9%. Rebleeding risk at 1 year was 2 per 1276 patient-years in the endovascular group versus 0 per 1081 patient-years in the surgical group.[4]

At 10 years, rebleeding was more likely after endovascular coiling than after neurosurgical clipping; however, the risk was small, and the probability of disability-free survival was significantly greater in the endovascular group than in the neurosurgical group. Other large trials show higher recanalization rate after coiling (20% according to Ferns et al., 2009).[5] Metaanalysis by Li et al. in 2013 suggested that endovascular treatment is associated with higher rates of rebleeding.[6] The six-year result of the Barrow ruptured aneurysm trial (BRAT trial 2015) suggested that complete aneurysm obliteration at 6 years was achieved in 96% (111/116) of the clipping group and in 48% (23/48) of the coiling group (P < 0.0001). Overall retreatment rates were 4.6% (13/280) for clipping and 16.4% (21/128) for coiling (P < 0.0001).[7] The outcomes for posterior circulation aneurysms continued to favor coiling. Subgroup analysis for saccular aneurysms shows there was no difference in outcome of intent-to-treat analysis. However, of the 178 clip-assigned patients with saccular aneurysms, 1 patient (<1%) was crossed over to coiling, and 64 (36%) of the 178 coil-assigned patients were crossed over to clipping.[8] The Cerebral Aneurysm Rerupture after Treatment (CARAT) Study suggested that the degree of aneurysm occlusion after treatment was strongly associated with risk of rerupture (overall risk: 1.1% for complete occlusion, 2.9% for 91% to 99% occlusion, 5.9% for 70% to 90%, 17.6% for <70%; P <0.0001 in univariate and multivariable analysis).[9] Overall risk of rerupture tended to be greater after coil embolization compared with surgical clipping (3.4% vs 1.3%; P <0.092).

Overall, patient-related factors (such as age and overall health), aneurysm-related factors (symptoms, size, location, configuration, and presence of an intracerebral hemorrhage), and the experience of the surgeon predict the complications and outcome. A number of aneurysms simply are not ideal for surgical management, including those in elderly patients, in patients with poor neurologic condition, and in patients presenting with cerebral vasospasm; aneurysms that are difficult to surgically access; and multiple aneurysms requiring multiple craniotomies for treatment. Many of these aneurysms are better treated by endovascular therapy because of recent advances in this discipline. Many aneurysms, however, still require surgical treatment. This includes fusiform, blister-like, very small, very large, thrombotic, and wide-necked aneurysms as well as those presenting with a clinically significant intracerebral hemorrhage. However, the endovascular treatment options have expanded in these cases as well.

Complications of Microsurgery

Direct Injury

Avoiding direct injury to the brain involves the use of surgical adjuncts, appropriate exposure, and brain relaxation. Minimizing the use of retractors to preserve veins is essential. Surgeons must be careful about brain protection during temporary occlusion. Judicious use of bypass procedures is an important skill in a surgeon's armamentarium. Intraoperative imaging with digital subtraction angiography or indocyanine green videoangiography is a proven adjunct to check for adequate occlusion of the aneurysm and distal patency of the vessels.

Incomplete Obliteration

Durability is the major advantage of surgical clip ligation of an aneurysm over current endovascular options. With the use of modern aneurysm clips, the risk of recurrence after appropriate clipping is very low. Indocyanine green videoangiography has provided beautiful fluorescent images of aneurysms before and after clipping.

Compromise of Parent Vessel

Complex clipping strategies can be used to completely obliterate aneurysms and to ensure the patency of perforating vessels and parent arteries. Some aneurysms simply are not suitable for either endovascular treatment or surgical clipping and require sacrifice of the parent artery and a bypass with either the saphenous vein or the radial artery to resupply the circulation eliminated by the sacrifice.

Intraoperative Rupture

Perhaps the most dramatic and potentially devastating complication of aneurysm surgery is intraoperative rupture (IOR). Sluzewski et al. noticed that the clinical outcome of IOR reflects an all-or-none phenomenon: Patients either do very well or die, which is probably related to the rapidity with which hemostasis can be achieved (or not) and intracranial pressure controlled (or not).[10]

As with most surgical complications, this one is better avoided than managed, but the vascular neurosurgeons must prepare for IOR in every surgery. Adequate exposure, sharp dissection, proximal control, and use of temporary clips are the primary means of avoiding IOR. Intraoperative tear of neck is more difficult to manage than rupture of dome. Barrow and Spetzler (2011) described a cotton-clipping technique in which a tear is covered with a piece of cotton and held in place with a suction device. The aneurysm clip can then be applied more distally on the cotton, using it as a bolster, preserving the patency.[11]

Complications of Endovascular Treatment

Intraoperative Rupture

An intraprocedural rupture may not always be evident on the angiographic images. Changes in the patient's vital signs and neurologic status can be a useful guide. A diminished or stagnant runoff of contrast from the internal carotid artery may reflect the pressure changes during the rupture of the aneurysm. Careful handling of the wire and catheter prevents potential rupture. Rupture of the aneurysm during coil placement can be seen as migration of coils into the subarachnoid space. The formation of a good "cage" early during the embolization procedure, in order to secure the aneurysm, is important. Aneurysms in the anterior communicating artery and those with a small dome size are likely to be risk factors for IOR.

Complications of Coil Embolization/Stent/Flow Diverter

The procedure-related morbidity and mortality are more for unruptured (~15%) aneurysms in comparison to ruptured ones (~10%). The thromboembolic complications related to the introducer catheter, the microcatheter, or the aneurysm itself may often be clinically silent. However, manifestation of stroke is not unlikely.

Compromise of the parent vessel or branch vessel may result from either inadvertent progressive coil packing in an anatomically hazardous pattern or from sudden prolapse of the coils into the parent artery due to coil instability; compromise also may occur during attempts to remove a damaged or ensnared coil. Balloon-assisted aneurysm coiling (using balloon inflation to temporarily remodel the neck of the aneurysm) can be helpful for wide-neck aneurysms; however, it may increase the risk of a thromboembolic phenomenon.[12] The commonly used stents (Neuroform or Enterprise) may be associated with thromboembolic events and institution of anti-platelet therapy should be confirmed before their use. Deploying stents (especially the Pipeline Embolization Device) in patients with tortuous vasculature is technically difficult and tri-axial catheter systems should be duly considered in such cases.

The introduction of flow diverters has revolutionized the field of aneurysm treatment. However, complications are not uncommon.

Zhou et al. published in 2017 a metaanalysis of all papers up to January 2016 discussing complications of flow diverters for treatment of intracranial aneurysms. The complication rate for unruptured intracranial aneurysms was significantly lower than that for ruptured intracranial aneurysms (14.6% vs 30.6%; P <0.05). The incidence of procedural technical complication was 9.4%. Poor stent opening was the major cause, followed by wire perforation. The operative complication rate was nearly double for posterior circulation aneurysms compared with anterior circulation aneurysms. The neurologic morbidity rate was 4.5%. The specific causes were ischemia > intracranial hemorrhages > rebleeding. The permanent morbidity rate and mortality rates were 3.7%

(95% confidence interval [CI] 2.5%–4.9%) and 2.8% (95% CI 1.2%–4.4%), respectively. In-stent thrombosis, stent migration, and delayed hemorrhage are other complications. Strict antiplatelet regimen, increasing experience of endovascular surgeons, and advancement of technology have improved the outcome.[13]

Postoperative Complications Common to Either Mode of Treatment

Vasospasm

Cerebral vasospasm remains a significant source of morbidity and mortality in patients with subarachnoid hemorrhage (SAH) after an aneurysmal rupture. It has been discussed in detail elsewhere in the present book. Nimodipine has been proven as a prophylactic agent since 1989.[14] Intraarterial milrinone has recently gained interest as a rescue agent. Endovascular balloon angioplasty is generally used when medication fails. Simvastatin in aneurysmal subarachnoid haemorrhage (STASH, 2014) trial did not detect any benefit in the use of simvastatin for long-term or short-term outcome in patients with aneurysmal SAH.[15]

Hydrocephalus

Hydrocephalus can occur in approximately one-fourth of patients, and its onset can be acute, within 48 hours after SAH or, rarely, chronic.

Electrolyte and Metabolic Imbalance

Hyponatremia is common after aneurysmal SAH. Hypernatremia, hypokalemia, and hypomagnesemia are rare but are associated with poor outcome.[16]

Neurosurgery for Arteriovenous Malformations

The Randomized Trial of Unruptured Brain AVMs (ARUBA) led to considerable controversy about the optimal treatment of arteriovenous malformation (AVM). Potts et al. analyzed the operative outcomes of 232 ARUBA-eligible patients with Spetzler-Martin grade I and II AVMs.[17,18] The outcomes were excellent with 97% of patients reporting improved or unchanged modified Rankin Scale (mRS). Complete obliteration was confirmed in 94% of cases. Their metaanalysis comparing surgery, radiosurgery, and endovascular treatment concluded that surgery is the preferred modality of treatment.

Increased surgical risk has been reported to be associated with increasing size, eloquent location, and the presence of deep venous drainage for patients with arteriovenous malformation of the brain. The presence of deep perforating arterial supply is also associated with an increased risk of surgical morbidity in high-grade AVMs. Treatment recommendations need to be individualized based on an understanding of individual patient factors and AVM morphology.

Intraoperative Complications

The so-called gliotic plane around an AVM may not be found in all cases. Therefore it cannot always be used as a guide. A bloodless, relatively avascular surgical plane may indicate dissection into the normal white matter. Coagulating feeders away from the nidus may impair normal perfusion to the brain. Feeders should be identified and secured at the entry point to the nidus. En passage vessels in the sylvian fissure and callosal region (distal middle cerebral artery and pericallosal branches, respectively) should be skeletonized, and only the side branches that clearly feed the AVM should be divided. The main trunks, if preserved, continue supplying the normal brain.

Controlling bleeding from deep perforators may often warrant following them into white matter. Packing the hemorrhage should be avoided for deep bleeding because it may cause deep hemorrhage resulting in significant damage. Micro-AVM clips are very useful for this purpose.

Excessive retraction can lead to transient deficit as well. Yasargil named this "temporary blocked syndrome" and suggested that its effects are similar to postictal deficit after an episode of seizure. Avoiding early surgery after hemorrhage (when significant edema is present), adequate positioning, and wide craniotomy minimize the injury.

Wide-based craniotomy also allows the surgeon to work around or in between the major veins without endangering the large bridging veins. Resection of a small amount of noneloquent brain often reduces the need for retraction, and also stretching of major veins.

The resections of AVMs in the temporal or occipital lobe may cause visual deficit due to damage of visual radiation fibers. Baskaya et al. suggested a transsylvian approach for anteromedial temporal AVMs, a subtemporal approach for small AVMs of the deep mid- and posterior temporal lobe, and an inferior temporal gyrus approach (staying underneath the optic radiation and avoiding excessive retraction of the temporal lobe) for more posterior and medial AVMs.[19] AVMs involving the roof and medial wall of the atrium can be approached through a transcortical posterior parietal lobule route. Yasargil advocates the posterior interhemispheric-transprecuneus approach to medial trigonal (parasplenial) AVMs.[20]

Premature occlusion of venous drainage can lead to intraoperative hemorrhage, so venous drainage should be preserved until the arterial supply is completely occluded. Abnormal thin feeding arteries may mimic draining veins. Looking for pulsation may help in identifying an artery. If a temporary clip is placed, the vein will collapse distally, whereas the artery will continue pulsating.

Postoperative Complications

Hemorrhage

Residual AVMs or unsecured hemostasis may lead to hemorrhage into the operative site. The small remnants of residual AVM are still arterialized with disconnection from venous drainage. Intraoperative angiogram or immediate postoperative angiogram is essential to rule out any residue.

Use of hypotension during surgery may reduce intraoperative bleeding, but it increases the risk of postoperative bleeding. Baskaya et al. suggest elevating the blood pressure 20 to 30 mm Hg higher than the patient's pressure after resection of the nidus.[19] Meticulous hemostasis should be achieved after this.

Maintaining blood pressure strictly below the level at which hemostasis was achieved would reduce the risk of hemorrhage during the immediate postoperative period.

Normal Perfusion Pressure Breakthrough (NPPB)

Normal perfusion pressure breakthrough (NPPB) was initially proposed by Spetzler et al. in 1978 to explain the presence of hemodynamic alterations upon restoration of normal tissue perfusion after AVM ablation.[21] They suggested that hypoperfusion could induce local vessels surrounding the nidus to chronically dilate and predispose the vascular territory to vasomotor paralysis. Upon restoration of normal perfusion after AVM resection, an impaired autoregulatory capacity may then be unable to compensate for increases in arterial flow and ultimately cause hyperemia, edema, or intracerebral hemorrhage. Debate remains on the significance of NPPB in the setting of hyperemic complications, and other mechanisms such as incomplete nidus obliteration, occlusive hyperemia, and increased capillary density have been implicated as contributing factors. Over the last 40 years, studies have suggested various techniques to reduce the incidence of edema and hemorrhage after AVM obliteration. Staged embolization of large AVMs, proximal arterial feeder ligation, and systemic hypotension have all been proposed to limit hyperperfusion injury. Generally, these protocols attempt to lower the potentially harmful elevated pressure in arterial feeders after partial nidus resection. Strict blood pressure control can be useful in the setting of complete AVM obliteration.

Venous Thrombosis

Stasis of blood flow in the venous system after resection of high-flow AVM can result in this rare complication. Staged embolization or staged ligation would reduce the flow in the venous system. Optimum maintenance of hydration during the intraoperative and postoperative period would prevent the collapse of veins. However, the neurologic deficit from venous thrombosis is often reversible, unlike arterial occlusion.

Vasospasm

Vasospasm is another rare complication of AVM because large subarachnoid clots in the basal cisterns are unlikely to occur after rupture of AVM, unlike SAH. However, as Yasargil notes, extensive dissection can result in this rare complication.

Retrograde Thrombosis of Feeding Arteries

Stagnation of arterial flow is common after surgical resection and may result in hypoperfusion. Old age, a large AVM, and marked dilation and elongation of feeding arteries are potential risk factors.

Seizures

Literature review states that New-onset seizures can occur in 6.5% to 22% of cases after resection of supratentorial AVM; however, Englot et al., in their series of 440 supratentorial AVM cases report a rate of only 3%.[22] It would be prudent to continue anti-seizure prophylaxis for 6 months.

Complications Specific for Endovascular Treatment

Endovascular treatment of AVM needs expertise. Excessive or early penetration of the venous side can lead to increased intraluminal pressure, resulting in hemorrhage. If it happens, the arterial side should be closed immediately or the patient should be planned for surgery at the earliest.

Wire navigation to a distal AVM is difficult and painstaking. Along with the microcatheter, multiple attempts impart stress on the vessel walls of the feeding arteries. A tear made by the microcatheter can lead to emboli formation. Reflux of embolic material into proximal branches is not uncommon.

Normal perfusion breakthrough bleeding can happen after substantial embolization. Retrograde thrombosis can be seen occasionally.

Direct Bypass for Moyamoya Disease or Complex Intracranial Aneurysms

Hyperperfusion Syndrome (HS) Induced Local Neurologic Impairment

This complication has gradually been recognized in recent years, and it is the most common complication of direct bypass in Moyamoya disease (MMD). Symptomatic HS is defined as the presence of a significant increase in cerebral blood flow (CBF) at the site of anastomosis that is responsible for the apparent neurologic signs. Fujimura and Tominaga reported that among 150 hemisphere surgeries of 106 consecutive MMD patients, the incidence of HS was 18% (27/150).[23] In 2012, Uchino et al. found that radiologic hyperperfusion occurred in 50% of MMD patients after surgery, and this rate was higher than previously thought.[24] Notably, adult patients are at a much higher risk of postoperative hyperperfusion than pediatric patients. The functional loss of cerebrovascular regulation due to long-term ischemia causes HS after superficial temporal artery to middle cerebral artery bypass in MMD. Uno et al. have suggested that blood pressure should be maintained within the normal range for the treatment of HS, with a systolic blood pressure of 120 to 140 mm Hg.[25] However, Ogasawara has set the target at a lower level (90 to 120 mm Hg). Minocycline can be a neuroprotective agent by effective control of HS.[26]

Hemorrhagic complications are not uncommon. Kazumata et al. found that most cases of postoperative hemorrhage occurred after combined revascularization for MMD either during surgery or within 4 weeks after surgery.[27]

Postoperative Infarction

Postoperative infarction can occur within the first postoperative day, but it has a high incidence within the first postoperative week. Hemodynamics should be kept stable after MMD direct bypass to prevent the occurrence of postoperative infarction. Schubert et al. advocated antiplatelet therapy in 2014, reporting that it does not increase the risk of hemorrhagic complications and that it might improve outcome.[28] In contrast, there have also been reports from Japan that do not support antiplatelet therapy.[29]

Others

- Complications of bypass graft vessels
- Postoperative bypass occlusion
- Reversible occlusion
- Bypass graft spasm
- Anastomotic aneurysm
- Local hypoperfusion
- Poor scalp healing and infection

Carotid Endarterectomy and Stenting for Carotid Stenosis

One of the earlier trials, Stent-Protected Angioplasty versus Carotid Endarterectomy (SPACE), suggested that carotid endarterectomy patients tended to have better outcomes in most of the 30-day end points compared with the angioplasty patients. Subgroup analysis suggested that patients less than 68 years of age had a lower periprocedural risk in the angioplasty group and that carotid endarterectomy had a lower periprocedural risk in those patients over 68 years.[30] However, recent reports suggest that carotid artery stenting can be performed safely in elderly patients, comparable to nonelderly patients.[31]

Another recent propensity score matching analysis based report suggested lower 30-day MACE (major adverse clinical events defined as stroke, transient ischemic attack, myocardial infarction, or death) and mid-term restenosis rates for carotid endarterectomy than for carotid artery stenting.[32]

Conclusion

Neurosurgeons, anesthesiologists, intensivists, and interventional neurosurgeon/neurologists painstakingly attempt to avoid complications of neurosurgical and endovascular procedures, but to some degree these are inevitable given the complexity of procedures. The comorbidities of a given patient also add to the difficulty.

Strict adherence to microsurgical and endovascular procedures to minimize the operative events is essential to minimize the complications, as is vigilant postoperative monitoring.

References

1. Levy E, Koebbe CJ, Horowitz MB, et al. Rupture of intracranial aneurysms during endovascular coiling: management and outcomes. *Neurosurgery*. 2001;49(4):807–813.
2. Molyneux AJ, Kerr RS, Yu LM, et al. International Subarachnoid Aneurysm Trial (ISAT) of neurosurgical clipping versus endovascular coiling in 2143 patients with ruptured intracranial aneurysms: a randomised comparison of effects on survival, dependency, seizures, rebleeding, subgroups, and aneurysm occlusion. *Lancet*. 2005;366(9488):809–817.
3. Michalak SM, Rolston JD, Lawton MT. Incidence and predictors of complications and mortality in cerebrovascular surgery: National trends from 2007 to 2012. *Neurosurgery*. 2016;79(2):182–192.
4. Molyneux A, Kerr R, Stratton I, et al. International Subarachnoid Aneurysm Trial (ISAT) of neurosurgical clipping versus endovascular coiling in 2143 patients with ruptured intracranial aneurysms: a randomised trial. *Lancet*. 2002;360(9342):1267–1274.
5. Ferns SP, Sprengers MES, Van Rooij WJ, et al. Coiling of intracranial aneurysms: a systematic review on initial occlusion and reopening and retreatment rates. *Stroke*. 2009;40(8):e523–e529.
6. Li H, Pan R, Wang H, et al. Clipping versus coiling for ruptured intracranial aneurysms: a systematic review and meta-analysis. *Stroke*. 2013;4:29–37.
7. Spetzler RF, McDougall CG, Zabramski JM, et al. The Barrow Ruptured Aneurysm Trial: 6-year results. *J Neurosurg*. 2015;123(3):609–617.
8. Spetzler RF, Zabramski JM, McDougall CG, et al. Analysis of saccular aneurysms in the Barrow Ruptured Aneurysm Trial. *J Neurosurg*. 2018;128(1):120–125.
9. Johnston SC, Dowd CF, Higashida RT, Lawton MT, Duckwiler GR, Gress DR. Predictors of rehemorrhage after treatment of ruptured intracranial aneurysms: the Cerebral Aneurysm Rerupture After Treatment (CARAT) study. *Stroke*. 2008;39(1):120–125.
10. Sluzewski M, Bosch JA, van Rooij WJ, Nijssen PCG, Wijnalda D. Rupture of intracranial aneurysms during treatment with Guglielmi detachable coils: incidence, outcome, and risk factors. *J Neurosurg*. 2001;94(2):238–240.
11. Barrow DL, Spetzler RF. Cotton-clipping technique to repair intraoperative aneurysm neck tear: a technical note. *Neurosurgery*. 2011;68(suppl 2):294–299.
12. Van Rooij WJ, Sluzewski M, Beute GN, Nijssen PC. Procedural complications of coiling of ruptured intracranial aneurysms: incidence and risk factors in a consecutive series of 681 patients. *AJNR Am J Neuroradiol*. 2006;27(7):1498–1501.
13. Zhou G, Su M, Yin Y-L, Li M-H. Complications associated with the use of flow-diverting devices for cerebral aneurysms: a systematic review and meta-analysis. *Neurosurg Focus*. 2017;42(6):E17.
14. Pickard JD, Murray GD, Illingworth R, et al. Effect of oral nimodipine on cerebral infarction and outcome after subarachnoid haemorrhage: British aneurysm nimodipine trial. *BMJ*. 1989;298:636–642.
15. Kirkpatrick PJ, Turner CL, Smith C, Hutchinson PJ, Murray GD. Simvastatin in aneurysmal subarachnoid haemorrhage (STASH): a multicentre randomised phase 3 trial. *Lancet Neurol*. 2014;13(7):666–675.
16. Wong JM, Ziewacz JE, Ho AL, et al. Patterns in neurosurgical adverse events: open cerebrovascular neurosurgery. *Neurosurg Focus*. 2012;33(5):E15.
17. Potts MB, Lau D, Abla AA, Kim H, Young WL, Lawton MT. UCSF Brain AVM Study Project. Current surgical results with low-grade brain arteriovenous malformations. *J Neurosurg*. 2015;122(4):912–920.
18. Mohr JP, Parides MK, Stapf C, et al. Medical management with or without interventional therapy for unruptured brain arteriovenous malformations (ARUBA): a multicentre, non-blinded, randomised trial. *Lancet*. 2014;383(9917):614–621.
19. Baskaya MK, Jea A, Heros RC, Javahary R, Sultan A. Cerebral arteriovenous malformations. *Clin Neurosurg*. 2006;53:114–144, Review.
20. Yaşargil MG, Jain KK, Antic J, Laciga R. Arteriovenous malformations of the splenium of the corpus callosum: microsurgical treatment. *Surg Neurol*. 1976;5(1):5–14.
21. Spetzler RF, Wilson CB, Weinstein P, Mehdorn M, Townsend J, Telles D. Normal perfusion pressure breakthrough theory. *Clin Neurosurg*. 1978;25:651–672.
22. Englot DJ, Young WL, Han SJ, McCulloch CE, Chang EF, Lawton MT. Seizure predictors and control after microsurgical resection of supratentorial arteriovenous malformations in 440 patients. *Neurosurgery*. 2012;71(3):572–580.
23. Fujimura M, Tominaga T. Lessons learned from Moyamoya disease: outcome of direct/indirect revascularization surgery for 150 affected hemispheres. *Neurol Med Chir (Tokyo)*. 2012;52(5):327–332.
24. Uchino H, Kuroda S, Hirata K, Shiga T, Houkin K, Tamaki N. Predictors and clinical features of postoperative hyperperfusion after surgical revascularization for Moyamoya disease: a serial single photon emission CT/positron emission tomography study. *Stroke*. 2012;43(10):2610–2616.
25. Uno M, Nakajima N, Nishi K, Shinno K, Nagahiro S. Hyperperfusion syndrome after extracranial-intracranial bypass in a patient with moyamoya disease—case report. *Neurol Med Chir (Tokyo)*. 1998;38(7):420–424.
26. Ogasawara K, Komoribayashi N, Kobayashi M, et al. Neural damage caused by cerebral hyperperfusion after arterial bypass surgery in a patient with moyamoya disease: case report. *Neurosurgery*. 2005;56(6):E1380.
27. Kazumata K, Ito M, Tokairin K, et al. The frequency of postoperative stroke in Moyamoya disease following combined revascularization: a single-university series and systematic review. *J Neurosurg*. 2014;121(2):432–440.
28. Schubert GA, Biermann P, Weiss C, et al. Risk profile in extracranial/intracranial bypass surgery—the role of antiplatelet agents, disease

pathology, and surgical technique in 168 direct revascularization procedures. *World Neurosurg*. 2014;82(5):672–677.
29. Yamada S, Oki K, Itoh Y, et al. Effects of surgery and antiplatelet therapy in ten-year follow-up from the Registry Study of Research Committee on Moyamoya disease in Japan. *J Stroke Cerebrovasc Dis*. 2016;25(2):340–349.
30. Eckstein HH, Ringleb P, Allenberg JR, et al. Results of the Stent-Protected Angioplasty versus Carotid Endarterectomy (SPACE) study to treat symptomatic stenoses at 2 years: a multinational, prospective, randomised trial. *Lancet Neurol*. 2008;7(10):893–902.
31. Nanto M, Goto Y, Yamamoto H, et al. Periprocedural outcomes of carotid artery stenting in elderly patients. *J Stroke Cerebrovasc Dis*. 2018;27(1):103–107.
32. Heo S-H, Yoon K-W, Woo S-Y, et al. Editor's Choice - Comparison of early outcomes and restenosis rate between carotid endarterectomy and carotid artery stenting using propensity score matching analysis. *Eur J Vasc Endovasc Surg*. 2017;54(5):573–578.

9

Intraoperative Rupture and Parent Artery Injury During Aneurysm Surgery

BRIAN M. HOWARD, DANIEL L. BARROW

HIGHLIGHTS

- Intraoperative rupture during intracranial aneurysm surgery is a stressful but manageable event.
- Successful management of intraoperative rupture requires the operator to stay calm and employ steps to clear the field of blood, limit continued bleeding, and clip the aneurysm.
- The neurologic outcome after aneurysm surgery complicated by intraoperative rupture is related to the reaction of the surgeon. If the surgeon rushes to blindly place clips on the aneurysm before the aneurysm is sufficiently dissected in an attempt to stop heavy bleeding, the tear may be made worse or the parent vessel may be irreparably damaged.

Background

As the proportion of intracranial aneurysms (IAs) treated by endovascular therapies rises, surgically treated patients will harbor more complex aneurysms.[1] Although the role of open microsurgical treatment of IAs remains, trainees and younger vascular neurosurgeons will be less experienced than their mentors. Experience is the ultimate tool in the surgeon's armamentarium to avoid complications and mitigate their potentially deleterious effects. Vascular neurosurgeons must develop strategies to hone microsurgical skills to keep the surgical treatment of IAs minimally disruptive in the combined microsurgical and endovascular era.[2]

Intraoperative rupture (IOR) and/or parent vessel injury (PVI) are among the most nerve-wracking and potentially devastating complications in the treatment of IAs. IOR occurs in as many as one-third of cases of microsurgically treated IAs and is more common when operating on ruptured aneurysms.[3–8] Aneurysm size, location, and morphology and the adherence of the fundus to surrounding structures are associated with IOR.[2,5,7,9] Patient outcomes after IOR are varied.[3–6,8,10] Rupture before opening the dura or arachnoid dissection is predictive of unfavorable outcomes.[3,6,10] Surgeon experience has been shown to have no effect on the rate of IOR,[5,7] but it is positively associated with improved outcomes, indicating "mental anticipation and technical repetition over time transform into efficiency, confidence and insight in the management of [IOR]."[7] IOR is inevitable; however, with adequate preparation and calm and decisive action, the surgeon can limit the possibility of IOR but also effectively manage the rupture while mitigating complications.

Anatomic Insights

Comprehensive understanding of the anatomy of IAs is imperative for prevention and management of IOR/PVI. The location of the aneurysm within the intracranial circulation determines the safest and most easily accessed sites of proximal control. The size and geometry of the aneurysm drive clipping strategy may increase the risk of IOR or PVI, and can dramatically influence the surgeon's ability to safely apply clips without injuring or occluding the parent artery, nearby perforators, or en passage vessels. Specific anatomic insights are noted throughout the ensuing text where appropriate.

Prevention

Prevention of IOR begins with patient selection. Surgical treatment of IAs is higher risk in many patient populations, including the elderly, those with multiple medical comorbidities, and those with subarachnoid haemorrhage and poor neurologic status or vasospasm. Atherosclerotic neck calcification makes IA surgery more difficult. Certain aneurysms are better treated endovascularly. With the advent of flow diversion, many surgically challenging IAs are successfully treated in this manner with less risk.[11] Ultimately, patient selection is the first line of defense against any surgical complication, including IOR.

Adequate bony exposure and a craniotomy that provides the most direct route to the aneurysm limit the need for brain retraction and provide adequate proximal control and maximal degrees of freedom to maximize clip application angle (Fig. 9.1). The pterional craniotomy is the workhorse of cerebrovascular surgery. When completed appropriately, the pterional approach provides a direct working corridor to most anterior circulation aneurysms as well as aneurysms that arise from the basilar artery apex (BAA) and superior cerebellar artery (SCA) origin. The entire anterior sylvian fissure is exposed, and the need for brain retraction is limited if the lesser wing of sphenoid is drilled completely flat. The modified orbito-zygomatic approach is sometimes necessary to visualize the BAA and distal basilar artery when the BAA is above the level of the posterior clinoid. A "half-and-half" approach provides the most versatile combination of angles of attack for many BAA and SCA aneurysms. In addition to performing a standard pterional craniotomy, the squamosal temporal bone is drilled flush with the floor of the middle fossa in the half-and-half approach, thereby granting access to the BAA through the optico-carotid cistern or

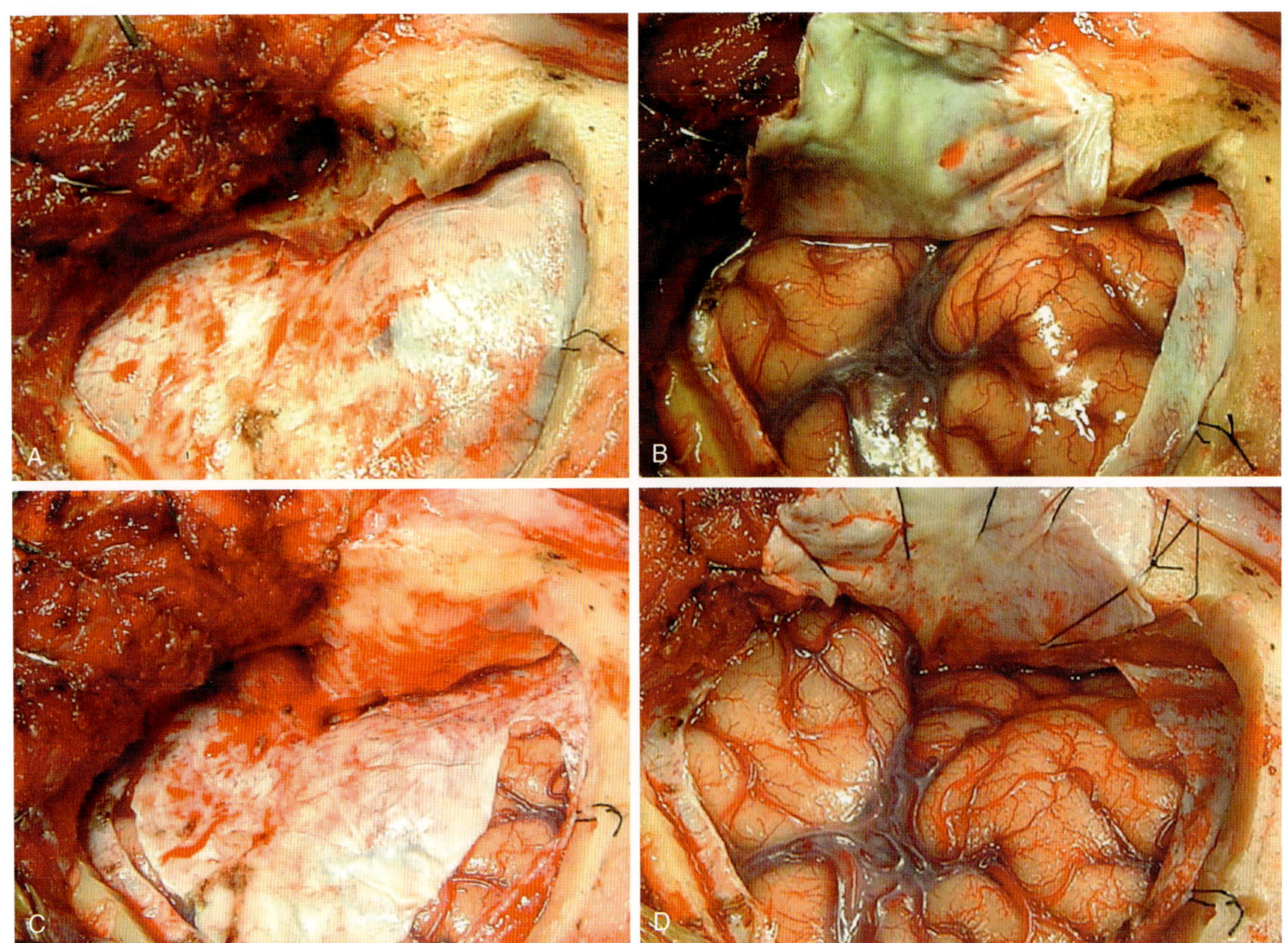

• **Fig. 9.1** Insufficient drilling of the lesser wing of sphenoid for pterional approach limits exposure of the sylvian fissure and cisterns associated with the vessels of the circle of Willis (A and B). Extensive drilling of the sphenoid wing exposes the entire sylvian fissure, provides a subfrontal corridor to the opticocarotid and oculomotor cisterns, limits the need for brain retraction, provides adequate proximal control, and maximizes degrees of freedom for clip application (C and D).

oculomotor triangle, a subtemporal approach, or a combination. Liberal drilling of the occipital condyle provides wide exposure to visualize posterior inferior cerebellar artery (PICA) aneurysms.

Meticulous arachnoid dissection is vital in the prevention of IOR/PVI. Adequate dissection of the arachnoid releases cerebrospinal fluid (CSF) from the cisterns. Egress of CSF in addition to administration of osmotic diuretics provides brain relaxation sufficient to limit the need for fixed retractors, which not only cause white matter injury, but also may lead to a tear in the dome of an aneurysm that is adherent to surrounding brain if retraction is overly aggressive. Microdissection should be completed sharply whenever possible, particularly when dissecting the neck of an IA. Forceful or blind blunt dissection of the neck of the aneurysm, the parent artery, and surrounding structures increases the risk of IOR/PVI.

Temporary clipping of the parent artery proximal to the inlet of an IA softens the aneurysm and can make final dissection and clip application safer. Temporary clipping is particularly useful in the setting of large or turgid aneurysms or for aneurysms where the orientation of the aneurysm neck and the origin of branch vessels, small perforating arteries, or surrounding cranial nerves is complicated and extensive dissection is required to define the anatomy. The surgeon must be mindful of the duration of parent vessel temporary occlusion to limit the possibility of irreversible ischemic injury. Several strategies can be employed, typically in concert, to protect the brain during temporary clipping, including hypothermia and pharmacologic burst suppression to limit metabolic demand from ischemic brain, and induced hypertension to maximize pial collateralization to the ischemic territory.

Modern aneurysm clips are available in a wide range of sizes and configurations, which makes clipping of IAs a versatile and durable treatment. Selection of the permanent clip(s) can have a profound effect on the likelihood of IOR/PVI. The risk of IOR increases each time an aneurysm clip is removed and reapplied. The most parsimonious combination of clips to completely occlude the IA should be used. The long axes of clip application and the parent vessel should be aligned as well as possible. Application of an aneurysm clip(s) parallel to the long axis of the parent artery limits stress on the arterial wall at the neck and increases the likelihood that the entire neck is obliterated, which limits the need for additional clip application. Additionally, angled, bayonetted, and right-angle clips all have lower closing force than straight clips and may lead to incomplete occlusion.[12] A well-thought-out, simple clipping strategy, executed deftly, maximizes the potential for complete occlusion and limits manipulation of the aneurysm, IOR, and PVI. Overall, IOR is better prevented than managed. Although IOR is inevitable, keeping to the principles of cerebrovascular surgery will limit the risk.

RED FLAGS

Patient-related:
- Atherosclerotic vessels
- Large and giant aneurysms
- Blister aneurysms
- Adherent en passage vessels

Surgeon-related:
- Inadequate exposure
- Failure to gain proximal control
- Clipping perpendicular to the long axis of the parent vessel
- Blind clipping
- Blunt arachnoid dissection
- Aggressive brain retraction

Management

Arguably, the most important attribute of the surgeon in the successful management of an IOR is unwavering calm. When IOR/PVI occurs, effective treatment relies on achieving two goals. First, the field must be cleared of blood. Second, the aneurysm must be definitively treated. The timing of aneurysm rupture in the course of surgery and the anatomic location of rupture also are important determinants of treatment. When IOR or PVI occurs, burst suppression should be induced to provide cerebral protection by lowering oxygen demand.

IOR before exposure of the aneurysm is uncommon but is potentially devastating and is associated with a high rate of morbidity and mortality.[3,6,10] Unfortunately, strategies to manage IOR before aneurysm exposure are limited. The surgeon must first clear the field of blood. This is best achieved using two large-bore suctions, one in the surgeon's nondominant hand and the other controlled by an assistant. Frequently, a jet of blood can be traced to the site of rupture. If possible, proximal control of the parent vessel should be achieved and a temporary clip placed to stem torrential hemorrhage. Once the site of IOR is located, cotton is placed over the ruptured portion of the aneurysm to control the extravasation of blood. As a consequence of its absorbency, loosely packed cotton serves as an ideal tamponade. Gentle pressure should be applied to the cotton, either with a suction tip or a retractor blade. Excessive force during tamponade may worsen the tear in the aneurysm or parent vessel and should be avoided. Although fixed retractors are almost never used in aneurysm surgery, we routinely set one up to assist in the event of an IOR. The self-retaining retractor can serve as a "third hand" to hold the cotton in place on the rent in the aneurysm, while the surgeon gains full use of both hands to complete microdissection and clip application. If the flow of blood is too brisk to clear effectively with suction alone, intravenous adenosine can be administered to induce temporary asystole, which typically lasts between 30 and 60 seconds and can yield enough time to locate and control the source of bleeding. Once relative hemostasis and proximal control have been achieved, the surgeon must efficiently dissect and apply permanent clips to the neck of the aneurysm.

IOR/PVI that occurs after proximal control has been achieved may occur for multiple reasons. Management of IOR/PVI after exposure of the aneurysm has been completed is directed toward the cause. IOR/PVI may occur before clip application, and the most common inciting events at this stage include excessive retraction on structures to which the dome of the aneurysm is affixed, or overly aggressive blunt or blind microdissection of the aneurysm neck or en passage vessels. If IOR/PVI occurs during dissection of the aneurysm and temporary parent vessel occlusion has not yet been utilized, a temporary clip should be placed on the parent vessel, if this is necessary to assist in controlling the hemorrhage. Temporary clipping to reduce the rate of extravasation followed by directed cotton tamponade and suction often easily controls the bleeding after proximal control is established. These actions give the surgeon adequate visualization to dissect the neck of the aneurysm and place permanent clips.

IOR/PVI may occur during clip application. Anecdotally, the most common reason for aneurysm rupture during clip application is inadequate neck dissection. When the neck has not been completely dissected, the operator uses the tips of the clip blades to bluntly dissect the remaining neck that was not previously freed. Moreover, this is often a blind maneuver by virtue of the fact that incomplete neck dissection occurs most often at the deepest aspect of the neck, which is difficult to visualize. Blind clipping in this scenario may lead to direct injury of the aneurysm neck, a tear in the parent vessel, laceration of a daughter sack, or avulsion or injury to an adjacent perforator. IOR can also occur with incomplete aneurysm occlusion. If the blades of the permanent clip do not completely cross the entire neck of the aneurysm, the hemodynamics change, sometimes producing an "inflow jet" that can lead to IOR. Incomplete clipping is often the result of blind clipping, or of the clipping of an aneurysm perpendicular to the long access of the parent vessel, in which case the length of the blades required to close the entire inlet of the aneurysm is underestimated. Particularly in the setting of aneurysms and parent vessels with extensive atherosclerosis, the rigidity of the walls of the aneurysm prevents complete closure of the clip blades, which can result in altered blood flow characteristics and IOR.

The treatment of IOR/PVI at the time of clip placement is focused on the cause. If the neck is incompletely obliterated, the clip can be opened slightly and advanced to span the entire neck. Alternatively, if the clip applied earlier to the aneurysm cannot be advanced further, an additional clip can be stacked parallel to the first clip to occlude the more distal neck. In the case of wide-necked or atherosclerotic aneurysms, if the clip does not close completely, a fenestrated clip can be applied to the distal neck to increase the closing pressure, and a shorter clip can then be placed within the fenestration to occlude the proximal neck. If the clip blades still do not close entirely, a clip with the strongest closing force should be used—i.e., straight rather than angled or bayonetted clips.

IOR/PVI rarely occurs after application of permanent clips. At this stage, IOR/PVI is the direct result of excessive torqueing of the clips to gain a view of relevant anatomy. After final clip placement, the aneurysm, parent artery, and surrounding neurovascular structures must be inspected to assure that the aneurysm is completely obliterated and that no perforating or en passage vessels or adjacent cranial nerves are impinged by the aneurysm clips. However, any manipulation of the permanent clips transmits force to the neck of the aneurysm and the interface with the parent vessel that can lead to injury. Care must be taken to limit manipulation of permanent clips when examining clip placement.

Once the aneurysm is secured after IOR/PVI, the temporary clip should be slowly opened, but not removed. The surgeon should pause briefly after the temporary clip has been opened to assure that no additional bleeding from the aneurysm is noted. If bleeding does occur when the temporary clip is released, it should be immediately reapplied and the aneurysm should be inspected.

Specific Anatomic Considerations

Most IA ruptures occur at the dome and, particularly after adequate aneurysm exposure, are easily controlled with the previously described methods. Sometimes, particularly during treatment of larger aneurysms, the fundus can be partially clipped below the site of rupture to control bleeding and to allow the surgeon to proceed to final clipping. Ruptures at the neck or at the interface of the neck and parent vessel are more difficult to manage. Often, the tissue is extremely fragile, and attempts to adjust clips either worsens the tear or occludes the parent vessel. Cotton-clipping is an effective way to occlude the aneurysm, but parent artery patency should be salvaged when the point of rupture is at the neck or the parent artery is injured at the interface with the aneurysm inlet.[13] A small piece of cotton is placed at the point of rupture, and a permanent clip is placed at the superior margin of the cotton, cheating toward the aneurysm side. The cotton distributes the closing force of the clip over a larger surface area than the clip alone, while leaving the parent vessel patent.

Blister aneurysms can be particularly treacherous to treat. The wall of the aneurysm and associated parent vessel is extremely thin, making these aneurysms prone to IOR and nearly impossible to occlude with standard clips. A Sundt-Kees clip (S-KC) can be applied to the parent vessel to treat such aneurysms. The S-KC is an encircling clip that envelops the aneurysm and parent artery. Although useful in emergent situations, S-KCs have several disadvantages. Pragmatically, the perfect size and length S-KC to adequately protect the aneurysm, while maintaining parent vessel patency and not overlapping perforators, is often lacking. An alternative strategy to treat blister aneurysms is Gor-Tex clip wrapping.[14] A piece of Gor-Tex is cut to span the exact length of parent artery required. If needed, slits can be cut into the Gor-Tex to allow unencumbered egress of essential perforators or branch vessels through the graft. The entire circumference of the parent vessel and blister aneurysm is surrounded by Gor-Tex, the tails are pulled snugly, and a 90-degree aneurysm clip is applied to secure the sling. The parent vessel should be slightly narrowed to ensure adequate protection from additional rupture of the blister aneurysm.

Posterior communicating artery (PCommA) aneurysms, particularly larger ones, can pose a challenge if IOR occurs. The space within the oculomotor triangle is often limited. IOR is likely to occur during dissection of the neck or surrounding structures. Often, the anterior choroidal artery (AchorA) is draped over the backside of PCommA aneurysms, and IOR may occur as a consequence of dissection of the AchorA from the aneurysm. IOR may also occur if the surgeon attempts to use a straight clip applied perpendicular to the long axis of the internal carotid artery (ICA). PCommA aneurysms project laterally or posterolaterally, and the surgeon's angle of approach to the oculomotor triangle via pterional craniotomy entices him or her to use a straight clip, which may lead to incomplete neck occlusion and IOR. Instead, an angled clip, or fenestrated angled clip for aneurysms that arise more ventrally, is favored to achieve parallel clipping.

To effectively control IOR when clipping anterior communicating artery (AcommA) aneurysms requires full understanding of the surrounding anatomy. The anatomy of the ACommA complex is highly variable, and bilateral inflow from the ipsi- and contralateral A1 segments can make achieving proximal control difficult, particularly for inferiorly directed aneurysms that may obscure the contralateral A1. Extensive dissection of the neck is often required to clip ACommA aneurysms to avoid injuring or occluding the recurrent artery of Heubner, other smaller medial lenticulostriate arteries, or hypothalamic and chiasmal perforators. The extent of dissection increases the risk of IOR/PVI. IOR may occur during clip placement, which can be partially blind as a result of obscuration by the ipsilateral A2 segment and gyrus rectus. If IOR occurs, proximal control of both A1 segments best mitigates the amount of extravasation. Removal of the inferomedial aspect of the gyrus rectus can aid in visualization and is well tolerated clinically. Resection of the gyrus rectus should be completed with suction and bipolar cautery and should be limited to the minimum necessary to avoid thermal injury to surrounding structures.

IOR when clipping middle cerebral artery (MCA) aneurysms is often easily controlled. Provided the sylvian fissure is widely opened, the proximal M1 segment should be readily accessible for temporary clipping. Premature rupture of MCA aneurysms often occurs when dissecting en passage vessels from the aneurysm neck or dome. MCA aneurysms are often nestled within the branches of the candelabra, making navigating to the aneurysm confusing, particularly when IOR occurs and the sylvian fissure fills with blood. Proximal control and cotton tamponade are effective tools to control IOR of MCA aneurysms, but the key to clipping in this location is careful and broad exposure of the sylvian fissure.

IOR may occur while approaching PICA aneurysms due to several factors. The fundus may be adherent to the cerebellar tonsils or clival dura depending on the direction the aneurysm points. Excessive retraction of the cerebellum should be avoided to avoid an avulsion tear of the dome. Bony exposure via a far lateral craniotomy allows for outstanding visualization of the foramen magnum, anterior medulla, lower clivus, lower cranial nerves, and PICA origin. IOR/PVI may occur during neck dissection if the aneurysm is entwined with the lower cranial nerves. Standard principles of proximal control and cotton tamponade apply to the management of PICA aneurysm IOR. The surgeon must remember that temporary clips must be placed on the vertebral artery both proximal and distal to the PICA origin to curtail the bleeding. Additionally, the surgeon must be sensitive to the directionality and precise location of final clip placement because the PICA is small and easily occluded by the clip.

SURGICAL REWIND

My Worst Case

The patient was a 32-year-old female who presented with subarachnoid haemorrhage. Angiography revealed a BAA aneurysm and a low-lying basilar artery. The interventional neuroradiologist felt that he could not safely and completely treat the aneurysm. Therefore the patient was brought to the operating room for a pterional craniotomy for microsurgical clip ligation of the aneurysm. The posterior clinoid was drilled to gain proximal control of the basilar artery. The posterior clinoid was cored using a high-speed drill and diamond burr. The supraclinoid ICA was accidentally severed with a curette that slipped off the posterior clinoid during removal of the remaining bone. The anterior clinoid was drilled, the distal dural ring opened sharply, and temporary aneurysm clips were placed on the proximal and distal stumps of the torn ICA. The ICA was repaired directly using 9-0 suture. ICG video angiography revealed patency of the ICA after repair. The BAA aneurysm was clipped without difficulty. The patient did well postoperatively. However, 48 hours after surgery the patient developed a right MCA syndrome. Computed tomography revealed a holohemispheric infarction from occlusion of the repaired ICA. Despite aggressive medical therapy to control cerebral edema and a large decompressive hemicraniectomy, the patient progressed to brain death (Fig. 9.2).

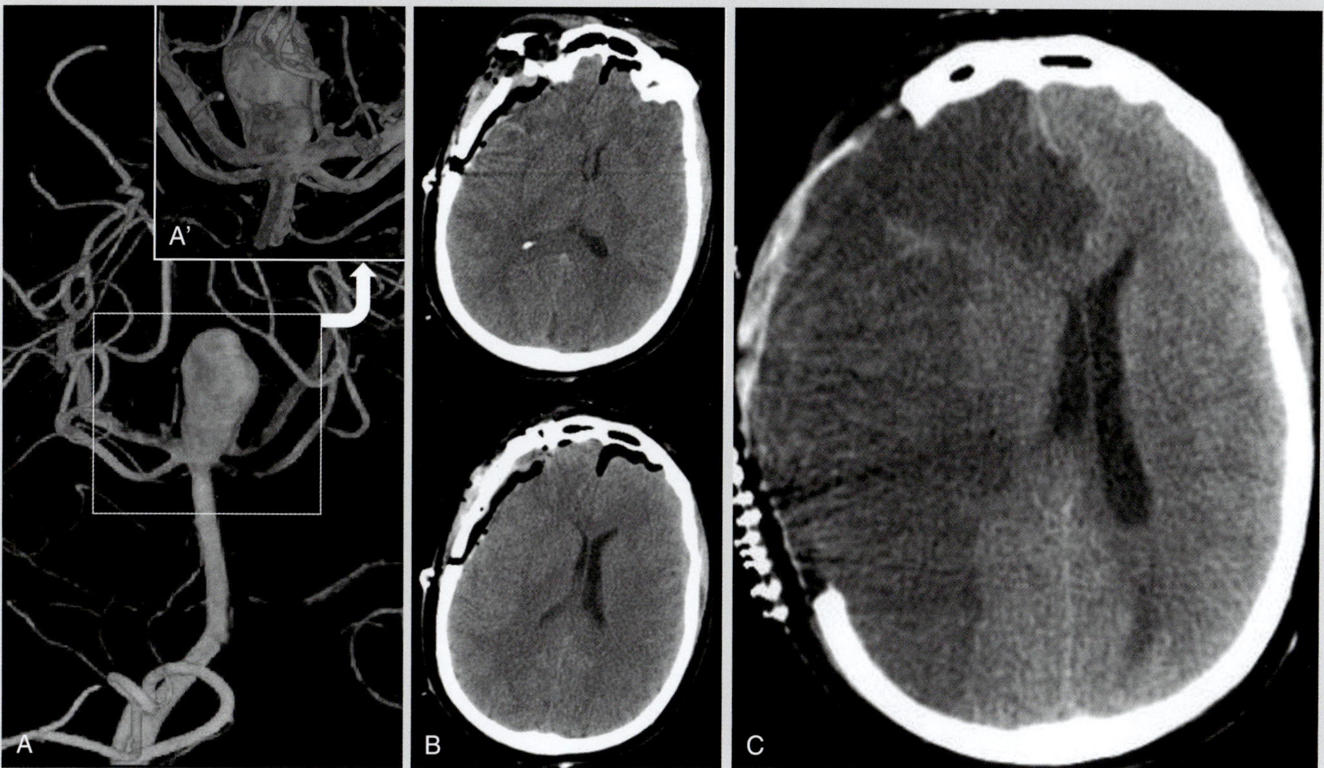

• **Fig. 9.2** Preoperative 3-D rotational angiography of a basilar artery apex aneurysm and a low-lying basilar artery (A and A′). The supraclinoid internal carotid artery (ICA) was inadvertently severed when a curette slipped off the posterior clinoid during removal. The ICA was repaired, and ICG video angiography revealed patency. The basilar artery apex aneurysm was clipped without difficulty. The patient did well postoperatively, and a computed tomography scan within 24 hours of surgery demonstrated expected postoperative changes, but no stroke (B). However, 48 hours after surgery, the patient developed a right middle cerebral artery syndrome. Computed tomography revealed a holohemispheric infarction from occlusion of the repaired ICA (C).

NEUROSURGICAL SELFIE MOMENT

IOR/PVI is a stressful but manageable event. Complication avoidance in the setting of IOR/PVI requires the operator to stay calm and employ steps to clear the field of blood, limit continued bleeding, and clip the aneurysm. The neurologic outcome after aneurysm surgery complicated by IOR is related less to the rupture and more to the reaction of the surgeon. If the surgeon rushes to blindly place clips on the aneurysm before the aneurysm is sufficiently dissected in an attempt to stop heavy bleeding, the tear may be made worse, or the parent vessel may be irreparably damaged.

References

1. Barrow DL, Cawley CM. Surgical management of complex intracranial aneurysms. *Neurol India*. 2004;52(2):156–162.
2. Schuette AJ, Barrow DL, Cohen-Gadol AA. Strategies to minimize complications during intraoperative aneurysmal hemorrhage: a personal experience. *World Neurosurg*. 2015;83(4):620–626.
3. Batjer H, Samson D. Intraoperative aneurysmal rupture: incidence, outcome, and suggestions for surgical management. *Neurosurgery*. 1986;18(6):701–707.
4. Elijovich L, Higashida RT, Lawton MT, et al. Predictors and outcomes of intraprocedural rupture in patients treated for ruptured

intracranial aneurysms: the CARAT study. *Stroke*. 2008;39(5):1501–1506.

5. Fridriksson S, Saveland H, Jakobsson KE, et al. Intraoperative complications in aneurysm surgery: a prospective national study. *J Neurosurg*. 2002;96(3):515–522.
6. Giannotta SL, Oppenheimer JH, Levy ML, Zelman V. Management of intraoperative rupture of aneurysm without hypotension. *Neurosurgery*. 1991;28(4):531–535, discussion 5–6.
7. Lawton MT, Du R. Effect of the neurosurgeon's surgical experience on outcomes from intraoperative aneurysmal rupture. *Neurosurgery*. 2005;57(1):9–15, discussion 9.
8. Sandalcioglu IE, Schoch B, Regel JP, et al. Does intraoperative aneurysm rupture influence outcome? Analysis of 169 patients. *Clin Neurol Neurosurg*. 2004;106(2):88–92.
9. Leipzig TJ, Morgan J, Horner TG, Payner T, Redelman K, Johnson CS. Analysis of intraoperative rupture in the surgical treatment of 1694 saccular aneurysms. *Neurosurgery*. 2005;56(3):455–468, discussion 455–68.
10. Schramm J, Cedzich C. Outcome and management of intraoperative aneurysm rupture. *Surg Neurol*. 1993;40(1):26–30.
11. Becske T, Brinjikji W, Potts MB, et al. Long-term clinical and angiographic outcomes following Pipeline Embolization Device treatment of complex internal carotid artery aneurysms: five-year results of the Pipeline for Uncoilable or Failed Aneurysms Trial. *Neurosurgery*. 2017;80(1):40–48.
12. Horiuchi T, Rahmah NN, Yanagawa T, Hongo K. Revisit of aneurysm clip closing forces: comparison of titanium versus cobalt alloy clip. *Neurosurg Rev*. 2013;36(1):133–137, discussion 7–8.
13. Barrow DL, Spetzler RF. Cotton-clipping technique to repair intraoperative aneurysm neck tear: a technical note. *Neurosurgery*. 2011;68(Operative suppl 2):294–299, discussion 9.
14. Barrow DL, Pradilla G, McCracken DJ. Intracranial blister aneurysms: clip reconstruction techniques. *Neurosurg Focus*. 2015;39(Video suppl 1):V20.

10

Cerebral Vasospasm: Complications and Avoidance

VERNARD S. FENNELL, ELAD I. LEVY

HIGHLIGHTS

- Multimodal management of cerebral vasospasm should include both medical and neuroendovascular options as part of the treatment paradigm.
- Correct application of intraarterial calcium channel antagonists should be the initial neuroendovascular treatment applied.
- Appropriate sizing of an intracranial-arterial balloon for angioplasty is crucial. Oversizing a balloon must be avoided to prevent potentially devastating sequelae.

Introduction

Subarachnoid hemorrhage as a result of aneurysm rupture (aSAH) is a worldwide phenomenon. The annual incidence is 9 per 100,000 persons (>30,000 cases) in the United States and is as high as 23.5 per 100,000 in Japan and 21.3 per 100,000 in Finland.[1] The incidence tends to be slightly higher in women than in men.[1] Cerebral vasospasm as a result of aSAH is a major source of morbidity and mortality and can occur in up to 70% of patients after aSAH.[2–4] The study of cerebral aneurysms as a simultaneously devastating and awe-inspiring intracranial disease process and key contributor in subarachnoid hemorrhage (SAH) has continued to progress since Symonds' description of hemorrhage within the subarachnoid space in 1923.[5] Initial treatments were surgically focused with wrapping by Dott in 1931, clip ligation by Dandy in 1938, and proliferation of the use of the operative microscope in the 1960s.[6–9] With the introduction of coil embolization by Guglielmi et al. in 1990, neuroendovascular therapy forever changed the treatment of cerebral aneurysms and subsequently the treatment of aSAH.[5]

Cerebral vasospasm continues to be the leading treatable cause of mortality and morbidity in patients with aSAH. Vasospasm has also been linked to nonaneurysmal sources such as skull-base tumor resection, meningitis, amygdalohippocampectomy, sexual intercourse, and even high consumption of black licorice.[10–14] However, aSAH initiates the most robust vasospastic response in the cerebral vasculature, which is what we will focus on in this chapter.

Cerebral vasospasm as a sequelae of aSAH was initially described in the literature by Ecker and Riemenschneider in 1951.[6] Allcock and Drake described vasospasm further in 1965.[15] Major advances in the perioperative management of vasospasm were spearheaded with the introduction of induced hypertension, hypervolemia, and hemodilution ("HHH" or "triple-H" therapy) in the 1960s.[5] Ongoing research evolves regarding the mitigation of the vasospastic effects of aSAH. An immense quantity of data has been studied and reported in the literature regarding cerebral vasospasm as a result of aSAH; however, no clear and definitive treatment paradigm has emerged.

Pathophysiology

Vasospasm after aSAH is typically seen 3 to 14 days after aneurysm rupture.[2,16] The biochemical and pathologic bases of cerebral vasospasm have been extensively studied and reviewed. Several hypotheses attempt to explain the pathogenesis and pathophysiology of vasospasm. Pasqualin and Findlay et al. revealed an increase in the production of protein kinase C (PKC) with an additional increase in the production of vasoconstricting prostaglandins and an inhibition of the production of prostacyclin (a vasodilator) as a partial contributor to the underlying pathophysiology.[17,18]

Takenaka et al. used rodent vascular smooth muscle cells as a model in conjunction with cerebrospinal fluid (CSF) from patients with aSAH.[19] They surmised that the subsequent increase in PKC led to excessive mobilization and intracellular activity of free calcium. They further theorized that increased PKC led to extracellular and intracellular influx into vascular smooth muscle, causing phosphorylation of contractile proteins and subsequent contraction of the vessels.

Experimental evidence exists to support the local depletion of nitric oxide (NO) as a major contributor in vasospasm, which is a crucial tonic dilator of intracranial arteries, by virtue of its activation of cyclic guanosine monophosphate (cGMP). Inactivation of NO by oxyhemoglobin or superoxide radicals may have a role in initiating or contributing to the vasospastic process.[20,21] Pluta used a primate model to study the role of oxyhemoglobin in the development of delayed cerebral vasospasm.[22] The author noted that oxyhemoglobin and its oxidized bilirubin metabolic fragments exert oxidative stress by damaging NO-producing neurons in the vessel walls. As a result, there is less available NO in the vessel wall. The vessel wall is unable to dilate appropriately, and constriction is then unopposed.[22] This may lead to the activation of calcium channels and of vasoactive proteins such as arachidonic acid to produce vasoactive lipids or, alternatively, bilirubin oxidation products that can precipitate vessel wall contraction.[23] Animal models have been instrumental in outlining the changes related to smooth muscle contractility.[24] aSAH can facilitate an increase in the availability, relative potency, and sensitivity of endothelin-1

(ET-1), which is a potent vasoconstrictor.[24] ET-1 levels rise in response to shear stress, hypoxia, catecholamines, insulin, and angiotensin II. ET-1 levels are subsequently counteracted by NO through the intermediary roles of endothelin-3, prostaglandin E2, and prostacyclin.[25]

Time Course

Some data indicate that cerebral vasospasm can occur in as many as 10% of patients within 3 days after aSAH. However, it is commonly accepted that cerebral vasospasm almost never occurs <3 days after aSAH.[26] The peak onset of vasospasm is quoted at day 6 to 10 post aSAH with a typical at-risk range of 3 to 14 days post aSAH.[18] There is the possibility of cerebral vasospasm up to 21 days post aSAH; however, this is uncommon.[18] The clinical manifestations of cerebral vasospasm are generally resolved within day 12 to 14. However, radiographic vasospasm, whether clinically significant or not, resolves much more slowly (within 3–4 weeks). Radiographic vasospasm has been identified in 20% to 100% of angiograms on post aSAH day 7. However, clinically evident vasospasm is typically seen in only approximately 30% of that same cohort of patients.[27] Vasospasm, as it pertains to the degree of aSAH, is associated with the presenting clinical grade as well as with the amount and location of blood present on the initial computed tomography (CT) scan.[28] CT results are currently one of the more widely used and reliable predictors of future vasospasm.[28,29] The clinical examination, coupled with regular monitoring by transcranial Doppler (TCD) imaging, is the most common and useful means of posthemorrhage surveillance as well as cerebral vasospasm diagnosis after aSAH.[30]

Treatment of Vasospasm

Medical Treatment

The most commonly used therapy for medical treatment of cerebral vasospasm is triple-H, or HHH, therapy.[2,31–33] The physiologic goals of the triple-H therapy paradigm are to augment blood flow by increasing intravascular volume while reducing viscosity.[2,34] Hypertension is often the modality initially employed, according to the literature, but also at our institution. It is achieved with vasopressor augmentation, most often by administering a low dose of phenylephrine or dopamine and titrating to blood pressure (BP) parameters to achieve the desired clinical or radiographic effect. The component of hemodilution in the triple-H therapy continues to be the least-defined aspect of the treatment. Enhancing the volume status can precipitate increases in cardiac output and peripheral vascular resistance, which translates into increased cerebral perfusion. However, it may also contribute to volume overloading and the associated sequelae.[2,35] A hematocrit goal of 30% to 35% is often suggested as an ideal balance to maximize oxygen-carrying capacity while limiting the negative effects of increased viscosity.[2,34,36] Instituting triple-H therapy should be cautiously considered given the risk profile. Cardiopulmonary failure, worsening of cerebral edema, renal failure, hyponatremia, and sepsis are all known complications associated with triple-H therapy.[2,37,38]

Despite a limited number of prospective clinical trials, triple-H therapy is widely used to varying degrees. At our institution, we more often employ hypertension as the initial medical modality instituted. As mentioned, hypervolemic therapy can have negative sequelae, whereas hypovolemia carries a known risk for delayed ischemia.[34,37] Euvolemia may have similar positive effects on vasospasm with a lower risk profile when compared with hypervolemia in triple-H therapy.[2,36,39] In a systematic review of the triple-H components, analysis suggested that induced hypertension as monotherapy may be more efficacious with respect to cerebral perfusion and blood flow than hemodilution or hypervolemia alone.[40] The American Heart Association (AHA) recommendations for triple-H therapy currently suggest maintaining euvolemia to prevent vasospasm and suggest induced hypertension for patients in active vasospasm.[41] However, the AHA recommendations advise against inducing hypervolemia without radiographic evidence of vasospasm.[41]

The role of calcium channel antagonists in the medical treatment of vasospasm associated with aSAH has been well studied.[5] However, most of the randomized controlled trials have been focused on treatment with nicardipine and nimodipine.[2,42] A metaanalysis of 16 studies including more than 3300 patients concluded that calcium channel antagonists reduced the risk of poor outcomes. The results were largely attributed to the administration of oral nimodipine, which is cemented as a nearly universal practice in the treatment of aSAH.[2,42] It is crucial to note that although nimodipine is widely used in the setting of aSAH and reduces the risk of poor outcome, it does not reverse angiographic vasospasm.[2,42] The effect of nimodipine is believed to be associated with a decrease in vessel resistance in the smaller arterial beds with associated pial collateral augmentation of flow.[2,43] There is also a reported effect of neuroprotection due to the reduction of calcium-mediated excitotoxicity.[2,43] Other calcium channel antagonists, such as nicardipine and fasudil, have been intently studied. Although they produce a variable effect on vasospasm, there is minimal effect on the overall clinical outcome.[44–47]

The success of calcium channel antagonists led to research with magnesium for cerebral vasospasm prophylaxis in the setting of aSAH.[48] Magnesium, like calcium, is also a divalent cation with tropism for voltage-dependent calcium channels. Magnesium may have some additional neuroprotective effects secondary to its inhibition of glutamate.[2,47] Much of the initial data with magnesium, albeit based on small sample sizes, showed trends toward improvements in Glasgow Outcome Scale (GOS) scores and TCD velocities.[49] Further studies showed nonstatistically significant trends toward improved outcomes. However, the results did show significant side effects, including hypocalcemia and hypotension.[50] Larger trials with magnesium did not provide clear evidence of effectiveness, and the side-effect profile remained constant.[51,52] In a metaanalysis that investigated seven trials and more than 2000 patients, no reduction of poor outcomes was established, prompting the authors to recommend against the use of intravenous (IV) magnesium for treatment or prophylaxis of cerebral vasospasm.[53] Numerous trials have been conducted to search for the ideal medical treatment for cerebral vasospasm.[2] Multiple studies investigating statins, endothelin receptor antagonists, NO, free radical scavengers, thromboxane inhibitors, antiinflammatory treatments, thrombolytics, and the search for other neuroprotective agents have not yielded any definitive medical treatment.[54–62]

Interventional Treatment

Microsurgery

Microsurgery is used for the acute treatment of appropriate aneurysms. Currently, there is no well-established open microsurgical treatment of vasospasm. Data support that microsurgical treatment for acutely ruptured aneurysms can yield good outcomes and that intraoperative measures can help reduce the incidence of vasospasm.[63]

Fenestration of the lamina terminalis in the microsurgical treatment of anterior communicating artery aneurysms has been reported to reduce the need for shunting from ~14% to 4.2% as well as reduce the frequency of vasospasm from 54.7% to 29.6% and ultimately improve outcome in ~34% to ~70% of patients.[63–65] Additional operative maneuvers that have been noted to further reduce the occurrence of vasospasm include clot removal, intracisternal injection of thrombolytics, and local application of vasodilators.

Neuroendovascular

Currently, there is no standard treatment paradigm for the endovascular treatment of cerebral vasospasm. Survey investigations have yielded a varying degree of identification and treatment of cerebral vasospasm.[66] Hollingworth et al. analyzed survey data from 344 physicians (177 US, 167 non-US) from 32 countries. Approximately half of the physicians had 10+ years of experience as well as a mix of low- and high-volume clinical practices. TCD ultrasound was the most commonly used screening modality by both US (70%) and non-US (53%) physicians.[66] Verapamil was the most common intraarterial (IA) first-line therapy in the United States, whereas nimodipine was the most common therapy used by non-US physicians. Balloon angioplasty was widely performed by 91% of US physicians and 83% of non-US physicians.[66]

Intensive endovascular treatment of vasospasm may result in favorable outcomes.[67] Mortimer et al. prospectively analyzed patients of similar aSAH grade (World Federation of Neurosurgical Societies Grade 1–2) presenting within 72 hours of SAH.[67] They identified those with no vasospasm and those with severe vasospasm (>50% luminal narrowing on cerebral angiogram). These authors noted no statistical difference in outcome for low-grade patients with no vasospasm versus low-grade patients with severe vasospasm who were treated with induced hypertension, IA verapamil, and transluminal balloon angioplasty. They concluded that maximal combined medical and endovascular treatment of severe vasospasm can produce favorable outcomes similar to those for aSAH patients who do not have vasospasm (90-day modified Rankin Scale [mRS] scores of 0–2, 88.2%; GOS scores of 4–5, 94%).

The use of IA verapamil as an adjunct to progressive and symptomatic medically managed vasospasm or as an addition to intraluminal balloon angioplasty is a constant at our institution. The addition of verapamil is a safe and effective means of endovascular management of vasospasm.[68] In their retrospective review of 34 procedures of IA verapamil infusion as an adjunct to balloon angioplasty, Feng et al. noted the relative safety and efficacy of the infusion.[69] They used IA verapamil in three settings: (1) before balloon angioplasty for prophylaxis against catheter-initiated vasospasm, (2) for treating mild vasospasm that did not warrant balloon angioplasty, and (3) for treating moderate to more severe vasospasm that could not be safely treated with balloon angioplasty. No clinically significant systemic changes (e.g., BP, heart rate) were observed after 10 minutes of verapamil administration. However, others did note systematic changes after IA verapamil infusion. Prospective in vivo data from Flexman et al. show that each 5 mg of IA verapamil is associated with a 3.5 mm Hg reduction in systemic mean arterial pressure and minimal cardiac chronotropic effects.[70] Stuart et al. noted that patients receiving high doses of IA verapamil (total dose ≥15 mg) had transient postprocedural increases in intracranial pressure (ICP) and brain glucose and reductions in cerebral perfusion pressure for up to 12 hours after administration.[71] The infusion rate should be cautiously monitored because rapid administration of IA verapamil can induce seizures.[72] We typically use 10 to 30 mg per vessel and infuse slowly over 3 to 4 min per 10 mg and have had minimal negative sequelae.

Nicardipine, a dihydropyridine calcium channel antagonist, has also been studied as an IA agent for the treatment of vasospasm.[68] It has advantages similar to those of verapamil in its relative tissue selectivity, which allows for minimal cardiac effects.[68,73] A great deal of the research that evaluated calcium channel antagonists as potential antispasmodic agents was generated by cardiothoracic research with coronary artery bypass grafts.[68,74] The initial results from He and Yang in their work with human radial arteries pointed to dihydropyridine calcium channel antagonists (nicardipine, nifedipine) as potentially more advantageous than verapamil or diltiazem in the treatment of vasospasm.[74] Additional rationale came from the intraoperative subarachnoid or intracisternal use of calcium channel antagonists in aSAH patients treated with microsurgery and an experimental SAH model in the rabbit.[75,76] Then, in a prospective, double-blinded trial of 125 patients conducted in 1983, Allen et al. showed that nimodipine improved outcomes of patients with aSAH.[35] Lavine et al. noted a more robust response to IA nicardipine than verapamil in ET-1–induced vasospasm in rabbits.[77] Badjatia et al. reported their results with IA nicardipine in 44 treated vessels in 18 patients.[78] They angiographically confirmed that nicardipine produced an immediate improvement in vessel caliber with no sustained cardiovascular sequelae.[78] However, these authors noted transient and some prolonged instances of elevated ICP post procedure as well as sustained improvements in TCD velocities as long as 4 days postinfusion.[78] Currently, Level 1 evidence does not exist to confirm which IA antispasmodic agent is more efficacious.

At our institution, we favor IA verapamil (10–30 mg per vessel, infused over 3–4 min per 10 mg) with or without balloon angioplasty in treating patients with aSAH-induced vasospasm that is refractory to medical management (see medical management section). Some centers favor balloon angioplasty only, as opposed to IA antispasmodics.[79]

Intraarterial balloon angioplasty remains the most definitive treatment of medically refractory cerebral vasospasm.[2,79] The initial investigations from Zubkov et al. included more than 100 vessels and helped establish the efficacy of balloon angioplasty.[80] The initial success rate with balloon angioplasty ranged from 30% to 90%.[81–84] Later, Hoh and Ogilvy noted a 62% success rate with balloon angioplasty in a case series review.[85] The best results associated with balloon angioplasty are seen in more proximal segments, particularly distal internal cerebral artery (ICA), M1 segment of the middle cerebral artery (MCA), and A1 segment of the anterior cerebral artery (ACA). Balloon angioplasty is avoided in more distal segments where the arterial wall is thinner.[81,86,87]

Although quite effective, balloon angioplasty for cerebral vasospasm may be associated with certain procedural caveats and limitations worth noting. Utilizing balloon angioplasty in a ruptured but unsecured aneurysm should be avoided given the risk of rerupture.[68] The potential complications of balloon angioplasty have been well noted in the literature. Vessel rupture, vessel perforation, thromboembolic events, intracranial hemorrhage, arterial dissection, reperfusion injury, and hemorrhage from unsecured aneurysms have been reported.[68] At our institution, we routinely infuse IA verapamil before balloon angioplasty to assist in navigation and to reduce the risk of procedural complications. We have used compliant, semicompliant, supercompliant, and noncompliant intracranial balloons in our practice. However, these can often vary in size. When sized appropriately, even noncompliant balloons can be safe and effective for angioplasty.[88] In a multicenter study,

Patel et al. reported on 165 angioplasty procedures using noncompliant balloons for SAH-induced vasospasm with improvement in 97% of cases without any procedure-related complications.[88] We also use compliant balloons for angioplasty. Stent retrievers have also been used to treat vasospasm in M1, M2, A1, and A2 segments with lasting (>24 h) radiographic success and without complication.[89] Particularly when using a noncompliant balloon, it is crucial that the balloon is sized appropriately. Use of a noncompliant balloon that is too large drastically increased the risk of vessel rupture. At our institution, with rare exceptions (see case example), it is our practice to avoid choosing a balloon larger than two-thirds the size of the native vessel. However, particularly when using a noncompliant balloon, we rarely size above a 2.25-mm diameter in the MCA.

We have also had early radiographic success in the use of stent retrievers in refractive vasospasm cases that had been maximally medically treated and treated maximally with IA calcium channel antagonists as well as balloon angioplasty. This version of adjunctive mechanical angioplasty is not widely used and may have good indications for those particularly refractory cases. There is, however, a need for additional study to appropriately elucidate the long-term clinical and radiographic outcomes.

Conclusion

Treatment of vasospasm associated with aSAH can be complex and fraught with potential complications from start to finish, as exemplified in the previous case illustration. The longtime course requires continual diligence to avoid potential complications. At present, no clear, consistent, and codified treatment of vasospasm is recommended in the literature, and as a result, research is robust and ever-advancing.

ILLUSTRATIVE CASE

A 25-year-old man with a history of congenital glaucoma with associated bilateral vision loss presented to our facility with a sudden and progressively worsening headache. The patient denied any recent or remote history of trauma. Other than his baseline lack of vision, the patient did not exhibit any focal neurologic deficits on the initial clinical examination. There was no nausea, emesis, or nuchal rigidity. The patient's vital signs were within normal limits.

CT and CT angiography of the head showed diffuse SAH with hydrocephalus noted and no evidence of arteriovenous malformation, arteriovenous fistula, or aneurysm. Lumbar puncture showed an opening pressure of 10 mm Hg with associated and expected xanthochromia. However, there was some apparent decrease in the caliber of the intracranial vasculature that was suggestive of vasospasm (Fig. 10.1A–E). Magnetic resonance imaging (MRI) of the brain and cervical spine with and without contrast material was also unremarkable. Initial digital subtraction angiography (DSA) did not reveal any evidence of arteriovenous malformation, arteriovenous fistula, or aneurysm or evidence of vasculitis (Fig. 10.2A–F). The patient was subsequently admitted to the neuroscience intensive care unit.

Daily TCD imaging of the intracranial vasculature was done to evaluate for vasospasm. The patient was started on oral nimodipine (60 mg every 4 hours), and systolic BPs were kept below 140 mm Hg. Daily TCD studies indicated a steady increase in mean velocity. On hospital day 5, an MCA/ICA Lindegaard ratio of 4.17 was noted on the right, suggestive of hyperemia, and a ratio of 5.29 was noted on the left, more suggestive of moderate spasm. His clinical examination was unremarkable for focal neurologic symptoms. He was then taken for DSA with IA verapamil infusion (10 mg in the right ICA, 20 mg in the left ICA, and 10 mg in the left vertebral artery) with improvement in vessel caliber. He had repeat DSA with IA verapamil (20 mg in the right ICA, 30 mg in the left ICA, and 10 mg in the left vertebral artery) for persistently elevated TCD mean velocity above 200 cm/s. He underwent repeat DSA with IA verapamil on hospital days 6 and 8. On hospital day 8, a 1.8 × 1.5-mm blister-type aneurysm was identified on the dorsal medial wall of the communicating segment of the ICA (Fig. 10.3A–D). A lumbar drain was placed in anticipation of possible CSF diversion. The opening pressure remained largely unchanged from that on the admission lumbar puncture. On hospital day 9, the patient was pretreated with aspirin (650 mg) and clopidogrel (600 mg); a Pipeline embolization device (PED; 3.75 × 20 mm; Medtronic, Minneapolis, MN) was placed in the left ICA (Fig. 10.4A). TCD values remained elevated above 200 cm/s on hospital day 10, with a stable clinical examination; the patient was taken for IA verapamil (20 mg in the right ICA, 30 mg in the left ICA) and again on day 11. On DSA completed on day 11, there was apparent migration of the previously placed PED. Subsequently, an additional PED was placed (Fig. 10.4B–D). The patient's spasm continued to be refractory, and he underwent repeated DSA with IA verapamil treatments (continued same infusion dose). On hospital day 16, the elevated TCD values were accompanied with right-upper-extremity drift. DSA with balloon angioplasty was planned; however, the DSA revealed, in addition to vasospasm, the presence of intraluminal thrombus (Fig. 10.5A and B). As a result of the thrombus, no balloon angioplasty was completed, and the patient was started on an IV infusion of heparin, with a goal partial thromboplastin time of 60 to 80 sec. The focal symptoms resolved, and the patient continued to receive multiple IA infusions of verapamil. The patient underwent a total of 22 diagnostic and/or treatment angiograms throughout his clinical course. He also had bilateral common femoral artery dissections with associated pseudoaneurysms that were of technical concern with respect to arterial access. In an attempt to maximize medical treatment, he was placed on a phenylephrine infusion for 26 days and norepinephrine infusion for 29 days for treatment of vasospasm, which resulted in a gastrointestinal ileus on hospital day 28. The patient underwent diagnostic gastrointestinal endoscopy to investigate his ileus. He complained of progressive abdominal pain post endoscopy. An abdominal radiograph revealed free air (Fig. 10.5C) and subsequent bowel perforation. The patient underwent open abdominal laparotomy with partial bowel resection and subsequently developed short-gut syndrome. On hospital day 30, with elevated TCD values with mean velocity >200 cm/s, he was successfully treated with balloon angioplasty using a 2.25 × 9-mm semicompliant balloon (Fig. 10.6A–C), with modest improvement on DSA (Fig. 10.6D) and improvement in clinical examination and mean TCD velocity. On hospital day 32, the patient had his most pronounced clinical symptoms, with mean TCD velocities >250 cm/s. He was taken for repeat balloon angioplasty; preprocedure DSA showed pronounced spasm (Fig. 10.6E) The decision was made to utilize a noncompliant balloon (3 × 12-mm NC Euphora, Medtronic) (Fig. 10.6F). There was intraprocedural M1 vessel rupture (Fig. 10.6G and H), which did not abate with repeat inflation of the balloon. The rupture was subsequently abated after sacrifice of the vessel via coil and liquid embolic occlusion (Fig. 10.6I).There was modest collateralization from the ipsilateral ACA and leptomeningeal collateral branches (Fig. 10.6J). The patient was intubated intraprocedurally, remained intubated, and subsequently required tracheostomy as well as percutaneous endoscopic gastrostomy tube placement. Diffuse subarachnoid, intraventricular, and intraparenchymal hemorrhage were noted on intraprocedural cone-beam CT; this finding was confirmed by postoperative noncontrast CT scan of the head (Fig. 10.6K and L). Clinically, the patient had dense right upper- and lower-extremity hemiplegia with expressive aphasia. He was eventually able to intermittently follow simple single-step commands. After prolonged negative-pressure wound vacuum-assisted closure of his abdominal surgical exposure, he was discharged to an intermediate skilled nursing facility.

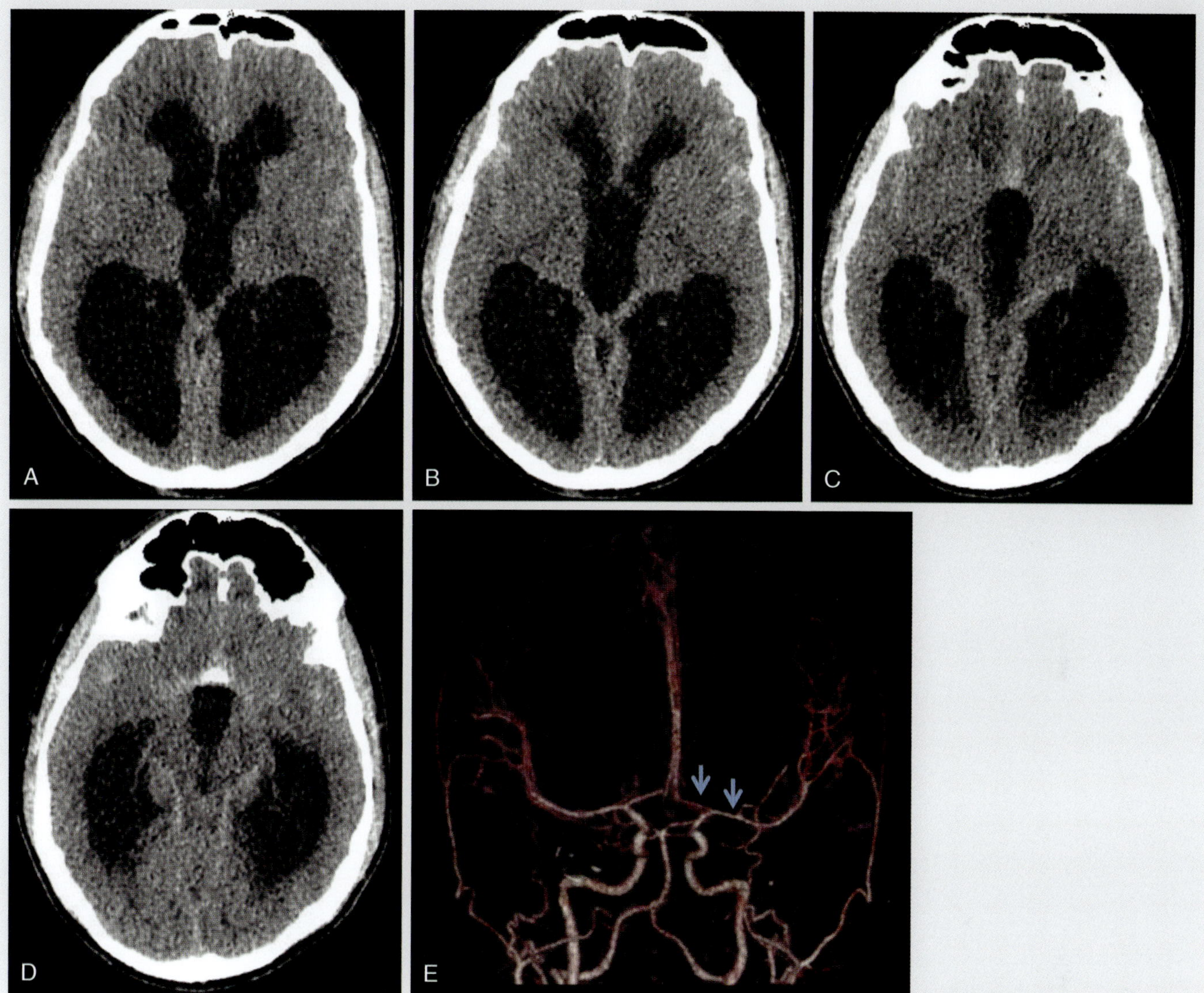

• **Fig. 10.1** CT images of the head showing symmetric dilation of the bilateral frontal horns, third ventricle, and ventricular atria with diffuse subarachnoid hemorrhage (A–D). CT angiography of the head with 3D reconstruction with no clear evidence of arteriovenous malformation, arteriovenous fistula, or aneurysm. There is some seemingly decreased caliber to the left A1 and M1 segments (arrows) (E).

This case is challenging on multiple fronts. There may be limited clinical utility in treating elevated intracranial velocities in the setting of minimal clinical features. It also highlights the risks of maximal medical treatment with respect to effects on visceral end organ ischemia as well as the associated surgical risks. Most importantly, this case highlights the need for appropriate sizing when using a noncompliant balloon. In a spastic vessel with a 1.5- to 2.0-mm diameter, an inappropriately sized compliant balloon is devastating and potentially fatal. Also highlighted is utilizing coil sacrifice of a vessel in the setting of vessel rupture. Balloon tamponade can be employed in intraprocedural aneurysm rupture with excellent results. However, the nature of a vessel rupture, usually over a larger linear or circumferential segment, is less likely to be effectively treated with balloon inflation in the setting of rupture.

Continued

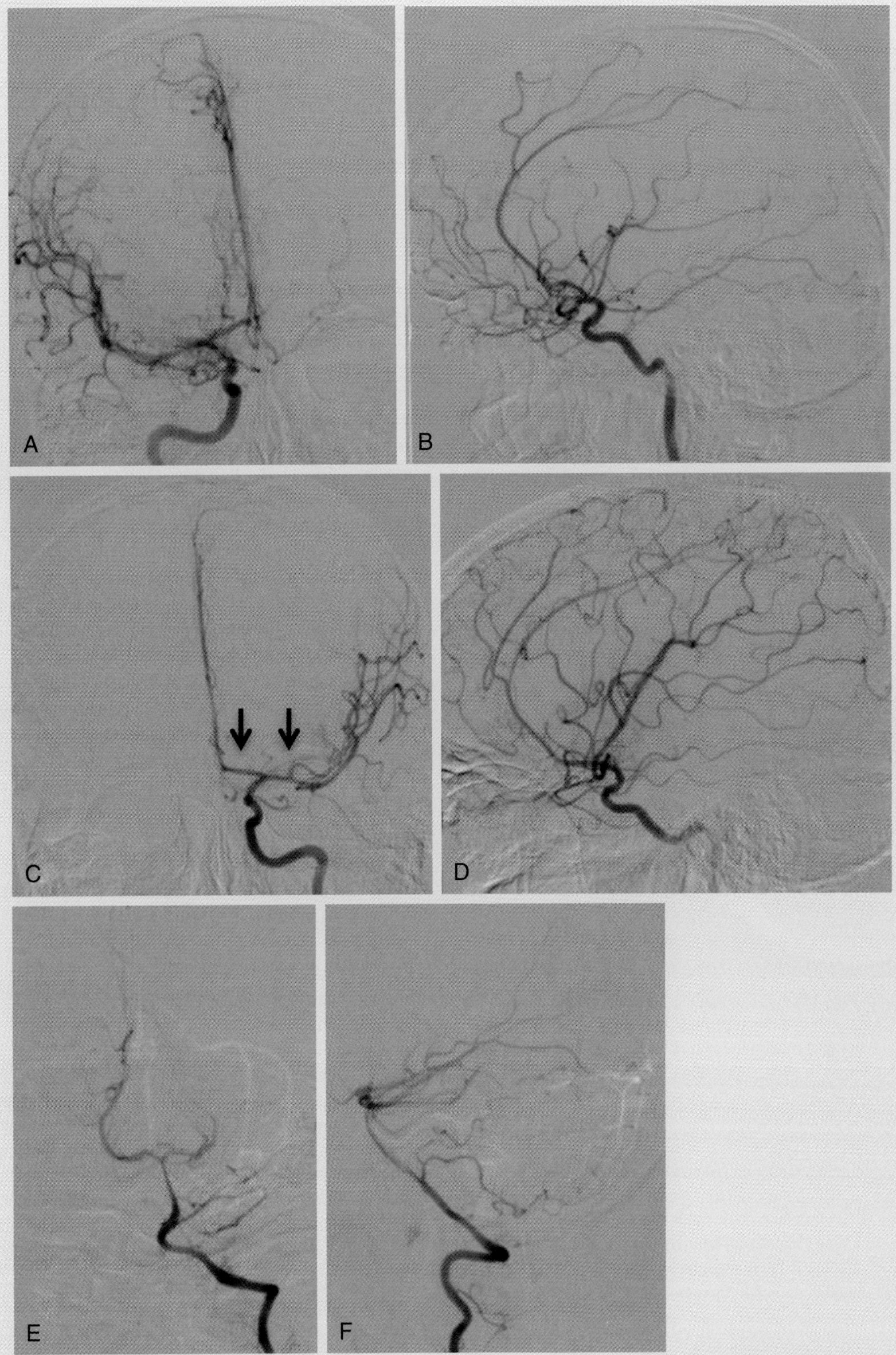

• **Fig. 10.2** Presenting diagnostic cerebral angiogram: right internal cerebral artery (ICA) injection, AP (A) and lateral (B) projections; left ICA injection, AP (C) and lateral (D) projections; left vertebral artery injection, AP (E) and lateral (F) projections. No aneurysm or offending vascular pathology was identified in this initial cerebral angiogram. Arrows indicate the region of decreased caliber of the left A1 and M1 segments.

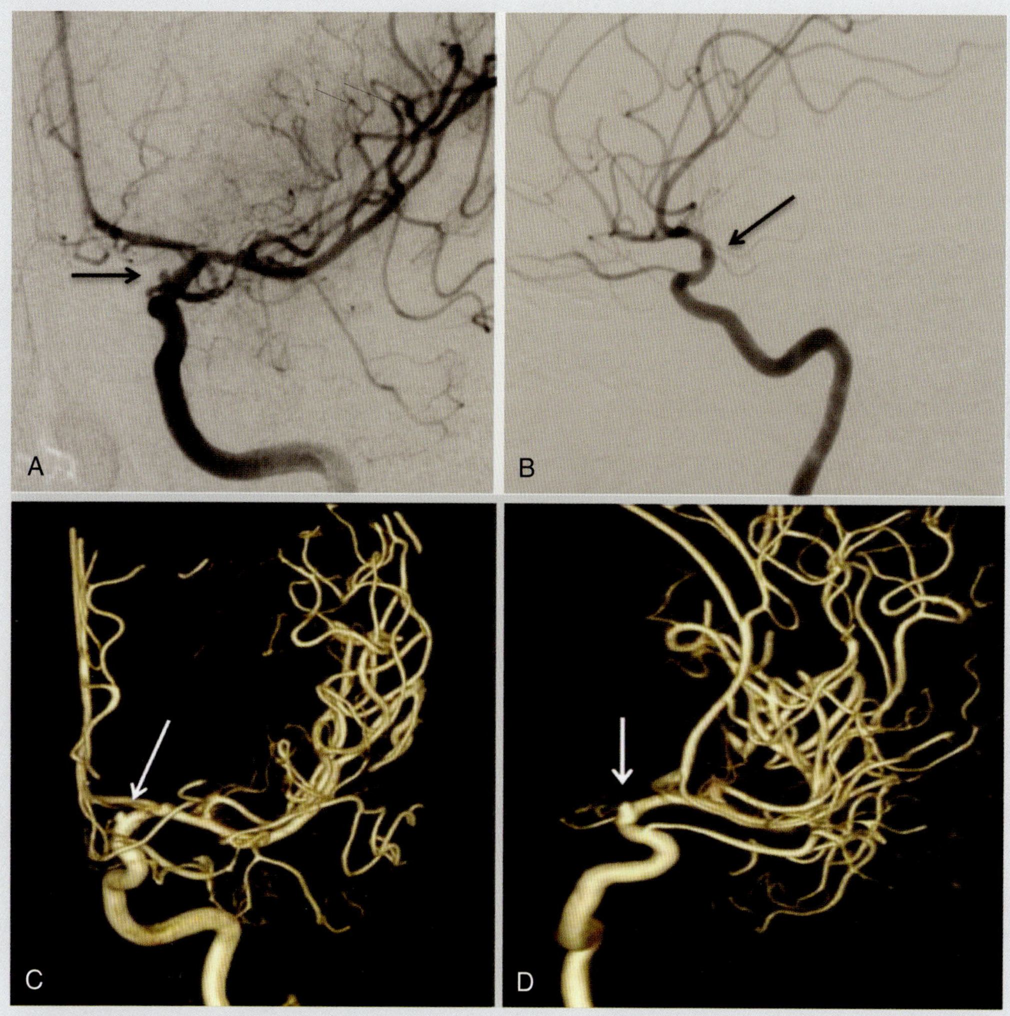

• **Fig. 10.3** Hospital day 8: Digital subtraction angiography (DSA), AP (A) and lateral (B) projections, identifying a blister-type aneurysm (arrows) in the left dorsal medial portion of the communicating segment of the internal cerebral artery (ICA) measuring 1.8 × 1.5 mm. 3D DSA demonstration of ICA aneurysm (arrows) (C and D).

Continued

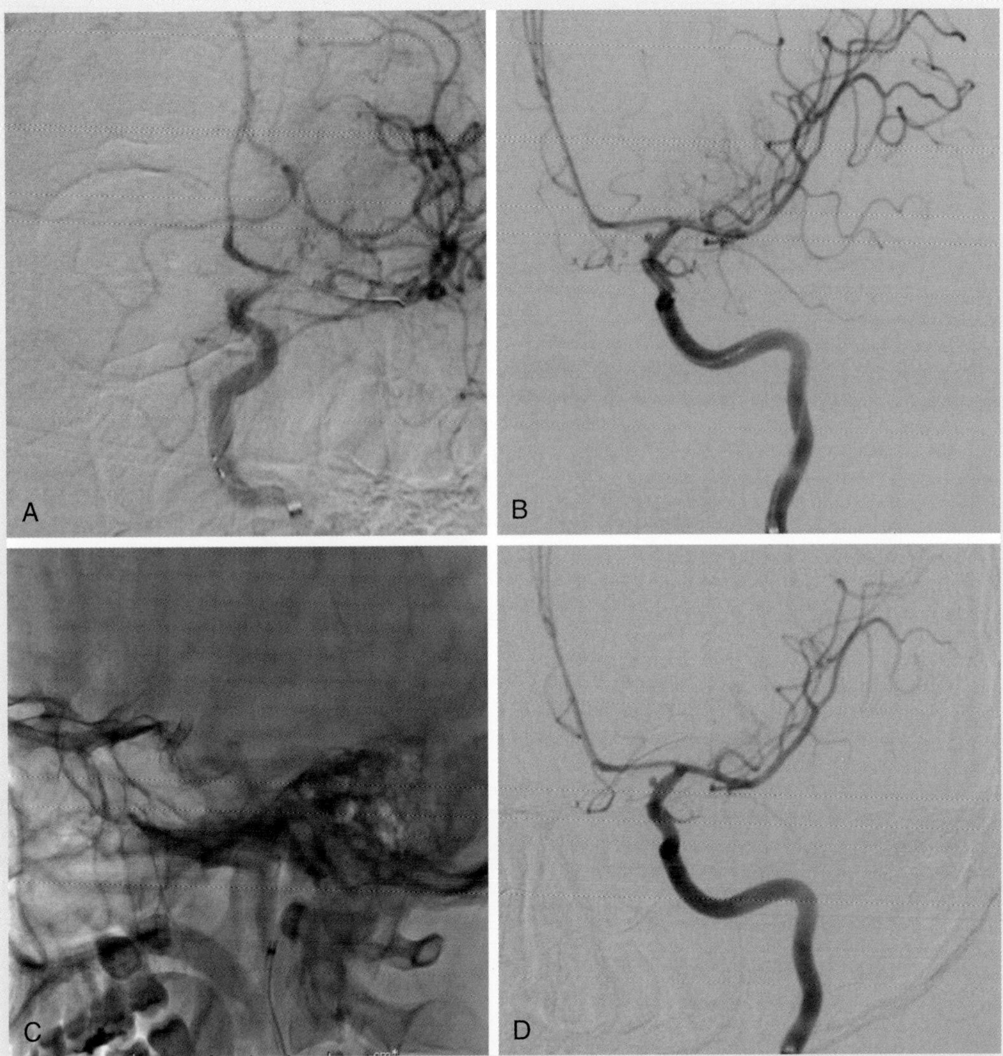

• **Fig. 10.4** Hospital day 9: Digital subtraction angiography (DSA) showing Pipeline embolization device (PED) (Medtronic, Minneapolis, MN) being placed in the left internal cerebral artery (A). Hospital day 11: Placement of a second PED after migration of the first PED (B). Single fluoroscopic still image of PED position (C). Follow-up DSA after PED deployment (D).

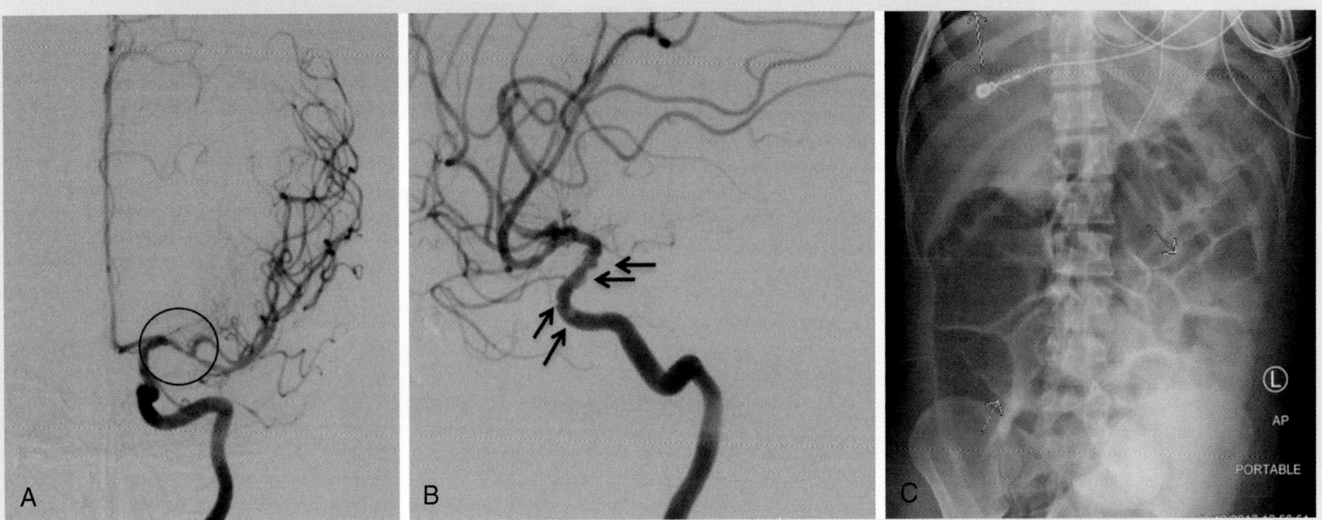

• **Fig. 10.5** Hospital day 16: Digital subtraction angiography showing vasospasm (circle) and intraluminal thrombus (arrows) (A and B). AP abdominal radiograph showing free air (arrows) (C).

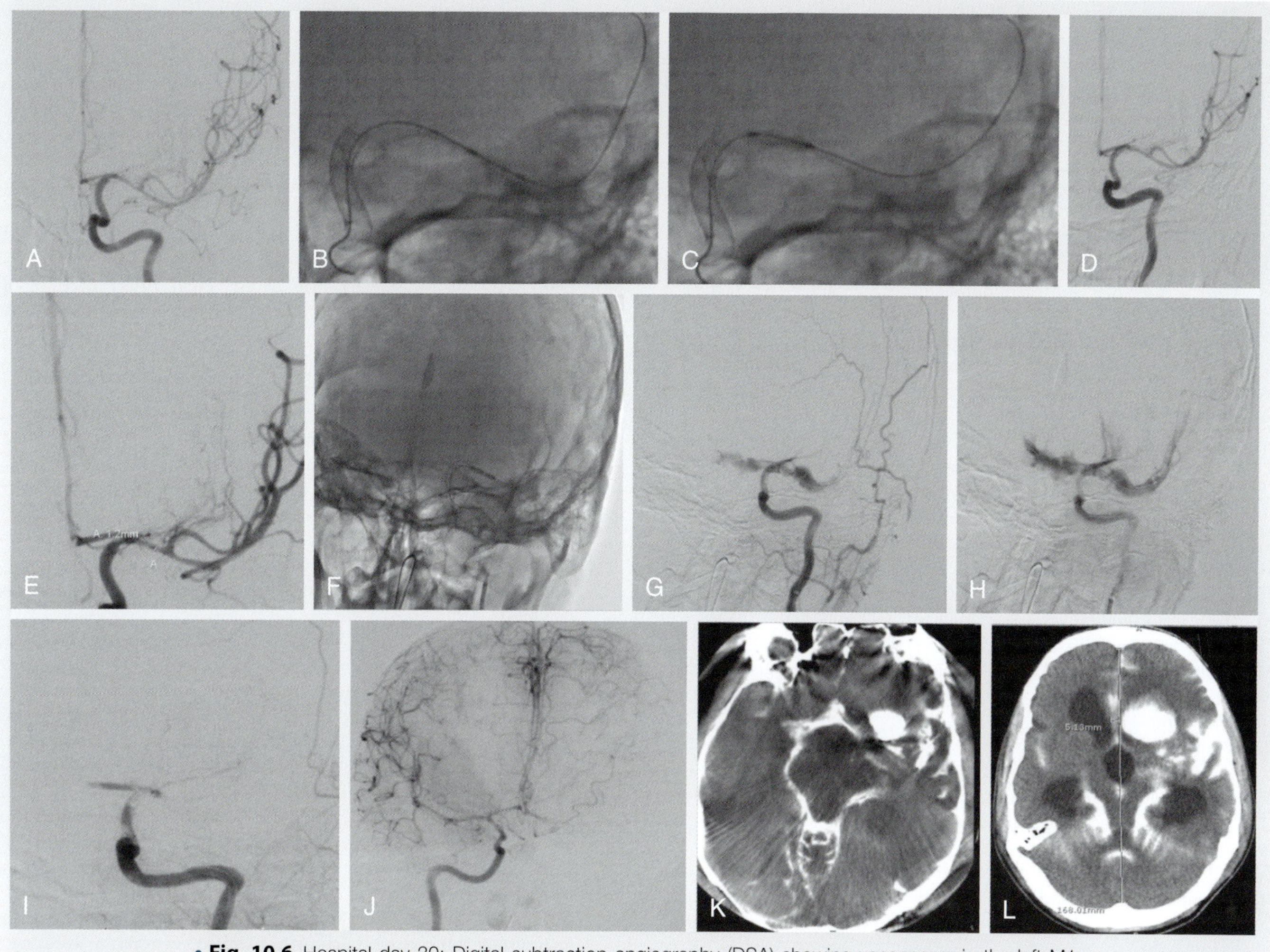

• **Fig. 10.6** Hospital day 30: Digital subtraction angiography (DSA) showing vasospasm in the left M1 and A1 segments (A). Single AP fluoroscopic still images with balloon (2.25 × 9-mm Gateway semicompliant balloon, Boston Scientific, Marlborough, MA) plasty locations (B and C). Modest improvement after balloon angioplasty (D). Hospital day 32: Pretreatment A1 and M1 stenosis with a 1.2-mm vessel diameter (E). Single AP fluoroscopic still image demonstrating position of balloon (F). Extravasation of contrast from ruptured M1 vessel (G and H). Left internal cerebral artery (ICA) DSA after coil and liquid embolic vessel sacrifice (I). Right ICA DSA with right-to-left cross filling and noted collateral flow (J). Intraprocedural angiography cone-beam CT image showing diffuse hemorrhage (K). Immediate postprocedural CT scan of the head with diffuse subarachnoid and intraparenchymal hemorrhage (L).

References

1. de Rooij NK, Linn FHH, van der Plas JA, et al. Incidence of subarachnoid haemorrhage: a systematic review with emphasis on region, age, gender and time trends. *J Neurol Neurosurg Psychiatry*. 2007;78:1365–1372.
2. Adamczyk P, He S, Amar AP, et al. Medical management of cerebral vasospasm following aneurysmal subarachnoid hemorrhage: a review of current and emerging therapeutic interventions. *Neurol Res Int*. 2013;2013:462491.
3. Gross BA, Rosalind Lai PM, Frerichs KU, et al. Treatment modality and vasospasm after aneurysmal subarachnoid hemorrhage. *World Neurosurg*. 2014;82:e725–e730.
4. Li H, Pan R, Wang H, et al. Clipping versus coiling for ruptured intracranial aneurysms: a systematic review and meta-analysis. *Stroke*. 2013;44:29–37.
5. Zhou J, Agarwal N, Hamilton DK, et al. The 100 most influential publications pertaining to intracranial aneurysms and aneurysmal subarachnoid hemorrhage. *J Clin Neurosci*. 2017;42:28–42.
6. Ecker A, Riemenschneider PA. Arteriographic demonstration of spasm of the intracranial arteries, with special reference to saccular arterial aneurysms. *J Neurosurg*. 1951;8:660–667.
7. Fletcher TM, Taveras JM, Pool JL. Cerebral vasospasm in angiography for intracranial aneurysms. Incidence and significance in one hundred consecutive angiograms. *Arch Neurol*. 1959;1:38–47.
8. Sundt TM Jr. Management of ischemic complications after subarachnoid hemorrhage. *J Neurosurg*. 1975;43:418–425.
9. Sundt TM Jr, Szurszewski J, Sharbrough FW. Physiological considerations important for the management of vasospasm. *Surg Neurol*. 1977;7:259–267.
10. Bejjani GK, Sekhar LN, Yost AM, et al. Vasospasm after cranial base tumor resection: pathogenesis, diagnosis, and therapy. *Surg Neurol*. 1999;52:577–583, discussion 83–84.
11. Chatterjee N, Domoto-Reilly K, Fecci PE, et al. Licorice-associated reversible cerebral vasoconstriction with PRES. *Neurology*. 2010;75:1939–1941.

12. Mandonnet E, Chassoux F, Naggara O, et al. Transient symptomatic vasospasm following antero-mesial temporal lobectomy for refractory epilepsy. *Acta Neurochir (Wien)*. 2009;151:1723–1726.
13. Popugaev KA, Savin IA, Lubnin AU, et al. Unusual cause of cerebral vasospasm after pituitary surgery. *Neurol Sci*. 2011;32:673–680.
14. Valenca MM, Valenca LP, Bordini CA, et al. Cerebral vasospasm and headache during sexual intercourse and masturbatory orgasms. *Headache*. 2004;44:244–248.
15. Allcock JM, Drake CG. Ruptured intracranial aneurysms—The role of arterial spasm. *J Neurosurg*. 1965;22:21–29.
16. Adams HP Jr. Calcium antagonists in the management of patients with aneurysmal subarachnoid hemorrhage: a review. *Angiology*. 1990;41:1010–1016.
17. Findlay JM, Macdonald RL, Weir BK. Current concepts of pathophysiology and management of cerebral vasospasm following aneurysmal subarachnoid hemorrhage. *Cerebrovasc Brain Metab Rev*. 1991;3:336–361.
18. Pasqualin A. Epidemiology and pathophysiology of cerebral vasospasm following subarachnoid hemorrhage. *J Neurosurg Sci*. 1998;42:15–21.
19. Takenaka K, Yamada H, Sakai N, et al. Induction of cytosolic free calcium elevation in rat vascular smooth-muscle cells by cerebrospinal fluid from patients after subarachnoid hemorrhage. *J Neurosurg*. 1991;75:452–457.
20. Fathi AR, Bakhtian KD, Pluta RM. The role of nitric oxide donors in treating cerebral vasospasm after subarachnoid hemorrhage. *Acta Neurochir Suppl*. 2011;110:93–97.
21. Wolf EW, Banerjee A, Soble-Smith J, et al. Reversal of cerebral vasospasm using an intrathecally administered nitric oxide donor. *J Neurosurg*. 1998;89:279–288.
22. Pluta RM. Delayed cerebral vasospasm and nitric oxide: review, new hypothesis, and proposed treatment. *Pharmacol Ther*. 2005;105:23–56.
23. Pluta RM, Hansen-Schwartz J, Dreier J, et al. Cerebral vasospasm following subarachnoid hemorrhage: time for a new world of thought. *Neurol Res*. 2009;31:151–158.
24. Kikkawa Y, Matsuo S, Kameda K, et al. Mechanisms underlying potentiation of endothelin-1-induced myofilament Ca(2+) sensitization after subarachnoid hemorrhage. *J Cereb Blood Flow Metab*. 2012; 32:341–352.
25. Levin ER. Endothelins. *N Engl J Med*. 1995;333:356–363.
26. Weir B, Grace M, Hansen J, et al. Time course of vasospasm in man. *J Neurosurg*. 1978;48:173–178.
27. Kassell NF, Sasaki T, Colohan AR, et al. Cerebral vasospasm following aneurysmal subarachnoid hemorrhage. *Stroke*. 1985;16:562–572.
28. Fisher CM, Kistler JP, Davis JM. Relation of cerebral vasospasm to subarachnoid hemorrhage visualized by computerized tomographic scanning. *Neurosurgery*. 1980;6:1–9.
29. Kistler JP, Crowell RM, Davis KR, et al. The relation of cerebral vasospasm to the extent and location of subarachnoid blood visualized by CT scan: a prospective study. *Neurology*. 1983;33:424–436.
30. Aaslid R, Markwalder TM, Nornes H. Noninvasive transcranial Doppler ultrasound recording of flow velocity in basal cerebral arteries. *J Neurosurg*. 1982;57:769–774.
31. Stachura K, Danilewicz B. Cerebral vasospasm after subarachnoid hemorrhage. Current possibilities of prevention and treatment. *Przegl Lek*. 2002;59:46–48.
32. Zhao B, Cao Y, Tan X, et al. Complications and outcomes after early surgical treatment for poor-grade ruptured intracranial aneurysms: a multicenter retrospective cohort. *Int J Surg*. 2015;23:57–61.
33. Zubkov AY, Rabinstein AA. Medical management of cerebral vasospasm: present and future. *Neurol Res*. 2009;31:626–631.
34. Sen J, Belli A, Albon H, et al. Triple-H therapy in the management of aneurysmal subarachnoid haemorrhage. *Lancet Neurol*. 2003; 2:614–621.
35. Allen GS, Ahn HS, Preziosi TJ, et al. Cerebral arterial spasm–a controlled trial of nimodipine in patients with subarachnoid hemorrhage. *N Engl J Med*. 1983;308:619–624.
36. Egge A, Waterloo K, Sjoholm H, et al. Prophylactic hyperdynamic postoperative fluid therapy after aneurysmal subarachnoid hemorrhage: a clinical, prospective, randomized, controlled study. *Neurosurgery*. 2001;49:593–605, discussion –6.
37. Solenski NJ, Haley EC Jr, Kassell NF, et al. Medical complications of aneurysmal subarachnoid hemorrhage: a report of the multicenter, cooperative aneurysm study. Participants of the Multicenter Cooperative Aneurysm Study. *Crit Care Med*. 1995;23:1007–1017.
38. Wartenberg KE, Schmidt JM, Claassen J, et al. Impact of medical complications on outcome after subarachnoid hemorrhage. *Crit Care Med*. 2006;34:617–623, quiz 24.
39. Loch Macdonald R. Vasospasm: my first 25 years-what worked? What didn't? What next? *Acta Neurochir Suppl*. 2015;120:1–10.
40. Dankbaar JW, Slooter AJ, Rinkel GJ, et al. Effect of different components of triple-H therapy on cerebral perfusion in patients with aneurysmal subarachnoid haemorrhage: a systematic review. *Crit Care*. 2010;14:R23.
41. Connolly ES Jr, Rabinstein AA, Carhuapoma JR, et al. Guidelines for the management of aneurysmal subarachnoid hemorrhage: a guideline for healthcare professionals from the American Heart Association/American Stroke Association. *Stroke*. 2012;43:1711–1737.
42. Dorhout Mees SM, Rinkel GJ, Feigin VL, et al. Calcium antagonists for aneurysmal subarachnoid haemorrhage. *Cochrane Database Syst Rev*. 2007;(3):CD000277.
43. Feigin VL, Rinkel GJ, Algra A, et al. Calcium antagonists in patients with aneurysmal subarachnoid hemorrhage: a systematic review. *Neurology*. 1998;50:876–883.
44. Barth M, Capelle HH, Weidauer S, et al. Effect of nicardipine prolonged-release implants on cerebral vasospasm and clinical outcome after severe aneurysmal subarachnoid hemorrhage: a prospective, randomized, double-blind phase IIa study. *Stroke*. 2007;38:330–336.
45. Flamm ES, Adams HP Jr, Beck DW, et al. Dose-escalation study of intravenous nicardipine in patients with aneurysmal subarachnoid hemorrhage. *J Neurosurg*. 1988;68:393–400.
46. Haley EC Jr, Kassell NF, Torner JC. A randomized controlled trial of high-dose intravenous nicardipine in aneurysmal subarachnoid hemorrhage. A report of the Cooperative Aneurysm Study. *J Neurosurg*. 1993;78:537–547.
47. Lu N, Jackson D, Luke S, et al. Intraventricular nicardipine for aneurysmal subarachnoid hemorrhage related vasospasm: assessment of 90 days outcome. *Neurocrit Care*. 2012;16:368–375.
48. Stippler M, Crago E, Levy EI, et al. Magnesium infusion for vasospasm prophylaxis after subarachnoid hemorrhage. *J Neurosurg*. 2006;105:723–729.
49. Veyna RS, Seyfried D, Burke DG, et al. Magnesium sulfate therapy after aneurysmal subarachnoid hemorrhage. *J Neurosurg*. 2002;96: 510–514.
50. Muroi C, Terzic A, Fortunati M, et al. Magnesium sulfate in the management of patients with aneurysmal subarachnoid hemorrhage: a randomized, placebo-controlled, dose-adapted trial. *Surg Neurol*. 2008;69:33–39, discussion 9.
51. van den Bergh WM, Algra A, van Kooten F, et al. Magnesium sulfate in aneurysmal subarachnoid hemorrhage: a randomized controlled trial. *Stroke*. 2005;36:1011–1015.
52. Wong GK, Chan MT, Boet R, et al. Intravenous magnesium sulfate after aneurysmal subarachnoid hemorrhage: a prospective randomized pilot study. *J Neurosurg Anesthesiol*. 2006;18:142–148.
53. Dorhout Mees SM, Algra A, Vandertop WP, et al. Magnesium for aneurysmal subarachnoid haemorrhage (MASH-2): a randomised placebo-controlled trial. *Lancet*. 2012;380:44–49.
54. Asano T, Takakura K, Sano K, et al. Effects of a hydroxyl radical scavenger on delayed ischemic neurological deficits following aneurysmal subarachnoid hemorrhage: results of a multicenter, placebo-controlled double-blind trial. *J Neurosurg*. 1996;84:792–803.
55. Kramer AH, Fletcher JJ. Statins in the management of patients with aneurysmal subarachnoid hemorrhage: a systematic review and meta-analysis. *Neurocrit Care*. 2010;12:285–296.
56. Lanzino G, Kassell NF, Dorsch NW, et al. Double-blind, randomized, vehicle-controlled study of high-dose tirilazad mesylate in women with aneurysmal subarachnoid hemorrhage. Part I. A cooperative

study in Europe, Australia, New Zealand, and South Africa. *J Neurosurg*. 1999;90:1011–1017.
57. Lynch JR, Wang H, McGirt MJ, et al. Simvastatin reduces vasospasm after aneurysmal subarachnoid hemorrhage: results of a pilot randomized clinical trial. *Stroke*. 2005;36:2024–2026.
58. Macdonald RL, Kassell NF, Mayer S, et al. Clazosentan to overcome neurological ischemia and infarction occurring after subarachnoid hemorrhage (CONSCIOUS-1): randomized, double-blind, placebo-controlled phase 2 dose-finding trial. *Stroke*. 2008;39:3015–3021.
59. Pluta RM, Oldfield EH, Bakhtian KD, et al. Safety and feasibility of long-term intravenous sodium nitrite infusion in healthy volunteers. *PLoS ONE*. 2011;6:e14504.
60. Suarez JI, Martin RH, Calvillo E, et al. The Albumin in Subarachnoid Hemorrhage (ALISAH) multicenter pilot clinical trial: safety and neurologic outcomes. *Stroke*. 2012;43:683–690.
61. Suzuki S, Sano K, Handa H, et al. Clinical study of OKY-046, a thromboxane synthetase inhibitor, in prevention of cerebral vasospasms and delayed cerebral ischaemic symptoms after subarachnoid haemorrhage due to aneurysmal rupture: a randomized double-blind study. *Neurol Res*. 1989;11:79–88.
62. Yanamoto H, Kikuchi H, Sato M, et al. Therapeutic trial of cerebral vasospasm with the serine protease inhibitor, FUT-175, administered in the acute stage after subarachnoid hemorrhage. *Neurosurgery*. 1992;30:358–363.
63. Alaraj A, Charbel FT, Amin-Hanjani S. Peri-operative measures for treatment and prevention of cerebral vasospasm following subarachnoid hemorrhage. *Neurol Res*. 2009;31:651–659.
64. Andaluz N, Zuccarello M. Fenestration of the lamina terminalis as a valuable adjunct in aneurysm surgery. *Neurosurgery*. 2004;55:1050–1059.
65. Komotar RJ, Hahn DK, Kim GH, et al. The impact of microsurgical fenestration of the lamina terminalis on shunt-dependent hydrocephalus and vasospasm after aneurysmal subarachnoid hemorrhage. *Neurosurgery*. 2008;62:123–132, discussion 32–34.
66. Hollingworth M, Chen PR, Goddard AJ, et al. Results of an international survey on the investigation and endovascular management of cerebral vasospasm and delayed cerebral ischemia. *World Neurosurg*. 2015;83:1120–1126.e1.
67. Mortimer AM, Steinfort B, Faulder K, et al. The detrimental clinical impact of severe angiographic vasospasm may be diminished by maximal medical therapy and intensive endovascular treatment. *J Neurointerv Surg*. 2015;7:881–887.
68. Mindea SA, Yang BP, Bendok BR, et al. Endovascular treatment strategies for cerebral vasospasm. *Neurosurg Focus*. 2006;21:E13.
69. Feng L, Fitzsimmons BF, Young WL, et al. Intraarterially administered verapamil as adjunct therapy for cerebral vasospasm: safety and 2-year experience. *AJNR Am J Neuroradiol*. 2002;23:1284–1290.
70. Flexman AM, Ryerson CJ, Talke PO. Hemodynamic stability after intraarterial injection of verapamil for cerebral vasospasm. *Anesth Analg*. 2012;114:1292–1296.
71. Stuart RM, Helbok R, Kurtz P, et al. High-dose intra-arterial verapamil for the treatment of cerebral vasospasm after subarachnoid hemorrhage: prolonged effects on hemodynamic parameters and brain metabolism. *Neurosurgery*. 2011;68:337–345, discussion 45.
72. Rahme R, Abruzzo TA, Zuccarello M, et al. Intra-arterial veramil-induced seizures: drug toxicity or rapid reperfusion? *Can J Neurol Sci*. 2012;39:550–552.
73. Bakris GL, Sarafidis PA, Weir MR, et al. Renal outcomes with different fixed-dose combination therapies in patients with hypertension at high risk for cardiovascular events (ACCOMPLISH): a prespecified secondary analysis of a randomised controlled trial. *Lancet*. 2010;375:1173–1181.
74. He GW, Yang CQ. Comparative study on calcium channel antagonists in the human radial artery: clinical implications. *J Thorac Cardiovasc Surg*. 2000;119:94–100.
75. Kasuya H, Onda H, Sasahara A, et al. Application of nicardipine prolonged-release implants: analysis of 97 consecutive patients with acute subarachnoid hemorrhage. *Neurosurgery*. 2005;56:895–902, discussion 895–902.
76. Vollmer DG, Takayasu M, Dacey RG Jr. An in vitro comparative study of conducting vessels and penetrating arterioles after experimental subarachnoid hemorrhage in the rabbit. *J Neurosurg*. 1992;77:113–119.
77. Lavine SD, Wang M, Etu JJ, et al. Augmentation of cerebral blood flow and reversal of endothelin-1-induced vasospasm: a comparison of intracarotid nicardipine and verapamil. *Neurosurgery*. 2007;60:742–748, discussion 8–9.
78. Badjatia N, Topcuoglu MA, Pryor JC, et al. Preliminary experience with intra-arterial nicardipine as a treatment for cerebral vasospasm. *AJNR Am J Neuroradiol*. 2004;25:819–826.
79. Brisman JL, Eskridge JM, Newell DW. Neurointerventional treatment of vasospasm. *Neurol Res*. 2006;28:769–776.
80. Zubkov YN, Nikiforov BM, Shustin VA. Balloon catheter technique for dilatation of constricted cerebral arteries after aneurysmal SAH. *Acta Neurochir (Wien)*. 1984;70:65–79.
81. Bejjani GK, Bank WO, Olan WJ, et al. The efficacy and safety of angioplasty for cerebral vasospasm after subarachnoid hemorrhage. *Neurosurgery*. 1998;42:979–986, discussion 86–87.
82. Coyne TJ, Montanera WJ, Macdonald RL, et al. Percutaneous transluminal angioplasty for cerebral vasospasm after subarachnoid hemorrhage. *Can J Surg*. 1994;37:391–396.
83. Eskridge JM, Newell DW, Pendleton GA. Transluminal angioplasty for treatment of vasospasm. *Neurosurg Clin N Am*. 1990;1:387–399.
84. Weir B, MacDonald L. Cerebral vasospasm. *Clin Neurosurg*. 1993;40:40–55.
85. Hoh BL, Ogilvy CS. Endovascular treatment of cerebral vasospasm: transluminal balloon angioplasty, intra-arterial papaverine, and intra-arterial nicardipine. *Neurosurg Clin N Am*. 2005;16:501–516, vi.
86. Dion JE, Duckwiler GR, Vinuela F, et al. Pre-operative micro-angioplasty of refractory vasospasm secondary to subarachnoid hemorrhage. *Neuroradiology*. 1990;32:232–236.
87. Higashida RT, Halbach VV, Dowd CF, et al. Intravascular balloon dilatation therapy for intracranial arterial vasospasm: patient selection, technique, and clinical results. *Neurosurg Rev*. 1992;15:89–95.
88. Patel AS, Griessenauer CJ, Gupta R, et al. Safety and efficacy of noncompliant balloon angioplasty for the treatment of subarachnoid hemorrhage-induced vasospasm: a multicenter study. *World Neurosurg*. 2017;98:189–197.
89. Bhogal P, Loh Y, Brouwer P, et al. Treatment of cerebral vasospasm with self-expandable retrievable stents: proof of concept. *J Neurointerv Surg*. 2017;9:52–59.

11

Complications of AVM Microsurgery; Steal Phenomenon and Management of Residual AVM

JAN-KARL BURKHARDT, ETHAN A. WINKLER, MICHAEL T. LAWTON

HIGHLIGHTS

- Careful patient selection, meticulous microsurgical technique, refined surgical strategy, and high-volume operative experience with arteriovenous malformations is key to prevent complications during microsurgical arteriovenous malformation resection.
- Intraoperative complications need to be addressed directly. When unintentional residual arteriovenous malformation is seen on postoperative angiography, reoperation is recommended within 48 hours.
- Arteriovenous malformation steal phenomenon caused by reduced blood flow in the surrounding healthy cortex is rare and can cause seizure, stroke, or other focal neurologic deficits, which may resolve after arteriovenous malformation resection.

Background

The microsurgical resection of an arteriovenous malformation (AVM) is a technically challenging endeavor. However, surgical resection remains the treatment modality with highest rates of cure and low rates of complication when compared with other treatments—including endovascular treatment or radiosurgery, despite the currently published ARUBA trial.[1–5] Careful patient and AVM subtype selection, meticulous microsurgical technique, precise surgical strategy, and surgical experience as well as a high AVM surgical volume are needed to prevent complications and to provide a favorable patient outcome.[6–8] Based on Spetzler-Martin (SM) grading and the supplementary SM grading system, patients are classified into subtypes and are risk stratified to effectively select appropriate patients for surgery.[7,8] In a multicenter validation study, the supplemented SM grading system was more precise than the SM grade for patient selection for surgery, with an acceptable surgical risk at 6 points or below.[9] The book *Seven AVMs* further describes how to subgroup AVMs based on locations and provides a nuanced stepwise approach to guide microsurgical resection to prevent complications and to achieve a complete AVM resection.[10] Despite adequate preparation and experience, unexpected things can happen during AVM surgery, requiring quick recognition and decisive action. Complications in AVM surgery include intraoperative AVM rupture, incomplete surgical resection with/without hemorrhage, and injury or occlusion of nonfeeding arteries causing stroke with/without clinical deficits, as well as delayed hemorrhage due to fragile deep feeding arteries.[11,12] These complications may occur immediately or may present in a delayed fashion. The rarely described AVM steal phenomenon due to reduced blood flow in the surrounding healthy cortex can cause seizure, stroke, or other focal neurologic deficits. This can also occur after AVM resection and might be due to the reorganization of blood distribution.

Anatomic Insights

Based on the SM grade or supplementary grade, the location of AVM (eloquent vs noneloquent), type of venous drainage (deep or superficial), size of the AVM (small or large), and additional features including nidus type (compact vs diffuse), patient age, and the presence of prior AVM-related hemorrhage are factors influencing the likelihood of complications and patient morbidity during or after AVM surgery. AVMs in eloquent locations—including the brainstem, thalamus, or primary motor or language cortices—are more prone to complications than those in other locations. This is in part due to brain retraction or misinterpretation and to sacrifice of feeding arteries with perforators, which may lead to acute infarction (Fig. 11.1).

RED FLAGS

- Complications will most likely happen if the draining vein is occluded too early. Draining veins should always be preserved until the end of the operation and should be sacrificed only in proportion to disruption of the arterial feeders.
- AVM border dissection too close to the nidus can result in residual AVM nidus and/or intra-/postoperative hemorrhage. Make sure to have enough distance to the nidus in noneloquent AVMs.
- Keep anesthesia involved: Always check blood pressure and estimated blood loss to stay on top of ongoing losses and remain one step ahead of the pathology.

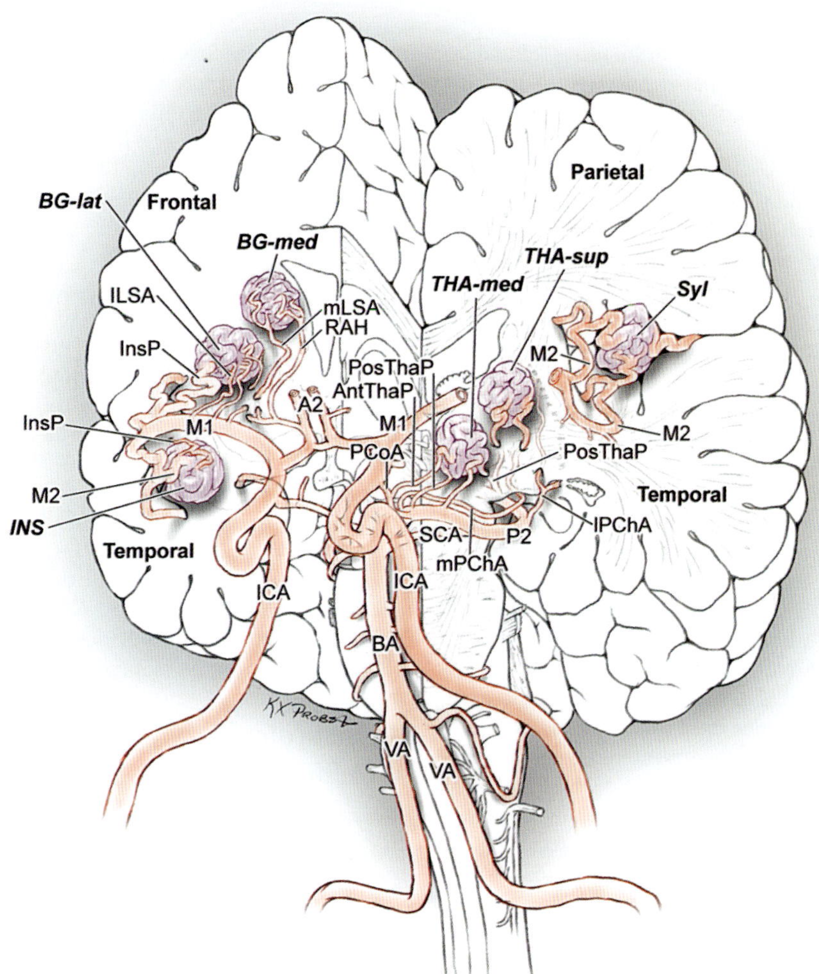

• **Fig. 11.1** Overview of deep AVM subtypes, which include pure sylvian (SYL), insular (INS), basal ganglial [lateral (BG-lat), and medial (BG-med)], and thalamic [superior (THA-sup) and medial (THA-med)], as seen in and anterior oblique, coronal cross-sectional view. (Fig. 15.4 from Lawton, Seven AVM's, Thieme 2014, pg 186.)

Risk Factors

Risk factors for complications in AVM surgery can be grouped into patient factors, AVM characteristics, and AVM location, which were described in the preceding subsection. Patient factors include age and cardiovascular and other medical comorbidities, which affect a patient's general surgical risk. Antiplatelet medication, anticoagulants, or conditions leading to an impaired coagulation increase the risk of hemorrhage perioperatively. High-risk AVM characteristics include the presence of aneurysms in the feeding arteries, nidus, or venous drainage. A large venous varix can mask the nidus or feeding arteries, and these dilatations need to be carefully dissected to prevent rupture. Other high-risk features are stenosis or narrowing of the draining vein, which can increase the pressure in the AVM nidus. AVMs reaching the ventricle often have small, fragile subcortical feeding arteries, which are difficult to coagulate and need to be clipped with small AVM/aneurysm clips.[12]

Prevention of Complication

Preoperative Prevention

Preoperative catheter angiography, magnetic resonance image (MRI)/MR angiogram, and/or computed tomography (CT) angiogram must be carefully evaluated to plan the surgical approach to maximize AVM exposure and minimize transgression of normal brain. The complex 3-dimensional angioarchitecture of the AVM, including the feeding arteries, nidus, and draining veins, must be carefully studied and high-risk features identified. A large craniotomy is warranted so that all of these features also may be confirmed and visualized intraoperatively. In addition to AVM-specific preoperative planning, all patients should undergo thorough medical evaluation to ensure safety with general anesthesia, cardiovascular stress, and the avoidance of coagulopathic conditions.

Perioperative Prevention

Patient positioning depends on AVM location by using standard non–skull-base and skull-base approaches if necessary. Surgical adjuncts including MR navigation, indocyanine green (ICG) angiography, and electrophysiologic monitoring are useful during AVM surgery. MR navigation can help plan the approach that minimizes transgression of normal brain and to provide guidance during the resection. Intraoperative electrophysiology, including motor evoked potentials (MEPs) and somatosensory evoked potentials (SEPs), provides valuable information to prevent strokes before definitive occlusion of vessels during surgery. Surgical resection should follow a systematic and stepwise surgical approach to standardize the resection without missing important aspects.[10] After large exposure, one must first identify feeding arteries and draining veins through careful subarachnoid dissection both to appreciate the 3-dimensional configuration of the lesion and to identify surgical planes. Wide pial dissection should be conducted in circumferential fashion around the AVM. During dissection, feeding arteries should be divided when encountered and draining veins preserved. After a large exposure of the AVM, the feeding artery/ies and draining vein/s are identified by subarachnoid dissection, which helps the surgeon to visualize the AVM nidus and surgical planes. While dividing the feeding arteries, the AVM borders are carefully encountered using a parenchymal circumferential dissection. The bottom border is always the last part to dissect, since deep small feeding arteries that may be difficult to control may be encountered. Therefore it is important to have enough space around the AVM to address these feeders to avoid intraoperative arterial AVM rupture. In a last step, the draining vein is cauterized, and the AVM is resected. ICG angiography might be useful to show AVM nidus residual or an early-filling vein as an indirect sign for AVM residual. Postoperative blood pressure should be kept in the low-normal range for 24 hours to prevent postoperative hemorrhage into the resection cavity.

Management

In general, the earlier the better is the rule for the management of AVM surgical complications—including postoperative hemorrhage and residual nidus. Intraoperative AVM rupture leads to a change of surgical strategy: An AVM resection needs to be finished as soon as possible to avoid blood loss. A take-back is painful for both the patient and the surgeon, but it is the treatment of choice in residual AVMs. Postoperative angiography is the gold standard to rule out residual AVM nidus and should be performed within 24 hours after surgery. If postoperative hemorrhage is suspected based on clinical examination, a noncontrast CT scan should be ordered. New neurologic deficits after surgery without a cause shown on CT or catheter angiography need MRI with diffusion-weighted imaging and/or electroencephalography to rule out postoperative stroke or seizure, respectively. In most cases direct postoperative neurologic deficits are only temporary due to steal phenomenon or irritation during surgery. If a postoperative stroke is identified, standard medical therapy should be initiated—including permissive hypertension—to facilitate restoration of regional cerebral perfusion loss.

Microsurgical Management of Residual AVM Nidus

In the case of a clearly documented AVM residual, the patient should be offered reoperation within 48 hours after the initial surgery. This is advantageous because the initial craniotomy is opened quickly without scar tissue, and the residual AVM nidus can be reached more easily than at later time points. Sometimes it is possible that postoperative catheter angiography does not show a true residual nidus but instead suspicious small vessels without a clear draining vein. In this situation it is reasonable to repeat an angiogram after 4 to 6 weeks to let the postoperative changes resolve. If there is evidence for an AVM residual on the follow-up angiography, reoperation should be considered.

Microsurgical Strategy in Intraoperative AVM Rupture

Intraoperative AVM rupture is an uncommon complication, occurring with a 5% frequency, and can be caused by either rupture due to arterial bleeding, nidal penetration, or premature venous occlusion.[12] Depending on the extent of hemorrhage, it is possible in some cases to control small amounts of bleeding with coagulation or clips, such as with small, unintended nidal penetration. In other scenarios with brisker rates of bleeding, such as early venous occlusion with AVM rupture, a change in surgical strategy must be implemented, and the AVM must be resected as quickly as possible to stop ongoing losses. No matter how severe the intraoperative AVM rupture is, it needs to be addressed immediately; otherwise, intraoperative AVM rupture can be devastating and ultimately fatal.[12] The so-called "commando resection" is an option of last resort when one is faced with impending or frank AVM rupture. It is not meant for simple arterial or venous bleeding or for minor nidal bleeding. Rupture of an AVM calls for decisive action, and the commando resection represents a point of no return. Measures explained in the prior subsections should be implemented to avoid intraoperative rupture.

SURGICAL REWIND

Intraoperative AVM Rupture (Fig. 11.2)

A 25-year-old man with a left medial parieto-occipital high-grade (Spetzler-Martin grade 5) AVM presented with a generalized seizure 10 years ago. Volume-staged radiosurgery was recommended during that time, and radiosurgery downgraded the AVM to a grade 2. Surgery was now recommended to cure the patient. Catheter angiography and MRI show this downgraded medial parieto-occipital AVM fed mainly through the posterior cerebral artery with a superficial drainage to the superior sagittal sinus (Fig. 11.2A and B). The patient was positioned in lateral position (left side down) to resect this AVM through an ipsilateral interhemispheric approach. During resection of the lateral border of the AVM (Fig. 11.2C), the nidus was penetrated unintentionally (Fig. 11.2D), which was controlled by suction and bipolar coagulation (Fig. 11.2E). In this case, these measures were enough to stop the intraoperative AVM bleeding (Fig. 11.2F), and the AVM was removed without complications (Fig. 11.2G) and with a dry resection cavity (Fig. 11.2H). Postoperative angiography showed complete resection of the AVM, and the patient was neurologically intact after surgery (Fig. 11.2I).

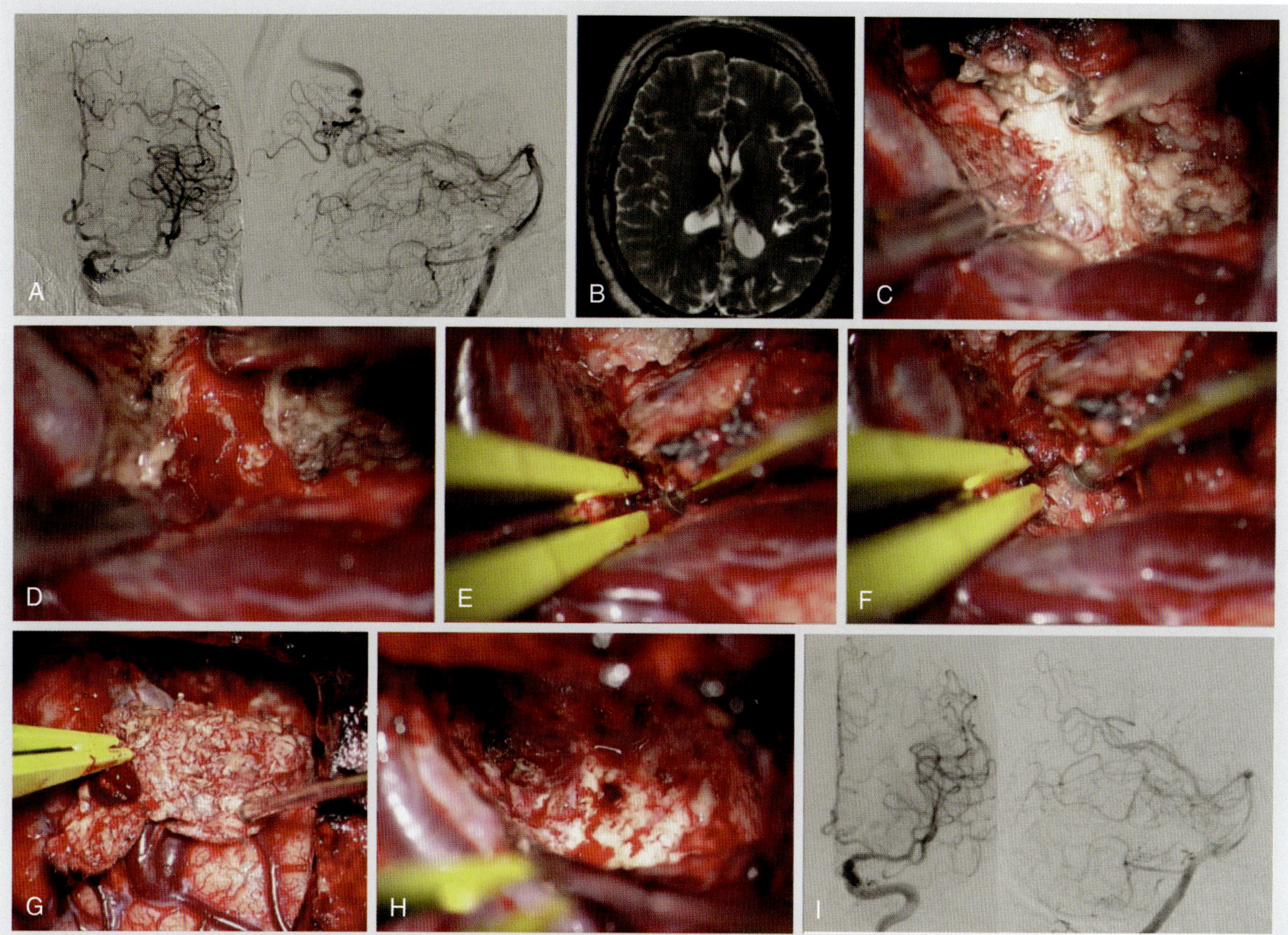

• **Fig. 11.2** Volume-staged radiosurgery downgraded left parieto-occipital AVM (Spetzler-Martin grade 2) in a 25-year-old male patient. Catheter angiography and MRI show this medial parieto-occipital AVM fed mainly through the posterior cerebral artery with a superficial drainage to the superior sagittal sinus (A and B). The patient was positioned in lateral position (left side down) to resect this AVM through an ipsilateral interhemispheric approach. During resection of the lateral border of the AVM (C), the nidus was partially opened (D), which was controlled by suction and bipolar coagulation (E). In this case, these measures were enough to stop the intraoperative AVM bleeding (F), and the AVM was removed without complications (G) and with a dry resection cavity (H). Postoperative angiography showed complete resection of the AVM, and the patient was neurologically intact after surgery (I).

NEUROSURGICAL SELFIE MOMENT

AVM surgery is the most demanding subspecialty in vascular neurosurgery and is reserved for experienced vascular neurosurgeons. A detailed knowledge of key anatomy, subtypes, surgical steps, and different surgical approaches is essential to avoid complications. The treatment of AVM complications should be tailored in each case to the site and type of complication to ensure patient safety. Intraoperative AVM rupture needs to be addressed directly; residual or postoperative symptomatic hemorrhage requires immediate reoperation, and steal phenomenon or stroke is treated with optimal medical management in the intensive care unit.

References

1. Bervini D, Morgan MK, Ritson EA, Heller G. Surgery for unruptured arteriovenous malformations of the brain is better than conservative management for selected cases: a prospective cohort study. *J Neurosurg*. 2014;121:878–890.
2. Lawton MT, Rutledge WC, Kim H, et al. Brain arteriovenous malformations. *Nat Rev Dis Primers*. 2015;1:15008.
3. Mohr JP, Parides MK, Stapf C, et al. Medical management with or without interventional therapy for unruptured brain arteriovenous malformations (ARUBA): a multicentre, non-blinded, randomised trial. *Lancet*. 2014;383:614–621.

4. Potts MB, Lau D, Abla AA, et al. Current surgical results with low-grade brain arteriovenous malformations. *J Neurosurg.* 2015;122:912–920.
5. van Beijnum J, van der Worp HB, Buis DR, et al. Treatment of brain arteriovenous malformations: a systematic review and meta-analysis. *JAMA.* 2011;306:2011–2019.
6. Davies JM, Kim H, Young WL, Lawton MT. Classification schemes for arteriovenous malformations. *Neurosurg Clin N Am.* 2012;23:43–53.
7. Lawton MT, Kim H, McCulloch CE, Mikhak B, Young WL. A supplementary grading scale for selecting patients with brain arteriovenous malformations for surgery. *Neurosurgery.* 2010;66:702–713, discussion 713.
8. Spetzler RF, Martin NA. A proposed grading system for arteriovenous malformations. *J Neurosurg.* 1986;65:476–483.
9. Kim H, Abla AA, Nelson J, et al. Validation of the supplemented Spetzler-Martin grading system for brain arteriovenous malformations in a multicenter cohort of 1009 surgical patients. *Neurosurgery.* 2015;76:25–31, discussion 31-22; quiz 32-23.
10. Lawton MT. *Seven AVMs.* San Francisco, CA: Thieme; 2014.
11. Reitz M, Schmidt NO, Vukovic Z, et al. How to deal with incompletely treated AVMs: experience of 67 cases and review of the literature. *Acta Neurochir Suppl.* 2011;112:123–129.
12. Torne R, Rodriguez-Hernandez A, Lawton MT. Intraoperative arteriovenous malformation rupture: causes, management techniques, outcomes, and the effect of neurosurgeon experience. *Neurosurg Focus.* 2014;37:E12.

12

Complications of Cerebral Bypass Surgery

SOPHIA F. SHAKUR, SEPIDEH AMIN-HANJANI, FADY T. CHARBEL

HIGHLIGHTS

- Cerebral bypass is a technically demanding surgery that can be fraught with several complications, including donor vessel injury, intraoperative bypass occlusion, postoperative bypass occlusion, and hemorrhage.
- Several management strategies can be implemented to address these complications.
- Adherence to a stereotyped step-by-step approach to this operation can result in consistent technical success.
- Incorporating blood flow measurements into decision-making during bypass surgery provides a tool to enhance the success of the operation.

Introduction

Extracranial-intracranial (EC-IC) bypass is used for flow replacement in the treatment of complex cerebral aneurysms or tumors that require vessel sacrifice, and for flow augmentation in the treatment of cerebral ischemia.[1] EC-IC bypass, however, is a technically demanding surgery that can be fraught with the potential for several complications, including donor vessel injury, intraoperative bypass occlusion, postoperative bypass occlusion, and hemorrhage. The overall morbidity and mortality rates in our own previously published series were 0% mortality and 4% morbidity, which are comparable to other reports of 0.6% to 4.3% mortality and 2.0% to 4.0% morbidity.[2–6] Our overall bypass patency rates for anterior and posterior circulation bypass are 90% and 83%, respectively, and are also similar to the patency rates documented by large clinical series.[3–5,7–10] Here we discuss the complications that can occur with cerebral bypass surgery as well as the associated preventive measures and management strategies.

Anatomic Insights

Superficial Temporal Artery

The superficial temporal artery (STA) to middle cerebral artery (MCA) bypass is considered the workhorse of cerebral revascularization. Indeed, the STA is an in situ native donor that has good flow-carrying capacity and can frequently be sufficient for flow replacement as well as flow augmentation.[2,11] Consequently, harvesting the STA is a technique that should be honed by cerebrovascular neurosurgeons.

The STA crosses the root of the zygoma, and then above the zygoma it divides into an anterior (frontal) and a posterior (parietal) branch (Fig. 12.1). The vessel runs parallel to the superficial temporal vein and in between the subcutaneous fat and temporalis muscle fascia. At the level of the zygoma, the diameter of the STA is approximately 3 mm.[12] The anterior and posterior branches are often similar in size, with a diameter measuring approximately 1.5 to 2 mm, although one branch can be dominant.

Doppler ultrasound is routinely used to map both branches of the STA after the patient's head has been placed in pins, because pinning can pull the skin and distort prior markings.[13] Additionally, dissection of the STA is performed under loupe or preferably microscope magnification with the surgeon and assistant seated. The skin incision is made with Colorado microneedle-tip monopolar cautery (Stryker Corp., Kalamazoo, MI) at a low setting of 8, allowing hemostasis of the skin edges while preventing skin edge necrosis. Once subcutaneous tissue is encountered, a blunt-tip curved hemostat is used to dissect down to the STA. Once the vessel is visualized, the hemostat is used to dissect proximally in the loose areolar plane above the vessel, and then the Colorado tip is used to open the skin to the tip of the hemostat as sequential dissection is performed proximally and distally along the STA.

Radial Artery

The radial artery is used as an autologous interposition graft in cerebral revascularization. Traditionally, it has been categorized as an "intermediate-flow" bypass. We have previously shown, though, that donor selection can be optimized with an algorithm based on intraoperative flow measurements.[14] In other words, a native donor (STA) may be found to carry sufficient flow for territory demand when a flow-based algorithm is used for donor selection, thereby circumventing the need for an interposition graft that requires a separate incision and an additional anastomosis, and that is associated with lower patency and higher morbidity rates.[14] The technique for harvesting the radial artery has been described in detail by Sekhar et al.[15] Preoperatively, an Allen test is performed to confirm patency of the palmar arch and to ensure adequate collateralization to the hand from the ulnar artery.

Saphenous Vein

The saphenous vein is used as an interposition graft in cerebral revascularization. This graft may be autologous or cadaveric in patients without available or suitable vein grafts.[16] Vein grafts have good patency rates overall but require higher flow rates of at least 40 to

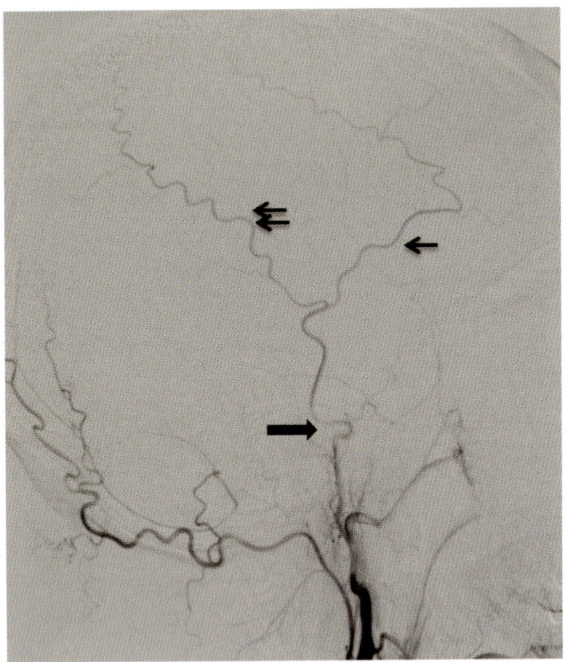

• **Fig. 12.1** Diagnostic cerebral angiogram, right external carotid artery injection, lateral projection, showing the course of the superficial temporal artery around the root of the zygoma (large arrow) and its division into an anterior (small single arrow) and a posterior branch (small double arrow).

50 mL/min to consistently maintain patency.[17,18] Advantages of a cadaveric over an autologous vein graft are its easy handling, quick availability, customizable diameter and length, and avoidance of an additional incision for graft harvesting. Disadvantages include the potential for lower long-term patency, theoretical risk of infection with transmissible diseases, possibility of chronic graft rejection, and cost.

The saphenous vein is harvested in the calf or thigh after preoperative ultrasound mapping to determine the size suitability of the vein.[14] The vein is then distended with heparinized saline using a Shiley balloon distention kit. The graft is tunneled preauricular through a 28-French chest tube to the neck. The proximal anastomosis is typically created to the common or external carotid artery in an end-to-side fashion after an arteriotomy is performed with an appropriately sized aortic punch device. The proximal anastomosis is occasionally created in an end-to-end fashion to the stump of the STA if the donor vessel is suitable. The distal anastomosis is made in an end-to-side fashion with the recipient branch.

RED FLAGS

- Atherosclerosis
- Interposition grafts (radial artery and saphenous vein)
- "Cut flow index" (CFI) <0.5
- Rapid thrombosis of the target aneurysm after bypass and distal occlusion

Prevention

Complication avoidance is key to performing a successful cerebral bypass. Cerebral bypass surgery is highly dependent on careful attention to technique at every stage of the operation, from donor vessel dissection to skin closure. Adherence to a stereotyped step-by-step approach to this operation, with decision-making regarding donor selection and bypass patency guided by intraoperative flow measurements, which our group described previously,[12] can result in consistent technical success.

Management of STA Injury

The STA can be injured during harvesting or during the craniotomy after dissection of the STA. STA injury, however, can be avoided by using microscope or loupe magnification, maintaining meticulous hemostasis, and using a round burr instead of a perforator drill bit.[13]

Injury to the superficial temporal vein rather than the artery should be recognized and managed appropriately because the STA may be inadvertently coagulated when attempting to control venous bleeding. Video 12.1 demonstrates a maneuver that can be applied to obtain venous hemostasis without risking injury to the STA. Once the vein is coagulated, it is important to cut any coagulated portion that might be draped over the STA and subsequently restrict flow through the donor vessel.

Injury to the STA itself can be ameliorated by using an amputated donor if the length remains suitable, using the uninjured anterior or posterior STA branch, or choosing a different donor vessel.

Management of Intraoperative Bypass Occlusion

The best management of intraoperative bypass occlusion is a preventive and preemptive strategy. Indeed, multiple preoperative and intraoperative steps can be taken to ensure patency of the cerebral bypass.[2,13] First, patients are instructed to take aspirin (325 mg) the day before surgery and are continued on aspirin postoperatively. Additionally, the STA is wrapped in a papaverine-soaked cottonoid during the craniotomy to protect it and to prevent or treat spasm caused by manipulation of the donor. Before the anastomosis is performed, the STA is flushed with heparinized saline through its cut end. Interposition grafts are distended before implantation to reduce the risk of later vasospasm, which can be particularly prevalent with radial artery grafts.[14,15] Care must be taken during tunneling of interposition grafts to avoid twisting and kinking; these grafts must be cut to a length that avoids tension on the anastomosis. At the same time, it must be taken into consideration that the elongation that occurs once the graft is distended with blood flow can lead to kinking of overly lengthy grafts. Attention to correct orientation of the vein graft with respect to its valves is also imperative.

It is also important to critically assess the suitability of a donor or recipient vessel before undertaking the bypass.[2] More specifically, iatrogenic injury to the donor during dissection or atheromatous changes within the STA should be appreciated. Video 12.2 shows an example of atheroma in the STA and demonstrates a technique to manage this problem by going more proximally on the STA. At the same time, the chosen recipient vessel should have a large enough diameter to allow adequate outflow to the graft. Our group previously outlined the use of a quantitative microvascular ultrasonic flow probe (Charbel Micro-Flowprobe; Transonics Systems, Inc., Ithaca, NY) and described the use of CFI to detect potential problems with the donor or recipient vessels.[2] Briefly, the technique entails measurement of the "cut flow" of the STA—that is, the maximal flow-carrying capacity after dissection and cutting the vessel open. Once the anastomosis has been completed, the flow in the donor STA is remeasured, and this bypass flow is compared with the cut flow to provide the CFI. When performed for flow augmentation, an index close to 1.0 indicates a highly successful bypass because it indicates that the donor graft is carrying its full capacity. A low index can indicate a problem with either the donor, the recipient, or the anastomosis that requires attention. For flow replacement bypass, cut flow measurement indicates the carrying capacity of the STA and its suitability as a donor that can replace the flow measured in the vessel to be sacrificed. After graft placement, whether the STA or interposition graft, measurement of the bypass flow indicates whether the graft has been successful in replacing the necessary flow to the revascularized territory.

Most importantly, intraoperative bypass occlusion must be recognized. Although visual inspection of the anastomosis should be done, the presence of pulsation can actually be misleading.[2] Intraoperative blood flow measurements, then, allow for a simple and accurate method to quantitatively assess bypass patency. If the bypass is found to be occluded intraoperatively, thrombectomy may be performed, and the anastomosis can be repeated, or a new anastomotic site can be chosen (Video 12.3).

Management of Postoperative Bypass Occlusion

Postoperative bypass occlusion is a rare occurrence because several preoperative and intraoperative steps can be taken to ensure patency of the bypass. First, the appropriate donor graft should be selected. For instance, vein grafts compared with other donors require higher flow rates to maintain patency.[16] Additionally, we have shown that the flow-based algorithm for donor selection in EC-IC bypass surgery for cerebral aneurysms results in sufficient flow for territory demand in the immediate, intermediate, and long-term postoperative periods.[11] Moreover, intraoperative quantitative assessment of the bypass can be used not only to discern a problem with the bypass so that corrective action can be taken, but also to predict the success of the bypass, with a CFI <0.5 indicative of higher risk of bypass occlusion or poor functioning.[2] Finally, closure of the craniotomy should be performed with care to prevent kinking or pressure on the donor vessel.[13] Typically, the dura is not closed, the burr hole is enlarged to accommodate the donor, the temporalis muscle is reapproximated loosely, and the skin is closed carefully to avoid injury to the donor. Postoperatively, pressure on the graft site anterior to the ear (by nasal cannula or glasses) must be avoided.

The status of the bypass should also be monitored postoperatively. At our institution, a diagnostic cerebral angiogram and quantitative magnetic resonance angiography scan using Non-invasive Optimal Vessel Analysis software (VasSol, Inc., Chicago, IL) are obtained postoperatively, and then both imaging modalities are used to interrogate bypass patency over time.[11,13]

Bypass occlusion in the early postoperative period is generally attributed to surgical technique, poor graft selection or function, and vasospasm.[19] On the other hand, bypass occlusion or stenosis in the late postoperative period is thought to be caused by intimal hyperplasia.[19–21] More specifically, the hemodynamic pattern at the junction of the donor and recipient vessels induces turbulence and high wall shear stress that results in endothelial injury and intimal hyperplasia.[21] Because blood flow rates are significantly higher in vein versus arterial grafts, vein grafts are more susceptible to intimal hyperplasia and stenosis.

If bypass occlusion is encountered postoperatively, surgical and endovascular rescue techniques can be implemented.[19,20] Surgical and endovascular bypass salvage methods, though, are both high-risk procedures. Consequently, bypass rescue is generally indicated in cases with progressive stenosis, stenosis >50%, or symptomatic stenosis. For early graft narrowing due to vasospasm, endovascular treatment with angioplasty is the treatment of choice. Early thrombosis of the graft, however, typically requires surgical repair; thrombectomy can be attempted, but often complete replacement of the graft is needed.[22] In the subacute or delayed setting, surgical repair of the bypass is particularly challenging, so endovascular techniques are considered the first-line management strategy for narrowed or stenotic bypass grafts.[19] Endovascular rescue techniques include balloon angioplasty and stenting. Several case series, including one published by our group, have demonstrated the safety and efficacy of endovascular rescue techniques for graft stenosis.[15,19,20] Surgical options to repair or replace the graft can be used if endovascular strategies fail.[22]

Management of Aneurysm Rupture After Bypass and Trapping

Giant cerebral aneurysms can be difficult to treat with standard microsurgery or endovascular techniques and thereby require more creative treatment strategies, such as parent artery occlusion with or without revascularization.[23–27] Complete trapping is likely the most definitive treatment, but partial trapping either proximally or distally is often technically more feasible or may be necessary to preserve perforators originating from the aneurysm.

However, aneurysm rupture can occur after bypass and partial trapping (see "Surgical Rewind: My Worst Case").[28,29] In these cases, patients can present with delayed rupture. This complication, therefore, is not related to the initial brief increase in intraluminal pressure but rather is likely attributed to inflammatory degradation of the aneurysm wall during rapid formation of a large thrombus. In fact, this mechanism has been used as an explanation for delayed aneurysm rupture after flow diversion treatment.[30–33]

If delayed rupture is encountered, the patient should be taken emergently to the operating room to secure the aneurysm as well as to perform hematoma evacuation and decompression, if necessary. We also suggest that complete trapping remains the optimal treatment strategy because it entirely excludes the aneurysm from the circulation. Additionally, if distal occlusion is performed and rapid thrombosis of the aneurysm is seen, immediate and complete aneurysm occlusion is warranted, even at the expense of perforator sacrifice, to avoid postoperative rupture.

SURGICAL REWIND

My Worst Case (Fig. 12.2)

A 54-year-old female presented with episodes of right-hand clumsiness and expressive aphasia for the last 6 months. A diagnostic cerebral angiogram revealed a giant left MCA aneurysm with all major MCA cortical branches and a few perforators arising directly from the aneurysm itself (Fig. 12.2A). The decision was made to treat the aneurysm using a bypass and distal vessel occlusion surgical strategy to preserve the perforators emanating from the aneurysm neck. First, a cadaveric saphenous vein graft was anastomosed to one of the MCA frontal branches using an end-to-side anastomosis. Then the frontal branch of the STA was anastomosed to the MCA temporal branch using an end-to-side anastomosis. Finally, the parietal

Continued

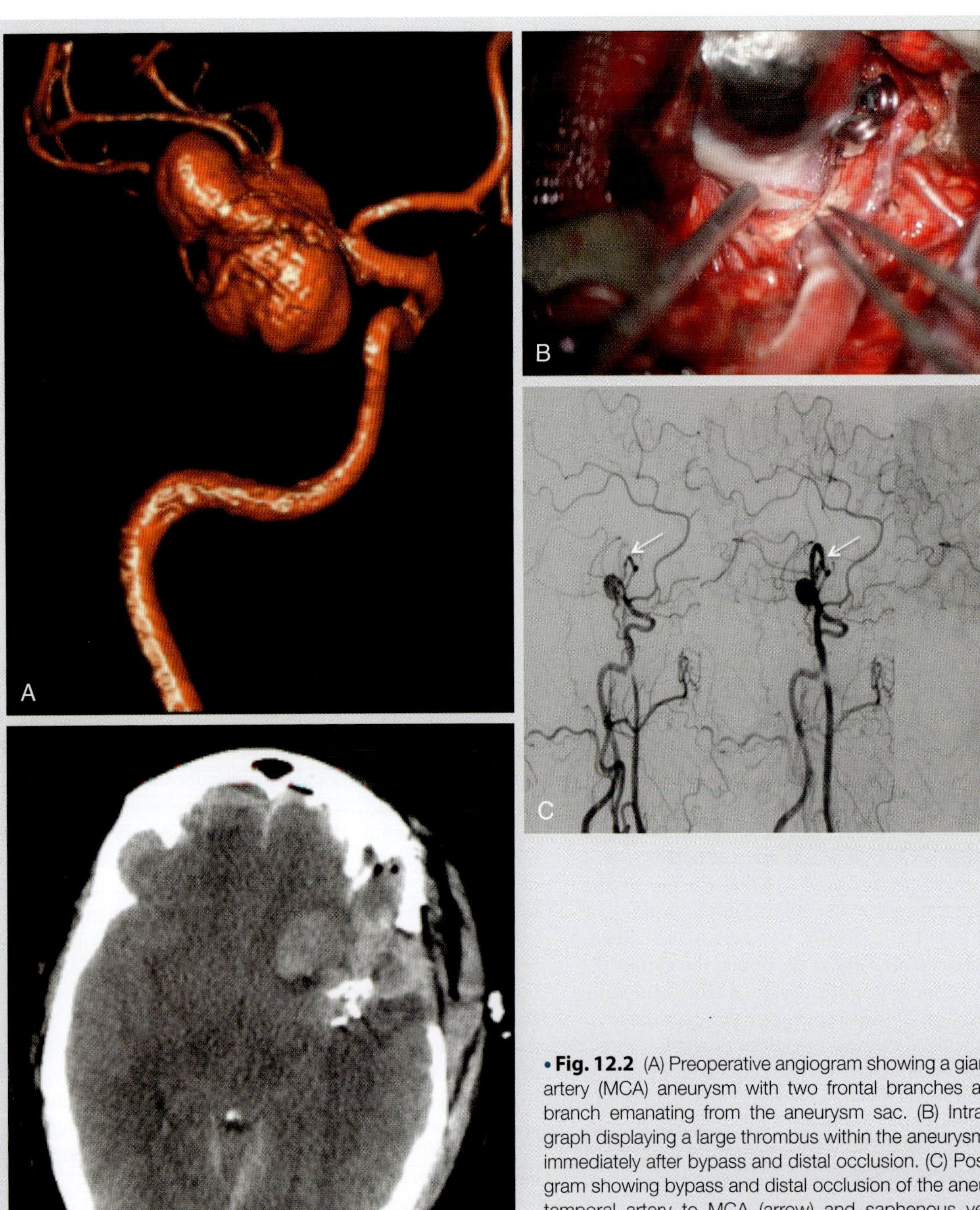

• **Fig. 12.2** (A) Preoperative angiogram showing a giant middle cerebral artery (MCA) aneurysm with two frontal branches and one temporal branch emanating from the aneurysm sac. (B) Intraoperative photograph displaying a large thrombus within the aneurysm and a perforator immediately after bypass and distal occlusion. (C) Postoperative angiogram showing bypass and distal occlusion of the aneurysm. Superficial temporal artery to MCA (arrow) and saphenous vein graft to MCA (arrow) bypasses are patent. There is also retrograde filling of an MCA frontal branch (dotted arrow), and part of the aneurysm sac is still seen to fill. (D) Computed tomography scan showing a large hematoma around the aneurysm clips and diffuse subarachnoid hemorrhage on postoperative day 2.

branch of the STA was anastomosed to the second MCA frontal branch, but this bypass thrombosed. Immediately after distal occlusion of the aneurysm, rapid thrombosis of the aneurysm as well as a large perforator was observed (Fig. 12.2B). Postoperatively, the patient intermittently followed commands on the left side but was weak on the right side. An angiogram performed on postoperative day 1 showed the two patent bypasses, retrograde filling of the second MCA frontal branch, and partial anterograde filling of the aneurysm sac (Fig. 12.2C). On postoperative day 2, however, the patient was found to have bilateral fixed and dilated pupils. A computed tomography scan showed a large hematoma around the aneurysm clips and diffuse subarachnoid hemorrhage (Fig. 12.2D). She was immediately taken to the operating room, where bleeding was seen from the thrombosed part of the aneurysm sac. The aneurysm was subsequently clipped and completely occluded. A temporal lobectomy and craniectomy were also performed. Unfortunately, her examination remained poor, and care was withdrawn on postoperative day 8.

NEUROSURGICAL SELFIE MOMENT

Cerebral bypass surgery can be undermined by several complications, including donor vessel injury, intraoperative bypass occlusion, postoperative bypass occlusion, and hemorrhage. Although numerous strategies are available to manage these complications, complication avoidance is key to performing a successful cerebral bypass. Cerebral bypass surgery is highly dependent on careful attention to technique at every stage of the operation, from donor vessel dissection to skin closure.

References

1. Charbel FT, Guppy KH, Ausman JI. Cerebral revascularization: superficial temporal middle cerebral artery anastomosis. In: Sekhar LN, Fessler RG, eds. *Atlas of Neurosurgical Techniques*. New York: Thieme; 2006.
2. Amin-Hanjani S, Du X, Mlinarevich N, Meglio G, Zhao M, Charbel FT. The cut flow index: an intraoperative predictor of the success of extracranial-intracranial bypass for occlusive cerebrovascular disease. *Neurosurgery*. 2005;56(suppl 1):75–85.
3. Chater N. Neurosurgical extracranial-intracranial bypass for stroke: with 400 cases. *Neurol Res*. 1983;5:1–9.
4. EC/IC Bypass Study Group. Failure of extracranial-intracranial arterial bypass to reduce the risk of ischemic stroke: results of an international randomized trial—EC/IC Bypass Study Group. *N Engl J Med*. 1985; 313:1191–1200.
5. Sundt TM Jr, Whisnant JP, Fode NC, Piepgras DG, Houser OW. Results, complications, and follow-up of 415 bypass operations for occlusive disease of the carotid system. *Mayo Clin Proc*. 1985;60: 230–240.
6. Samson DS, Boone S. Extracranial-intracranial (EC-IC) arterial bypass: past performance and current concepts. *Neurosurgery*. 1978;3: 79–86.
7. Gratzl O, Schmiedek P, Spetzler RF, Steinhoff H, Marguth F. Clinical experience with extra-intracranial arterial anastomosis in 65 cases. *J Neurosurg*. 1976;44:313–324.
8. Onesti ST, Solomon RA, Quest DO. Cerebral revascularization: a review. *Neurosurgery*. 1989;25:618–629.
9. Ausman JI, Diaz FG, Vacca DF, Sadasivan B. Superficial temporal and occipital artery bypass pedicles to superior, anterior inferior, and posterior inferior cerebellar arteries for vertebrobasilar insufficiency. *J Neurosurg*. 1990;72:554–558.
10. Hopkins LN, Budny JL. Complications of intracranial bypass for vertebrobasilar insufficiency. *J Neurosurg*. 1989;70:207–211.
11. Rustemi O, Amin-Hanjani S, Shakur SF, Du X, Charbel FT. Donor selection in flow replacement bypass surgery for cerebral aneurysms: quantitative analysis of long-term native donor flow sufficiency. *Neurosurgery*. 2016;78:332–342.
12. Pinar YA, Govsa F. Anatomy of the superficial temporal artery and its branches: its importance for surgery. *Surg Radiol Anat*. 2006;28:248–253.
13. Charbel FT, Meglio G, Amin-Hanjani S. Superficial temporal artery-to-middle cerebral artery bypass. *Neurosurgery*. 2005;56(suppl 1):186–190.
14. Amin-Hanjani S, Alaraj A, Charbel FT. Flow replacement bypass for aneurysms: decision-making using intraoperative blood flow measurements. *Acta Neurochir (Wien)*. 2010;152:1021–1032.
15. Sekhar LN, Duff JM, Kalavakonda C, Olding M. Cerebral revascularization using radial artery grafts for the treatment of complex intracranial aneurysms: techniques and outcomes for 17 patients. *Neurosurgery*. 2001;49:646–659.
16. Mery FJ, Amin-Hanjani S, Charbel FT. Cerebral revascularization using cadaveric vein grafts. *Surg Neurol*. 2009;72:362–368.
17. Bremmer JP, Verweij BH, Klijn CJ, van der Zwan A, Kappelle LJ, Tulleken CA. Predictors of patency of excimer laser-assisted nonocclusive extracranial-to-intracranial bypasses. *J Neurosurg*. 2009; 110:887–895.
18. Regli L, Piepgras DG, Hansen KK. Late patency of long saphenous vein bypass grafts to the anterior and posterior cerebral circulation. *J Neurosurg*. 1995;83:806–811.
19. Ramanathan D, Ghodke B, Kim LJ, Hallam D, Herbes-Rocha M, Sekhar LN. Endovascular management of cerebral bypass graft problems: an analysis of technique and results. *AJNR Am J Neuroradiol*. 2011;32:1415–1419.
20. Qahwash O, Alaraj A, Aletich V, et al. Endovascular intervention for delayed stenosis of extracranial-intracranial bypass saphenous vein grafts. *J Neurointerv Surg*. 2013;5:231–236.
21. Haruguchi H, Teraoka S. Intimal hyperplasia and hemodynamic factors in arterial bypass and arteriovenous grafts: a review. *J Artif Organs*. 2003;6:227–235.
22. Ramanathan D, Temkin N, Kim LJ, Ghodke B, Sekhar LN. Cerebral bypasses for complex aneurysms and tumors: long-term results and graft management strategies. *Neurosurgery*. 2012;70: 1442–1457.
23. Kivipelto L, Niemela M, Meling T, Lehecka M, Lehto H, Hernesniemi J. Bypass surgery for complex middle cerebral artery aneurysms: impact of the exact location in the MCA tree. *J Neurosurg*. 2014; 120:398–408.
24. Nussbaum ES, Madison MT, Goddard JK, Lassig JP, Janjua TM, Nussbaum LA. Remote distal outflow occlusion: a novel treatment option for complex dissecting aneurysms of the posterior inferior cerebellar artery. Report of 3 cases. *J Neurosurg*. 2009;111: 78–83.
25. Amin-Hanjani S, Chen PR, Chang SW, Spetzler RF. Long-term follow-up of giant serpentine MCA aneurysm treated with EC-IC bypass and proximal occlusion. *Acta Neurochir (Wien)*. 2006;148: 227–228.
26. Esposito G, Fierstra J, Regli L. Distal outflow occlusion with bypass revascularization: last resort measure in managing complex MCA and PICA aneurysms. *Acta Neurochir (Wien)*. 2016;158:1523–1531.
27. van Doormaal TP, van der Zwan A, Verweij BH, Han KS, Langer DJ, Tulleken CA. Treatment of giant middle cerebral artery aneurysms with a flow replacement bypass using the excimer laser-assisted nonocclusive anastomosis technique. *Neurosurgery*. 2008;63:12–20.
28. Scott RM, Liu H-C, Yuan R, Adelman L. Rupture of a previously unruptured giant middle cerebral artery aneurysm after extracranial-intracranial bypass surgery. *Neurosurgery*. 1982;10:600–603.
29. Anson JA, Stone JL, Crowell RM. Rupture of a giant carotid aneurysm after extracranial-to-intracranial bypass surgery. *Neurosurgery*. 1991;28:142–147.
30. Ikeda H, Ishii A, Kikuchi T, et al. Delayed aneurysm rupture due to residual blood flow at the inflow zone of the intracranial paraclinoid internal carotid aneurysm treated with the Pipeline embolization device: histopathological investigation. *Interv Neuroradiol*. 2015;21: 674–683.
31. Hampton T, Walsh D, Tolias C, Fiorella D. Mural destabilization after aneurysm treatment with a flow-diverting device: a report of two cases. *J Neurointerv Surg*. 2011;3:167–171.
32. Siddiqui AH, Kan P, Abla AA, Hopkins LN, Levy EI. Complications after treatment with pipeline embolization for giant distal intracranial aneurysms with or without coil embolization. *Neurosurgery*. 2012;71:E509–E513.
33. Kulcsar Z, Houdart E, Bonafe A, et al. Intra-aneurysmal thrombosis as a possible cause of delayed aneurysm rupture after flow-diversion treatment. *AJNR Am J Neuroradiol*. 2011;32:20–25.

13 Complications of the Surgery for Cavernomas

MIGUEL A. ARRAEZ, BIENVENIDO ROS, CINTA ARRAEZ

HIGHLIGHTS

- The most frequent complication in cavernoma surgery is the damage of the surrounding central nervous tissue during resection and/or during the approach to the lesion.
- Cavernomas are benign lesions that frequently have a favorable course. The first step in prevention of postoperative complications is the appropriate selection of the surgical candidate.
- To avoid complications in cavernoma surgery, the selection of the entry point in eloquent areas and meticulous technique are of paramount importance.

Background

Cavernomas are vascular cavernomatous (cavernous angiomas) lesions histologically characterized by abnormal vessels with large capillaries. There is little or no cerebral brain tissue in the lesion. The natural course of cavernous malformations is rather unpredictable.[1] The malformations may arise in and outside the central nervous system. Cerebrum, cerebellum, brainstem, and spinal cord are common sites of origin. Multiplicity of lesions is not rare ("cavernomatosis"), and there is also great disparity in size and locations. "De novo" lesions are seen in some instances as well as familial cases. Bleeding is the most devastating presentation, sometimes leading to death in the first episode.[2]

Cavernomatous lesions can lead to bleeding in a variable fashion irrespective of the location. Symptoms and clinical deficit will be in accordance to the severity of the hemorrhage and neurologic territory. Supratentorial cavernomas may provoke seizures. The risk of hemorrhage (rehemorrhage) and the presence of seizures are the most frequent reasons to undertake surgical removal. The risk for hemorrhage is estimated between 0.6% and 5% (annual rate). Among those who bleed, 30% will rebleed over time. There is some assumption according to which once the cavernoma bleeds, the risk of rebleeding will persist for life. This is considered the major indication for surgery because the severity of the clinical deficit would increase over time due to further episodes of hemorrhage. Another reason for surgery is epilepsy in certain contexts. Also de novo cavernomas or growing lesions should be removed.[3] Radiosurgery has also been advocated as a treatment modality for cavernoma,[4] not without debate. Large metaanalysis studies conclude that long-term effects for stereotactic radiosurgery are unknown.[5]

Brainstem cavernomas can produce a great variety of symptoms and neurologic deficit according to the location. Long tract involvement and cranial nerve dysfunction are very frequent. At the spinal cord, cavernomas have the same consideration as mentioned earlier, with the exception of seizures. Symptoms and neurologic deficit are related to spinal cord dysfunction. Lesions at the superficial pial layer can be removed without major postoperative consequences. Small lesions anteriorly placed are the most problematic for excision.

Cavernomas are associated with venous anomalies, sometimes very prominent. Venous anomaly is the current denomination, after having been very frequently reported as venous angiomas[6] for many years. Unlike some other vascular malformations at the central nervous system, far from being removed or coagulated during surgery, these structures must be preserved to maintain normal venous drainage and to avoid venous infarction.[7] Some authors do consider the coexistence of a cavernoma and a venous anomaly a risk factor for rebleeding.[8]

The Choice of the Surgical Candidate for Cavernoma Removal

It has been extensively assumed that surgery is the best option to treat symptomatic cavernomas, even in difficult areas like the brainstem. This opinion is not unanimously accepted,[9] showing that the decision is usually controversial and varies according to surgeons, institutions, and published articles. The decision must be made on a case-to-case basis that balances the risks of surgery and the experience of the surgical team against the natural history of the disease.

Bleeding is one of the indications for surgery. The recommendation for surgery is influenced by the estimated risk of future bleeding (that is, the natural history of the lesion), the neurologic injury predicted to occur with such a hemorrhage, and the patient's clinical situation with special attention to neurologic condition, age, and the size and location of the lesion. Intralesional bleeding is a very common finding and doesn't itself represent an indication for surgery. Acute extralesional hemorrhage is considered a clear sign of the potential aggressiveness of the lesion. Mass effect due to hemorrhage is a formal indication for removal of the clot along with cavernoma excision, which sometimes must be done in emergency basis. The decision also must be individualized after assessing a combination of different factors. One of them is the timing of the first episode of bleeding, and another is the age of the patient. Surgical removal should not be encouraged for older patients with very late bleeding. Early bleeding and younger patients would lead toward a more aggressive attitude because outcome is linked to the rate of further episodes of rebleeding.[10]

Another important parameter is the location of the cavernoma. Cavernomas in "eloquent" areas are poorer candidates. Some series have published rates as high as 47% impairment after surgery in such "eloquent" areas (optic pathways, brainstem, motor and speech area).[11] This anatomic fact must be combined with the cavernoma's size and its deep or superficial location. Small cavernomas can be a problem regarding intraoperative identification and also postoperative morbidity. Bigger and superficial lesions would have less chance for neurologic morbidity.

Another important consideration for surgery is epilepsy. The lack of control of epilepsy in spite of medical treatment, a situation that is not infrequent when the lesion is harbored at the temporal lobe, is a formal indication. Another reason to advise the surgical excision of cavernoma is the attempt to "cure" epilepsy, removing the cause in the context of surgery of focal epilepsy. This would allow for discontinuation of the antiepileptic drug, which is of paramount importance when the patient is very young. Microsurgical resection of cavernomas responsible for intractable epilepsy is very much linked to the debate about the extent of tissue surrounding the cavernoma that needs to be removed to achieve the best outcome for epilepsy, which in some series is as high as 87% seizure-free.[12]

A third indication for surgery on cavernomas is the progressive growth of the lesion (after preexisting lesion or "the de novo appearance") and/or recurrence.

General Principles of Cavernoma Surgery to Avoid Morbidity

Once the decision has been made to perform cavernoma surgery, several principles and rules must be considered. Regarding the surgical approach, supratentorial or cerebellar lesions usually need standard craniotomies centered in the malformation. Brainstem cavernomas may require sophisticated skull base techniques to get access to the malformation. Lesions at the cerebrum and cerebellum may require entrance through the sulcus and/or linear incisions. The brainstem requires entrance through the already recognized "safe entry points" and/or an elongated puncture point. As a general rule, the direction of the entrance is given establishing a line connecting the center of the lesions with the point where the cavernoma is abutting with the pial surface ("two points").[13] A small window to the cavernous malformation is created, with the direction of access defined by the safest anatomic corridor possible.[14]

The essence of the avoidance of neurologic morbidity (the most worrisome complication) is the preservation of the white and gray matter surrounding the cavernomatous malformation. The configuration of the cavernoma includes a more or less definable cleavage plane (gliosis and/or hemosiderin) that is the real clue for neurologic preservation. Bulky lesions need previous intralesional removal to achieve a very good preservation of this plane. Racemose and very irregular tumors can make the preservation of the surrounding tissue difficult.

As an ancillary intraoperative procedure, neurophysiologic neuromonitoring is nowadays crucial for the resection of these lesions in eloquent areas.[15] The standard neurophysiologic techniques (cortical and subcortical mapping, cranial nerves, motor evoked potentials (PEM), somatosensory evoked potentials (SSEP)) are complemented by fourth ventricle mapping when the removal requires the penetration of such an eloquent anatomy at the brainstem.

Complications Related to Operative Technique (and Their Avoidance)

The Lesion Doesn't Appear

This frustrating intraoperative complication was more common before the era of the intraoperative image. Deep cavernomas need intraoperative imaged-guided resection, among them neuronavigation. This technique can help anywhere in the central nervous system. At the brainstem it can help find the most suitable point for entrance.[16] Ultrasonography can be also used in the cerebrum, cerebellum, and spinal cord. Smaller lesions are, of course, more problematic. Even with an intraoperative image, the lesion can be missed because the displacement of the white matter during the subcortical penetration can displace the cavernoma in its vicinity.

Neurologic Deficit After a Wrong Approach and/or Wrong Entry Point

These neurologic complications may arise when the direction of the approach given by the craniotomy/osteotomy (the surgical approach, in a general sense) is not appropriate and implies excessive retraction and/or distortion of the cortical or subcortical brain, brainstem, or spinal cord. The standard supratentorial or suboccipital craniotomies give a very straightforward route to lesions of the cerebrum and cerebellum. Sulcal navigation offers the best chance for gray and white matter preservation. The vicinity of the motor cortex, speech areas, and pyramidal tracts deserves special interest and the application of the current intraoperative refinements and armamentarium.[16]

Brainstem lesions represent by far the most challenging operations. Brainstem cavernous malformations are associated with higher hemorrhagic rates and poorer neurologic outcome.[17,18] Immediate postoperative impairment can be 35% to 45%,[13] and long-term morbidity is no less than 15% in a metaanalysis of 1390 patients.[17,19] The concept of a "safe entry zone"[20] is crucial at the brainstem.

Cavernomas at the posterior medullary region can be entered through the median, paramedian, and lateral sulcus (similar to intramedullary tumors). When the cavernoma is anteriorly placed at the medulla, a far lateral approach must be taken to get the antero-lateral safe entry point at the medulla: the retro-olivary sulcus, particularly between the exit of the XII nerve and first cervical root. This approach allows maneuvering in front of the lower cranial nerves. Transclival endoscopic approaches would expose anteriorly the intradural foramen magnum area. The dorsal pontine region does allow the fourth ventricle to be entered through the median sulcus. Another entry point is the so-called pericollicular area (supra- and infrafacial triangles). The latter route avoids the nuclei and paths of the VI and VII nerves.[21] The ventral/ventrolateral pontine brainstem can be approached through several surgical strategies: the simple retrosigmoid approach, the transpetrous approach, and the presigmoid approach.[22] There are two main safe entry zones: One of them is the peritrigeminal area, right in front of the exit of the V nerve. This entrance is just lateral to the corticospinal tract. The other safe entry zone is the exit between the V and VII cranial nerves, which is very accessible through a retrosigmoid craniotomy. The supratonsillar approach has been described to reach the inferior cerebellar peduncle. The ventral mesencephalon can be approached through a frontotemporal craniotomy with the addition of a zygomatic osteotomy. Because cerebral peduncles do contain the corticospinal tracts in a very tight fashion (unlike the anterior pontine region, in which the corticospinal tract is found to be very loose), morbidity after surgery at this level can be very high. The subtemporal approach can also be useful for certain intrinsic anterior or lateral mesencephalic lesions. The subthalamic lateral mesencephalon can be approached looking for the safe entry zone called the lateral mesencephalic sulcus, bounded by the lateral mesencephalic vein. This entrance needs a suboccipital craniotomy with the addition of a supratentorial osteotomy allowing for upper retraction of the transverse sinus and (sometimes) cutting and opening of the tentorium according to its shape and conformation (paramedial suboccipital supratentorial approach). Thus the lateral mesencephalic sulcus can be approached.[23] The opening of the lateral mesencephalic sulcus leads to the junction of corticospinal and lemniscal tracts. The dorsal mesencephalon/tectal plate can be reached through a supracerebellar-infratentorial approach, a suboccipital-transtentorial approach, or a combination of both. The collicular plate can be penetrated through the infracollicular safe entry zone.[20] In spite of the presumed high morbidity when dealing with brainstem structures, a very acceptable postoperative morbidity has been published.[24]

At the spinal cord, strict intramedullary cavernomas must be approached in a fashion similar to that of any other kind of tumor inside the spinal cord.[17] When the tumor abuts the surface, the lesion itself provides the access. In spite of that, a superficial cavernoma at the spinal cord does not seem to show a better outcome than deeper lesions.[25] One important consideration must be made in regard to pure anteriorly placed cavernomas. For these cases, a ventral approach to the spinal cord through a vertebrectomy has been sometimes indicated.[26] Anterior cavernomas have the added problem of the vicinity of the spinal anterior artery.

Intraoperative Bleeding

Cavernous angiomas have been classically defined as occult malformations at angiography. In spite of this, not infrequently one of several arterial feeders of variable diameter can be identified during surgery. This can be the explanation for why some of them tend to rebleed, occasionally in a profuse manner (Fig. 13.1). Intraoperative rupture and bleeding can be a big problem in areas like the brainstem or in deep-brain areas like the thalamus, leading to increased postoperative morbidity.[27,28] The intraoperative identification of feeders in such a crucial anatomic region is not easy. Preoperative angiography can help in some cases, providing useful information[29] if high vascularity is suspected. Normal venous anatomy and any suspected venous anomaly must be preserved during the procedure.

Timing for Surgery

Timing for cavernoma surgery is a very important aspect of the management of these malformations. Emergency-based surgery must be done only in case of neurologic deterioration, which fortunately happens only in a very restricted percentage of cases.[30] This ultra-early surgery carries, of course, obvious risk and also the possibility of having remaining fragments in the hemorrhagic bed that later on can rebleed. Surgical timing appeared to influence the treatment results. Mathiesen et al.[31] compared patients who underwent surgery within 1 month after the latest hemorrhage with those who underwent surgery at a later time. Transient neurologic deterioration was detectable in 15 of 17 patients who were treated later and in only 4 of 12 patients who were treated early. Bruneau et al.[32] published their series of patients with "early" surgery after a first episode of bleeding at the brainstem with rather good results (improvement of more than 90%), thus avoiding the postoperative morbidity of the "delayed" surgery and preventing further bleeding. In spinal cord surgery for cavernoma, surgery within the first 3 months is also followed by a better outcome.[25] Several publications have shown late surgery to be significantly associated with worse outcomes, but timing for surgery has also to be considered under the difficulty of every case. Some authors advocate waiting for the second bleeding before surgery, trying thus to avoid the 30% to 60% initial morbidity and the 15% late morbidity in eloquent areas like the brainstem.[17]

It is clear that early surgery can prevent further episodes of bleeding. On top of that, delayed surgery may increase postoperative morbidity due to the modification of the cleavage plane of dissection over time. A few weeks the after initial bleeding, the cavernoma malformation can be sourrounded by a very easy plane for dissection. In a later stage, a hard-gliotic tissue makes the dissection from nervous tissue riskier (Fig. 13.2). Because in this chronic stage after hematoma organization, gliosis is very adherent to normal tissue.[17] This is of great importance at the brainstem and in eloquent supratentorial structures. In summary, the timing for surgery is a factor to be taken into account to avoid postoperative morbidity.

Recurrence of Hemorrhage After Cavernoma Surgery

Recurrence of bleeding after initial surgery is directly related to incomplete previous resection. It is not infrequent that the logical explanation is the difficulty of the area being operated on (i.e., brainstem) and/or the difficulty of the procedure (surgery done on an emergency basis).[33] Obviously, those factors are clearly linked to the surgical technique. Although the global rate of rebleeding in cavernoma surgery is considered very low (less than 1%),[19] when a remnant is left in the surgical field, there is a high probability for rebleeding: 62% of residual lesions will bleed.[17] This is a very important problem because the operation would not achieve its goal: diminishing the probability of further bleeding to zero. Detection of remnants after surgery is of course crucial. In regard to that, recent publications have stated that early postoperative magnetic resonance imaging (MRI) after cavernoma surgery is often hampered by imaging artifacts creating false positive results, therefore rendering the patient ineligible for resection control. However, the reliability of a negative result on an early postoperative T2-weighted MRI is relatively high regarding both cavernomatous malformation and hemosiderin remnants.[34] These considerations have to be taken into account for the appropriate follow-up in cavernoma surgery.

SURGICAL REWIND

My Worst Case (Fig. 13.1)

A 31-year-old male was admitted due to progressive loss of balance and tetraparesis. Magnetic resonance imaging (MRI) showed a pontine lesion with mass effect and edema (A–C) suggesting cavernoma. The neurologic condition of the patient declined rapidly, and the patient underwent an operation on an emergency basis. The lesion was approached through the fourth ventricle (opening of the median sulcus). The lesion blew up and bled copiously without identifiable vessels, making hemostasis really difficult. Finally, hemostasis was achieved and the lesion resected. Fortunately, the patient did not relapse to his preoperative condition. Postoperative MRI (D–F) showed a remaining lesion that is under close follow-up. "D" shows linear-vascular images suggesting vessels nearby the remaining tumor. This case illustrates the potential difficulty of cavernoma surgery (increased in the acute stage) and the frustrating effect of the incomplete resection.

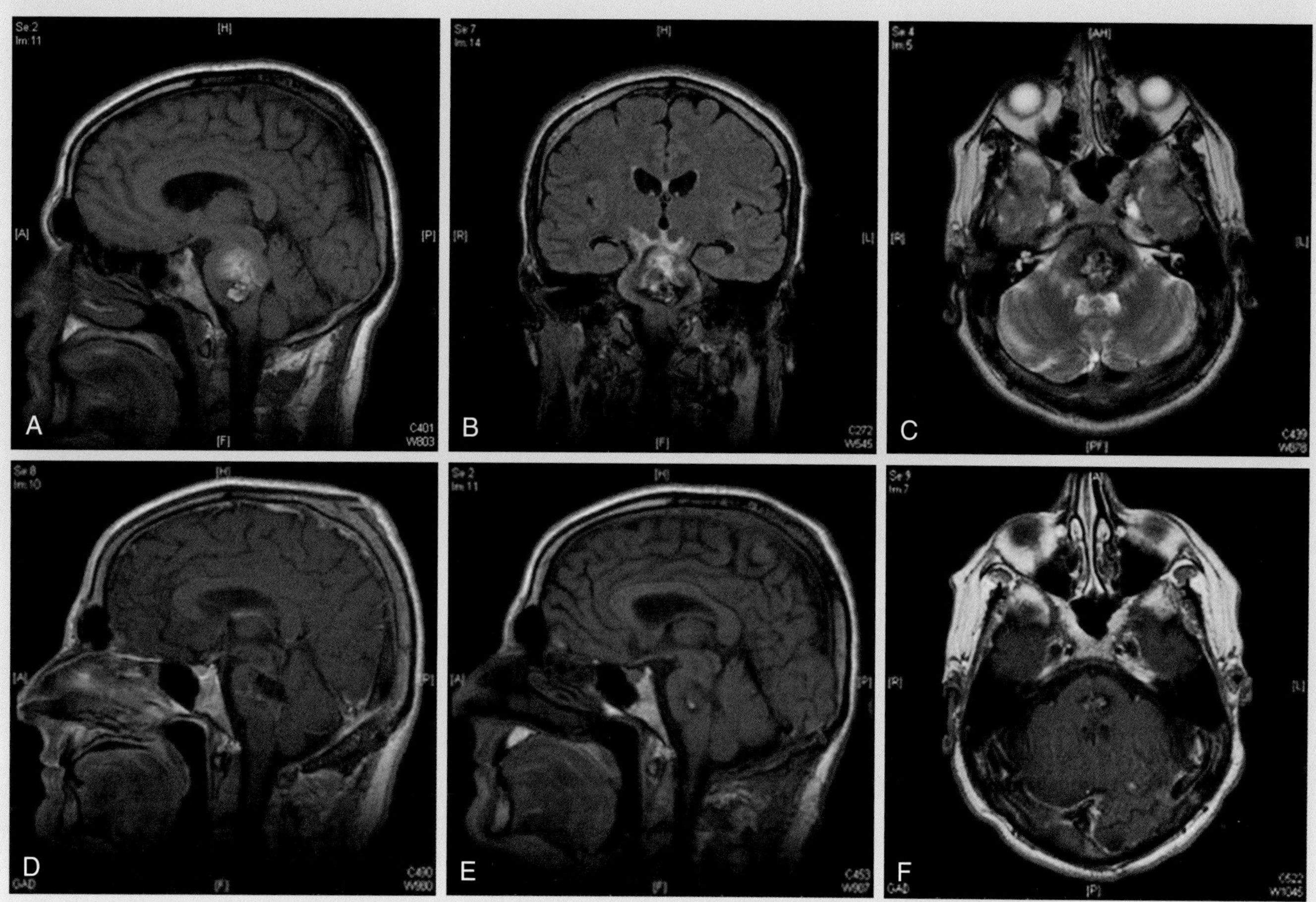

• **Fig. 13.1**

Continued

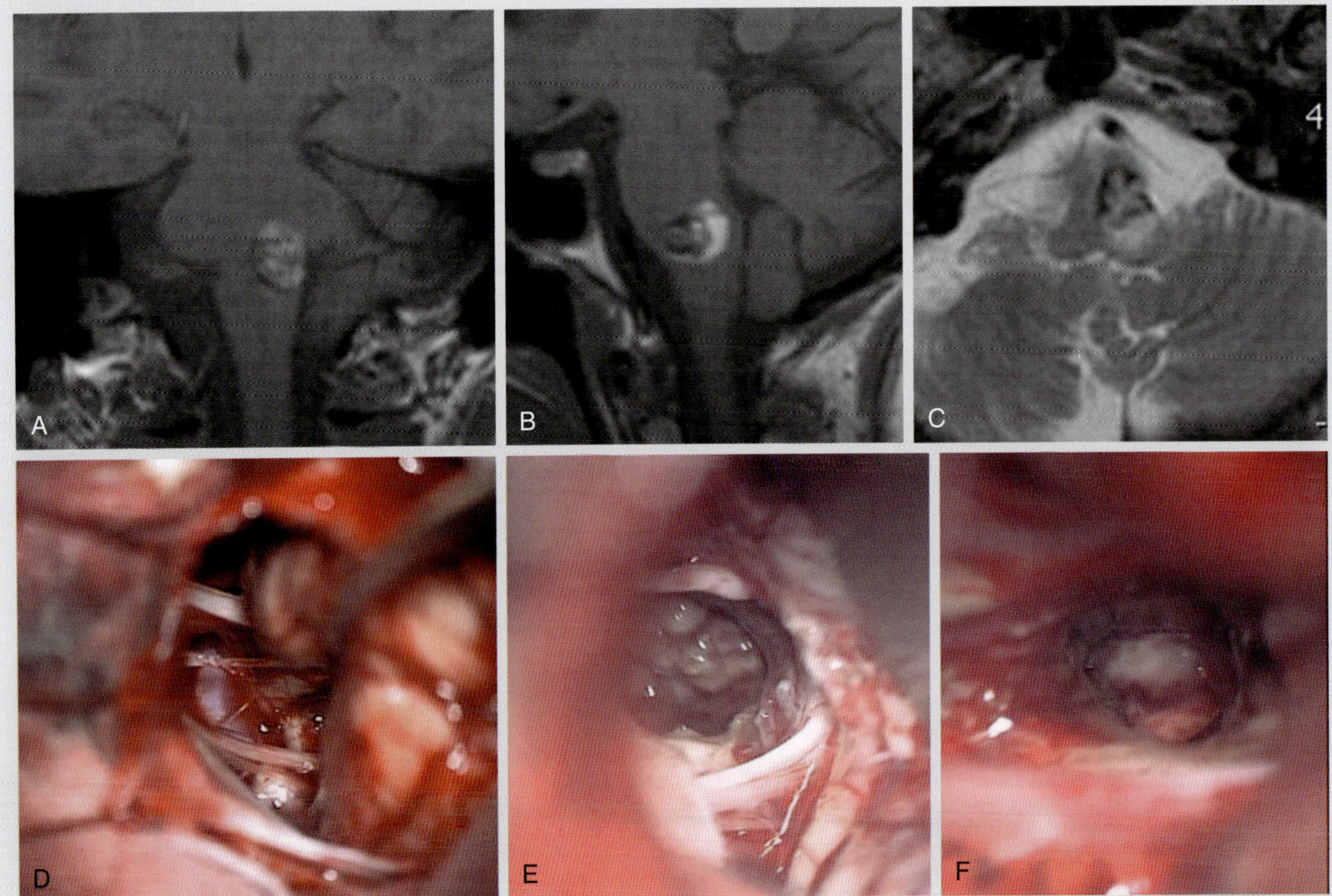

• **Fig. 13.2** A 46-year-old female with recurrent episodes of right hemiparesis, hemidysesthesia, and diplopia. (A–C) Magnetic resonance imaging shows cavernous angioma at the anterior ponto-medullary region. (D) Surgical procedure (retrosigmoid approach) with exposure of the lesion between nerves IX and X. (E) Gliotic tissue is seen consistently around the lesion, making the identification of the plane of cleavage and/or any remaining tumor difficult (Video 13.1). (F) Final intraoperative image after resection of this surrounding tissue. Postoperative course had increase of the preoperative neurologic deficit due to white matter damage during the procedure. The patient had been operated on after several episodes of minor bleeding in a "later" stage. This case illustrates the importance of the cleavage plane and the implication of "late" surgery in cavernoma surgery.

RED FLAGS

- Tailored decisions. Try to ascertain the natural history of the cavernoma for every patient.
- Judicious evaluation of the presumed impact of possible further bleedings in the neurologic condition.
- Surgery of higher risk in brainstem, spinal cord, deep locations, and eloquent cortex.
- Never omit intraoperative neurophysiologic monitoring and neuronavigation in difficult cases.
- Eloquent areas need very careful preoperative planning. Use combined osteotomies and skull base techniques when necessary.
- Neurologic morbidity is related to the entry zone (always look for safe entry zones!) and to the management of the cleavage plane around the lesion.
- The remaining lesion makes the big effort of the operation and the suffering of the patient useless.
- Timing for surgery: neither too early nor too late.

References

1. Abla AA, Lekovic GP, Turner JD, de Oliveira JG, Porter R, Spetzler RF. Advances in the treatment and outcome of brainstem cavernous malformation surgery: a single-center case series of 300 surgically treated patients. *Neurosurgery*. 1999;68(2):403–414.
2. Dey M, Turner MS, Wollmann R, Awad IA. Fatal "hypertensive" intracerebral hemorrhage associated with a cerebral cavernous angioma: case report. *Acta Neurochir (Wien)*. 2011;153(2):421–423.
3. Gangemi M, Maiuri F, Donati PA, Sigona L. Rapid growth of a brainstem cavernous angioma. *Acta Neurol (Napoli)*. 1993;15(2):132–137.
4. Lu XY, Sun H, Xu JG, Li QY. Stereotactic radiosurgery of brainstem cavernous malformations: a systematic review and meta-analysis. *J Neurosurg*. 2014;120(4):982–987.
5. Poorthuis MH, Klijn CJ, Algra A, Rinkel GJ, Al-Shahi Salman R. Treatment of cerebral cavernous malformations: a systematic review and meta-regression analysis. *J Neurol Neurosurg Psychiatry*. 2014;85(12):1319–1323.

6. Scamoni C, Dario A, Basile L. The association of cavernous and venous angioma. Case report and review of the literature. *Br J Neurosurg.* 1997;11(4):346–349.
7. Detwiler PW, Porter R, Lawton MT, Spetzler RF. Detection of delayed cerebral vasospasm, after rupture of intracranial aneurysms by magnetic resonance angiography. *Neurosurgery.* 1997;41:997–998.
8. Abdulrauf SI, Kaynar MY, Awad IA. A comparison of the clinical profile of cavernous malformations with and without associated venous malformations. *Neurosurgery.* 1999;44:41–47.
9. Tarnaris A, Fernandes RP, Kitchen ND. Does conservative management for brain stem cavernomas have better long-term outcome? *Br J Neurosurg.* 2008;22(6):748–757.
10. Menon G, Gopalakrishnan CV, Rao BR, Nair S, Sudhir J, Sharma M. A single institution series of cavernomas of the brainstem. *J Clin Neurosci.* 2011;18(9):1210–1214.
11. Wostrack M, Shiban E, Harmening K, et al. Surgical treatment of symptomatic cerebral cavernous malformations in eloquent brain regions. *Acta Neurochir (Wien).* 2012;154(8):1419–1430.
12. Van Gompel JJ, Marsh WR, Meyer FB, Worrell GA. Patient-assessed satisfaction and outcome after microsurgical resection of cavernomas causing epilepsy. *Neurosurg Focus.* 2010;29(3):E16.
13. Brown AP, Thompson BG, Spetzler RF. The twopoint method: evaluating brainstem lesions. *BNI Q.* 1996;12:20–24.
14. Mai JC, Ramanathan D, Kim LJ, Sekhar LN. Surgical resection of cavernous malformations of the brainstem: evolution of a minimally invasive technique. *World Neurosurg.* 2013;79(5–6):691–703.
15. Matsuda R, Coello AF, De Benedictis A, Martinoni M, Duffau H. Awake mapping for resection of cavernous angioma and surrounding gliosis in the left dominant hemisphere: surgical technique and functional results: clinical article. *J Neurosurg.* 2012;117(6):1076–1078.
16. Slotty PJ, Ewelt C, Sarikaya-Seiwert S, Steiger HJ, Vesper J, Hänggi D. Localization techniques in resection of deep seated cavernous angiomas – review and reevaluation of frame based stereotactic approaches. *Br J Neurosurg.* 2013;27(2):175–180.
17. Gross BA, Batjer HH, Awad IA, Bendok BR, Du R. Brainstem cavernous malformations: 1390 surgical cases from the literature. *World Neurosurg.* 2013;80(1–2):89–93.
18. Washington CW, McCoy KE, Zipfel GJ. Update on the natural history of cavernous malformations and factors predicting aggressive clinical presentation. *Neurosurg Focus.* 2010;29:E7.
19. Qiao N, Ma Z, Song J, et al. A systematic review and meta-analysis of surgeries performed for treating deep-seated cerebral cavernous malformations. *Br J Neurosurg.* 2015;29(4):493–499.
20. Giliberto G1, Lanzino DJ, Diehn FE, et al. Brainstem cavernous malformations: anatomical, clinical, and surgical considerations. *Neurosurg Focus.* 2010;29(3):E9.
21. Strauss C, Romstöck J, Fahlbusch R. Pericollicular approaches to the rhomboid fossa. Part II. Neurophysiological basis. *J Neurosurg.* 1999;91(5):768–775.
22. Hauck EF, Barnett SL, White JA, Samson D. The presigmoid approach to anterolateral pontine cavernomas. Clinical article. *J Neurosurg.* 2010;113(4):701–708.
23. Recalde RJ, Figueiredo EG, de Oliveira E. Microsurgical anatomy of the safe entry zones on the anterolateral brainstem related to surgical approaches to cavernous malformations. *Neurosurgery.* 2008;62(3 suppl 1):9–15.
24. Dukatz T, Sarnthein J, Sitter H, et al. Quality of life after brainstem cavernoma surgery in 71 patients. *Neurosurgery.* 2011;69(3):689–695.
25. Badhiwala JH, Farrokhyar F, Alhazzani W, et al. Surgical outcomes and natural history of intramedullary spinal cord cavernous malformations: a single-center series and meta-analysis of individual patient data: Clinic article. *J Neurosurg Spine.* 2014;21(4):662–676.
26. Santoro A, Innocenzi G, Bellotti C, Cancrini A, Delfini R, Cantore GP. Total removal of an intramedullary cavernous angioma by transthoracic approach. *Ital J Neurol Sci.* 1998;19(3):176–179.
27. Kon T, Mori H, Hasegawa K, Nishiyama K, Tanaka R, Takahashi H. Neonatal cavernous angioma located in the basal ganglia with profuse intraoperative bleeding. *Childs Nerv Syst.* 2007;23(4):449–453.
28. Lekovic GP, Gonzalez LF, Khurana VG, Spetzler RF. Intraoperative rupture of brainstem cavernous malformation. Case report. *Neurosurg Focus.* 2006;21(1):e14.
29. Mori H, Koike T, Endo S, et al. Tentorial cavernous angioma with profuse bleeding. Case report. *J Neurosurg Pediatr.* 2009;3(1):37–40.
30. Avci E, Oztürk A, Baba F, Karabağ H, Cakir A. Huge cavernoma with massive intracerebral hemorrhage in a child. *Turk Neurosurg.* 2007;17(1):23–26.
31. Mathiesen T, Edner G, Kihlström L. Deep and brainstem cavernomas: a consecutive 8-year series. *J Neurosurg.* 2003;99(1):31–37.
32. Bruneau M, Bijlenga P, Reverdin A, et al. Early surgery for brainstem cavernomas. *Acta Neurochir (Wien).* 2006;148(4):405–414.
33. Kikuta K, Nozaki K, Takahashi JA, Miyamoto S, Kikuchi H, Hashimoto N. Postoperative evaluation of microsurgical resection for cavernous malformations of the brainstem. *J Neurosurg.* 2004;101(4):607–612.
34. Chen B, Göricke S, Wrede K, et al. Reliable? The value of early postoperative magnetic resonance imaging after CCM surgery. *World Neurosurg.* 2017;5:1878–1887.

14

Complications of Carotid Endarterectomy

STACEY QUINTERO WOLFE, JAMES L. WEST, KYLE M. FARGEN, JOHN A. WILSON

HIGHLIGHTS

- Carotid endarterectomy is a safe, effective, and durable procedure with a complication rate approximating 2% to 4% in recent studies.
- Patient selection is the single most important factor in complication avoidance.
- Although uncommon, complications of carotid endarterectomy can be devastating unless promptly recognized and corrected.

Background

Throughout its history, carotid endarterectomy (CEA) has been a safe and effective means of preventing stroke due to carotid artery disease. The procedure was first shown to reduce incidence of stroke in patients with symptomatic carotid artery stenosis in a randomized multicenter trial in 1969. The North American Symptomatic Carotid Endarterectomy Trial (NASCET), a non-blinded, multicenter randomized controlled trial, was halted in 1991 after interim analysis of 659 patients with high-grade stenosis (>70%) revealed a 17% absolute risk reduction of ipsilateral stroke at 18 months in those undergoing CEA compared with medical management.[1] The European counterpart to NASCET, the European Carotid Surgery Trial (ECST), similarly demonstrated an 11.6% absolute risk reduction of stroke at 3 years after surgery in patients with symptomatic, high-grade (80% or greater) stenosis.[2] Studies have also suggested that CEA is superior to medical management in patients with asymptomatic carotid stenosis. Most notably, the Asymptomatic Carotid Atherosclerosis Study (ACAS) was a prospective, randomized, multicenter trial that enrolled 1662 patients and showed an estimated 5-year risk reduction of stroke or death of 6% in those with greater than 60% stenosis undergoing CEA compared with medical management.[3]

CEA has remained the mainstay treatment for carotid artery stenosis because of its effectiveness, durability, and low complication rate. Most series report a periprocedural complication rate approximating 2.3 to 4.3.[4,5] Even in the most recent trials comparing modern minimally invasive endovascular techniques, carotid angioplasty and stenting (CAS), to CEA, CEA has a safety profile equivalent to that of CAS and may be associated with a lower risk of stroke.[5] This chapter will review the periprocedural and postprocedural complications of CEA with a focus on techniques to mitigate or avoid complications.

Anatomic Insights

Standard exposure for CEA involves dissection medial to the sternocleidomastoid muscle with dissection in an avascular plane to find the carotid sheath. This is then opened and the jugular mobilized laterally to identify the carotid artery, and the vagus nerve is identified as well. When exposing the carotid artery, one must be aware of the close proximity of a number of cranial nerves or their branches, including the vagus, the recurrent laryngeal, and the hypoglossal nerve as well as the marginal mandibular branch of the facial nerve (Fig. 14.1). Cranial neuropathy has been reported at a rate of 5% to 8% according to recent multicentered trials, including CREST and NASCET.[1,5–7] In general, these are the result of neuropraxic traction injuries which will improve or resolve with time.

The most common cranial nerve palsy is a hypoglossal nerve injury, which accounts for more than half of all cranial neuropathies after CEA, according to one recent study.[6] The hypoglossal nerve is routinely identified during surgery because it usually crosses the internal carotid artery (ICA) and external carotid artery a few centimeters above the bifurcation. It is helpful to identify the superior root of the ansa cervicalis and follow it superiorly to its branch point from the hypoglossal. Occasionally, the hypoglossal nerve may be hidden or fixed behind the facial vein, and injury can occur when dividing the facial vein is attempted. Dissection carried along the entire length of the nerve to allow medial mobilization is helpful in preventing traction injury, as is sectioning the ansa cervicalis if the nerve is tethered.

The marginal mandibular branch of the facial nerve is also at risk during CEA. The marginal mandibular branch typically runs along the inferior aspect of the jaw and is at risk for neuropraxic injury via compression from retractors. To avoid this, retractors should be placed superficially, and care should be taken to maintain retractor blades without excessive direct compression at the angle of the jaw. If injury is encountered, patients can be reassured that this palsy typically resolves over the course of weeks to months. Clinically, marginal mandibular palsy can mimic a postoperative ischemic event but will always be ipsilateral to the CEA. A thorough neurologic examination, clearly ruling out any other neurologic deficits to exclude stroke, is of key importance when attributing facial droop to marginal mandibular palsy.

The vagus nerve lies posterolateral to the carotid in the carotid sheath and can be inadvertently injured when exposing and

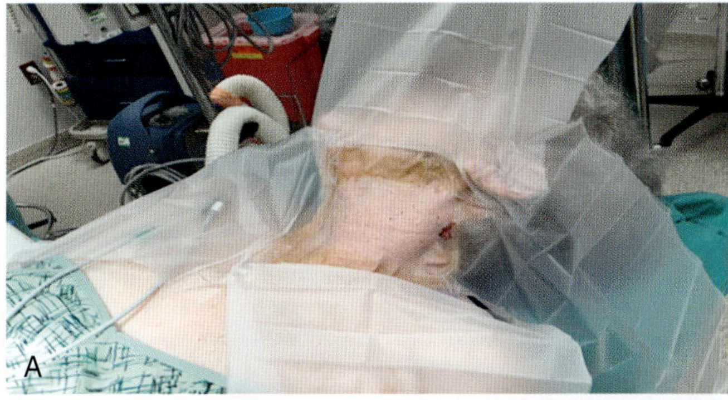

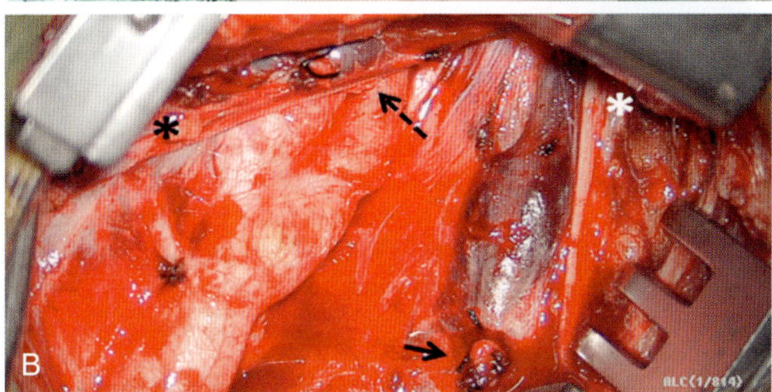

• **Fig. 14.1** Anatomic Considerations. Anatomic Considerations. (A) Demonstrates typical positioning. Important considerations include: position patient with ipsilateral side on the edge of the OR table, with the head at the top of the OR table and then place a shoulder roll between the shoulder blades to aid with neck extension. (B) Intraoperatively, care should be taken to identify important neurovascular structures and protect them, such as the ansa cervicalis (black asterisk), the typical location of the hypoglossal nerve (dotted arrow), the branch of the spinal accessory nerve to the sternocleidomastoid muscle (white asterisk), typical region of the marginal mandibular (underneath the retractor blade superiorly, and the jugular vein with ligated facial vein (solid arrow).

attempting to separate the carotid artery and the internal jugular vein or when clamping the carotid artery. Injury can lead to hoarseness, which, depending on the mechanism of injury, often recovers over the course of months. Careful identification of the vagus nerve once the carotid sheath is entered as a routine part of the exposure minimizes the risk of vagal nerve injury. The recurrent laryngeal nerve lies in the tracheoesophageal groove and is also prone to traction injury if the medial blade of the retractor is placed too deeply.

The key to minimizing or avoiding cranial nerve complications altogether lies in a solid understanding of the anatomy encountered during the exposure of the carotid artery. Armed with this knowledge, the surgeon can avoid almost all of the more serious cranial nerve injuries.

RED FLAGS

- Preoperative Risk Reduction: Patient selection
  - Patients with anatomic red flags such as previous neck radiation, previous neck surgery, high carotid bifurcation, or a contralateral carotid occlusion should be carefully evaluated.
- Perioperative Risk Reduction: Intraoperative technique and early recognition
  - Intraoperative monitoring techniques such as regional anesthesia with awake neurologic examination, EEG, somatosensory evoked potential (SSEP), transcranial Doppler.
  - Changes in mental status or focal neurologic deficits during cross-clamp may be overcome with proper increase in blood pressure or shunting.
  - Identify intraoperative carotid occlusion by backbleeding.
  - Ensure there is no chance of dissection flap with careful plaque removal and inspection.
- Postoperative Risk Reduction: Early recognition and treatment
  - Expanding neck hematomas demand prompt recognition and treatment at bedside with early involvement of anesthesia.
  - Preventing intraparenchymal reperfusion hemorrhage postoperatively necessitates precise blood pressure management.
  - Stroke can be a devastating complication of surgery, and prompt recognition is paramount because it is often reversible if caught early.

Complication Prevention: Patient Selection

The first step in complication avoidance is appropriate preoperative patient selection. The NASCET and ACAS trials firmly established CEA as superior to best medical management for both symptomatic and asymptomatic carotid atherosclerotic disease in the early 1990s; however, medical management has improved since that time with the evolution of statins and antiplatelet drugs. CREST-2 is currently enrolling patients to answer the question of best treatment for asymptomatic carotid stenosis in the modern era. Certain patients carry a high surgical risk, such as those with previous neck radiation, previous carotid disease, severe heart or lung disease, a high carotid bifurcation or plaque extension above C2, and/or contralateral carotid occlusion, and CAS is noninferior to CEA in this population.[8] 2016 data shows that CAS is also noninferior to CEA for patients <80 years of age with asymptomatic stenosis ≥70%,[9] with an experienced endovascular surgeon and use of an embolic protection device. Given the slightly higher risk of stroke in CAS and its impact on quality of life, CEA may be preferred over CAS in symptomatic patients without high surgical risk factors.

Perioperative Complication Prevention and Management

Dissection Flap

It is imperative to ensure that the plaque is removed completely with a smooth transition to the normal intima. An intimal flap can lead to dissection of blood between the endothelial and muscular layers, leading to occlusion or stenosis of the artery. This is best prevented by performing an arteriotomy of the ICA of sufficient length to allow adequate visualization and dissection of the distal end of the plaque. The plaque can usually be feathered out by careful circumferential dissection with an instrument such as a Rhoton round knife. If the plaque fragments, ring forceps should be used to ensure complete removal under magnified vision. On occasion, there may be an edge of the plaque that does not feather out and is not a completely smooth transition to normal intima. In this case, a 7-0 or 8-0 Prolene suture should be used to tack the flap at its most proximal edge. The suture knot must of course be outside the vessel lumen, which can be accomplished by using a double-armed suture. The bite must be small to prevent kinking or stenosis of the artery. At times several tiny sutures should be used, rather than one suture with a larger bite. On the unusual occasion that the plaque continues distally and maximum cranial exposure has been obtained with mobilization of the digastric belly, it may be necessary to secure the remaining plaque with a mosquito or ring forceps and sharply pull to release the plaque. Although this may cause some angst on the part of the surgeon, it has proven successful and without complication on a number of cases in our experience. Should this maneuver be required, it may be advisable to use dual antiplatelet agents for 6 weeks after the endarterectomy.

Intraoperative Ischemia

The use of shunting in CEA is a topic of controversy. Some surgeons use shunts for all cases, whereas others use this technique selectively in the case of neurologic decline. Both are well supported in the literature and are dependent on the surgeons' training and preference.

Both methods have benefits as well as potential complications. Use of a shunt carries risk of embolization of distal debris or air as well as the risk of distal dissection as demonstrated in Surgical Rewind, "My Worst Case". Ensuring that the artery is opened distal to the plaque and that the shunt is appropriately backbled will help prevent these complications. In 754 patients undergoing CEA with selective shunting, 32.6% had a new lesion on diffusion-weighted magnetic resonance imaging compared with 4.2% of the nonshunted patients, although 80% of these were asymptomatic.[10]

In the case of CEA with selective shunting, a shunt is employed only if the patient develops ischemia with impairment of neurologic function during the period of carotid cross-clamp. Numerous monitoring techniques for the detection of cerebral ischemia have been described. We prefer a neurologic examination in a patient who is awake and under local anesthesia due to its high sensitivity and specificity for ischemic impairment. This may manifest as alteration in level of consciousness, agitation, hemiplegia, or aphasia. Other techniques such as EEG, SSEP, or transcranial Doppler have also been successfully employed for monitoring patients under general anesthesia. During temporary carotid occlusion, maintaining systemic blood pressure between 160 and 200 systolic, or 20% above baseline, can help maintain perfusion through the maximally dilated vasculature of the ischemic brain. Ensuring careful dissection around the carotid body can help prevent bradycardia and hypotension, which can be augmented by the injection of local anesthetic into the carotid body. Preoperative recognition of the patency of the anterior communicating or posterior communicating arteries can help predict whether a shunt will be needed; however, in the senior author's experience (JAW) using regional anesthetic, 4.9% of patients required shunting (n = 325, unpublished data). In fact, only 23.3% of patients with a contralateral occlusion required shunting in this series. Prior to incising the carotid, neurologic testing should be performed after 30 to 60 seconds of ICA clamp time. A carotid shunt should always be immediately available, and the surgeon and surgical team should be familiar with its use.

Intraoperative Carotid Occlusion

Intraoperative carotid occlusion is a potentially catastrophic complication that must be recognized promptly and followed immediately by corrective actions. Intraoperative occlusion is evaluated by backbleeding the ICA before final closure of the suture line, which also allows for egress of any remaining air and/or microdebris. If there is no backflow, additional heparin is given with an activated clotting time (ACT) to confirm that the patient is appropriately anticoagulated. We aim for a goal ACT of 225 to 250. The distal suture line should be immediately reopened and the lumen inspected for clot, debris, or a backwalled suture. When flow is reestablished, the ICA clip is replaced and the ICA sutured and backbled again just before the final suture is tied. If there is no flow, a Valsalva and suction should be performed with the ICA clip off to dislodge potential clot. Should this fail to result in brisk backbleeding, a 3-French Fogarty catheter can be passed distally, inflated gently, and pulled back to remove any clot, followed by backbleeding.

If the reason for thrombosis is not mechanical (i.e., a backwalled suture), addition of a second antiplatelet agent such as clopidogrel should be considered because certain patients demonstrate relative insensitivity to aspirin, with a 34% incidence of normal collagen/epinephrine closure times on PGY100 testing in patients with cerebrovascular ischemic symptoms.[11]

Postoperative Complication Prevention and Management

Ischemic Event

Postprocedural stroke after CEA is a devastating event. Prompt recognition of ischemic symptoms and workup of the etiology cannot be overstated, because urgent treatment of ischemia may be reversible and prevent permanent tissue damage. Possible etiologies must be considered and ruled out by the treating surgeon, with the mindset that time is brain and the quickest route to the diagnosis and treatment is best. Etiologies for post-CEA ischemia include carotid thrombosis at the operative site due to technical error or aspirin insensitivity, distal thromboembolization, or relative hypoperfusion. Additionally, cerebral hyperperfusion is a rare but well-documented cause of neurologic symptoms after CEA.

Emergent imaging is usually the most appropriate first step to assess for carotid occlusion or stenosis, or intimal flap and dissection. If imaging as described below cannot be accomplished expeditiously, immediate return to the operating room for exploration of the operative site should be considered. If the operative bed cannot be examined in a satisfactory manner via ultrasound, or if no obvious abnormalities are identified, we recommend emergent computed tomography (CT) angiogram with perfusion study, which will allow for assessment of intracranial hemorrhage, cervical carotid thrombosis, and tandem intracranial thromboemboli as well as ischemic penumbra. If distal large-vessel occlusion is confirmed, we recommend emergent angiogram for cervical and intracranial embolectomy with angioplasty/stenting if needed. If there is cervical carotid intraluminal thrombus, dissection, or occlusion, immediate return to the operating room with revision of CEA is advised, with stepwise exploration as described in the previous section (Fig. 14.2). If there is no evidence of stenosis or occlusion but imaging is suggestive of hypoperfusion, we recommend increasing systolic blood pressure to 160 to 180 mm Hg or 20% above baseline as well as ruling out significant anemia or hypovolemia. If perfusion imaging suggests cerebral hyperperfusion, strict normotension is recommended.

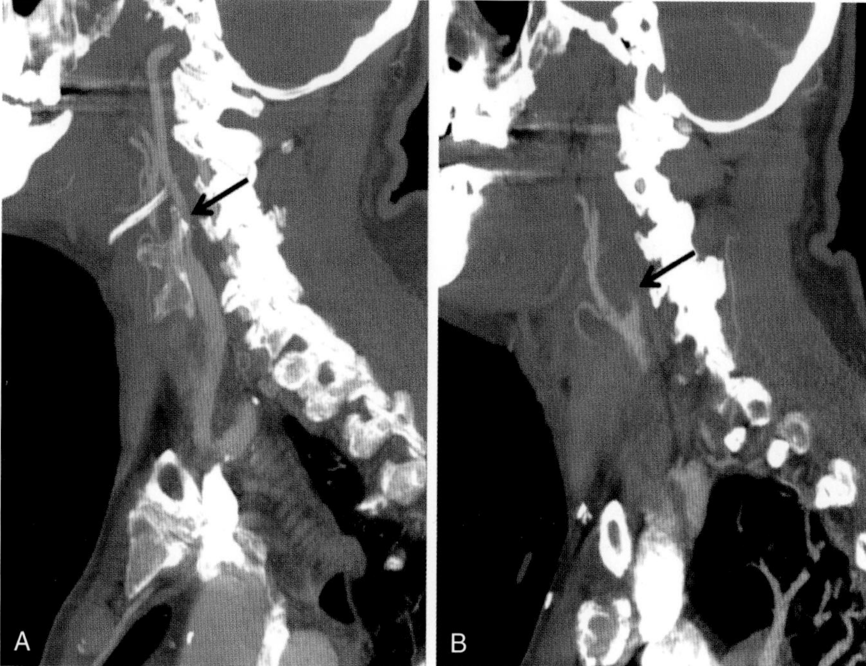

• **Fig. 14.2** Postoperative Thrombosis. Postoperative carotid thrombosis from an aspirin non-responder. 70-year-old male who underwent a right carotid endarterectomy for high-grade stenosis measuring 90%, of the right internal carotid artery from which he had had multiple embolic strokes two days prior (A). He did well and was taken to the recovery room and approximately an hour and one-half after the procedure he became relatively hypotensive with systolic blood pressure of 90 mm Hg and then acutely stopped moving his left side. He was taken emergently for a CTA head and neck, which showed a complete occlusion of the right internal carotid artery at the suture line, but no tandem intracranial occlusion (B). He was then emergently taken back to the operating room for exploration. He was heparinized with an ACT of 250 and the suture line reopened. He was given a Valsalva and suction applied to the distal carotid with expulsion of a large thrombus. Once good back-bleeding was demonstrated, we reclosed the suture line primarily. He awoke from general anesthesia neurologically intact. He was loaded with Plavix 450 mg and continued on Plavix for 3 months.

Intracranial Hemorrhage

Cerebral hemorrhage or cerebral hyperperfusion after CEA occurs in less than 1% of the CEA population. Perioperative hypertension is a significant risk factor in the potential development of intracranial hemorrhage, likely related to impairment of the normally cerebral-protective carotid sinus reflex. Independent of hypertension, Sundt et al. demonstrated increased cerebral blood flow after CEA, likely related to impaired cerebral autoregulation of the blood-brain barrier after a prolonged period of relative cerebral ischemia.[12] This increase in cerebral blood flow in a region of the brain with already impaired autoregulation can lead to potential for hemorrhage when combined with anticoagulation and antiplatelets.

Prevention is the key to managing hyperperfusion because consequences can be permanent and severe. Patient complaint of headache in the postoperative period is unusual and should raise the level of suspicion. Strict attention to perioperative hemodynamics and blood pressure control is paramount. Specifically, maintenance of the systolic blood pressure within the normal confines of cerebral autoregulation ameliorates the negative effects of impaired autoregulation. Systolic blood pressure is maintained at 110 to 160 mm Hg utilizing intravenous medications as necessary in the ICU overnight after CEA. The following morning patients resume their normal home medication regimen in order to maintain normotension after discharge.

Neck Hematoma

Expanding neck hematoma is an uncommon but dangerous postoperative complication associated with CEA. Reported rates of symptomatic neck hematoma range from 1% to 8%. Neck hematoma has been associated with both perioperative hypertension and clopidogrel usage.[13] In a recent large series, the average time from surgery completion to return to the operating room was 6 hours for symptomatic, progressive neck hematomas.[14]

Immediate recognition and establishment of a secure airway at bedside is the mainstay of care. An airway that cannot be secured may require prep of the wound and reopening at bedside to release hematoma, with the anesthesia team standing by to intubate. Early involvement of anesthesia for airway management is important. Per the anesthesia literature, the vast majority of hematoma patients, over 70%, were safely intubated with simple direct laryngoscopy, and evacuation of the hematoma facilitated direct laryngoscopic intubation in the remainder of patients who initially had difficult airways.[14] This complication, although emergent with the potential for rapid decompensation, is one that can be safely managed with early aggressive care and vigilance.

Myocardial Infarction

Perioperative myocardial infarction continues to be a significant source of perioperative morbidity in the CEA population, with a reported rate of approximately 2% to 3%.[5] This is an inherent risk as patients with carotid disease develop atherosclerotic disease in multiple vascular territories. Additionally, perioperative changes in hemodynamics from anesthesia, including: potential expansion of intravascular volume from perioperative fluid overload, increased catecholamine production with increased myocardial oxygen demand, hemodynamic changes from carotid manipulation and altered autoregulation are potential cardiac stressors.

Close attention must be paid to preoperative symptoms such as chest pain and shortness of breath as well as to preoperative evaluation by cardiology. Additionally, in the perioperative window, close attention to patient symptoms and a low threshold to order basic chest pain workup, including ECG and troponins, can ensure prompt diagnosis of cardiac events.

Regional Versus General Anesthesia

Carotid stenosis and cerebrovascular disease place the body at risk for dysautoregulation, which may be further disrupted by general anesthesia. Perioperative blood pressure control, heart rate, and cerebral perfusion are significantly impacted by the induction of general anesthesia, and hemodynamic swings may be mitigated with regional anesthesia in the form of a superficial cervical plexus block (JAW, unpublished data[15]). A recent review of 4558 patients undergoing CEA showed a twofold higher percentage of any morbidity (8.7% vs 4.2%) in patients having general anesthesia versus a regional block, as well as longer length of stay and increased rate of readmission, although there was no difference in stroke or myocardial infarction.[15]

Delayed Complication Prevention and Management

Carotid Restenosis

Delayed stenosis after CEA may occur regardless of technique used. Although the incidence is low, restenosis may place patients at risk for future stroke and may require repeat surgical or endovascular treatment. Although etiologies may vary according to the initial pathology and surgical conditions, typically early restenosis lesions are secondary to intimal hyperplasia, whereas the majority of late lesions appear to be primarily reaccumulation of atherosclerotic material. A recent review of 1782 CEAs showed that the rate for ipsilateral restenosis ≥70% was 3.4%, 6.5%, 10.2% at 2, 5 and 10 years, respectively, with no significant difference between patch angioplasty vs primary closure.[16] However, primary closure decreases clamping time, which may decrease overall perioperative risk and has been found to have very low restenosis rates, even approaching 0%.[17] Primary closure has been our institutional preference except in the rare case of very small vessel caliber, with similarly low restenosis rates. No significant risk factors for delayed restenosis have been convincingly established in the literature; however, continued smoking appears to be associated with an increased risk for restenosis.

Evaluation for intervention when restenosis is identified is multifactorial. Clearly, the increased complexity of treating a restenosis needs to be considered and weighed against the consequences of not intervening. The criteria used in the recent literature are symptomatic stenosis exceeding 50% caliber reduction, or asymptomatic restenosis exceeding 70% to 80% stenosis.[18]

Surgically, repeat CEA is made more challenging by previous scar tissue, but accepted options for reoperation include primary endarterectomy, patch angioplasty, or replacement of the severely diseased segment with a vein graft. If a plane can be clearly established and the artery is otherwise healthy, a repeat endarterectomy can be considered. A number of authors recommend patch angioplasty if a clear plane cannot be established or if there is concern that overall vessel caliber is too small. If the artery lumen is significantly damaged, another potential salvage option is interposition graft using harvested saphenous vein. Cranial nerves may be at greater risk in repeat CEA.

Endovascular intervention for angioplasty and stenting of the restenosis has been shown as noninferior, often with a better risk profile.[8] A recent metaanalysis examining revision CEA versus carotid stenting for restenosis found that revision CEA carries a higher risk of cardiac complications, whereas stenting had a higher rate of subsequent restenosis.[18] There still exists no Level 1 evidence for either option, and in general we opt for carotid stenting for carotid restenosis in the majority of our patient population.

SURGICAL REWIND

My Worst Case

Carotid Dissection and Restenosis

A 75-year-old female presented with progressive asymptomatic left carotid stenosis measuring 75% by CT angiogram. Upon clamping of the left ICA, she developed aphasia and hemiplegia, and a Pruitt-Inahara shunt was placed. The distal balloon was inadvertently overinflated, with concern for a dissection. Urgent postoperative angiography showed a dissection and pseudoaneurysm, which was treated with a stent (A). On routine follow-up 2 years later, she had progressive increase in the left ICA velocities with restenosis measuring 75% (B). She was taken for successful angioplasty and stent, and complete resolution of the previous dissection and pseudoaneurysm was confirmed (C).

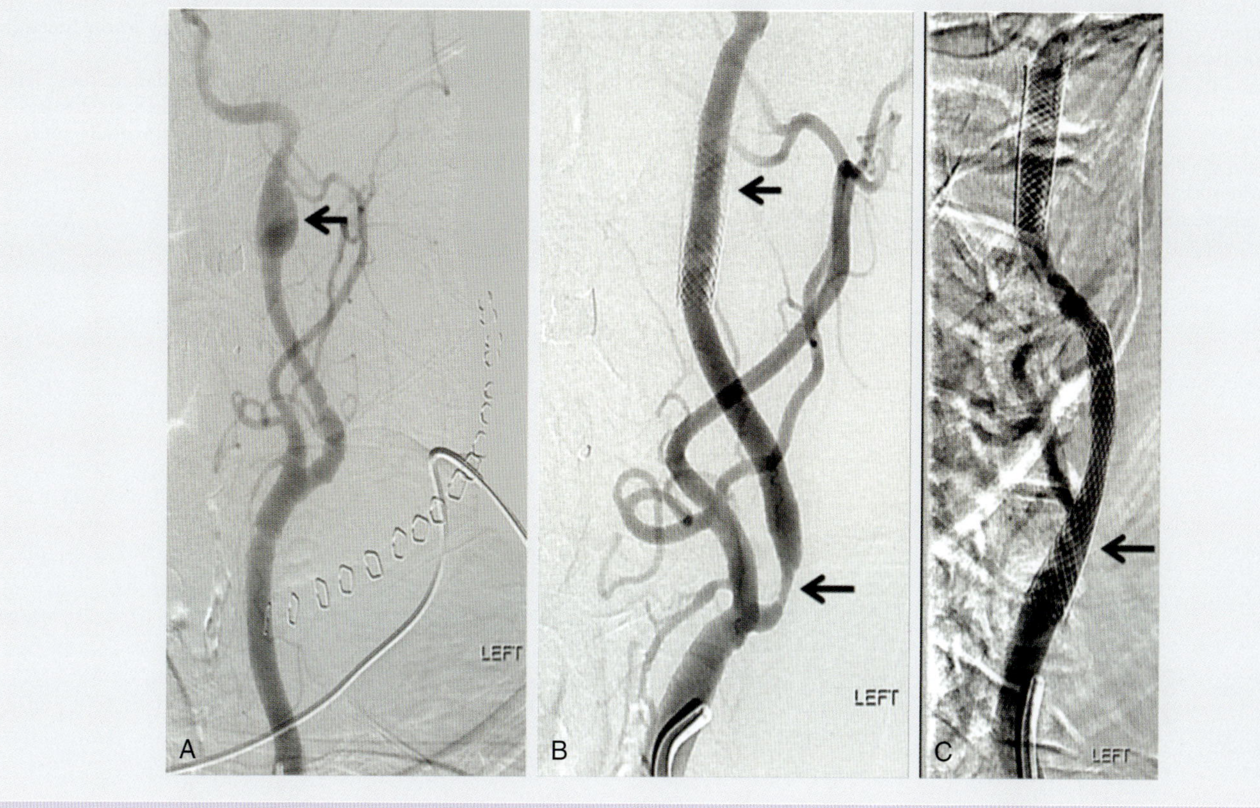

NEUROSURGICAL SELFIE MOMENT

- If acute postoperative thrombosis or occlusion is encountered, bring the patient back to the operating room immediately; open the carotid suture line, and use your suction as you have anesthesia perform a Valsalva to dislodge clot.
- If progressive feathering leads to a plaque that terminates too cranially to access, grip the ends of the plaque with hemostats and pull briskly to dislodge the remaining plaque.
- If a postoperative neck hematoma is expanding, have anesthesia attempt intubation; if unable to intubate, open the incision at the bedside to evacuate hematoma immediately.
- If a patient develops a sudden postoperative deficit in the immediate perioperative window concerning for stroke, obtain a CT angiogram head and neck to rule out carotid occlusion versus tandem occlusion.

References

1. Committee NS. NASCET: North American Symptomatic Carotid Endarterectomy Trial. *Stroke*. 1991;22(6):711–720.
2. Farrell B, Fraser A, Sandercock P, et al. Randomised trial of endarterectomy for recently symptomatic carotid stenosis: final results of the MRC European Carotid Surgery Trial (ECST). *Lancet*. 1998; 351(9113):1379–1387.
3. Executive Committee for the Asymptomatic Carotid Atherosclerosis Study. ACAS. Endarterectomy for asymptomatic carotid artery stenosis. *JAMA*. 1995;273(18):1421–1428.
4. Bonati LH, Dobson J, Featherstone RL, et al. Long-term outcomes after stenting versus endarterectomy for treatment of symptomatic carotid stenosis: the International Carotid Stenting Study (ICSS) randomised trial. *Lancet*. 2015;385(9967):529–538.
5. Brott TG, Hobson RW, Howard G, et al; for CREST Investigators. Stenting versus endarterectomy for treatment of carotid-artery stenosis. *N Engl J Med*. 2010;363(1):11–23.
6. Cunningham EJ, Bond R, Mayberg MR, et al. Risk of persistent cranial nerve injury after carotid endarterectomy. *J Neurosurg*. 2004;101(3):445–448.
7. Fokkema M, de Borst GJ, Nolan BW, et al. Clinical relevance of cranial nerve injury following carotid endarterectomy. *Eur J Vasc Endovasc Surg*. 2014;47(1):2–7.
8. Yadav JS, Wholey MH, Kuntz RE, et al. Protected carotid-artery stenting versus endarterectomy in high-risk patients. *N Engl J Med*. 2004;351(15):1493–1501.
9. Rosenfield K, Matsumura JS, Chaturvedi S, et al; for ACT I Investigators. Randomized trial of stent versus surgery for asymptomatic carotid stenosis. *N Engl J Med*. 2016;374(11):1011–1020.
10. Orlicky M, Vachata P, Bartos R, et al. A selective carotid artery shunting for carotid endarterectomy: prospective MR DWI monitoring of embolization in a group of 754 patients. *J Neurol Surg A Cent Eur Neurosurg*. 2015;76(2):89–92.
11. Grundmann K, Jaschonek K, Kleine B, et al. Aspirin non-responder status in patients with recurrent cerebral ischemic attacks. *J Neurol*. 2003;250(1):63–66.
12. Sundt TM, Sharbrough FW, Piepgras DG, et al. Correlation of cerebral blood flow and electroencephalographic changes during carotid endarterectomy: with results of surgery and hemodynamics of cerebral ischemia. *Mayo Clin Proc*. 1981;56(9): 533–543.
13. Baracchini C, Gruppo M, Mazzalai F, et al. Predictors of neck bleeding after eversion carotid endarterectomy. *J Vasc Surg*. 2011;54(3): 699–705.

14. Shakespeare WA, Lanier WL, Perkins WJ, et al. Airway management in patients who develop neck hematomas after carotid endarterectomy. *Anesth Analg*. 2010;110(2):588–593.
15. Hussain AS, Mullard A, Oppat WF, et al. Increased resource utilization and overall morbidity are associated with general versus regional anesthesia for carotid endarterectomy in data collected by the Michigan Surgical Quality Collaborative. *J Vasc Surg*. 2017;66(3):802–809.
16. Avgerinos ED, Go C, Ling J, et al. Carotid artery disease progression and related neurologic events after carotid endarterectomy. *J Vasc Surg*. 2016;64(2):354–360.
17. Zenonos G, Lin N, Kim A, et al. Carotid endarterectomy with primary closure: analysis of outcomes and review of the literature. *Neurosurg*. 2012;70:646–654.
18. Tu J, Wang S, Huo Z, et al. Repeated carotid endarterectomy versus carotid artery stenting for patients with carotid restenosis after carotid endarterectomy: systematic review and meta-analysis. *Surgery*. 2015;157(6):1166–1173.

15

Skull Base Surgery Complications: An Overview

VINAYAK NARAYAN, ANIL NANDA

"All said and done, it is the final result that counts, and having been brought up to believe that convalescence is shortened by attention to the technical details while the patient is on the operating-table, I have no dread of a long section."

HARVEY CUSHING

HIGHLIGHTS

- The main goal of all skull base approaches, whether microscopic or endoscopic, is to minimize the brain retraction by optimum bone resection.
- The common complications of skull base surgery are vascular injuries, cerebrospinal fluid leak, cranial nerve palsy, wound infection, meningitis, hydrocephalus, vision changes, and cosmetic issues.
- The understanding of the relevant surgical anatomy, patience and meticulous maneuvering at each step of surgery, anticipation of complication, and the ability to manage the complication are the key factors for optimizing the surgical outcome.

Introduction

Skull base surgeries have evolved over a long period in response to meeting the necessity of treating complex tumors and vascular pathologies while avoiding retraction injuries to normal neurologic structures. Numerous pathologic processes arise within the skull base or extend there by direct growth. The main goal of all skull base approaches, whether microscopic or endoscopic, is to minimize the brain retraction by optimum bone resection. The widespread use of endoscopic surgical techniques in addition to advanced microsurgical skull base techniques in current times has advanced the frontiers of skull base neurosurgery.

The prevention and management of complications are an important cornerstone of skull base surgery. The complications at the skull base may be quite hazardous and usually occur due to errors in choosing the right approach or selecting the patient, or even due to technical gaffes. A myriad of complications can be encountered in skull base surgeries. The common complications are vascular injuries, cerebrospinal fluid (CSF) leak, cranial nerve palsy, wound infection, meningitis, hydrocephalus, vision changes, and cosmetic issues. The breakthroughs in radiologic imaging, advances in neuroanesthesia, and the conceptual progress in surgical techniques and intraoperative monitoring lead to the convergent evolution of this neurosurgical subspecialty. This chapter provides an overview of the major complications encountered in microsurgical and endoscopic skull base surgery and radiosurgery.

Vascular Complications

Vascular complications are the most feared complications of skull base surgeries. They can result from many causes. The infiltration of tumor to the adjacent vasculature, error in surgical technique, prior radiotherapy, inadequate preoperative imaging or interventions like cerebral angiogram or embolization, and nonoptimal use of neuronavigation or micro-Doppler are a few of them.[1] A variety of skull base lesions can encircle the major vascular structures and lead to their narrowing. Cavernous meningioma and petroclival meningioma, which can encircle the internal carotid artery (ICA) and basilar artery, respectively, are classical examples. Pituitary adenoma and chordoma and chondrosarcoma tumors can also invade the major vascular structures like the ICA and basilar artery.

Tumors like the giant medial sphenoid wing meningioma are better evaluated with a preoperative angiogram. It provides information on the course of the ICA in relation to the tumor and associated tumor feeders and offers the opportunity to perform preoperative tumor embolization and collateral circulation assessment. Most patients may be able to tolerate ICA sacrifice based on intraoperative carotid endarterectomy studies.[2] Depending on the possible anticipated complication of the artery/vein, the patient should be well prepared for possible bypass surgery or sinus reconstruction surgery. Knowing the relevant anatomy and the safe handling techniques for the critical neurovascular structures is essential to avoiding such complications.

CSF Leak

CSF leak is a very common complication after skull base surgery due to the close communication of the cisterns with most of the skull base approaches. The incidence of CSF leak in endonasal skull base surgeries ranges from 2% to 64% and ranges from 3% to 26.7% in vestibular schwannoma surgeries.[3–5] It can range from 4% to 17% in any posterior fossa surgery.[6] The major complications arising as a result of CSF leak are meningitis, ventriculitis, and brain abscess, which may increase the duration of hospital stay, readmission rate, and mortality risk. Craniopharyngioma usually has a higher rate of intraoperative CSF leak relative to other tumor pathologies.[7] The incidence of pseudomeningocele after posterior fossa surgery varies between 15% and 28%.[8] The most common factors associated with such leaks are inadequate dura and wound closure or healing, wound infection, raised intracranial pressure, and opened air petrous cells that have not been occluded. The basic strategies to prevent CSF leak are watertight dural closure and meticulous sealing of opened air cells. Multilayered closure involving fat or muscle patch, along with nasoseptal flap and bony reconstruction with placement of lumbar drain, is helpful in avoiding the postoperative CSF leak in endoscopic skull base surgeries. The Hadad-Bassagasteguy flap (HBF), a neurovascular pedicled flap of the nasal septum mucoperiosteum and mucoperichondrium based on the nasoseptal artery, seems to be advantageous for the reconstruction of the cranial base after endonasal cranial base surgery.[9] The rate of CSF leak can be further reduced by plugging the leaking site with small pieces of fat sealed with fibrin glue.[10] Early detection of CSF leak and avoiding raised intracranial pressure (ICP) are the important precautions to be taken for avoiding this serious complication.

Cranial Nerve Palsy

Cranial nerve deficits are commonly seen after skull base surgeries. We reported 44% cranial neuropathies in our series of 50 patients who underwent surgical treatment for petroclival meningioma.[6] The most common cranial nerve deficit after surgery was oculomotor nerve dysfunction, followed by facial weakness. Transient cranial nerve dysfunction was noted in 41% of patients. The facial nerve may be injured while performing the transposition of the nerve during transcochlear approach. Premeatal cerebellopontine angle meningiomas have been reported to be associated with poorer postoperative facial nerve function than retromeatal tumors.[11] In our series of patients operated on for cavernous meningioma, we noted that 54% of patients developed postoperative cranial nerve deficits, among which oculomotor palsy was the most common (24.6%).[12] At the last follow-up, complete recovery was noted in 62.5% of patients. Two patients developed transient deterioration in their vision due to the manipulation of the optic nerve, which recovered completely at their first clinical follow-up. Two patients (0.06%) had swallowing dysfunction after the surgery. The meticulous handling of the tumor, avoiding cauterization in close proximity to the cranial nerve, and early identification of the nerve and its gentle mobilization are the measures that help to prevent postoperative cranial nerve deficits.

Other Complications

The other complications after skull base surgery include operative site hematoma, cosmetic deformity, pulsatile enophthalmos (after orbitozygomatic osteotomy surgeries), wound infection, and temporomandibular and palatal complications. Apart from microscopic/endoscopic skull base surgeries, radiosurgery of the skull base lesions also carries the risk of postprocedural complications. A few of them include hydrocephalus, hypopituitarism, worsening of vision, stroke, radiation necrosis, and carotid stenosis.[13,14] The optimization of marginal and maximal radiation dose in stereotactic radiosurgery (SRS) may help to avoid most of these complications.

Conclusion

The nuances in current skull base surgery involving both microscopic and endoscopic approaches are rapidly developing and provide a wide circumferential access to the entire skull base. However, the complication rate is still a matter of concern. Understanding the relevant surgical anatomy, meticulous maneuvering at each step of surgery, anticipating complications, and managing the complications skillfully are the key factors for optimizing the surgical outcome.

References

1. Gardner PA, Snyderman CH, Fernandez-Miranda JC, Jankowitz BT. Management of major vascular injury during endoscopic endonasal skull base surgery. *Otolaryngol Clin North Am*. 2016;49(3):819–828.
2. Modica PA, Tempelhoff R, Rich KM, Grubb RL. Computerized electroencephalographic monitoring and selective shunting: influence on intraoperative administration of phenylephrine and myocardial infarction after general anesthesia for carotid endarterectomy. *Neurosurgery*. 1992;30(6):842–846.
3. Patel PN, Stafford AM, Patrinely JR, et al. Risk factors for intraoperative and postoperative cerebrospinal fluid leaks in endoscopic transsphenoidal sellar surgery. *Otolaryngol Neck Surg*. 2018; 158(5):952–960.
4. Hoffman RA. Cerebrospinal fluid leak following acoustic neuroma removal. *Laryngoscope*. 1994;104(1):40–58.
5. Rodgers GK, Luxford WM. Factors affecting the development of cerebrospinal fluid leak and meningitis after translabyrinthine acoustic tumor surgery. *Laryngoscope*. 1993;103(9):959–962.
6. Nanda A, Javalkar V, Banerjee AD. Petroclival meningiomas: study on outcomes, complications and recurrence rates. *J Neurosurg*. 2011;114(5):1268–1277.
7. Karnezis TT, Baker AB, Soler ZM, et al. Factors impacting cerebrospinal fluid leak rates in endoscopic sellar surgery. *Int Forum Allergy Rhinol*. 2016;6(11):1117–1125.
8. Manley GT, Dillon W. Acute posterior fossa syndrome following lumbar drainage for treatment of suboccipital pseudomeningocele. *J Neurosurg*. 2000;92(3):469–474.
9. Kassam AB, Thomas A, Carrau RL, et al. Endoscopic reconstruction of the cranial base using a pedicled nasoseptal flap. *Neurosurgery*. 2008;63(1 suppl 1):ONS44–ONS52.
10. Ludemann WO, Stieglitz LH, Gerganov V, Samii A, Samii M. Fat implant is superior to muscle implant in vestibular schwannoma surgery for the prevention of cerebrospinal fluid fistulae. *Neurosurgery*. 2008;63(1 suppl 1):ONS38–ONS42.
11. Schaller B, Merlo A, Gratzl O, Probst R. Premeatal and retromeatal cerebellopontine angle meningioma. Two distinct clinical entities. *Acta Neurochir (Wien)*. 1999;141(5):465–471.
12. Nanda A, Thakur JD, Sonig A, Missios S. Microsurgical resectability, outcomes, and tumor control in meningiomas occupying the cavernous sinus. *J Neurosurg*. 2016;125(2):378–392.
13. Sheehan JP, Starke RM, Mathieu D, et al. Gamma Knife radiosurgery for the management of nonfunctioning pituitary adenomas: a multicenter study. *J Neurosurg*. 2013;119(2):446–456.
14. Pollock BE, Nippoldt TB, Stafford SL, Foote RL, Abboud CF. Results of stereotactic radiosurgery in patients with hormone-producing pituitary adenomas: factors associated with endocrine normalization. *J Neurosurg*. 2002;97(3):525–530.

16

Complications in Anterior Cranial Fossa Surgery

FRANCESCO TOMASELLO, ALFREDO CONTI, FILIPPO F. ANGILERI, SALVATORE M. CARDALI, DOMENICO LA TORRE, ANTONINO F. GERMANÒ

Background

A variety of neurosurgical disorders affect the anterior cranial base and require an anterior cranial fossa approach. As neurosurgeons, we usually deal with the treatment of benign neoplasms, in particular meningiomas. Nonetheless, other common neurosurgical pathologies include traumatic injuries, craniofacial malformations (i.e., hypertelorism, craniosynostosis), cerebrospinal fluid (CSF) fistulas, and vascular lesions (i.e., arterio-venous fistulas). Although surgery of benign lesions of the anterior cranial fossa is a relatively common procedure, tumors like meningiomas can reach huge sizes and encase vital neurovascular structures, making surgery in the area a real challenge.

Furthermore, the anterior cranial base is also involved by malignant tumors. With some notable exceptions (leukemia, lymphoma, myeloma, metastases), malignant neoplasms are treated surgically but require adjuvant radiation or chemotherapy. Malignant lesions are generally challenging lesions that require a multidisciplinary approach to achieve an en bloc resection with margins of uninvolved tissue after broad circumferential exposure whenever possible.[1] Indications for surgical treatment of malignant tumors are influenced by the extent of the lesion taken together with clinical data, including age and performance. Surgical morbidity must be weighed against the anticipated natural course of the lesion and results of nonsurgical treatments, when applicable.

Here we briefly describe the transcranial approaches to the anterior cranial fossa and discuss complications commonly encountered in anterior cranial fossa surgery and their avoidance.

How I Do Anterior Cranial Fossa Surgery

Cushing originally described a unilateral frontal craniotomy.[2] This approach evolved to a bifrontal craniotomy and transbasal approach in the descriptions made by Dandy.[3] In both cases, however, a resection of the frontal lobes was necessary. Later, Tonnis reported his successful experience with the bifrontal approach while preserving the brain tissue. The introduction of the operating microscope in the 1970s and the refinement of surgical instruments improved the ability of neurosurgeons to carefully work on the skull base.[3] The unilateral and bifrontal craniotomies have been further modified, and craniofacial approaches have been used to treat tumors invading the nasal cavity and/or paranasal sinuses. The endoscope, which has been available for a long time for the treatment of other neurosurgical entities, was introduced recently in the treatment of selected anterior cranial fossa tumors.[4]

The selection of the most appropriate approach depends on multiple factors, including surgeon's preference and experience, tumor size and location, extent of dural attachment, and relation with the surrounding neurovascular structures. Antero-lateral approaches provide enough exposure to control the tumor, its base, and relevant neurovascular structures and to interrupt the tumor blood supply early on. Also, brain retraction and manipulation of critical neurovascular structures can be minimized using a unilateral subfrontal or pterional approach. Transbasal approaches should be reserved for cases in which a wider access to the skull base is desirable and bone resection and subsequent cranial base reconstruction are necessary because of tumor extension to paranasal sinuses. We briefly describe a few approaches that can be safely used to deal with all the lesions involving the anterior cranial fossa and beyond (Fig. 16.1).

Pterional Approach

A right pterional approach is usually performed to minimize manipulation of the dominant frontal lobe. The patient is therefore placed in the supine position, with his or her head fixed in a Mayfield three-pin head holder. The head is then rotated 30 to 60 degrees toward the left side and extended to help a spontaneous retraction of the frontal lobe from the skull base. After a fronto-temporal skin incision, the skin flap and the underlying temporalis fascia/muscle are elevated and reflected anteriorly as separate layers. According to the original description by Yasargil et al.,[5] an interfascial dissection of the temporalis muscle can be performed to preserve the frontal branch of the facial nerve.[6] Otherwise, the anterior retraction of temporalis muscle with the skin flap also can be performed, sparing the frontal branch of the facial nerve effectively.

The standard pterional craniotomy is usually slightly modified for the anterior skull base. The craniotomy is performed to be 2/3 frontal and 1/3 temporal (Fig. 16.2). An essential step of the approach is the high-speed drilling of the lesser sphenoidal wing and, even more important, the flattening of any ridge over the orbital roof to gain the necessary view on the midline.

After opening of the dura, by microsurgical technique, the sylvian fissure is sharply dissected and widely opened, and the optic-carotid cistern is fenestrated, allowing the further release of CSF and brain relaxation. With a minimal frontal lobe retraction, the tumor can be exposed and excised (Figs. 16.3 and 16.4).

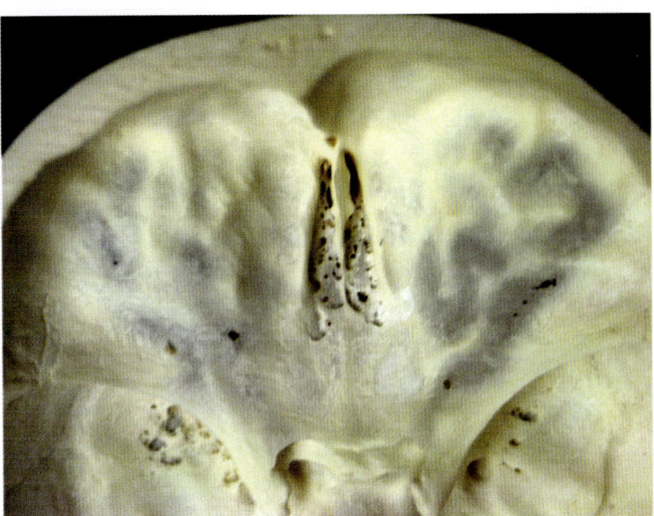

• **Fig. 16.1** Overview of bony landmarks of anterior cranial base as seen from an intracranial perspective.

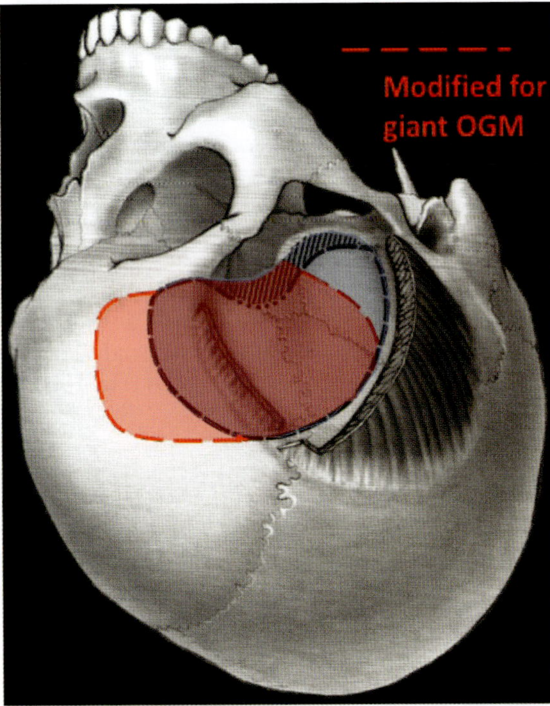

• **Fig. 16.2** Schematic drawing of a pterional craniotomy with slight modification for giant olfactory groove meningiomas. Red line demonstrates the area of craniotomy allowing transsylvian and subfrontal routes in the same approach.

Tumor Resection

Especially for meningioma of the olfactory groove, the typical lesion in the area, a minimal initial debulking of the lesion provides a better exposure of the basal dura through a transtumoral route.[7–9] Dural feeding arteries must be identified, coagulated, and divided. Tumor debulking is then performed. Internal carotid artery bifurcation is identified at the posterolateral aspect of the tumor, with subsequent identification of the anterior cerebral artery complex, ipsilateral carotid artery, optic chiasm, and both optic nerves. All these neurovascular structures must be carefully dissected and decompressed. Falx opening and crista galli drilling allows contralateral tumor control when using a unilateral approach and identification of contralateral olfactory nerve. The dorsal aspect of the tumor is eventually exposed and excised. When appropriate, the operating table can be tilted to change head rotation and, accordingly, to allow a better exposure of the contralateral distal anterior cerebral artery and the surrounding brain tumor interface.[7–9] In cases of optic canal involvement, this needs to be unroofed intradurally and the tumor removed (Video 16.1).

After tumor removal, the fronto-basal dura is cauterized and, when possible, reconstructed by using fascial graft or commercially available dura substitutes sealed with fibrin glue.

Subfrontal Transbasal Approach

This approach often combines maxillofacial and neurosurgical teams, and the details of the surgical technique have been described elsewhere.[10,11] In brief, with the head extended and fixed in a three-pin head holder, a modified zig-zag bicoronal skin incision is performed. The supraorbital nerves are dissected free; periorbital tissue, beneath both of the orbital roofs, is separated, and a bifrontal craniotomy is performed. Supraorbital and fronto-naso-orbital osteotomies are performed in addition to a bifrontal craniotomy including the frontal sinus. A two-piece osteotomy is obtained eventually. In all the cases the frontal sinus must be cranialized. With the aid of a surgical microscope, the dura of the anterior cranial base is dissected free from the underlying bone, and the dural basal vessels are then coagulated and divided. This step allows an early devascularization of the tumor. Therefore the dura is opened and the tumor excised by a standard microsurgical technique. The basal dura is resected, and after circumferential osteotomies, the cribriform plate is removed en bloc. Any hyperostotic or involved bone is drilled away. The mucosa of the sinus is then stripped until the sinus is cleaned out. After obtaining a good hemostasis, the dura is grafted by commercially available dural substitutes. Finally, the galeal-pericranial flap is secured with single sutures to the basal dura or, when applicable, to the basal bone lying on the frontal anterior fossa to carpet its floor. No additional structural support, such as bone graft, is needed.[11,12] A lumbar drainage is positioned immediately before surgery and can be kept in place for 5 days, allowing CSF drainage (approximately 50 mL every 8 hours). Prophylactic antibiotics are administered intravenously until the lumbar drainage is removed. Postoperatively, a mild compressive dressing is kept in place for 48 hours to avoid subcutaneous blood and fluid collection.

Supraorbital Approach

Introduced by Reisch and Perneczky[13] and van Lindert et al.,[14] the supraorbital approach has gained increasing success after several refinements.[13–18] The approach can be used to operate on most situations in which the classical pterional approach would be used. There are almost no craniotomy-related complications with this approach. Nevertheless, it is not suitable in certain lesions requiring a more temporal exposure.

The skin incision is performed along the eyebrow without shaving since previous studies have shown no increased risk of infection and better cosmetic result.[13–18] The medial limit of the skin incision is the notch of the supraorbital nerve that must be preserved to avoid bothersome numbness of the forehead. The incision is made through the skin and dermis, just superficial to the orbicularis oculi, pericranium, and temporalis fascia. This layer is important

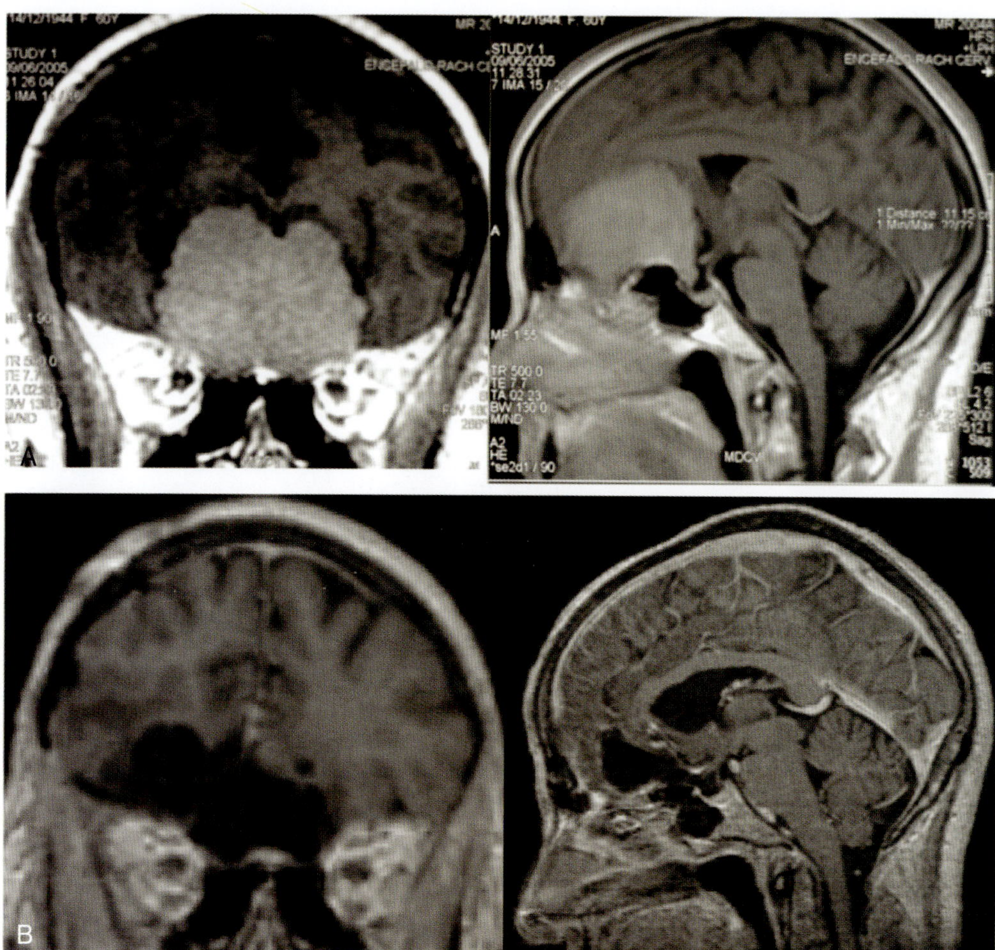

• **Fig. 16.3** (A) preoperative contrast-enhanced magnetic resonance imaging (MRI) in coronal and sagittal view of a huge olfactory groove meningioma. (B) postoperative contrast-enhanced MRI in coronal and sagittal view showing gross total removal with relative sparing of frontal lobes using a right pterional craniotomy.

for closure purposes as well as for an optimal cosmetic result. Dissection continues for approximately 1.5 to 2 cm superior to the supraorbital ridge. The pericranium is incised medially beginning lateral to the supraorbital nerve. Pericranial dissection continues in a "C"-shaped fashion extending approximately 1.5 to 2 cm superior to the supraorbital ridge and laterally to the superior temporal line. The pericranial flap is reflected inferiorly and retracted out of the way with a suture. The craniotomy is made after bluntly dissecting a small portion of temporalis muscle and fascia at the superior temporal line and drilling a burr hole on the lateral aspect of the exposure below the temporalis, for cosmetic reasons. Care must be taken not to cause damage to the frontalis branch of the facial nerve coursing in the temporalis fascia at this level.

The craniotomy is then performed. A first cut is done starting from the burr hole along the orbital rim up to just laterally to the supraorbital notch. The second cut, again starting from the lateral burr hole, makes a superior arch to meet the medial edge of the first cut. It is important to ensure a frontal craniotomy of at least 1.5 to 2 cm in width to avoid difficulties in manipulating micro-instruments. It is also important to identify any breach of the frontal sinus, because this can be a source of CSF leak if not adequately addressed. With this approach, the use of vascularized pericranial flaps to repair fistulas or reconstruct the skull base is precluded.

The dura is then dissected off the orbital roof. At this point, the inner table of the inferior edge of the craniotomy is drilled with any ridge of the orbital roof. This not only improves visualization, but also allows greater access of instruments during the procedure. The outer table is left intact to preserve cosmetics. The dura is opened and reflected inferiorly. The microscope is brought into the field, the frontal lobe is lightly retracted with a cottonoid, and the optic-chiasmatic cistern is opened to allow CSF egress to facilitate brain relaxation. At the end of the procedure, the dural leaflets are reapproximated and sutured in a running fashion. The craniotomy bone flap is repositioned with care to restore the supraorbital ridge. The pericranium and muscle flap are then closed primarily. Interrupted and absorbable sutures are used in the dermis, and a 5-0 Prolene suture is placed on the skin without any knots and removed in 7 to 10 days.

Complications and Management

Postoperative complications of anterior cranial fossa surgery can be classified as brain-related and non-brain-related. Most serious complications of cranial base surgery are brain-related,[19] and their prevention and management demand neurosurgical expertise.

Direct brain injury, contusion, or edema. Brain manipulation, especially from excessive or prolonged brain retraction, can lead

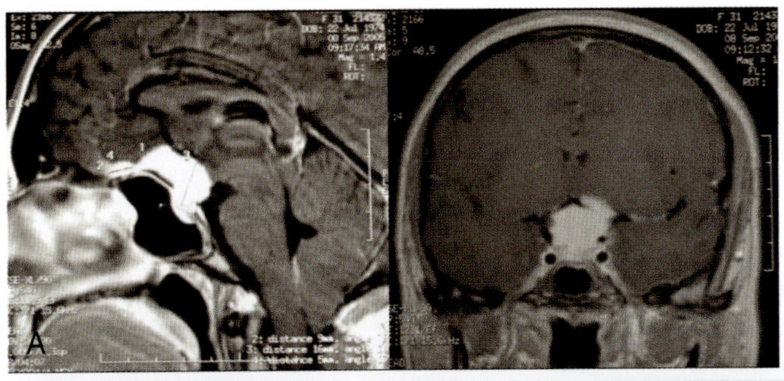

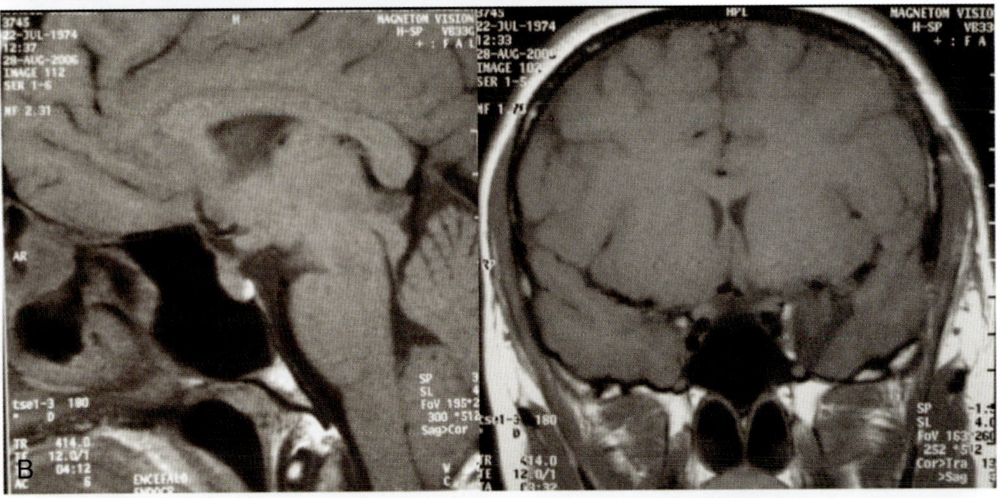

• **Fig. 16.4** (A) preoperative contrast-enhanced magnetic resonance imaging (MRI) in coronal and sagittal view of a tuberculum sellae meningioma with left A1 encasement. (B) postoperative contrast-enhanced MRI in coronal and sagittal view showing gross total removal using a right pterional craniotomy.

to cerebral edema or contusion and consequent dysfunction, which typically involves the frontal lobes. This can eventually result in a severe encephalomalacia and to stable deficits of speech, memory, and cognitive and intellectual functions.[8] Such injuries may also predispose to the occurrence of epilepsy. These complications can and must be avoided or minimized. Frontal lobe damage is best prevented by the combination of different techniques. One major issue is the use of self-retaining retractors for prolonged periods. In particular, the use of a unilateral approach on the right side may reduce the manipulation of the left frontal lobe while still allowing an early control of bilateral neurovascular structures.[8,9] Generally speaking, it should be considered that an optimal microsurgical technique allows progressive brain relaxation and access to the brain without a self-retaining retractor. Alternatively, a transbasal approach and craniofacial disassembly allow a lesser need for significant brain manipulation, but of course adding a risk for other complications. Of utmost importance is gaining space through intraoperative "brain relaxation" by positioning a lumbar drainage, early and wide opening of the cisterns, and using specific anesthesiology techniques including a totally intravenous anesthesia, neuroprotective agents, and hyperventilation.[20,21] Preoperative high-dose steroid administration would reduce the effects of brain manipulation.

Pneumocephalus may occur as a sudden event or as a gradual onset in the early postoperative period. An acute pneumocephalus may sometimes occur after a strain, for example after a patient's attempt to blow his or her nose, so insufflating air through the dural closure if the paranasal sinuses had been inadvertently opened and thus communicate with the intracranial compartment. A rapid-onset pneumocephalus may cause intracranial mass effect (tension pneumocephalus) with confusion and progressive neurologic deterioration. On the other hand, pneumocephalus may also develop slowly, that is, as a result of overdrainage of CSF from a lumbar spinal drain, with a siphoning effect drawing air upward from the nasal cavity. Preventive measures therefore include keeping patients intubated or tracheotomized until the patient is alert enough to follow instructions, and the judicious use of spinal drainage at a conservative rate and for short duration. In most patients after cranial base surgery, the lumbar catheter is allowed to drain 25 to 50 mL every 8 hours and is removed after 24 to 72 hours. When pneumocephalus is suspected, prompt computed tomography (CT) assessment is necessary. Small collections of air may simply be observed, whereas larger ones may require decompression, by re-exploration and reinforcement of the reconstruction. In cases of acute-onset pneumocephalus, administration of 100% oxygen is a useful adjunctive measure to enhance reabsorption of the intracranial air. Lumbar subarachnoid CSF drainage should be, clearly, discontinued.

CSF fistula is another rather common complication of anterior cranial fossa surgery. Infection is the unavoidable consequence of prolonged CSF leakage. CSF leak usually presents as clear rhinorrhea but may also cause the patient to complain of a salty taste in the throat. If there is doubt as to the nature of a nasal discharge, the presence of glucose and beta-2 transferrin assay may be used to confirm or rule out the presence of CSF. For small-volume leaks, which are by far more common, observation and continued spinal drainage (or serial lumbar spinal taps) are usually sufficient to stop the outflow. For high-volume leaks (grossly apparent rhinorrhea) or those that are persistent, careful sinonasal endoscopy and CT cisternography will be necessary to attempt to localize the fistula site (frontal, ethmoidal, sphenoidal), after which operative repair is frequently needed. In some situations, the original repair simply needs to be revised; in others, additional vascularized tissue may be needed to obliterate the fistula site. Such tissues may include temporalis muscle, galeal, or free microvascular flaps (i.e., rectus abdominis). In selected cases the closure may be augmented by the judicious use of free autogenous fat grafts or fibrin glue. The risk of reconstructive failure is substantially decreased if the original repair is done using vascularized local tissues. We strongly advocate the preventive preparation of a large galeal-pericranial flap.[11] If the frontal sinus is violated, the mucosa must be stripped and the posterior wall of the sinus drilled to cranialize the cavity. The pericranial flap is then reflected on the skull base and sutured to the fronto-basal dura as much posteriorly as possible. The empty spaces are then filled with fibrin sealant. This repair warrants a high probability of successful isolation of the intracranial compartment from the paranasal cavities.

Central nervous system infections, including meningitis and brain abscess, may also occur. These complications can lead to extreme neurologic morbidity or death. Preventive measures include the use of perioperative antibiotics, strict adherence to sterile technique, minimization of dural exposure to the aerial tract, and meticulous attention to reconstruction as outlined earlier. Treatment consists of antimicrobial agents (intravenously and sometimes intrathecally[22]) and surgical exploration when necessary to drain abscesses or to obliterate sources of continued bacterial contamination.

Cerebrovascular complications are the major concern in the perioperative period. These events may have several causes. Carotid pseudoaneurysmal rupture may occur as a result of excessive adventitial dissection. This complication is usually sudden and fatal and does occur intraoperatively. Nevertheless, it can occur postoperatively and may sometimes be preceded by a sentinel bleed, which, if recognized, can allow time for prompt treatment (re-exploration and bypass or permanent internal carotid artery [ICA] occlusion).

Thrombotic ICA occlusion or *embolism* into distal vessels can cause stroke and death. Careful surgical technique when working close to the ICA and cautious postoperative anticoagulation in high-risk patients may decrease embolic phenomena. Although the incidence of stroke in anterior cranial base surgery is low, it is a source of considerable morbidity when it does occur. We advocate the use of an anterolateral approach for an early identification of key vascular structures, which are important in very large tumors or in those extending in the parasellar area.

Morbidity can be reduced by an immediate and robust intervention and rehabilitation approach. Intervention after stroke occurrence should include control of hemodynamic factors affecting cerebral blood flow to prevent extension of the infarct. Surgical treatment includes a decompressive craniectomy if mass effect is evident and life-threatening. Essential medical measures include airway and oxygenation maintenance, fluid and electrolyte balance, and nutritional support.

Cranial nerve deficits. Sacrifice of olfactory nerves is a common complication of anterior cranial fossa surgery. It is often regarded as a minor disability, but anosmia can definitely impact the quality of life (i.e., patients no longer enjoy eating) and can even be a life-threatening condition because anosmic patients are unable to smell potentially dangerous odors, such as gas leaks or smoke. In the performance of a pterional or subfrontal approach, standard techniques may be insufficient to guarantee anatomic preservation of the olfactory nerve after frontal lobe elevation. Early identification and arachnoidal dissection of the nerve may reduce the rate of postoperative olfaction compromise. The opening of the subarachnoidal space should be performed in a postero-anterior direction to allow early visualization of the olfactory bulb and its dissection. The arachnoidal dissection should be performed with sharp instruments while avoiding any traction on the posterior portion of the olfactory tract. Such maneuvers allow for an overall mobilization of the nerve of 25 to 35 mm in length, which enables a greater degree of the frontal lobe retraction window up to 15 mm, while maintaining olfactory nerve integrity. Any compression exerted by the retractor should also be avoided to spare the microvasculature lying on the dorsal surface of the nerve.[23]

Deficits of cranial nerves II, III, IV, and VI lead to visual disability of variable degree, depending on the extent of surgical trauma and nerve involvement by the disease process itself. Dense palsies of the extraocular muscles seldom recover completely. Patients in whom such deficits are predictable should therefore be prepared for loss of binocular vision before surgery is undertaken. Loss of visual acuity is a potential complication of anterior cranial base surgery but is unusual unless the optic nerves are compromised preoperatively. In these patients, recovery of optic nerve function is difficult to predict.

SURGICAL REWIND

My Worst Clinical Case

A 38-year-old man was admitted for the treatment a huge recurrent anterior cranial base meningioma extending to the paranasal sinus (Fig. 16.5). The patient was operated on through a bifrontal craniotomy with a transbasal approach. The recurrent tumor and a newly diagnosed right clinoidal meningioma were removed in the same procedure. The anterior cranial base defect was reconstructed by means of a wide vascularized galeal-pericranial flap. The early postoperative period was uneventful. About 1 month later, the patient returned in an outpatient follow-up evaluation, declaring previous clear fluid dropping from the right naris with spontaneous resolution in a couple of days. Postoperative endoscopic endonasal exploration revealed good mucosal regrowth without clear signs of CSF leakage. 18 months later, the patient presented with bacterial meningitis requiring intensive care unit admission and management. The patient recovered with mild neurologic sequelae preventing full-time return to his job. After that episode a subclinical anterior cranial base CSF leak was suspected. Operation was simulated by virtual endoscopy, and the CSF leak point was hypothesized (Fig. 16.6 and Video 16.2). With the aid of intrathecal fluorescein injection, the CSF leakage point was identified and repaired by multilayer reconstruction using autologous and heterologous material. A Foley catheter was kept in place for 5 days to sustain the reconstruction and aid the sealing process (Video 16.3). At 1-year follow-up from the last operation, the patient does not present any CSF leak or other infective episodes, but he is still moderately disabled. The last MR scan does not reveal any recurrent or residual tumor (Fig. 16.7).

Continued

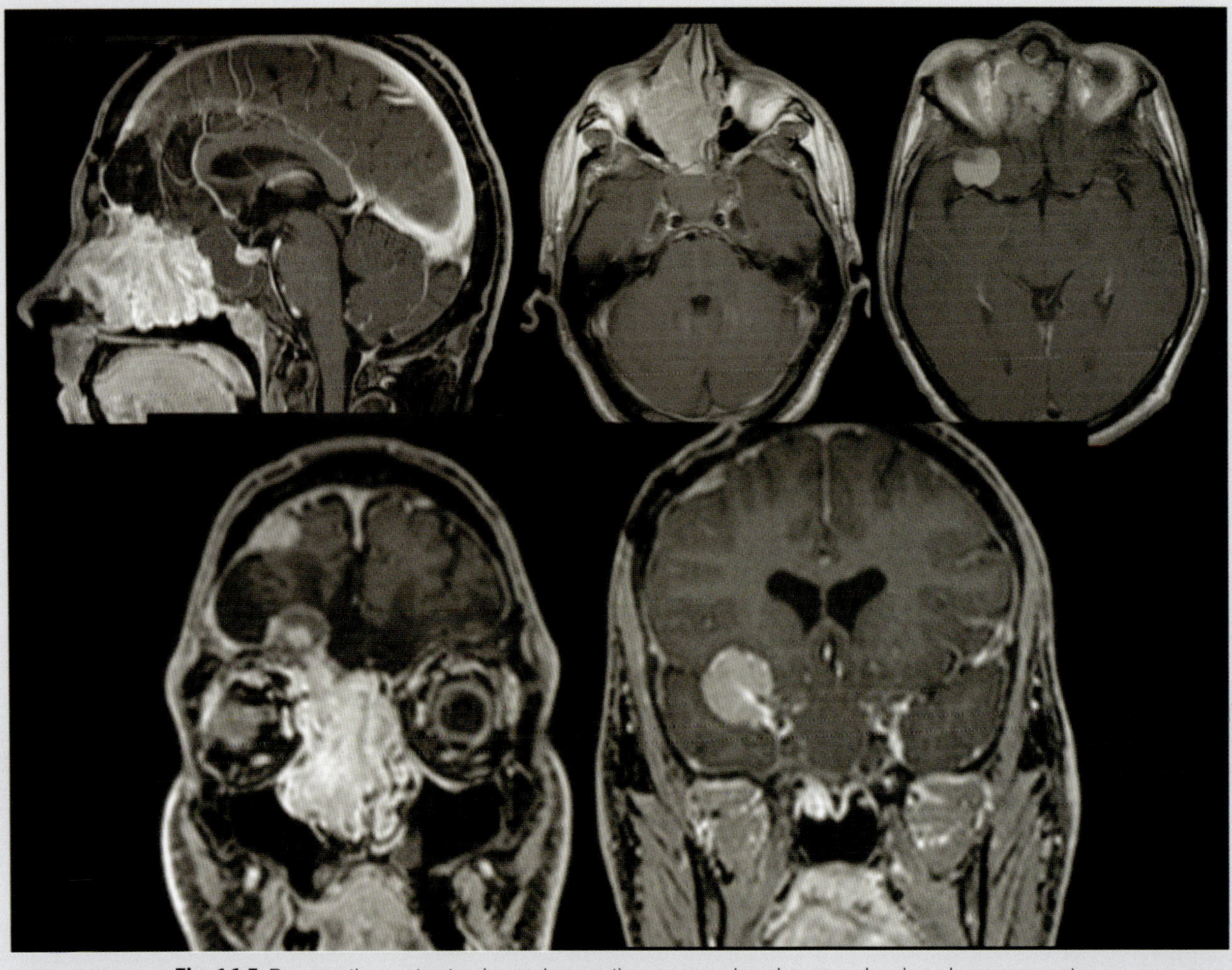

• **Fig. 16.5** Preoperative contrast-enhanced magnetic resonance imaging scan showing a huge recurrent anterior cranial base meningioma extending to the paranasal sinus and a right clinoidal meningioma.

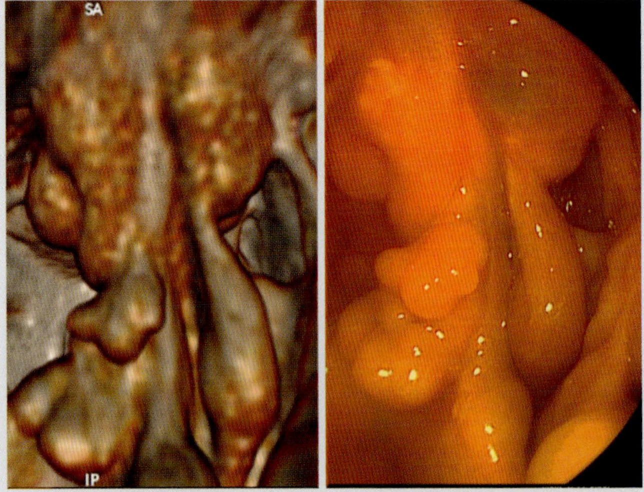

• **Fig. 16.6** Virtual endoscopy image (left) and intraoperative (right) picture demonstrating basic anatomy of anterior cranial base as seen from below.

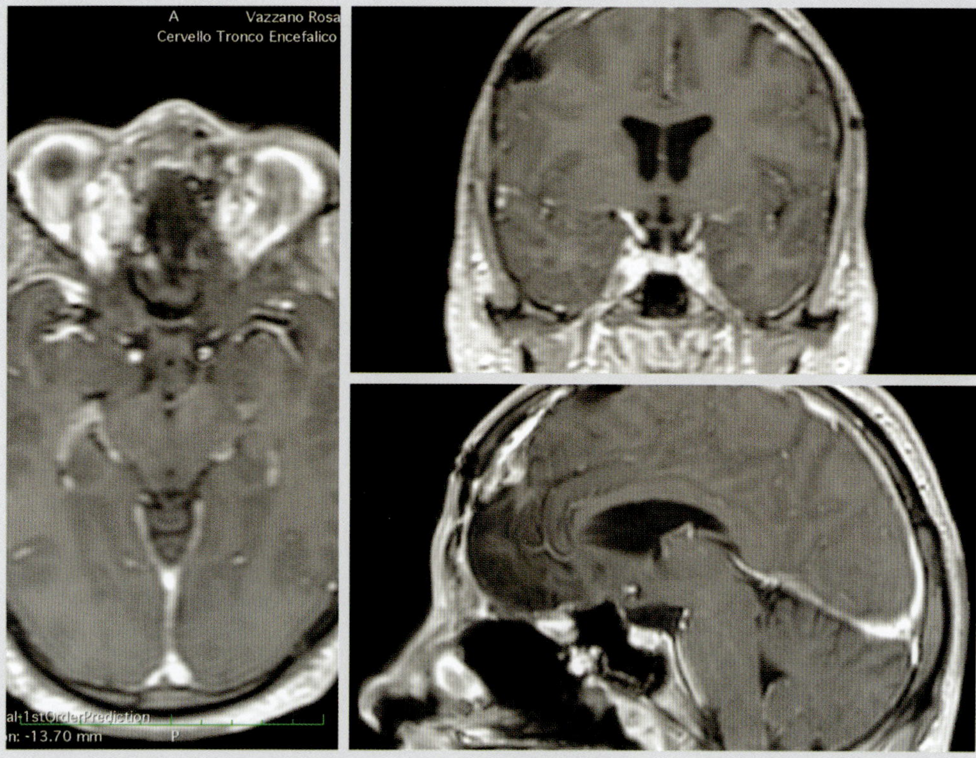

• **Fig. 16.7** Postoperative magnetic resonance imaging scan showing complete excision of the tumor and anterior cranial base reconstruction.

References

1. Ganly I, Patel SG, Singh B, et al. Complications of craniofacial resection for malignant tumors of the skull base: report of an international collaborative study. *Head Neck.* 2005;27(6):445–451.
2. Cushing H. *Meningiomas, Their Classification, Regional Behaviour, Life History and Surgical End Results.* Springfield, IL: Charles C. Thomas; 1938.
3. Morales-Valero SF, Van Gompel JJ, Loumiotis I, Lanzino G. Craniotomy for anterior cranial fossa meningiomas: historical overview. *Neurosurg Focus.* 2014;36(4):E14.
4. de Divitiis E, Esposito F, Cappabianca P, Cavallo LM, de Divitiis O. Tuberculum sellae meningiomas: high route or low route? a series of 51 consecutive cases. *Neurosurgery.* 2008;62(3):556–563, discussion 556–563.
5. Yasargil MG, Antic J, Laciga R, Jain KK, Hodosh RM, Smith RD. Microsurgical pterional approach to aneurysms of the basilar bifurcation. *Surg Neurol.* 1976;6(2):83–91.
6. Yasargil MG, Reichman MV, Kubik S. Preservation of the frontotemporal branch of the facial nerve using the interfascial temporalis flap for pterional craniotomy. Technical article. *J Neurosurg.* 1987;67(3):463–466.
7. d'Avella D, Salpietro FM, Alafaci C, Tomasello F. Giant olfactory meningiomas: the pterional approach and its relevance for minimizing surgical morbidity. *Skull Base Surg.* 1999;9(1):23–31.
8. Tomasello F, Angileri FF, Grasso G, Granata F, De Ponte FS, Alafaci C. Giant olfactory groove meningiomas: extent of frontal lobes damage and long-term outcome after the pterional approach. *World Neurosurg.* 2011;76(3–4):311–317, discussion 255–258.
9. Tomasello F, de Divitiis O, Angileri FF, Salpietro FM, d'Avella D. Large sphenocavernous meningiomas: is there still a role for the intradural approach via the pterional-transsylvian route? *Acta Neurochir (Wien).* 2003;145(4):273–282, discussion 82.
10. Feiz-Erfan I, Spetzler RF, Horn EM, et al. Proposed classification for the transbasal approach and its modifications. *Skull Base.* 2008;18(1):29–47.
11. Siniscalchi EN, Angileri FF, Mastellone P, et al. Anterior skull base reconstruction with a galeal-pericranial flap. *J Craniofac Surg.* 2007;18(3):622–625.
12. Romano F, Catalfamo L, Siniscalchi EN, et al. Complex craniofacial trauma resulting from fireworks blast. *J Craniofac Surg.* 2008;19(2):322–327.
13. Reisch R, Perneczky A. Ten-year experience with the supraorbital subfrontal approach through an eyebrow skin incision. *Neurosurgery.* 2005;57(suppl 4):242–255, discussion 242–255.
14. van Lindert E, Perneczky A, Fries G, Pierangeli E. The supraorbital keyhole approach to supratentorial aneurysms: concept and technique. *Surg Neurol.* 1998;49(5):481–489, discussion 9–90.
15. Cheng CM, Noguchi A, Dogan A, et al. Quantitative verification of the keyhole concept: a comparison of area of exposure in the parasellar region via supraorbital keyhole, frontotemporal pterional, and supraorbital approaches. *J Neurosurg.* 2013;118(2):264–269.
16. Dare AO, Landi MK, Lopes DK, Grand W. Eyebrow incision for combined orbital osteotomy and supraorbital minicraniotomy: application to aneurysms of the anterior circulation. Technical note. *J Neurosurg.* 2001;95(4):714–718.
17. Reisch R, Perneczky A, Filippi R. Surgical technique of the supraorbital key-hole craniotomy. *Surg Neurol.* 2003;59(3):223–227.

18. Telera S, Carapella CM, Caroli F, et al. Supraorbital keyhole approach for removal of midline anterior cranial fossa meningiomas: a series of 20 consecutive cases. *Neurosurg Rev*. 2012;35(1):67–83, discussion 83.
19. Janecka IP, Sen CN, Sekhar LN, Nuss DW. Facial translocation for cranial base surgery. *Keio J Med*. 1991;40(4):215–220.
20. Conti A, Iacopino DG, Fodale V, Micalizzi S, Penna O, Santamaria LB. Cerebral haemodynamic changes during propofol-remifentanil or sevoflurane anaesthesia: transcranial Doppler study under bispectral index monitoring. *Br J Anaesth*. 2006;97(3):333–339.
21. Iacopino DG, Conti A, Battaglia C, et al. Transcranial Doppler ultrasound study of the effects of nitrous oxide on cerebral autoregulation during neurosurgical anesthesia: a randomized controlled trial. *J Neurosurg*. 2003;99(1):58–64.
22. Cascio A, Conti A, Sinardi L, et al. Post-neurosurgical multidrug-resistant Acinetobacter baumannii meningitis successfully treated with intrathecal colistin. A new case and a systematic review of the literature. *Int J Infect Dis*. 2010;14(7):e572–e579.
23. Cardali S, Romano A, Angileri FF, et al. Microsurgical anatomic features of the olfactory nerve: relevance to olfaction preservation in the pterional approach. *Neurosurgery*. 2005;57(suppl 1):17–21, discussion 17–21.

17 Complications in Middle Cranial Fossa Surgery

AQUEEL PABANEY, VINAYAK NARAYAN, ANIL NANDA

HIGHLIGHTS

- The middle cranial fossa approach is a versatile skull base approach that is utilized to address small intracanalicular vestibular schwannomas, petroclival meningiomas, midbasilar/anterior inferior cerebellar artery aneurysms, and medial temporal bone lesions.
- Common complications encountered with the middle cranial fossa approach include facial palsy, seizures, cerebrospinal fluid leak, hearing loss from injury to the cochlea or labyrinth, and internal carotid injury.
- Complications can be avoided by use of lumbar drain, intraoperative monitoring, neuronavigation, and careful examination of patient imaging.

Introduction

The main indications for the middle cranial fossa (MCF) approach include removal of a small, predominantly intracanalicular vestibular schwannoma (VS), exposure of the labyrinthine and upper tympanic segments of the facial nerve for decompression, vestibular nerve section, and repair of superior semicircular canal dehiscence.[1] Historically, the MCF approach offers some of the highest hearing preservation rates, but it can also place the facial nerve between the surgeon and the tumor, potentially leading to a higher risk of postoperative facial weakness.[1,2] In some cases, this configuration results in the need for blind dissection. This route also requires some retraction on the temporal lobe, with the ensuing potential risk of postoperative seizures and speech disturbances, while providing a limited view of the cerebellopontine (CP) angle. The MCF approach is poorly tolerated by the elderly because extradural dissection of the adherent dura in this specific population may be difficult.[1] This approach is suggested for younger patients with smaller tumors that harbor the predominant component of their growth within the internal auditory canal (IAC). Specifically, tumors that involve the fundus of the IAC, a location to which access and visualization are restricted during the retrosigmoid trajectory, are good candidates for the MCF route.[3] Overall, the MCF approach provides a limited working window into the posterior fossa. This limitation is complicated by the presence of the facial nerve within the surgeon's view and restricts the surgeon's ability to resect large tumors. The retrosigmoid option, on the other hand, provides a more panoramic view of the tumor in the CP angle cisterns and its relationship to the surrounding neurovascular structures.[4]

Anatomic Insights

Several structures must be identified when utilizing the MCF approach. These structures include the arcuate eminence, the tegmen tympani, the greater superficial petrosal nerve (GSPN), the internal carotid artery (ICA), the middle meningeal artery (MMA) exiting the foramen spinosum, the mandibular division of the trigeminal nerve (V3) exiting the foramen ovale, the petrous apex (Kawase's quadrilateral space), and the true petrous ridge with superior petrosal sinus (SPS).

This approach is performed after a temporal craniotomy is completed.[2,5] Craniotomy is placed two-thirds in front of and one-third behind the IAC. An extradural approach is maintained, and the temporal lobe dura is elevated from the middle fossa floor in a posterior to anterior direction. It is important to avoid working from lateral to medial in the anterior aspect (i.e., medial to the root of the zygoma) to avoid inadvertently damaging or putting traction on the GSPN. The nerve lies in the major petrosal groove and is covered by a thin layer of periosteum. Working from lateral to medial across the floor in this area risks lifting the nerve out of the groove, potentially resulting in traction on the nerve and therefore the geniculate ganglion. This is a potential mechanism for facial nerve injuries in these approaches. Regardless of the dural elevation technique, it is critical to understand the GSPN location in the middle fossa floor and to leave the nerve in its groove, protecting it from inadvertent traction. Safe bone removal centers on properly identifying the orientation of the IAC, deep to the meatal plane and petrous ridge. A number of methods have been described for this elemental task. We prefer to visualize axis lines along the GSPN and the arcuate eminence. These axes form an angle, which is then bisected. The bisection line of this angle is an approximation of the IAC position in the bone.

RED FLAGS

- Anatomic variations (e.g., pneumatization of petrous bone)
- Dehiscent bone overlying the ICA
- Previous surgery or radiation therapy
- Dominant temporal lobe and inadequate relaxation of the brain

Prevention

Several maneuvers can be undertaken to avoid major complications in the MCF approach. First, a thorough study of the patient's computed tomography (CT) and magnetic resonance imaging (MRI) scans of the temporal bone should be undertaken and a morphometric analysis performed. Secondly, an intraoperative lumbar drain should be used to achieve optimal brain relaxation. Neuronavigation and neuromonitoring should be used generously to ascertain the location of the various neurovascular structures mentioned above. Drilling should be performed with plenty of irrigation to avoid heat-related injury to facial and vestibulocochlear nerves.

Facial Nerve Function Preservation

Facial nerve functional preservation serves as the best indicator of quality of life after VS resection by any route. The MCF approach is ideal for small, intracanalicular tumors that do not extend more than 1 cm into the CP angle.[1] The facial nerve can be damaged during this approach by making blind moves to dissect the tumor. During the MCF approach for larger tumors, the facial nerve is often located between the surgeon and the tumor; this topography places the facial nerve at a greater risk for damage. Use of neuromonitoring and the exercise of great patience and caution can yield excellent outcomes. The facial nerve can also be damaged due to inadvertent traction on the GSPN while elevating the dura off the MCF floor. The surgeon can minimize the risk of this type of injury by lifting the dura in a posterior-to-anterior direction. As mentioned above, thermal injury to the facial nerve can be prevented by generous irrigation while drilling.

Hearing Preservation

The MCF approach is preferable for hearing preservation in patients with smaller tumors (<1.5 cm extension into the CP angle).[1] The MCF approach provides a limited window into the posterior fossa, and the potentially blind dissection necessitated by the presence of the facial nerve in the surgeon's field of view may limit the resection of larger tumors and allow damage to the cochlear portion of cranial nerve VIII and its vasculature during resection.

CSF Leakage

CSF leak is a relatively common complication with any operative approach utilized to resect VS (retrosigmoid, MCF, or translabyrinthine). CSF leaks after the MCF approach can occur with concurrent violation of the tegmen tympani and dura, inability to pack the IAC appropriately after tumor resection with adipose tissue, or violation of mastoid or vestibular apparatus. CSF leak can be prevented by using bone wax to wax the air cells and by sealing all potential sites that could serve as fistulous connections for CSF egress.[1,6]

Postoperative Headache

Headaches are generally more common after the retrosigmoid approach compared with the MCF approach.[7] Patients usually complain of pain with chewing after the MCF approach due to temporalis muscle dissection. Avoiding use of electrocautery for muscle dissection and rather using instruments to elevate the muscle off the temporal bone, along with preservation of its periosteum and blood supply, can reduce postoperative pain with mastication. Some centers advocate giving patients chewing gum postoperatively to reduce edema and atrophy in the temporalis muscle.

SURGICAL REWIND

My Worst Case

A 53-year-old man is diagnosed with left petrous apex cyst after having the symptom of headache without any focal deficit. He was planned for surgery in view of his persistent symptom. He underwent left transzygomatic craniotomy and decompression of the cyst, and the procedure was uneventful. Postoperatively he developed left ptosis with LMN facial paresis (House-Brackmann grade IV) associated with reduced sensation on the left cheek. Postoperative imaging revealed a resolving cyst with good hemostasis. He was discharged with a steroid, artificial tears, and analgesic medications along with facial physiotherapy (preoperative and postoperative images are shown in Fig. 17.1).

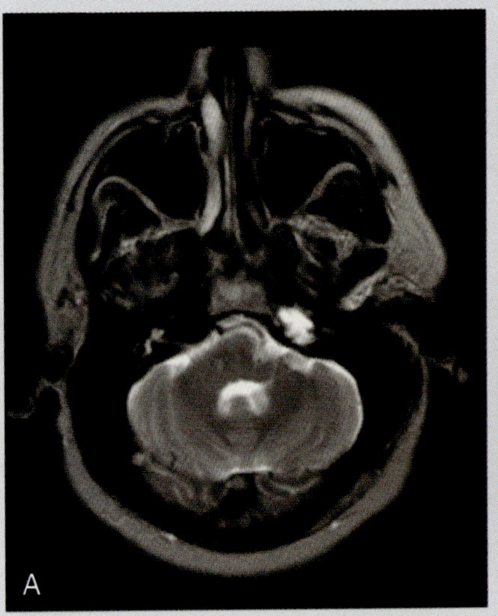

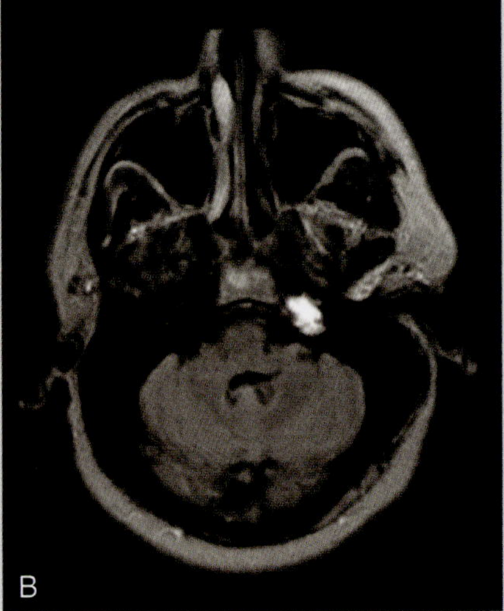

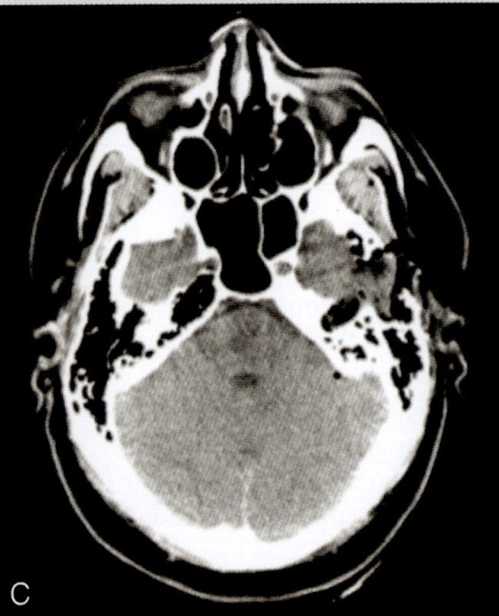

• **Fig. 17.1** (A) Preoperative T2-weighted MRI, (B) preoperative FLAIR MRI, and (C) postoperative CT imaging.

NEUROSURGICAL SELFIE MOMENT

Complications during the MCF approach are not uncommon but are avoidable if the above-mentioned precautions are kept in mind. The most common complications are secondary to technical errors or lack of anatomic familiarity. Facial nerve injury is the most devastating complication associated with this approach and can be prevented by careful patient selection, technical finesse, understanding of anatomy, and generous use of neuromonitoring modalities.

References

1. Ansari SF, Terry C, Cohen-Gadol AA. Surgery for vestibular schwannomas: a systematic review of complications by approach. *Neurosurg Focus*. 2012;33(3):E14.
2. Angeli S. Middle fossa approach: indications, technique, and results. *Otolaryngol Clin North Am*. 2012;45(2):417–438.
3. Lambert PR. House: "surgical exposure of the internal auditory canal and its contents through the middle cranial fossa." *Laryngoscope*. 1996;106(10):1195–1198.
4. Samii M, Matthies C. Management of 1000 vestibular schwannomas (acoustic neuromas): surgical management and results with an emphasis on complications and how to avoid them. *Neurosurgery*. 1997;40(1): 11–21.
5. Diaz Day J. The middle fossa approach and extended middle fossa approach. *Oper Neurosurg*. 2012;70(2 Suppl Operative):192–201.
6. Kulwin CG, Cohen-Gadol AA. Technical nuances of resection of giant (> 5 cm) vestibular schwannomas: pearls for success. *Neurosurg Focus*. 2012;33(3):E15.
7. Schessel DA, Nedzelski JM, Rowed D, Feghali JG. Pain after surgery for acoustic neuroma. *Otolaryngol Head Neck Surg*. 1992;107(3): 424–429.

18
Complications in Posterior Cranial Fossa Surgery

ROBERT S. HELLER, CARL B. HEILMAN

HIGHLIGHTS

- Posterior fossa meningiomas can completely encase or densely adhere to perforating arteries from the basilar artery and its branches. Dissecting small blood vessels from within a meningioma is extremely treacherous and can easily lead to disastrous results.
- Patients having received prior radiation therapy to a petroclival meningioma are likely to have significant adhesions between the meningioma and the brainstem. Attempting to dissect such a meningioma off the brainstem when adherent is fraught with danger.
- Take advantage of good dissection planes when able. However, do not attempt to dissect a completely encased or adherent perforating blood vessel out of a petroclival meningioma.

Background

Surgery within the posterior cranial fossa requires a detailed anatomic understanding of the relevant vascular and neural structures to minimize the risk of inadvertent injury. Dissection near or on vital neural structures must be performed delicately because undue tension can lead to traction injury on the brainstem. Inadvertent loss of a single perforating artery from the vertebrobasilar vasculature can lead to a brainstem infarct. Several studies have identified a low but consistent rate of postoperative brainstem infarction from 0.5% to 0.75% of cases.[1–3] Vascular complications remain the greatest source of permanent postoperative morbidity after surgery in the posterior fossa.[4] Though these are rare complications, the neurologic deficits they produce can be devastating.

Anatomic Insights

Neural

The posterior cranial fossa contains several vital neural structures that are relatively intolerant to excessive manipulation and trauma. Handling of the cerebellum should be performed gently to avoid contusion of the cerebellar hemisphere, which can result in uncontrolled swelling. Appropriate patient positioning, as described later, decreases venous congestion in the cerebellum and brainstem, thus aiding in retraction.

Knowledge of the course of the cranial nerves through the posterior fossa is important in predicting their location during surgery. Tumor resection within the posterior fossa often requires piecemeal removal of the target lesion while working in between the cranial nerves. The trigeminal nerve exits the pons on the anterolateral surface and moves rostrally toward Meckel's cave. The abducens nerve exits the brainstem at the pontomedullary sulcus and courses rostrally to Dorello's canal. The facial nerve, nervus intermedius, and vestibulocochlear nerve exit the ventrolateral brainstem adjacent to each other approximately 2 to 3 mm rostral to the glossopharyngeal rootlets and course laterally into the internal auditory canal. The glossopharyngeal, vagus, and spinal accessory nerves exit the medulla lateral to the inferior olive and course anteriorly toward the jugular foramen.[5] It is necessary to perform dissection and tumor removal in between these nerves to prevent unintended cranial nerve palsies.

Obtaining appropriate brain relaxation is key to reducing morbidity in posterior fossa surgery. Historically, many surgeons advocated for preoperative placement of a lumbar subarachnoid drain to achieve adequate cerebrospinal fluid drainage; this practice has been shown to slightly increase the risk of drain-associated complications without decreasing other operative risks.[6]

Advancements in inhalational and intravenous anesthetics, hyperosmolar therapy with mannitol and hypertonic saline, and moderate hyperventilation have all resulted in improved control of brain relaxation. Intraoperatively, piercing the arachnoid membrane covering the foramen magnum on the suboccipital surface of the cerebellum as a first step after dural opening facilitates significant cerebrospinal fluid egress and results in excellent brain relaxation.[7–9]

Arterial

The vertebral arteries join in the posterior fossa anterior to the brainstem to form the basilar artery. This junction occurs caudal to the level of the pontomedullary sulcus.[10] The last major branch of the vertebral artery is the posterior inferior cerebellar artery (PICA), which has an extradural origin in up to 20% of cases. Rhoton identified that the extradural PICA, unlike cases of intradural PICA origin, remained lateral and posterior to the medulla without providing a perforator branch to the anterior brainstem.[11]

The basilar artery runs along the ventral surface of the brainstem in the basilar sulcus before bifurcating into the posterior cerebral arteries at the level of the rostral mesencephalon. The major named arterial branches of the basilar artery are the anterior inferior cerebellar artery (AICA) and the superior cerebellar artery (SCA).[12] Either artery can have a duplicated origin, and the SCA may receive contribution from the posterior cerebral artery.[13]

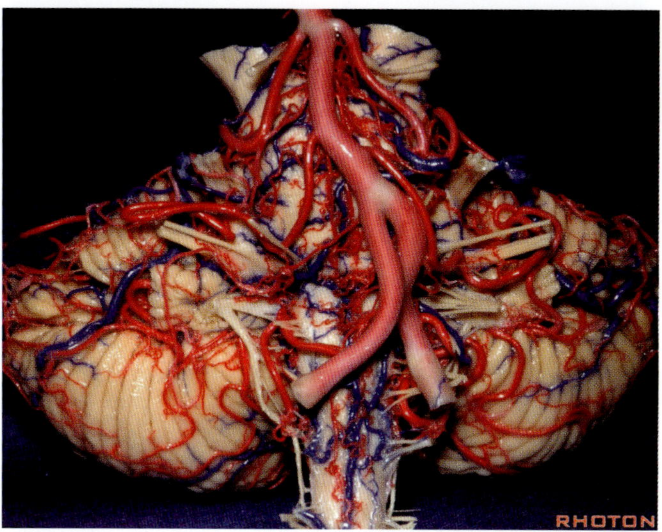

• **Fig. 18.1** Ventral view of the posterior fossa after anatomic dissection removing all of the bony anatomy. The basilar artery is anterior to the brainstem, with multiple small feeder vessels seen coursing toward the brainstem itself. Starting from rostral, cranial nerves III through XII are viewed as they exit the brainstem.

Anatomic studies of cadaveric specimens have identified wide variability in the number and caliber of small perforating arteries that arise from the basilar artery, AICA, and SCA (Fig. 18.1). Perforators off the basilar artery range in number from 5 to 20 with diameters from 80 to 940 mcm. These arteries are divided into short paramedian arteries that supply the medial brainstem and long circumferential arteries that supply the lateral brainstem. Importantly, all of these arteries arise from the dorsal surface of the basilar artery.[10,14,15] The variability among brainstem perforators and their parent vessels is matched by the finding that perforator arteries tend to penetrate the brainstem itself at relatively constant locations along the anterolateral surface.[16]

Ventral or ventrolateral displacement of the basilar artery from the basilar sulcus into the prepontine cistern is occasionally seen in cases of posterior fossa tumors extending to the midline. In these situations, the small perforator arteries emanating from the dorsal side of the basilar artery are stretched, and they can be encased within the tumor itself. Occasionally a meningioma will encase the basilar artery with much displacement. The presence of an arachnoidal plane separating the perforators from the meningioma is variable, but its presence does aid in careful dissection and preservation of these small arteries.

Venous

Venous drainage of the posterior cranial fossa consists of several anastomotic pathways, and sacrifice of small cerebellar draining veins to aid in retraction or visualization is generally considered to be a safe maneuver. The superior petrosal vein, also known as Dandy's vein, is found in the rostral aspect of the cerebellopontine angle as it courses toward its junction with the superior petrosal sinus. The superior and inferior petrosal sinuses are found within the dura along the petrous ridge and temporal bone, respectively, and as such do not usually pose as risks to surgery within the posterior fossa.

Ensuring adequate venous drainage during patient positioning is critical to lower venous pressure during surgery. Elevation of the head above the level of the heart using reverse Trendelenburg is useful for encouraging cerebral outflow and maintaining adequate venous drainage to the heart. Prevention of excessive flexion or rotation of the head and neck ensures patency of both jugular veins and also reduces venous congestion.[9]

RED FLAGS

- History of prior surgery
- History of prior radiation therapy
- Displacement of the basilar artery out of the basilar sulcus
- Peritumoral edema (T2/FLAIR hyperintensity in the adjacent brainstem and cerebellum)
- Cystic component of the tumor adjacent to the brainstem
- Circumferential encasement of posterior circulation arteries and their branches

Prevention

Careful preoperative planning is vital in prevention of posterior cranial fossa complications. Diligent study of preoperative neuroimaging can identify risk factors such as complete encasement of the basilar artery, encasement of AICA, encasement of SCA, or brainstem edema suggesting tumor adherence.

Management

Perforator Artery Injury

The small caliber of the perforator arteries emanating from the dorsal basilar artery precludes the option of direct suture repair in cases of injury. Arteries that have been severed should be coagulated to prevent free hemorrhage. Perforator arteries that are anatomically intact but bleeding from a small arteriotomy are not to be coagulated. Rather, hemorrhage should be controlled by direct pressure held over the point of injury using a hemostatic agent and possibly a cotton patty. Hemostatic agents such as Surgicel (Ethicon, Somerville, NJ) or Gelfoam (Pfizer, New York, NY) soaked in thrombin are effective adjuvants if needed. Once hemorrhage has been controlled, the surgeon should allow the artery to rest and can continue the operation at other sites. If the target pathology is adherent to a perforating artery or arteries, we advise cessation of resection before removing all gross pathology to prevent critical injury and ischemia.

Circumferential encasement of the posterior circulation arteries and their branches poses an additional surgical challenge. Occasionally these arteries are contained in a cleft surrounded by the tumor capsule that aids in dissection. Appreciation of the small branches emanating from the artery is easier in these cases, thus leading to a greater ability to preserve them. Full 360-degree encasement of an artery by tumor can lead to difficulty in determining whether small branches are tumor-feeder arteries or brainstem perforators, and sacrifice of these arteries carries risk.

In cases of a perforator artery that has been bluntly injured and is under vasospasm, the surgeon can apply papaverine directly to the artery to encourage continued blood flow and reduce the risk of ischemia. Risk factors for vasospasm include larger tumor size, prolonged operative time, and greater blood loss.[17]

Traction Injury to the Brainstem

Large tumors of the cerebellopontine angle and posterior cranial fossa often lead to deformation of the adjacent cerebellum and brainstem. Removal of these tumors is often fraught by the lack of a safe dissection plane between the tumor and the brainstem. Although peritumoral edema has been theorized to correlate with absence of a safe dissection plane between tumor and brainstem, one small report identified this finding to be correlated only with increased vascularity in the tumor bed and thus increased risk of postoperative hemorrhage.[18]

Aggressive tumor manipulation can lead to traction injury of the brainstem, or even dissection into the brainstem itself. Cystic vestibular schwannomas may have significant adhesions between the cyst wall and the brainstem and nerves, increasing the risk of injury to the adjacent structure.[19,20] In cases of pathologies with dense adhesions to the brainstem, dissection should be carried out using traction and countertraction. Using microbayonet forceps or a similar instrument, the brainstem is held in its anatomic position while the tumor is dissected away. This maneuver prevents undue manipulation and pulling on the brainstem.

Patients treated previously with radiation therapy have been documented to have an increase in number and severity of adhesions between the tumor capsule and the brainstem/cranial nerves in up to 69% of cases.[21] Residual or recurrent tumors undergoing surgery are also at higher risk of brainstem or nerve injury due to adhesions, which can be partially ameliorated by selection of a different operative approach than the initial operation.[22] Subtotal resection should be considered in cases of severe adhesions to avoid unintended neurologic injury.

SURGICAL REWIND

My Worst Cases

Case 1 (Fig. 18.2)

This patient is a 27-year-old man with a history of a left frontal "ganglioglioma with glioblastomatous changes" resected at the age of 18 months. He was treated with postoperative whole brain radiation therapy. This treatment left him developmentally delayed with a severe right hemiparesis, but throughout his life he was able to ambulate with a limp. He re-presented at the age of 24 years with a presumed radiation-induced clival meningioma. Clinically he had worsening headaches and mild bilateral sixth cranial nerve palsies. Neuroimaging confirmed a petroclival meningioma eccentric to the right measuring 3 cm in greatest diameter. There was

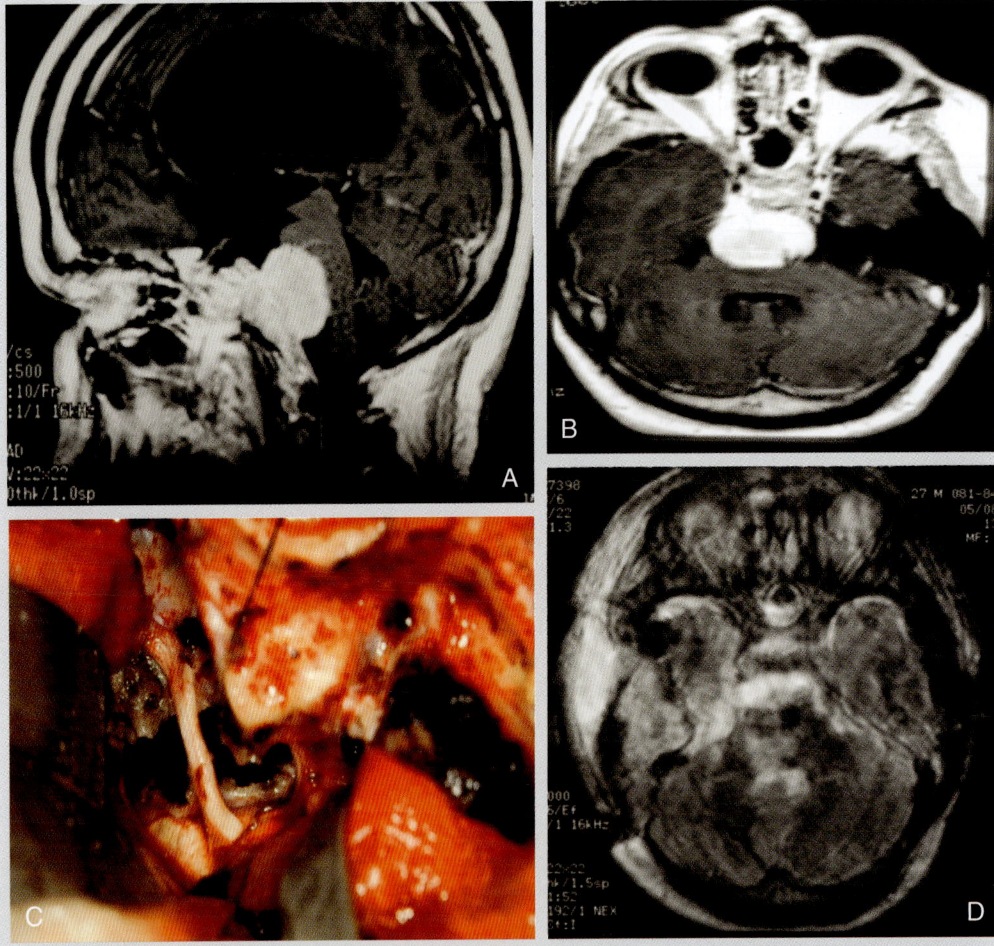

• **Fig. 18.2** Sagittal (A) and axial (B) post–gadolinium T1-weighted magnetic resonance (MR) images demonstrate a large petroclival meningioma with posterior displacement of the brainstem. Intraoperative photograph (C, rostral to the left) obtained at the completion of resection demonstrates the position of the trigeminal nerve and facial-vestibulocochlear nerve complex within the cerebellopontine angle. In between the trigeminal nerve and VII–VIII complex, a rim of tumor capsule is seen densely adherent to the surface of the pons. Postoperative T2-weighted axial MR (D, image quality degraded by patient motion) shows hyperintensity within the pons consistent with edema.

severe atrophy of the left midbrain peduncle. He was followed initially, but the tumor grew, and he developed increasing difficulty with ambulation. Surgery was recommended by a posterior transpetrosal approach.

During surgery the central aspect of the clival meningioma was debulked. There was significant arachnoidal thickening and adhesions in the prepontine cistern presumably due to the meningioma and prior radiation therapy. The tumor capsule was densely adherent to the belly of the pons and the basilar artery. I tried repeatedly to dissect the tumor capsule off the pons to achieve a complete resection. Ultimately but a little too late, I decided that this tumor could not be dissected off the ventral brainstem due to adherence of the meningioma to the pons.

Postoperatively, the patient failed to regain normal consciousness. He had an unreactive right pupil, a complete right ophthalmoplegia, and right decerebrate posturing. Neuroimaging showed no mass lesions but did demonstrate edema within the right side of the pons consistent with traction injury or perhaps perforator injury during the operation. Ultimately, he required tracheostomy and jejunostomy placement and was discharged to rehab on postoperative day 30. By 6 months' follow-up, his examination had improved to being awake and alert with the beginnings of functional movements of his left hand and leg. He died a few years later due to complications of pneumonia. He never regained the ability to ambulate.

Case 2 (Fig. 18.3)

A 55-year-old woman presented with headaches, paresthesias of the left face, and mild left facial weakness. Neuroimaging confirmed a left petroclival meningioma extending from Meckel's cave to the superior aspect of the jugular foramen with significant compression of the brainstem. There was edema of the left midbrain and pons. After careful discussion of the options, the patient was taken to the operating room for a left posterior transpetrosal approach. The posterior cerebral artery was partially encased and the SCA completely encased by the tumor. During surgery these vessels were both carefully dissected out of the tumor so that the superior aspect of the tumor capsule could be dissected off the brainstem to improve the extent of removal. Small vessels that had been parasitized by the meningioma were coagulated and divided. Postoperatively, the patient was slow to wake from anesthesia and initially had a left facial palsy and right hemiparesis. As she continued to wake, she demonstrated left-sided dysmetria and dysarthric speech. Neuroimaging showed an infarct in the dorsolateral midbrain (including the superior cerebellar peduncle) due to loss of a perforator branch off the left superior cerebellar artery. Although she can walk with assistance and is living at home, she remains unstable when ambulating and has left upper-extremity dysmetria and severely dysarthric speech.

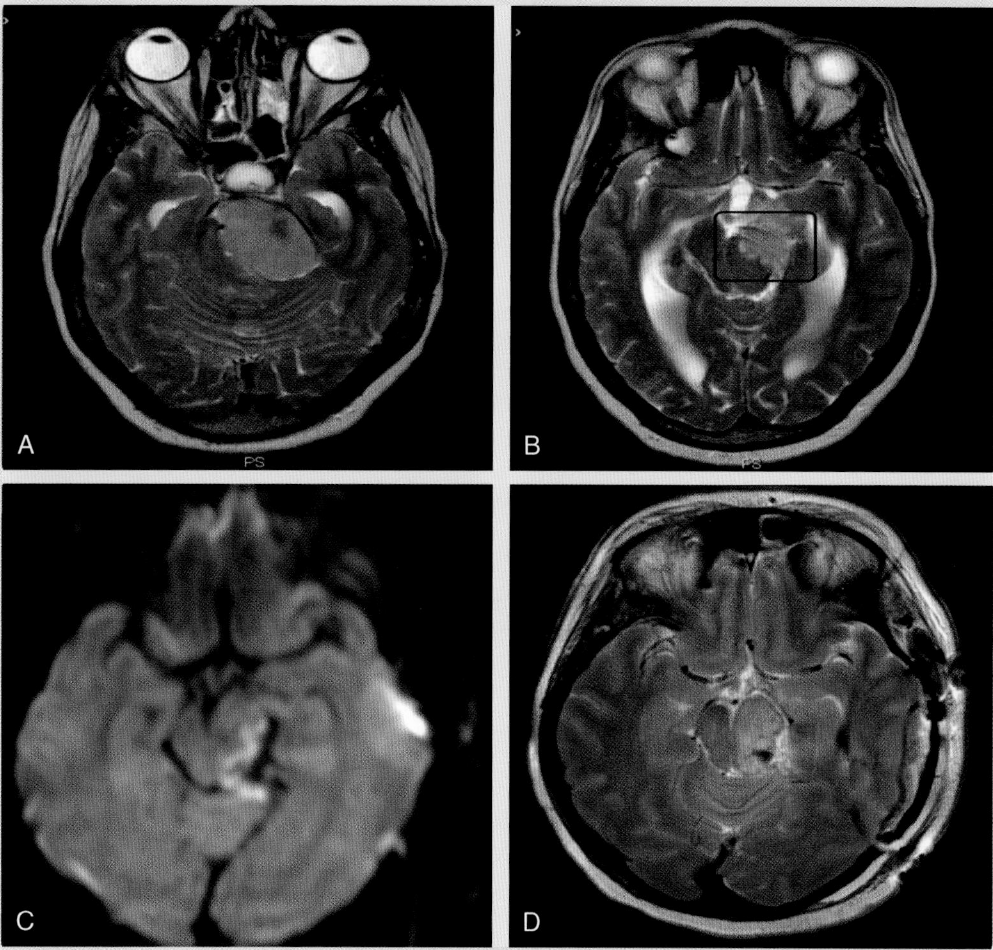

• **Fig. 18.3** Axial T2-weighted magnetic resonance (MR) images (A and B) of a case of petroclival tumor similar to that of the patient described in Case 2. Preoperative source images for Case 2 were not available for digitization. There is a large left petroclival meningioma with posterior displacement of the brainstem and internal calcifications (hypointensity in A). The posterior cerebral and superior cerebellar arteries are seen coursing through the middle of the tumor (B, black box). Postoperative diffusion-weighted MR sequence from the patient in Case 2 (C) demonstrates acute infarct and marginal ischemia in the midbrain and vermis. Axial T2 MR image (D) highlights significant edema with the entire left half of the midbrain.

NEUROSURGICAL SELFIE MOMENT

The surgical removal of a petroclival meningioma is extremely difficult. Constant internal deliberation or mental dialogue is required throughout the surgery about whether it is wiser to continue with the resection or stop with a subtotal resection. It cannot be overemphasized how difficult a decision this can be. On the one hand, there is no benefit of a small partial resection of a petroclival meningioma, often referred to as a "peek and shriek." If a surgical resection is undertaken, the brainstem should be decompressed. On the other hand, loss of a single brainstem perforator cannot be undone.

If small arteries are present within a cleft along the edge of a meningioma, it is reasonable to try to dissect these vessels off the tumor capsule so that a more complete tumor resection can be accomplished. However, if small arteries are completely encased within a posterior fossa meningioma, or if the plane along the vessel is poor, it is wiser to be satisfied with a subtotal resection. In cases where a meningioma is fused to the belly of the pons, perhaps due to prior radiation, the surgeon should be satisfied with a subtotal resection. The patient is the prize, not the postoperative magnetic resonance image.

References

1. Kunert P, Dziedzic T, Nowak A, Czernicki T, Marchel A. Surgery for sporadic vestibular schwannoma. Part I: General outcome and risk of tumor recurrence. *Neurol Neurochir Pol.* 2016;50:83–89.
2. Darrouzet V, Martel J, Enee V, Bebear JP, Guerin J. Vestibular schwannoma surgery outcomes: our multidisciplinary experience in 400 cases over 17 years. *Laryngoscope.* 2004;114:681–688.
3. Sade B, Mohr G, Dufour JJ. Vascular complications of vestibular schwannoma surgery: a comparison of the suboccipital retrosigmoid and translabyrinthine approaches. *J Neurosurg.* 2006;105:200–204.
4. Roche PH, Ribeiro T, Fournier HD, Thomassin JM. Vestibular schwannomas: complications of microsurgery. *Prog Neurol Surg.* 2008;21:214–221.
5. Rhoton AL Jr. The cerebellopontine angle and posterior fossa cranial nerves by the retrosigmoid approach. *Neurosurgery.* 2000;47:S93–S129.
6. Crowson MG, Cunningham CD 3rd, Moses H, Zomorodi AR, Kaylie DM. Preoperative lumbar drain use during acoustic neuroma surgery and effect on CSF leak incidence. *Ann Otol Rhinol Laryngol.* 2016;125:63–68.
7. Prabhakar H, Singh GP, Anand V, Kalaivani M. Mannitol versus hypertonic saline for brain relaxation in patients undergoing craniotomy. *Cochrane Database Syst Rev.* 2014;(7):CD010026.
8. Fang J, Yang Y, Wang W, et al. Comparison of equiosmolar hypertonic saline and mannitol for brain relaxation during craniotomies: a meta-analysis of randomized controlled trials. *Neurosurg Rev.* 2017;doi: 10.1007/s10143-017-0838-8.
9. Elhammady MS, Telischi FF, Morcos JJ. Retrosigmoid approach: indications, techniques, and results. *Otolaryngol Clin North Am.* 2012;45:375–397, ix.
10. Pai BS, Varma RG, Kulkarni RN, Nirmala S, Manjunath LC, Rakshith S. Microsurgical anatomy of the posterior circulation. *Neurol India.* 2007;55:31–41.
11. Fine AD, Cardoso A, Rhoton AL Jr. Microsurgical anatomy of the extracranial-extradural origin of the posterior inferior cerebellar artery. *J Neurosurg.* 1999;91:645–652.
12. Martin RG, Grant JL, Peace D, Theiss C, Rhoton AL Jr. Microsurgical relationships of the anterior inferior cerebellar artery and the facial-vestibulocochlear nerve complex. *Neurosurgery.* 1980;6:483–507.
13. Hardy DG, Peace DA, Rhoton AL Jr. Microsurgical anatomy of the superior cerebellar artery. *Neurosurgery.* 1980;6:10–28.
14. Mercado R, Santos-Franco J, Ortiz-Velazquez I, Gomez-Llata S. Vascular anatomy of the foramen of vicq d'azyr: a microsurgical perspective. *Minim Invasive Neurosurg.* 2004;47:102–106.
15. Marinkovic SV, Gibo H. The surgical anatomy of the perforating branches of the basilar artery. *Neurosurgery.* 1993;33:80–87.
16. Grand W, Budny JL, Gibbons KJ, Sternau LL, Hopkins LN. Microvascular surgical anatomy of the vertebrobasilar junction. *Neurosurgery.* 1997;40:1219–1223, discussion 1223–1215.
17. Rahimpour S, Friedman AH, Fukushima T, Zomorodi AR. Microsurgical resection of vestibular schwannomas: complication avoidance. *J Neurooncol.* 2016;130:367–375.
18. Samii M, Giordano M, Metwali H, Almarzooq O, Samii A, Gerganov VM. Prognostic significance of peritumoral edema in patients with vestibular schwannomas. *Neurosurgery.* 2015;77:81–85, discussion 85–86.
19. Thakur JD, Khan IS, Shorter CD, et al. Do cystic vestibular schwannomas have worse surgical outcomes? systematic analysis of the literature. *Neurosurg Focus.* 2012;33:E12.
20. Nair S, Baldawa SS, Gopalakrishnan CV, Menon G, Vikas V, Sudhir JB. Surgical outcome in cystic vestibular schwannomas. *Asian J Neurosurg.* 2016;11:219–225.
21. Nonaka Y, Fukushima T, Watanabe K, Friedman AH, Cunningham CD 3rd, Zomorodi AR. Surgical management of vestibular schwannomas after failed radiation treatment. *Neurosurg Rev.* 2016;39:303–312, discussion 312.
22. Freeman SR, Ramsden RT, Saeed SR, et al. Revision surgery for residual or recurrent vestibular schwannoma. *Otol Neurotol.* 2007;28:1076–1082.

19

Complications of Chiari Malformation Surgery

ANIL NANDA, BHAVANI KURA

HIGHLIGHTS

- Watertight dural closure and careful wound closure in multiple layers are imperative to prevent cerebrospinal fluid leak and pseudomeningocele.
- Avoid vascular or brainstem injury with sharp, midline dissection within the subarachnoid space and with the judicious lysis of adhesions.
- Prompt treatment of cerebrospinal fluid leak, infection, or hydrocephalus can prevent further complications.

Background

Three types of Chiari malformations were described by Hans Chiari (1851–1916) in 1891,[1,2] and half a century later in 1950, W. James Gardner described the surgical treatment by posterior fossa decompression (PFD).[3] After yet another half century, the pathogenesis of the disease remains unclear. Although bony decompression for Chiari malformations is routine, there is still no consensus on the optimal surgical techniques, which may or may not include dural opening, expansile duraplasty, use of autologous or synthetic graft, arachnoid opening and dissection, and tonsillar reduction.[4–7] Patients have 70.3% clinical improvement postoperatively whether or not the surgery included duraplasty.[8] The reported rate of complications ranges from 2.4% to greater than 20% in various studies, and the complications can vary based on the invasiveness of the surgery.[9–13] There has been no direct comparison of posterior fossa decompression with duraplasty (PFDD) and without duraplasty (PFD), but several studies and a metaanalysis indicate that patients who underwent PFD had a higher reoperation rate but a lower rate of cerebrospinal fluid (CSF) related complications than those who underwent PFDD.[8,13–15] CSF leak or pseudomeningocele is typically the most common complication when duraplasty is performed, but others include wound infection, meningitis, hydrocephalus, need for reoperation, craniocervical instability, and cerebellar sag.

Anatomic Insights

Inside the dura and arachnoid, the cerebellar tonsils are visible bilaterally and the uvula superiorly. The tela choroidea and inferior medullary velum make up the inferior part of the roof of the fourth ventricle and can be seen when the tonsils are retracted laterally.[16] The posterior inferior cerebellar artery (PICA) has a complicated and variable course. It usually arises from the vertebral artery but can arise from the basilar artery; it may also be absent on one side, or duplicate. The location of the origin may vary as well from the extradural vertebral artery below the foramen magnum to the vertebrobasilar junction.[17,18] It travels dorsally around the medulla and passes by, or through, the hypoglossal, glossopharyngeal, vagus, and accessory nerves, then enters the cerebellomedullary fissure, making a caudal loop at the inferior pole of the tonsil.[19] The caudal loop of the PICAs is noted to be inferiorly displaced in angiograms performed on patients with Chiari malformation, due to the tonsillar herniation.[20,21] Perforating arteries arise from the PICA as it passes around the medulla. Vermian branches of PICA or the tonsils sometimes lie in a more medial position and cause obstruction of the foramen of Magendie.[22]

Risk Factors

Several factors predict favorable or unfavorable outcomes after PFD for Chiari malformation. Young age at time of surgery and signs of paroxysmal intracranial hypertension are associated with favorable outcomes. Better preoperative status also indicates a better prognosis.[12] Prior history of Chiari decompression, arachnoiditis, older age at time of surgery, and long-tract signs are associated with unfavorable outcomes.[12,23] Young age at the time of initial surgery, complex bony foramen magnum anatomy, and syndromic craniosynostosis are associated with reoperation.[24]

Several studies have found associations between the type of dural graft used and frequency of need for reoperation, CSF leak, and aseptic meningitis, but the results have varied from study to study, and more optimal results have been reported for both allogenic and autologous graft materials.[25,26] Untreated hydrocephalus is associated with increased incidence of CSF leak or pseudomeningocele. Klippel-Feil syndrome, atlantoaxial assimilation, and basilar invagination can be predictive of craniocervical instability.[10,27]

Prevention

Imaging should be examined closely preoperatively. Surgeons can get an idea of the extent of bone removal required. The torcular and transverse sinuses may be low-lying, especially in Chiari II malformation, and should be avoided during bone removal. Hydrocephalus, which can contribute to a higher rate of CSF leak, can be treated with CSF diversion before a decompression. Anomalies associated with Chiari malformation—Klippel-Feil syndrome, atlantoaxial assimilation, and basilar invagination—can indicate possible craniocervical instability.[10,27] Some surgeons routinely obtain preoperative cervical x-rays. Patients may need posterior occipitocervical stabilization, possibly preceded by ventral decompression. Instability should also be kept in mind postoperatively because rapid treatment can prevent neurologic damage.

Adequate bone removal at the foramen magnum, and possible duraplasty and careful arachnoid exploration and dissection, may prevent the persistence or recurrence of symptoms. If a duraplasty is not performed, the dural band at the foramen magnum and outer dural layer should be incised to help prevent the need for reoperation. Intraoperative ultrasound can also help identify whether additional decompression is required.[28] If the dura is opened, blood and debris should be kept out of the subarachnoid space because they could lead to aseptic meningitis or adhesions and scar formation. Arachnoid dissection should be limited to the midline and should be sharp only, to avoid damaging perforators and cranial nerves. For the same reason, tonsillar reduction should be limited to coagulation or subpial removal rather than resection. Rather than cause brainstem injury by manipulation of the medulla and obex, dense adhesions between the tonsils and brainstem may need to be left in place.[9]

The dural graft should be carefully sutured in a watertight fashion; a Valsalva maneuver after closure can help identify gaps in the closure. Meticulous closure of the fascia and soft tissues also helps prevent CSF leak. If a CSF leak occurs postoperatively, the incision can initially be resutured and managed conservatively, but imaging to assess for hydrocephalus should be obtained if the problem persists. Timely treatment of a CSF leak can help prevent postoperative infection. Preoperative antibiotics, intraoperative sterile technique, and management of risk factors such as diabetes should be standard for infection prevention, as well as prompt treatment when an infection is identified. A postoperative infection can lead to a possible recurrence of preoperative symptoms due to inflammation and subsequent scarring.[29]

Management

Intraoperatively, the transverse sinus may be lacerated during the craniectomy. Additional bone removal may be needed to better visualize the injury, which can be repaired by suturing with a small piece of muscle. Dural venous lakes can be clipped to stop bleeding.[28] An operative site hemorrhage large enough to necessitate reoperation for hematoma evacuation rarely occurs but is a consideration with a poor postoperative neurologic examination.[30]

Patients may develop fever, headache, nausea, vomiting, and malaise postoperatively. A lumbar puncture should be done to send CSF for culture, and antibiotics may be started. Aseptic meningitis can occur as a result of irritation from blood and debris; it is generally treated with symptomatic management and steroids after bacterial meningitis has been ruled out. If bacterial meningitis or wound infection is diagnosed, in addition to antibiotics, treatment may require replacement of the dural graft.[28] The type of graft used for duraplasty has been linked to the incidence of need for reoperation, CSF leak, and aseptic meningitis, but varying results have been reported for different dural grafts with regard to these complications.[25,26]

CSF leak and pseudomeningocele are the most commonly observed complications. Even if the arachnoid is not intentionally opened intraoperatively, it can be torn during dural opening, and CSF leaks can still occur.[9] Initially, a leak can be managed conservatively with a dressing and additional sutures, but if the leak persists, imaging should be obtained and examined for hydrocephalus. If hydrocephalus is present, it must be treated with CSF diversion, or the leak will persist. In the absence of hydrocephalus, a leak can be treated with lumbar drainage and/or reoperation with revision of the duraplasty and improved soft tissue closure.[31] A pseudomeningocele similarly can be treated with conservative measures at first if there is no evidence of hydrocephalus, and small pseudomeningoceles may resolve without any intervention. With a persistent pseudomeningocele, the duraplasty should be repaired or replaced. Hydrocephalus can also present after a PFD without an accompanying CSF leak and can be delayed months postoperatively.[9] It may be possible to observe for development of symptoms, but placement of a shunt should be performed for symptomatic patients or those with worsening imaging findings.

When the preoperative symptoms persist or recur, imaging should be obtained. Mild recurrent symptoms may be followed initially. If compression is still evident on magnetic resonance imaging (MRI), reoperation is likely needed. Based on the imaging and intraoperative findings and the extent of the initial surgery, the second surgery could include additional bone removal, a more expansile duraplasty, wide lysis of adhesions, and coagulation of the tonsils.[30] Reoperation can be technically challenging due to adhesions and scar formation, and intraarachnoid dissection must be performed meticulously.

An overly aggressive decompression can lead to the rare complication of cerebellar sag, in which the cerebellum herniates into the area of decompression when the craniectomy extends too far laterally.[28,30,32] Patients present with symptoms of cerebellar or brainstem compression or return of syrinx several weeks to months postoperatively. For patients with signs of increased intracranial pressure, the surgical treatment includes placement of a ventriculopleural shunt. The other intervention is a revision with cranioplasty to partially reconstruct the posterior fossa. Occasionally, both are required.

Patients presenting with pain and progressive neurologic deficits after Chiari decompression may have craniocervical instability evident on MRI and cervical x-rays. Surgical treatment involves occipitocervical fusion stabilization.

SURGICAL REWIND

My Worst Case

A 45-year-old woman presented to the clinic with headaches due to Chiari I malformation (Fig. 19.1A). She underwent suboccipital craniectomy and C1 laminectomy. She developed a CSF leak, which was repaired in the operating room and also treated with lumbar drainage. With continued leak, the patient had a ventriculoperitoneal shunt placed for hydrocephalus. She had resolution of her preoperative headaches but began to complain of radicular pain and paresthesias, then weakness and difficulty walking. Her imaging revealed a cervicothoracic syrinx that increased in size and adhesions with crowding of the foramen magnum (Fig. 19.1B and C). She underwent redo decompression and C1,2 laminectomy, which was technically difficult due to scarring. Her postoperative head computed tomography (CT) (Fig. 19.1D) revealed intraventricular hemorrhage (IVH). She had respiratory difficulty and eventually required intubation, but initially she was neurologically stable. After a decline in mental status, a head CT was obtained and an external ventricular drain (EVD) was placed for hydrocephalus. Her mental status improved and the EVD was later removed, but the patient could not be taken off the ventilator and required tracheostomy. She later returned to the hospital because of decreased responsiveness, and another EVD was placed for recurrent hydrocephalus seen on head CT. She developed IVH after the EVD placement. Her neurologic status remained poor despite continued treatment, and eventually the family chose to withdraw care.

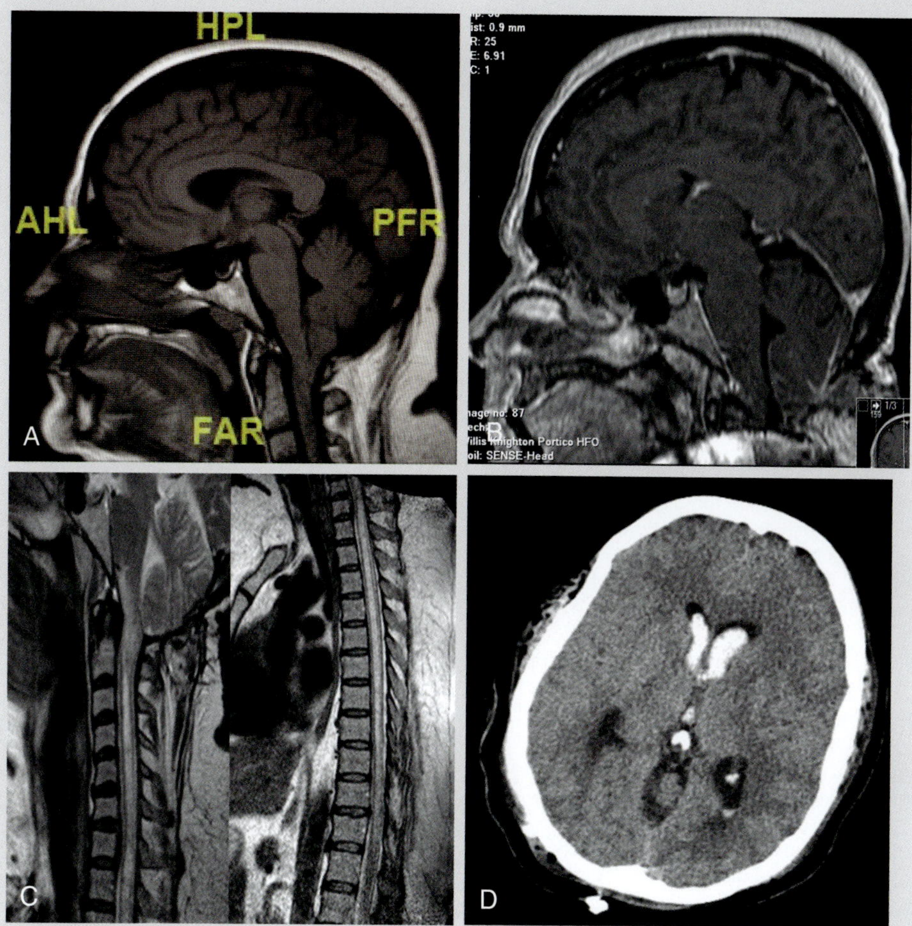

• **Fig. 19.1** Preoperative brain magnetic resonance image (MRI) (A) showing Chiari I malformation. Brain MRI (B) and cervical and thoracic spine MRIs (C) showing extensive syrinx before redo decompression. Postoperative head computed tomography scan (D) with intraventricular hemorrhage after second decompression surgery.

NEUROSURGICAL SELFIE MOMENT

Patients undergoing decompression surgery for Chiari malformations can have multiple complications. With preoperative planning and careful intraoperative technique, poor outcomes can often be avoided. Complications can still occur, but their rapid diagnosis and treatment are essential to preventing exacerbation and the development of further problems.

References

1. Massimi L, Peppucci E, Peraio S, Di Rocco C. History of Chiari type I malformation. *Neurol Sci*. 2011;32(suppl 3):S263–S265.
2. Loukas M, Noordeh N, Shoja MM, Pugh J, Oakes WJ, Tubbs RS. Hans Chiari (1851-1916). *Childs Nerv Syst*. 2008;24:407–409.
3. Gardner WJ, Goodall RJ. The surgical treatment of Arnold-Chiari malformation in adults: an explanation of its mechanism and importance of encephalography in diagnosis. *J Neurosurg*. 1950;7(3):199–206.
4. Haroun RI, Guarnieri M, Meadow JJ, Kraut M, Carson BS. Current opinions for the treatment of syringomyelia and Chiari malformations: survey of the Pediatric Section of the American Association of Neurological Surgeons. *Pediatr Neurosurg*. 2000;33(6):311–317.
5. Schijman E, Steinbok P. International survey on the management of Chiari I malformation and syringomyelia. *Childs Nerv Syst*. 2004; 20(5):342–348.
6. Javalkar V, Nanda A. Congenital Chiari malformations. In: Nanda A, ed. *Principles of Posterior Fossa Surgery*. New York, NY: Thieme; 2012:57–67.
7. Alden TD, Ojemann JG, Park TS. Surgical treatment of Chiari I malformation: indications and approaches. *Neurosurg Focus*. 2001;11(1):1–5.
8. Durham SR, Fjeld-Olenec K. Comparison of posterior fossa decompression with and without duraplasty for the surgical treatment of

Chiari malformation type I in pediatric patients: a meta-analysis. *J Neurosurg Ped*. 2008;2:42–49.
9. Klekamp J. Surgical Treatment of Chiari I malformation – analysis of intraoperative findings, complications, and outcome for 371 foramen magnum decompressions. *Neurosurg*. 2012;71(2):365–380.
10. Tubbs RS, Beckman J, Naftel RP, et al. Institutional experience with 500 cases of surgically treated pediatric Chiari malformation type I. *J Neurosurg Pediatr*. 2011;7(3):248–256.
11. McGirt MJ, Garces-Ambrossi GL, Parker S, et al. Primary and revision suboccipital decompression for adult Chiari I malformation: analysis of long-term outcomes in 393 patients: 924. *Neurosurg*. 2009;65(2):408–409.
12. Aghakhani N, Parker F, David P, et al. Long-term follow-up of Chiari-related syringomyelia in adults: analysis of 157 surgically treated cases. *Neurosurgery*. 2009;64(2):308–315, discussion 315.
13. Hankinson TC, Tubbs RS, Oakes WJ. Surgical decision-making and treatment options for Chiari malformations in children. In: Quinones-Hinojosa A, ed. *Schmidek & Sweet Operative Neurosurgical Techniques: Indications, Methods, and Results*. 6th ed. Philadelphia, PA: Elsevier/Saunders; 2012:695–700.
14. Lu VM, Phan K, Crowley SP, Daniels DJ. The addition of duraplasty to posterior fossa decompression in the surgical treatment of pediatric Chiari malformation type I: a systematic review and meta-analysis of surgical and performance outcomes. *J Neurosurg Ped*. 2017; 20(5):439–449.
15. Forander P, Sjavik K, Solheim O, et al. The case for duraplasty in adults undergoing posterior fossa decompression for Chiari I malformation: a systematic review and meta-analysis of observational studies. *Clin Neurol and Neurosurg*. 2014;125:58–64.
16. Cavalcanti DD, Preul MC, Kalani YS, Spetzler RF. Microsurgical anatomy of safe entry zones to the brainstem. *J Neurosurg*. 2016;124:1359–1376.
17. Rhoton AL. The cerebellar arteries. *Neurosurgery*. 2000;47(suppl 3): S29–S68.
18. Rhoton AL. The foramen magnum. *Neurosurgery*. 2000;47(suppl 3): S155–S193.
19. Matsushima K, Yagmurlu K, Kohno M, Rhoton AL. Anatomy and approaches along the cerebellar-brainstem fissures. *J Neurosurg*. 2016;124:248–263.
20. Mascitelli JR, Ben-Haim S, Paramasivam S, Zarzour HK, Rothrock RJ, Bederson JB. Association of a distal intradural-extracranial posterior inferior cerebellar artery aneurysm with Chiari type I malformation: case report. *Neurosurg*. 2015;77:660–665.
21. Rhoton AL. Microsurgery of Arnold-Chiari malformation in adults with and without hydromyelia. *J Neurosurg*. 1976;45(5):473–483.
22. Dlouhy BJ, Dawson JD, Menezes AH. Intradural pathology and pathophysiology associated with Chiari I malformation in children and adults with and without syringomyelia. *J Neurosurg Pediatr*. 2017;20(6):526–541.
23. Chotai S, Medhkour A. Surgical outcomes after posterior fossa decompression with and without duraplasty in Chiari malformation-I. *Clin Neur and Neurosurg*. 2014;125:182–188.
24. Sacco D, Scott RM. Reoperation for Chiari malformations. *Pediatr Neurosurg*. 2003;39:171–178.
25. Parker SR, Harris P, Cummings TJ, George T, Fuchs H, Grant G. Complications following decompression of Chiari malformation type I in children: dural graft or sealant? *J Neurosurg Ped*. 2011;8:177–183.
26. Attenello FJ, McGirt MJ, Garces-Ambrossi GL, Chaichana KL, Carson B, Jallo GI. Suboccipital decompression for Chiari I malformation: outcome comparison of duraplasty with expanded polytetrafluoroethylene dural substitute versus pericranial graft. *Childs Nerv Syst*. 2009;25:183–190.
27. Smith JS, Shaffrey CI, Abel MF, Menezes AH. Basilar invagination. *Neurosurg*. 2010;66(suppl 3):A39–A47.
28. Menezes AH. Chiari I malformations and hydromyelia – complications. *Pediatr Neurosurg*. 1991-92;17:146–154.
29. Heiss J, Oldfied EH. Management of Chiari malformations and syringomyelia. In: Quinones-Hinojosa A, ed. *Schmidek & Sweet Operative Neurosurgical Techniques: Indications, Methods, and Results*. 6th ed. Philadelphia, PA: Elsevier/Saunders; 2012:2072–2080.
30. Mazzola CA, Fried AH. Revision surgery for Chiari malformation decompression. *Neurosurg Focus*. 2003;15(3):1–8.
31. Dubey A, Sung WS, Shaya M, et al. Complications of posterior cranial fossa surgery – an institutional experience of 500 patients. *Surg Neurol*. 2009;72(4):369–375.
32. Tubbs RS, Oakes WJ. Syringomyelia, Chiari malformations and hydromyelia. In: Youmans JR, Winn HR, eds. *Youmans and Winn Neurological Surgery*. Philadelphia, PA: Elsevier/Saunders; 2011:1531–1540.

20

Primary Brain Lesion Resection Complications: An Overview and Malignant Brain Swelling After Resection of Superior Sagittal Sinus Meningioma

VINAYAK NARAYAN, VIJAY AGARWAL, MICHAEL J. LINK, ANIL NANDA

HIGHLIGHTS

- The overall incidence of complications associated with primary brain tumor resection worldwide ranges from 20% to 35%.
- These complications can be broadly divided into neurologic, regional, and systemic complications.
- The surgery of superior sagittal sinus meningioma carries high risk of complications.
- Due to the advancements in neuroimaging, neuroanesthesia, and surgical adjunct precision in modern times, gross total resection of a primary brain tumor can be performed without significant complications.
- The careful selection of patients, a proper surgical plan, meticulous operative technique, anticipation of a complication, and the precautions to avoid the same are the main keys to a good surgical outcome.

Introduction

The surgical management of brain tumors has taken a paradigm shift over the last century from the Cushing era of cytoreduction surgery to the present golden period of advanced tumor surgery. Neurosurgical adjuncts such as cortical mapping, frameless stereotaxy, and intraoperative magnetic resonance imaging (MRI) play a huge role in the safe resection of primary brain tumors with absent or minimal complications. The objectives of brain tumor resection are the establishment of exact histopathologic diagnosis, neurologic recovery, and prolongation of patient survival. The overall incidence of complications associated with primary brain tumor resection worldwide ranges from 20% to 35%.[1–4] This chapter throws light on a variety of complications associated with resection of primary brain lesions, its classification, diagnostic methods, and management strategies.

The definition of complication in primary brain tumor surgery is mostly subjective. Most surgical series define the adverse events as complications without giving due regard to whether they are expected.[1–3,5] Apart from the surgeon's knowledge and skill, there are various factors directly or indirectly involved in the incidence of a complication. The patient's age, physical/neurologic status, previous treatment, tumor size and location, extent of resection, availability of monitoring/operative navigational devices, and histopathologic characteristics are a few of them.[3] The neurosurgeon should have good acumen on all tumor-related complications because it helps in better counseling of the patient and family, both before and after surgery.

Classification of Neurosurgical Complications

A neurosurgical complication is not a single entity. It encompasses a spectrum of surgical complications as well as medical complications that may happen in the perioperative period[3] (Table 20.1). Sawaya et al. provide a rational framework for categorizing complications associated with brain tumor surgery.[3] In this classification pattern, the neurosurgery-related complications are broadly organized into neurologic, regional, and systemic complications.[3] Neurologic complications are adverse events that directly impair motor, sensory, language, or visual functions (e.g., hematoma, vascular injury, edema), whereas regional complications are related either to the wound (e.g., infection, pseudomeningocele) or to the brain (e.g., seizures, hydrocephalus), but they are not associated with any

TABLE 20.1 Summary of the Complications Associated With Primary Brain Tumor Surgery

Neurologic	Regional	Systemic
Motor deficit	Hydrocephalus	Pulmonary embolism
Sensory deficit	Seizure	Deep vein thrombosis
Aphasia/dysphasia	Pneumocephalus	Pneumonia
Visual field deficit	Wound infection	Urinary infection
	Meningitis	Sepsis
	Brain abscess	Myocardial infarction
		Gastrointestinal bleed
		Electrolyte disturbances

Courtesy Winn HR. *Youmans Neurological Surgery,* 6th edition, Surgical Complications of Brain Tumors and Their Avoidance. Elsevier Saunders, 2011, Philadelphia.

neurologic deficits. Systemic complications include more generalized medical conditions (e.g., thromboembolism, pneumonia). Neurologic complications are the most common cause of postoperative mortality. These three complications can be further subclassified into major and minor complications based on the severity, duration of deficit, and need of reexploration surgery.

Complications and Strategy for Their Avoidance

Neurologic Complications

The incidence of a new neurologic deficit (minor or major) after craniotomy for intrinsic tumor ranges from 10% to 25% in many surgical series.[1,3–4] Several predictors of adverse neurologic outcome have been described in previous surgical series: age older than 60 years, Karnofsky Performance Scale (KPS) score less than 60, deep tumor location, and tumor in proximity to eloquent brain areas.[1–3,5] The surgical strategy must be ideally planned based on these factors.

The main causes for neurologic complications are direct brain parenchymal injury, brain edema, vascular injury, and hematoma. The wrong localization of the tumor in relation to the adjacent eloquent brain areas is the main reason for inadvertent brain injury. Brain edema is also a notorious cause of neurosurgical morbidity. The predisposing factors for postoperative brain edema include excessive brain retraction and subtotal resection of the tumors, commonly high-grade gliomas. The incidence rate of vascular injury associated with primary brain tumor surgery is around 1% to 2%.[1] A major venous occlusion can result in a hemorrhagic stroke where the neurologic manifestations may be delayed, whereas an arterial occlusion or injury can have an immediate catastrophic effect. The probable difference between these two problems is that in the former case, there can be a gradual recovery over a period of time, whereas in the latter it may permanently affect the patient's quality of life. Postoperative hematomas, including subdural and extradural hematomas, cause neurologic deficits in 1% to 5% of patients; they are usually detected in the early postoperative period when the patient develops altered sensorium, seizures, or focal neurologic deficit.[1–3]

The conventional knowledge of the tumor in relation to the normal brain and precise eloquent areas as well as the tumor's identification/confirmation using various adjuncts such as cortical mapping, frameless stereotactic navigation, intraoperative MRI, or awake stimulation helps to a great extent in avoiding direct brain injury.[4,6–8] Similarly, excessive brain retraction can be minimized by proper positioning of the patient, hyperventilation, high-dose corticosteroids, diuretics, and intermittent retractor placement. Frameless stereotaxy also helps in determining the optimal surgical trajectory and reduces the need for prolonged retraction and consequent cerebral edema.[7] The gross total resection of a malignant glioma is associated with reduced postoperative edema/hematoma (wounded glioma syndrome) and the resulting morbidity compared with its partial-resection counterparts.[1,3,9] The risk of vascular injury while performing surgery can be reduced by the strong anatomic suspicion of the location of vascular structures, early identification of arteries and veins, judicious sacrifice of draining veins, careful and intermittent retraction, surgery along the subpial plane, and careful use of an ultrasonic aspirator. Most of the operative site hematomas can be avoided by careful preoperative preparation, meticulous operative technique, and vigilant postoperative care.

Regional Complications

Regional complications are events associated with the surgical site (e.g., infection, pseudomeningocele) or the brain (e.g., seizures, hydrocephalus, pneumocephalus) without any neurologic deficits.[3] A complication occurs in 1% to 5% of patients undergoing craniotomy for removal of intrinsic brain tumors.[1,2–4] Redo surgery and radiotherapy are two plausible factors that can lead to wound infection.[4,5] The tumor proximity to the motor cortex and a history of preoperative epilepsy are the strongest predictors for seizures.[10] Local factors such as degree of cortical injury, prolonged retraction while performing the operation, and postoperative edema/hematoma as well as systemic factors such as hyponatremia and acidosis influence the incidence of postoperative seizures.[2,10] Even though there is a controversy regarding the administration of prophylactic antiepileptics, most surgical series demonstrated a lower frequency of seizures in patients who received phenytoin either before or during surgery.[11–13] Postoperative seizures must be managed aggressively with intravenous (IV) lorazepam, phenytoin, and IV fluids, and computed tomography (CT) imaging must be done to rule out a structural cause.

The risk of postoperative infections ranges from 1% to 2%, and it can extend from superficial to deep, involving bone, meninges, and brain parenchyma.[3,14] The most common microbes involved are *Staphylococcus aureus* and *S. epidermidis,* although nosocomial infections can happen also with Gram-negative organisms.[14] The predisposing factors for wound infection are proximity to paranasal sinus, presence of foreign body, prolonged surgery, corticosteroid administration, cerebrospinal fluid fistula, previous surgery, and cytotoxic therapy.[3,5,14] The administration of prophylactic antibiotics and meticulous wound closure help in reducing the incidence of postoperative wound infection.[14]

Systemic Complications

The incidence of medical complications ranges from 5% to 10% of patients undergoing craniotomy and removal of primary brain tumor.[3] The spectrum of medical complications includes deep venous thrombosis, pulmonary embolism, myocardial infarction, infection, gastrointestinal hemorrhage, and electrolyte disturbances, of which the most frequent is deep venous thrombosis.[3,15] The predisposing factors are elderly population, poor KPS score, preexisting medical conditions, prolonged surgery, and bed rest.

Several perioperative mechanical and pharmacologic prophylactic measures can reduce the risk of thromboembolic events. The use of elastic stockings and compression boots and the administration of minidose heparin (5000 units subcutaneously twice a day) or low-molecular-weight heparin after craniotomies are some of them.[16–20] The neurosurgeon should keep a vigilant eye in the postoperative period to avoid or minimize the aforementioned complications to a great extent.

Next is an example of primary brain tumor; superior sagittal sinus (SSS) meningioma and the complications associated with its resection are discussed.

Neurosurgical Complications After Resection of Superior Sagittal Sinus Meningioma

The treatment of meningiomas that invade the intracranial venous system remains a significant and controversial challenge for neurosurgeons.[21] Specifically, damage to the major dural venous sinuses, the deep cerebral veins, and the vein of Labbé, among others, can lead to major complications such as seizures, hemorrhage, sinus occlusion, corticovenous thrombosis, and regional or diffuse brain swelling.[22,23] These complications can lead to significant morbidity and mortality. Meningiomas in the parasagittal region comprise 21% to 31% of all intracranial meningiomas.[21,22] Invasion of the SSS is common with these lesions and increases the risk of subtotal resection and thus recurrence. Meningiomas along the SSS range from 14.8% to 33.9% in the anterior third, from 44.8% to 70.4% in the middle third, and from 9.2% to 29.6% in the posterior third of the sinus.[21] Those lesions involving the posterior two-thirds of the SSS pose a substantially increased risk, whereas the previous literature has supported the sacrifice of the anterior one-third, with minimal consequence.

There is a current lack of large published series of parasagittal meningiomas that invade the SSS. Due to this, there are no accepted guidelines for the management of these lesions or their complications, and treatment paradigms vary significantly between institutions.

Anatomic Insights

Venous Anatomy

The intracranial venous system can be divided into a superficial and a deep system (Fig. 20.1). The superficial system is comprised of the sagittal sinuses and cortical veins. The deep system drains the deep gray structures via the internal cerebral veins, basal veins of Rosenthal, vein of Galen, and the straight sinus. The SSS, the lateral sinuses (including the transverse and sigmoid sinus), and the cavernous sinus are the most frequently thrombosed dural sinuses, followed by the straight sinus and vein of Galen.[24] Studies have shown a permanent morbidity range of 6% to 20% from cerebral venous thrombosis, although prognosis is thought to be better than for arterial stroke.[25,26] Detailed evaluation of the venous sinuses and information on patency are best obtained via a venous MR angiogram, CT venography, or a digital subtraction angiography with late venous phases.

Dural Sinuses

Superficial veins of both hemispheres drain via the SSS, which starts at the foramen cecum and runs posteriorly toward the internal occipital protuberance, at which point it joins the straight and lateral sinuses to form the torcular Herophili. The SSS increases in size from anterior to posterior and ranges in width from 4.3 to

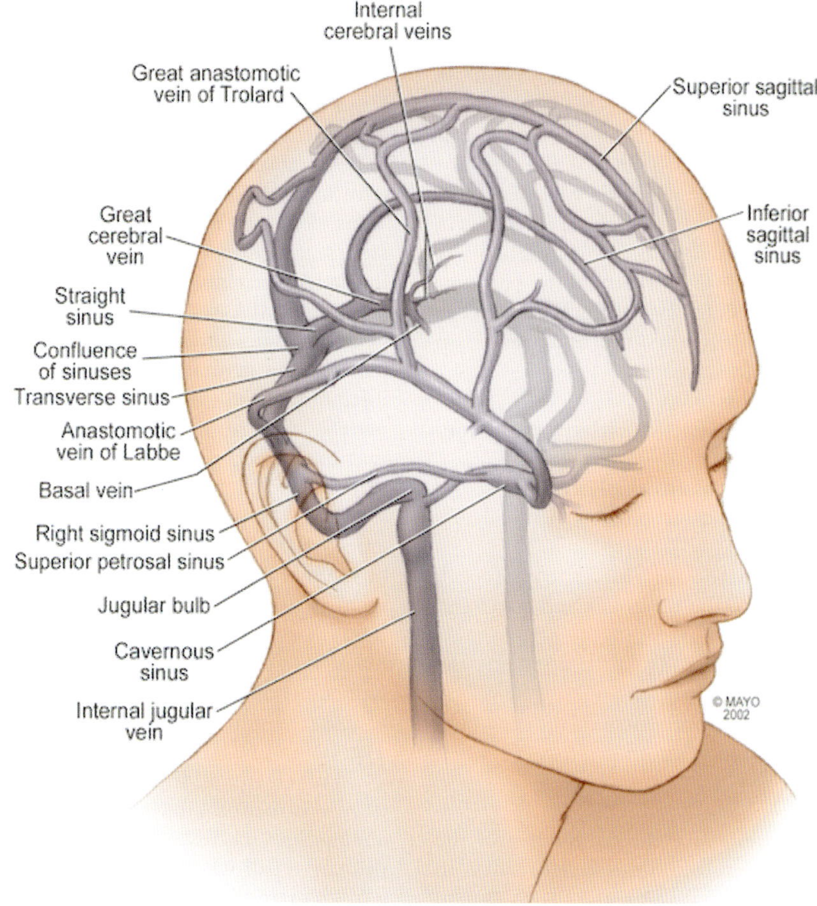

• **Fig. 20.1** Venous anatomy. (Copyright © Mayo 2002.)

9.9 mm.[27] As mentioned, the sacrifice of the anterior one-third of the SSS is usually well tolerated, but complications can include akinetic mutism, short-term memory deficits, or personality changes from compromise of prefrontal afferent drainage. At times, this anterior portion is narrow or absent, replaced by two superior cerebral veins.[21] The middle one-third of the SSS drains the central group of cortical veins, and, as such, its sacrifice has the potential to cause bilateral hemiplegia or akinesia. A good landmark for division of the anterior and middle one-third of the SSS is the coronal suture. Occlusion of the posterior one-third of the SSS, or the torcular Herophili, carries a significant risk of potentially fatal diffuse brain edema. Fibrous septa at the inferior angle of the sinus, in addition to turbulent flow from draining superficial cortical veins, are felt to account for a greater risk of SSS thrombosis. The SSS, along with the other dural venous sinuses, receives blood from diploic, meningeal, and emissary veins. This accounts for the frequent occurrence of cerebral venous thrombosis as a complication of infectious pathologies, such as in cavernous sinus thrombosis in facial infections, lateral sinus thrombosis in chronic otitis media, and sagittal sinus infection in scalp infections. Because the dural sinuses contain the pacchionian or arachnoid granulations, thrombosis can lead to intracranial hypertension and papilledema.

The Superficial Veins of the Brain

The superficial veins can be classified into three categories: (1) midline afferents to the SSS, (2) inferior cerebral afferents to the transverse sinus, or (3) superficial sylvian afferents to the cavernous sinus. Midline afferents are primarily encountered when using interhemispheric approaches. Sacrifice of the midline central group of veins within 2 cm posterior to the coronal suture carries a significant risk. Other small-caliber midline veins can be taken with minimal risk. The vein of Trolard, or the superior anastomotic vein, is the primary connecting midline afferent and usually enters into the SSS in the postcentral region. Inferior cerebral veins are cortical bridging veins that primarily channel into the basal sinuses or the deep venous system. Small-caliber veins in this system can usually be sacrificed with minimal consequence if they do not contribute significantly to the Labbé system. The vein of Labbé, or inferior anastomotic vein, connects the superficial sylvian vein and the transverse sinus. Injury to the vein of Labbé, particularly in the dominant hemisphere, can cause an infarct in the posterior hemisphere with severe, permanent neurologic deficit. The superficial sylvian vein is formed from the connection of the temporosylvian veins and enters into the cavernous sinus.

Important superficial veins include:

- Superior cerebral veins: drain the superior surface; empty into the SSS
- Superficial middle cerebral vein: drains the lateral surface of each hemisphere; empties into the cavernous or sphenopalatine sinuses
- Inferior cerebral veins: drain the inferior aspect of each cerebral hemisphere; empty into the cavernous and transverse sinuses.
- Superior anastomotic vein (vein of Trolard): connects the superficial middle cerebral vein and the SSS
- Inferior anastomotic vein (vein of Labbé): connects the superficial middle cerebral vein and the transverse sinus

The Deep Veins of the Brain

The deep veins of the brain drain into the confluence of the Galen complex, which, in turn, drains into the straight sinus. In addition to the paired internal cerebral veins, the Galen system also receives the paired basilar veins of Rosenthal (which begins at the anterior perforated substance by the union of the anterior cerebral vein, the middle cerebral vein, and the striate vein); the veins from the corpus callosum, the cerebellum, and the occipital cortex; and the vermian precentral vein. The deep veins are often encountered when operating in the lateral ventricle, third ventricle, and pineal region. The great cerebral vein of Galen is approximately 1 to 2 cm long and passes posterosuperiorly behind the splenium of the corpus callosum in the quadrigeminal cistern. Injury or occlusion of the vein of Galen can have catastrophic consequences. There have been case reports of ligation of the vein of Galen without significant clinical sequelae, but this is likely due to the development of collateral circulation and to the significant anatomic variation of the vein of Galen and its tributaries.[28,29]

Surgical Resection of SSS Meningiomas

Meningiomas invading the SSS remain a challenging lesion for neurosurgeons. They can be difficult to resect completely and carry significant risk of morbidity, including intraoperative and postoperative hemorrhage, sinus occlusion, and corticovenous thrombosis.[22] Although subtotal resection is associated with a high rate of recurrence, absolute care must be taken to preserve the collateral channels at all steps of the surgery.[30–32]

Venous invasion by the meningioma can range from invasion of the outer surface of the venous wall to complete invasion and occlusion of the sinus. The first detailed classification scheme was proposed by Merrem and Krause et al. and then later modified by Bonnal and Brotchi et al.[33] A simplified version was proposed by Sindou and Hallacq in 1998.[23] This classification included the categorization described later.

With the advent of microsurgical techniques, intracranial dural venous sinus reconstruction became possible. In 1971, Kapp et al. used an autogenous great saphenous vein and shunt device to reconstruct the SSS.[32] This was followed by Marks et al. in 1986 and Sakaki et al. in 1987.[30,34] Reconstructive materials have included autologous great saphenous vein, neck superficial veins, Dacron, and silicone tubing.[35–37] Sindou and Hallacq reported a series of 47 meningiomas: 41 of the sagittal sinus, 4 of the transverse sinus, and 2 torcular.[23] A gross total resection was achieved in all cases. Thirty-nine patients were reported as having good outcomes and resumed their previous activities, whereas five patients had permanent neurologic deficit due to central venous infarction (all in the middle one-third of the sagittal sinus). Three patients died from brain swelling; all three involved meningiomas totally occluding the sinus, and in all three patients resection was achieved without sinus reconstruction. Nine patches, six Gore-Tex bypasses, and nine autologous vein bypasses were employed. The authors recommended the following: excision of the outer layer of sinus wall and coagulation of dural attachment in Type 1, removal of intraluminal fragment and repair of dural defect with a patch in Type 2, resection of sinus wall and repair by patch graft in Type 3, repair by patch or bypass with saphenous or external jugular vein graft in Type 4, and removal of involved portion of sinus and restoration by venous bypass in Types 5 and 6.

Mathiesen et al. supported the practice of sagittal sinus repair or reconstruction after resection by invasive meningiomas when attempting a macroscopic radical removal.[38] They proposed a direct primary repair when resecting just an invaded edge; closure with a patch graft of dural, falcine, or pericranial tissue when resecting one to two invaded walls; and using an interposition venous graft when resecting three sinus walls. In this prospective study of 100 patients, the authors had good to excellent outcomes in 94 patients but found that microscopic radical resection was difficult to achieve. Gamma Knife radiosurgery was used as an adjunct in patients with tumors of low proliferative index, and the authors felt that tumor control was better when Gamma Knife radiosurgery was used as a primary treatment strategy than when it was employed only after tumor progression.

Over time, however, extensive reconstruction of the SSS after meningioma resection has played a diminishing role. In 2014, Mantovani et al. reported on the management of meningiomas invading the major dural venous sinuses.[39] The authors reported on 38 patients who underwent operations for meningioma resection: 26 patients with lesions in the SSS, 5 with lesions in the torcular Herophili, 5 with lesions in the transverse sinus, and 2 with lesions in the sigmoid sinus. Twenty-seven patients had World Health Organization (WHO) Grade I meningiomas, and 11 had WHO Grade II meningiomas. In 50% of cases (13 patients), the sinus was completely occluded. A gross total resection was achieved in 86.9% of patients. Sinus reconstruction was performed in 21 cases: 13 by direct suture and 8 using a patch. Postoperatively, the sinus was found to be patent in 52.4% of patients and narrowed in 33.3% of patients. Correspondingly, an occlusion rate of 14.3% was found. No deaths were reported, and one major postoperative complication occurred. Further diminishing the role of sinus reconstruction, DiMeco et al. reported on their surgical experience in 108 cases of meningiomas invading the SSS.[22] Thirty patients with meningiomas completely occluding the SSS had complete resection of the involved portion of sinus, and Simpson Grade I or II resection was achieved in 100 patients. Two perioperative deaths were noted. Serious complications included brain swelling in 9 patients (8.3%) and postoperative hematoma in 2 patients (1.85%). At a mean follow-up of 79.5 months, tumor recurrence was noted in 15 patients (13.9%). The authors concluded that if extreme care is taken to preserve cortical veins, good results are achieved without reconstruction of the sinus.

Surgical management of meningiomas of the SSS remains controversial. Resection should be offered to those with symptoms or with lesions that exhibit growth. Close examination of preoperative imaging for extent of SSS invasion is essential to guide the surgeon's goals of care. After exposure or injury of the sagittal sinus during meningioma surgery, the patient is at risk for intraoperative excessive blood loss or air embolism. In most cases, injury is controllable with packing by Surgicel, Gelfoam, and microsurgical patties. Care should be taken with injectable thrombotic agents to avoid inadvertent occlusion. If there is planned resection of a portion of the SSS during surgery, a preoperative formal angiogram may be very helpful in evaluating the collateral venous anatomy to avoid inadvertently interrupting critical pathways.

Complications of Venous Injury

The risk of postoperative seizures after craniotomy is a well-recognized phenomenon.[40] They are generally classified into three categories based on time interval: immediately postoperatively, occurring within 24 hours; early seizures, within 1 week; and late seizures, 1 week or more after the craniotomy.[41] Immediately postoperative seizures occur in approximately 4.3% of craniotomy patients.[42] Patients with supratentorial meningiomas or supratentorial low-grade gliomas are at a much higher risk than patients with lesions in various other intracranial locations.[40,43–52] Generalized tonic-clonic seizures are the most common postoperative seizure noted in the neurologic intensive care unit, but a high index of suspicion must be maintained because some patients will present with neurologic deterioration and decreased level of consciousness rather than with convulsions.

Literature regarding the benefit of prophylactic treatment with antiepileptics in brain tumor patients is inconsistent.[43,53,54] Furthermore, the exact choice of antiepileptic agent remains controversial. Phenytoin, phenobarbital, carbamazepine, valproic acid, zonisamide, and levetiracetam have all been used for the prevention of early postoperative seizures with varying results.[40] However, inadequate dosing is common, and caregivers must be vigilant about maintaining appropriate levels.[42,55] Seizures manifesting from a reversible primary source such as cerebral edema, intracranial hemorrhage, meningitis, or infection should be addressed by aggressively reversing the source.

SURGICAL REWIND

My Worst Case

This is the case of 52-year-old woman who was referred for treatment of petroclival and SSS meningiomas invading into and occluding the SSS at the level of the coronal suture (Fig. 20.2). She was asymptomatic until approximately 1 year prior, when she noted the onset of right face tingling and the onset of headache centered over the right orbit. She did not note face pain, weakness, or numbness. She also noted a distant history of right-sided hearing loss. Approximately 4 months before presentation she developed diplopia with a right lateral gaze palsy. She subsequently underwent Gamma Knife radiosurgery to treat her right cavernous sinus Meckel's cave meningioma (marginal dose of 14 Gy and a maximum dose of 28 Gy to a volume of 9.1 cm^3) (Fig. 20.3). After Gamma Knife treatment her diplopia resolved, and she had no new symptoms. A cerebral angiogram confirmed that the SSS was completely occluded at the site of the tumor, with collateral venous circulation around the tumor.

Approximately 3 months after Gamma Knife therapy, she underwent a bifrontal craniotomy for complete resection of her meningioma involving the anterior one-third of the SSS and overlying bone. At the time of craniotomy, extensive venous bleeding was noted arising from collateral veins and the SSS at the posterior margin of the tumor. This was controlled with Gelfoam soaked in thrombin, bipolar coagulation, and 5-0 monofilament suture. There were no other adverse events during tumor resection, and she did not require blood transfusion. Immediately upon awakening from anesthesia, she was noted to have difficulty speaking. A CT scan showed a small intraparenchymal hematoma in the medial left frontal lobe beneath the tumor resection. The patient was taken to the neurosurgery intensive care unit for postoperative monitoring. She continued to follow commands but had a complete motor aphasia. She had some difficulty with following commands with the tongue and mouth.

On postoperative day 2, she suffered a generalized seizure. She was taken to the CT scanner for a repeat scan, which revealed some new circumferential hemorrhage around the previous hematoma as well as increased edema around the hematoma with minimal left-to-right shift (Fig. 20.4). The patient recovered and was able to move three of her four extremities purposefully and without motor deficit. Her left lower extremity

Continued

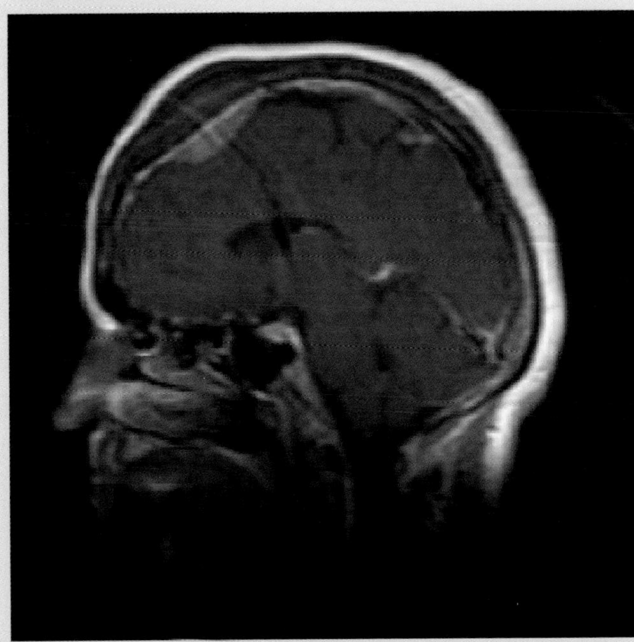

• **Fig. 20.2** Sagittal magnetic resonance image of the brain with contrast showing a meningioma invading and occluding the superior sagittal sinus at the level of the coronal suture.

was weak. It was intended to reload the patient with phenytoin; however, it was written as a per oral order, and she did not receive it because she was not deemed safe for oral intake.

Four hours after her seizure, she suffered a respiratory arrest felt possibly secondary to another seizure. She was apneic with desaturation, and she was intubated. She also required resuscitation for hypotension during this episode. Once hemodynamically stable, she was taken to the CT scanner, which showed increased size of her hematoma and diffuse cerebral edema. An intracranial pressure monitor was placed in the left frontal area with readings in the range of 110 to 120 mm Hg. She was taken to the operating room for a left frontal lobectomy and decompressive hemicraniectomy. Gross herniation was noted. She was taken back to the intensive care unit and subsequently progressed to clinical brain death.

In the case presented here, even though the anterior one-third of the SSS was completely occluded by the tumor, both frontal lobes were draining via cortical collaterals and then entering the SSS at the posterior margin of the tumor. These veins were injured during the craniotomy and subsequently sacrificed to control the bleeding. In retrospect, performing a small craniectomy with a diamond burr over this area would have been much safer than elevating a large bone flap that put these veins at risk. The immediate frontal lobe dysfunction also should have been an indication that there was a vascular problem and that the patient would be at risk of increased intracranial pressure. Finally, after her initial generalized seizure, anticonvulsant therapy should have been aggressively pursued. Likely, after the initial seizure she hypoventilated, which increased her PCO_2 and cerebral blood flow with aggravation of already elevated ICP from insufficient venous drainage of the frontal lobes.

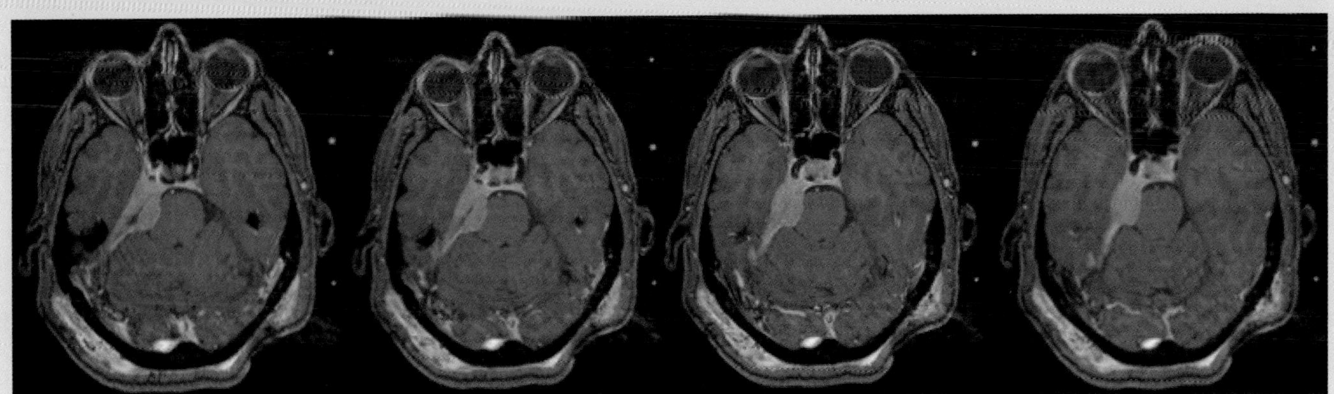

• **Fig. 20.3** Axial magnetic resonance image of the brain with contrast showing the right cavernous sinus Meckel's cave meningioma that was treated with Gamma Knife therapy.

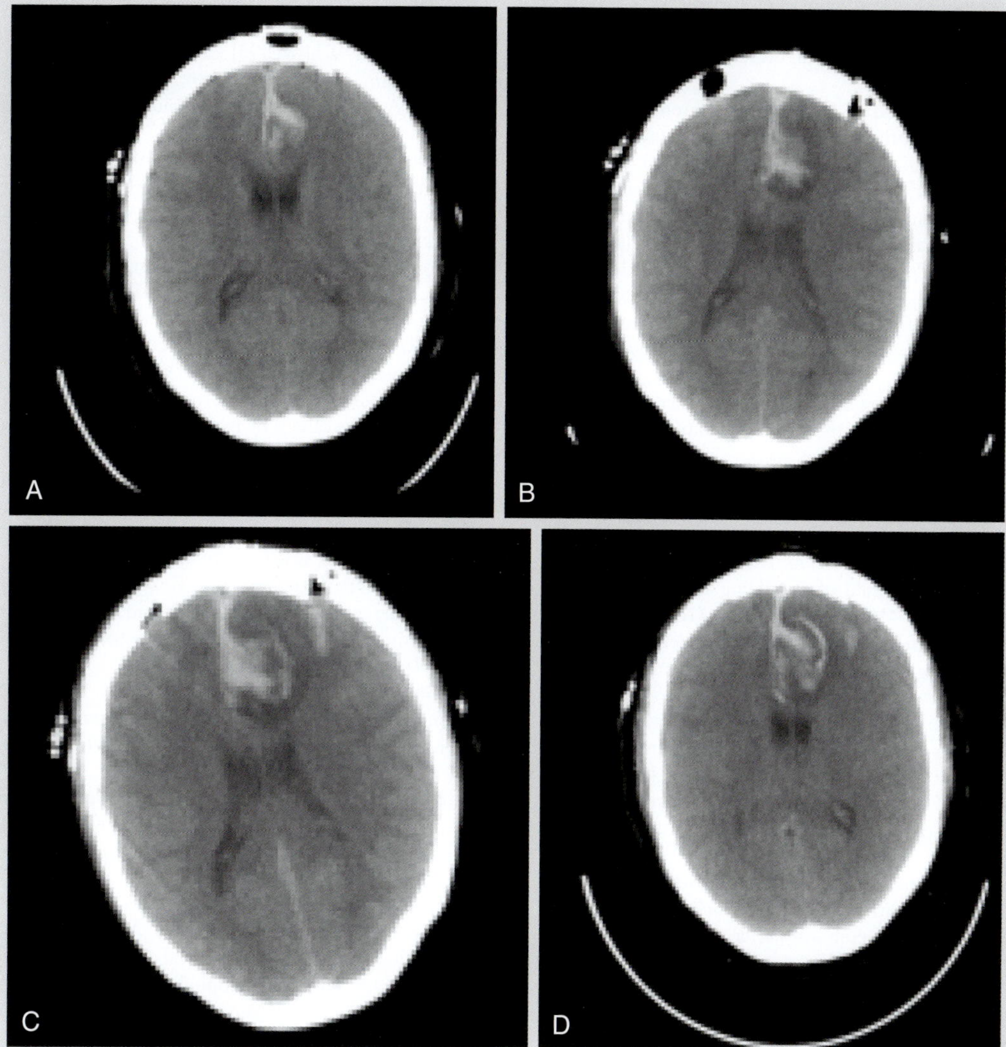

• **Fig. 20.4** (A) Computed tomography (CT) scan of the brain without contrast directly from the operating room showing hemorrhage in surgical resection bed. (B) Repeat CT scan of the brain without contrast showing blossomed blood products and edema. (C) CT scan of the brain without contrast taken post-seizure showing continued increased hemorrhage and edema. (D) CT scan of the brain taken after apneic arrest showing diffuse cerebral edema and graying of the gray–white matter border.

NEUROSURGERY SELFIE MOMENT

Due to advancements in neuroimaging, neuroanesthesia, and surgical adjunct precision in modern times, gross total resection of a primary brain tumor can be performed without significant complications. The careful selection of patients, a proper surgical plan, meticulous operative technique, anticipation of a complication and the precautions to avoid the same are the main keys to a better outcome.

Venous injury during resection of SSS meningiomas can have severe consequences. It is imperative to closely examine preoperative imaging for patency of the sagittal sinus and orientation of collateral flow. Due to the high recurrence rate, aggressive surgical resection is warranted, but the collateral flow must be vigilantly maintained. If resection of the SSS is undertaken, the anterior one-third is felt to pose the least risk of new neurologic morbidity. After injury or resection of a portion of the SSS, close observation must be maintained for the onset of seizures or brain edema. Early intervention is critical in the event of complications arising from dural venous compromise.

References

1. Fadul C, Wood J, Thaler H, Galicich J, Patterson RH, Posner JB. Morbidity and mortality of craniotomy for excision of supratentorial gliomas. *Neurology*. 1988;38(9):1374–1379.
2. Cabantog AM, Bernstein M. Complications of first craniotomy for intra-axial brain tumour. *Can J Neurol Sci*. 1994;21(3):213–218.
3. Sawaya R, Hammoud M, Schoppa D, et al. Neurosurgical outcomes in a modern series of 400 craniotomies for treatment of parenchymal tumors. *Neurosurgery*. 1998;42(5):1044–1055, discussion 1055–1056.
4. Taylor MD, Bernstein M. Awake craniotomy with brain mapping as the routine surgical approach to treating patients with supratentorial intraaxial tumors: a prospective trial of 200 cases. *J Neurosurg*. 1999;90(1):35–41.
5. Vorster SJ, Barnett GH. A proposed preoperative grading scheme to assess risk for surgical resection of primary and secondary intraaxial supratentorial brain tumors. *Neurosurg Focus*. 1998;4(6):e2.
6. Berger MS, Ojemann GA, Lettich E. Neurophysiological monitoring during astrocytoma surgery. *Neurosurg Clin N Am*. 1990;1(1):65–80.

7. Bohinski RJ, Kokkino AK, Warnick RE, et al. Glioma resection in a shared-resource magnetic resonance operating room after optimal image-guided frameless stereotactic resection. *Neurosurgery.* 2001;48(4):731–42.
8. Black PM, Alexander E, Martin C, et al. Craniotomy for tumor treatment in an intraoperative magnetic resonance imaging unit. *Neurosurgery.* 1999;45(3):423–431, discussion 431–433.
9. Ciric I, Ammirati M, Vick N, Mikhael M. Supratentorial gliomas: surgical considerations and immediate postoperative results. Gross total resection versus partial resection. *Neurosurgery.* 1987;21(1):21–26.
10. Kvam DA, Loftus CM, Copeland B, Quest DO. Seizures during the immediate postoperative period. *Neurosurgery.* 1983;12(1):14–17.
11. Boarini DJ, Beck DW, VanGilder JC. Postoperative prophylactic anticonvulsant therapy in cerebral gliomas. *Neurosurgery.* 1985; 16(3):290–292.
12. Lee ST, Lui TN, Chang CN, et al. Prophylactic anticonvulsants for prevention of immediate and early postcraniotomy seizures. *Surg Neurol.* 1989;31(5):361–364.
13. North JB, Penhall RK, Hanieh A, Frewin DB, Taylor WB. Phenytoin and postoperative epilepsy. A double-blind study. *J Neurosurg.* 1983;58(5):672–677.
14. Narotam PK, van Dellen JR, du Trevou MD, Gouws E. Operative sepsis in neurosurgery: a method of classifying surgical cases. *Neurosurgery.* 1994;34(3):409–415, discussion 415–416.
15. Brandes AA, Scelzi E, Salmistraro G, et al. Incidence of risk of thromboembolism during treatment of high-grade gliomas: a prospective study. *Eur J Cancer.* 1997;33(10):1592–1596.
16. Bucci MN, Papadopoulos SM, Chen JC, Campbell JA, Hoff JT. Mechanical prophylaxis of venous thrombosis in patients undergoing craniotomy: a randomized trial. *Surg Neurol.* 1989;32(4):285–288.
17. Cerrato D, Ariano C. Fiacchino F. Deep vein thrombosis and low-dose heparin prophylaxis in neurosurgical patients. *J Neurosurg.* 1978;49(3):378–381.
18. Agnelli G, Piovella F, Buoncristiani P, et al. Enoxaparin plus compression stockings compared with compression stockings alone in the prevention of venous thromboembolism after elective neurosurgery. *N Engl J Med.* 1998;339(2):80–85.
19. Nurmohamed MT, van Riel AM, Henkens CM, et al. Low molecular weight heparin and compression stockings in the prevention of venous thromboembolism in neurosurgery. *Thromb Haemost.* 1996;75(2):233–238.
20. Macdonald RL, Amidei C, Lin G, et al. Safety of perioperative subcutaneous heparin for prophylaxis of venous thromboembolism in patients undergoing craniotomy. *Neurosurgery.* 1999;45(2):245–51.
21. Selcuk Peker MNP. Meningiomas: a comprehensive text. In: Fahlbusch R, ed. *Management of Superior Sagittal Sinus Invasion in Parasagittal Meningiomas.* Philadelphia, PA: Saunders Elsevier; 2010.
22. DiMeco F, Li KW, Casali C, et al. Meningiomas invading the superior sagittal sinus: surgical experience in 108 cases. *Neurosurgery.* 2008; 62:1124–1135.
23. Sindou M, Hallacq P. Venous reconstruction in surgery of meningiomas invading the sagittal and transverse sinuses. *Skull Base Surg.* 1998;8:57–64.
24. Sasidharan PK. Cerebral vein thrombosis misdiagnosed and mismanaged. *Thrombosis.* 2012;2012:210676.
25. Canhao P, Ferro JM, Lindgren AG, Bousser MG, Stam J, Barinagarrementeria F. Causes and predictors of death in cerebral venous thrombosis. *Stroke.* 2005;36:1720–1725.
26. Ferro JM, Canhao P, Stam J, Bousser MG, Barinagarrementeria F. Prognosis of cerebral vein and dural sinus thrombosis: results of the International Study on Cerebral Vein and Dural Sinus Thrombosis (ISCVT). *Stroke.* 2004;35:664–670.
27. Andrews BT, Dujovny M, Mirchandani HG, Ausman JI. Microsurgical anatomy of the venous drainage into the superior sagittal sinus. *Neurosurgery.* 1989;24:514–520.
28. Youssef AS, Downes AE, Agazzi S, Van Loveren HR. Life without the vein of Galen: clinical and radiographic sequelae. *Clin Anat.* 2011;24:776–785.
29. Chaynes P. Microsurgical anatomy of the great cerebral vein of Galen and its tributaries. *J Neurosurg.* 2003;99:1028–1038.
30. Marks SM, Whitwell HL, Lye RH. Recurrence of meningiomas after operation. *Surg Neurol.* 1986;25:436–440.
31. Ricci A, Di Vitantonio H, De Paulis D, et al. Parasagittal meningiomas: our surgical experience and the reconstruction technique of the superior sagittal sinus. *Surg Neurol Int.* 2017;8:1.
32. Kapp JP, Gielchinsky I, Petty C, McClure C. An internal shunt for use in the reconstruction of dural venous sinuses. Technical note. *J Neurosurg.* 1971;35:351–354.
33. Bonnal J, Brotchi J. Surgery of the superior sagittal sinus in parasagittal meningiomas. *J Neurosurg.* 1978;48:935–945.
34. Sakaki T, Morimoto T, Takemura K, Miyamoto S, Kyoi K, Utsumi S. Reconstruction of cerebral cortical veins using silicone tubing. Technical note. *J Neurosurg.* 1987;66:471–473.
35. Oka K, Go Y, Kimura H, Tomonaga M. Obstruction of the superior sagittal sinus caused by parasagittal meningiomas: the role of collateral venous pathways. *J Neurosurg.* 1994;81:520–524.
36. Parker JW, Gaines RW Jr. Long-term intravenous therapy with use of peripherally inserted silicone-elastomer catheters in orthopaedic patients. *J Bone Joint Surg Am.* 1995;77:572–577.
37. Wei XLZ, Lin S. Reconstruction of sagittal sinus after total resection of parasagittal meningioma. *Chn J Neurosurg.* 1994;313–315.
38. Mathiesen T, Pettersson-Segerlind J, Kihlstrom L, Ulfarsson E. Meningiomas engaging major venous sinuses. *World Neurosurg.* 2014;81:116–124.
39. Mantovani A, Di Maio S, Ferreira MJ, Sekhar LN. Management of meningiomas invading the major dural venous sinuses: operative technique, results, and potential benefit for higher grade tumors. *World Neurosurg.* 2014;82:455–467.
40. Manaka S, Ishijima B, Mayanagi Y. Postoperative seizures: epidemiology, pathology, and prophylaxis. *Neurol Med Chir (Tokyo).* 2003;43:589–600.
41. Jennett WB. Early traumatic epilepsy. Definition and identity. *Lancet.* 1969;1:1023–1025.
42. Kvam DA, Loftus CM, Copeland B, Quest DO. Seizures during the immediate postoperative period. *Neurosurgery.* 1983;12:14–17.
43. Gokhale S, Khan SA, Agrawal A, Friedman AH, McDonagh DL. Levetiracetam seizure prophylaxis in craniotomy patients at high risk for postoperative seizures. *Asian J Neurosurg.* 2013;8:169–173.
44. Hwang SL, Lin CL, Lee KS, et al. Factors influencing seizures in adult patients with supratentorial astrocytic tumors. *Acta Neurochir (Wien).* 2004;146:589–594.
45. Pace A, Bove L, Innocenti P, et al. Epilepsy and gliomas: incidence and treatment in 119 patients. *J Exp Clin Cancer Res.* 1998;17:479–482.
46. Kahlenberg CA, Fadul CE, Roberts DW, et al. Seizure prognosis of patients with low-grade tumors. *Seizure.* 2012;21:540–545.
47. Chaichana KL, Pendleton C, Zaidi H, et al. Seizure control for patients undergoing meningioma surgery. *World Neurosurg.* 2013;79:515–524.
48. Das RR, Artsy E, Hurwitz S, et al. Outcomes after discontinuation of antiepileptic drugs after surgery in patients with low grade brain tumors and meningiomas. *J Neurooncol.* 2012;107:565–570.
49. Suri A, Mahapatra AK, Bithal P. Seizures following posterior fossa surgery. *Br J Neurosurg.* 1998;12:41–44.
50. Chadduck W, Adametz J. Incidence of seizures in patients with myelomeningocele: a multifactorial analysis. *Surg Neurol.* 1988;30:281–285.
51. Copeland GP, Foy PM, Shaw MD. The incidence of epilepsy after ventricular shunting operations. *Surg Neurol.* 1982;17:279–281.
52. Dan NG, Wade MJ. The incidence of epilepsy after ventricular shunting procedures. *J Neurosurg.* 1986;65:19–21.
53. Temkin NR. Antiepileptogenesis and seizure prevention trials with antiepileptic drugs: meta-analysis of controlled trials. *Epilepsia.* 2001;42:515–524.
54. Pulman J, Greenhalgh J, Marson AG. Antiepileptic drugs as prophylaxis for post-craniotomy seizures. *Cochrane Database Syst Rev.* 2013;(2):CD007286.
55. Yeh JS, Dhir JS, Green AL, Bodiwala D, Brydon HL. Changes in plasma phenytoin level following craniotomy. *Br J Neurosurg.* 2006;20:403–406.

21

Complications After Glioma Surgery

ALEXA N. BRAMALL, ALLAN FRIEDMAN, JOHN H. SAMPSON

HIGHLIGHTS

- Complications after glioma surgery can be characterized as local or direct, regional, and systemic.
- White matter structures are often overlooked but are important to consider when planning surgery for gliomas and may be mapped using modalities such as diffusion tensor imaging (DTI).
- Awake craniotomy is preferred to asleep surgery when a tumor is in close proximity to eloquent cortex and may significantly reduce postoperative deficits.

Introduction

Residual tumor volume and extent of resection (EOR) are important predictors of long-term survival in glioblastoma patients,[1,2] and mounting evidence also supports the role of gross total resection in the survival of patients with low-grade gliomas (LGGs).[3–5] Nonetheless, the risk of surgical complications must be weighed against the benefits of obtaining a gross total resection, especially for tumors in close proximity to eloquent brain. A recent review of 16,530 patients undergoing surgery for malignant gliomas reported in the nationwide inpatient sample database found at least one surgical complication in 3.4% of patients with a 4.5% risk in patients for hospital-associated complications such as surgical site infection.[6] Complication rates are affected by a myriad of factors including but not exclusive to tumor characteristics, surgeon experience, patient comorbidities, age, and operative resources.[7] It is therefore of critical importance to identify ways to minimize operative risk. Complications may be classified as primary/direct (due to resection of tissue) or secondary/indirect and may further be categorized by severity, chronology (acute, subacute, delayed), or geography (local, regional, systemic).[8] Complications may be minor or potentially debilitating and have an enormous impact on a patient's quality of life.[9] The classification scheme used in the following chapter characterizes complications as local versus regional versus systemic. Local complications arise from resection of cortex or tracts within or in close proximity to eloquent brain and include examples such as motor weakness due to damage to the primary motor cortex as well as stroke from vessel sacrifice and postoperative hematomas. Regional complications include seizures, cerebrospinal fluid (CSF) leaks, pneumocephalus, meningitis, delirium, and hygroma. Systemic complications include but are not limited to deep vein thromboses (DVTs), pulmonary emboli (PEs), acute kidney injury (AKI), sepsis, and pneumonia (Table 21.1).

Anatomic Insights

White and Gray Matter

A knowledge of brain anatomy is critical in neurosurgery. The risk of postoperative neurologic deficits is influenced by tumor location and neighboring anatomy, including white matter, gray matter, and vessel architecture. Gliomas are heterotopically diverse and can arise anywhere in the brain, although there is a predilection for the frontal lobe.[10] LGGs are also geographically diverse but may be more commonly identified in "secondary functional areas," or directly adjacent to eloquent brain, especially near the supplementary motor area (SMA) and insula.[11] Some tumors are compact and appear to displace functional brain. Other tumors are more diffuse and may contain critically important functioning brain tissue. Consistent with diffusion tensor magnetic resonance imaging (MRI) fiber tractography studies, the highly invasive nature of high-grade gliomas allows these tumors to easily disrupt surrounding tissue.[12]

Language is complex and can manifest as difficulty with expression, comprehension, prosody, pitch, volume, and intonation.[13] Invasion of gliomas into the language centers or damage of these areas during surgery can lead to linguistic deficits in the perisylvian regions of the dominant lobe, or impairment in the emotional or rhythm elements of speech in the nondominant lobe. Essential language-related white matter tracts include the superior longitudinal fasciculus, the arcuate fasciculus, and the inferior fronto-occipital fasciculus (Fig. 21.1). The subcallosal and aslant fasciculus connect the SMA with the caudate nucleus and inferior frontal gyrus, respectively. Disruption of these pathways can result in difficulty initiating speech. In the perisylvian white matter, disruption of the anterior limb of the superior longitudinal fasciculus results in dysarthrias, whereas disruption of the more medial arcuate fasciculus results in phonologic paraphasias. The inferior fronto-occipital fasciculus is part of the inferior sagittal striatum in the temporal lobe, and passes through the temporal stem terminating in the middle frontal gyrus, inferior frontal gyrus, and orbital frontal cortex. Injury of this fasciculus results in difficulty with visual naming and semantic paraphasias. Additionally, the inferior longitudinal fasciculus connects the occipital lobe with the basal temporal lobe. Injury to this fasciculus on the language-dominant side can result in reading difficulty. With respect to gray matter structures, damage to the inferior frontal gyrus, the superior temporal gyrus, the supramarginal gyrus, the angular gyrus, and any interconnections between these regions can result in language impairment.

The optic radiation transmits visual information from the retina to the visual cortex and emanates from the lateral geniculate nucleus.

TABLE 21.1 Classification of Complications of Glioma Surgery as Local, Regional, or Systemic

CLASSIFICATION OF COMPLICATIONS		
Local	**Regional**	**Systemic**
• Stroke • Postoperative hematoma • Direct intraoperative injury resulting in deficits in speech, motor, sensory, cognitive function • Cerebral edema	• Seizures • CSF leaks • Pneumocephalus • Meningitis • Hydrocephalus • Delirium • Subdural hygroma • Wound infection	• Deep vein thrombosis • Pulmonary embolism • Acute kidney injury • Sepsis • Pneumonia • Urinary tract infection • Myocardial infarction

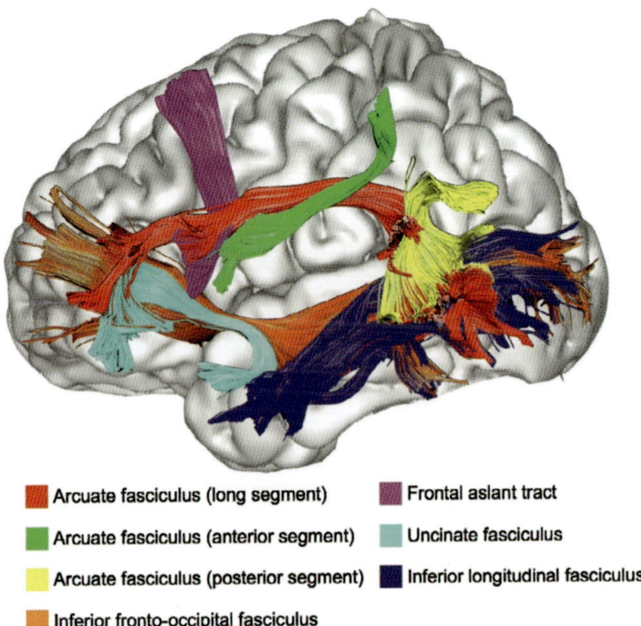

• **Fig. 21.1** Tractography reconstruction of the major association pathways involved in auditory processing and language.[14] (Courtesy of Maffei C, Soria G, Prats-Galino A, Catani M. Imaging white-matter pathways of the auditory system with diffusion imaging tractography. *Handb Clin Neurol.* 2015;129:277–288.)

The anterior bundle mediating information from the inferior retina, which forms part of the superior visual field, passes lateral to the temporal horn, doubling back to join the central and posterior bundles. The three bundles pass lateral to the atrium of the ventricle in the inferior sagittal striatum, and damage to any of these fibers may cause visual field deficits. The first branch of the superior longitudinal fasciculus connects in the superior parietal lobule with the dorsal premotor cortex. Disruption of this pathway results in optic ataxia, a condition in which visually guided movements are impaired.

The SMA is a region rostral to the primary motor cortex on the mesial hemispheric surface, and damage to this area in the language-dominant hemisphere is characterized by global akinesia of the contralateral limb with preserved muscle strength and mutism.[15,16] Unlike damage in other parts of the brain, SMA deficits are generally temporary and resolve within weeks to months. The incidence of SMA-related deficits in one series of 27 patients harboring gliomas in the SMA was 26%, with resolution by 6-month follow-up examination.[17] The main motor tract or the corticospinal tract passes from the motor cortex to the posterior limb of the internal capsule deep to the sensory face area, and damage to these areas may cause contralateral motor deficits when the injury occurs above the pyramidal decussation. Injury to the dorsolateral frontal lobe, prefrontal cortex, and orbitofrontal cortex can lead to impairments in planning and executive function, verbal memory or spatial memory, and impulse control and social behavior, respectively. Within the posterior fossa, damage to the flocculonodular lobe, the vermis, or the cerebellar hemispheres can lead to alterations in eye movement and gross balance, gait and locomotion, and coordination and precise motor control.[13]

Cognitively, neuropsychological studies demonstrate that many glioma patients have subtle deficits before surgery.[18] Neurocognitive worsening is common in the immediate postoperative period (specifically in language and executive function domains), and in the months after surgery, recovery to preoperative levels of cognition is variable. As expected, cognitive deficits are highly correlated with tumor location.[18,19]

Vascular

Injury to arteries and veins can also lead to irreparable deficits consistent with the vascular territory supplied. The frequency of direct vascular injury is estimated in the range of 1% to 2%.[20] Arterial injuries are frequently evident in the immediate postoperative period, whereas venous injuries typically present days later, resulting in congestive edema, hemorrhage, and seizures. In a recent report using the nationwide inpatient sample from 2002 to 2011,[6] the incidence of iatrogenic stroke approached 10%, but it has been reported to be as high as 31% when reviewing postoperative MRI scans.[21] Tumors located in the insula, operculum, and superior temporal lobe are at higher risk for new restricted diffusion areas on postoperative MRI.[22]

Multiple vascular structures may be compromised during surgery. Gliomas can surround major vessels such as the anterior, middle, and posterior cerebral arteries and smaller cortical vessels. Perforating vessels, the thalamostriate vessels, branches of the anterior choroidal artery, and posterior branches of the middle cerebral artery that irrigate the motor fibers in the corona radiata and internal capsule may be engulfed by tumor. Thalamostriate vessels are frequently engulfed by tumors of the insula as the vessels pass from the sylvian fissure through the uncinate fasciculus to the basal ganglia. Branches of the anterior choroidal artery passing to the posterior perforating substance may be adherent to the uncus of the temporal lobe. Small branches of the middle cerebral artery passing through the central sulcus or the posterior portion of the superior circular sulcus around the insula provide a blood supply to the corticospinal tract in the corona radiate, and disruption of these vessels may lead to motor deficits in addition to other neurologic impairments.

RED FLAGS

- Highly vascularized tumors and tumors in close proximity to a major sinus
- Lesions located in close proximity to or within critically important structures
- Patients with a high number of medical comorbidities
- Patients with a history of antiplatelet or anticoagulant use

Prevention

Complications Resulting From Tumor Resection

Neurologic deficits are associated with worse overall outcomes and decreased longevity. However, there are a number of imaging modalities and technologies that may aid in preoperative or intraoperative planning to improve EOR, especially for complex gliomas in challenging locations. Examples include diffusion tensor imaging, which can be used to delineate white matter tracts and build a three-dimensional map for preoperative visualization.[23] Task-based functional MRI (fMRI) can also be used to identify cortical and subcortical areas of activation corresponding to eloquent brain (Fig. 21.2).

Modalities such as intraoperative MRI (iMRI), 5-aminolevulinic acid (5-ALA) fluorescence, and intraoperative ultrasound may also be helpful for identifying tumor margins. iMRI, although expensive and potentially time-consuming, has been shown to result in greater EOR and progression-free survival (PFS) compared with conventional neuronavigation.[2,24] Although conventional neuronavigation is helpful for initial localization of tumor and optimization of the surgical approach, accuracy is affected by slice thickness of cross-sectional imaging, tracking modality, image to patient registration, and especially brain shift during surgery.[25] Newer neuronavigation platforms will have the capacity to combine multimodal imaging including fMRI and DTI with MRI data to further improve preoperative planning.

Dyes such as 5-ALA and fluorescein have also been shown to enhance EOR.[27,28] The utility of ALA was demonstrated in a randomized controlled trial of 243 patients undergoing surgery for high-grade glioma. Patients receiving ALA had a significantly higher rate of gross total resection (65% vs 36%) and a higher rate of 6-month PFS (41.7% vs 21%).[29] Intraoperative ultrasound[30] can be easily combined with any of the other described techniques and has been shown to increase the probability of obtaining a gross total resection, especially for lesions that are solitary and subcortical.[30]

Awake craniotomy with intraoperative mapping has been shown to significantly reduce postoperative neurologic deficits,[31] although stringent patient selection is a key to success. Electrical stimulation of the brain during surgery with the patient awake or asleep has become a regular part of the surgeon's armamentarium and is used to delineate the borders of safe tumor resection. The value of intraoperative mapping in preserving neurologic function has

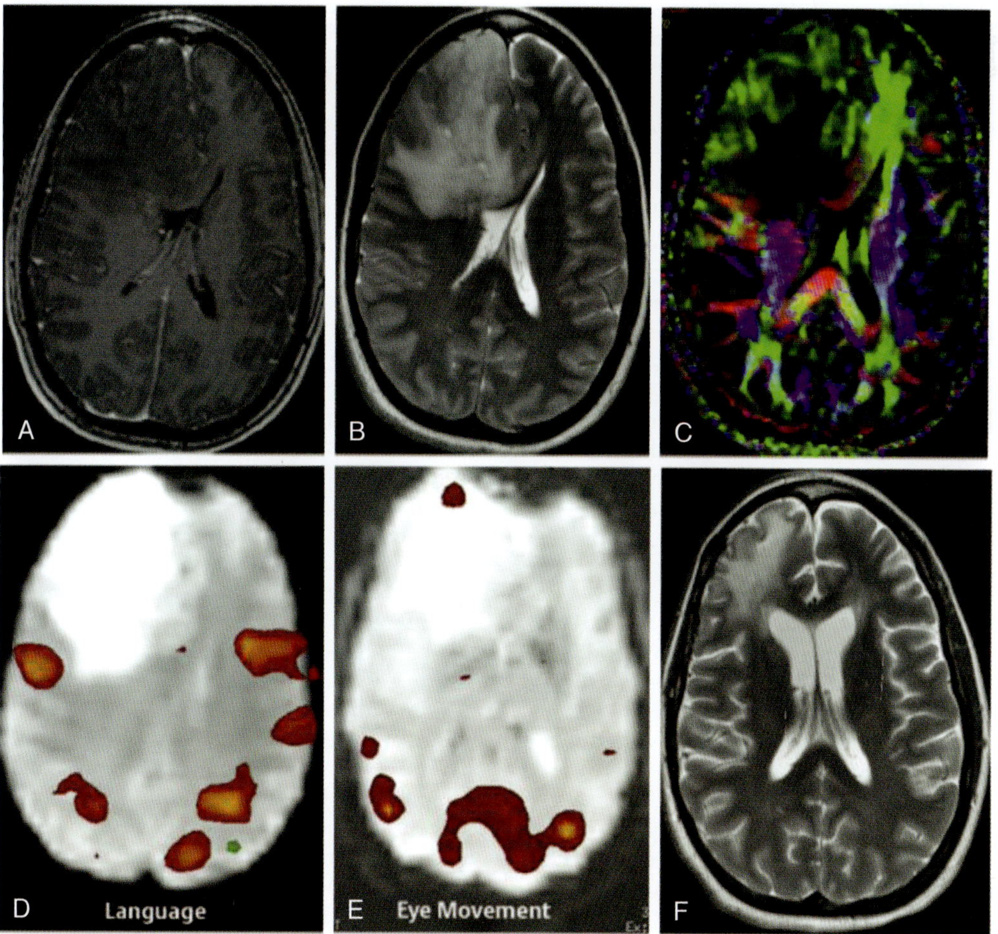

• **Fig. 21.2** Functional magnetic resonance imaging (MRI) in operative planning. (A) Axial T1-weighted MRI with contrast showing a nonenhancing isointense mass lesion of the right frontal lobe with mass effect and midline shift. (B) Same hyperintense lesion on T2-weighted sequence. (C) Functional MRI showing displacement of different white matter tracts. (D and E) Functional MRI showing the language and eye movement area in relation to the tumor. Notice the close relation with the right eye movement area (E). (F) One-year follow-up MRI showing complete resection and no recurrence.[26] (Fig. 19.2 from Nader, Scott, Abdulrahman, Levy, Neurosurgery Tricks of the Trade – Cranial, Thieme 2013, pg 74.)

been reported by a number of surgeons. A literature review of 90 reports published between 1990 and 2010 demonstrates a significant decrease in postoperative neurologic deficits and a significant increase in the rate of gross total resections when intraoperative stimulation was used.[32] Awake craniotomy is well tolerated by patients but is not infallible, because persistent neurologic deficits can still occur despite negative mapping. Whether these deficits are the result of ischemia, cortical function confined in the depth of a sulcus, damaged white matter tracts, or some other mechanism is uncertain.

In addition to minimizing damage to eloquent brain, it is also important to prevent injury to the vascular structures that supply eloquent brain. Malignant gliomas are highly vascular tumors and subsist in a highly proangiogenic milieu.[33] To prevent complications resulting from damage to vascular structures in the brain, preoperative computed tomography (CT) angiography or MR angiography to identify the location of vessels embedded within tumor tissue may be helpful for preoperative planning. For tumors encasing critical arteries of veins, tumor tissue may have to be left behind. To minimize the risk of stroke from vasospasm, papaverine-soaked Gelfoam may be placed on arteries if they appear to be in spasm after tumor dissection.

Disruption of the vascular supply around a tumor may lead to iatrogenic stroke, which has been shown to increase hospital mortality 9-fold.[6] It should be noted that small areas of restricted diffusion are not uncommon on postoperative MRI scans. Whether this is due to disruption of blood flow or contusion is uncertain. Nonetheless, disruption of large arteries such as M_4 branches of the middle cerebral artery can lead to areas of ischemia beyond the tumor. These branches have a propensity to lie within the sulci of the brain. As with an arteriovenous malformation, the surgeon is wise to open the sulci, coagulate the branches supplying the tumor, and preserve the main trunks that go on to supply normal brain. When operating on what looks to be a compact malignant tumor, it is not uncommon to identify large vessels in the sulci surrounding the tumor. When operating on low-grade tumors in the brain surrounding the sylvian fissure, the surgeon should debulk the tumor through openings in the crest of the gyri, preserving the pial vessels passing beyond the tumor. Low-grade tumor emanating from the insula may break through the pia and engulf M2 and M3 branches within the sylvian fissure. Using a subpial dissection, large branches within the sulci can be spared.

Regional Complications

Seizures, postoperative edema, hematoma, infection, and CSF leak are examples of more frequent regional complications and occur at a rate approximately between 1% and 10%. Excess brain retraction and residual tumor can result in significant postoperative edema which may not reach its peak until several days after surgery. Local edema may manifest as a focal neurologic deficit, but severe edema can result in life-threatening trans-tentorial herniation. Postoperative edema can be minimized by limiting brain retraction during surgery. Residual tumor, especially residual high grade tumor, is a nidus for postoperative swelling and hemorrhage, and therefore as much of the tumor as possible should be resected without causing new postoperative deficits. Postoperative steroids seem to mitigate postsurgical edema, but appear to be associated with an increased risk of infection.[34] Head elevation and osmotic agents may be necessary when postoperative edema is severe.

Postoperative hematomas causing deficits occur 1% to 5% of the time and may be influenced by coagulation status, hemostasis, age, comorbid medical conditions, and oftentimes residual tumor.[6] Consequently, careful preoperative evaluation including analysis of coagulation status and review of the patient's history, combined with meticulous hemostasis at the conclusion of a case, may help mitigate the risk of postoperative hematomas.

To prevent seizures, antiepileptic drugs may be administered during the pre- and postoperative period; however, the efficacy of seizure prophylaxis is controversial.[35] In our practice, we typically add seizure prophylaxis for supratentorial tumors. To reduce perioperative infections, adherence to sterile technique is also important, including the use of clippers instead of shaving for hair removal,[36] preoperative glycemic control,[37] intraoperative antibiotics, careful wound closure, normothermia,[38] and the changing of dressings when saturated. High extracellular glucose concentrations have been shown to inhibit neutrophil function; in general, the administration of insulin in the perioperative period to maintain blood glucose <180 mg/dL is recommended for the prevention of infection.[37] CSF leaks are more common with posterior fossa tumors, and the incidence may be reduced with meticulous dural closure. Postoperative incisional pain is also very common and can be alleviated by administering pregabalin in the preoperative setting. A recent randomized controlled trial showed that administering 150 mg BID of pregabalin during the perioperative period reduced preoperative anxiety, improved sleep quality, and reduced perioperative pain scores,[39] and we are currently using this for a vast majority of our preoperative craniotomy patients.

Systemic Complications

The risk of systemic complications such as DVT, PE, myocardial infarction, and pneumonia can also be reduced through good clinical practice behaviors. Surgical complications are associated with a significantly higher risk of general medical complications. Patients who end up with a surgical complication have a significantly higher rate of comorbidities before surgery. In a review of 20,000 glioma patients, the risk for cardiac complications was 0.7%, 0.5% for respiratory complications, 0.8% for deep wound infection, 0.6% for deep venous thromboses (DVTs), 3.1% for pulmonary embolus (PE), and 1.3% for acute renal failure (ARF).[40] DVT prophylaxis initiated on postoperative day 1,[41] close monitoring of respiratory status and oral intake, promotion of measures such as incentive spirometry, and judicious but appropriate use of intravenous fluids can help mitigate these risks.

There are a number of measures that may be taken to reduce the risk of postoperative systemic complications. Venous thromboembolism (VTE) rates are higher for postoperative cranial glioma patients (3.5%) than patients with other types of cancers. The risk can be reduced with the use of both mechanical and chemical prophylaxis; the combination of intermittent pneumatic compression devices with heparin prophylaxis is more effective in preventing VTE than either method alone.[42,43] One retrospective review showed that there was no statistically significant increase in hemorrhagic complications but a reduction in the rate of DVTs from 16% to 9% when subcutaneous heparin was administered either 24 or 48 hours postoperatively.[44] Blood pressure control can reduce the risk of postoperative hemorrhage; in general, systolic blood pressure in the first 24 hours after surgery is maintained at <140 mm Hg systolic.[45] In our practice we generally maintain systolic blood pressure for all postoperative craniotomy patients less than 160 mm Hg and start chemical prophylaxis 24 hours after surgery.

Management

All postoperative glioma patients should be monitored with frequent neurologic examinations. Immediate CT head without contrast should be performed for patients presenting with unexpected neurologic deficits to rule out common etiologies such as postoperative hematoma, stroke, or hydrocephalus. If a head CT is negative and the deficit persists, EEG monitoring may be indicated to rule out seizures, or MRI to rule out stroke. Due to the frequent incompatibility of EEG leads with MRI, MRI is often performed before the placement of EEG monitoring hardware to rule out acute stroke.

Stages of stroke on CT scan can be divided into the acute (<24 hours), subacute (24 hours to 5 days), and chronic (weeks) stages, characterized by cytotoxic edema causing loss of normal gray/white matter differentiation and effacement of cortical sulci, vasogenic edema resulting in hypoattenuation on CT, and loss of brain matter with hypoattenuation, respectively.[46] In general, CT is not sensitive enough to reliably detect hyperacute stroke within the first 6 hours, and MRI may be indicated.[47] MRI diffusion is used to detect acute changes within minutes of stroke onset, and once a hemorrhagic stroke has been excluded by CT, MR diffusion improves stroke detection from 50% to more than 95%.[46] In the first week after a stroke, diffusion weighted imaging (DWI) and its correlate apparent diffusion coefficient (ADC) images appear hyper- and hypointense, respectively, and ADC images therefore help to identify areas of acute infarction from vasogenic edema. The diffusion and ADC abnormalities will begin to reverse as the stroke moves from the acute to the subacute phase.[46] As previously mentioned, it is common to see hyperintense DWI lesions surrounding the resection cavity postoperatively, and the size of the lesion may sometimes correlate with postoperative neurologic deficits. Although neurologic deficits due to direct injury to the brain are likely irreversible, current guidelines for ischemic injury recommend a 15% reduction in blood pressure within the first 24 hours only in cases where BP exceeds 220/120 mm Hg[48]; otherwise, in cases of stroke, blood pressure should be allowed to rise to facilitate cerebral perfusion.

A postoperative hematoma may necessitate further surgery; however, postoperative hematomas that are small may be observed over time with repeat imaging and close blood pressure monitoring, frequent neurologic checks, and cessation of any anticoagulation or reversal of existing coagulopathy. The recent ATACH-2 trial showed that intensive blood pressure lowering in patients with intracerebral hemorrhage to 110–139 mm Hg did not reduce death and disability compared with a standard target of 140–179 mm Hg.[49] If there is significant mass effect and risk of brain herniation, operative intervention after temporizing measures such as the administration of mannitol or hypertonic saline may be considered. Although both agents provide brain relaxation, hypertonic saline has been shown to be slightly superior to mannitol.[50] Placement of an external ventricular drain for immediate decompression or hydrocephalus is indicated in patients with symptomatic enlarging ventricles.

The administration of aspirin for ischemic injury or therapeutic doses of heparin for patients with DVT or PE is especially controversial during the immediate postoperative period. Although no good guidelines currently exist, one study examined 30 patients administered therapeutic anticoagulation for DVT or PE 12 days after surgery on average, and none exhibited hemorrhagic complications.[51] Twenty of these patients received therapeutic doses of anticoagulation between postoperative days 2 and 7.

Pneumocephalus, seizures, and edema are common regional complications. Pneumocephalus is typically managed by placing the patient in the Fowler position of 30 degrees, avoiding Valsalva maneuver, and administering an oxygen mask for 100% O_2.[52] CSF leaks can be treated with lumbar drainage if there is no intracranial mass effect, which may be continued 3 to 5 days after cessation of the leak to allow for adequate healing. However, persistent CSF leaks that communicate outside the epidermis require surgical intervention. There are many antiepileptic agents available to treat seizures; however, there is support for leviratecam as both an effective and generally safe first choice, and we use it frequently in our practice. Postoperative edema is typically treated with steroids such as dexamethasone.

Management of systemic complications for surgical glioma patients is similar to that for other postsurgical patients. DVT/PE is treated with therapeutic anticoagulation, and the timing of initiation may be variable depending on the number of days from surgery. When the risk of intracranial hemorrhage is high, a temporary vena cava filter should be considered. In one study comparing 92 patients who received an inferior vena cava filter versus 92 patients who received therapeutic anticoagulation, there was no significant difference in the incidence of PE, which was between 3% and 7%, respectively.[53] AKI is treated with fluid resuscitation and the removal of renal toxic medications, pneumonia and sepsis with antibiotics and fluid resuscitation as required, and the treatment of delirium involves eliminating pro-cholinergic medications and reducing frequent interruptions and decreasing environmental stimulation. Delirium is especially a problem in the elderly and can result in longer hospital stays and higher rates of major complications.[54] A study evaluating the incidence and risk factors of delirium in neurosurgical patients greater than 70 years of age showed an incidence of 21.4% by postoperative day 3.[55] Risk factors for delirium included previous history of dementia, abnormal preoperative glucose levels, preexistent diabetes, longer operation time, and severe pain requiring the use of opioids.[55] Satisfactory pain control with minimal use of opioid medications and strict preoperative glucose control may therefore be quite helpful to reduce the risk of delirium.

SURGICAL REWIND

My Worst Case

This 45-year-old father of two presented with a partial complex seizure beginning with left hand numbness. An MRI demonstrated a nonenhancing lesion involving the lower motor and sensory strips of the right cerebral hemisphere, and an awake craniotomy was performed to monitor motor function intraoperatively.

The tumor was found to have superiorly displaced the motor hand area. The resection proceeded, slowly resecting the tumor while stimulating for the motor fibers assumed to pass medial to the posterior part of the tumor. Although these fibers could not be located with electrical stimulation, the patient developed left hand and wrist weakness in a subacute fashion. A postoperative MRI demonstrated restricted diffusion medial to the tumor. Quite possibly, a perforating vessel originating from an M4 branch of the middle cerebral artery and supplying the corona radiate was sacrificed during the surgery.

Fortunately, the patient made a nice recovery of his hand function over the next 3 months, but his MRI continued to show signs of the stroke even 7 years later (Fig. 21.3).

Continued

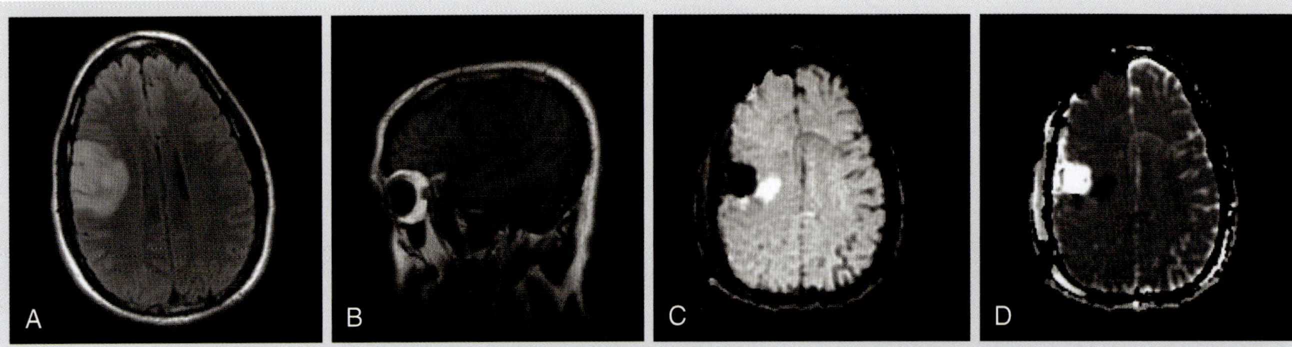

• **Fig. 21.3** (A) An axial flair-weighted magnetic resonance imaging demonstrates the right-sided tumor involving motor and sensory areas. (B) A sagittal T1-weighted image demonstrates the inferior superior extent of the tumor. (C) A diffusion-weighted image demonstrates the area of restricted diffusion medial to the resection cavity and extending into the corona radiate. (D) Apparent diffusion coefficient (ADC) map of resection cavity confirming restricted diffusion.

NEUROSURGICAL SELFIE MOMENT

Brain tumor surgery is a delicate art and must be approached with an understanding and appreciation for cerebral anatomy and function. Neuronavigation and the development of intraoperative visual aids have nonetheless made surgery safer. Postoperatively, craniotomy patients should be monitored with frequent neurologic examinations. The frequency of complications can be reduced through awareness of the risks, clinical vigilance, and an attention to detail.

References

1. Grabowski MM, Recinos PF, Nowacki AS, et al. Residual tumor volume versus extent of resection: predictors of survival after surgery for glioblastoma. *J Neurosurg*. 2014;121(5):1115–1123.
2. Li P, Qian R, Niu C, Fu X. Impact of intraoperative MRI-guided resection on resection and survival in patient with gliomas: a meta-analysis. *Curr Med Res Opin*. 2017;33(4):621–630.
3. Ius T, Isola M, Budai R, et al. Low-grade glioma surgery in eloquent areas: volumetric analysis of extent of resection and its impact on overall survival. A single-institution experience in 190 patients: clinical article. *J Neurosurg*. 2012;117(6):1039–1052.
4. Hollon T, Hervey-Jumper SL, Sagher O, Orringer DA. Advances in the surgical management of low-grade glioma. *Semin Radiat Oncol*. 2015;25(3):181–188.
5. Aghi MK, Nahed BV, Sloan AE, Ryken TC, Kalkanis SN, Olson JJ. The role of surgery in the management of patients with diffuse low grade glioma: a systematic review and evidence-based clinical practice guideline. *J Neurooncol*. 2015;125(3):503–530.
6. De la Garza-Ramos R, Kerezoudis P, Tamargo RJ, Brem H, Huang J, Bydon M. Surgical complications following malignant brain tumor surgery: an analysis of 2002–2011 data. *Clin Neurol Neurosurg*. 2016;140:6–10.
7. Cabantog AM, Bernstein M. Complications of first craniotomy for intra-axial brain tumour. *Can J Neurol Sci*. 1994;21(3):213–218.
8. Dindo D, Demartines N, Clavien PA. Classification of surgical complications: a new proposal with evaluation in a cohort of 6336 patients and results of a survey. *Ann Surg*. 2004;240(2):205–213.
9. Landriel Ibanez FA, Hem S, Ajler P, et al. A new classification of complications in neurosurgery. *World Neurosurg*. 2011;75(5–6):709–715, discussion 604–611.
10. Larjavaara S, Mantyla R, Salminen T, et al. Incidence of gliomas by anatomic location. *Neuro Oncol*. 2007;9(3):319–325.
11. Duffau H, Capelle L. Preferential brain locations of low-grade gliomas. *Cancer*. 2004;100(12):2622–2626.
12. Wei CW, Guo G, Mikulis DJ. Tumor effects on cerebral white matter as characterized by diffusion tensor tractography. *Can J Neurol Sci*. 2007;34(1):62–68.
13. Campbell WW. *DeJong's The Neurologic Examination*. Lippincott Williams & Wilkins; 2005.
14. Maffei C, Soria G, Prats-Galino A, Catani M. Imaging white-matter pathways of the auditory system with diffusion imaging tractography. *Handb Clin Neurol*. 2015;129:277–288.
15. Potgieser AR, de Jong BM, Wagemakers M, Hoving EW, Groen RJ. Insights from the supplementary motor area syndrome in balancing movement initiation and inhibition. *Front Hum Neurosci*. 2014;8:960.
16. Nachev P, Kennard C, Husain M. Functional role of the supplementary and pre-supplementary motor areas. *Nat Rev Neurosci*. 2008;9(11):856–869.
17. Russell SM, Kelly PJ. Incidence and clinical evolution of postoperative deficits after volumetric stereotactic resection of glial neoplasms involving the supplementary motor area. *Neurosurgery*. 2003;52(3):506–516, discussion 15–16.
18. Satoer D, Visch-Brink E, Dirven C, Vincent A. Glioma surgery in eloquent areas: Can we preserve cognition? *Acta Neurochir (Wien)*. 2016;158(1):35–50.
19. Noll KR, Wefel JS. Response to "From histology to neurocognition: the influence of tumor grade in glioma of the left temporal lobe on neurocognitive function". *Neuro Oncol*. 2015;17(10):1421–1422.
20. Warnick P, Mai I, Klein F, et al. Safety of pancreatic surgery in patients with simultaneous liver cirrhosis: a single center experience. *Pancreatology*. 2011;11(1):24–29.
21. Gempt J, Forschler A, Buchmann N, et al. Postoperative ischemic changes following resection of newly diagnosed and recurrent gliomas and their clinical relevance. *J Neurosurg*. 2013;118(4):801–808.
22. Dutzmann S, Gessler F, Bink A, et al. Risk of ischemia in glioma surgery: comparison of first and repeat procedures. *J Neurooncol*. 2012;107(3):599–607.
23. Nimsky C, Ganslandt O, Fahlbusch R. Implementation of fiber tract navigation. *Neurosurgery*. 2007;61(1 suppl):306–317, discussion 17–18.
24. Swinney C, Li A, Bhatti I, Veeravagu A. Optimization of tumor resection with intra-operative magnetic resonance imaging. *J Clin Neurosci*. 2016;34:11–14.
25. Orringer DA, Golby A, Jolesz F. Neuronavigation in the surgical management of brain tumors: current and future trends. *Expert Rev Med Devices*. 2012;9(5):491–500.

26. Nader R, Gragnaniello C, Berta SB, Sabbagh AJ, Levy, ML. In: Conerly K, ed. *Neurosurgery Tricks of the Trade Cranial.* New York, NY: Thieme Medical Publishers Inc.; 2014.
27. Mansouri A, Mansouri S, Hachem LD, et al. The role of 5-aminolevulinic acid in enhancing surgery for high-grade glioma, its current boundaries, and future perspectives: a systematic review. *Cancer.* 2016;122(16):2469–2478.
28. Neira JA, Ung TH, Sims JS, et al. Aggressive resection at the infiltrative margins of glioblastoma facilitated by intraoperative fluorescein guidance. *J Neurosurg.* 2017;127(1):111–122.
29. Stummer W, Pichlmeier U, Meinel T, et al. Fluorescence-guided surgery with 5-aminolevulinic acid for resection of malignant glioma: a randomised controlled multicentre phase III trial. *Lancet Oncol.* 2006;7(5):392–401.
30. Mahboob S, McPhillips R, Qiu Z, et al. Intraoperative ultrasound-guided resection of gliomas: a meta-analysis and review of the literature. *World Neurosurg.* 2016;92:255–263.
31. Brown T, Shah AH, Bregy A, et al. Awake craniotomy for brain tumor resection: the rule rather than the exception? *J Neurosurg Anesthesiol.* 2013;25(3):240–247.
32. Byrne RW. *Functional Mapping of the Cerebral Cortex: Safe Surgery for Eloquent Brain.* Berlin: Springer; 2015.
33. Giusti I, Delle Monache S, Di Francesco M, et al. From glioblastoma to endothelial cells through extracellular vesicles: messages for angiogenesis. *Tumour Biol.* 2016;37(9):12743–12753.
34. Kostaras X, Cusano F, Kline GA, Roa W, Easaw J. Use of dexamethasone in patients with high-grade glioma: a clinical practice guideline. *Curr Oncol.* 2014;21(3):e493–e503.
35. Meng L, Weston SD, Chang EF, Gelb AW. Awake craniotomy in a patient with ejection fraction of 10%: considerations of cerebrovascular and cardiovascular physiology. *J Clin Anesth.* 2015;27(3): 256–261.
36. Mangram AJ, Horan TC, Pearson ML, Silver LC, Jarvis WR. Guideline for prevention of surgical site infection, 1999. Hospital Infection Control Practices Advisory Committee. *Infect Control Hosp Epidemiol.* 1999;20(4):250–278, quiz 79–80.
37. Ehlers AP, Khor S, Shonnard N, et al. Intra-wound antibiotics and infection in spine fusion surgery: a report from Washington State's SCOAP-CERTAIN Collaborative. *Surg Infect (Larchmt).* 2016;17(2):179–186.
38. Scott EM, Buckland R. A systematic review of intraoperative warming to prevent postoperative complications. *AORN J.* 2006;83(5):1090–1104, 1107–1113.
39. Shimony N, Amit U, Minz B, et al. Perioperative pregabalin for reducing pain, analgesic consumption, and anxiety and enhancing sleep quality in elective neurosurgical patients: a prospective, randomized, double-blind, and controlled clinical study. *J Neurosurg.* 2016;125(6):1513–1522.
40. Jensen RL. Predicting outcomes after glioma surgery: model behavior. *World Neurosurg.* 2015;84(4):894–896.
41. Smith TR, Lall RR, Graham RB, et al. Venous thromboembolism in high grade glioma among surgical patients: results from a single center over a 10 year period. *J Neurooncol.* 2014;120(2): 347–352.
42. Cote DJ, Smith TR. Venous thromboembolism in brain tumor patients. *J Clin Neurosci.* 2016;25:13–18.
43. Agnelli G, Piovella F, Buoncristiani P, et al. Enoxaparin plus compression stockings compared with compression stockings alone in the prevention of venous thromboembolism after elective neurosurgery. *N Engl J Med.* 1998;339(2):80–85.
44. Khaldi A, Helo N, Schneck MJ, Origitano TC. Venous thromboembolism: deep venous thrombosis and pulmonary embolism in a neurosurgical population. *J Neurosurg.* 2011;114(1):40–46.
45. Monisha K, Levine J, Schuster J, Kofke AW. *Neurocritical Care Management of the Neurosurgical Patient.* Philadelphia, PA: Elsevier; 2017.
46. Birenbaum D, Bancroft LW, Felsberg GJ. Imaging in acute stroke. *West J Emerg Med.* 2011;12(1):67–76.
47. Bryan RN, Levy LM, Whitlow WD, Killian JM, Preziosi TJ, Rosario JA. Diagnosis of acute cerebral infarction: comparison of CT and MR imaging. *AJNR Am J Neuroradiol.* 1991;12(4):611–620.
48. Bowry R, Navalkele DD, Gonzales NR. Blood pressure management in stroke: five new things. *Neurol Clin Pract.* 2014;4(5): 419–426.
49. Qureshi AI, Palesch YY, Barsan WG, et al. Intensive blood-pressure lowering in patients with acute cerebral hemorrhage. *N Engl J Med.* 2016;375(11):1033–1043.
50. Prabhakar H, Singh GP, Anand V, Kalaivani M. Mannitol versus hypertonic saline for brain relaxation in patients undergoing craniotomy. *Cochrane Database Syst Rev.* 2014;(7):CD010026.
51. Scheller C, Rachinger J, Strauss C, Alfieri A, Prell J, Koman G. Therapeutic anticoagulation after craniotomies: Is the risk for secondary hemorrhage overestimated? *J Neurol Surg A Cent Eur Neurosurg.* 2014;75(1):2–6.
52. Dabdoub CB, Salas G, Silveira Edo N, Dabdoub CF. Review of the management of pneumocephalus. *Surg Neurol Int.* 2015;6:155.
53. Zektser M, Bartal C, Zeller L, et al. Effectiveness of inferior vena cava filters without anticoagulation therapy for prophylaxis of recurrent pulmonary embolism. *Rambam Maimonides Med J.* 2016;7(3).
54. Marcantonio ER, Goldman L, Mangione CM, et al. A clinical prediction rule for delirium after elective noncardiac surgery. *JAMA.* 1994;271(2):134–139.
55. Oh YS, Kim DW, Chun HJ, Yi HJ. Incidence and risk factors of acute postoperative delirium in geriatric neurosurgical patients. *J Korean Neurosurg Soc.* 2008;43(3):143–148.

22

Complications of Surgery for Pituitary Tumors

JOSEPH R. KEEN, NELSON M. OYESIKU

HIGHLIGHTS

- Depending on certain preexisting factors, the transcranial approach may be more favorable compared with a transnasal approach.
- Optic apparatus and pituitary axis injuries are rare but devastating.
- Visual deterioration and pituitary dysfunction are more common with a transcranial approach.
- The approach should be tailored to the position of the optic chiasm relative to the tuberculum sella and the tumor.
- Careful perioperative monitoring and management of vision and pituitary hormone status are imperative.

Background

The transsphenoidal approach revolutionized pituitary surgery and not only has become the mainstay for treating sellar pathology but also continues to evolve as expanded, endonasal approaches are continuously being developed to access tumors beyond the original limits. However, up to 10% of pituitary tumor cases still present with factors that make a transcranial approach necessary.[1,2] These include (1) difficult-to-access suprasellar, parasellar, or retrosellar/retroclival extension, (2) involvement or encasement of circle of Willis vasculature or the optic apparatus, (3) "dumbbell-shaped" tumors with significant constriction of the diaphragma sellae, (4) brain invasion or cerebral edema, (5) firm, fibrotic tumor consistency, (6) previous surgery or radiation therapy, (7) coexistent nearby aneurysm, (8) "kissing" carotids, (9) predominantly cavernous sinus involvement, and (10) inaccessible subfrontal extension.[1–4]

The goal of surgery is maximal resection to decompress neurovascular structures without causing or worsening neurologic and endocrinologic dysfunction. Compared with the endonasal, transsphenoidal route, the transcranial approach is associated with higher rates of anterior pituitary dysfunction, diabetes insipidus (DI), visual deterioration, and hypothalamic injury.[1] Mortality was 2.3% (6 of 259 patients) in one series[1] and 10.6% (7 of 66 patients) in a systematic review of three other studies, compared with 2.0% and 0% for microscopic and endonasal transsphenoidal resection, respectively.[5] Although there may be a selection bias that shifts larger tumors with less favorable prognoses and high complications rates into transcranial series, the risk of visual deterioration, hypopituitarism, and permanent DI is 22.9%, 9.1%, and 9.1%, respectively, for the transcranial approach compared with 0.8%, 9.5%, and 8.7%, respectively, for microscopic transsphenoidal, and 0.0%, 1.1%, and 4.7%, respectively, for endoscopic transsphenoidal.[5]

This chapter will discuss iatrogenic injury to the optic and pituitary apparatuses, which can lead to dreaded vision and hormonal dysfunction.

Anatomic Insights

Common Transcranial Approaches

An ideal transcranial approach offers the shortest distance with the widest corridor to access the tumor. The subfrontal approach is most commonly used to access the supra- and parasellar regions. From medial to lateral, craniotomies include bifrontal interhemispheric, unilateral frontal, frontoorbital, and frontotemporal. The most relevant neurovascular structures encountered during these approaches are the optic apparatus (nerves, chiasm, tracts), the pituitary gland and stalk, and circle of Willis vessels (internal carotid artery [ICA], anterior cerebral artery [ACA], middle cerebral artery [MCA]), including perforators (hypothalamic perforators as well as inferior and superior hypophyseal arteries).

Relevant Operative Anatomy (Fig. 22.1)

One of the first structures encountered in open pituitary surgery by the subfrontal approach is the ipsilateral optic nerve, which should serve as a landmark to find neighboring structures. The ICA resides inferolaterally, which can be followed posteriorly until it bifurcates into the ACA and MCA. Whereas the MCA courses laterally out of the surgical field and typically does not pose an obstacle, the ACA curves superomedially over the optic nerve and chiasm and is intimately involved in this approach. Following the optic nerve posteromedially leads to the chiasm and contralateral optic nerve. The lamina terminalis lies posterior to the chiasm and, depending on tumor size, may be thinned and displaced along with the optic apparatus. Deep and medial to the ipsilateral optic nerve and inferior to the optic chiasm resides the pituitary stalk, which extends through the diaphragma sellae into the gland within the sella turcica. Important perforators to be preserved are the superior and inferior hypophyseal arteries, arising from the medial and meningohypophyseal arterial trunks, respectively. These are critical perforators to the pituitary and optic apparatuses.[6]

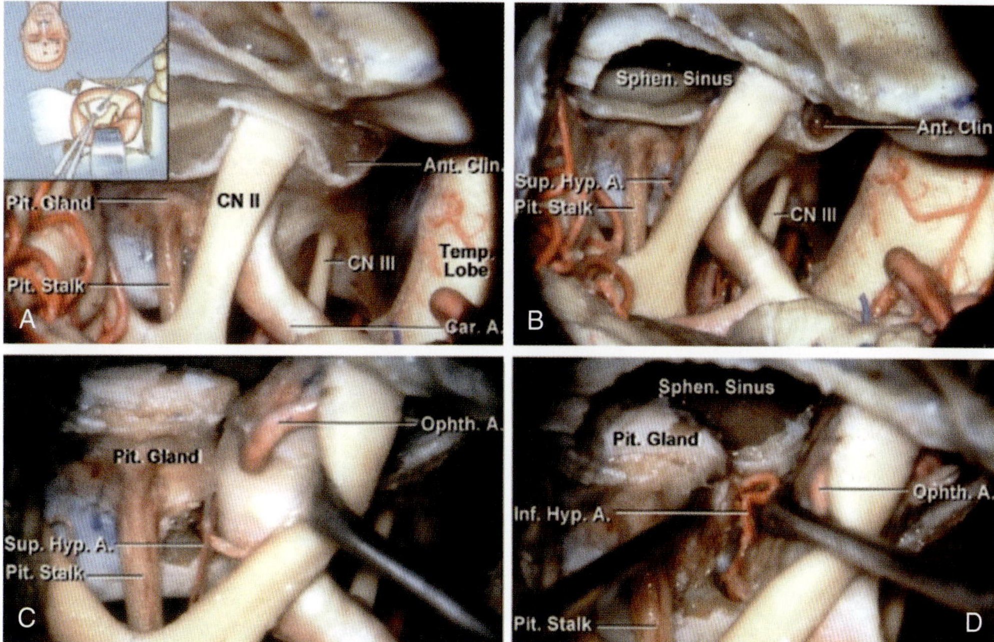

• **Fig. 22.1** Subfrontal exposure of the suprasellar region provided by a right frontal craniotomy. (A) Frontal lobe has been retracted to expose the right optic nerve with the right internal carotid artery inferolateral and the pituitary stalk deep and medial as it descends into the gland. (B) Planum sphenoidale has been removed to expose the sphenoid sinus. The superior hypophyseal artery is identified inferior and medial to the optic nerve arising from the medial aspect of the supraclinoid carotid and passing to the pituitary stalk. (C) The anterior sellar wall has been removed to demonstrate the anterior and posterior surfaces of the pituitary gland. (D) The pituitary gland is displaced to the left, demonstrating the inferior hypophyseal artery arising from the meningohypophyseal trunk of the intracavernous carotid. (Courtesy of The Rhoton Collection, Neurosurgery, Oxford University Press).

A key factor in the outcome of a transcranial pituitary surgery involves the relationship of the optic chiasm to the tuberculum sella and, consequently, the pituitary tumor. Bergland et al. described three scenarios: (1) normal position over the diaphragma sellae, (2) prefixed, in which the chiasm overlies the tuberculum sella, and (3) postfixed, in which it overlies the dorsum sella (Fig. 22.2).[7] A normal or postfixed chiasm offers a corridor in which the tumor resides anterior to the chiasm in between the optic nerves and provides access to the tuberculum sella region. A prefixed chiasm necessitates an approach that will provide access to the inferior aspects of the third ventricle through the lamina terminalis and tumor resection within the opticocarotid triangle. Whereas a subfrontal approach is sufficient for the previous scenarios, a bifrontal interhemispheric approach is recommended if there is more significant retrosellar extension.[2]

An additional consideration is that tumors, especially large macroadenomas, frequently distort the normal neurovascular anatomy, obliterate the cisterns, and stretch and displace the optic apparatus against the bony compartments and foramina. Great care must be taken to minimize retraction on these compromised structures.

Mechanisms of Injury

Short of transecting the optic chiasm or nerve, a common mechanism of injury involves a stretch or crush injury, which incites a proinflammatory cascade that not only damages retinal ganglion and support cells but also exacerbates vascular compromise to, and venous congestion within, the nerve or retina.[8] A less obvious injury involves inadvertent devascularization as a result of coagulating or disrupting shared blood supply between the nerve and the tumor. Injury to any part of the optic apparatus can lead to a corresponding visual field deficit.

The pituitary apparatus is likewise vulnerable to these types of injuries, but there is an additional risk of being resected along with tumor tissue, especially in cases of large macroadenomas with substantial perisellar extension, where normal tissue is obscured and significantly distorted. Stalk and posterior pituitary injury leads to DI, whereas anterior pituitary injury manifests as hypopituitarism requiring complete or partial hormone replacement.

RED FLAGS

- Prefixed optic chiasm.
- Significant supra- and parasellar extension.
- Evidence of invasion and brain edema can lead to hypothalamic injury.
- Firm, fibrotic tumor consistency.
- Shared blood supply with critical neurovascular structures.
- Significantly distorted/displaced neurovascular complexes.
- Redo surgeries with significant scarring and adhesions.

Prevention of Complication

Neuroimaging must be carefully evaluated to establish that there are preexisting factors that make the transcranial route, as opposed to an endonasal approach, the best approach. Magnetic resonance imaging with and without contrast, as well as pituitary protocol,

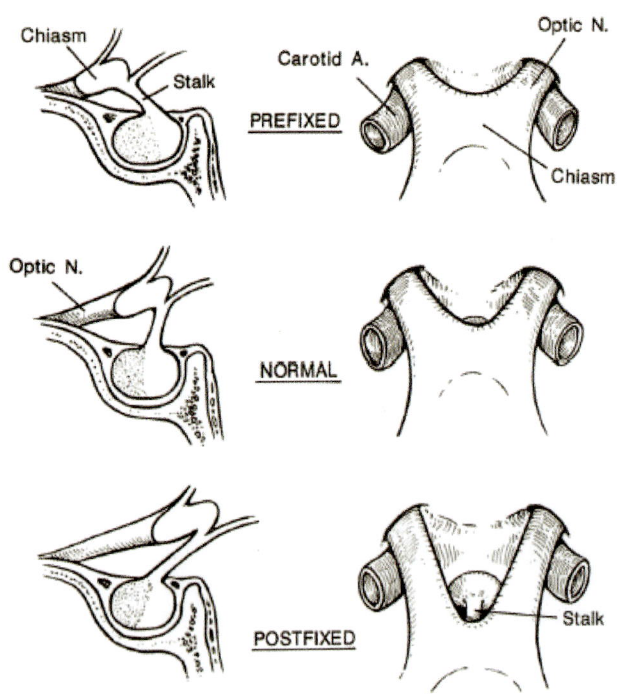

• **Fig. 22.2** Sagittal (left) and superior axial (right) views of the sellar region showing the optic nerve and chiasm and the pituitary stalk and gland as well as the carotid arteries. The top illustration demonstrates a "prefixed" chiasm, which overlies the tuberculum sella. The middle illustrates a normal chiasm over the diaphragm, and the bottom illustration demonstrates a "postfixed" chiasm situated above the dorsum sella. (Courtesy The Rhoton Collection, Neurosurgery, Oxford University Press).

will best demonstrate the position of the chiasm relative to the tuberculum (i.e., normo-, pre-, and postfixed) and the tumor to design a craniotomy and approach that will offer the shortest distance to the pathology while minimizing interference from neighboring critical structures. A head computed tomography (CT) scan will provide details about the bony compartments, and both modalities can be used to register the patient's cranium with navigation.

Given that pituitary tumor–related emergencies are rare, all pituitary tumor patients ideally should be evaluated preoperatively by endocrinology, even if admitted urgently, so that a full endocrine workup can be performed or a previous one can be reviewed to determine what laboratory tests and hormone replacements will be needed. Although all anterior pituitary hormone levels need to be assessed, the following are the most critical in the perioperative period. Prolactin levels should be known because even macroprolactinomas with optic nerve compression should undergo a pharmacologic trial first. This is because rapid shrinkage with normalization of vision can often occur within days, obviating the need for surgery. Free T4 is important because a substantially low free T4 is a requirement for perioperative levothyroxine and can be associated with increased morbidity and mortality, including anesthesia difficulties and myxedema coma. If free T4 is severely low, surgery should be postponed if possible. Patients for whom there is a concern for Cushing's disease may undergo a cosyntropin stimulation test (CST) and have a fasting morning cortisol level drawn. If the CST is abnormal (peak cortisol level <18 μg/dL) or fasting morning cortisol is <12 μg/dL, 100 mg of IV hydrocortisone should be given at anesthesia induction and 100 mg 12 hours later for the first 24 hours, followed by 50 mg every 12 hours on postoperative day 2. By postoperative day 3, most patients can switch to PO hydrocortisone so that the patient can take 20 mg in the morning and 10 mg in the afternoon daily for 5 days, and then 15 mg each morning and 5 mg each afternoon for maintenance until a 6-week follow-up visit, at which point the CST will be repeated without the morning hydrocortisone dose. Empiric use of hydrocortisone in all patients is unnecessary and has not been shown to improve outcomes, and it may impair healing and raise glucose levels. Lastly, all patients with optic nerve compression or visual field deficits need to have formal visual field testing by ophthalmology, the results of which could guide resection strategy.

Management

Operative Considerations

Choosing the Approach

Much of complication avoidance is achieved by carefully planning an operative approach that addresses the pathology while accounting for distortion of normal anatomy and anatomic variants. One should choose the approach that provides the shortest distance to the para- or suprasellar area of interest and provides the greatest exposure to maneuver within the confines of critical neurovascular structures with the least amount of retraction and manipulation. Typically, a frontotemporal craniotomy with a subfrontal approach suffices in the majority of cases.

Rhoton describes four main corridors that can be used for tumor resection. (1) The subchiasmatic approach between the optic nerves and below the chiasm is the most common because the majority of tumors elevate the chiasm and enlarge this space. (2) The opticocarotid approach is directed between the carotid artery and the optic nerve when tumors protrude through the space between the optic nerve and the carotid artery and are difficult to reach via the subchiasmatic corridor. When the chiasm is prefixed, the tumor can be accessed through a (3) lamina terminalis approach. In the event that the chiasm is prefixed with a large portion of tumor within the sphenoid sinus, a (4) transfrontal-transsphenoidal approach, in which the planum sphenoidale is drilled off from above to enter the sphenoid sinus, can be used when an endonasal approach is contraindicated.[6]

Operative Techniques

Efforts to reduce brain or cranial nerve retraction provide subtle advantages that can minimize injury. Rotating the head approximately 25 to 35 degrees contralaterally with slight extension allows the frontal lobe to fall posteriorly away from the anterior skull base, and using lumbar or ventricular drainage can help facilitate relaxation of the frontal lobe. Whenever possible, the tumor should be approached from the nondominant side, but in cases of severe unilateral visual compromise, it may be approached on the side of more severe dysfunction to minimize risking injury to the functional side. It has been suggested that the best method to avoid disrupting the microvascular supply is to decompress the functional optic nerve from below, which tends to be more feasible by approaching from the contralateral side.[1]

To enhance frontal lobe mobility and to minimize retraction, the sylvian fissure is opened as described by Yasargil.[9] MCA M3 and M2 segments are followed to the ICA bifurcation and optic nerve within their corresponding cisterns. Opening the cisterns and draining cerebrospinal fluid provides further brain relaxation necessary to achieve a wide exposure to understand the anatomic relationship of the optic and pituitary apparatuses, vascular structures, and the tumor.

Efforts should be made to identify and preserve the various subtle planes involved with the tumor. Frequently the tumor has elevated and significantly thinned the diaphragma sellae. This should be incised meticulously so that the underlying ultrathin rim of pituitary gland, or pseudocapsule of the tumor, can be preserved and entered. To avoid inadvertent injury to neurovascular structures around the tumor, it should be debulked maximally from within, allowing for the eventual manipulation and rolling-in of the tumor walls. One must resist the urge to manipulate the tumor outside the capsule before debulking, which could inadvertently traction cranial nerves or disrupt critical perforators. Microsurgical principles with sharp dissection should be employed instead of blunt dissection. An ultrasonic aspirator will facilitate tumor removal without undo manipulation.

Postoperative Management

Postoperative management varies depending on the underlying functional status of the pituitary tumor, but all patients should be closely managed in a multidisciplinary fashion by neurosurgery, endocrinology, ENT, and ophthalmology.

Optic Nerve Injury

This rare but devastating injury can lead to permanently impaired visual acuity and field deficits as well as complete blindness. Literature is nonexistent for treatment of iatrogenic optic apparatus injury; however, studies pertaining to traumatic optic neuropathy in the setting of head injury have linked steroids to improved microcirculation, energy metabolism, postinjury histology, and functional outcomes.[8] A retrospective study demonstrated that patients treated with intravenous followed by oral corticosteroids had better visual outcome compared with those under conservative management but found also that continuation was beneficial only in patients with immediate visual improvement.[10] Furthermore, methylprednisolone injections combined with optic nerve decompression resulted in better outcomes without major risks.[11] Though it is difficult to extrapolate from the traumatic optic neuropathy data, a trial of steroids (e.g., Decadron taper from 6 mg every 6 hours over 2 weeks) may be of benefit but must be weighed against the known adverse effects of steroid use (gastrointestinal bleeding, impaired wound healing, psychiatric disturbances, pneumonia, sepsis).

Pituitary Axis Injury

Diabetes Insipidus. Disrupted water regulation can result from injury to the pituitary stalk, posterior pituitary gland, or hypothalamus and can manifest as a result of decreased antidiuretic hormone (ADH) release (leading to DI) or excess ADH release (leading to syndrome of inappropriate ADH, or SIADH).[12–14] Postoperatively, the patient should be closely monitored in an ICU for DI and the need for hormone replacement. Fluid balance should be monitored hourly with urine specific gravity measurements every 4 hours and anytime urine output is greater than 250 mL/hr. Serial serum and urine sodium and osmolality should be obtained at least every 8 hours to help distinguish between normal diuresis, DI, or SIADH. Patients should have access to free water and be encouraged to drink according to their thirst response. The criteria for DI include urine output greater than 250 mL/hr over 1 to 2 hours and a specific gravity less than 1.005. If DI develops and the patient is not able to keep up with fluid losses with IV and oral fluid replacement, vasopressin (5 U aqueous IV/IM/SQ q hr PRN) can be administered, or desmopressin injections (0.5–1 mL [2–4 µg] SQ/IV daily in 2 divided doses) can be titrated to urine output. The patient can be switched to intranasal desmopressin (100 µg/mL, range 0.1–0.4 mL [10–40 µg] intranasally BID PRN) once nasal packings are removed. Endocrinology should be involved from the outset.

Anterior Pituitary Hormone Dysfunction. In the event of stalk or anterior pituitary injury, a patient can develop either partial or total hypopituitarism. However, the most critical hormones to be monitored and replaced, if necessary, are cortisol, adrenocorticotropic hormone (ACTH), and thyroid (free T4, thyroid-stimulating hormone). One of the most concerning, and potentially life-threatening, conditions is central adrenal insufficiency due to loss of mineralocorticoid and glucocorticosteroid production. Clinically this manifests as severe lethargy, altered level of consciousness, severe electrolyte abnormalities, and severe volume depletion leading to hypotension and tachycardia. Prompt diagnosis and replacement with exogenous steroids are imperative. Other gonadal and growth hormone axis hormones are evaluated several weeks after surgery and are typically not replaced in the immediate postoperative period.

SURGICAL REWIND

My Worst Case (Fig. 22.3)

A 26-year-old male underwent a right frontotemporal craniotomy for gross total resection of a residual suprasellar Rathke's cleft cyst causing displacement of a prefixed optic chiasm. The suprasellar component was retroinfundibular, enhanced mildly, and was initially part of a bilobed cystic-solid mass that was partially resected during an initial endonasal, transsphenoidal approach performed several years earlier. At that time, the intrasellar cyst was drained but became disconnected from the suprasellar component as a result of dense adherence of the rostral aspect of the cyst wall to the pituitary gland, which impeded access the suprasellar space. During the transcranial approach, the firm suprasellar component was found to be subchiasmatic; it had elevated the optic chiasm and thinned the lamina terminalis substantially. The lamina terminalis was opened and the mass debulked and resected without obvious complications. Postoperatively, the patient was neurologically intact but developed DI requiring a Pitressin drip. On postoperative day 3, the patient became acutely unresponsive, stopped following commands, and developed bilaterally dilated and nonreactive pupils. A STAT head CT scan demonstrated diffuse cerebral edema causing sulcal and cisternal effacement (Fig. 22.4). An external ventricular drain was placed, and the patient was found to be hyponatremic after a precipitous drop in sodium to 125 mmol/L, likely secondary to overcorrection of DI. The Pitressin drip was discontinued, hypertonic saline was given, and sodium eventually normalized as well as the patient's neurologic examination. Though there was no need for ventriculoperitoneal shunting, he developed pituitary-related adrenal cortical insufficiency, hypothyroidism, and hypogonadism, requiring hydrocortisone, levothyroxine, and testosterone replacement.

Continued

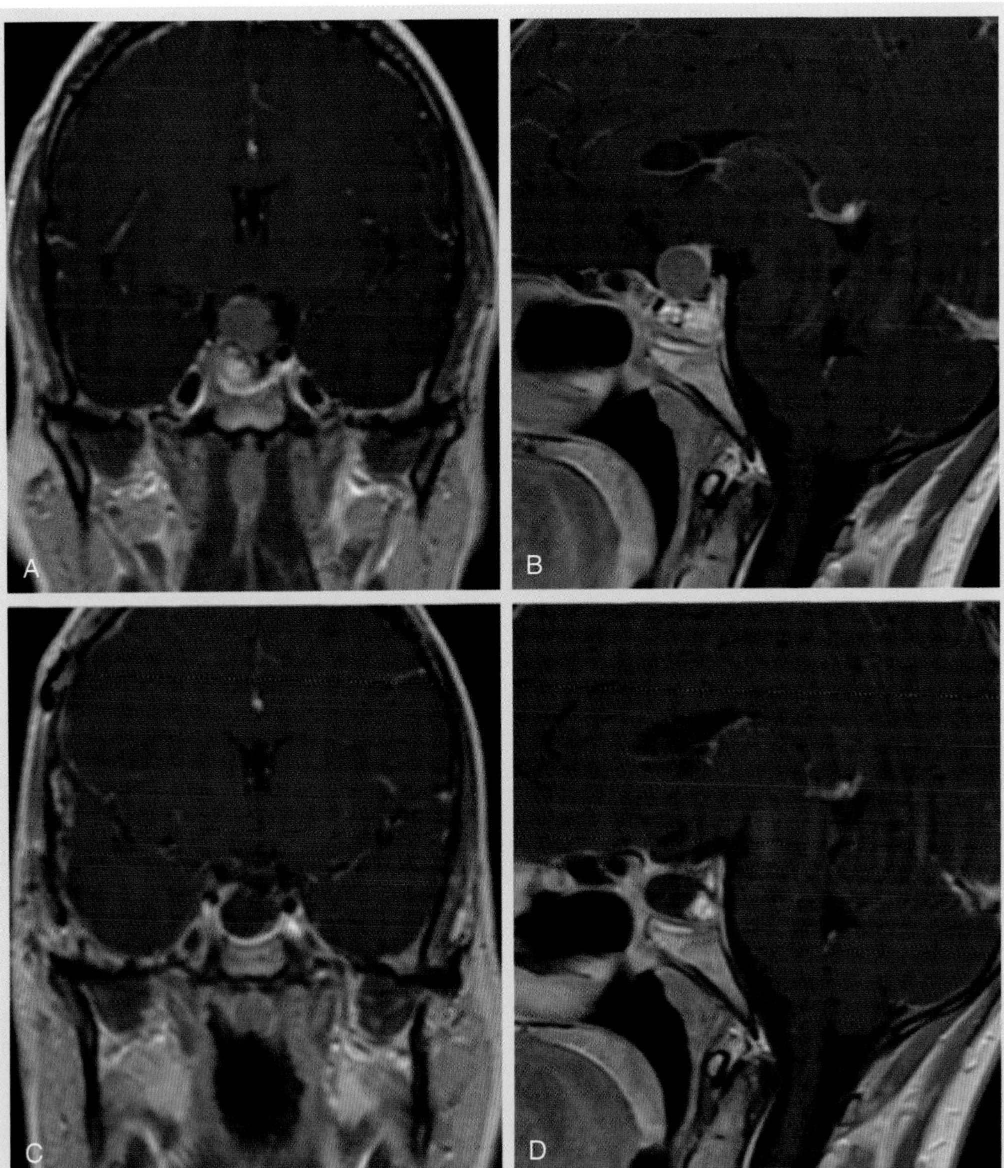

• **Fig. 22.3** Postcontrast magnetic resonance images demonstrate the mildly enhancing residual suprasellar component of a previously resected bilobed cystic-solid Rathke's cleft cyst. (A) Preoperative coronal image demonstrates mild displacement of the overlying optic chiasm by the suprasellar mass. (B) Preoperative sagittal image demonstrates that the mass is suprasellar and disconnected from the sella. (C and D) 3-month postoperative coronal and sagittal images demonstrate gross total resection with preservation of the optic chiasm and pituitary stalk.

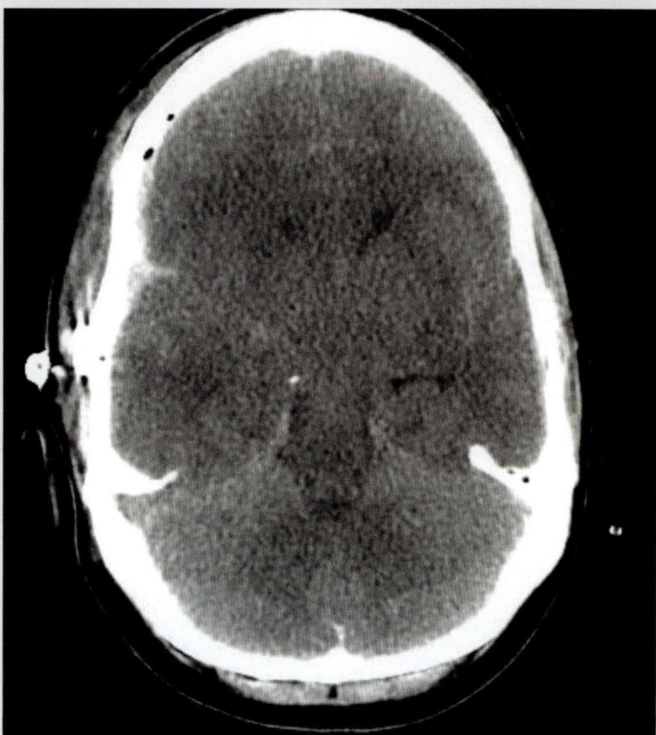

• **Fig. 22.4** Noncontrast head computed tomography shows diffuse cerebral edema and effacement of the basal cisterns. There is also mild enlargement of the left temporal horn.

NEUROSURGICAL SELFIE MOMENT

Despite the advantages of transnasal routes, a small proportion of pituitary tumors require a transcranial approach, depending on several preexisting factors. Careful preoperative evaluation of imaging will help guide the appropriate approach, and detailed knowledge of the normal and distorted anatomy is essential to avoid complications. Because optic and pituitary apparatus injuries are devastating, patients should undergo meticulous pre- and postoperative monitoring and management to avoid or minimize the effects of vision loss and pituitary hormone dysfunction. Preserving the subtle planes involved with pituitary tumor surgery, combined with meticulous microscopic dissection, will minimize both direct and indirect injury.

References

1. Buchfelder M, Kreutzer J. Transcranial surgery for pituitary adenomas. *Pituitary*. 2008;11(4):375–384.
2. Pratheesh R, Rajaratnam S, Prabhu K, Mani SE, Chacko G, Chacko AG. The current role of transcranial surgery in the management of pituitary adenomas. *Pituitary*. 2013;16(4):419–434.
3. Zada G, Du R, Laws ER. Defining the "edge of the envelope": patient selection in treating complex sellar-based neoplasms via transsphenoidal versus open craniotomy. *J Neurosurg*. 2011;114(2):286–300.
4. Youssef AS, Agazzi S, van Loveren HR. Transcranial surgery for pituitary adenomas. *Neurosurgery*. 2005;57(suppl 1):168–175, discussion 168–175.
5. Komotar RJ, Starke RM, Raper DMS, Anand VK, Schwartz TH. Endoscopic endonasal compared with microscopic transsphenoidal and open transcranial resection of giant pituitary adenomas. *Pituitary*. 2012;15(2):150–159.
6. Rhoton AL. The sellar region. *Neurosurgery*. 2002;51(suppl 4):S335–S374.
7. Bergland RM, Ray BS, Torack RM. Anatomical variations in the pituitary gland and adjacent structures in 225 human autopsy cases. *J Neurosurg*. 1968;28(2):93–99.
8. Kumaran AM, Sundar G, Chye LT. Traumatic optic neuropathy: a review. *Craniomaxillofac Trauma Reconstr*. 2015;8(1):31–41.
9. Yasargil MG. *Microneurosurgery*. Stuttgart: Georg Thieme; 1984.
10. Lee KF, Muhd Nor NI, Yaakub A, Wan Hitam WH. Traumatic optic neuropathy: a review of 24 patients. *Int J Ophthalmol*. 2010; 3(2):175–178.
11. Rajiniganth MG, Gupta AK, Gupta A, Bapuraj JR. Traumatic optic neuropathy: visual outcome following combined therapy protocol. *Arch Otolaryngol Head Neck Surg*. 2003;129(11):1203–1206.
12. Prete A, Corsello SM, Salvatori R. Current best practice in the management of patients after pituitary surgery. *Ther Adv Endocrinol Metab*. 2017;8(3):33–48.
13. Nemergut EC, Dumont AS, Barry UT, Laws ER. Perioperative management of patients undergoing transsphenoidal pituitary surgery. *Anesth Analg*. 2005;101(4):1170–1181.
14. Kristof RA, Rother M, Neuloh G, Klingmüller D. Incidence, clinical manifestations, and course of water and electrolyte metabolism disturbances following transsphenoidal pituitary adenoma surgery: a prospective observational study. *J Neurosurg*. 2009;111(3): 555–562.

23

Thalamic and Insular Tumors: Minimizing Deficits

SHAWN L. HERVEY-JUMPER, MITCHEL S. BERGER

HIGHLIGHTS

- Insular and thalamic intrinsic brain tumors pose perioperative risk due to their proximity to functional cortical and subcortical pathways and neurovascular structures.
- Preservation of M2 insular and lenticulostriate arteries is critical to prevent postoperative stroke.
- Cortical and subcortical mapping to identify language and motor sites, particularly the posterior limb of the internal capsule, limits the risk of postoperative deficits.

Introduction

The role of surgery in the treatment of intrinsic brain tumors is to establish the correct histologic and molecular diagnosis, relieve mass effect, and provide maximal safe resection to improve both overall and progression-free survival. Nearly 50% of tumors are within difficult-to-access areas, with either presumed functional significance or close association with vascular structures. Surgical decisions therefore must balance reduction of tumor volume with avoidance of important neurovascular structures. Gliomas are the most common primary intrinsic brain tumor. The majority of gliomas are located in the cerebral hemispheres; however, 6.4% are located within the deep structures of the cerebrum, including primarily the insula and thalamus.[1,2] Tumors within the insula and thalamus remain a challenge to manage given proximity to functionally significant areas and intimate relationship with vascular structures. Surgical techniques such as awake craniotomy with cortical and subcortical mapping permit maximal extent of resection while minimizing postoperative morbidity.[3,4] Intraoperative violation of cortical and subcortical functional pathways may lead to immediate neurologic sequelae, negatively impacting quality of life and survival. Additionally, injuries to branches of the middle cerebral artery or lenticulostriate arteries are well reported and often have catastrophic consequences, which can range from (1) stroke to (2) hemorrhage, (3) vasospasm, or (4) thrombosis. This chapter will discuss surgical approaches for intrinsic brain tumors located within the thalamus and insula.

Indications for Surgery

Gliomas and brain metastasis are the most common deep-seated intrinsic brain tumors, with the most robust body of literature in support of maximal safe resection. There are four histologic grades for gliomas recognized by the World Health Organization (WHO). Grade I tumors have minimal proliferative potential and circumscribed growth. WHO grade II gliomas include diffuse astrocytoma, pleomorphic xanthoastrocytoma, and oligodendroglioma. These tumors have low mitotic activity; however, given their infiltrative nature, they have a tendency to recur, albeit most commonly near the site of initial presentation. WHO grade III gliomas, such as anaplastic astrocytoma, display nuclear anaplasia and increased cellularity. Glioblastomas are WHO grade IV gliomas and represent the most common primary brain tumor in adults. Numerous studies have examined the relationship between extent of resection and volume of residual tumor, overall survival, progression-free survival, and time to malignant transformation among patients with low- and high-grade gliomas.[2,5–26] Although no class I data exist, the majority of published reports suggest that greater extent of resection improves overall survival and progression-free survival, and lengthens the time to malignant transformation.

Anatomic Insights and Surgical Approach

Intrinsic brain tumors within the insula or thalamus were previously considered inoperable due to the high risk of perioperative complications. However, a combination of improved microsurgical techniques, neuroanesthesia, and advanced structural and functional imaging permit greater access to many insular and thalamic tumors. Surgical approach and technical considerations for tumors within the insula and thalamus are discussed in this chapter.

Approaches to the Insula

Opercular landmarks at the cerebral surface may be beneficial to localize structures within the insula. The insula is a triangular-shaped structure within the sylvian fissure, which lies deep to the frontal, parietal, and temporal lobes. The optimal approach to insular lesions may require either splitting the sylvian fissure or resecting the overlying operculum; therefore it's critical to know both sylvian fissure anatomy and cortical opercular landmarks. The sylvian fissure consists of a central stem in addition to horizontal, anterior ascending, and posterior rami. The longest portion of the sylvian fissure is the posterior ramus, which extends posterior and superior and terminates in the inferior parietal lobule. The anterior horizontal and anterior ascending rami are shorter and divide the inferior frontal gyrus into the pars opercularis, orbitalis, and triangularis. The insular surface faces laterally and is enclosed by the anterior and posterior limiting (also known as circular) sulci. The limiting sulcus has anterior, superior, and inferior parts.[27]

The insular cortex is composed of an anterior limen insula, central sulcus, three anterior short gyri, and two posteriorly placed long gyri. The central sulcus of the insula is a continuation of the central sulcus of the cerebral hemispheres. Two anterior sulci separate the three short gyri, and a single sulcus separates the two long posterior gyri. The insular pole is located at the anteroinferior edge of the insula, where the short gyri converge to form a rounded area lateral to the limen. The insular apex is the highest and most prominent laterally projecting area on the insular convexity. Lying underneath the cortical surface of the pars opercularis is the superior portion of the anterior and middle short insular gyri. Posteriorly, the supramarginal gyrus overlies the superior limiting sulcus and the superior portion of the posterior long gyri. The limen insula overlies the uncinate fasciculus.[27,28] Additionally, the anterior perforated substance lies medial to the limen. The middle cerebral artery bifurcates at the limen insula, forming M2 branches, which overlay the insular surface.

Insular tumors are among the most challenging neurosurgical lesions to manage. Tumor location and hemisphere of language dominance determine whether a transcortical or transsylvian approach should be considered.[28] Patients are put in a semilateral position with the head parallel to the floor.[29] For tumors located predominantly above or below the sylvian fissure, the vertex of the head is positioned 15 degrees toward the floor. The craniotomy is tailored based on tumor location and involvement of the overlying frontal or temporal operculum. Insular tumors may be approached based on their location within four zones. The sylvian line divides the insular cortex into dorsal and ventral parts. The foramen of Monro divides the insula into rostral and caudal portions, creating four zones.[4] The transcortical exposure offers the maximal insular exposure with the widest surgical window and surgical freedom.[28] The insular surface is exposed and surgical resection continues as the vessels of the sylvian fissure are skeletonized, which creates "surgical windows." The resection is continued by working under the sylvian fissure along the uncinate fasciculus. Cortical and subcortical sensorimotor and language mapping may be utilized, particularly for posterior zone 2 and 3 tumors. The suprasylvian lenticulostriate arteries must be identified and preserved, and subcortical motor mapping of the corticospinal tract marks the medial border of the resection.

Approaches to the Thalamus

The choice of surgical approach for thalamic tumor resection balances tumor location, vascularity, and the location of the posterior limb of the internal capsule. Thalamic tumors are relatively rare, representing 2% of all brain tumors.[30] Although lesions in this location have historically been surgically treated with stereotactic biopsy alone, advanced structural imaging and microsurgical techniques have allowed for surgical resection with acceptable perioperative morbidity. The surgical corridor of choice uses the shortest route to the tumor avoiding the internal capsule and normal thalamus. These decisions are made based on careful study of preoperative axial and coronal magnetic resonance imaging (MRI) with addition of diffusion tensor imaging (DTI) tractography. Operative approaches include (1) middle temporal gyrus approach, (2) occipital transtentorial approach, (3) middle frontal gyrus approach, (4) transcallosal approach, and (5) combined approaches.[30]

Surgical resection is reserved for contrast-enhancing tumors with clear margins on preoperative imaging. Nonenhancing tumors with poorly defined margins should be treated with biopsy alone given their propensity to have functional tissue within the lesion. Surgical approach is based on tumor location (anterior or posterior within the thalamus) and proximity to the posterior limb of the internal capsule. The middle temporal gyrus approach is used predominantly for posterolateral tumors close to the temporal horn of the lateral ventricle. The occipital transtentorial approach offers maximal exposure for posterior medially placed thalamic tumors in close proximity to the third ventricle. The middle frontal gyrus approach is used for anterolateral thalamic tumors extending superiorly into the frontal lobe. The transcallosal approach is rarely used but is saved for anteromedial thalamic tumors. The majority of deep-seated intrinsic tumors cause anterolateral displacement of the posterior limb of the internal capsule, making the middle temporal gyrus corridor the common approach. After a temporal corticectomy, the tumor is approached through the lateral ventricle along the posterolateral margin of the tumor. Upon reaching the temporal horn of the lateral ventricle, the tumor is approached through the choroidal fissure. This approach ensures an entry corridor inferior to the insula and posterior to the internal capsule.

Complications

Surgery for intrinsic brain tumors within the insula and thalamus carries risk of developing postoperative medical and surgical complications. Neurologic complications may produce visual field, motor, sensory, cognitive, or language deficits.[31] They result from violation of functional cortical and subcortical pathways, cerebral edema, hematoma, or vascular injury. In most series, the risk of a new neurologic deficit after craniotomy for resection of a thalamic or insular tumor ranges from 10% to 25%. These risks increase with older age, deep tumor location, tumor proximity to functional regions, and a low Karnofsky Performance Scale score at presentation. Neurologic complications can be minimized by individualizing the surgical approach based on anatomic and functional imaging, cortical mapping techniques, minimizing excessive brain retraction, meticulous hemostasis, and early identification of major vascular structures.

Additional complications are related to the surgical wound and surrounding brain parenchyma. These events include surgical wound infections, pneumocephalus, cerebrospinal fluid (CSF) leaks, hydrocephalus, seizure, brain abscess/cerebritis, meningitis, and pseudomeningocele. These complications occur in 1% to 5% of patients undergoing craniotomy for resection of an intrinsic brain tumor, and happen more readily in patients over the age of 65 years and in those undergoing reoperation. Posterior fossa location and reoperations are associated with a higher rate of pseudomeningocele, CSF fistula, and hydrocephalus. Postoperative wound infections occur in 1% to 2% of patients after supratentorial craniotomy, most commonly from *Staphylococcus* or *Staphylococcus* species. The risk of postoperative seizures after supratentorial craniotomy is 0.5% to 5%.

Complication Avoidance

Neurologic deficits from insular and thalamic tumors are highly variable and depend on tumor location and extent of disease. Preoperative clinical evaluation includes baseline motor and language assessments for dominant-hemisphere tumors. DTIs for white matter tracts and task-based functional brain MRI are helpful adjuvants to decrease perioperative morbidity (Fig. 23.1).[32,33] Preoperative imaging provides information regarding tumor location,

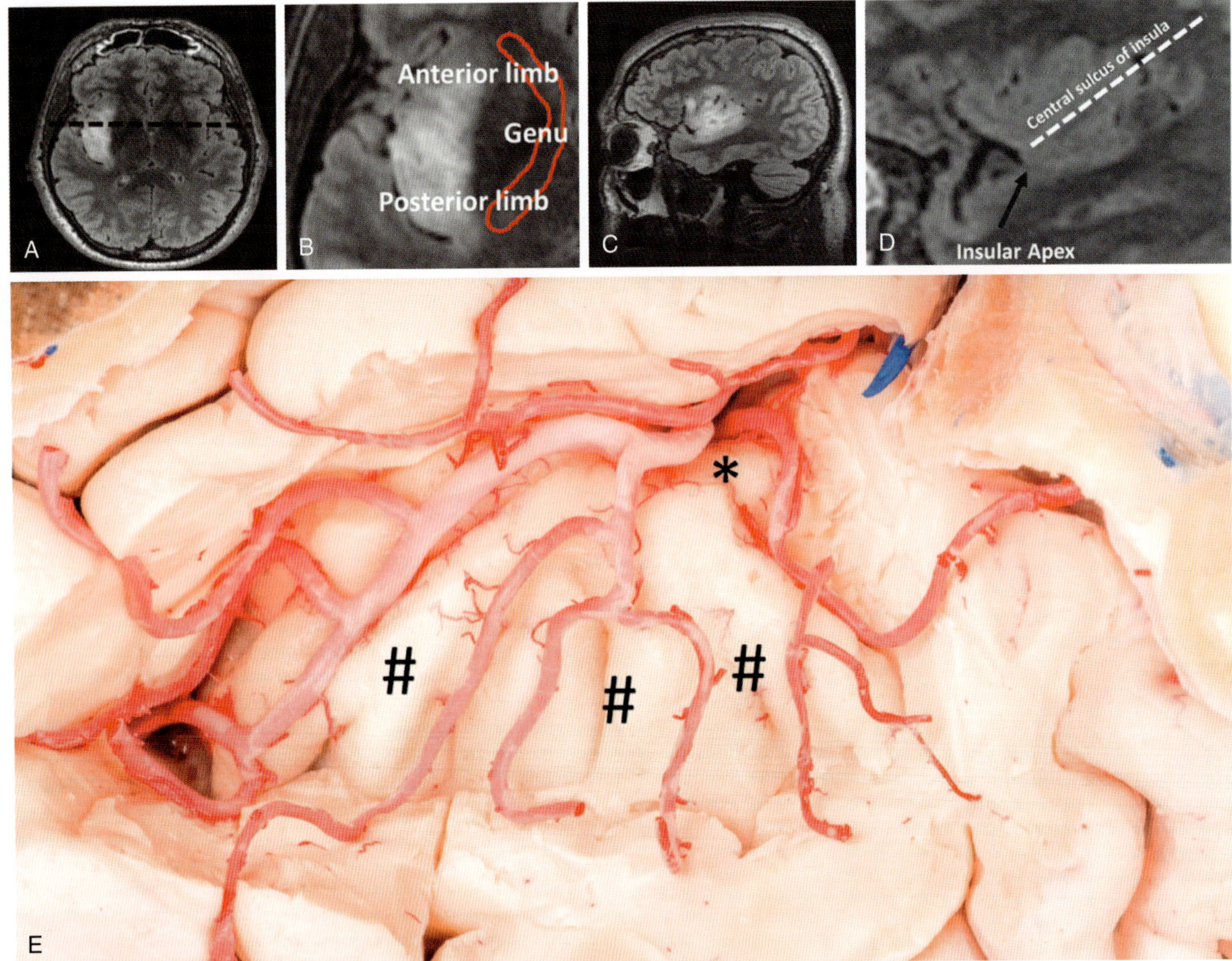

• **Fig. 23.1** (A) Axial fluid-attenuated inversion recovery (FLAIR) magnetic resonance imaging (MRI) shows zone 2 insular glioma with the majority of the mass posterior to the foramen of Monro, according to Berger-Sanai classification system. (B) Magnified view reveals proximity of the insular mass to the posterior limb of the internal capsule (outlined in red). (C) Sagittal FLAIR MRI reveals anterior short and posterior long insular gyri, which upon further magnification (D) illustrates the central sulcus of the insula. (E) Cadaveric dissection inverted for surgical views shows the insular apex (*) in addition to operative "windows" between M2 vessels, through which tumor resection occurs (#).

vascularity, mass effect, peritumoral edema, and proximity to areas of potential functional significance. Additionally, MRIs can be reconstructed to create three-dimensional neuronavigation models for use during surgery. Functional MRI uses blood oxygenation level–dependent signal to identify cortical regions of activation with 85% sensitivity for language and 92% sensitivity for motor areas.[34,35] Similarly, DTI defines the structure of white matter tracts surrounding a tumor and is commonly used in the planning of both surgical and radiation therapy.[36–38]

RED FLAGS

- Large infiltrative tumors
- Significant mass effect
- Lesions infiltrating basal ganglia and deep nuclei
- Previous radiation therapy
- Patients presenting with neurologic deficits

Avoiding Functional Cortical and Subcortical Pathways

The management of intrinsic brain tumors begins with surgery aimed at establishing the pathologic diagnosis and maximal safe resection. Corticosteroids are commonly used preoperatively to reduce symptoms of mass effect and peritumoral vasogenic edema during surgery. Though timing and dose of corticosteroids vary by surgeon preference, a common regimen for adults is 4 to 6 mg of dexamethasone intravenously or by mouth every 6 hours for 48 hours before surgery. Patients presenting with seizures should be initiated on an anticonvulsant, especially if considering intraoperative mapping.[31,39,40] Direct cortical stimulation mapping allows for the identification of language, motor, and sensory function during surgery.[4] Direct stimulation mapping is the gold standard for identification and preservation of functional areas, which are critical when determining a function-free corridor. Cortical stimulation depolarizes a focal area of brain, which excites local neurons via diffusion of current using both orthodromic and antidromic propagation. Bipolar or monopolar stimulation may be used. Bipolar stimulation using a 2-mm tip with 5 mm of separation allows for local diffusion and more precise mapping.[41] Mapping begins with a stimulation current of 1.5 to 2 mA and increases to a maximum of 6 mA if necessary. A constant current generator delivers 1.25-ms biphasic square waves in 4-s trains at 60 Hz. Electrocorticography is used to detect after-discharge potentials and subclinical seizures, which improves both safety and accuracy. Motor sites are identified as slowing of movement with active mapping or involuntary movement with passive mapping. Cortical language sites are tested at least three times, and a positive site is defined as the inability to count, name objects, or read words during stimulation in at least two of three trials.[42] Positive language sites include speech arrest, anomia, and alexia. Speech arrest is defined as discontinuation in number counting without simultaneous motor response.[42]

Maintaining an Intralesional Resection

When approaching insular and thalamic tumors, an intralesional resection is critical given surrounding neurovascular structures. Working through narrow surgical corridors, it may be difficult to remain within the tumor and avoid functional areas. The nonfluorescent amino acid precursor 5-ALA produces an accumulation of fluorescent porphyrins (mainly protoporphyrin IX) in high-grade gliomas.[43] Exogenous 5-ALA results in accumulation of intracellular fluorescent protoporphyrins in high-grade glioma, which peaks 4 to 6 hours after administration and remains elevated for 12 hours.[44] The active metabolite protoporphyrin IX has an absorption band strongest in the 380 ± 420-nm spectrum, emitting red fluorescence at 635 and 704 nm in the brain. A long-pass filter mounted to the surgical microscope allows for tumor visualization as the operator switches between white and violet light. Thorough removal of all fluorescent tumor improves 6-month and overall survival in malignant glioma without an increase in postoperative neurologic deficits.[43] This approach is particularly useful for insular and thalamic gliomas.

Avoiding Vascular Injury

The M2 branches of the middle cerebral artery supply the insula and arise from the superior, inferior, and middle trunks of the middle cerebral artery. Short insular perforator arteries may be sacrificed because they supply only the insular cortex; however, the three to five main insular arteries should be maintained throughout resection. After passing over the insular surface, these vessels continue to supply the extreme capsule and claustrum. Additionally, the lenticulostriate artery branches off the main M1 trunk, which supplies the substantia innominate, putamen, globus pallidus, caudate, and internal capsule after penetrating the anterior perforating substance. Preservation of these vessels is critical to prevent stroke (particularly involving the posterior internal capsule).

Conflicts of Interest

Shawn L. Hervey-Jumper and Mitchel S. Berger declare that they have no conflicts of interest.

SURGICAL REWIND

My Worst Case

A 44-year-old male presented with new-onset seizure and was found to have a nonenhancing brain mass concerning for glioma located within zone 1 of the insula on the left. The patient was scheduled for an awake language and motor mapping craniotomy for tumor resection. Tumor was "woody" and firm in consistency. The resection began through three windows into the subinsular space with motor mapping and monitoring during the resection. During follow-up motor mapping, it was determined that the patient was no longer able to move his right arm or leg, with associated facial asymmetry. Papaverine was used intraoperatively, and all insular arteries were inspected. The lenticulostriate artery along the proximal M1 vessel was encased in tumor and never found throughout the case. On postoperative day 2, patient had complete right-sided flaccid paralysis with 3+ deep tendon reflexes. On postoperative day 4, patient began to have a flicker of movement in toes and proximal thigh. Postoperative MRI diffusion-weighted images showed a small area of restricted diffusion within the posterior limb of the internal capsule. Patient returned to clinic 2 months later able to ambulate with 4-/5 right biceps and triceps but continued to have severe functional limitations in the right hand.

References

1. Larjavaara S, Mantyla R, Salminen T, et al. Incidence of gliomas by anatomic location. *Neuro Oncol.* 2007;9:319–325.
2. Smith JS, Chang EF, Lamborn KR, et al. Role of extent of resection in the long-term outcome of low-grade hemispheric gliomas. *J Clin Oncol.* 2008;26:1338–1345.
3. Hervey-Jumper SL, Berger MS. Role of surgical resection in low- and high-grade gliomas. *Curr Treat Options Neurol.* 2014;16:284.
4. Hervey-Jumper SL, Li J, Lau D, et al. Awake craniotomy to maximize glioma resection: methods and technical nuances over a 27-year period. *J Neurosurg.* 2015;123:325–339.
5. Claus EB, Horlacher A, Hsu L, et al. Survival rates in patients with low-grade glioma after intraoperative magnetic resonance image guidance. *Cancer.* 2005;103:1227–1233.
6. Ito S, Chandler KL, Prados MD, et al. Proliferative potential and prognostic evaluation of low-grade astrocytomas. *J Neurooncol.* 1994;19:1–9.
7. Ius T, Isola M, Budai R, et al. Low-grade glioma surgery in eloquent areas: volumetric analysis of extent of resection and its impact on overall survival. A single-institution experience in 190 patients: clinical article. *J Neurosurg.* 2012;117:1039–1052.
8. Johannesen TB, Langmark F, Lote K. Progress in long-term survival in adult patients with supratentorial low-grade gliomas: a population-based study of 993 patients in whom tumors were diagnosed between 1970 and 1993. *J Neurosurg.* 2003;99:854–862.
9. Karim AB, Maat B, Hatlevoll R, et al. A randomized trial on dose-response in radiation therapy of low-grade cerebral glioma: European Organization for Research and Treatment of Cancer (EORTC) Study 22844. *Int J Radiat Oncol Biol Phys.* 1996;36:549–556.
10. Leighton C, Fisher B, Bauman G, et al. Supratentorial low-grade glioma in adults: an analysis of prognostic factors and timing of radiation. *J Clin Oncol.* 1997;15:1294–1301.
11. Lote K, Egeland T, Hager B, et al. Survival, prognostic factors, and therapeutic efficacy in low-grade glioma: a retrospective study in 379 patients. *J Clin Oncol.* 1997;15:3129–3140.
12. Nakamura M, Konishi N, Tsunoda S, et al. Analysis of prognostic and survival factors related to treatment of low-grade astrocytomas in adults. *Oncology.* 2000;58:108–116.
13. Nicolato A, Gerosa MA, Fina P, Iuzzolino P, Giorgiutti F, Bricolo A. Prognostic factors in low-grade supratentorial astrocytomas: a

uni-multivariate statistical analysis in 76 surgically treated adult patients. *Surg Neurol.* 1995;44:208–221, discussion 221–223.
14. North CA, North RB, Epstein JA, Piantadosi S, Wharam MD. Low-grade cerebral astrocytomas. Survival and quality of life after radiation therapy. *Cancer.* 1990;66:6–14.
15. Peraud A, Ansari H, Bise K, Reulen HJ. Clinical outcome of supratentorial astrocytoma WHO grade II. *Acta Neurochir (Wien).* 1998;140:1213–1222.
16. Philippon JH, Clemenceau SH, Fauchon FH, Foncin JF. Supratentorial low-grade astrocytomas in adults. *Neurosurgery.* 1993;32: 554–559.
17. Rajan B, Pickuth D, Ashley S, et al. The management of histologically unverified presumed cerebral gliomas with radiotherapy. *Int J Radiat Oncol Biol Phys.* 1994;28:405–413.
18. Sanai N, Berger MS. Glioma extent of resection and its impact on patient outcome. *Neurosurgery.* 2008;62:753–764, discussion 264–266.
19. Scerrati M, Roselli R, Iacoangeli M, Pompucci A, Rossi GF. Prognostic factors in low grade (WHO grade II) gliomas of the cerebral hemispheres: the role of surgery. *J Neurol Neurosurg Psychiatry.* 1996;61:291–296.
20. Shaw E, Arusell R, Scheithauer B, et al. Prospective randomized trial of low- versus high-dose radiation therapy in adults with supratentorial low-grade glioma: initial report of a North Central Cancer Treatment Group/Radiation Therapy Oncology Group/Eastern Cooperative Oncology Group study. *J Clin Oncol.* 2002;20:2267–2276.
21. Shibamoto Y, Kitakabu Y, Takahashi M, et al. Supratentorial low-grade astrocytoma. Correlation of computed tomography findings with effect of radiation therapy and prognostic variables. *Cancer.* 1993;72:190–195.
22. Snyder LA, Wolf AB, Oppenlander ME, et al. The impact of extent of resection on malignant transformation of pure oligodendrogliomas. *J Neurosurg.* 2014;120:309–314.
23. van Veelen ML, Avezaat CJ, Kros JM, van Putten W, Vecht C. Supratentorial low grade astrocytoma: prognostic factors, dedifferentiation, and the issue of early versus late surgery. *J Neurol Neurosurg Psychiatry.* 1998;64:581–587.
24. Vecht CJ, Avezaat CJ, van Putten WL, Eijkenboom WM, Stefanko SZ. The influence of the extent of surgery on the neurological function and survival in malignant glioma. A retrospective analysis in 243 patients. *J Neurol Neurosurg Psychiatry.* 1990;53:466–471.
25. Whitton AC, Bloom HJ. Low grade glioma of the cerebral hemispheres in adults: a retrospective analysis of 88 cases. *Int J Radiat Oncol Biol Phys.* 1990;18:783–786.
26. Yeh SA, Ho JT, Lui CC, Huang YJ, Hsiung CY, Huang EY. Treatment outcomes and prognostic factors in patients with supratentorial low-grade gliomas. *Br J Radiol.* 2005;78:230–235.
27. Tanriover N, Rhoton AL Jr, Kawashima M, Ulm AJ, Yasuda A. Microsurgical anatomy of the insula and the sylvian fissure. *J Neurosurg.* 2004;100:891–922.
28. Benet A, Hervey-Jumper SL, Sanchez JJ, Lawton MT, Berger MS. Surgical assessment of the insula. Part 1: surgical anatomy and morphometric analysis of the transsylvian and transcortical approaches to the insula. *J Neurosurg.* 2016;124:469–481.
29. Sanai N, Polley MY, Berger MS. Insular glioma resection: assessment of patient morbidity, survival, and tumor progression. *J Neurosurg.* 2010;112:1–9.
30. Sai Kiran NA, Thakar S, Dadlani R, et al. Surgical management of thalamic gliomas: case selection, technical considerations, and review of literature. *Neurosurg Rev.* 2013;36:383–393.
31. Chang SM, Parney IF, Huang W, et al. Patterns of care for adults with newly diagnosed malignant glioma. *JAMA.* 2005;293:557–564.
32. Deng X, Zhang Y, Xu L, et al. Comparison of language cortex reorganization patterns between cerebral arteriovenous malformations and gliomas: a functional MRI study. *J Neurosurg.* 2015;122:996–1003.
33. Ille S, Sollmann N, Hauck T, et al. Combined noninvasive language mapping by navigated transcranial magnetic stimulation and functional MRI and its comparison with direct cortical stimulation. *J Neurosurg.* 2015;123:212–225.
34. Bogomolny DL, Petrovich NM, Hou BL, Peck KK, Kim MJ, Holodny AI. Functional MRI in the brain tumor patient. *Top Magn Reson Imaging.* 2004;15:325–335.
35. Nimsky C, Ganslandt O, Von Keller B, Romstock J, Fahlbusch R. Intraoperative high-field-strength MR imaging: implementation and experience in 200 patients. *Radiology.* 2004;233:67–78.
36. Alexander AL, Lee JE, Lazar M, Field AS. Diffusion tensor imaging of the brain. *Neurother.* 2007;4:316–329.
37. Bello L, Gambini A, Castellano A, et al. Motor and language DTI Fiber Tracking combined with intraoperative subcortical mapping for surgical removal of gliomas. *Neuroimage.* 2008;39:369–382.
38. Berman JI, Berger MS, Chung SW, Nagarajan SS, Henry RG. Accuracy of diffusion tensor magnetic resonance imaging tractography assessed using intraoperative subcortical stimulation mapping and magnetic source imaging. *J Neurosurg.* 2007;107:488–494.
39. Chang EF, Potts MB, Keles GE, et al. Seizure characteristics and control following resection in 332 patients with low-grade gliomas. *J Neurosurg.* 2008;108:227–235.
40. Lima GL, Duffau H. Is there a risk of seizures in "preventive" awake surgery for incidental diffuse low-grade gliomas? *J Neurosurg.* 2015;122:1397–1405.
41. Nathan SS, Sinha SR, Gordon B, Lesser RP, Thakor NV. Determination of current density distributions generated by electrical stimulation of the human cerebral cortex. *Electroencephalogr Clin Neurophysiol.* 1993;86:183–192.
42. Sanai N, Mirzadeh Z, Berger MS. Functional outcome after language mapping for glioma resection. *N Engl J Med.* 2008;358:18–27.
43. Stummer W, Pichlmeier U, Meinel T, et al. Fluorescence-guided surgery with 5-aminolevulinic acid for resection of malignant glioma: a randomised controlled multicentre phase III trial. *Lancet Oncol.* 2006;7:392–401.
44. Stummer W, Reulen HJ, Novotny A, Stepp H, Tonn JC. Fluorescence-guided resections of malignant gliomas–an overview. *Acta Neurochir Suppl.* 2003;88:9–12.

24 Complications of Surgery for Pineal Region Tumors

RANDY S. D'AMICO, JEFFREY N. BRUCE

HIGHLIGHTS

- Gross total resection decreases the risk for postoperative hemorrhage and should be pursued in the absence of contraindications.
- Pupil abnormalities, difficulty focusing or accommodating, impaired extraocular movements, and limited upward gaze are postoperative deficits that are frequently encountered after surgery for pineal lesions. These deficits are typically transient.
- Great care should always be taken to avoid damage to the deep cerebral veins.
- Acute cerebellar swelling from venous infarct is an unpredictable and potentially deadly complication of supracerebellar infratentorial approaches to the pineal region.
- In the setting of acute postoperative cerebellar swelling, rapid decompression and/or removal of hematoma and infarcted cerebellum may be the only way to efficiently treat and save a patient.
- The use of fixed retractors should be minimized whenever possible.

Background

The pineal region gives rise to a heterogeneous group of neoplastic and nonneoplastic lesions. Neurosurgical intervention—ranging from biopsy to complete resection—remains vital to the management of pineal region tumors.[1–4] In particular, aggressive surgical resection facilitates accurate diagnosis, the reduction of mass effect, and the management of associated symptoms such as hydrocephalus. Management strategies centered around aggressive resection, in conjunction with advances in microsurgical techniques, neuroanesthesia, postoperative critical care, and chemotherapy/radiotherapy, have resulted in excellent long-term outcomes for patients with benign pathologies and in improved long-term prognoses for patients with malignant tumors.[5]

The pineal region is an anatomically complex and surgically intimidating environment. Located deep and centrally within the posterior incisural space, the pineal gland is in close proximity to the cerebellum, collicular plate, bilateral pulvinars, and critical deep cerebrovascular structures.[6] As a result, the complete, safe resection of pineal lesions remains among the most challenging of neurosurgical procedures.

Fortunately, a variety of adaptable surgical approaches to the pineal region have been developed.[5,7,8] Each approach takes into consideration the relevant anatomic relationships of the region, the location of the blood supply to the lesion, and the extent of resection goals of the surgery. Furthermore, each approach offers unique mitigation of the risks to critical adjacent structures. Although the availability of a variety of surgical approaches, in combination with advances in microsurgical techniques, has made the surgical management of pineal lesions safer, surgery for pineal region tumors remains complex and fraught with potential pitfalls, with permanent morbidity ranging from 1.0% to 20.0%, and reported mortality rates ranging from 0.7% to 4.0% (Table 24.1) in large series.[1–4]

Anatomic Insights

Hemorrhage

Postoperative hemorrhage into an incompletely resected tumor (Fig. 24.1) is the most serious complication after pineal surgery.[1–5] Risk of postoperative hemorrhage is closely associated with the nature of the tumor and its malignant potential, with a higher incidence after subtotal resections of soft, vascular malignant pineal parenchymal tumors.[1-5,9] Notably, the risk of postoperative hemorrhage remains over several postoperative days, and careful surveillance with frequent neurologic assessment is critical. Whereas small hemorrhages without significant mass effect can usually be managed conservatively, large hemorrhages may require immediate evacuation and are associated with a greater risk of mortality.[4] Importantly, any hemorrhage can result in obstructive hydrocephalus requiring urgent cerebrospinal fluid (CSF) diversion.

Hydrocephalus

Pineal lesions are commonly diagnosed in the setting of progressive symptomatic hydrocephalus, and the majority of patients require preoperative CSF diversion.[1,2] Accepted methods of preoperative CSF diversion include temporary solutions such as external ventricular drain (EVD) insertion, or permanent solutions such as ventriculoperitoneal shunt (VPS) insertion or endoscopic third ventriculostomy (ETV). Regardless of the surgeon's choice of CSF diversion, postoperative air, blood, or operative debris after resection of a pineal tumor can result in blockage of a preexisting VPS or EVD catheter, or ventriculostomy. This is particularly worrisome because acute hydrocephalus can result in rapid neurologic deterioration and major morbidity. In cases of acute hydrocephalus after

TABLE 24.1 Pineal Complications

Author	Year	*n*	Approach	Severe/Permanent Morbidity	%	Mortality (%)
Bruce and Stein[1]	1995	160	SCIT	EOM dysfunction	16.0	4.0
			IHTC	Hemorrhage	6.0	
			OTT	Altered mental status	5.0	
				Ataxia	3.0	
				Hemianopsia	1.0	
				Paraparesis/quadriparesis	1.0	
Konovalov and Pitskhelauri[3]	2003	287	OTT	EOM dysfunction	31.0	1.8
			SCIT	Hemorrhage	11.0	
			Subchoroidal	Meningoencephalitis	6.0	
			Fourth ventricle	Hemianopsia	4.0	
Hernesniemi et al.[2]	2008	119	SCIT	Ataxia	1.7	0
			OTT	Vision changes	1.6	
				Hemiparesis	0.8	
Qi et al.[4]	2014	143	OTT	Hemorrhage	3.5	0.7
				Hemianopsia	3.5	
				Parinaud syndrome	2.1	
				Hemiparesis	2.1	
				Altered mental status	1.4	

SCIT, Supracerebellar infratentorial; *IHTC,* interhemispheric transcallosal; *OTT,* occipital transtentorial; *EOM,* extraocular movements.

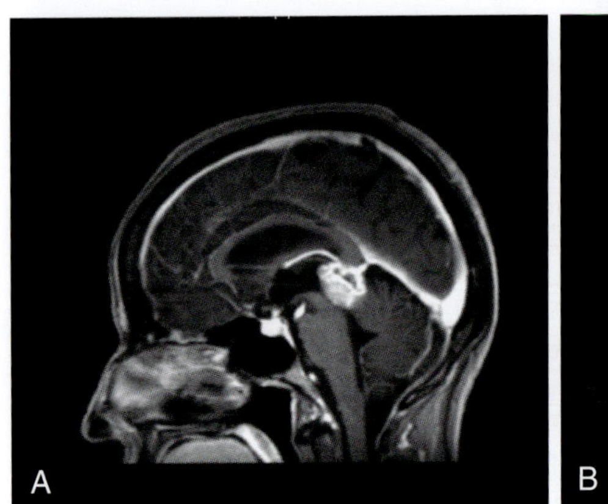

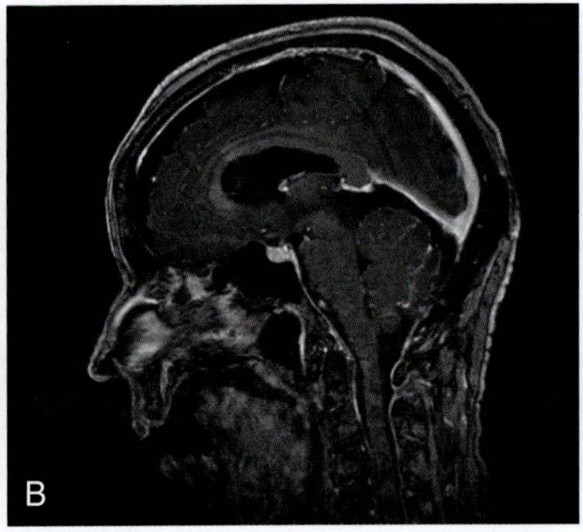

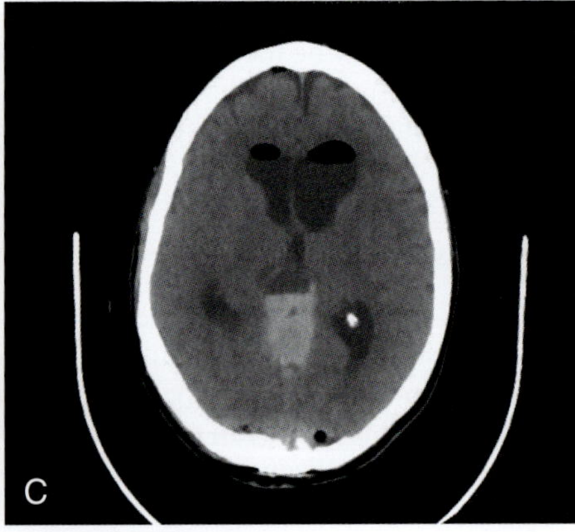

• **Fig. 24.1** Postoperative hemorrhage. This case represents a 65-year-old female who presented for resection of a pineal lesion. Preoperative contrast-enhanced T1-weighted magnetic resonance imaging (MRI) demonstrated what was ultimately diagnosed as a pineal parenchymal tumor of intermediate differentiation (A). The patient underwent uncomplicated tumor resection via a supracerebellar infratentorial approach in the seated position. The patient did well initially and postoperative MRI revealed gross total resection of her tumor (B). On postoperative day 2, the patient developed tachypnea and was diagnosed with massive bilateral pulmonary emboli requiring anticoagulation. On postoperative day 6, while therapeutic on her anticoagulation, she developed headache and nausea progressing to lethargy and left facial weakness. Urgent computed tomography imaging demonstrated acute hemorrhage into the surgical bed with extension into the third and fourth ventricles and associated hydrocephalus, as well as a small epidural hematoma at the site of the craniotomy (C). Anticoagulation was reversed, and an external ventricular drain (EVD) was emergently inserted with improvement of her neurologic symptoms. Given the size of her pulmonary emboli, her cardiopulmonary status, and contraindication to systemic anticoagulation, the patient underwent successful thoracotomy for thrombectomy. During her recovery, her EVD was subsequently transitioned to endoscopic third ventriculostomy and weaned successfully. She has since returned to her preoperative neurologic baseline.

pineal surgery in patients with previous CSF diversion, urgent replacement of an EVD, revision of VPS, or exploration of the previous ventriculostomy should be considered.[5]

In asymptomatic or nonhydrocephalus patients, the surgical resection of a pineal lesion communicates the third ventricle with the quadrigeminal cistern and may preclude the need for permanent CSF diversion. As a result, these patients often do not undergo preoperative definitive management of their hydrocephalus in hopes that resection of the pineal region tumor will prevent the future development of hydrocephalus. However, the presence of intraoperative or postoperative hemorrhage, air, or debris into the ventricular system after pineal region tumor resection can similarly result in the blockage of natural CSF egress with the subsequent development of acute hydrocephalus. Postoperative surveillance is again critical because this group of patients may similarly require urgent temporary or permanent CSF diversion.

Third Ventricle, Brainstem, and Cerebellum

Pineal lesions may cause mass effect on the posterior third ventricle anteriorly, the quadrigeminal plate inferiorly, and the cerebellum posteriorly. Dissection of lesions off the quadrigeminal plate commonly results in pupil abnormalities, difficulty with focusing or accommodating, impaired extraocular movements, and limited upward gaze.[1,10] Permanent impairment is rare. However, normal function may take several months to return, or sometimes as long as a year, and patients should be counseled accordingly. A residual mild limitation of upgaze is common but bears little clinical significance. Although the fourth cranial nerve originates on the posterior midbrain, it generally arises caudal to the tumor origin and is rarely identified or injured during resection.

Impaired consciousness can result from manipulation of brain adjacent to the third ventricle. This impairment is typically transient with return to normal mental status occurring usually over several days after surgery. Significant manipulation of the brainstem can also result in cognitive impairment or, rarely, akinetic mutism.[1–5,7]

Cerebellar manipulation frequently results in mild ataxia postoperatively that resolves over several days. Of greater clinical significance, cerebellar venous infarction with acute cerebellar swelling is a rare and dangerous complication that may cause a rapid clinical decline with high risk of morbidity and mortality due to associated obstructive hydrocephalus or mass effect on the brainstem. This is further discussed below.

Arterial

The pineal gland receives its blood supply from the medial and lateral posterior choroidal branches of the posterior cerebral artery (PCA), and through anastomoses between the pericallosal arteries, the PCA, and the superior cerebellar artery (SCA).[11,12] Both the PCA and SCA and their branches course through the posterior incisural space.[6] The PCA bifurcates into the calcarine and parieto-occipital arteries within the posterior incisural space before crossing above the free edge of the tentorium. Typically, branches of the PCA supply structures above the level of the superior colliculus, whereas branches of the SCA supply structures at or below the inferior colliculus.[6] Damage to the trunks of the PCA or the SCA is rare during surgery for pineal lesions given their caudal location in relation to the tumor. The main arterial risk is to the small perforating branches of the PCA, the SCA, and the choroidal arteries that enter the borders of the quadrigeminal cistern and supply the colliculi, thalamus, and pineal gland itself. In general, choroidal vessels along the tumor capsule are dissected if amenable. However, their preservation is not mandatory if they are simply supplying the choroid plexus.[5]

Venous

The pineal gland is located just anterior to the vein of Galen and is surrounded by many of its large tributaries, including the internal cerebral and basal veins of Rosenthal. Additional nearby veins include the anterior calcarine vein, the posterior pericallosal vein, the collicular veins, and the pineal veins.[6] The risk of significant venous injury varies with approach. Supratentorial approaches require the surgeon to work carefully around the convergence of the deep cerebral veins, where injury can result in venous infarction of the thalamus, hypothalamus, or midbrain. Infratentorial approaches are more suitable for protecting the deep cerebral veins, because the surgeon accesses the pineal gland from a space beneath the bilateral basal veins of Rosenthal.

Two significant venous convergences must still be carefully navigated with infratentorial approaches. Superior cerebellar hemispheric veins and inferior cerebellar hemispheric veins frequently join to form bridging veins that drain large parts of the cerebellum into the tentorial sinuses. Whereas lateral bridging veins may be avoided with midline or off-midline approaches, midline veins may need to be retracted or sacrificed to reach the quadrigeminal cistern and the pineal gland. There is considerable variability in the site of these veins, and available preoperative imaging should be thoroughly reviewed before planning a particular surgical approach.

Once the arachnoid of the quadrigeminal cistern is dissected during infratentorial approaches, a second significant venous convergence that blocks access to the pineal region is identified. The superior vermian vein and the precentral cerebellar vein approach the vein of Galen inferiorly in the midline. The superior vermian vein and the precentral cerebellar vein may need to be retracted or are often sacrificed with midline supracerebellar infratentorial (SCIT) approaches to the pineal region. Importantly, when the precentral cerebellar vein must be sacrificed, it should be divided peripherally to avoid back propagation of thrombosis into the vein of Galen and occlusion of critical collateral circulation, because rare but devastating injuries have been reported.[13]

In general, sacrificing the superior vermian, precentral cerebellar, and hemispheric or vermian bridging veins has been considered relatively safe as long as the collateral circulation of each vein is preserved.[2,14–16] Unfortunately, sacrificing even a limited number of these veins may cause acute or subacute postoperative cerebellar swelling due to venous infarction and/or hemorrhagic conversion (Fig. 24.2). This serious complication may rapidly progress to a life-threatening condition because of mass effect on the brainstem or direct venous infarct of the brainstem.[13,17] This rare and unpredictable complication is thought to be the result of venous insufficiency in a small subset of patients who cannot tolerate the sacrifice of bridging veins in the cerebellum.

The use of cerebellar self-retaining retractors during surgery may further increase the risk of cerebellar swelling by causing local ischemia, cerebellar contusions with resultant venous congestion, or even rupture of superficial bridging veins.[9] The presence of obstructive hydrocephalus or a tight posterior fossa may further contribute to the clinical picture.[18] Rapid decompression and/or removal of hematoma and infarcted cerebellum is the only way to efficiently treat and save a patient in this situation.

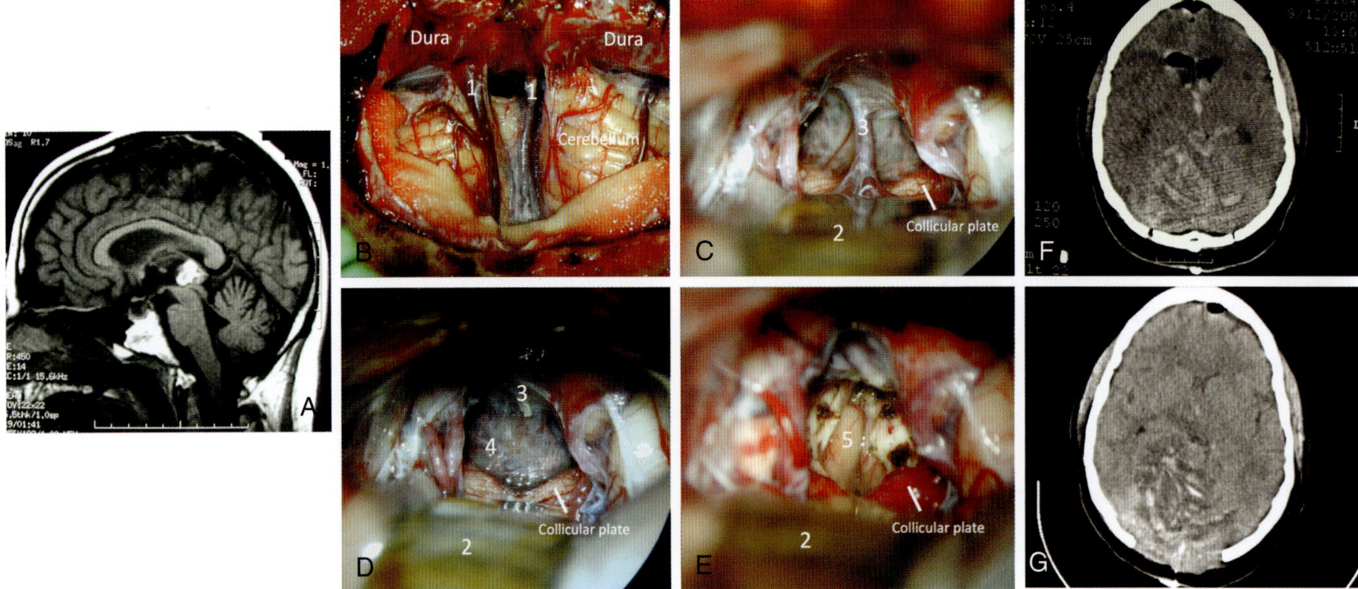

• **Fig. 24.2** Postoperative cerebellar swelling. A 29-year-old female with a history of recurrent headaches presented with acute-onset CN IV palsy, causing diplopia and tinnitus in her left ear, and was found to have a hemorrhagic pineal mass (shown here on noncontrast T1-weighted sagittal magnetic resonance imaging): (A) causing aqueductal stenosis and mild hydrocephalus. The patient underwent an uncomplicated supracerebellar infratentorial approach in the sitting position (B–E). (B) shows the superficial cerebellum after dural opening. Two medial superficial cerebellar bridging veins (1) were identified and sacrificed. Next, the adhesions between the cerebellum and the tentorium were sharply dissected, expanding the operative corridor, and a retractor (2) was placed, permitting clear visualization of the precentral cerebellar vein (3) as shown in (C). The precentral cerebellar vein was subsequently sacrificed, improving visualization of the arachnoid of the quadrigeminal cistern (4) as shown in (D). The lesion was completely removed, and the third ventricle and bilateral medial thalami (5) were clearly visualized and clear of residual tumor, as shown in (E). Postoperatively, the patient did well and was awake, alert, and conversant. Approximately 4 hours postoperatively, the patient was found unresponsive and cyanotic and was emergently intubated. Immediate computed tomography scan demonstrated an acute right cerebellar hemorrhagic infarction with associated mass effect causing severe brainstem compression (F). The patient was taken emergently back to the operating room for decompressive craniectomy (G) and external ventricular drain insertion. Postoperatively, the patient underwent aggressive medical management of persistently elevated intracranial pressures. Unfortunately, the patient remained respirator dependent, quadriplegic, and with a neurologic examination consistent with a locked-in syndrome. Ultimately, the patient's neurologic status did not improve, and she made the decision with her family to withdraw supportive care. Care was withdrawn according to her wishes, and the patient subsequently died. Final pathology was consistent with a hemorrhagic pineal cyst.

Complications Associated With Surgical Approaches

Supracerebellar Infratentorial Approach

The SCIT approach is the most commonly utilized infratentorial approach to the pineal region.[1–3] Performed most frequently in the sitting position, the SCIT capitalizes on the effects of gravity to naturally retract the cerebellum and minimize pooling fluids. The approach provides a relaxed, anatomically neutral midline corridor to the pineal region. As mentioned above, infratentorial approaches require navigation through two sets of venous convergences. Great effort must be taken to minimize the sacrifice of lateral bridging veins responsible for draining large portions of the cerebellum to avoid disruption of the extensive collateral circulation and prevent cerebellar venous infarct and swelling. Fixed rigid retractors are necessary initially, but their use should be minimized as CSF is released. Thick bridging veins and lateral hemispheric bridging veins should be avoided. Similarly, it is critical to avoid injury to the deep cerebral veins.

Complications associated with the sitting position include the potential for air embolism, systemic hypotension (Fig. 24.3), pneumocephalus, and subdural hematomas due to cortical collapse in the setting of significant hydrocephalus suddenly relieved by tumor resection.[1] Air embolism can be anticipated intraoperatively by a drop in end-tidal CO_2 monitoring or by precordial Doppler. Flooding the field with irrigation, applying bilateral jugular vein compression, and obliterating the point of air entrainment usually resolve further air entry, and a central venous catheter is sometimes placed as a way to withdraw intravascular air if clinically indicated.

The incidence of cortical collapse can be reduced by preoperative CSF diversion by ETV or VPS insertion because this allows the ventricular system to accommodate over several days before the resection. Cortical collapse can occur in varying degrees, and

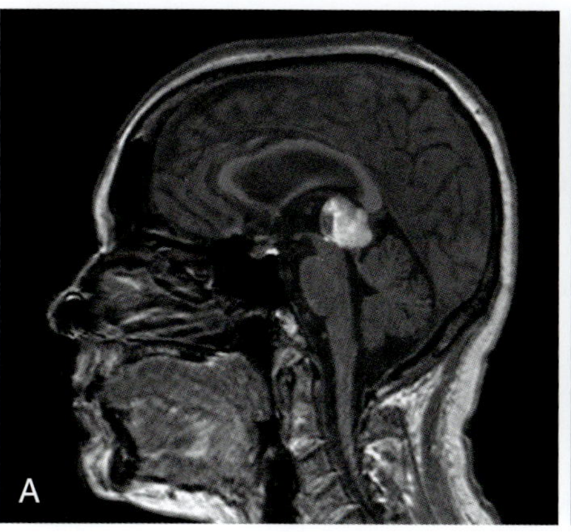

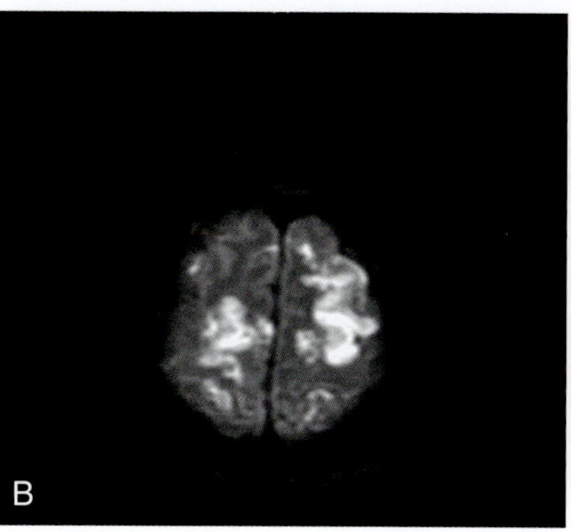

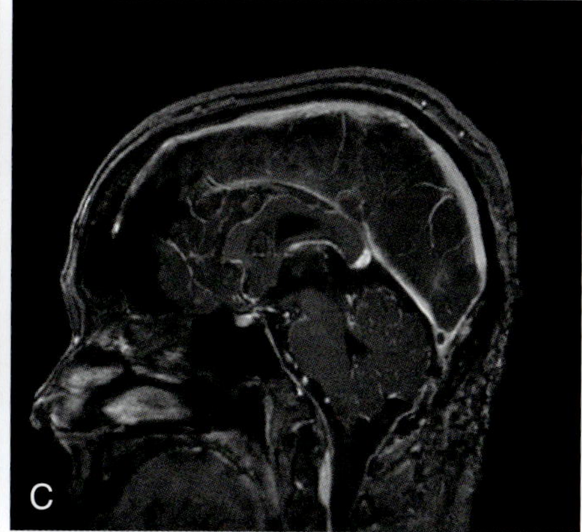

• **Fig. 24.3** Postoperative stroke after intraoperative hypotension in the sitting position. This case represents a 56-year-old female who presented with nausea, ataxia, and fatigue secondary to hydrocephalus caused by a pineal gland lesion. Preoperative contrast-enhanced T1-weighted magnetic resonance imaging (MRI) demonstrated what ultimately was diagnosed as a melanoma metastasis to the pineal gland (A). The patient underwent tumor resection via a supracerebellar infratentorial approach in the seated position. Intraoperatively, the patient experienced a period of hypotension for which she required multiple fluid boluses and pressors. Postoperatively, the patient was slow to return to her baseline neurologic status. Postoperative computed tomography imaging demonstrated normal postoperative changes and pneumocephalus. Postoperative MRI revealed bilateral middle cerebral artery distribution watershed infarcts due to the period of intraoperative hypotension (B), and gross total resection (C). After a prolonged course, the patient returned to her preoperative mental status with residual bilateral lower-extremity weakness.

although it is striking on postoperative imaging, it gradually improves without major neurologic complication.

Occipital Transtentorial Approach

The occipital transtentorial (OTT) approach is the most commonly utilized supratentorial approach and follows a natural corridor between the falx medially, the tentorium inferiorly, and the medial occipital lobe laterally.[4] The OTT requires the surgeon to work past the deep cerebral veins that remain at significant risk during the procedure, because instruments are manipulated between them during tumor removal. The most notable complication of OTT approaches is a transient, and sometimes permanent, postoperative hemianopsia due to excessive retraction on the occipital lobe.[19,20] As with infratentorial approaches, permanent morbidity is reduced by avoiding rigid retraction when possible. Although a significant degree of fixed retraction is initially necessary to provide adequate working space in the interhemispheric fissure, proper head position, mannitol, reverse-Trendelenburg bed position, and progressive CSF drainage during surgery permit removal of the fixed retractors as the operative corridor relaxes and becomes easily accessible. There are few bridging veins encountered during an OTT approach. Although sacrifice should be avoided when possible, deficits after sacrifice of these veins have not been serious or permanent in large series.[4] Cutting the tentorium entails some risk of damage to the deep venous structures given their close relationship to the tentorium, and Doppler ultrasound is typically employed to facilitate safe identification of the straight sinus.

Interhemispheric Transcallosal

The interhemispheric transcallosal (IHTC) approach is an alternative supratentorial approach that develops an operative corridor along the parieto-occipital junction, between the falx medially, the medial cerebral hemisphere laterally, and through the posterior corpus callosum. Complications of the IHTC approach are primarily the result of retraction injury of the parietal lobe, or damage or division of bridging veins, which can cause mild contralateral hemiparesis or astereognostic deficits due to venous congestions or infarction.[5,21] Although these effects are typically transient, sacrifice of more than one bridging vein should be avoided if possible. Unlike the OTT approach, the IHTC approach has not been associated with visual field defects. Rare disconnection syndromes have been reported with dissection of the corpus callosum.[22] Similarly, splenial incisions may rarely cause hemialexia.[21]

RED FLAGS

- Complications are more common in previously irradiated patients, patients with invasive tumors, and those who were progressively symptomatic preoperatively.
- A drop in end-tidal CO_2 is a sign of possible air embolism and demands the surgeon's attention.
- Radiographic findings suggestive of a malignant vascular tumor should inform the surgeon of a higher risk of postoperative hemorrhage.
- Evidence of cerebellar swelling intraoperatively should raise concerns over venous congestion.
- Swelling and progressive encroachment of the operative field by brain may suggest pneumocephalus and warrant placement of a supratentorial burr hole to equalize intracranial compartment pressures.
- Tumor encasement of part of or the entire Galenic venous convergence requires extra care to avoid injury to these veins.

Prevention of Complications

The heterogeneous population of pineal lesions presents with great morphologic variability and varied involvement of adjacent structures. As a result, the surgeon must tailor operative strategies specifically to each case he encounters.[9] Defining the goals and indications for surgical intervention helps avoid a high-risk surgical procedure in some situations. For instance, patients with imaging suggestive of small, nonprogressive low-grade gliomas or a pineal cyst may be observed initially with serial scans. Furthermore, most germ cell tumors are exquisitely sensitive to radiation and therefore do not necessarily warrant immediate surgical intervention. Similarly, certain metastatic tumors may be managed with radiation and Gamma knife radiosurgery, depending on the underlying pathology and prognosis of the patient.

Thorough review of available imaging provides details regarding the size, extent, and vascularity of the lesion. In addition, the surgeon can identify the presence of hydrocephalus and evaluate the involvement of adjacent neurovascular structures. The deep vascular structures, including the internal cerebral veins, the basal vein of Rosenthal, the precentral cerebellar veins, and the superficial vermian vein, should be clearly visualized on preoperative magnetic resonance imaging (MRI).[15] It is equally important to look for superficial bridging veins arising from the cerebellum.[23] However, whether sacrifice of a superficial bridging vein will lead to cerebellar swelling, infarction, or hemorrhage remains unpredictable. Importantly, the angle of tentorium and straight sinus should always be noted because this might influence approach, and the volume of the posterior fossa must be considered in cases of postoperative cerebellar swelling and the potential for brainstem compression.[18]

Neurosurgeons must be proficient with various surgical approaches to the pineal region and knowledgeable of their specific potential risks and benefits. In addition, great consideration must be given to the position of the patient because unique risks and benefits are associated with specific patient positions. For instance, patients undergoing resection in the sitting position should be positioned with the knees bent slightly to avoid stretch injury to the sciatic nerve. The trunk and neck should be flexed as much as needed to orient the tentorium parallel with the floor while maintaining patency of the endotracheal tube as well as venous return via the jugular veins.

With any operative approach described, great care must be taken to spare bridging veins when possible. As the operating microscope remains focused on the pineal region during tumor resection, superficial veins remain out of focus and at risk for injury by passing instruments or excess retraction. This is particularly critical during infratentorial approaches, where venous infarction can have devastating effects. Lateral supracerebellar approaches have been described and may minimize the risk and sacrifice of bridging veins when indicated.[24] The use of a retractor should be minimized when possible to avoid stretch injury to bridging veins or compression and contusion of the underlying brain.[1,13,15] Thoughtful positioning can often use gravity in addition to the surgical release of CSF to assist in natural retraction, reducing the need for fixed, rigid retraction. When necessary, surgical approaches to pineal lesions must be designed to limit venous sacrifice to the smallest number of the smallest veins.

Surgical manipulation of tumor attached to or encasing the Galenic veins requires particular care. In general, tumor debulking should begin in the central or lower tumor region to avoid initial contact with the deep cerebral veins. Once the tumor size is reduced, gentle microsurgical dissection can proceed with care to avoid mechanical damage to the tributaries of the vein of Galen. Small residual tumor should be carefully cauterized and left behind if it does not readily separate from these veins.

Management of Injuries

Careful and frequent neurologic examination for possible hemorrhage, cerebellar swelling, or progressive hydrocephalus should occur over several postoperative days. However, in the immediate postoperative period, a reliable neurologic examination can often be difficult to obtain because transient postoperative lethargy and mild cognitive impairment commonly accompany pineal region surgery. Clinicians should have a low threshold for obtaining a computed tomography (CT) scan that easily identifies acute blood, hydrocephalus, pneumocephalus, or completed infarction. Whereas small hemorrhages without significant associated mass effect can be managed conservatively, large hemorrhages may need emergent evacuation, depending on the patient's clinical condition.

Acute hydrocephalus can occur intraoperatively, where it manifests as progressive brain swelling into the operative field due to CSF outflow obstruction; it can also occur postoperatively after hemorrhage, causing obstruction of normal CSF outflow, obstruction of a previously placed VPS or EVD catheter, or blockage of a previous ETV site. Regardless of its etiology, the presence of hydrocephalus should be managed with temporary or permanent CSF diversion, or with revision of previously placed permanent CSF diversion as indicated.

Intraoperative injury to adjacent arteries and veins is rare. Because the deep location of the pineal gland often precludes two surgeons working together, the operating surgeon must divert torrential bleeding using a large-bore suction while simultaneously visualizing the injury site. Standard maneuvers for obtaining hemostasis should be employed. Normal blood pressure parameters should be maintained to ensure adequate cerebral perfusion. Packing agents should be attempted, including: Gelfoam (Pfizer, New York, NY); oxidized cellulose packing thrombin-gelatin matrix; and fibrin glue, applied with mild pressure with a cottonoid. Overpacking should be avoided. Ultimately, ligation or cauterization is usually necessary for significant unremitting arterial injury, which predisposes the patient to ischemic stroke within the relevant vascular distribution. Similarly, the deep cerebral veins should be ligated or cauterized if uncontrollable bleeding unresponsive to standard techniques is encountered. There is some evidence that one internal cerebral vein can be sacrificed safely but that interruption of two would likely greatly increase the risk of a devastating infarction.[25] Great care to preserve as many of these critical neurovascular structures as possible should be taken.

In the setting of significant cerebellar swelling during a supracerebellar approach, an initial survey of the superficial bridging veins should be performed. If possible, CSF should be evacuated from the cisterna magna or the third ventricle. Hyperventilation and treatment with medical management with hypertonic solutions may be attempted. As a last resort, resection of cerebellar tissue can facilitate decompression. Determining that the craniotomy is large enough before closure and leaving the bone flap off ensure adequate decompression. Acute postoperative cerebellar swelling is similarly managed acutely with medical management, but with a low threshold for rapid decompression and/or removal of hematoma and infarcted cerebellum, because this is the most efficient way to treat and save a patient.

In the setting of cortical collapse with subdural hematoma, or of significant tension pneumocephalus, a supratentorial burr hole may be drilled to equalize supratentorial and infratentorial pressures.

SURGICAL REWIND

My Worst Case

A 29-year-old female with a history of recurrent headaches presented with acute-onset cranial nerve IV (CN IV) palsy causing diplopia, and tinnitus in her left ear. MRI showed a hemorrhagic pineal mass with associated hydrocephalus (Fig. 24.2). The patient underwent an uncomplicated SCIT approach in the sitting position for resection of the lesion. During the procedure, only the medial superficial cerebellar bridging veins and the precentral cerebellar vein were sacrificed to facilitate visualization of the lesion within the quadrigeminal cistern as per our standard approach. The lesion was completely removed with sacrifice of only a few additional small choroidal feeding vessels. Postoperatively, the patient was taken to the neurologic intensive care unit (NICU), where she was awake, alert, and fully conversant with excellent eye movements and strength. Approximately four hours postoperatively, she was found unresponsive and cyanotic, and she was emergently intubated. Immediate CT scan demonstrated a large left cerebellar hemorrhagic infarct causing mass effect, brainstem compression, and upward herniation, as well as intraventricular hemorrhage and hydrocephalus. The patient was taken emergently back to the operating room, where an EVD was placed and a decompressive craniectomy was performed. Postoperatively, the patient underwent aggressive medical management of persistently elevated intracranial pressures. Unfortunately, despite aggressive management, she remained respirator dependent, quadriplegic, and with a neurologic examination consistent with a locked-in syndrome due to extension of the infarction into the brainstem. Ultimately, the patient's neurologic status did not improve, and she made the decision with her family to withdraw supportive care. Care was withdrawn, and the patient died according to her wishes. Final pathology was consistent with a hemorrhagic pineal cyst.

NEUROSURGICAL SELFIE MOMENT

The pineal region is anatomically complex and gives rise to a highly diverse group of lesions. Surgical intervention remains a mainstay of effective treatment for both benign and malignant pineal lesions, and a variety of surgical approaches have been designed to treat tumors based on their histology and location. Advances in microsurgical techniques have enabled surgeons to achieve safe and complete resections of the majority of lesions that arise within the pineal region with excellent long-term prognoses for nearly all patients with benign tumors and for a large percentage of patients with malignant tumors. However, although morbidity rates are low and mortality rates have significantly improved from the early days of pineal surgery, a deep understanding of the anatomic associations of the region in the context of the particular approach and position chosen is paramount to successful pineal region surgery. Special attention should be given to preservation of critical deep neurovascular structures, and postoperative surveillance for catastrophic hemorrhage or significant cerebellar swelling is critical.

References

1. Bruce JN, Stein BM. Surgical management of pineal region tumors. *Acta Neurochir (Wien)*. 1995;134(3–4):130–135.
2. Hernesniemi J, Romani R, Albayrak BS, et al. Microsurgical management of pineal region lesions: personal experience with 119 patients. *Surg Neurol*. 2008;70(6):576–583.
3. Konovalov AN, Pitskhelauri DI. Principles of treatment of the pineal region tumors. *Surg Neurol*. 2003;59(4):250–268.
4. Qi S, Fan J, Zhang XA, Zhang H, Qiu B, Fang L. Radical resection of nongerminomatous pineal region tumors via the occipital transtentorial approach based on arachnoidal consideration: experience on a series of 143 patients. *Acta Neurochir (Wien)*. 2014;156(12):2253–2262.
5. Sonabend AM, Bowden S, Bruce JN. Microsurgical resection of pineal region tumors. *J Neurooncol*. 2016;130(2):351–366.
6. Matsuo S, Baydin S, Gungor A, et al. Midline and off-midline infratentorial supracerebellar approaches to the pineal gland. *J Neurosurg*. 2017;126(6):1984–1994.
7. Bruce JN, Ogden AT. Surgical strategies for treating patients with pineal region tumors. *J Neurooncol*. 2004;69(1–3):221–236.
8. Kennedy BC, Bruce JN. Surgical approaches to the pineal region. *Neurosurg Clin N Am*. 2011;22(3):367–380, viii.
9. Bertalanffy H. Avoidance of postoperative acute cerebellar swelling after pineal tumor surgery. *Acta Neurochir (Wien)*. 2016;158(1):59–62.
10. Little KM, Friedman AH, Fukushima T. Surgical approaches to pineal region tumors. *J Neurooncol*. 2001;54(3):287–299.
11. Quest DO, Kleriga E. Microsurgical anatomy of the pineal region. *Neurosurgery*. 1980;6(4):385–390.
12. Yamamoto I, Kageyama N. Microsurgical anatomy of the pineal region. *J Neurosurg*. 1980;53(2):205–221.
13. Kanno T. Surgical pitfalls in pinealoma surgery. *Minim Invasive Neurosurg*. 1995;38(4):153–157.
14. Hart MG, Santarius T, Kirollos RW. How I do it–pineal surgery: supracerebellar infratentorial versus occipital transtentorial. *Acta Neurochir (Wien)*. 2013;155(3):463–467.
15. Kodera T, Bozinov O, Surucu O, Ulrich NH, Burkhardt JK, Bertalanffy H. Neurosurgical venous considerations for tumors of the pineal region resected using the infratentorial supracerebellar approach. *J Clin Neurosci*. 2011;18(11):1481–1485.
16. Rey-Dios R, Cohen-Gadol AA. A surgical technique to expand the operative corridor for supracerebellar infratentorial approaches: technical note. *Acta Neurochir (Wien)*. 2013;155(10):1895–1900.
17. Stein BM. The infratentorial supracerebellar approach to pineal lesions. *J Neurosurg*. 1971;35(2):197–202.
18. Hasegawa M, Yamashita J, Yamashima T. Anatomical variations of the straight sinus on magnetic resonance imaging in the infratentorial supracerebellar approach to pineal region tumors. *Surg Neurol*. 1991;36(5):354–359.
19. Lapras C, Patet JD, Mottolese C, Lapras C Jr. Direct surgery for pineal tumors: occipital-transtentorial approach. *Prog Exp Tumor Res*. 1987;30:268–280.
20. Asgari S, Engelhorn T, Brondics A, Sandalcioglu IE, Stolke D. Transcortical or transcallosal approach to ventricle-associated lesions: a clinical study on the prognostic role of surgical approach. *Neurosurg Rev*. 2003;26(3):192–197.
21. Yagmurlu K, Zaidi HA, Kalani MY, Rhoton AL Jr, Preul MC, Spetzler RF. Anterior interhemispheric transsplenial approach to pineal region tumors: anatomical study and illustrative case. *J Neurosurg*. 2018;128(1):182–192.
22. Duffau H, Khalil I, Gatignol P, Denvil D, Capelle L. Surgical removal of corpus callosum infiltrated by low-grade glioma: functional outcome and oncological considerations. *J Neurosurg*. 2004;100(3):431–437.
23. Ueyama T, Al-Mefty O, Tamaki N. Bridging veins on the tentorial surface of the cerebellum: a microsurgical anatomic study and operative considerations. *Neurosurgery*. 1998;43(5):1137–1145.
24. Kulwin C, Matsushima K, Malekpour M, Cohen-Gadol AA. Lateral supracerebellar infratentorial approach for microsurgical resection of large midline pineal region tumors: techniques to expand the operative corridor. *J Neurosurg*. 2016;124(1):269–276.
25. Chaynes P. Microsurgical anatomy of the great cerebral vein of Galen and its tributaries. *J Neurosurg*. 2003;99(6):1028–1038.

25

Complications Associated With Surgery for Intracranial Infectious Lesions: Brain Abscess, Tuberculosis, Hydatid Disease, Neurocysticercosis

AMEY R. SAVARDEKAR, DHANANJAYA I. BHAT, INDIRA DEVI BHAGAVATULA

HIGHLIGHTS

- The complications associated with dealing with any intracranial space-occupying lesion are also inherent to intracranial infectious lesions. In addition, there are certain issues that need special mention.
- Unlike tumors, infectious space-occupying lesions may or may not contain active disease-causing pathogens, and hence spillage of contents into the surrounding normal brain carries risk of intracranial dissemination and should be avoided at all costs.
- It should always be borne in mind that surgery is an adjunct to treat the infectious lesion and that the mainstay always remains the antimicrobial or antihelminthic agents. With this dictum, the surgeon should aim at keeping the surgical intervention to a minimum and avoid complications as a rule.
- Long-term follow-up is mandated in spite of complete resolution of the infection due to the potential seizure risk in these patients. Scarring of the brain due to perilesional scar tissue formation occurring in infectious lesions acts as the seizure focus.

Brain Abscess

Introduction

Pyogenic brain abscess (PBA) is a focal collection of pus within the brain.[1] The incidence of PBAs is 8% of intracranial masses in the developing countries, whereas in the West the incidence is 1% to 2%, with male predominance.[2] The overall occurrence of brain abscess does not appear to have changed significantly in the antibiotic era. The presenting features of brain abscess depend on the size and intracranial location of the lesions, the virulence of the infecting agents, the immunologic status of the host, and the cerebral edema caused by the expanding intracranial mass lesion.[1] The usual treatment combines antimicrobial therapy, serial imaging studies, and surgical drainage. Surgical treatment can be either aspiration of brain abscess content or surgical excision of abscess capsule.[3]

Complications

Surgery for PBA is performed with the dual aim of obtaining microbiologic confirmation of the offending organism and decompressing the space-occupying lesion to relieve pressure on the surrounding normal brain. The argument for "craniotomy and excision" versus "stereotactic aspiration" is still contentious.[2,4] Eloquent and deep location, size, multiplicity, and radiologic characteristics of the abscess play an important role in guiding treatment strategy. Complications arising from the treatment also matter. Aspiration of brain abscess has low surgery-related morbidity and mortality rates; however, this comes at the cost of high post-aspiration relapse rates (up to 32%), and such a relapse necessitates reaspiration.[2] Computed tomography (CT)–guided stereotactic aspiration is a modality accurate to within a few millimeters with a diagnostic yield of 95%, is associated with transient morbidity in only 5% of patients, and is highly effective in the definitive drainage of abscesses. Epilepsy is a common posttreatment sequel of brain abscess occurring in 30% to 50% of patients. Seizure frequency is reportedly highest in the fourth and fifth years after diagnosis. Nielsen et al. reported high incidence of seizures with frontal lobe abscesses.[5] Some studies have suggested a trend toward a lower incidence of seizures and other sequelae in those treated by aspiration as opposed to excision.[2]

Intraventricular rupture of brain abscess (IVROBA) is a potentially fatal complication of PBA and can occur iatrogenically during excision or manipulation of the deep wall of the brain abscess.[6] Capsule formation and ring enhancement on imaging studies are generally thinner and less complete on the ventricular side of the abscess, and this may result in a false plane of dissection resulting in inadvertent but disastrous rupture of the abscess into the ventricle. Ill-formed medial abscess wall is probably due to the relatively poor vascularity of the deep white matter and reduced migration of fibroblasts into that area. Mortality rates after IVROBA have been reported to range between 39% and 80%.[6] Individualized approach to iatrogenic IVROBA with intrathecal and intravenous antibiotic therapy, cerebrospinal fluid (CSF) diversion (if under high pressure), and close monitoring of clinical status, CSF reports, and CT scan findings is vital to achieving a satisfactory outcome in such patients.

Prevention

Standard precautions for avoiding complications while operating on intracranial space-occupying lesions should be adhered to while dealing with PBA. Special care should be taken to avoid spillage of contents into the ventricles to prevent IVROBA, which carries an unacceptably high morbidity and mortality. For stereotactic aspiration, it is imperative to plan an appropriate trajectory to avoid the ventricles. For craniotomy and excision, the medial/deep wall of the abscess deserves special mention. Its thickness and intactness as well as its relation to the ventricular wall should be meticulously studied on the preoperative radiology. If the medial wall is too close (<1 cm) to the ventricular wall, or if it is ill-formed, it would be prudent to proceed with subtotal abscess wall resection to prevent an inadvertent breach in the ventricular wall.

Due to the high incidence of seizures, all patients with supratentorial brain abscess should be given prophylactic anticonvulsant coverage in the perioperative period and should be continued in the postoperative period for at least one year.[2] The anticonvulsant should be tapered if the electroencephalography shows no epileptogenic activity. Patients having intractable seizures may sometime respond to temporal lobe resection or resection of the seizure focus.

Tubercular Infections

Introduction

Infection of the central nervous system (CNS) by *Mycobacterium tuberculosis* is invariably secondary to a primary focus elsewhere in the body and is one of the most devastating clinical manifestations of tuberculosis.[7] CNS tuberculosis manifests as meningitis, cerebritis, tuberculous abscesses, or tuberculomas and accounts for approximately 1% of all cases of tuberculosis.[8] Presently, surgery is rarely used as a treatment modality for CNS tuberculosis. With the availability of specific magnetic resonance imaging (MRI) sequences, diagnosis of intracranial tuberculomas can be obtained with reasonable accuracy based on radiology.[9] Hence, indications for surgery/biopsy per se have decreased. The two forms of CNS tuberculosis infections that are most often managed surgically are tuberculomas and tuberculous meningitis with hydrocephalus.[10]

At present, indications for surgery for a suspected case of tuberculoma are: uncertain diagnosis, paradoxical increase in size of the lesion while on medication for tuberculosis, and tuberculomas with mass effect causing raised intracranial pressure (ICP).[11]

Complications and Prevention

With the use of modern techniques, the mortality and morbidity of surgery for tuberculosis are negligible.[9] A trial of antitubercular therapy should always be considered before surgery is attempted, especially in the absence of raised ICP. When surgery is indicated, the approach needs to be conservative rather than risk an undesirable neurologic deficit. The patient should be started on antitubercular chemotherapy, preferably a few days before surgery, if the patient is not already on it. Administration of preoperative corticosteroids is also desirable. No attempt should be made to excise large tuberculomas en masse. Piecemeal removal or initial debulking does not increase the risk of meningitis if the patient is covered with antitubercular drugs. Subtotal or partial excision of lesions situated in or near eloquent areas is justified in order to prevent neurological deficits. No attempt should be made to aggressively excise tuberculomas attached to vital structures like the brainstem or the major dural venous sinuses. Endoscopy has a role in management of associated hydrocephalus and can be used to do third ventriculostomy, fenester the septum pellucidum, break loculations, and reduce the need for multiple shunts.

Hydatidosis

Introduction

Cerebral hydatid cysts constitute approximately 2% of all hydatid cysts occurring in the body, and account for approximately 2% of all intracranial mass lesions occurring in humans.[12] Cerebral cysts are mostly solitary (90%) and predominantly supratentorial, with 60% to 70% located in or around the middle cerebral artery territory. Due to their slow growth, the surrounding normal tissue adapts to the chronic compression, and the symptoms are noted only after a prolonged latent period. Chronicity of the illness may also be due to the lack of cerebral edema in the surrounding brain. The average size of a cerebral hydatid cyst ranges from 6 to 10 cm, but 5% reach a diameter of 20 cm. Enucleation of the intact cyst/cysts remains the treatment of choice for cerebral hydatid cysts.[13] The aim of surgery is to excise the cyst intact without spillage of hydatid fluid and to preserve the surrounding brain parenchyma as much as possible. Surgical treatment is complemented with perioperative medical management in the form of albendazole.

Complications

Complications of surgery for intracranial hydatid are likely in two settings: very large cyst [giving rise to sudden intracranial decompression on excision and leading to subdural hematoma (SDH), contusions, seizures] and inadvertent rupture of cyst (spillage of hydatid fluid into the surrounding normal brain, leading to dissemination).[13]

Tuzun et al., in their review of 25 pediatric patients operated for cerebral hydatid cysts, review the complications related to cerebral hydatid cyst surgery. Intraoperative cyst rupture occurred in three (12%) patients.[14] Pneumocephalus developed in three (12%) patients. Subdural effusion occurred in five (20%) patients, whereas subdural effusion plus porencephalic cyst occurred in two, hemorrhage in two, epidural hematoma in one, and porencephalic cyst in four patients. After inadvertent intraoperative rupture, the cyst bed was irrigated with 20% saline.[14] No anaphylactic reaction developed. Seizure was not observed. Recurrence of cerebral hydatid cyst was observed in only one (4%) patient who experienced intraoperative cyst rupture and underwent reoperation for the cyst extirpation. However, the location of the recurrence was in a site opposite that of the first cysts.

Intraoperative cyst rupture is the most common and serious complication, which can lead to widespread dissemination followed by severe inflammatory or anaphylactic response. Seizure, subdural effusion, porencephalic cyst, hemorrhage, pneumocephalus, hydrocephalus, stroke, eosinophilic meningitis, and transient neurologic deficits are the postoperative complications that were reported in the literature. Ciurea et al. reported their experience of 27 pediatric cases with cerebral hydatid cyst in 1995.[15] Epilepsy, paresis, subdural effusion, ventricular dilatation, and recurrence were the postoperative complications, and operative mortality was very low with only one death. Subdural effusion or hematoma is a well-known complication of cranial operations that also occurs after surgery for cerebral hydatid cyst. The ICP is high when a hydatid cyst exists in the brain parenchyma. This drops rapidly after the removal of the cyst. This low pressure causes the brain to sag away from the calvarium, opening up the subdural space (Fig. 25.1). Vessels traversing the subdural space get stretched, resulting in transudation of fluid from the intravascular compartment to the subdural space. This is the probable pathogenesis of subdural effusion in such cases.

Prevention

The craniotomy should be large, and the cyst wall be exposed by a series of radiating cortical incisions, as described in Dowling's technique.[16] It is advisable to cover the surrounding exposed brain with lints soaked in normal saline to prevent contamination of the surrounding brain by accidental rupture of the cyst. A thin cyst wall, periventricular location, and microadhesions to the surrounding brain tissue were the main surgical problems resulting in rupture in about 12% of cases, causing distal deposit of secondary cysts elsewhere on follow-up. If accidental rupture of the cyst occurs, irrigation with hypertonic saline (3%) is recommended in the hope of destroying the scolices in the operative field through osmotic desiccation.

Rapid decompression caused by evacuation of a large cyst may result in disturbances in autoregulatory mechanisms, which need to be watched for in the postoperative period. Occasionally, when there is previous spillage or added infection, the cyst becomes adherent to the surrounding brain, and removal without rupture becomes difficult. Regular monitoring is essential for detection of delayed recurrences (26.6%) in patients with primary cyst rupture.

Neurocysticercosis

Introduction

Cysticidal drugs, namely albendazole and praziquantel, are the primary modality of treatment for all forms of neurocysticercosis.[17] Surgery per se has been indicated in only a few situations, for example the following: indefinite diagnosis, cysts causing tumor-like effects (edema and/or mass effect) that are refractory to medical treatment, hydrocephalus, and intraventricular cysticerosis.[17–19] Stereotactic excisional biopsy/open craniotomy and cyst removal are recommended in cases of a single giant cortical cyst or large clumps exhibiting tumor-like behavior, if the lesion is in a surgically accessible area, is producing progressive deficits, or is not responding to cysticidal therapy.[17] This approach may also be used when diagnosis is uncertain—e.g., a single small enhancing lesion with atypical features—and when the lesion is worsening or not responding to cysticides, or when there are multiple lesions. Supratentorial decompressive craniectomy is undertaken when the pseudotumor type of edema is refractory to medical treatment, particularly in the disseminated variety of the disease frequently seen in India.[17] For intraventricular and subarachnoid forms of neurocysticercal cysts (NCC), the surgical procedure may include shunting for hydrocephalus, cyst removal or excision through a posterior fossa craniotomy for fourth ventricle/subarachnoid cysts, and supratentorial open or stereotactic craniotomy for subarachnoid third or lateral ventricle cysts.[18,20,21]

Complications and Prevention

The advent of new surgical techniques have decreased morbidity and mortality associated with surgical procedures for neurocysticercosis.[17] Minimally invasive techniques have been shown to be effective as a principal strategy in many cases that are complemented with cysticidal therapy.[22,23] Some authors state that patients with ventricular

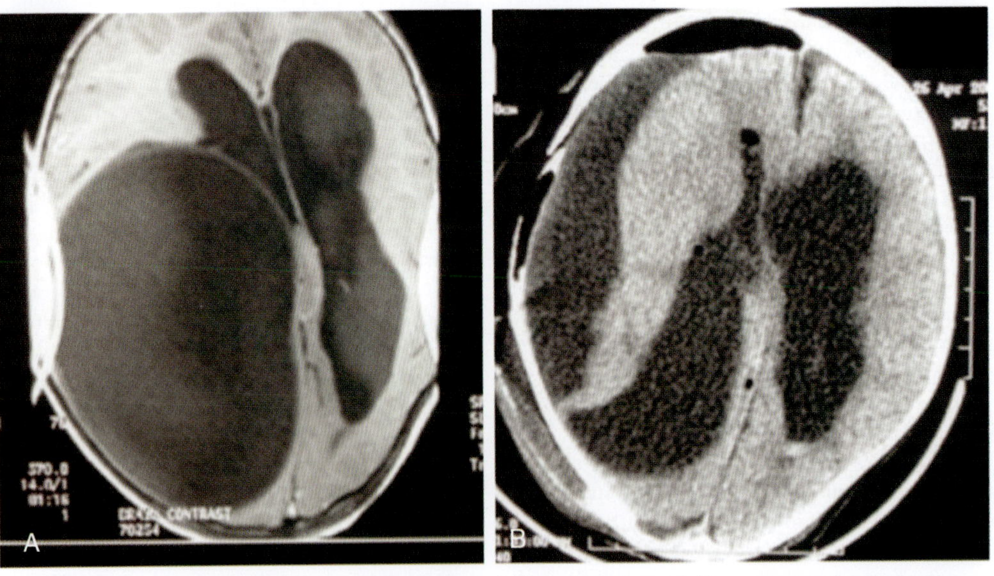

• **Fig. 25.1** (A) Axial section of contrast-enhanced T1-weighted magnetic resonance imaging scan showing a large hydatid cyst at the left atrium of the lateral ventricle. (B) Postoperative axial computed tomography scan showing complete cyst removal, but with the development of subdural hygroma on the right side.

or subarachnoid cysticerci, or with the parenchymatous racemose form of the disease, should be treated surgically with endoscopy or with highly selective minimally invasive microsurgery initially, if the risk-benefit assessment is favorable.[19,23] Bergsneider et al. reported a series of 10 patients with intraventricular cysticercal cysts presenting with hydrocephalus. Combined endoscopic removal of the cysts with a third ventriculostomy and/or a septal pellucidotomy produced excellent results.[22] They advocate endoscopic removal of cysts as the primary therapy for intraventricular cysticercosis, as it enabled them to avoid shunts in this setting.

Detritus of the cysticerci are capable of inducing an inflammatory response in the ependyma. Hence, shunt is associated with a high percentage of complications like blockage and infection. Shunt obstruction rate is 50% within the first 4 months. Khade et al., in their review of the literature, concluded that of patients who had undergone surgical resection of a single intraventricular lesion, those who received postoperative antihelminthic therapy had a significantly lower risk of developing delayed hydrocephalus (18.8%, vis-à-vis 59.1% for those who did not receive medical therapy).[24] In this way, it is possible to avoid the severe inflammatory reaction after pharmacologic treatment and rupture of the cyst. Intermittent long-term prednisolone therapy after ventriculo-peritoneal shunt reduces shunt malfunction and may improve the functional status of the patient.[17]

SURGICAL REWIND

My Worst Case

A 5-year-old boy was brought to the emergency room with a history of multiple right focal motor seizures, progressive right upper and lower limb weakness, fever since 2 weeks, and altered sensorium of 1-day duration. On examination, the child was drowsy, localizing with right-sided hemiparesis [British Medical Research Council (MRC) grade: 3/5]. CT scan of the head and MRI of the brain revealed multiple small ring-enhancing lesions located in the bilateral cerebral hemisphere with large peripherally enhancing left frontal lesions with perilesional edema and mass effect (Fig. 25.2). The initial impression was tubercular infection due to the endemic nature of the disease. Other possibilities considered included neuroblastoma with metastases. Chest radiography was also done, which showed no positive findings. Human immunodeficiency virus (HIV) enzyme immunoassay test was negative.

The patient was treated with an empiric antitubercular regimen, anticonvulsants, and steroids. Because the patient's neurologic status did not improve on medical management, he underwent a left frontal craniotomy and decompression of the lesion. Postoperative CT brain showed good decompression of the lesion with no evidence of operative site bleed. Histopathologic examination was suggestive of tuberculoma (Fig. 25.3). After surgery, the patient improved in sensorium and was conscious, obeying on discharge.

At discharge, the patient was advised to continue antitubercular therapy, steroids, and anticonvulsant. He presented to the emergency room 10 days after discharge with multiple episodes of seizure followed by altered sensorium. On evaluation, CT brain showed evidence of bleed in left frontal

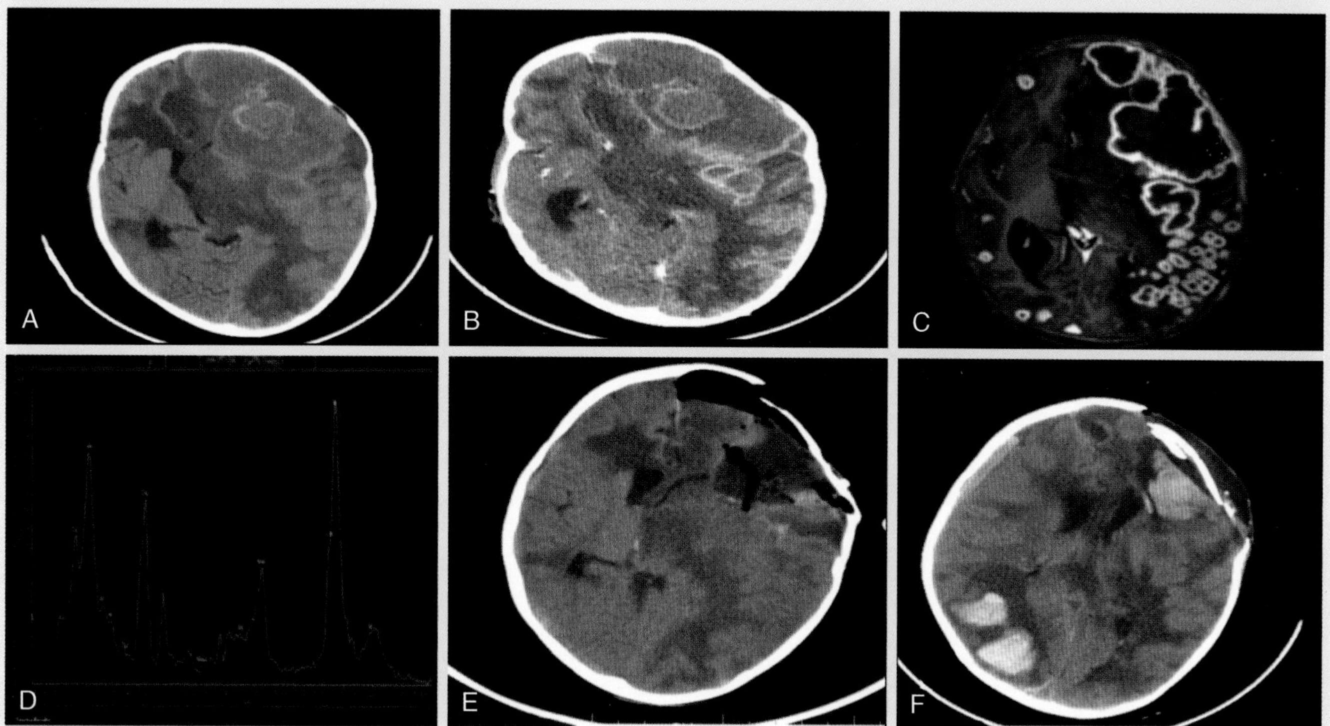

• **Fig. 25.2** (A and B) Computed tomography (CT) brain plain and contrast showing multiple cerebral cortical tuberculoma with perilesional edema. (C) Contrast magnetic resonance imaging showing giant tuberculoma with multiple miliary tuberculoma. (D) MR spectroscopy showing raised lipid and lactate peak. (E) Postoperative CT brain showing good decompression of left frontal tuberculoma. (F) CT brain showing areas of cortical bleed.

Continued

and right parieto-occipital region. His biochemistry revealed normal coagulation profile and mild derangement of liver enzymes. In view of the possibility of drug-induced hepatotoxicity, isoniazid, rifampicin, and pyrazinamide were withheld, and he was started on ofloxacin along with streptomycin. Isoniazid and rifampicin were restarted after normalization of liver enzymes in a phased manner. Patient improved on medical management and was conscious, obeying on discharge. He was advised to continue antitubercular therapy, anticonvulsant, and steroid.

Literature shows very few case reports of tuberculous meningitis patients complicated by intraventricular, intracerebral, and subarachnoid hemorrhage. It has been ascribed to aneurysmal rupture after the formation of mycotic aneurysms, or to nonaneurysmal rupture as a consequence of weakening of the vessel wall by the granulomatous inflammation. The perilesional hemorrhage in close opposition to a tuberculoma, the venular necrosis, fibrin deposition, and neutrophil infiltration could be a manifestation of acute hemorrhagic leucoencephalitis.[25] It has rapid evolution with significant morbidity and mortality. It has been suggested that this could be an immune-mediated reaction to damaged vascular basement membrane, or release of mycobacterial proteins from death bacilli after starting chemotherapy.[26] We also considered that hepatotoxicity induced by antitubercular therapy could be responsible for the bleed, but coagulation profiles were normal, and the patient did not have any bleeding tendencies.

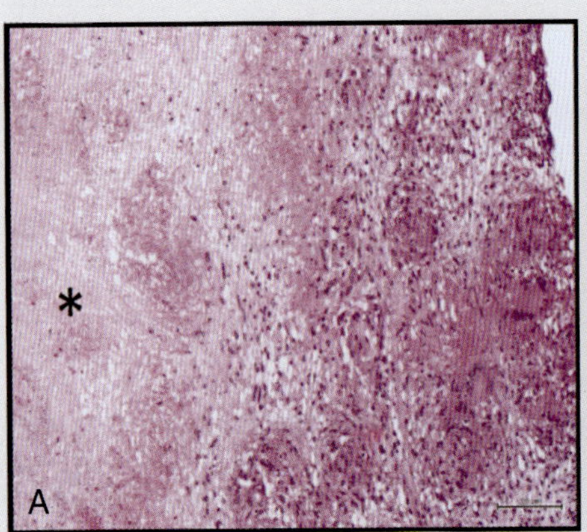

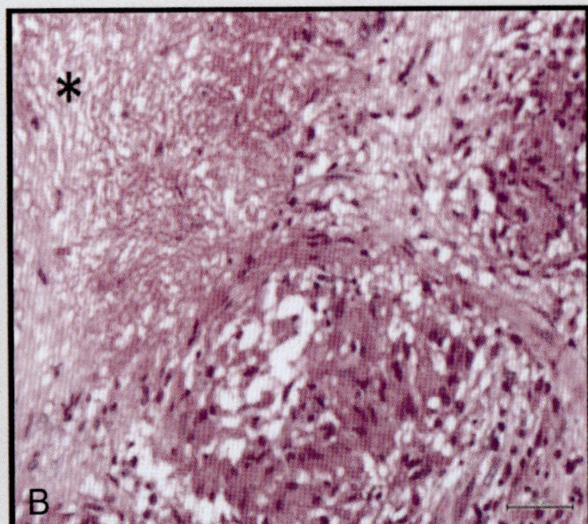

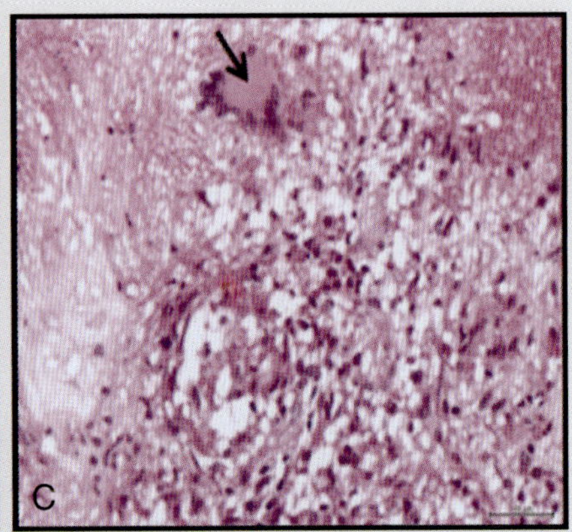

• **Fig. 25.3** Microphotograph showing (A) Hematoxylin and eosin (H&E) ×100 showing epithelioid cell granuloma with Langhans-type giant cells (asterisk). (B) H&E ×200: Epithelioid cell granuloma with caseous necrosis (arrow). (C) H&E ×200: Langhans-type giant cells (asterisk).

NEUROSURGICAL SELFIE MOMENT

The study of neurosurgical literature regarding surgical intervention for intracranial infections teaches us the philosophy of avoiding surgery until mandatory and of being as conservative as possible in the event of a mandatory surgical intervention, because antimicrobial or antihelminthic therapy is the mainstay of treatment. Biding by this philosophy helps minimize complications arising from surgery for intracranial infections. Additionally, administering antimicrobial chemotherapy and perioperative steroids as well as avoiding spillage of intralesional contents and using minimally invasive techniques can help limit complications.

References

1. Nielsen H, Gyldensted C, Harmsen A. Cerebral abscess. Aetiology and pathogenesis, symptoms, diagnosis and treatment. A review of 200 cases from 1935-1976. *Acta Neurol Scand.* 1982;65(6):609–622.
2. Dharkar SR, Sardana VR, Purohit D. Brain abscess. In: *Ramamurthy and Tandon's Textbook of Neurosurgery*. 3rd ed. New Delhi: Jaypee Brothers Medical Publishers (P) Ltd; 2012:695–707.
3. Aras Y, Sabanci PA, Izgi N, et al. Surgery for pyogenic brain abscess over 30 years: evaluation of the roles of aspiration and craniotomy. *Turk Neurosurg.* 2016;26(1):39–47.
4. Boviatsis EJ, Kouyialis AT, Stranjalis G, Korfias S, Sakas DE. CT-guided stereotactic aspiration of brain abscesses. *Neurosurg Rev.* 2003;26(3):206–209.
5. Nielsen H, Harmsen A, Gyldensted C. Cerebral abscess. A long-term follow-up. *Acta Neurol Scand.* 1983;67(6):330–337.
6. Savardekar AR, Krishna R, Arivazhagan A. Spontaneous intraventricular rupture of pyogenic brain abscess: a short series of three cases and review of literature. *Surg Neurol Int.* 2016;7(suppl 39):S947–S951.
7. Tandon PN, Pande A. Tuberculosis of the central nervous system. In: *Ramamurthy and Tandon's Textbook of Neurosurgery*. 3rd ed. New Delhi: Jaypee Brothers Medical Publishers (P) Ltd; 2012: 725–741.
8. Mohindra S, Savardekar A, Gupta R, Tripathi M, Rane S. Tuberculous brain abscesses in immunocompetent patients: a decade long experience with nine patients. *Neurol India.* 2016;64(1):66–74.
9. Patir R, Bhatia R, Tandon PN. Surgical management of tuberculous infections of the nervous system. In: Sweet S, ed. *Operative Neurosurgical Techniques: Indications, Methods and Results*. 5th ed. Philadelphia, PA: Elsevier; 2006.
10. Bhagwati SN, Parulekar GD. Management of intracranial tuberculoma in children. *Childs Nerv Syst.* 1986;2(1):32–34.
11. Indira B, Panigrahi MK, Vajramani G, Shankar SK, Santosh V, Das BS. Tuberculoma of the hypothalamic region as a rare case of hypopituitarism: a case report. *Surg Neurol.* 1996;45(4):347–350.
12. Mohindra S, Savardekar A, Gupta R, Tripathi M, Rane S. Varied types of intracranial hydatid cysts: radiological features and management techniques. *Acta Neurochir (Wien).* 2012;154(1):165–172.
13. Izci Y, Tuzun Y, Secer HI, Gonul E. Cerebral hydatid cysts: technique and pitfalls of surgical management. *Neurosurg Focus.* 2008;24(6):E15.
14. Tuzun Y, Solmaz I, Sengul G, Izci Y. The complications of cerebral hydatid cyst surgery in children. *Childs Nerv Syst.* 2010;26(1): 47–51.
15. Ciurea AV, Vasilescu G, Nuteanu L, Carp N. Cerebral hydatid cyst in children. Experience of 27 cases. *Childs Nerv Syst.* 1995;11(12):679–685.
16. Carrea R, Dowling E Jr, Guevara JA. Surgical treatment of hydatid cysts of the central nervous system in the pediatric age (Dowling's technique). *Childs Brain.* 1975;1(1):4–21.
17. Sharma BS, Sarat Chandra P. Cysticercosis. In: *Ramamurthy and Tandon's Textbook of Neurosurgery*. 3rd ed. New Delhi: Jaypee Brothers Medical Publishers (P) Ltd; 2012:777–793.

18. Colli BO, Martelli N, Assirati JA Jr, Machado HR, de Vergueiro Forjaz S. Results of surgical treatment of neurocysticercosis in 69 cases. *J Neurosurg*. 1986;65(3):309–315.
19. Colli BO, Carlotti CG Jr, Assirati JA Jr, Machado HR, Valenca M, Amato MC. Surgical treatment of cerebral cysticercosis: long-term results and prognostic factors. *Neurosurg Focus*. 2002;12(6):e3.
20. Zee CS, Segall HD, Destian S, Ahmadi J, Apuzzo ML. MRI of intraventricular cysticercosis: surgical implications. *J Comput Assist Tomogr*. 1993;17(6):932–939.
21. Apuzzo ML, Dobkin WR, Zee CS, Chan JC, Giannotta SL, Weiss MH. Surgical considerations in treatment of intraventricular cysticercosis. An analysis of 45 cases. *J Neurosurg*. 1984;60(2):400–407.
22. Bergsneider M, Holly LT, Lee JH, King WA, Frazee JG. Endoscopic management of cysticercal cysts within the lateral and third ventricles. *J Neurosurg*. 2000;92(1):14–23.
23. Psarros TG, Krumerman J, Coimbra C. Endoscopic management of supratentorial ventricular neurocysticercosis: case series and review of the literature. *Minim Invasive Neurosurg*. 2003;46(6):331–334.
24. Khade P, Lemos RS, Toussaint LG. What is the utility of postoperative antihelminthic therapy after resection for intraventricular neurocysticercosis? *World Neurosurg*. 2013;79(3–4):558–567.
25. Dastur DK, Udani PM. The pathology and pathogenesis of tuberculous encephalopathy. *Acta Neuropathol*. 1966;6(4):311–326.
26. Dastur DK, Dave UP. Ultrastructural basis of the vasculopathy in and around brain tuberculomas. Possible significance of altered basement membrane. *Am J Pathol*. 1977;89(1):35–50.

26

Management of Facial Nerve Injury in Vestibular Schwannoma

JOSHUA D. HUGHES, MICHAEL J. LINK

HIGHLIGHTS

- In the current era of vestibular schwannoma surgery, the rate-limiting step to gross total resection, especially in tumors ≥3.0 centimeters, is the course and integrity of the facial nerve.
- Even with a combination of meticulous microsurgical technique and intraoperative electromyography, injury to the facial nerve can still occur.
- In instances in which the nerve is anatomically intact, reanimation with anastomotic techniques should be deferred in favor of a course of postoperative observation to see how much function is regained.

Introduction

Since its inception, surgery for vestibular schwannoma (VS) has striven for a balance between complete tumor removal and satisfactory patient outcomes. At the turn of the 20th century, mortality was the major obstacle to extirpation, but as the era and surgical technique progressed, mortality rates declined precipitously, and reducing loss of function, especially with regard to the facial nerve, became the focus of improvement.[1-4] In the current era of VS surgery, the rate-limiting step to gross total resection, especially in tumors ≥3.0 centimeters, is the course and integrity of the facial nerve.[5] Even with a combination of meticulous microsurgical technique and intraoperative electromyography (EMG), injury to the facial nerve can still occur. We present a case of facial nerve injury and discuss anatomic factors that lead to such an injury, as well as management strategies to take when it occurs.

Discussion

The early history of VS surgery was devoted to balancing patient operative survival and extent of resection. In 1913, using finger dissection, some of the earliest case series of VS removal reported operative mortality rates between 67% and 84%.[1,2,4] Finding this unacceptably high, Cushing endorsed internal debulking of VS without removing the capsule and reported a mortality rate of 10% to 15%, though this increased to 54% at 5 years secondary to tumor recurrence.[1,4] Dandy further refined VS surgery with intratumoral decompression followed by extracapsular dissection with an operative mortality rate of 10.9% in 1941. Not long after, using a similar technique, Horrax and Poppen reported a 5-year mortality rate of 12.7%.[1]

While mortality rates declined, morbidity rates remained high due to cranial nerve injury, particularly of the facial nerve. Although the first successful gross total resection of a VS with preservation of the facial nerve was reported by Cairns in 1931,[1] it could not be accomplished on a routine basis; it was not until the microsurgical revolution led by House, Hitselberger, Kurze, and Yasargil in the 1960s[1,4] and the introduction of intraoperative EMG monitoring in 1979[6] that facial nerve preservation became routinely achievable. Currently, rates of mortality are less than 1%,[7] and facial nerve dysfunction rates are between 3% and 43%, depending on tumor size.[8]

Even with these advances, sometimes the surgeon and patient must choose between complete tumor resection and risk of permanent facial nerve dysfunction. Factors that influence this are tumor size, the degree to which the nerve fibers are spread out by the tumor, and the location of the facial nerve relative to the tumor.[6,9,10] The most common location of the facial nerve is anterior to the tumor in over 75% of patients,[11] which means the tumor bulk is posterior to the facial nerve and the nerve is not encountered until most of the tumor is removed. In addition, an anterior course of the nerve means that it does not have to be protected while dissecting the tumor away from the medial interface of the tumor and cerebellum. When the course of the facial nerve is on the posterior surface of the tumor, it is encountered earlier in the surgery and must be protected while removing the bulk of the tumor.

In the presented case, the facial nerve was taking a course over the superomedial portion of the tumor that put it in close relationship to two large veins: the veins of the cerebellopontine fissure and the middle cerebellar peduncle.[12] This course is unusual and present in approximately 1% of tumors.[11] After debulking the tumor, as the tumor capsule was being separated from the cerebellum and brainstem, heavy bleeding was encountered from one of these two aforementioned veins. It is very common in our experience that these veins become quite engorged with even medium-sized VS as they and the adjacent brainstem get compressed by the tumor, and the tumor may drain into these veins, increasing their flow and pressure. Despite the course of the facial nerve being known, inadvertent injury to the facial nerve with the bipolar occurred, resulting in a proximal conduction block. The rest of the tumor was safely removed, resulting in complete tumor resection and an anatomically intact, but nonfunctioning, nerve.

In instances where the facial nerve is completely severed during surgery, there is no question that reconstruction with an end-to-end

SURGICAL REWIND

My Worst Case

A 40-year-old female presented with right-sided hearing loss, imbalance, and tinnitus, all of which had grown progressively worse over the preceding year. An audiogram showed sensorineural hearing loss on the right with a pure-tone average of 55 decibels and a word recognition score of 25%. An MRI revealed an approximately 3.1-cm tumor in the right cerebellopontine angle consistent with VS. Given the size and age of the patient, treatment was recommended with microsurgical resection through a retrosigmoid craniotomy. She underwent surgery 2 months after presentation.

The patient was placed under general anesthesia with endotracheal intubation. Intraoperative monitoring of cranial nerves V, VII, VIII, X, and XI was utilized. After positioning in a left lateral decubitus position, a semilunar incision was marked out approximately three fingerbreadths medial to the digastric notch. The scalp was incised and moved laterally while the nuchal musculature was mobilized inferiorly. A burr hole was made over the junction of the transverse and sigmoid sinus, and a bone flap was turned. The dura was opened in a semilunar fashion. The ninth, tenth, and eleventh cranial nerves were identified inferiorly as well as the inferior pole of the tumor, and the arachnoid over the tumor was released from inferior to superior. The posterior pole of the tumor was stimulated at 3.0 milliamps without response from the facial nerve. The tumor was then internally debulked and rolled superiorly. The eighth cranial nerve fibers were identified and cut because they were splayed out over the posterior portion of the tumor, which allowed visualization of cranial nerve VII at the brainstem. Further internal debulking of the tumor was performed, and as the tumor capsule was being mobilized from the lateral aspect of the cerebellum and brainstem, a significant amount of venous bleeding occurred from a large venous tributary. It was thought to be away from the course of the facial nerve and was controlled with bipolar cautery. Shortly after, a conduction block in the facial nerve occurred. The remaining tumor in the cerebellopontine angle was removed. The facial nerve was taking a course over the superior pole of the tumor before entering the acoustic meatus. Distal to the conduction block, the nerve stimulated at 0.2 milliamps. The posterior part of the acoustic meatus was drilled away, and the remaining portion of the tumor was removed for a gross total resection. Careful inspection showed that the facial nerve was intact but that it would not conduct proximal to the area of the bipolar injury. A 3-mm nerve support supplement tube was placed over this region and coated in dural sealant. The dura was closed primarily, the bone flap replaced, and the wound closed in anatomic layers.

Postoperatively, the patient had House-Brackmann VI right facial weakness and some mild right V3 numbness. She was discharged home on postoperative day 4. At 3 months postoperatively, the patient continued to have House-Brackmann VI right facial weakness, and an MRI showed gross total resection of the tumor. At 1 year postoperatively, the patient had improved to House-Brackmann IV right facial weakness. Her improvement started about 7 months from surgery with the right corner of her mouth and then with the right eye at about 9 months. She also noticed altered taste sensation and some watering of her eye with olfactory stimulation. Two and a half years from surgery, she continued with House-Brackmann IV right facial weakness, and MRI showed no evidence of recurrent tumor.

anastomosis or interposition graft should be attempted during or shortly after surgery.[13] However, there is some debate regarding an anatomically intact but electrically diminished or unresponsive nerve, with some endorsing resection of the damaged section and immediate reconstruction[14] and others delaying reinnervation for at least 1 year to determine whether the nerve recovers.[15,16] In our institutional series of 11 patients with anatomically intact but nonstimulating nerves, we found that 64% of patients improved to at least House-Brackmann grade III in less than 1 year from surgery.[17] Because these results are on par or better than those seen with reinnervation, we do not perform immediate facial nerve reconstruction of any type until a year from surgery if the nerve is anatomically contiguous.

NEUROSURGICAL SELFIE MOMENT

Remarkable progress has been made in VS surgery over the past century with the advances in both surgical technique and technology. Although permanent facial nerve dysfunction after surgery is the exception, not the norm, injury can still occur. In instances in which the nerve is anatomically intact, reanimation with anastomotic techniques should be deferred in favor of a course of postoperative observation to see how much function is regained.

References

1. Akard W, Tubbs RS, Seymour ZA, Hitselberger WE, Cohen-Gadol AA. Evolution of techniques for the resection of vestibular schwannomas: from saving life to saving function. *J Neurosurg*. 2009;110(4): 642–647.
2. Koerbel A, Gharabaghi A, Safavi-Abbasi S, Tatagiba M, Samii M. Evolution of vestibular schwannoma surgery: the long journey to current success. *Neurosurg Focus*. 2005;18(4):e10.
3. Machinis TG, Fountas KN, Dimopoulos V, Robinson JS. History of acoustic neurinoma surgery. *Neurosurg Focus*. 2005;18(4):e9.
4. Ramsden RT. The bloody angle: 100 years of acoustic neuroma surgery. *J R Soc Med*. 1995;88(8):464P–468P.
5. Gurgel LG, Dourado MR, Moreira TD, et al. Correlation between vestibular test results and self-reported psychological complaints of patients with vestibular symptoms. *Braz J Otorhinolaryngol*. 2012;78(1):62–67.
6. Delgado TE, Bucheit WA, Rosenholtz HR, Chrissian S. Intraoperative monitoring of facila muscle evoked responses obtained by intracranial stimulation of the facila nerve: a more accurate technique for facila nerve dissection. *Neurosurgery*. 1979;4(5):418–421.
7. McClelland S 3rd, Kim E, Murphy JD, Jaboin JJ. Operative mortality rates of acoustic neuroma surgery: a national cancer database analysis. *Otol Neurotol*. 2017;38(5):751–753.
8. Ansari SF, Terry C, Cohen-Gadol AA. Surgery for vestibular schwannomas: a systematic review of complications by approach. *Neurosurg Focus*. 2012;33(3):E14.
9. Deguine O, Maillard A, Bonafe A, el Adouli H, Tremoulet M, Fraysse B. Pre-operative and per-operative factors conditioning long-term facial nerve function in vestibular schwannoma surgery through translabyrinthine approach. *J Laryngol Otol*. 1998;112(5):441–445.
10. Rivas A, Boahene KD, Bravo HC, Tan M, Tamargo RJ, Francis HW. A model for early prediction of facial nerve recovery after vestibular schwannoma surgery. *Otol Neurotol*. 2011;32(5):826–833.
11. Sampath P, Rini D, Long DM. Microanatomical variations in the cerebellopontine angle associated with vestibular schwannomas (acoustic neuromas): a retrospective study of 1006 consecutive cases. *J Neurosurg*. 2000;92(1):70–78.
12. Rhoton AL Jr. Microsurgical anatomy of the brainstem surface facing an acoustic neuroma. *Surg Neurol*. 1986;25(4):326–339.

13. Samii M, Matthies C. Management of 1000 vestibular schwannomas (acoustic neuromas): the facial nerve – preservation and restitution of function. *Neurosurgery*. 1997;40(4):684–694.
14. Samii M, Turel KE, Penkert G. Management of seventh and eighth nerve involvement by cerebellopontine angle tumors. *Clin Neurosurg*. 1985;32:242–272.
15. Arriaga MA, Luxford WM, Atkins JS Jr, Kwartler JA. Predicting long-term facial nerve outcome after acoustic neuroma surgery. *Otolaryngol Head Neck Surg*. 1993;108(3):220–224.
16. Fenton JE, Chin RY, Fagan PA, Sterkers O, Sterkers JM. Predictive factors of long-term facial nerve function after vestibular schwannoma surgery. *Otol Neurotol*. 2002;23(3):388–392.
17. Carlson ML, Van Abel KM, Schmitt WR, Driscoll CL, Neff BA, Link MJ. The anatomically intact but electrically unresponsive facial nerve in vestibular schwannoma surgery. *Neurosurgery*. 2012;71(6):1125–1130, discussion 1130.

27 Complications in Vestibular Schwannoma Patients

AJAY NIRANJAN, EDWARD MONACO III, L. DADE LUNSFORD

HIGHLIGHTS

- Auditory nerve function can be preserved in the majority of patients regardless of tumor volume. Rates of serviceable hearing preservation range from 49% to 79% in published studies.
- With the current Gamma Knife radiosurgery technique, facial nerve function can be preserved in almost all (99%) patients.
- Vestibular schwannoma radiosurgery leads to improved quality of life.

Background

During the last three decades, stereotactic radiosurgery (SRS) has become a widely preferred surgical strategy to manage patients with small- to moderate-size vestibular schwannomas (VSs). Long-term results from multiple international studies have established the Leksell Gamma Knife® (GK) method to perform SRS as a more effective and safer method to manage VS, compared with the older techniques that require craniotomy and attempt tumor removal. This has become especially important now that such tumors are frequently detected earlier. Patients with episodic disequilibrium, asymmetric hearing, episodes of vertigo, or tinnitus should now get an appropriate magnetic resonance imaging (MRI) with and without contrast agents with sufficient resolution of the internal auditory canal to exclude the possibility of a VS. Ironically, since the introduction of SRS, patients with early detection are now often counseled to simply wait and observe their tumor until the tumor volume has progressed significantly. Unfortunately, such treatment delay is often associated with worsened outcomes, regardless of the interventional strategy.

The goals of VS radiosurgery are to control tumor growth, preserve cranial nerve function, and rapidly return the patient to work. With current techniques, useful hearing is preserved in the majority of patients, and the facial nerve are preserved in almost all patients.[1] Preservation of auditory and facial nerve function is related to various factors that include dose planning and dose delivery technique, margin dose, tumor volume, and cranial nerve function at the time of the procedure. It is important to understand the published outcome data as a means to refute the disinformation often provided to patients with VS who are evaluating SRS as an option: (1) It will damage your hearing and face. (2) It will fail, and your tumor will grow. (3) When it fails, your tumor will be stuck and your nerves will be cut when it requires removal. (4) Even if it works for a brief period of time, the risk of getting cancer caused by radiation of the brain is too high. This report will describe the current outcomes patients and their referring doctors may expect after VS Gamma Knife stereotactic radiosurgery (GKRS).

Anatomic Insights

The radiosurgery dose plan should be highly conformal, especially at the anterior margin of the VS, because the facial and cochlear nerve complexes are generally considered to be stretched along the anterior-superior and anterior-inferior sides of the tumor, respectively (Fig. 27.1A and B). Although there is no clear consensus on the sensitivity of the cochlea, it is important to minimize the amount of radiation falloff on the cochlea.

Prevention

Conformal Gamma Knife Radiosurgery Technique to Prevent Cranial Nerve Complications

Complete 3-D coverage of the tumor with sparing of facial and cochlear nerves and the cochlea is given priority during dose planning. This is achieved with the use of multiple small-volume isocenters, beam weighting, and beam plug patterns to spare the cochlea and brainstem. A series of 4-mm isocenters are used to create a tapered isodose plan to conform to the intracanalicular portion of the tumor. Current GK models (LGK Icon® and LGK Perfexion®) allow for selective beam channel sector (24 beams) blocking that can be used to enhance dose falloff (selectivity) and to create sharp falloff of the energy deposited in the cochlea. Planning is typically performed by the neurosurgeon in consultation with a radiation oncologist and medical physicist. The oncologist often performs tumor contouring, and the physicist can calculate the conformality (how well the 3-D plan conforms to the tumor margin at the prescription isodose) as well as the selectivity (how rapidly the dose falls off outside of the tumor). It is thus both conformality and selectivity that set the GK planning apart from other radiation tools and that allows the surgical procedure to be performed in a single session. Technologies that fractionate radiation therapy to such tumors do so because poor conformality and selectivity require dividing dose delivery into multiple sessions to maintain safety.

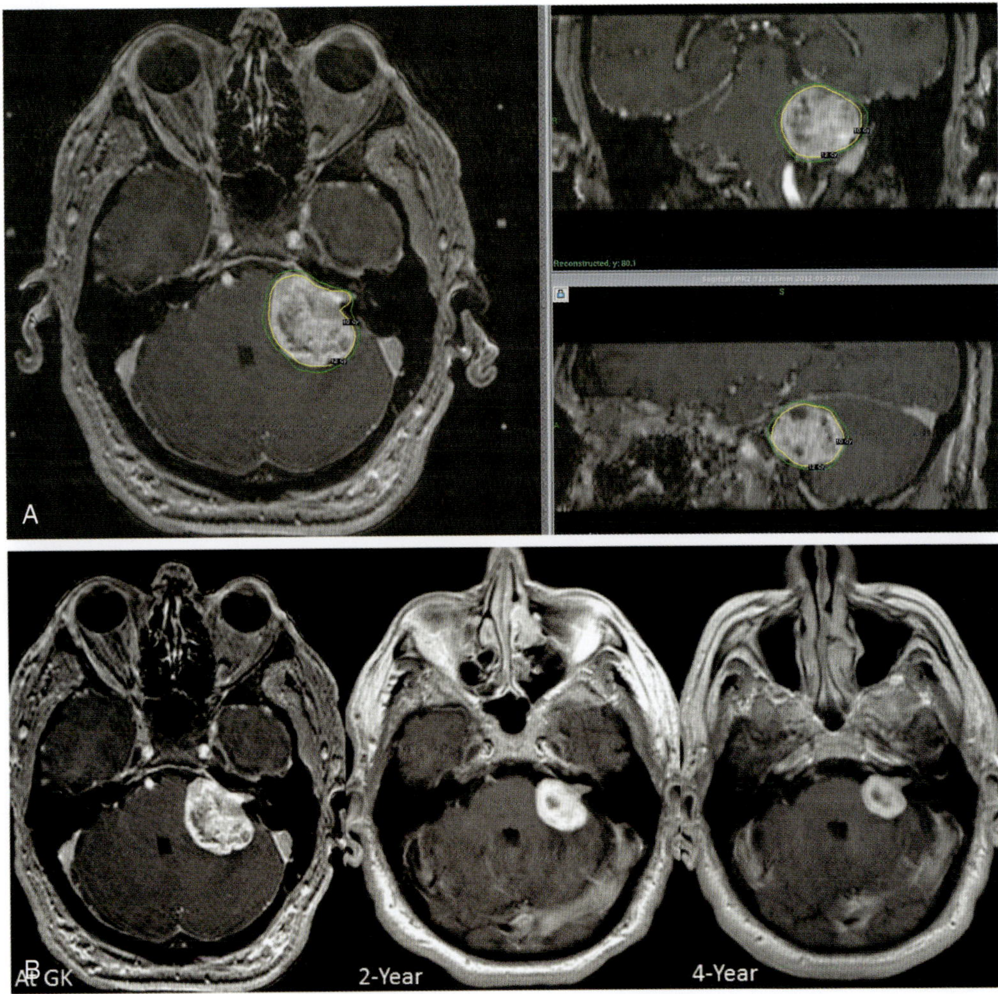

• **Fig. 27.1** (A) Conformal Gamma Knife dose plan projected on a contrast-enhanced axial magnetic resonance imaging (MRI) with coronal and sagittal reformation. (B) Contrast-enhanced axial MRI showing significant regression in vestibular schwannoma at 2- and 4-year follow-up after radiosurgery.

In Gamma Knife® radiosurgery (GKS), a dose of 12 to 12.5 Gy is typically prescribed to the isodose line that conforms to the tumor margin. This margin dose is associated with a low complication rate and a high rate of tumor control. After the margin dose is prescribed, the dose falloff on the cochlea and brainstem are checked to keep them below tolerance level. The dose–volume histograms of tumor, cochlea, and brainstem are evaluated to document minimum tumor dose and to check the volumes of the cochlea and brainstem. At our center we attempt to keep the cochlear dose below 4.2 Gy in patients with preserved hearing.

RED FLAGS

1. **Large Tumors:** Large tumors with symptomatic mass effect on the brainstem are not candidates for radiosurgery as the primary management. Partial tumor resection followed by planned radiosurgery offers the best chance of preserving facial and cochlear function in such patients.
2. **Cystic Tumors:** There is a misconception among some physicians that cystic tumors do not respond to radiosurgery and therefore should not be offered radiosurgery. On the contrary, the fact is that cystic VS often responds with significant tumor regression.
3. **Higher Margin Doses:** Margin doses higher than 13 Gy are not needed for VS radiosurgery. Higher doses are associated with higher risk of facial and auditory nerve complication.
4. **Tumor Expansion:** Follow-up MRI shows some tumor expansion after radiosurgery in about 5% of patients. These patients should be followed using serial MRIs and should not be rushed to surgery.

Clinical Results

Hearing Preservation

Published VS radiosurgery studies show that rates of serviceable hearing preservation range from 49% to 79% (Table 27.1). In a study by Flickinger et al., the 5-year actuarial rates of hearing level preservation and speech preservation were 75.2% and 89.2%, respectively, for patients (n = 89) treated with a 13-Gy tumor margin dose.[2] Kano et al. evaluated factors related to hearing preservation in 77 VS patients.[3] At a median of 20 months after SRS, serviceable hearing was preserved in 71%. Among the patients who had Gardner-Robertson (GR) Class I hearing before radiosurgery, 89% retained serviceable hearing. Significant prognostic factors for serviceable hearing preservation were GR Class I hearing, a patient age younger than 60 years, an intracanalicular tumor,

TABLE 27.1 **Published Reports With Serviceable Hearing Preservation**

First Author	Year	Marginal Doses	Follow-up Months, Median/Mean (Range)	Serviceable Hearing Preservation %
Flickinger[29]	2004	13 (12–13)	24 (12–115)	78.6
Pollock[30]	2006	12.2	42 (12–62)	63
Chopra[31]	2007	13 (12–13)	68 (12–143)	57
Regis[32]	2007	12	≥24	60
Niranjan[33]	2008	13 (10–18)	28 (12–144)	64.5
Kano[34]	2009	12.5 (12–13)	20 (6–40)	71
Myrseth[35]	2009	12	24	68
Tamura[36]	2009	12 (9–13)	48 (36–132)	78
Kim[37]	2010	12 (11–15)	36 (9–81)	68
Delbrouck[38]	2011	12	≥12	66
Kim[39]	2011	12 (12–13)	25 (6–48)	61
Massager[40]	2011	12	43 (24–96)	79
Boari[4]	2014	13 (11–15)	60 (36–1530)	49
Lipski[6]	2015	11.5 (11–12)	48 (24–84)	77
Mousavi[10]	2015	12.5 (12–13)	65 (12–183)	67
Horiba[9]	2016	11.9 (11–12)	56 (24–99)	57
Akpinar[12]	2016	12.5 (11.5–13)	59 (10–168)	79

and a smaller tumor volume. A cochlear dose of less than 4.2 Gy to the central cochlea was significantly correlated with better hearing preservation of the same GR class.

Boari et al. reviewed 152 VS patients with 10-year audiologic follow-up after GKRS using a median margin dose of 13 Gy (range, 11–15 Gy).[4] In patients with GR Class I hearing, hearing preservation was 71% and reached 93% among cases of GR Class I hearing in patients younger than 55 years. This study suggests that younger GR Class I patients have a significantly higher probability of retaining functional hearing even at the 10-year follow-up.

Baschnagel et al. studied the effect of cochlear dose on serviceable hearing preservation.[5] Forty patients with VS with serviceable hearing were treated using GKS with a median marginal dose of 12.5 Gy (range, 12.5–13 Gy) to the 50% isodose volume. The median cochlear maximum and mean doses were 6.9 and 2.7 Gy, respectively. The 1-, 2-, and 3-year actuarial rates of maintaining serviceable hearing were 93%, 77%, and 74%, respectively. Patients who received a mean cochlear dose less than 3 Gy had a 2-year hearing preservation rate of 91% compared with 59% in those who received a mean cochlear dose of 3 Gy or greater. In this study a mean cochlear dose less than 3 Gy was associated with higher serviceable hearing preservation.

Lipski et al. analyzed 126 patients with VS who were treated with GKRS using a mean marginal dose of 11.5 Gy (range, 11–12 Gy).[6] Impairment of hearing compared with its pretreatment level was revealed in 12%, 13%, and 16% of patients at 1 year, 2 years, and 3 years after radiosurgery, respectively. Overall, 77% of patients with pre-GK serviceable hearing maintained it 3 years after GKRS. Klijn et al. treated VS patients with GKRS using a median marginal dose of 11 Gy.[7] Preservation of serviceable hearing was evaluated in a subgroup of 71 patients with serviceable hearing at baseline. Actuarial 3- and 5-year hearing preservation rates were 65% and 42%, respectively. In a recent study Schumacher et al. used low-dose (11.0 Gy) GKRS in 30 patients with VSs.[8] At a median follow-up time of 42 months, serviceable hearing was preserved in 50% of patients. Only higher mean and maximum dose to the cochlea significantly decreased the proportion of patients with serviceable hearing. Horiba et al. evaluated the outcome of low-dose GKS for VSs.[9] Patients underwent treatment with a mean marginal dose of 11.9 Gy (range, 11–12 Gy). The doses for the cochlea were kept below 4 Gy. Out of 49 patients with serviceable hearing before GKS, 28 (57%) demonstrated its preservation at the time of the last follow-up.

Mousavi et al. studied the impact of pre-GK hearing status on hearing preservation rates after GKRS. These authors analyzed 68 VS patients with GR class I hearing.[10] Twenty-five patients had no subjective hearing loss (group A), and 43 patients reported subjective hearing loss (group B) before GKRS. Three years after GKRS, serviceable hearing (GR grade I or II) was preserved in 100% of patients in group A compared with 81% at 1 year, 60% at 2 years, and 57% at 3 years after GKRS for group B patients. Patients without subjective hearing loss had higher rates of grade I or II hearing preservation. To identify the candidates with a high chance of hearing preservation, Mousavi et al. retrospectively analyzed 166 patients who had pre-GK audiograms showing GR class I hearing.[11] These patients were subclassified into Class I-A (no subjective hearing loss, 53 patients) and class I-B (subjective hearing loss, 113 patients). Class I-B was further divided into two groups: class I-B1 (56 patients) if the difference in pure tone average (PTA) in the affected ear was ≤10 dB compared with the unaffected ear, and class I-B2 (57 patients) if the difference in PTA was >10 dB. The 5- and 10-year rates of serviceable hearing preservation for Class I-A were 100% and 92%, respectively. The 5- and 10-year rates of serviceable hearing preservation for Class I-B1 were 71% and 57%, respectively. The 5- and 10-year rates of serviceable hearing preservation for Class I-B2 were 26% and 26%, respectively. This study suggested that hearing preservation in patients with small VSs with pre-GK normal hearing (GR class I) was significantly better if SRS was performed before subjective hearing loss was reported. In patients who reported subjective hearing loss, the difference in PTA between the affected ear and the unaffected ear was an important factor in long-term hearing preservation.

In a recent study Akpinar et al. studied the impact of an observation period in patients with a small VS who present with normal hearing.[12] The 5- and 10-year preservation rates of serviceable hearing for patients treated early were 89% and 86%, respectively. The 5- and 10-year preservation rates of serviceable hearing for patients treated later were 66% and 66%, respectively. This study suggested that early intervention using GKS results in better hearing preservation rates.

Yang et al. reviewed the published literature on the GKS for VS patients.[13] These authors evaluated 45 articles that represented 4234 patients. At a median follow-up of 35 months, an overall hearing preservation rate was 51%, regardless of radiation dose, patient age, or tumor volume. Lower margin doses (≤13 Gy) were associated with better (60.5%) hearing preservation rates. Patients with smaller tumors (average tumor volume ≤1.5 cc) had a higher hearing preservation rate (62%) compared with patients harboring larger tumors.

Yomo et al. compared the post-SRS hearing deterioration with the natural course of hearing deterioration due to the tumor itself.[14] A group of 154 patients with unilateral VS was conservatively monitored for more than 6 months and then treated with GKS. The annual hearing decrease rate was measured before and after radiosurgery. The mean dose prescribed to the tumor margins was 12.1 Gy. The mean annual hearing decrease rates before and after GKS were 5.39 dB/year and 3.77 dB/year, respectively ($p > 0.05$). A maximum cochlear dose of less than 4 Gy was found to be the only prognostic factor for hearing preservation. This study demonstrated the absence of an increase in annual hearing decrease rate after radiosurgery as compared with the natural history.

Overall long-term studies suggest that hearing can be preserved in the majority of patients who present with small- to medium-size tumors and good or normal hearing.

Facial Nerve Preservation

With the current technique, facial nerve function can be preserved in almost all patients (Table 27.2). In an analysis of VS radiosurgery using current techniques (MR based dose planning, a 13 Gy or less tumor margin dose), Flickinger et al. reported a 0% risk of new facial weakness numbness (5-year actuarial rates). A higher margin dose (>14 Gy) was associated with 5-year actuarial rates of 2.5% risk of new onset facial weakness.[2] None of the patients who had radiosurgery for intracanalicular tumors developed new facial or trigeminal neuropathies.

Chung et al. retrospectively studied 195 patients with VS who had GKRS using multiisocenter dose planning with a prescription dose of 11 to 18.2 Gy on the 50% to 94% isodose located at the tumor margin.[15] Two patients (1%) experienced a temporary facial palsy. Hasegawa et al. evaluated long-term outcome after VS radiosurgery.[16] The median follow-up period was 12.5 years. Of 287 patients treated with a margin dose of 13 Gy or less, 3 (1%) developed facial palsy (2 with transient palsy and 1 with persistent palsy after a second GKRS procedure). The actuarial 10-year facial nerve preservation rate was 97% in the high marginal dose group (>13 Gy) and 100% in the low marginal dose group (≤13 Gy).

In a prospective study, van Eck and Horstmann investigated the role of lower central dose (maximum, 20 Gy) while maintaining a margin dose of 13 Gy. One out of 95 patients suffered transient facial nerve impairment.[17] Lipski et al. reported 3% of patients with transitory impairment of the facial nerve function in a study of 126 patients with VS who were treated with GKRS using a mean marginal dose of 11.5 Gy (range, 11–12 Gy).[6] In a study by Klijn et al., 420 patients underwent GKRS for VS with a median marginal dose of 11 Gy.[7] Four patients (1.0%) reported new or increased permanent facial weakness. Tveiten et al. studied patient-reported outcomes after VS management.[18] This study included 247 treated with GKS, and 144 with microsurgery. Almost 20%

TABLE 27.2 Published Reports With Facial Nerve Deficit

First Author	Year	Marginal Doses	# of Patients With Facial Deficit	% Facial Deficit
Flickinger[29]	2004	13 (12–13)	0	0
Niranjan[33]	2008	13 (10–18)	0	0
Chung[15]	2013	11–18.2	2 (transient)	1
Hasegawa[16]	2013	12.5	3 (2 transient)	1
Van Eck[17]	2013	13	1	1
Lipski[6]	2015	11.5	4 (transient)	3
Klijn[7]	2016	11	4	1
Horiba[9]	2016	11.9	1 (transient)	1

of the patients treated with microsurgery had an objective decline in facial nerve function, whereas only 2% in the GKS group had a decline in facial nerve function.

Compared with surgical resection, preservation of facial nerve function is very high after GKRS. With current techniques, less than 1% of patients are expected to develop transient facial nerve dysfunction.

Auditory and Facial Nerve Preservation in Younger Patients

Radiosurgery has been shown to be a very effective management strategy for younger patients with VSs. In a study of 55 younger patients managed with GKRS Lobato-Polo et al. reported preserved serviceable hearing in 100%, 93%, and 93% of patients at 3, 5, and 10 years, respectively.[19] A margin dose of 13 or less was significantly associated with hearing preservation ($p = 0.017$). None of the patients treated with doses lower than 13 Gy experienced facial neuropathy.

Auditory and Facial Nerve Preservation in Patients With Larger Tumors

SRS is an established management option for patients with small- and medium-size VSs. However, radiosurgery has been performed for several patients with larger tumors who either refused surgery or were found to be high risk for resection due to comorbidities. Yang et al. studied 65 patients with larger VS (3–4 cm in diameter, median tumor volume 9 mL) who underwent radiosurgery.[20] Serviceable hearing was preserved in 82% of patients. van de Langenberg et al. evaluated outcome in large VSs in 33 patients who had GK.[21] The preservation of serviceable hearing and facial nerve function was achieved in 58% and 91% of patients, respectively, with any facial neuropathy being transient. Primary GKS for large VSs leads to acceptable rates of hearing preservation. Milligan et al. analyzed 22 patients who had undergone GKS for VSs larger than 2.5 cm in the posterior fossa diameter.[22] The median treated tumor volume was 9.4 cc (range, 5.3–19.1 cc). The median maximum posterior fossa diameter was 2.8 cm (range, 2.5–3.8 cm). The median tumor margin dose was 12 Gy (range, 12–14 Gy). The 3-year actuarial rate of freedom from new facial neuropathy and preservation of functional hearing were 92% and 47%, respectively. At 5 years post-GKS, these rates decreased to 85% and 28%, respectively. These studies suggest that single-session radiosurgery is a successful treatment for the majority of patients with larger VS. The cranial nerve morbidity of GKS was significantly lower than that typically achieved via resection of larger VS. The value of radiosurgery in selected patients with large tumors is encouraging. However, all the options should be discussed with the patient, and an individualized decision should be made after considering the patient's wishes and goals and the surgeon's experience.

Cystic Vestibular Schwannomas

Patients with cystic VS are often told that these tumors do not respond well to SRS. Bowden et al. recently reviewed the outcome of radiosurgery in cystic VSs.[23] Despite the myth that cystic VSs do not respond to SRS, this study documented that macrocystic VSs have the greatest chance of tumor regression after SRS. Overall, tumor control in this study was 99.4% at 2 years and 96.4% at 5 years. The median percentage regression in volume was 79% for macrocystic and 43% for microcytic, compared with 35% for homogeneously enhancing tumors. In this group the 2- and 5-year serviceable hearing preservation rates were 82.2% and 61.5%. There was no significant difference in auditory outcomes between the groups. Post-SRS facial nerve function was assessed using the House–Brackman scale. Compared with pre-SRS, two additional patients developed facial weakness (1 grade II and 1 grade III).

Oncogenesis

Many patients seeking information about the options for VS management are told by consultants that even if GKRS is effective, they have a high chance of developing cancer caused by exposure to radiation. Cahan's criteria of radiation-related neoplasms state that the patient must develop the tumor within the field of radiation, that the tumor must be of a different histology, and that a period of time must elapse before the development of the secondary tumor.[24] Patel and Chiang recently reviewed the literature on this topic and noted that 36 patients fit the criteria among over 100,000 patients treated by GKRS worldwide over a 40-year period.[25] Pollock et al. reviewed 1142 patients and reported a 0% risk of radiation-induced tumor at 15 years. Malignant transformation was reported in 1 of 358 VSs (0.3%) at a median of 4.9 years.[26] To put this into perspective, the risk of death after craniotomy for a VS is estimated to be 1/500 to 1/1000 at centers of microsurgical excellence. Patients should be told that the estimated risk of tumor oncogenesis varies between 1/1000 and 1/100,000 radiosurgical cases.

Resection After GKRS

The final source of confusion to many VS patients lies in the report they receive that after radiosurgery fails, the tumor will be stuck to the brainstem and cranial nerves, posing serious risks of brain or nerve injury because of difficulty of resection. This misconception seems to have originated in the otology literature, which initially failed to differentiate various radiation therapy techniques from GKRS. Wide-field fractionated radiation therapy may result in such scarring. In centers with both GK radiosurgical and microsurgical experience, no clear relationship has been found between prior radiosurgery and difficulty in subsequent resection.[27] It is important for patients and referring physicians to recall that less than 2% of patient who undergo GKRS will require microsurgical intervention because of sustained growth after the procedure.

Quality of Life

GKRS is an outpatient procedure that allows patients to resume their prior life within 12 hours of the procedure's completion. For patients with imbalance or disequilibrium, such symptoms may persist but are generally mild. They reflect the loss of unilateral vestibular input in a complex system that requires vision, two functional ears, and intact dorsal column function. Neither surgery nor radiosurgery can make a dysfunctional vestibular nerve work. Most patients make lifestyle adjustments so that disequilibrium, rare vertiginous events, and even tinnitus, when present, are compensated. A recent experience from Norway further defined the improved quality of life that GKRS patients experience compared with those who underwent microsurgery.[28]

SURGICAL REWIND

My Worst Case (Fig. 27.2)

A 64-year-old man presented with tinnitus and diminished right ear hearing. His brain MRI showed right-sided intracanalicular VS. He underwent GKS with 12.5-Gy margin dose. His 6-month and 1.5-year follow-up MRI showed a stable tumor. However, a 3-year imaging follow-up showed tumor growth (Fig. 27.2).

Management: This patient underwent second radiosurgery without any complication for management of tumor progression. Persistent tumor growth requiring intervention can be expected in about 2% of VSs treated with GKS. About half of these cases are eligible for repeat radiosurgery, and others can be treated with microsurgery.

In the case of unexpected hearing loss or facial dysfunction, we recommend a short course of oral corticosteroids and an MRI to evaluate the tumor response. The majority of the time, this sudden cranial nerve dysfunction can be reverted.

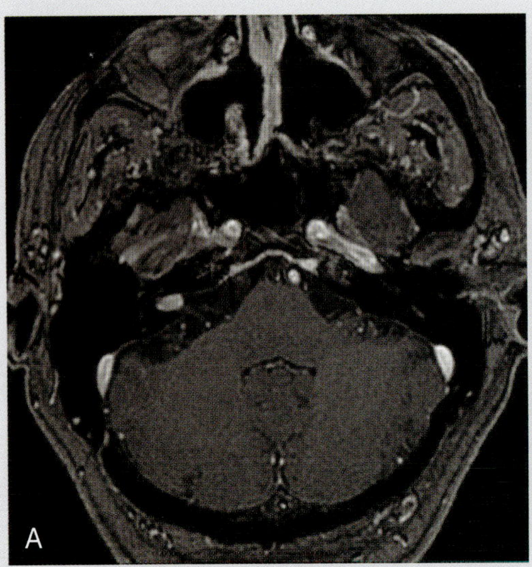

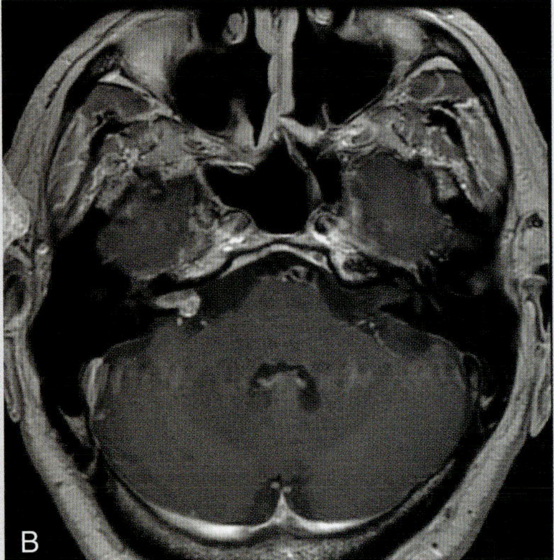

• **Fig. 27.2** (A) Contrast-enhanced axial magnetic resonance imaging showing intracanalicular vestibular schwannoma at the time of radiosurgery. (B) Tumor remained stable for 2 years; however, tumor progression was documented at 3-year follow-up.

NEUROSURGICAL SELFIE MOMENT

The long-term outcome data for single-session radiosurgery using 12- to 13-Gy margin dose is available from several institutions. Radiosurgery is now considered the first-line management option for the majority of patients with small- to medium-size acoustic VSs who desire facial and auditory nerve preservation. Surgery may be needed for patients with larger tumors associated with symptomatic mass effect (headache, ataxia, and imbalance). Such surgery should aim to debulk the mass and preserve existing cranial nerve function. SRS can be used to achieve long-term tumor control, along with high rates of facial and auditory function preservation. GKRS remains the best procedure to perform for patients with small- to moderate-size VSs, and even for patients with larger tumors not associated with symptomatic mass effect (headache and severe imbalance).

References

1. Lunsford LD, Niranjan A, Flickinger JC, Maitz A, Kondziolka D. Radiosurgery of vestibular schwannomas: summary of experience in 829 cases. *J Neurosurg*. 2005;102(suppl):195–199.
2. Flickinger JC, Kondziolka D, Niranjan A, Maitz A, Voynov G, Lunsford LD. Acoustic neuroma radiosurgery with marginal tumor doses of 12 to 13 Gy. *Int J Radiat Oncol Biol Phys*. 2004;60:225–230.
3. Kano H, Kondziolka D, Khan A, Flickinger JC, Lunsford LD. Predictors of hearing preservation after stereotactic radiosurgery for acoustic neuroma. Clinical article. *J Neurosurg*. 2009;111:863–873.
4. Boari N, Bailo M, Gagliardi F, et al. Gamma Knife radiosurgery for vestibular schwannoma: clinical results at long-term follow-up in a series of 379 patients. *J Neurosurg*. 2014;121(suppl):123–142.
5. Baschnagel AM, Chen PY, Bojrab D, et al. Hearing preservation in patients with vestibular schwannoma treated with Gamma Knife surgery. *J Neurosurg*. 2013;118:571–578.
6. Lipski SM, Hayashi M, Chernov M, Levivier M, Okada Y. Modern Gamma Knife radiosurgery of vestibular schwannomas: treatment concept, volumetric tumor response, and functional results. *Neurosurg Rev*. 2015;38:309–318, discussion 318.
7. Klijn S, Verheul JB, Beute GN, et al. Gamma Knife radiosurgery for vestibular schwannomas: evaluation of tumor control and its predictors in a large patient cohort in The Netherlands. *J Neurosurg*. 2016;124:1619–1626.
8. Schumacher AJ, Lall RR, Lall RR, et al. Low-dose Gamma Knife radiosurgery for vestibular schwannomas: tumor control and cranial nerve function preservation after 11 Gy. *J Neurol Surg B Skull Base*. 2017;78:2–10.
9. Horiba A, Hayashi M, Chernov M, Kawamata T, Okada Y. Hearing preservation after low-dose Gamma Knife radiosurgery of vestibular schwannomas. *Neurol Med Chir (Tokyo)*. 2016;56:186–192.
10. Mousavi SH, Kano H, Faraji AH, et al. Hearing preservation up to 3 years after Gamma Knife radiosurgery for Gardner-Robertson class I patients with vestibular schwannomas. *Neurosurgery*. 2015;76:584–590, discussion 590–581.

11. Mousavi SH, Niranjan A, Akpinar B, et al. Hearing subclassification may predict long-term auditory outcomes after radiosurgery for vestibular schwannoma patients with good hearing. *J Neurosurg.* 2016;125:845–852.
12. Akpinar B, Mousavi SH, McDowell MM, et al. Early radiosurgery improves hearing preservation in vestibular schwannoma patients with normal hearing at the time of diagnosis. *Int J Radiat Oncol Biol Phys.* 2016;95:729–734.
13. Yang I, Sughrue ME, Han SJ, et al. A comprehensive analysis of hearing preservation after radiosurgery for vestibular schwannoma: clinical article. *J Neurosurg.* 2013;119(suppl):851–859.
14. Yomo S, Carron R, Thomassin JM, Roche PH, Regis J. Longitudinal analysis of hearing before and after radiosurgery for vestibular schwannoma. *J Neurosurg.* 2012;117:877–885.
15. Chung WY, Liu KD, Shiau CY, et al. Gamma Knife surgery for vestibular schwannoma: 10-year experience of 195 cases. *J Neurosurg.* 2013;119(suppl):87–97.
16. Hasegawa T, Kida Y, Kato T, Iizuka H, Kuramitsu S, Yamamoto T. Long-term safety and efficacy of stereotactic radiosurgery for vestibular schwannomas: evaluation of 440 patients more than 10 years after treatment with Gamma Knife surgery. *J Neurosurg.* 2013;118:557–565.
17. van Eck AT, Horstmann GA. Increased preservation of functional hearing after Gamma Knife surgery for vestibular schwannoma. *J Neurosurg.* 2013;119(suppl):204–206.
18. Tveiten OV, Carlson ML, Goplen F, et al. Patient- versus physician-reported facial disability in vestibular schwannoma: an international cross-sectional study. *J Neurosurg.* 2017;127(5):1015–1024.
19. Lobato-Polo J, Kondziolka D, Zorro O, Kano H, Flickinger JC, Lunsford LD. Gamma Knife radiosurgery in younger patients with vestibular schwannomas. *Neurosurgery.* 2009;65:294–300, discussion 300–291.
20. Yang HC, Kano H, Awan NR, et al. Gamma Knife radiosurgery for larger-volume vestibular schwannomas. Clinical article. *J Neurosurg.* 2011;114:801–807.
21. van de Langenberg R, Hanssens PE, Verheul JB, et al. Management of large vestibular schwannoma. Part II. Primary Gamma Knife surgery: radiological and clinical aspects. *J Neurosurg.* 2011;115:885–893.
22. Milligan BD, Pollock BE, Foote RL, Link MJ. Long-term tumor control and cranial nerve outcomes following Gamma Knife surgery for larger-volume vestibular schwannomas. *J Neurosurg.* 2012;116:598–604.
23. Bowden G, Cavaleri J, Monaco E III, Niranjan A, Flickinger J, Lunsford LD. Cystic vestibular schwannomas respond best to radiosurgery. *Neurosurgery.* 2017;81(3):490–497.
24. Cahan WG, Woodard HQ, Higinbotham NL, Stewart FW, Coley BL. Sarcoma arising in irradiated bone: report of eleven cases. 1948. *Cancer.* 1998;82:8–34.
25. Patel TR, Chiang VL. Secondary neoplasms after stereotactic radiosurgery. *World Neurosurg.* 2014;81:594–599.
26. Pollock BE, Link MJ, Stafford SL, Parney IF, Garces YI, Foote RL. The risk of radiation-induced tumors or malignant transformation after single-fraction intracranial radiosurgery: results based on a 25-year experience. *Int J Radiat Oncol Biol Phys.* 2017;97:919–923.
27. Regis J, Pellet W, Delsanti C, et al. Functional outcome after Gamma Knife surgery or microsurgery for vestibular schwannomas. *J Neurosurg.* 2002;97:1091–1100.
28. Varughese JK, Wentzel-Larsen T, Pedersen PH, Mahesparan R, Lund-Johansen M. Gamma Knife treatment of growing vestibular schwannoma in Norway: a prospective study. *Int J Radiat Oncol Biol Phys.* 2012;84:e161–e166.
29. Flickinger JC, Kondziolka D, Niranjan A, Maitz A, Voynov G, Lunsford LD. Acoustic neuroma radiosurgery with marginal tumor doses of 12 to 13 Gy. *Int J Radiat Oncol Biol Phys.* 2004;60:225–230.
30. Pollock BE, Driscoll CL, Foote RL, et al. Patient outcomes after vestibular schwannoma management: a prospective comparison of microsurgical resection and stereotactic radiosurgery. *Neurosurgery.* 2006;59:77–85, discussion 77–85.
31. Chopra R, Kondziolka D, Niranjan A, Lunsford LD, Flickinger JC. Long-term follow-up of acoustic schwannoma radiosurgery with marginal tumor doses of 12 to 13 Gy. *Int J Radiat Oncol Biol Phys.* 2007;68:845–851.
32. Regis J, Roche PH, Delsanti C, et al. Modern management of vestibular schwannomas. *Prog Neurol Surg.* 2007;20:129–141.
33. Niranjan A, Mathieu D, Flickinger JC, Kondziolka D, Lunsford LD. Hearing preservation after intracanalicular vestibular schwannoma radiosurgery. *Neurosurgery.* 2008;63:1054–1062, discussion 1062–1053.
34. Kano H, Kondziolka D, Khan A, Flickinger JC, Lunsford LD. Predictors of hearing preservation after stereotactic radiosurgery for acoustic neuroma. *J Neurosurg.* 2009;111:863–873.
35. Myrseth E, Moller P, Pedersen PH, Lund-Johansen M. Vestibular schwannoma: surgery or Gamma Knife radiosurgery? A prospective, nonrandomized study. *Neurosurgery.* 2009;64:654–661, discussion 661–653.
36. Tamura M, Carron R, Yomo S, et al. Hearing preservation after Gamma Knife radiosurgery for vestibular schwannomas presenting with high-level hearing. *Neurosurgery.* 2009;64:289–296, discussion 296.
37. Kim CH, Chung KW, Kong DS, et al. Prognostic factors of hearing preservation after Gamma Knife radiosurgery for vestibular schwannoma. *J Clin Neurosci.* 2010;17:214–218.
38. Delbrouck C, Hassid S, Choufani G, De Witte O, Devriendt D, Massager N. Hearing outcome after Gamma Knife radiosurgery for vestibular schwannoma: a prospective Belgian clinical study. *B-ENT.* 2011;7(suppl 17):77–84.
39. Kim JW, Kim DG, Paek SH, et al. Efficacy of corticosteroids in hearing preservation after radiosurgery for vestibular schwannoma: a prospective study. *Stereotact Funct Neurosurg.* 2011;89:25–33.
40. Massager N, Lonneville S, Delbrouck C, Benmebarek N, Desmedt F, Devriendt D. Dosimetric and clinical analysis of spatial distribution of the radiation dose in Gamma Knife radiosurgery for vestibular schwannoma. *Int J Radiat Oncol Biol Phys.* 2011;81:e511–e518.

28 Complications of Posterior Fossa Tumors: Ependymoma/ Medulloblastoma/Pilocytic Astrocytoma

FREDERICK A. BOOP, JIMMY MING-JUNG CHUANG

HIGHLIGHTS

- Cautions for resection of these tumors will vary depending upon the location of the tumor.
- Medulloblastomas most arise from the roof of the fourth ventricle, pushing downward into the ventricle. 35% of medulloblastoma invade the floor of the fourth ventricle and the brainstem. This tumor debulking may lead to a "floor of the fourth syndrome" which includes an ipsilateral nuclear palsy of cranial nerves VI and VII and a contralateral hemiparesis.
- Juvenile pilocytic astrocytomas arise within the cerebellar hemispheres and are usually separated from the ventricle by the ependyma. A variant of the cerebellar astrocytoma actually arises from the brainstem and is dorsally exophytic into the ventricle. Such tumors exit the brainstem, pulling functional tissue up as they grow dorsally. The inexperienced surgeon may shave these tumors off with inadvertently injuring the brainstem in the process.
- Ependymomas take origin from the ependymal lining of the ventricle. Those arising from the floor of the fourth ventricle derive blood supply from multiple small perforating vessels arising from the brainstem. These vessels must be meticulously coagulated and cut, as avulsing them may cause them to retract and bleed into the brainstem. A variant of the ependymoma arises from ependymal rests at the lateral margin of the foramen of Luschka and grows out the foramen into the cerebellopontine angle. These tumors often encase the lower cranial nerves as well as the vertebra-basilar complex, and may invade the side of the pons.

Introduction

The incidence of brain tumors in children is 2.6 to 4 per 100,000.[1] Half of the brain tumors found in childhood occur in the posterior fossa, with medulloblastoma, juvenile pilocytic astrocytoma (JPA), and ependymoma being the big three.[2] Tumors of the fourth ventricle offer a unique challenge to the neurosurgeon because they lie deep in the brain in close proximity to a number of vital structures. Posterior fossa surgery involves greater morbidity and mortality and has a wider variety of complications than surgery in the supratentorial region. In addition, multiple reviews have shown that the single most important determinant of survival in children with posterior fossa tumors is the extent of surgical resection. The pediatric neurosurgeon must achieve a maximal safe resection.

Thus surgery for pediatric posterior fossa tumors is important not only to the survival but also to the quality of the survival. To date there is no study to report the true complication rate of pediatric posterior fossa surgery. Sawaya et al. classified the complications associated with craniotomy into three major categories: neurologic, regional, and systemic complications.[3] In this article, we focus mainly on neurologic and regional complications associated with posterior fossa surgery for children with ependymoma, medulloblastoma, and pilocytic astrocytoma. We also review the causes of delayed diagnosis and the precautions that can be taken in the preoperative and intraoperative period to minimize complications (Fig. 28.1).

Delayed Diagnosis or Misdiagnosis of Posterior Fossa Tumor

Previous studies have indicated that delays in the diagnosis of childhood brain tumors may be much longer than those associated with other pediatric neoplasms.[4,5] Dobrovoljac et al. found the median prediagnostic symptomatic interval (PSI) was 60 days, with a parental delay of 14 days and a doctor's delay of 30 days. Only 33% of brain tumors were diagnosed within the first month after the onset of signs and symptoms.[6] In children older than 2 years, most common initial complaints were headache, nausea/vomiting, seizures, squint/diplopia, ataxia, and behavioral changes. In children younger than 2 years, the most common initial presenting symptoms were seizures, vomiting, head tilt, and behavior changes. These signs and symptoms are nonspecific, thus making the diagnosis early in the course often difficult.

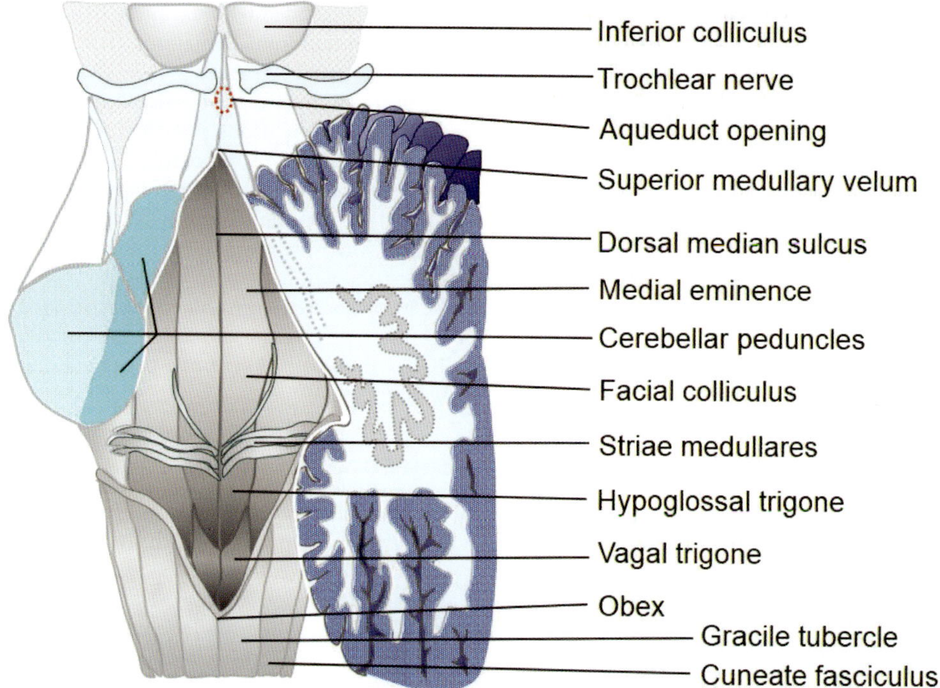

• **Fig. 28.1** The fourth ventricle lies dorsal to the pons and medulla and ventral to the cerebellum. It extends from the cerebral aqueduct to the obex. The fourth ventricle has an anterior floor with a characteristic diamond shape, named the rhomboid fossa, and a posterior tent-shaped roof. The entire floor is divided into right and left halves by the dorsal median sulcus. At its widest part, the floor is crossed transversely by glistening white fibers, the stria medullaris. The medial eminence presents as an oval swelling in the pontine part of the floor at the level of the superior fovea, the facial colliculus. From the inferior fovea, the medullary part of the floor divides into two triangles: the hypoglossal triangle above and the vagal triangle below.

The mean age at presentation of children with medulloblastoma or ependymoma is 5 years or less, whereas the mean age at presentation of the child with a JPA is 9 years. JPAs often exhibit a long history of ataxia and elevated intracranial pressure (ICP) resulting from gradual obstructive hydrocephalus. Neck pain may be a presenting symptom in cases of chronic tonsillar herniation. Medulloblastomas may produce symptoms and signs similar to those for pilocytic astrocytoma, but because they are malignant tumors and grow more rapidly, the time course of progression is usually over weeks rather than months. Ependymomas typically arise from the floor of the fourth ventricle. Nausea and vomiting as a result of irritation of the "vomiting center" near the obex is often an initial symptom. Progressive headaches usually herald the evidence of a brain tumor in children; however, headaches may be experienced by 5% to 30% of elementary school children. Most children with headache as an initial symptom of a brain tumor will show additional signs and symptoms within a relatively short period. In the study of the Childhood Brain Tumor Consortium with 3276 patients, less than 3% of children with headache caused by a brain tumor had no other abnormality on neurologic examination.[7]

An earlier diagnosis of pediatric posterior fossa brain tumor has not been seen since the popularity of computed tomography and magnetic resonance imaging (MRI). Only a high degree of suspicion, a detailed clinical history, and a targeted neurologic examination lead to more accurate and timely diagnosis.

Presurgical Precautions

Although most children present with ventricular obstruction and symptoms of increased ICP, the vast majority can be observed in an intensive care setting and do not require placement of an emergent shunt, third ventriculostomy, or external ventricular drain (EVD). Within 12 hours of initiating intravenous steroids, most children will recognize improvement in nausea/vomiting or headache, allowing surgery to be performed on an elective basis. There are rare cases in which a child declined neurologically and had to be operated on emergently, but such cases are uncommon.

Most children with posterior fossa tumors do not require permanent shunts. The need for external ventricular drainage is determined at the time of surgery based on the turgor of the dura after the craniectomy. Again, the majority of children do not require external ventricular drainage, even though the ventricles may appear quite enlarged on preoperative imaging.

Intraoperative Precautions

Several age-dependent factors enter into the decision-making of positioning, anesthesia, and postoperative care. They are discussed in the following subsections.

Blood Transfusion

The major challenge of tumor surgery in young children is that of blood loss. The circulating blood volume of a young child is estimated at 70 cc per kilogram body weight. Loss of more than 1.5 blood volumes runs the risk of a coagulopathy. The anesthesiologist should begin replacement early when it becomes apparent that a transfusion will be necessary. Washed red blood cells are less likely to cause intraoperative problems with hyperkalemia in the child requiring large volumes of blood. Irradiated red blood cells may be given to reduce the likelihood of viral transmission to a compromised host, especially if the child is likely to require chemotherapy after surgery.

Positioning and Fixation

There are three possibilities for positioning: prone, lateral decubitus, or sitting. Each of the positions requires the head to be pinned as long as the patient is more than 2 years old. Use of pins in infants can lead to skull penetration producing depressed skull fracture, pneumocephalus, dural laceration, hematoma, or postoperative abscess. Posterior fossa surgery in children younger than 2 is probably safer if the child is in the prone position with the face down on a padded horseshoe headrest. It is important to adjust the width of the horseshoe to ensure that there is no pressure on the eyes. In this position, malar eminences or the forehead area is at risk to get pressure sores. Placing rest-on foam over the face, with the adhesive side to the skin, may help avoid pressure injury. For children over 3 years of age, the pediatric pins are utilized but tightened to only 40 pounds of pressure per inch until the pins penetrate the outer table of the skull. It is important for the pin placement to avoid the thin squamous temporal bone and shunt tubing, if present.

Prone position or concorde position (prone with neck flexed) affords many ergonometric advantages such as better visualization, better exposure, greater surgeon comfort, and minimized risk of air embolus. The most significant disadvantage of the prone position is venous congestion that can lead to more significant blood loss and soft tissue swelling of the face. This congestion can be improved by elevating the head above the level of the heart. In the prone position, care must be taken to protect the pressure points—such as the ulnar nerve at the elbow, the common peroneal nerve across fibular head, and the lateral femoral cutaneous nerve at the iliac crest—to avoid skin breakdown and compression neuropathy. Two longitudinal padded rolls are placed under the patient, and the knees and ankles are padded.

In the lateral decubitus position, the patient is lying on his side. This allows superior visualization in the lateral recesses or cerebello-pontine angle. The disadvantage of the lateral position is that the anatomy is not centered, so the surgeon must visualize all anatomic structures as rotated. The patient is placed on his side with a soft roll placed in the axilla of the dependent arm to prevent brachial plexus injury or vascular compression, and the dependent leg is padded with special attention paid to the fibular head of the upper leg to avoid peroneal palsy.

The sitting position with the patient positioned sitting upright offers a clear operative field because blood and cerebrospinal fluid (CSF) drain out of the operative site. Some studies also showed better lower cranial nerve preservation in the sitting position.[8] However, there are many risks to the sitting position. The most significant dangers are cardiovascular instability and hypotension, venous air embolism (VAE), and subdural hematoma. Precordial Doppler ultrasonic flow and end-tidal CO_2 should be monitored throughout the case for detecting VAE. In adult studies, the incidence of end-tidal CO_2–detected VAE is up to 15.2% compared with only 1.4% in the prone position.[8] If the child has a shunt, it should be occluded before surgery in a sitting position to decrease the risk of subdural hematoma. For the same reason, mannitol should be used with caution in the sitting position because it has been implicated in the development of subdural hematomas. Other risks of the sitting position include tension pneumocephalus, cervical myelopathy, thermal loss (especially in children), surgeon discomfort, and the rapid escape of CSF from the ventricular system. When applying the head holder, the pin sites must be covered with Vaseline gauze to minimize entry of air. If air embolism occurs, the wound should be packed with a saline-soaked sponge, the head lowered immediately, and the atrial catheter aspirated by anesthesia to attempt to remove the embolus from the left atrium. If the embolus is severe, the patient should be placed in the left decubitus position.

Selection of Surgical Approach

The safest and most direct approach to the fourth ventricle is the midline suboccipital approach. In children, the dura is not firmly adherent to the skull, so it is safe to drill close to or even on top of the major venous sinuses. The superior and lateral limits of the craniotomy are the transverse and sigmoid sinuses. Inferiorly, the craniotomy should always include the posterior edge of the foramen magnum to prevent laceration of the brain against the closed bony rim when cerebellar elements are retracted downward or if hematoma or swelling should occur postoperatively. To expose the posterior arch of C1, monopolar cautery should be used with caution when dissecting the soft tissue over C1 (especially at the superolateral surface) to prevent vertebral artery injury. In infants or young children, C1 is often cartilaginous, and the dorsal arch does not fuse until age 3 years. C1 laminectomy is helpful for lesions that herniate through the foramen magnum. It is important to remember that extending a laminectomy below C2 in young children increases the risk of swan neck deformity.[9]

All techniques for dural incision require crossing the occipital and annular sinuses, which may be very large in infants under age 2 years. If there is significant bleeding from the midline occipital sinus, it should be controlled with obliquely placed hemostatic clips or suture ligatures. The arachnoid is opened next over the cisterna magna to allow drainage of CSF. Gentle separation of the cerebellar tonsils will expose the cerebello-medullary fissure through the opened vallecula, giving an unimpeded view of the inferior roof of the fourth ventricle. The locations of the vermian branches of posterior inferior cerebellar artery (PICA) should be carefully dissected out because they are often tethered to the tonsils and the walls of the cerebello-medullary fissure. If there is a limitation of this exposure when approaching the rostral portion of the fourth ventricle, incising the inferior vermis of the cerebellum and retracting the two halves of the vermis may provide a greater working angle in this area and a better visualization of the midline inferior portion of the superior medullary velum and fastigium. If there is extension of the tumor through one of the foramina of Luschka into the cerebello-pontine cistern, the ipsilateral tonsil and cerebellar hemisphere can be retracted dorsally to expose it. Sometimes it is necessary to do a secondary retromastoid approach to completely resect the tumor.

Techniques for intradural exposure and resection of the tumor will vary depending upon the location and size of the tumor. Medulloblastomas can be found within the cerebellar hemisphere, but most arise from the roof of the fourth ventricle, pushing downward into the ventricle; 35% invade the brainstem, often at the obex or the floor of the fourth ventricle. If the ventricular floor is invaded by tumor, caution must be taken in manipulation of the tumor as it is debulked to avoid "floor of the fourth syndrome," which includes an ipsilateral nuclear palsy of cranial nerves VI and VII and a contralateral hemiparesis. Irritation of the obex can induce persistent postoperative vomiting and present an aspiration risk.

JPAs arise within the cerebellar hemispheres and are usually separated from the ventricle by the ependyma. On some occasions, however, they also invade the floor of the fourth ventricle. A variant of the cerebellar astrocytoma actually arises from the brainstem and is dorsally exophytic into the ventricle or laterally into the cerebello-pontine angle. Such tumors exit the brainstem, pulling functional tissue up with them as they grow dorsally, much like the sides of a volcano. The inexperienced surgeon may be inclined to shave off these tumors flush with the floor of the ventricle or with the side of the stem, inadvertently injuring the brainstem in the process.

Ependymomas, by definition, take origin from the ependymal lining of the ventricle. They must be debulked carefully as the capsule is dissected away from neural tissue. Those arising from the floor of the fourth ventricle derive their blood supply from multiple small perforating vessels arising from the brainstem. These vessels must be meticulously coagulated and cut, because avulsion may cause them to retract and bleed into the brainstem. If they do, they should not be pursued. Gentle, regulated suction, gentle irrigation, and time will allow them to stop oozing without injuring the brainstem. A variant of the ependymoma arises from ependymal rests at the lateral margin of the foramen of Luschka and grows out the foramen into the cerebello-pontine angle. These tumors often encase the lower cranial nerves as well as the vertebro-basilar complex, and may invade the side of the pons. This tumor is one of the most formidable posterior fossa tumors for the surgeon. The skin incision begins midline but curves up behind the ear on the involved side. This allows bony removal across the midline, up to the torcular herophili, and around to the sigmoid sinus of the involved side. By gently elevating the involved cerebellar hemisphere and opening the telovelar space (cerebello-medullary fissure), one can dissect out the entire tumor and accomplish a gross total resection. One-third of these children may require temporary tracheostomies and gastrostomies, but most of them can be decannulated by 6 months postoperatively.

Intraoperative Monitoring

Intraoperative monitoring during posterior fossa surgery may be helpful if there is danger of violating the brainstem or cranial nerves. In addition, children are as much at risk of neurologic deterioration during various neurosurgical procedures as adults, and benefit as much from intraoperative monitoring.[10] Neurophysiologic monitoring consists of two main categories of techniques: monitoring techniques and mapping techniques. Monitoring is the identification of the source of surgically induced neurophysiologic changes, allowing prompt correction of the cause before permanent neurologic impairment occurs. Mapping includes those techniques that allow the functional identification and preservation of anatomically important nervous tissue.[11]

Monitoring refers to the continuous assessment of the functional integrity of neural pathways. The common option for direct monitoring of brainstem function is brainstem auditory-evoked potentials (BAEP). This technique produces five waves that correspond to the proximal cochlear nerve, the distal cochlear nerve, the cochlear nucleus, the superior olivary complex, and the lateral lemniscus/inferior colliculus in response to auditory stimulation. Evidence of pontomesencephalic transmission of the impulses implies that the brainstem has not been compromised. Another monitoring technique, somatosensory evoked potentials (SSEP), follows sensory signals through the medial lemniscus, tracing the pathway more laterally. Due to its distance from the floor of the fourth ventricle, SSEP is less sensitive than BAEP. Mapping with direct stimulation of the facial nerve or facial nucleus can be used to identify the integrity of cranial nerve fibers or the safe entry zones for entering the brainstem.

Finally, it is important to mention that intraoperative monitoring tends to cause the surgeon to leave more tumor behind. Recognizing that the most important predictor of survival in pediatric posterior fossa tumors is currently a gross or near-total resection, the neurosurgeon relying on intraoperative monitoring must still accomplish this goal, or the tumor will likely progress and the child will die.

Complication During the Postoperative Period

Resectable Residual Tumor

Although resectable residual tumor is not a real surgical complication, we have to remember that the single most important determinant of outcome for the majority of cases of pediatric medulloblastoma/ependymoma/pilocytic astrocytoma is the extent of surgical resection. The pediatric neurosurgeon must achieve a maximal safe resection.

Multiple reviews of outcomes of children with posterior fossa tumors have demonstrated that, regardless of histology, the extent of resection is the most important predictor of outcome. In trials of ependymoma and medulloblastoma, a gross total resection or near-total resection has been shown to double the 5-year survival of the child compared with a lesser resection.[12–15] This concept is currently being questioned for certain molecular subtypes of medulloblastoma and may not remain as important as new targeted molecular therapies come into play.[16]

It has been our practice to inform the parents preoperatively that the child will undergo a postoperative MRI within 48 hours of surgery, and that if this scan demonstrates any resectable residual tumor, the child will be returned to the operating room to remove that remnant. This is true unless the surgeon stopped the initial resection because of excessive vascularity or invasion of critical structures.

Hydrocephalus

Eighty percent of children with posterior fossa tumors have hydrocephalus at the time of presentation due to obstruction of the fourth ventricle. As such, the management of hydrocephalus is usually the first intervention. In the past, many patients with tumors and hydrocephalus underwent temporizing preoperative shunting at presentation to treat hydrocephalus and make tumor resection elective. Sainte-Rose et al. have advocated endoscopic third ventriculostomy at presentation rather than shunting.[17] However, more recently it has been observed that preoperative dexamethasone results in significant alleviation of the symptoms and a reduction in vomiting within 24 to 48 hours. Given this, an appropriate alternative to permanent shunting is perioperative external ventricular drainage, especially if a patient presents with lethargy or obtundation. When an EVD is placed in the face of a large posterior fossa mass, consideration must be given to the possibility of upward herniation, and the rate and quantity of CSF drainage must be carefully monitored. Most of the time, CSF diversion, either temporary or permanent, is not required, and the hydrocephalus resolves once the tumor is removed. The height of an EVD can be gradually increased in the postoperative period, and in most cases the EVD can be successfully removed within a week to 10 days postoperatively.

Today, only about 10% to 20% of patients with cerebellar and posterior fossa tumors require permanent shunting. Risk factors for shunt dependence include younger age, larger preoperative ventricle size, more extensive tumors, and the presence of metastatic disease.[18,19] CSF diversion is rarely required in children older than age 10. When persistent hydrocephalus is present, either ventriculo-peritoneal shunting or endoscopic third ventriculostomy can be considered.[20] If a shunt is required for a malignant tumor, there may be an increased risk of extraneural metastasis through the shunt tubing (especially to the peritoneum).[21]

Pneumocephalus

Pneumocephalus in the ventricles and subdural space is not uncommon after fourth ventricular surgery, especially when patients are operated upon in the sitting position. It frequently results from overdrainage of CSF through an EVD during surgery. If tension pneumocephalus is recognized intraoperatively, the patient should be placed in Trendelenburg position and the operative bed irrigated to replace air with the irrigating fluid. Symptomatic postoperative tension pneumocephalus can be treated with a small frontal burr hole to relieve the pressure caused by the trapped air. Intraventricular air may cause ventriculo-peritoneal shunt malfunction due to an air lock within the valve.

Vascular Injury

Injury to major vessels is rare with fourth ventricular surgery. The most likely artery to be injured is PICA. Most patients with PICA injury present with postoperative flocculonodular lobe dysfunction causing nausea, vomiting, nystagmus, vertigo, and inability to stand or walk without appendicular dysmetria (Fig. 28.2).

Venous infarction is rare even if veins are sacrificed due to diffuse anastomosis of the venous system in this region. One or two veins near the tonsils, vermis, and inferior roof can be safely sacrificed. Medial retraction of the cerebellar hemisphere to expose the lateral recess and cerebello-pontine cistern can stretch bridging veins to the sigmoid sinus, but it is seldom necessary to sacrifice these. Most venous infarctions of the posterior fossa have occurred after sacrifice of the petrosal veins or veins of the cerebello-mesencephalic fissure (including the precentral cerebellar vein).

Postoperative Pseudomeningoceles

Postoperative pseudomeningoceles affect 15% to 28% of all children with posterior fossa tumors.[22,23] Normally, these small collections

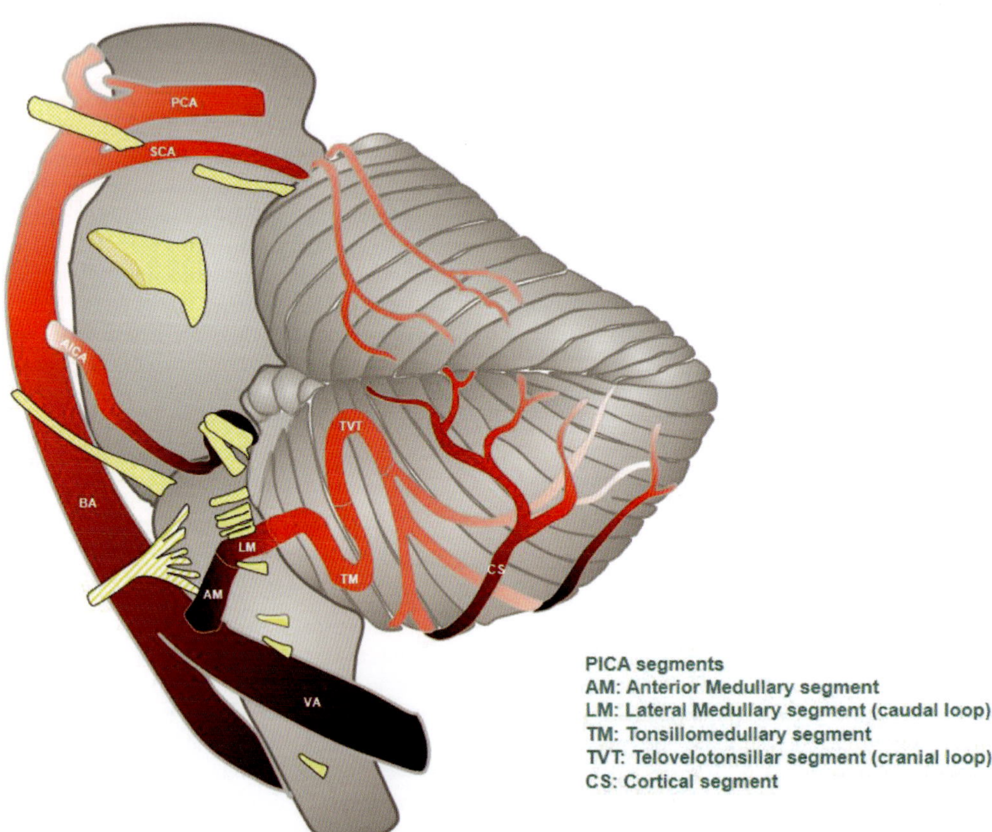

• **Fig. 28.2** The posterior inferior cerebellar artery, originating from the vertebral artery, courses around the medulla oblongata from the anterior to the posterior aspects of the brainstem. Then it passes through the cerebello-medullary fissure between the tonsil and the roof of the fourth ventricle, reaches the cerebellar hemispheric and vermian surfaces, and finally supplies the suboccipital surface.

of fluid are self-limited and may respond well to serial lumbar punctures. Occasionally they can enlarge, putting the closure under tension, and may eventually produce a CSF leak, which carries a risk of meningitis. Pseudomeningoceles may be a manifestation of hydrocephalus and in some cases may require a permanent CSF diversion to resolve.

Incisional Cerebrospinal Fluid Leaks

CSF leakage is a common complication associated with posterior fossa surgery. Leaks usually occur in the early stage of the postoperative period. CSF rhinorrhea and otorrhea are very rare in pediatric posterior fossa surgery. In the case of incisional CSF leak, they are often secondary to a failed watertight dural closure. Some adult studies have found that the size of the tumor appears to have a positive correlation to the incidence of CSF leakage.[24] The use of tissue glue, dural grafting, and external ventricular drainage have been advocated as helpful but without proof that they decrease the incidence of CSF leak.[25] If a CSF leak is a manifestation of hydrocephalus, permanent CSF diversion may be required.

Aseptic Meningitis

The syndrome of aseptic meningitis, also called posterior fossa fever, is characterized by spiking fever and meningismus after posterior fossa surgery. This has been particularly true for epidermoids or dermoids that rupture intraoperatively, leaking cholesterol cyst fluid into the ventricles. It also occurs rarely after resection of astrocytoma or medulloblastoma. Patients usually present about 1 week after surgery with fever, headache, meningismus, and irritability. CSF analysis generally shows increased pleocytosis, hypoglycorrhachia, elevated protein, and negative CSF cultures. It can be difficult in some cases to differentiate aseptic meningitis from true bacterial meningitis, which should always be carefully excluded before assuming the diagnosis of aseptic meningitis. The condition resolves with steroids or antiinflammatory medications and serial lumbar punctures to remove bloody CSF.[26]

Cranial Nerve Palsies

Cranial VI and VII Palsy ("Floor of the Fourth" Syndrome)

Transient or permanent cranial nerve palsies sometimes occur after surgery of the fourth ventricle. These deficits are usually immediately evident in the recovery room. The most common deficit is cranial VI and VII palsy caused by disruption of the nerve fibers coursing under the fourth ventricular floor along the facial colliculus where the intrapontine course of the facial nerve loops around the abducens nucleus. The nucleus of the abducens nerve (CN VI) is located in the dorsomedial pons just beneath the floor of the fourth ventricle. Fibers from the facial nucleus (CN VII) run dorsomedially toward the floor of the fourth ventricle, making an acute bend around the abducens nucleus. If this area is invaded by tumor, caution must be taken in manipulation of the tumor as it is debulked to avoid "floor of the fourth syndrome," which includes an ipsilateral palsy of cranial nerves VI and VII and a contralateral hemiparesis. Even gentle diathermy with low-current bipolar can produce a partial paralysis with total or near-total recovery. Likewise, entering the floor of the fourth ventricle through the midline should be avoided, because the medial longitudinal fasciculus courses just under the ependymal, and disruption of these fibers will lead to a permanent, and potentially bilateral, intranuclear ophthalmoplegia. By staying at least 4 mm off midline, this complication can be avoided.

In most cases, patients with temporary facial weakness should be treated with artificial tears to prevent corneal desiccation. Temporary tarsorrhaphy or gold-weight implantation in the upper eyelid may be a more permanent solution. Permanent weakness has been treated with facial-hypoglossal anastomosis, which can partially restore upper eyelid function. Abducens palsy is best treated with an eye patch to prevent diplopia (or amblyopia if the patient is under 5 years of age); if the condition persists beyond 6 months, eye muscle surgery may be appropriate (Fig. 28.3).

Low Cranial Nerve Palsy

Cranial nerve XII palsy can occur from injury to the hypoglossal trigone. In instances such as the dorsally exophytic brainstem tumors or the cerebello-pontine angle ependymomas, in which the tumor invades the inferior floor of the fourth ventricle or involves the lower cranial nerves, children are at risk for aspiration pneumonitis in the acute postoperative period. Although less common than facial palsy, this is a very serious complication. Patients present with dysarthria, swallowing apraxia, central rhonchi, and continuous drooling. In these instances, it has been our practice to keep the children intubated and sedated overnight after surgery. On the day after surgery, if the child is wide awake, the ENT team is present in the intensive care unit and inspects the vocal cords and pharyngeal motility by fiber-optic endoscopy at the time of extubation. Children with an abnormal examination are maintained on nasogastric feeds and receive nothing by mouth until a formal swallowing study can be performed. When an abnormal examination is combined with cranial nerve VII or IX/X deficits, even aggressive treatment with tracheostomy and feeding tubes may not prevent serious complications due to aspiration. For those with vocal cord paralysis or insensate pharynges, we have been quick to recommend tracheostomy and gastrostomy. This routine has prevented all but one death in affected children (Fig. 28.4).

Skewed Ocular Deviation

Skewed ocular deviation is a rare condition that is sometimes seen after fourth ventricular surgery during which the aqueductal opening is manipulated. This usually occurs with damage to the region of the cerebral aqueduct. It is thought to occur because vertical yoking of eye movements involves pathways that pass through the periaqueductal gray matter in the mesencephalic tegmentum. This condition usually resolves within weeks after surgery and can be avoided by gentleness when working around the aqueduct (Fig. 28.5).

Posterior Fossa Syndrome

The most common postoperative complication is the posterior fossa syndrome, also referred to as cerebellar mutism or pseudobulbar palsy. One of the earlier reports of posterior fossa syndrome was by Wisoff and Epstein.[27] It is characterized by the delayed onset of mutism, emotional lability, and supranuclear lesions that occur 12 to 72 hours after resection of a posterior fossa tumor. In a prospective Children's Cancer Group questionnaire-based study, approximately 22% of patients developed posterior fossa syndrome postoperatively; however, these cases were rated as moderate to severe, suggesting that the incidence of milder cases may be much

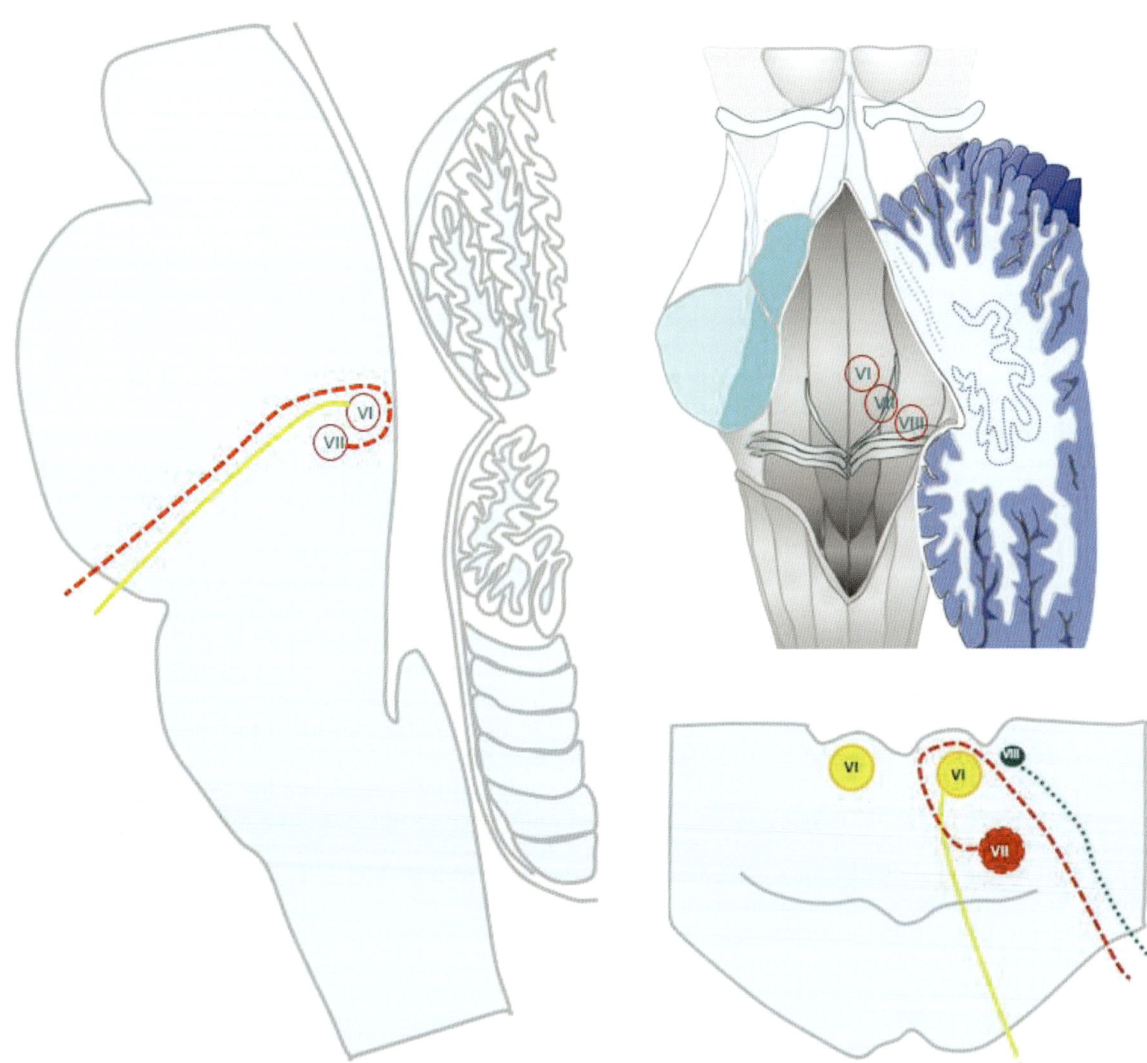

• **Fig. 28.3** The nucleus of the abducens nerve (CN VI) is located in the dorsomedial pons just beneath the floor of the fourth ventricle. Fibers from the facial nucleus (CN VII) run dorsomedially toward the floor of the fourth ventricle, making an acute bend around the abducens nucleus. If this area is invaded by tumor, caution must be taken in manipulation of the tumor as it is debulked to avoid "floor of the fourth syndrome," which includes an ipsilateral palsy of cranial nerves VI and VII and a contralateral hemiparesis.

higher.[28] The syndrome has been seen in intraventricular approaches to lesions near the brainstem, but it has also been described after a supracerebellar infratentorial approach to the pineal region and a retromastoid lateral cerebellar approach to the side or front of the brainstem.

Posterior fossa syndrome is characterized by a triad of (1) decreased production of speech or mutism, (2) cerebellar dysfunction including ataxia and axial hypotonia, and (3) neurobehavioral affective symptoms such as emotional lability, irritability, and apathy.[29] Patients who initially awaken from surgery speaking and moving well appear to present with global confusion, disorientation, combativeness, paranoia, or visual hallucinations. They are generally alert and will follow simple commands, but will sometimes refuse to speak or will present scanning speech. Oro-facial apraxia, drooling, dysphagia, pharyngeal dysfunction, and flat affect are common, but there is no actual weakness; hence the term pseudobulbar palsy. Fecal and urinary incontinence have been observed in up to 60% of patients.[30]

The cause of the syndrome is poorly understood. Because of the delay in onset, it had been suggested that edema from operative manipulation might play a role. However, there is evidence that perturbations in the proximal dentothalamocortical pathway as a result of the midline tumor and/or surgical resection are causative.[31]

Some studies have attempted to correlate tumor size with the development of posterior fossa syndrome; however, results of these studies have been inconclusive. Surgical approaches that avoid splitting the cerebellar vermis do not seem to prevent development of the posterior fossa syndrome.[30] There is also recent evidence of presurgical language impairment as a primary risk factor for development of the posterior fossa syndrome; children without a presurgical language deficit did not develop mutism, suggesting that the technical aspects of surgery are unlikely to be causative.[32]

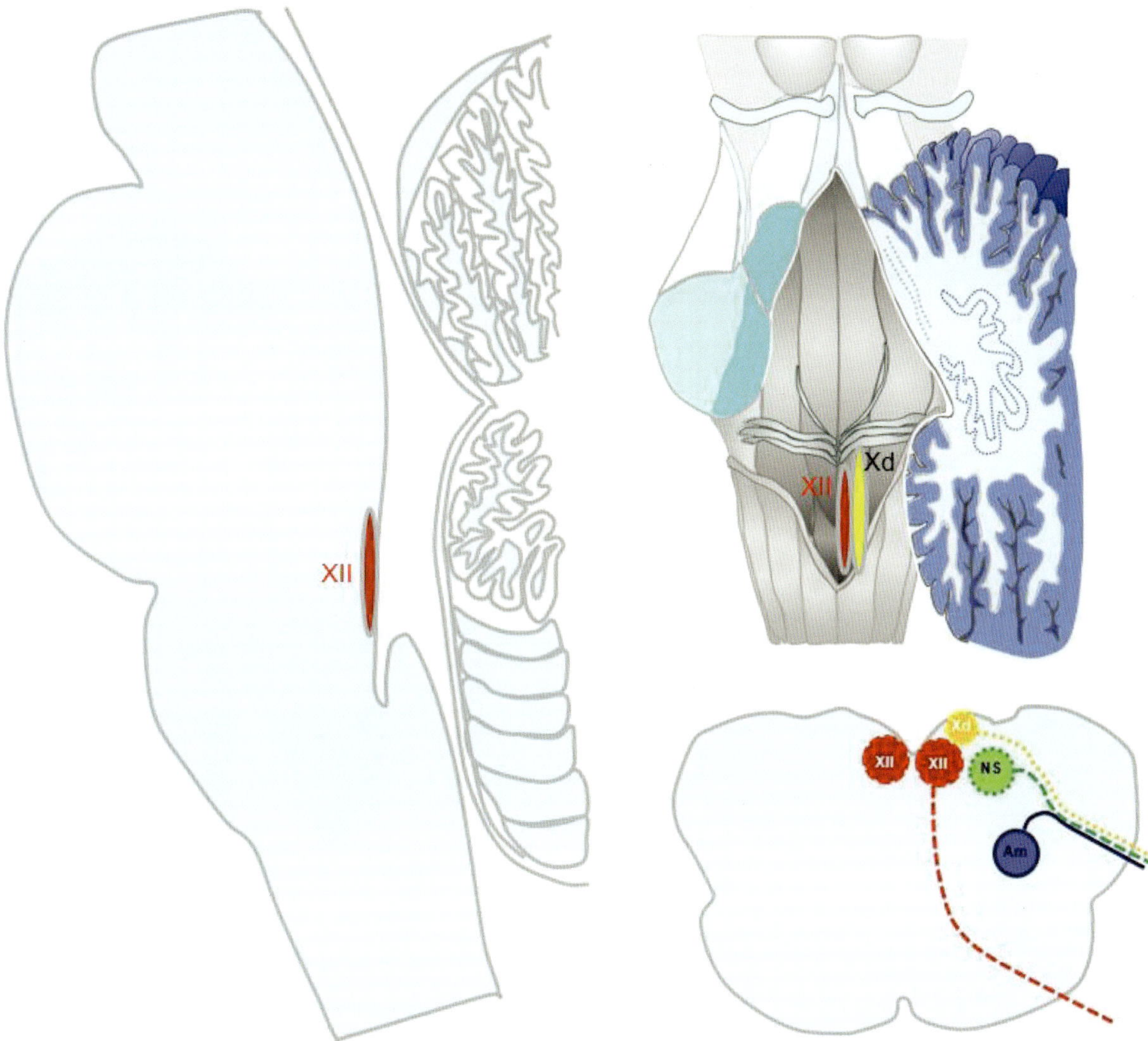

• **Fig. 28.4** The prominent hypoglossal nucleus lies near the midline in the dorsal medullary gray matter. It is approximately 2 cm long. Its rostral part lies beneath the hypoglossal trigone in the floor of the fourth ventricle. The vagal nucleus (also known as the dorsal motor nucleus of the vagus) lies dorsolateral to the hypoglossal nucleus. The nucleus solitarius lies ventrolateral to the vagal nucleus.

The outcome of posterior fossa syndrome is variable. Typically, the child recovers from mutism at a mean of 8.3 weeks; however, a residual ataxic dysarthria is common. Indeed, speech impairments were present in 95% of patients with moderate or severe mutism 1 year postoperatively.[33] Earlier authors felt that the syndrome always resolved within 6 months or a year of surgery. More recent studies have demonstrated that all of these children have long-term cognitive impairments and emotional problems.[34] Neuropsychiatric deficits in patients with posterior fossa syndrome, such as deficits in receptive language, memory, cognitive function, and executive function, suggest that multidisciplinary rehabilitation is required in these patients.[30] There are no available modalities for either the treatment or prevention of posterior fossa syndrome. An intensive multidisciplinary rehabilitation program involving neurologists, physiatrists, and oncologists as well as speech, occupational, and physical therapists is required to manage the global neurologic dysfunction observed in these patients.

Seizure

Generalized and focal seizures have been reported in 5.9% of pediatric patients after posterior fossa surgery. The incidence is higher in faster-growing tumors and in the presence of ventricular drainage or shunting and venous air embolism. Late-onset seizures may be related to remote hemorrhage, meningitis, or hydrocephalus.[35] Children less than 3 years of age appear to be at increased risk, with the seizure commonly being secondary to postoperative hyponatremia.

Dyspraxia

Ipsilateral limb ataxia, dysmetria, dysdiadokinesis, and hypotonia usually result from damage to the cerebellar hemisphere, especially the dentate nucleus, which is located along the superolateral margin of the roof of the fourth ventricle adjacent to the upper pole

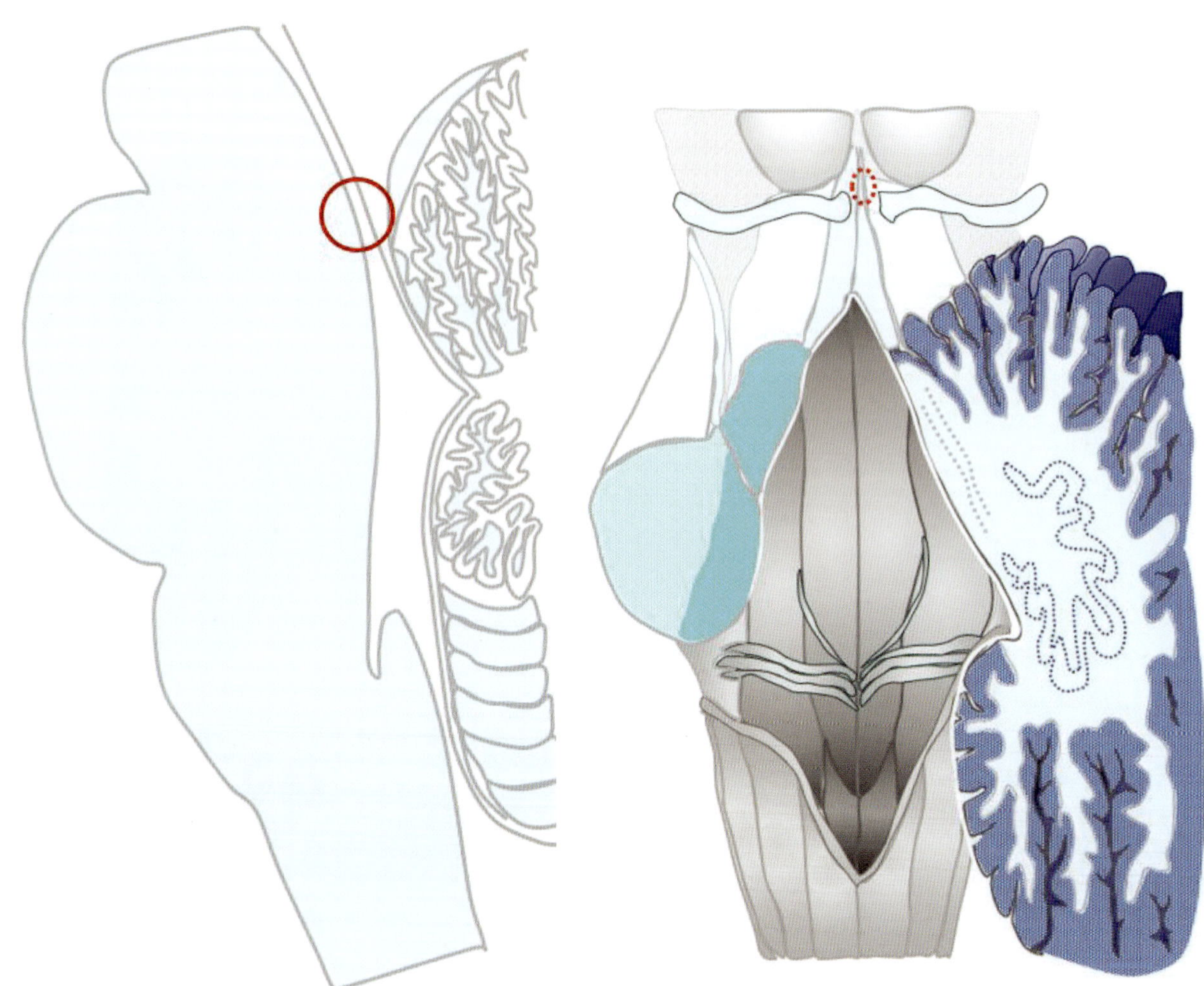

• **Fig. 28.5** Cerebral aqueduct. The canal passes through the periaqueductal gray matter in the mesencephalic tegmentum. Notice that the cerebral aqueduct is located immediately ventral to the corpora quadrigemina in the midbrain tectum and is surrounded by the central gray matter. The midbrain region ventral to the aqueduct is the tegmentum, which contains important structures such as the red nucleus and reticular formation nuclei.

of the tonsil. Most injuries to the dentate nucleus occur during dissection of a hemispheric tumor. Retraction during dissection of the superior vermis can injure the superior cerebellar peduncle, producing similar symptoms. Most patients recover well within a few months with only a minor residual intention tremor that does not interfere with activities of daily living (Fig. 28.6).

Complications of Adjuvant Therapy

Radiation Therapy

Craniospinal radiation (CSI) is an essential adjuvant treatment for medulloblastomas due to this tumor's potential for leptomeningeal spread. The standard postoperative CSI regimen is 36 Gy to the entire neuraxis, with a boost to the posterior fossa to a total dose of 54 Gy.[36] However, CSI can be associated with long-term central nervous system toxicities. Acute postradiation effects consist of drowsiness, nausea, and headaches. Late changes include cognitive impairment, growth abnormalities, hypopituitarism, severe sensorineural hearing loss, moyamoya syndrome, and secondary neoplasms (gliomas, meningiomas).[37] A risk-adapted therapeutic strategy has been employed due to adverse sequelae of full-dose radiation seen in the last 20 years. High-risk patients typically receive the standard-dose CSI plus adjuvant chemotherapy. The average-risk patients receive reduced-dose CSI (23.4 Gy) in combination with adjuvant chemotherapy.[38]

Another method being investigated for maximizing target radiation dose and reducing toxicity to adjacent normal brain is the use of conformal boost radiotherapy limited to the tumor bed alone.[39] Another newer choice is proton radiation therapy (PRT). It is increasingly being used for patients with medulloblastoma in an effort to reduce treatment-related sequelae by delivering equivalent tumor control while reducing the late effects of radiation.[40] The best treatment option for ependymoma is surgical resection followed by focal radiotherapy to the tumor bed, although there are no randomized prospective studies available yet. CSI is employed only for patients with metastatic disease at presentation. The volume of focal irradiation is currently one of the primary

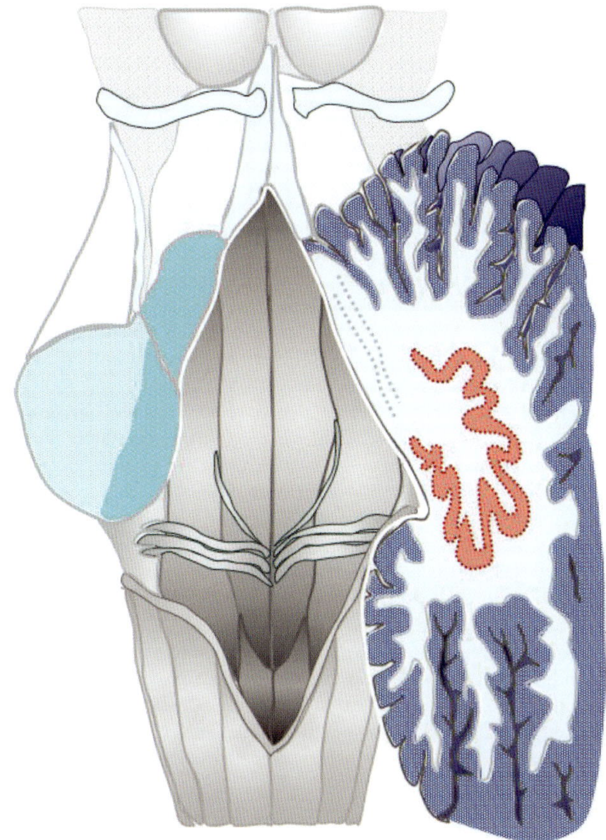

• **Fig. 28.6** The dentate nucleus is a cluster of neurons located within the deep white matter of each cerebellar hemisphere. The dorsal region of the dentate nucleus is involved in motor function.

SURGICAL REWIND

My Worst Cases

Case 1

An 11-year-old girl went to clinic with chief complaint of vomiting once or twice per week for two months. Neurological examination revealed significant dysmetria and clumsy tandem gait. Brain magnetic resonance imaging (MRI) revealed a globular mass lesion measuring 4.3 cm × 4.4 cm × 3.8 cm in diameter in the fourth ventricle with obstructive hydrocephalus. Sub-occipital craniotomy for near-total excision of the tumor was performed. During the surgery, the tumor was noted to invade the floor of the 4th ventricle just above the obex. Despite leaving a carpet of tumor along the floor of the 4th ventricle, there was continued bleeding from tumor vessels arising from the floor of the 4th ventricle and efforts to achieve hemostasis included bipolaring vessels on the floor of the 4th ventricle. After the surgery, pathology report confirmed the diagnosis of medulloblastoma. However, bursts of vomiting about 10 times per day developed after the surgery. Postoperative swallowing impairment was also noted. These caused to episoides of aspiration pneumonia. Finally, tracheostomy and gastrostomy were done for serious complications due to aspiration.

Case 2

A previously healthy 3-year-old girl presented with frequent falling and occasional headache. Neurological examination revealed mild truncal ataxia without focal neurological deficit. Brain MRI showed a very large heterogeneously enhancing posterior fossa tumor centered in the fourth ventricle with no evidence of spinal metastasis. Sub-occipital craniotomy for near-total excision of the tumor was performed. For surgical exposure, the lower two-thirds of the vermis was split in the midline. Pathology confirmed classic medulloblastoma M0. Postoperatively, the patient was awaked and followed commands. The next days, she is noted to be irritable, mutism and unable to talk or sit up. Postoperative MR imaging showed no evidence of residual tumor. Her mutism symptoms improved significantly by 1 month, with continuing speech therapy and occupational therapy. At her 2-month follow-up, she demonstrated persistent mild dysarthria, ataxia, and left-sided dysmetria. At last follow-up, 45 months after tumor resection, she continues to have mild dysarthria, dysmetria, hypotonia, and wide-based gait with poor school performance.

clinical questions and is modified by newer focal irradiation techniques and the choice of PRT.[41]

Chemotherapy

Different chemotherapy regimens have been developed for high-risk medulloblastoma patients as well as average-risk patients. Current investigations attempt to determine the optimal timing and dosage of adjuvant therapies to maximize efficacy and minimize toxicity. These modalities are also modified according to the molecular subtype of the medulloblastoma. Chemotherapy has been associated with a variety of adverse events such as fatigue, nausea, vomiting, loss of appetite, stomatitis, myelosuppression, and infection. Some studies have found greater hematologic toxicity when chemotherapy was combined with radiation therapy compared with radiotherapy alone.[42] Less common side effects include nephrotoxicity, hepatotoxicity, cardiomyopathy, urinary bladder, sensorineural hearing loss, acute myelogenous leukemia, or pulmonary fibrosis, depending on the agent used.

The strategy of high-dose myeloablative chemotherapy followed by hematopoietic stem cell rescue has been tried as an option for recurrent disease, high-risk patients, those with disseminated disease, or children less than 36 months of age, in which we try to avoid radiotherapy.[43] However, higher transplant-related toxicity and 5% to 10% mortality due to the toxic effects of high-dose chemotherapy have been reported in multiple studies. Better patient selection (complete remission before transplantation, total resection ...) can reduce the transplant-related mortality.[44,45]

Conclusion

Surgery is the mainstay of treatment for the child with a posterior fossa tumor. For those with a pilocystic astrocytoma, surgery alone can guarantee a cure and the chance to lead a normal life. For posterior fossa ependymoma, complete resection promises the best chance for extended survival in children. Even for those with medulloblastoma, major advances in therapy have occurred over the last decade such that 5-year progression-free survival has improved from 35% to 80%. The neurosurgeon has a significant role to play in the management of posterior fossa tumors in children.

However, posterior fossa tumor surgery does involve greater morbidity and mortality and has a wider variety of complications than surgery in the supratentorial compartments. These complications may be avoided with careful perioperative planning and a full understanding of the patient's history, neurologic findings, and imaging studies; meticulous microsurgical dissection and complete knowledge of neuroanatomy are also necessary. Therefore each hospital should know its own incidence of complications; in that way, each institution can provide specific strategies to minimize their occurrence.

References

1. Legler JM, Ries LA, Smith MA, et al. Cancer surveillance series: brain and other central nervous system cancers: recent trends in incidence and mortality. *J Natl Cancer Inst.* 1999;91:1382–1390.
2. Schoenberg BS, Schoenberg DG, Christine BW, Gomez MR. The epidemiology of primary intracranial neoplasms of childhood. A population study. *Mayo Clin Proc.* 1976;51:51–56.
3. Sawaya R, Hammoud M, Schoppa D. Neurosurgical outcomes in a modern series of 400 craniotomies for treatment of parenchymal tumors. *Neurosurgery.* 1998;42(5):1044–1055.
4. Edgeworth J, Bullock P, Bailey A, Gallagher A, Crouchman M. Why are brain tumours still being missed? *Arch Dis Child.* 1996;74:148–151.
5. Saha V, Love S, Eden T, Micallef-Eynaud P, MacKinlay G. Determinants of symptom interval in childhood cancer. *Arch Dis Child.* 1993;68(6):771–774.
6. Dobrovoljac M, Hengartner H, Boltshauser E, Grotzer MA. Delay in the diagnosis of paediatric brain tumours. *Eur J Pediatr.* 2002;161(12):663–667.
7. The Childhood Brain Tumor Consortium. The epidemiology of headache among children with brain tumor. *J Neurooncol.* 1991;10:31–46.
8. Rath GP, Bithal PK, Chaturvedi A, Dash HH. Complications related to positioning in posterior fossa craniectomy. *J Clin Neurosci.* 2007;14(6):520–525.
9. Steinbok P, Boyd M, Cochrane D. Cervical spine deformity following craniotomy and upper cervical laminectomy for posterior fossa tumors in children. *Childs Nerv Syst.* 1989;5:25–28.
10. Harper CM, Nelson KR. Intraoperative electrophysiological monitoring in children. *J Clin Neurophysiol.* 1992;9:342–356.
11. Sala F, Krzan MJ, Deletis V. Intraoperative neurophysiological monitoring in pediatric neurosurgery: why, when, how? *Childs Nerv Syst.* 2002;18:264–287.
12. Albright AL, Wisoff JH, Zeltzer PM, Boyett JM, Rorke LB, Stanley P. Effects of medulloblastoma resections on outcome in children: a report from the Children's Cancer Group. *Neurosurgery.* 1996;38:265–271.
13. Zeltzer PM, Boyett JM, Finlay JL, et al. Metastasis stage, adjuvant treatment, and residual tumor are prognostic factors for medulloblastoma in children: conclusions from the Children's Cancer Group 921 randomized phase III study. *J Clin Oncol.* 1999;17:832–845.
14. Merchant TE, Mulhern RK, Krasin MJ, et al. Preliminary results from a phase II trial of conformal radiation therapy and evaluation of radiation-related CNS effects for pediatric patients with localized ependymoma. *J Clin Oncol.* 2004;22:3156–3162.
15. Desai KI, Nadkarni TD, Muzumdar DP, Goel A. Prognostic factors for cerebellar astrocytomas in children: a study of 102 cases. *Pediatr Neurosurg.* 2001;35:311–317.
16. Thompson EM, Hielscher T, Bouffet E, et al. Prognostic value of medulloblastoma extent of resection after accounting for molecular subgroup: a retrospective integrated clinical and molecular analysis. *Lancet Oncol.* 2016;17(4):484–495.
17. Sainte-Rose C, Cinalli G, Roux FE, et al. Management of hydrocephalus in pediatric patients with posterior fossa tumors: the role of endoscopic third ventriculostomy. *J Neurosurg.* 2001;95:791–797.
18. Riva-Cambrin J1, Detsky AS, Lamberti-Pasculli M. Predicting postresection hydrocephalus in pediatric patients with posterior fossa tumors. *J Neurosurg Pediatr.* 2009;3(5):378–385.
19. Lee M, Wisoff JH, Abbott R, Freed D, Epstein FJ. Management of hydrocephalus in children with medulloblastoma: prognostic factors for shunting. *Pediatr Neurosurg.* 1994;20:240–247.
20. Morelli D, Pirotte B, Lubansu A, et al. Persistent hydrocephalus after early surgical management of posterior fossa tumors in children: is routine preoperative endoscopic third ventriculostomy justified? *J Neurosurg.* 2005;103(suppl):247–252.
21. Berger MS, Baumeister B, Geyer JR, Milstein J, Kanev PM, LeRoux PD. The risks of metastases from shunting in children with primary central nervous system tumors. *J Neurosurg.* 1991;74:872–877.
22. Steinbok P, Singhal A, Mills J, Cochrane DD, Price AV. Cerebrospinal fluid (CSF) leak and pseudomeningocele formation after posterior fossa tumor resection in children: a retrospective analysis. *Childs Nerv Syst.* 2007;23(2):171–174, discussion 175.
23. Parizek J, Sercl M, Michl A, et al. Posterior fossa duraplasty in children: remarks on surgery and clinical and CT follow-up. *Childs Nerv Syst.* 1994;10:444–449.
24. Fishman AJ, Marrinan MS, Golfinos JG, et al. Prevention and management of cerebrospinal fluid leak following vestibular schwannoma surgery. *Laryngoscope.* 2004;114:501–505.
25. Steinbok P, Singhal A, Mills J, Cochrane DD, Price AV. Cerebrospinal fluid (CSF) leak and pseudomeningocele formation after posterior fossa tumor resection in children: a retrospective analysis. *Childs Nerv Syst.* 2007;23(2):171–174, discussion 175.
26. Carmel PW1, Greif LK. The aseptic meningitis syndrome: a complication of posterior fossa surgery. *Pediatr Neurosurg.* 1993;19(5):276–280.
27. Wisoff JH, Epstein FJ. Pseudobulbar palsy after posterior fossa operation in children. *Neurosurgery.* 1984;15:707–709.
28. Robertson PL, Muraszko KM, Holmes EJ, et al. Children's Oncology Group. Incidence and severity of postoperative cerebellar mutism syndrome in children with medulloblastoma: a prospective study by the Children's Oncology Group. *J Neurosurg.* 2006;105(suppl):444–451.
29. Siffert J, Poussaint TY, Goumnerova LC, et al. Neurological dysfunction associated with postoperative cerebellar mutism. *J Neurooncol.* 2000;48:75–81.
30. Pollack IF, Polinko P, Albright AL, Towbin R, Fitz C. Mutism and pseudobulbar symptoms after resection of posterior fossa tumors in children: incidence and pathophysiology. *Neurosurgery.* 1995;37:885–893.
31. Morris EB, Phillips NS, Laningham FH, et al. Proximal dentatothalamocortical tract involvement in posterior fossa syndrome. *Brain.* 2009;132:3087–3095.
32. Di Rocco C, Chieffo D, Frassanito P, Caldarelli M, Massimi L, Tamburrini G. Heralding cerebellar mutism: evidence for pre-surgical language impairment as primary risk factor in posterior fossa surgery. *Cerebellum.* 2011;10:551–562.
33. Robertson PL, Muraszko KM, Holmes EJ, et al. Children's Oncology Group. Incidence and severity of postoperative cerebellar mutism syndrome in children with medulloblastoma: a prospective study by the Children's Oncology Group. *J Neurosurg.* 2006;105(suppl):444–451.
34. Steinbok P, Cochrane DD, Perrin R, Price A. Mutism after posterior fossa tumour resection in children: incomplete recovery on long-term follow-up. *Pediatr Neurosurg.* 2003;39:179–183.
35. Suri A, Mahapatra AK, Bithal P. Seizures following posterior fossa surgery. *Br J Neurosurg.* 1998;12(1):41–44.
36. Bloom HJ, Wallace EN, Henk JM. The treatment and prognosis of medulloblastoma in children. A study of 82 verified cases. *Am J Roentgenol Radium Ther Nucl Med.* 1969;105:43–62.
37. Jenkin D. The radiation treatment of medulloblastoma. *J Neurooncol.* 1996;29:45–54.
38. Packer RJ, Goldwein J, Nicholson HS, et al. Treatment of children with medulloblastomas with reduced-dose craniospinal radiation therapy and adjuvant chemotherapy: a Children's Cancer Group Study. *J Clin Oncol.* 1999;17:2127–2136.
39. Douglas JG, Barker JL, Ellenbogen RG, et al. Concurrent chemotherapy and reduced-dose cranial spinal irradiation followed by conformal posterior fossa tumor bed boost for average-risk medulloblastoma: efficacy and patterns of failure. *Int J Radiat Oncol Biol Phys.* 2004;58:1161–1164.
40. Eaton BR, Esiashvili N, Kim S. Clinical outcomes among children with standard-risk medulloblastoma treated with proton and photon radiation therapy: a comparison of disease control and overall survival. *Int J Radiat Oncol Biol Phys.* 2016;94(1):133–138.

41. Merchant TE, Fouladi M. Ependymoma: new therapeutic approaches including radiation and chemotherapy. *J Neurooncol.* 2005;75:287–299.
42. Kortmann RD, Kuhl J, Timmermann B, et al. Postoperative neoadjuvant chemotherapy before radiotherapy as compared to immediate radiotherapy followed by maintenance chemotherapy in the treatment of medulloblastoma in childhood: results of the German prospective randomized trial HIT '91. *Int J Radiat Oncol Biol Phys.* 2000;46:269–279.
43. Gajjar A, Chintagumpala M, Ashley D, et al. Risk-adapted craniospinal radiotherapy followed by high-dose chemotherapy and stem-cell rescue in children with newly diagnosed medulloblastoma (St Jude Medulloblastoma-96): long-term results from a prospective, multicentre trial. *Lancet Oncol.* 2006;7:813–820.
44. Graham ML, Herndon JE II, Casey JR, et al. High-dose chemotherapy with autologous stem-cell rescue in patients with recurrent and high risk pediatric brain tumors. *J Clin Oncol.* 1997;15:1814–1823.
45. Pérez-Martínez A, Lassaletta A, González-Vicent M. High-dose chemotherapy with autologous stem cell rescue for children with high risk and recurrent medulloblastoma and supratentorial primitive neuroectodermal tumors. *J Neurooncol.* 2005;71(1):33–38.

29

Craniopharyngioma: Complications After Microsurgery

WILLIAM B. LO, JAMES T. RUTKA

HIGHLIGHTS

- Endocrinologic abnormality, visual deficit, cranial nerve palsy, obesity, and neuropsychological disturbances are the most common surgical complications in transcranial microsurgery for craniopharyngioma.
- Careful study of preoperative imaging is essential for deciding the most appropriate microsurgical approach, assessing hypothalamic involvement, and anticipating the relationship between the tumor and surrounding neurovascular structures.
- The tumor capsule and the Liliequist's membrane provide safe tissue planes for dissection.
- Similar medium-term outcome between gross total resection versus subtotal resection with adjuvant radiotherapy means that patients' functional outcome should not be compromised to achieve complete section.

Background

Craniopharyngioma is an uncommon tumor arising from the embryonic squamous cells of the craniopharyngeal duct (Rathke's pouch) at the suprasellar region. It is benign but locally aggressive. Management of this entity is challenging and requires a multidisciplinary approach. Surgical resection remains the mainstay of treatment. However, it carries significant risks due to the deep-seated midline location and the proximity to important neurovascular structures.[1,2] There has been an increased use of the extended endoscopic endonasal approach in the last two decades.[3–6] However, transcranial microsurgery continues to be an important approach for large tumors with lateral extension, vascular encasement, and significant peripheral calcification and in children less than 3 years of age whose sphenoid sinus is conchal and not fully pneumatized and the basicranium is small. The transcranial approaches are broadly divided into midline anterior (interhemispheric, unilateral subfrontal/bifrontal) and frontolateral (pterional-frontotemporal and modified orbitozygomatic), lateral (combined petrosal and subtemporal), and transcallosal or transventricular intraventricular approaches.[1,2,7–9] Posterior approaches for retrochiasmatic tumor have been described, and stereotactic aspiration and decompression surgery with Ommaya reservoir are routinely used for cystic tumors, but these will not be discussed in further detail. All transcranial approaches carry the risks of brain retraction, vascular injury, pituitary stalk disturbance, optic nerve (ON) manipulation for tumor exposure, and difficulty of accessing the infrachiasmatic portion, superior pole, and posterior fossa extension of the tumor.[5] In large series, the proportion of patients experiencing at least one complication ranges between 53% and 79.4%.[5–7] The main intra- and postoperative complications include: endocrinologic, electrolyte, ophthalmologic, neurologic, vascular, metabolic, infective, hydrocephalus, long-term cognitive impairment, and nonneurosurgical complications. Historically, complete excision was advocated because it offered the best outcome.[2,10] However, the 10-year outcome is not different between gross total resection versus subtotal resection followed by adjuvant radiotherapy.[9] Therefore, microsurgery with the aim of debulking and sparing important anatomic structures, thereby reducing morbidities, is a safe and efficacious treatment option.

Anatomic Insights

Arterial

The suprasellar arterial relationships are complex because this region contains all the parts of the circle of Willis (Fig. 29.1A).[11] The anterior part of the craniopharyngioma is usually supplied by perforators from the anterior communicating artery (AComA) and the proximal anterior cerebral artery (ACA), the lateral part from the posterior communicating artery (PComA), and the intrasellar part from intracavernous meningohypophyseal arteries. It is not usually supplied by the posterior cerebral (PCA) and basilar arteries (BA).[12]

1. *Internal carotid artery*: The ICA courses inferior, then lateral to the ON and chiasm, sending perforating branches to the ON, chiasm, tract, and the floor of the third ventricle. These branches can be obstacles to the surgical approach through the triangle formed by the ICA, ACA, and the ON. The ICA also gives rise to the superior hypophyseal artery, which courses medially toward the tuber cinereum to form a ring around the infundibulum with its opposite mate (Fig. 29.1A).
4. *Posterior communicating artery*: The PComA branches penetrate the floor between the optic chiasm and the cerebral peduncle to supply the thalamus, hypothalamus, subthalamus, and internal capsule.
6. *Anterior cerebral artery*: The origin and the course of the ACA are highly variable.[13] Normally, it arises from the ICA inferior to the anterior perforated substances (APS) and courses anteromedially superior to the ON and chiasm toward the interhemispheric fissure, where it joins the opposite ACA via the AComA.

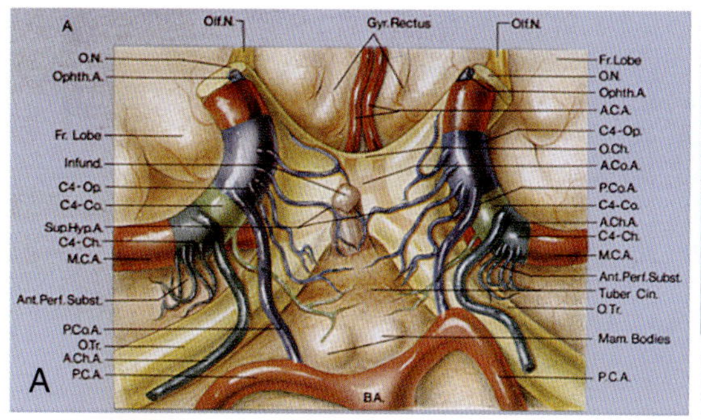

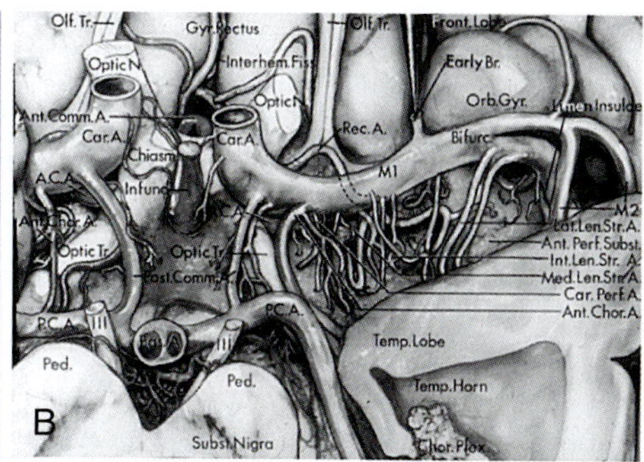

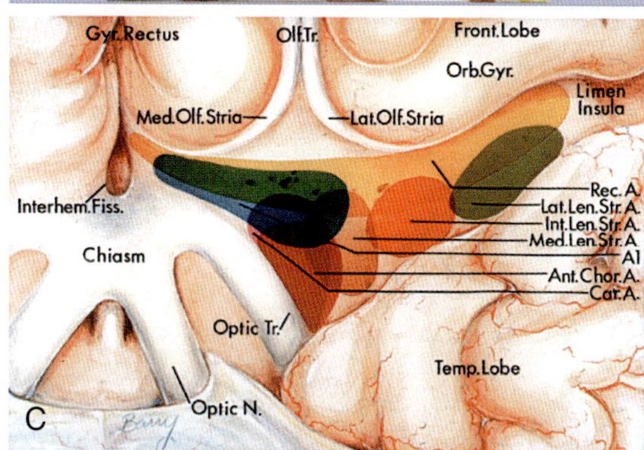

• **Fig. 29.1** (A) The circle of Willis and perforating branches of the internal carotid artery (ICA), inferior view. The circle of Willis is formed by the bilateral C4 segments of the internal carotid arteries and the anterior cerebral arteries (A.C.A.), joined by the anterior communicating artery (A.Co.A.) and the posterior communicating arteries (P.Co.A.), which connect to the posterior cerebral arteries (P.C.A.), themselves branches of the basilar artery (B.A.). The ICA perforating branches relevant to craniopharyngioma surgery include the superior hypophyseal arteries (Sup.Hyp.A.), which arise from the ophthalmic segment and extend to the infundibulum of the pituitary gland. The perforating branches of the communicating segment of ICAs reach the optic tracts, floor of the third ventricle, and the area around the mammillary bodies (Mam.Bodies). The perforating branches arising from the choroidal segment pass superiorly and enter the anterior perforated substance (Ant.Perf.Subst.). (B) Arteries entering the left anterior perforated substance (APS), inferior view. The anterior perforating substance extends anteriorly to the medial and lateral olfactory straie, posteriorly to the optic tract and temporal lobe, laterally to the limen insulae, and medially to the interhemispheric fissure, superior to the optic chiasm. The internal carotid (Car.A.), anterior choroidal (Ant.Chor.A.), and anterior and middle cerebral arteries (M1 and M2) give rise to the branches to the APS. ICA and AChA branches enter the posterior half of the central portion; the MCA branches, also called the lenticulostriate arteries, enter the middle and posterior part of the lateral half; the A1 branches enter the medial half related to the optic apparatus; and the recurrent artery (Rec.A.) sends branches into the anterior two-thirds across the mediolateral extent. (C) Site of entry of branches of the ICA, AChA, ACA, and MCAs into the left APS, by colors. The anatomic territories are as described in B. Blue: territory of branches arising from A1 segment of ACA; Purple: ICA (Car.A.); Red: AChA (Ant. Chor.A.); Brown, orange, green: medial (Med.), intermediate (Int.), and lateral (Lat.) lenticulostriate arteries (Len.Str.A.) arising from MCA; Yellow: recurrent artery (Rec.A.). As seen on the B and C, there are minimal anastomoses and overlap between these groups of arteries, and thus their preservation during surgery is important. (A, Reproduced with permission from Gibo H, Lenkey C, Rhoton AL. Microsurgical anatomy of the supraclinoid portion of the internal carotid artery. *J Neurosurg.* 1981. 55[4]:560–574.[11] B and C, Reproduced with permission from Rhoton AL. The supratentorial arteries. *Neurosurgery.* 2002;51 [suppl 4]:53–120.[14])

The AComA is usually related to the chiasm. Displacement of the chiasm against the anterior ACAs can lead to visual impairment before that caused by direct compression by the tumor. The perforating branches from the ACA and AComA supply the anterior wall of the third ventricle, hypothalamus, fornix, septum pellucidum, and striatum. The recurrent branch enters the APS.

7. *Middle cerebral artery*: The MCA originates at the medial end of the sylvian fissure, lateral to the optic chiasm.[14] It courses 1 cm posterior and parallel to the sphenoid ridge, sending the lenticulostriate arteries to the APS.
8. *Anterior perforating arteries*: Of all the arterial systems at risk, the anterior perforating arteries are perhaps the most feared if interrupted during craniopharyngioma surgery. These arteries are the group that enters the brain through the APS (Fig. 29.1A–C), arising from the ICA, anterior choroidal artery, ACA, and MCA.[14] There are minimal anastomoses and overlap between these groups of arteries, and thus their preservation during surgery is important.
9. *Basilar artery*: The BA bifurcates to form the two PCAs. Proximally, they send thalamoperforating arteries to supply the posterior part of the third ventricular floor and the lateral walls.

Venous

The veins in the suprasellar region drain mainly to the bilateral basal veins. They are generally small and do not usually present as obstacles to operative approaches to the suprasellar region and the lower part of the third ventricle. The internal cerebral vein originates at the foramen of Monro and courses in the velum interpositum, which forms the roof of the third ventricle.

Because the anatomy is highly variable between individuals, and because it can be distorted by the expansile craniopharyngioma, the vascular relationships should be studied carefully from cross-sectional imaging.

Third Ventricle and Hypothalamus

The inferior lateral walls and the floor of the third ventricle are formed by the hypothalamus. Thus, manipulation of the walls can cause hypothalamic dysfunction, including altered consciousness, metabolic disturbance, temperature control, and hypophyseal secretion. Injury to the columns of the fornix in the walls can lead to memory impairment.[15] The roof is formed by four layers: one neural layer formed by the fornix and two membraneous layers of tela choroidea, which contains the layer velum interpositum, where the internal cerebral veins reside.

Position of Optic Chiasm to the Sella

The "normal" optic chiasm overlies the diaphragma sellae and pituitary gland (70%), the prefixed chiasm overlies the tuberculum sellae (10%); and the postfixed chiasm overlies the dorsum sellae (10%)[13] (Fig. 29.2). Several anatomic configurations limit the exposure to the suprasellar region in the transcranial approach: (1) a prefixed chiasm, (2) a normal chiasm with a small window between the tuberculum and the chiasm, and (3) a superior protruding tuberculum sellae. There are several surgical strategies to circumvent these obstacles. A transfrontal-transsphenoidal exposure is achieved by opening through the tuberculum and planum sphenoidale. If the chiasm is prefixed and the tumor is identified through a thinned-out anterior third ventricular wall, it can be accessed by opening the lamina terminalis. An expanded space between the ICA and ON caused by a lateral or parasellar extension of tumor can also provide a surgical corridor.

A good understanding of the relationship between the ON, the ICA, and the anterior clinoid process (AC) is essential for craniopharyngioma surgery in the sellar/parasellar regions.[15] Both the ON and the ICA are medial to the ACP. The ICA exits from the cavernous sinus and courses posterolaterally, whereas the ON travels posteromedially toward the chiasm.[15]

Classifications for Tumor Locations

Craniopharyngiomas are found typically in the infundibulo-hypophyseal axis in the sella and suprasellar area, and may grow in any direction. Several systems have been described to classify their location and anatomy. Most are topographically based and aid surgeons in choosing the optimal operative approaches. Some also have predictive value in surgical outcome.[16]

The classifications are mostly based on (1) the vertical extension of the tumor or (2) its relation with normal anatomic structures including the sella turcica, optic chiasm, infundibulum, and ventricles. The main classifications are listed in Table 29.1, and Fig. 29.2 is the diagrammatic representation of Yaşargil et al.'s classification.[2] A prechiasmatic tumor extends from the sella into the subfrontal spaces. A retrochiasmatic tumor displaces the pituitary

TABLE 29.1 Summary of Anatomic and Other Classifications of Craniopharyngioma

Authors and Year	Basis of Classification	Classification
Ciric and Cozzens 1980[39]	Developmental and microsurgical relation.	• Intrapial intraventricular • Partially intrapial • Extrapial intraarachnoid • Extrapial, partially extraarachnoid (dumbbell) • Extrapial extraarachnoid intrasellar
Konovalov 1983[40]	In relation to surgical management.	• Endosuprasellar • Suprasellar-extraventricular • Intraventricular
Yaşargil et al 1990[2]	Relation with diaphragm sellae and ventricle.	a: Purely intrasellar-infradiaphragmatic b: Intra- and suprasellar, infra- and supradiaphragmatic c: Supradiaphragmatic, parachiasmatic, extraventricular d: Intra- and extraventricular e: Paraventricular in respect to the third ventricle f: Intraventricular
Hoffman 1994[17]	Relation with sella turcica and chiasm.	• Sellar • Prechiasmatic • Retrochiasmatic • Giant
Samii and Tatagiba 1997[12]	Anatomic, radiologic.	• Intrasellar • Infundibulum-tuberian • Intraventricular • Dumbbell-shaped

TABLE 29.1 Summary of Anatomic and Other Classifications of Craniopharyngioma—Cont'd

Authors and Year	Basis of Classification	Classification
Samii and Samii 2000[41]	Tumor vertical extension.	I: Intrasellar or infradiaphragmatic II: Occupying the cistern with/without an intrasellar component III: Lower half of the third ventricle IV: Upper half of the third ventricle V: Reaching the septum pellucidum or lateral ventricles
Matsuo et al 2014[42]	Relation with anatomic structures.	Relation with diaphragm: • Subdiaphragmatic with competent • Subdiaphragmatic with incompetent • Supradiaphragmatic Relation with stalk: • Preinfundibular • Transinfundibular • Retroinfundibular • Intraventricular • Not identify Relation with optic nerve: • Prechiasmatic type • Retrochiasmatic type • Other (pure intrasellar) Tumor extension: • Third ventricle • Interpeduncular cistern • Prepontine cistern • Frontal base • Cavernous sinus Sphenoid sinus: • Sellar type • Presellar type • Concha type
Pascual et al 2004[43]	Relation with third ventricle floor, only applicable to tumors involving the third ventricle area.	• Pseudointraventricular: suprasellar tumor pushing the intact third ventricle floor upward • Secondarily intraventricular craniopharyngioma: suprasellar mass breaking through the third ventricle floor and invading the third ventricle cavity • Nonstrictly intraventricular craniopharyngioma: intraventricular mass within the third ventricle cavity and floor, the latter being replaced by the tumor • Strictly intraventricular craniopharyngioma: intraventricular mass completely located within the third ventricle cavity and with the intact floor lying below its inferior surface
Wang et al 2005[44]	Level of origin and the competence of the diaphragm sellae.	• Subdiaphragmatic with competent diaphragm sellae • Subdiaphragmatic with incompetent diaphragm sellae • Supradiaphragmatic
Kassam et al 2008[45]	Relation with infundibulum, relevant to expanded endonasal approach.	I: Preinfundibular II: Transinfundibular III: Retroinfundibular (IIIa: extending into the third ventricle, IIIb: extending into the interpeduncular cistern) IV: Isolated to the third ventricle and/or optic recess
Fatemi et al 2009[46]	Anatomic extension of tumor, for comparison of endonasal and supraorbital approaches.	• Retrochiasmal • Sellar and suprasellar • Cavernous sinus invasion • Far lateral extension
Pan et al 2011[47]	Intraoperative and histologic classification of intraventricular tumor, third ventricle floor anatomy; no preoperative MRI correlation.	A: Purely intraventricular with pedicle attachment to third ventricle floor B: Intrathird ventricle tumors with wide-based attachment but a dissectible boundary C: Intrathird ventricle floor tumors with an undissectible wide, tight attachment

Continued

TABLE 29.1 Summary of Anatomic and Other Classifications of Craniopharyngioma—Cont'd

Authors and Year	Basis of Classification	Classification
Qi at al 2011[48]	Histologic findings and intraoperative tumor-membrane relationship around the pituitary stalk, leading to a proposed theory of four basic growth patterns. Aim to supplement existing classifications.	• Infradiaphragmatic • Extraarachnoidal • Intraarachnoidal (subdivided to growth within the fibrous or trabecular components of the arachnoid sleeve) • Subarachnoidal
Šteňo et al 2014[49]	Relation to sellae and third ventricle.	• Intrasellar/intrasellar and suprasellar • Suprasellar extraventricular • Intraventricular and extraventricular
Pan et al 2016[16]	Site of tumor origin and tumor development. This simplifies the earlier classification by Qi et al 2011[48] and is more practical.	I: Infrasellar/infradiaphragmatic II: Suprasellar subarachnoid extraventricular III: Suprasellar subpial ventricular
Jeswani et al 2016[7]	Based on Kassam et al 2008.[45]	Type I: Preinfundibular Type II: Transinfundibular Type III: Retroinfundibular

Adapted from Lubuulwa J, Lei T. Pathological and topographical classification of craniopharyngiomas: a literature review. *J Neurol Surg Reports.* 2016;77:e121–e127.

stalk anteriorly and the chiasm anterosuperiorly, resulting in a falsely prefixed ON. A subchiasmatic tumor displaces the chiasm superiorly and the pituitary stalk posteriorly.[12] However, because the tumor growth pattern is often complex, not every tumor fits into a group neatly, and the suggested surgical approach by the scheme does not replace the careful study of the preoperative images.

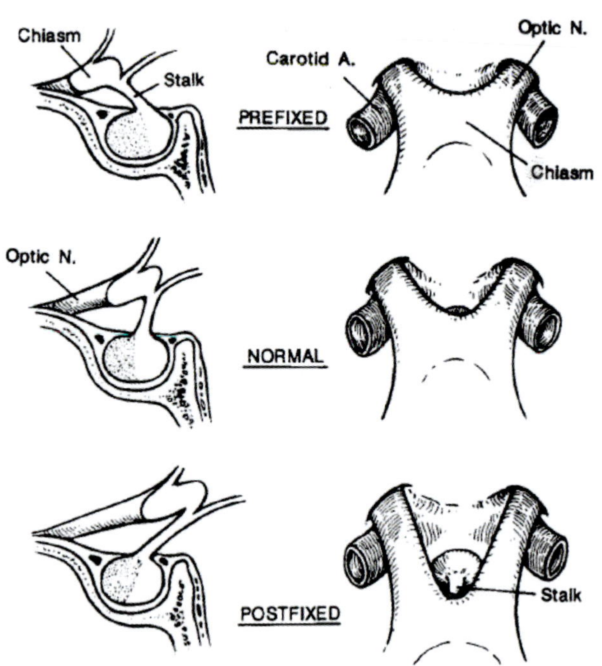

• **Fig. 29.2** Classification of the position of the chiasm in relationship to the osseous anatomy, as demonstrated by the sagittal sections and superior views of the sellar region showing the optic nerve (Optic N.), chiasm, and carotid artery (Carotid A.). The prefixed chiasm is located above the tuberculum; the normal chiasm above the diaphragm; the postfixed chiasm above the dorsum. (Reproduced with permission from Rhoton AL. Anatomy of the pituitary gland and sellar region. In: Thapar K, Kovacs K, Scheithauer B, Lloyd RV, eds. *Diagnosis and Management of Pituitary Tumors.* 1st ed. Humana Press New York; 2001: 13–40.[15])

RED FLAGS

- Prefixed chiasm
- Large tumor with lateral extension
- Tumor encasing the ICA
- Tumor adherent to the pituitary stalk
- Hypothalamic infiltration
- Recurrent tumor
- Previous radiation therapy

Prevention of Complication

Preoperative Prevention

Early surgical resection when the tumor is small reduces complication rates.[2] The MR images must be carefully studied to understand the relationship between the craniopharyngioma and the surrounding neurovascular structures. In particular, attention to the coronal magnetic resonance imaging (MRI) sequences through the hypothalamus will typically reveal the dominant side of attachment. The anatomic classifications can help in choosing the most appropriate surgical approach. A thorough endocrinologic evaluation should be undertaken.

Perioperative Prevention

Regardless of the approach, neuronavigation is particularly helpful for planning the incision, craniotomy, and route of dissection down to the tumor and for ensuring that the lateral extensions are reached and resected. In general, the tumor capsule should be kept in its continuity to define the resection plane and allow traction to the remaining tumor, maximizing the chance of total resection. The Liliequist's membrane is always intact at the primary surgery and serves as a useful barrier to the BA and brainstem.[17] If the tumor is very adherent or intimately associated with important neurovascular structures and the hypothalamus, or if the tumor capsule is intimately associated with blood vessels, e.g., at the infundibulum, it should be left in situ. Fusiform dilatation of the ICA is a well-recognized vascular sequela. This can be caused by surgical manipulation of the vessel without intraoperative vascular injury. Prevention of dissemination of tumor cystic contents reduces the risk of aseptic meningitis, hydrocephalus and, in theory, ectopic recurrence. The specific operative risks vary depending on the approaches[18]:

Midline Anterior Approaches: Subfrontal Transbasal (Uni- or Bilateral) or Frontobasal Interhemispheric Approach

This is suitable for midline prechiasmatic and suprasellar tumors with anterior third ventricular extension (Fig. 29.3A and B).[12,17,19–20] In the supine position with the head extended, the frontal lobes fall away from the anterior fossa floor. This reduces the frontal lobe retraction required. If the tumor is retrochiasmatic, the bone flap can be extended to the pterion, usually the right side. The dura is opened just superior to the supraorbital ridge. The olfactory nerves are preserved by careful dissection and gentle elevation of the frontal lobe(s). An alternative is the interhemispheric approach, which offers a higher olfactory nerve preservation rate. The chiasmatic and opticocarotid cisterns over the ONs and chiasm are sharply divided to allow drainage of cerebrospinal fluid (CSF), retraction of the frontal lobe, and full access to the chiasmatic cistern. This approach offers a clear view and control of the ONs and ICAs, ACAs, A1 branches, and both walls of the third ventricle and the interpeduncular cistern.[8] For a prechiasmatic tumor, it would be visualized between the two ONs. Aspiration of a cystic tumor can help move the chiasm away from the tuberculum to open up the surgical window. If the tumor has a large calcified area or extends into the sella or the sphenoid sinus, drilling of the tuberculum sellae can create more room for the calcified portions to be delivered. The tumor is debulked using an ultrasonic surgical aspirator and gentle aspiration for the solid and cystic components, respectively. The tumor is dissected from the ICAs and their branches (including those supplying the diencephalon) and the ONs. Once free, the tumor can be gently pulled by its capsule and extracted from the third ventricle floor. If identifiable, the gliotic layer can be used as the dissection plane between the tumor and the hypothalamus. Sometimes, due to the invasive papillary periphery of the tumor, differentiating tumor, gliotic tissue, and normal brain tissue can be challenging. If there is only unilateral hypothalamic involvement, total tumor resection leads to fewer long-term complications. If there is bilateral involvement, the risk is higher, and so a less aggressive approach should be taken. A dental mirror is useful to inspect the sella turcica and the undersurface of the optic apparatus.[1]

A retrochiasmatic tumor can be accessed through the lamina terminalis and/or between the opticocarotid triangle, although this approach is less suitable for a patient with a truly prefixed chiasm (Fig. 29.3E).[21–24] Once the lamina terminalis is opened, the tumor is debulked from a superior-inferior direction. After this, the tumor capsule is dissected carefully from the walls of the hypothalamus. Almost always the craniopharyngioma has a distinct attachment to one side of the hypothalamus. Careful study of the preoperative image prepares the neurosurgeon to tackle this attachment. As soon as the ependyma of the third ventricle is identified, micropatties are used to maintain the tumor capsule–ventricular wall plane. The capsule should be preserved initially and truncated with care to prevent it from retracting out of view. Gentle traction on the capsule can also deliver a large portion of the retrochiasmatic tumor. If the pituitary stalk is involved and the neurosurgeon decides to sacrifice it, it is preferable to section it distally, which offers a higher chance of preserving antidiuretic hormone production than a more proximal section or pulling the stalk with the tumor.[12] For a residual tumor adherent to the tuber cinereum, the lamina terminalis is opened and a patty inserted into and pushed down on the third ventricle floor, for the tumor to be accessed between the ONs.

After careful hemostasis, a meticulous closure with reconstitution of the anatomic layers is essential to prevent CSF leak and hematoma formation.[1]

Frontolateral Approaches: Pterional-Frontotemporal and Orbitozygomatic

The pterional approach is the most common approach, either on its own or in combination with a different approach (Fig. 29.3A and C).[2] It provides the shortest distance to the tumor and is suitable for intrasellar, suprasellar, prechiasmatic and, particularly, retrochiasmatic tumors and for patients with prefixed chiasms.[17] It allows access to all parts of even large tumors via dissection through the prechiasmatic, opticocarotid, carotid-oculomotor, supracarotid triangles, and the lamina terminalis. The sylvian fissure is widely opened, and CSF is drained. Excessive frontal and temporal lobe retraction is avoided to prevent ischemia. Craniopharyngiomas are usually subarachnoid tumors, and thus all attempts should be made to free them from the surrounding structures, e.g., nerves, vessels, and infundibulum, which also have their own arachnoid layers. The tumor is vascularized by the branches of the ICAs, but large parts of it have little or no blood supply. The technique is similar to that of the subfrontal approach. The tumor resection should be carried out with stepwise internal decompression and dissection of the capsular-arachnoid plane. The infundibulum can be displaced and compressed, often posterior to the tumor, and thus it is difficult to identify and preserve.[2] Sharp dissection around the infundibulum is preferred to electrocauterization.

The orbitozygomatic approach offers a wider exposure for the posterior clinoid, basilar apex, and suprasellar region. Removing the orbital rim provides a better inferior-to-superior ("looking-up") angle to the hypothalamic and suprasellar region and to the third ventricular portion through the lamina terminalis.[25]

Interhemispheric-Transcallosal and Transcortical-Transventricular Approach

The interhemispheric-transcallosal approach is suitable for cranio-pharyngiomas protruding or arising within the third ventricle and projecting into the lateral ventricle (Fig. 29.3A and D). Cortical vessels and bridging veins, and vessels on the medial aspect of the frontal lobe and the corpus callosum, should be preserved to avoid ischemic complications.[2,26] Brain retraction with a fixed malleable brain retractor of 15 mm from the midline is sufficient. Distinguishing the cingulate gyrus from the corpus callosum may require tracing of the callosomarginal arteries to their origin anterior to the corpus callosum. The corpus callosum is often thinned out to 3 to 5 mm due to hydrocephalus. A callosal incision 1 to 2 cm posterior to the tip of the genu of <2.5 cm reduces the risk of disconnection syndrome. Vessels crossing between the pericallosal arteries may be sacrificed only if they are observed not to penetrate the cingulum. The lateral ventricle is entered. It is preferable to approach the tumor

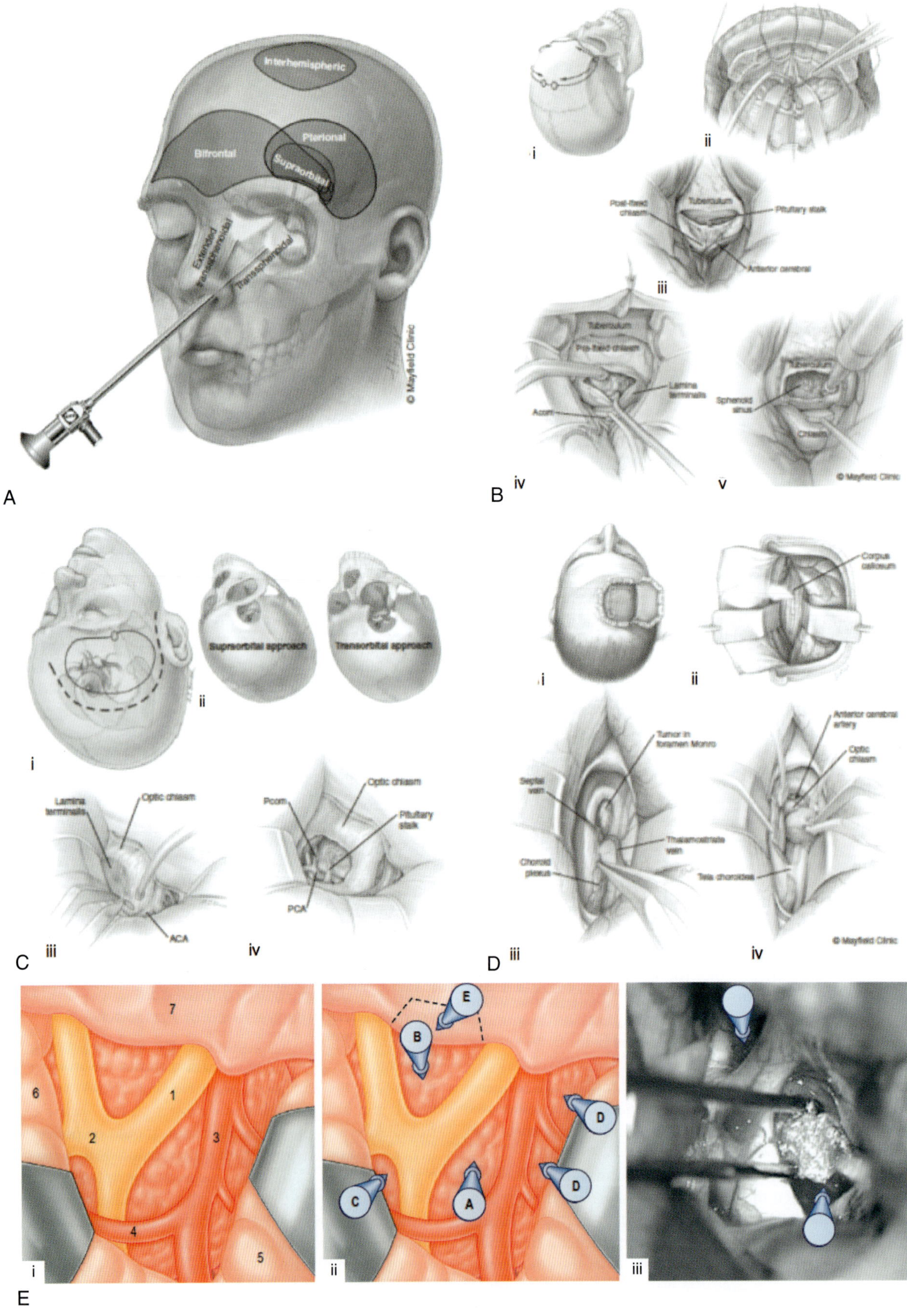

Interhemispheric
Pterional
Bifrontal
Supraorbital
Extended transsphenoidal
Transsphenoidal
© Mayfield Clinic
A
i
ii
Post-fixed chiasm
Tuberculum
Pituitary stalk
Anterior cerebral
iii
Tuberculum
Pre-fixed chiasm
Lamina terminalis
Acom
Sphenoid sinus
Chiasm
© Mayfield Clinic
B iv
v
i
ii
Supraorbital approach
Transorbital approach
Lamina terminalis
Optic chiasm
ACA
Pcom
Optic chiasm
Pituitary stalk
PCA
C iii
iv
i
ii
Corpus callosum
Tumor in foramen Monro
Septal vein
Thalamostriate vein
Choroid plexus
Anterior cerebral artery
Optic chiasm
Tela choroidea
© Mayfield Clinic
D iii
iv
7
6
1
2
3
4
5
i
E
B
D
C
A
D
ii
iii
E

• **Fig. 29.3** Cranial approaches to craniopharyngioma. **(A)** Artist's sketch of various approaches: bifrontal interhemispheric, pterional, interhemispheric transcallosal and endoscopic transsphenoidal. (Reproduced with permission from: Theodosopoulos P, Sughrue M, McDermott M. Craniopharyngioma. In: Quiñones-Hinojosa A, ed. Schmidek and Sweet: Operative neurosurgical techniques. 6th ed. Philadelphia, PA: Saunders/Elsevier; 2012. pp 292–302[20]). **(B)** The bifrontal approach is suitable for suprasellar pre-chiasmatic craniopharyngioma. **i:** Burr holes are made over the bilateral pterions and on both sides of the anterior superior sagittal sinus. The burr holes are joined up with a craniotome to raise a single bone flap. **ii:** The dura is opened bilaterally and the superior sagittal sinus is ligated and divided. The falx deep to the division is cut and released. Adhesions around the olfactory tracts are dissected, allowing the frontal lobes to fall backwards aided by gravity or to be gently retracted. **iii:** The anterior cerebral arteries and optic chiasm are identified. **iv:** For a retrochiasmatic tumor, the lamina terminalis is opened to allow access. **v:** For a tumor with sellar extension, the tuberculum can be drilled away to maximize the surgical corridor. **(C)** The pterional approach is the commonest approach. **i:** A cutaneous flap is raised from a curved incision. A single burr hole is made at the anterior aspect of the superior temporal line, and a bone flap is created. **ii:** The supraorbital and transorbital approaches are demonstrated. Removing the orbital rim offers an improved inferior-to-superior "looking-up" angle to the hypothalamic, suprasellar and third ventricular regions. **iii:** Through the transsylvian approach, the optic nerves and chiasmatic cisterns are identified. Small vessels are coagulated and the lamina terminalis is opened. **iv:** The suprasellar and third ventricular components of the tumor can be removed through the lamina terminalis with the preservation of the pituitary stalk. **(D)** The interhemispheric transcallosal approach. **i:** A bone flap, typically two-thirds anterior and one-third posterior to the right coronal suture, is made. **ii:** The frontal lobe is held in place with a brain retractor 1.5 cm from the falx. The pericallosal arteries and corpus callosum are identified. A 2.5 cm callosotomy is made. **iii:** The foramen of Monro is confirmed by the normal anatomy of the thalamostriate vein and choroid plexus. Approach through the dilated foramen is preferred although a subchoroidal dissection can be done to improve exposure. This is achieved after coagulation of the choroid plexus and thalamostriate vein and opening the choroidal fissure **(iv)**. **(E)** Schematic drawing demonstrating the various surgical corridors available via the right pterional approach. **i:** (1) optic nerve, (2) optic chiasm, (3) right internal carotid artery, (4) right anterior cerebral artery (A1), (5) temporal lobe being retracted, (6) frontal lobe being retracted, (7) tuberculum sella. **ii:** Surgical corridors: (A) between the optic nerve and chiasm medially and internal carotid artery laterally, (B) prechiasmatic, (C) retrochiasmatic, (D), lateral to the internal carotid artery, (E) drilling away and through the tuberculum sella. **iii:** intraoperative image demonstrating the prechiasmatic corridor and tumor removal between the optic apparatus and internal carotid artery. (Reproduced with permission from: Maartens N, Kaye A. Craniopharyngiomas. In: Kaye AH, Laws ER, Jr, eds. Brain tumors: an encyclopedic approach. Philadelphia, PA: Saunders/Elsevier; 2011. pp 807–830[21]).

through the dilated foramen of Monro. Initial internal decompression can be achieved by aspiration of the cystic or solid parts of the tumor, or piecemeal extirpation of the calcified portions. This enables dissection of the tumor from the wall of the third ventricle. Further exposure could be via the subchoroidal approach posteriorly or via the interforniceal approach and aided by coagulation and sectioning of the thalamostriate vein.[27] The column of the fornix anterior to the foramen of Monro, anterior commissure, choroid plexus, choroidal arteries, and septal and internal cerebral veins should also be identified and preserved. A septostomy allows communication of the lateral ventricles and dissection of possible adhesions of the tumor at the contralateral foramen of Monro. The aqueduct of Sylvius should be protected from obstruction with blood by the placement of patties. Preservation of the ventricular walls and floor and infundibulum are paramount to prevent severe morbidity, and therefore leaving residual tumor attached to the third ventricle floor is probable.[28] Damage to the fornices and the diencephalic nuclei is implicated in memory impairment and should be avoided.[29]

The transcortical-transventricular approach is more suitable when the tumor is projecting up and out through the foramen of Monro and there is ventriculomegaly.[1] It avoids cortical retraction but carries a higher risk of seizures. After a right frontal corticotomy, an external ventricular drain can be inserted to the foramen of Monro to guide subsequent dissection into the lateral ventricle.

Combined Approaches

The subfrontal approach offers a less lateral view than the pterional approach. The pterional approach offers limited view of the contralateral opticocarotid triangle and retrocarotid space and does not offer visualization of tumors extending superoposteriorly into the third ventricle, even if the lamina terminalis is opened. Similarly, the transcallosal approach does not allow clear access to the anterosuperior part of the tumor inferior to the optic chiasm. Therefore a combined or staged approach should be considered for large tumors involving multiple anatomic spaces.

Management

In addition to the nuances in surgical techniques discussed above, the management of three intra- and postoperative complications require special attention.

Fusiform Dilatation of the Internal Carotid Artery (FDCA)

This unusual vascular complication can occur during surgery by manipulation of the ICA with no laceration. Its incidence is 2.4%. It occurs ipsilateral to the surgical approach and is not related to the degree of resection, hypothalamic involvement, or radiation.[30] The median time interval between surgery and diagnosis is 0.79 year. The speculated cause is "hyperplasia mechanism", where microdamage to the adventitia from surgical manipulation triggers a healing process of the adventitia and vasa vasorum. In a registry of 583 patients, none of the 14 patients with FDCA exhibited decreased survival rate or functional capacity after a median follow-up of 9.7 years. FDCA can therefore be considered as a sequela of craniopharyngioma surgery with minimal consequence. Treatment, including clipping, coiling, and bypass surgery, should be reserved for symptomatic cases and lesions that are rapidly evolving on serial imaging.[31]

Hypothalamic Dysfunction and Morbid Obesity

Due to the anatomic proximity, 35% of patients with craniopharyngioma have some hypothalamic dysfunction at the time of diagnosis, including obesity, disturbed circadian rhythm, behavioral changes, and imbalance in regulation of thirst, body temperature, heart rate, and blood pressure. Of these patients, 12% to 19% are obese. After treatment, 65% to 80% of patients are morbidly obese, which is associated with poorer survival and quality of life.[32] The cause of obesity includes impairment of energy metabolism due to tumor involvement or treatment-related injury to the medial hypothalamus, complicated by daytime sleepiness, neurologic and visual deficits, reduced physical activity, and psychosocial difficulty. So far, diet, exercise, and pharmacologic treatment remain unsatisfactory. Bariatric surgery is controversial due to its legal and ethical implications. Preoperative posterior hypothalamic involvement remains the only independent risk factor for severe obesity. In these cases, the aim of surgery should be maximal resection with preservation of the hypothalamus.[33–35]

Ectopic Recurrence

Ectopic recurrence of craniopharyngioma is an uncommon but well-recognized sequela, occurring in 0% to 4.7% of all cases, accounting for 7% to 27% of all recurrences.[36,37] Sixty cases have been described, of which 33 are by "seeding" along the surgical tract and 27 are disseminated along the CSF pathway to a distant location. No surgical risk factors have been identified, and radiotherapy is not protective against the occurrence.[38] However, several surgical techniques reduce the theoretic risk:

1. Protect the surgical field with patties prior to resection.
2. Aspirate the cyst fluid early to minimize the contamination of the surgical field with tumor fluid.
3. Reduce the use of ultrasonic aspirator and irrigation during resection.
4. Keep the tumor capsule intact to avoid spreading of tumor cells.
5. Extensively irrigate the surgical field after resection.

The mean time between first surgery and ectopic recurrence is 6.8 years. Therefore close follow-up is essential to diagnose when the recurrence is small and thus surgical resection is less challenging.

SURGICAL REWIND

My Worst Cases

Case 1 (Fig. 29.4A–F)

A 10-year-old girl presented with a 1-month history of worsening headache, nausea, vomiting, and blurred vision. Computed tomography and MRI suggested a retrochiasmatic cystic craniopharyngioma extending to the foramen of Monro and causing obstructive hydrocephalus of the right lateral ventricle (Fig. 29.4A–C). There was calcification. Her preoperative visual acuity and endocrine status were normal. The patient underwent a bifrontal craniotomy, right supraorbital osteotomy, and gross total removal of the tumor through an interhemispheric, trans-lamina terminalis approach. The tumor capsule was well defined and dissected circumferentially off the third ventricular wall, the left side coming off more readily than the right. The subchiasmatic portion of the tumor was removed. The infundibulum was identified so it could be displaced anteriorly and preserved.

Postoperatively, she did not develop new neurologic or ophthalmologic deficit. She developed panhypopituitarism including diabetes insipidus, requiring hormone replacement and DDAVP. Postoperative MRIs confirmed complete resection, no hypothalamic injury, and no recurrence (Fig. 29.4D–F). In the second postoperative month, she developed hyperphagia syndrome and subsequently became obese. From 12 to 17 years of age, she was on growth hormone. At 14 years old, she started estrogen therapy. Her peak body mass index was 41.5 kg/m^2.[28] With diet control, this stabilized at 35.4 kg/m^2 at 18 years old.

In spite of the preservation of the hypothalamus and infundibulum intraoperatively and on follow-up imaging, hypothalamic dysfunction and hypopituitarism can occur.

Case 2 (Fig. 29.4G–P)

A 9-year-old boy presented with progressive visual loss in his left eye and was found to have optic atrophy and papilledema. MRI revealed a calcified suprasellar lesion extending into the third ventricle and the left cerebellopontine angle (CPA) (Fig. 29.4G and H). He underwent a left extended frontal craniotomy and tumor resection via a subfrontal approach. The tumor wrapped around the left MCA; it was dissected off the MCA and other vessels easily. The left tumor-hypothalamus tissue plane was indistinct, and resection was less aggressive on this side. Despite a densely calcified lesion, a near total resection was achieved with the highest power of ultrasonic aspirator. The boy took 2 weeks to recover from drowsiness secondary to hypothalamic manipulation. He developed a left third nerve palsy, right hemiparesis, and panhypopituitarism requiring complete hormone replacement. One year later, surveillance MRI showed a progressed CPA residual tumor, left basal ganglia infarct, and a right ICA aneurysmal dilatation (Fig. 29.4I–L). He underwent a left temporal craniotomy and tumor resection via a subtemporal approach with splitting of the tentorium. A gross total resection was achieved with a few fragments of calcium left in situ (Fig. 29.4M). The ICA dilatation was conservatively managed and remained stable in subsequent imaging. One year later, on surveillance scan, the prepontine cistern cystic tumor recurred, extending down the clivus (Fig. 29.4N and O). He underwent re-exploration of the temporal craniotomy and insertion of Ommaya reservoir into the adherent cyst. During the following 18 months, he underwent 10 aspirations. At 13 years old, he had some residual left vagal and hypoglossal palsy. The tumor solid component initially progressed but eventually stabilized, so radiotherapy was held off. At 17½ years old, he had a mild right hemiparesis, was blind in the left eye and in the temporal field of the right eye, had a left eye adduction palsy and facial numbness, and was mildly obese and on testosterone replacement (Fig. 29.4P).

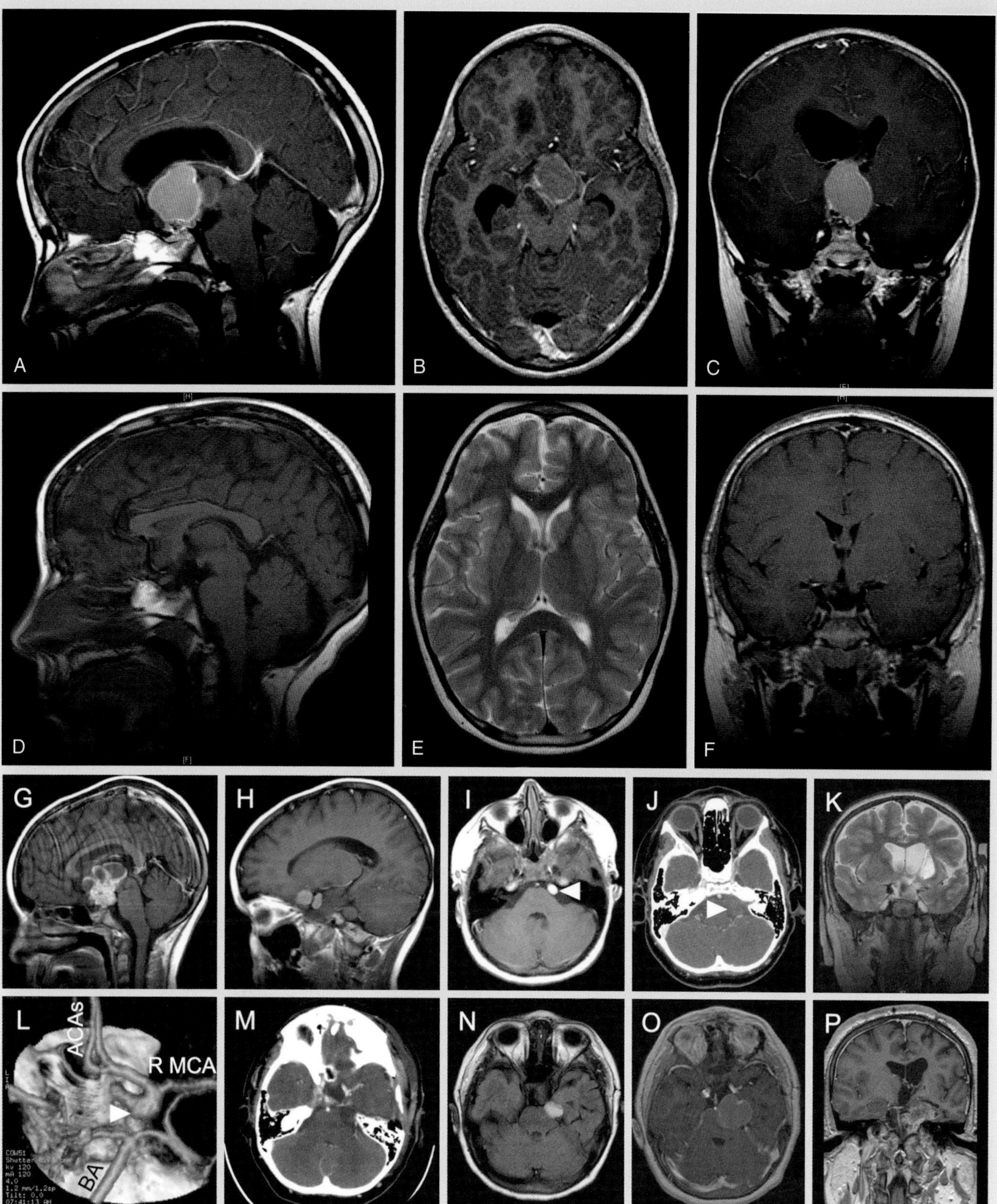

• **Fig. 29.4** *Case 1*: (A–C) Preoperative magnetic resonance image (MRI) of a 10-year-old girl, demonstrating a retrochiasmatic cystic tumor extending up to foramina of Monro, causing obstructive hydrocephalus of the right lateral ventricle. (D–F) Two-month postoperative MRI demonstrating no residual tumor and no hypothalamic injury. *Case 2*: (G and H) midsagittal and left parasagittal MRI demonstrating a complex suprasellar tumor extending into the third ventricle, prepontine and mesencephalic cisterns, and left cerebellopontine angle. (I and J) Serial MRI/computed tomography (CT) scan at 8, 12, and 13 months after operation showing progressive growth of left cerebellopontine angle (CPA) tumor from 10, 20, to 25 mm in its maximal dimension (arrowheads). (K) MRI at 12 months showing left basal ganglia infarct and right ICA aneurysmal dilatation. (L) CT angiogram showing ICA aneurysm dilatation of 6 mm (arrowhead). (M) Complete resection of CPA tumor after the second surgery. (N and O) Progressive growth of prepontine cyst over 18 months after the second surgery. (P) Stabilized tumor at 8 years after first presentation. *ACAs,* Anterior cerebral arteries; *R MCA,* right middle cerebral artery; *BA,* basilar artery.

NEUROSURGICAL SELFIE MOMENT

Microsurgery for craniopharyngioma carries significant risks. Careful study of the preoperative images is essential to plan the surgical approach, maximize visibility and resection, minimize risks, and anticipate pathologic anatomy. Care should be taken not to compromise the small blood vessels. Gross total resection should not be performed at the expense of injury to the hypothalamus.

References

1. Alli S, Isik S, Rutka JT. Microsurgical removal of craniopharyngioma: endoscopic and transcranial techniques for complication avoidance. *J Neurooncol.* 2016;130(2):1–9.
2. Yaşargil MG, Curcic M, Kis M, Siegenthaler G, Teddy PJ, Roth P. Total removal of craniopharyngiomas. Approaches and long-term results in 144 patients. *J Neurosurg.* 1990;73(1):3–11.
3. Cavallo LM, Solari D, Esposito F, Villa A, Minniti G, Cappabianca P. The role of the endoscopic endonasal route in the management of craniopharyngiomas. *World Neurosurg.* 2014;82(6):S32–S40.
4. Elliott RE, Jane JA, Wisoff JH. Surgical management of craniopharyngiomas in children: meta-analysis and comparison of transcranial and transsphenoidal approaches. *Neurosurgery.* 2011;69(3):630–643.
5. Wannemuehler TJ, Rubel KE, Hendricks BK, et al. Outcomes in transcranial microsurgery versus extended endoscopic endonasal approach for primary resection of adult craniopharyngiomas. *Neurosurg Focus.* 2016;41(6):E6.
6. Zaidi HA, Chapple K, Little AS. National treatment trends, complications, and predictors of in-hospital charges for the surgical management of craniopharyngiomas in adults from 2007 to 2011. *Neurosurg Focus.* 2014;37(5):E6.
7. Jeswani S, Nuño M, Wu A, et al. Comparative analysis of outcomes following craniotomy and expanded endoscopic endonasal transsphenoidal resection of craniopharyngioma and related tumors: a single-institution study. *J Neurosurg.* 2016;124(3):627–638.
8. Liu JK, Sevak IA, Carmel PW, Eloy JA. Microscopic versus endoscopic approaches for craniopharyngiomas: choosing the optimal surgical corridor for maximizing extent of resection and complication avoidance using a personalized, tailored approach. *Neurosurgery.* 2016;41 (6):E5.
9. Yang I, Sughrue ME, Rutkowski MJ, et al. Craniopharyngioma: a comparison of tumor control with various treatment strategies. *Neurosurg Focus.* 2010;28(4):E5.
10. Hoffman HJ, De Silva M, Humphreys RP, Drake JM, Smith ML, Blaser SI. Aggressive surgical management of craniopharyngiomas in children. *J Neurosurg.* 1992;76(1):47–52.
11. Gibo H, Lenkey C, Rhoton AL. Microsurgical anatomy of the supraclinoid portion of the internal carotid artery. *J Neurosurg.* 1981;55(4):560–574.
12. Samii M, Tatagiba M. Surgical management of craniopharyngiomas: a review. *Neurol Med Chir (Tokyo).* 1997;37(2):141–149.
13. Renn WH, Rhoton AL. Microsurgical anatomy of the sellar region. *J Neurosurg.* 1975;43:288–298.
14. Rhoton AL. The supratentorial arteries. *Neurosurgery.* 2002;51(4 suppl):53–120.
15. Rhoton AL. Anatomy of the pituitary gland and sellar region. In: Thapar K, Kovacs K, Scheithauer B, Lloyd RV, eds. *Diagnosis and Management of Pituitary Tumors.* Humana Press; 2001:13–40.
16. Pan J, Qi S, Liu Y, et al. Growth patterns of craniopharyngiomas: clinical analysis of 226 patients. *J Neurosurg Pediatr.* 2016;17: 1–16.
17. Hoffman HJ. Surgical management of craniopharyngioma. *Pediatr Neurosurg.* 1994;21(suppl 1):44–49.
18. Hofmann BM, Höllig A, Strauss C, Buslei R, Buchfelder M, Fahlbusch R. Results after treatment of craniopharyngiomas: further experiences with 73 patients since 1997. *J Neurosurg.* 2012;116(2):373–384.
19. Cook DJ, Rutka JT. Craniopharyngioma: neurosurgical management. In: Hanna EY, DeMonte F, eds. *Comprehensive Management of Skull Base Tumors.* New York, NY: CRC Press; 2008.
20. Maartens N, Kaye A. Craniopharyngiomas. In: Kaye AH, Laws ER Jr, eds. *Brain Tumors: An Encyclopedic Approach.* Philadelphia, PA: Saunders/Elsevier; 2011.
21. Theodosopoulos P, Sughrue M, McDermott M. Craniopharyngioma. In: Quiñones-Hinojosa A, ed. *Schmidek and Sweet: Operative Neurosurgical Techniques.* 6th ed. Philadelphia, PA: Saunders/Elsevier; 2012.
22. Carmel PW. Tumours of the third ventricle. *Acta Neurochir (Wien).* 1985;75(1–4):136–146.
23. Liu JK, Christiano LD, Gupta G, Carmel PW. Surgical nuances for removal of retrochiasmatic craniopharyngiomas via the transbasal subfrontal translamina terminalis approach. *Neurosurg Focus.* 2010;28(4):E6.
24. Silva PS, Cerejo A, Polónia P, Pereira J, Vaz R. Trans-lamina terminalis approach for third ventricle and suprasellar tumours. *Clin Neurol Neurosurg.* 2013;115(9):1745–1752.
25. Golshani KJ, Lalwani K, Delashaw JB, Selden NR. Modified orbitozygomatic craniotomy for craniopharyngioma resection in children. *J Neurosurg Pediatr.* 2009;4(4):345–352.
26. Sugita K, Kobayashi S. Preservation of large bridging veins during brain retraction. Technical note. *J Neurosurg.* 1982;57(6):856–858.
27. Hirsch J, Zouaoui A, Renier D, Pierre-Kahn A. A new surgical approach to the third ventricle with interruption of the striothalamic vein. *Acta Neurochir (Wien).* 1979;47:135–147.
28. Behari S, Banerji D, Mishra A, et al. Intrinsic third ventricular craniopharyngiomas: report on six cases and a review of the literature. *Surg Neurol.* 2003;60(3):245–252.
29. Catani M, Dell'Acqua F, Thiebaut de Schotten M. A revised limbic system model for memory, emotion and behaviour. *Neurosci Biobehav Rev.* 2013;37(8):1724–1737.
30. Hoffmann A, Warmuth-Metz M, Lohle K, et al. Fusiform dilatation of the internal carotid artery in childhood-onset craniopharyngioma: multicenter study on incidence and long-term outcome. *Pituitary.* 2016;19(4):422–428.
31. Wang L, Shi X, Liu F, Qian H. Bypass surgery to treat symptomatic fusiform dilation of the internal carotid artery following craniopharyngioma resection: report of 2 cases. *Neurosurg Focus.* 2016;41(6):E17.
32. Müller HL. Craniopharyngioma and hypothalamic injury: latest insights into consequent eating disorders and obesity. *Curr Opin Endocrinol Diabetes Obes.* 2016;23(1):81–89.
33. Elowe-Gruau E, Beltrand J, Brauner R, et al. Childhood craniopharyngioma: hypothalamus-sparing surgery decreases the risk of obesity. *J Clin Endocrinol Metab.* 2013;98(6):2376–2382.
34. Müller HL, Gebhardt U, Teske C, et al. Post-operative hypothalamic lesions and obesity in childhood craniopharyngioma: results of the multinational prospective trial KRANIOPHARYNGEOM 2000 after 3-year follow-up. *Eur J Endocrinol.* 2011;165(1):17–24.
35. Puget S, Garnett M, Wray A, et al. Pediatric craniopharyngiomas: classification and treatment according to the degree of hypothalamic involvement. *J Neurosurg.* 2007;106(1 suppl):3–12.
36. Du C, Feng CY, Yuan J, Yuan X. Ectopic recurrence of pediatric craniopharyngiomas after gross total resection: a report of two cases and a review of the literature. *Child's Nerv Syst.* 2016;32(8):1523–1529.
37. Elliott RE, Moshel YA, Wisoff JH. Surgical treatment of ectopic recurrence of craniopharyngioma. Report of 4 cases. *J Neurosurg Pediatr.* 2009;4(2):105–112.
38. Elfving M, Lundgren J, Englund E, Strömblad LG, Erfurth EM. Ectopic recurrence of a craniopharyngioma in a 15-year-old girl 9 years after surgery and conventional radiotherapy: Case report. *Child's Nerv Syst.* 2011;27(5):845–851.
39. Ciric I, Cozzens J. Craniopharyngiomas: transsphenoidal method of approach for the virtuoso only? *Clin Neurosurg.* 1980;27:169–187.
40. Konovalov AN. Microsurgery of tumours of diencephalic region. *Neurosurg Rev.* 1983;6(2):37–41.

41. Samii M, Samii A. Surgical management of craniopharyngiomas. In: Schmidek H, ed. *Schmidek Sweet Oper. Neurol. Tech. Indic. Methods, Results*. 4th ed. Philadelphia: WB Saunders; 2000:489–502.
42. Matsuo T, Kamada K, Izumo T, Nagata I. Indication and limitations of endoscopic extended transsphenoidal surgery for craniopharyngioma. *Neurol Med Chir (Tokyo)*. 2014;54:974–982.
43. Pascual JM, González-Llanos F, Barrios L, Roda JM. Intraventricular craniopharyngiomas: topographical classification and surgical approach selection based on an extensive overview. *Acta Neurochir (Wien)*. 2004;146(8):785–802.
44. Wang KC, Hong SH, Kim SK, Cho BK. Origin of craniopharyngiomas: implication on the growth pattern. *Child's Nerv Syst*. 2005;21(8–9):628–634.
45. Kassam AB, Gardner PA, Snyderman CH, Carrau RL, Mintz AH, Prevedello DM. Expanded endonasal approach, a fully endoscopic transnasal approach for the resection of midline suprasellar craniopharyngiomas: a new classification based on the infundibulum. *J Neurosurg*. 2008;108(4):715–728.
46. Fatemi N, Dusick JR, De Paiva Neto MA, Malkasian D, Kelly DF. Endonasal versus supraorbital keyhole removal of craniopharyngiomas and tuberculum sellae meningiomas. *Neurosurgery*. 2009;64(suppl 5):41–45.
47. Pan J, Qi S, Lu Y, et al. Intraventricular craniopharyngioma: morphological analysis and outcome evaluation of 17 cases. *Acta Neurochir (Wien)*. 2011;153(4):773–784.
48. Qi S, Lu Y, Pan J, Zhang X, Long H, Fan J. Anatomic relations of the arachnoidea around the pituitary stalk: relevance for surgical removal of craniopharyngiomas. *Acta Neurochir (Wien)*. 2011;153(4): 785–796.
49. Šteňo J, Bízik I, Šteňo A, Matejčík V. Recurrent craniopharyngiomas in children and adults: long-term recurrence rate and management. *Acta Neurochir (Wien)*. 2014;156(1):113–122.

30

Complications Associated With Cerebrospinal Fluid Diversion

JAMES A. STADLER III, HAMIDREZA ALIABADI, GERALD A. GRANT

HIGHLIGHTS

- Endoscopic third ventriculostomy complications include hemorrhage, neurologic deficits, and failure of the ventriculostomy.
- Ventricular shunt complications can be broadly categorized as infections, mechanical failures of the shunt, and long-term complications.
- Careful preoperative planning and meticulous surgical techniques may help prevent complications related to cerebrospinal fluid diversion.
- Potential complications should be investigated thoroughly to allow for appropriate treatment as needed.

Background

Cerebrospinal fluid (CSF) diversion is important, and often lifesaving, in the treatment of several common disorders, including hydrocephalus, intracranial hypertension, and CSF leaks or fistulas. When possible, treatment of hydrocephalus starts with correcting the underlying pathology. Reestablishment of physiologic CSF circulation and absorption, via either removal of the anatomic obstruction or creation of alternative fluid pathways, should be a primary consideration for these patients. When these options cannot be achieved, CSF may also be diverted using implanted shunts. Many surgical options allow for treatment to be individualized to patient-specific anatomic and pathologic factors, and with each technique there are known potential complications. The relative risks of these surgical options must be discussed with patients and their families as treatment plans are developed.

Anatomic Insights

Endoscopic Third Ventriculostomy

Endoscopic third ventriculostomy (ETV) should be considered for patients with obstructive hydrocephalus and favorable ventricular anatomy. Entry point and trajectory through the frontal horn of the lateral ventricle are determined preoperatively by careful review of the imaging. A straight line from the floor of the third ventricle through the foramen of Monro can be extended to allow measurements in sagittal and coronal planes at the surface for optimization of skin incision (Fig. 30.1). Neuronavigation may be considered for more challenging cases. An adequate prepontine space to avoid the basilar artery, a large enough lateral and third ventricle to insert the neuroendoscope through the foramen of Monro without injuring the fornix, and lack of significant intraventricular or subarachnoid adhesions on imaging are also reassuring as an ETV is planned.

Understanding of intraventricular anatomy is critical for surgeons performing an ETV. Within the lateral ventricle, the foramen of Monro is identified in association with the choroid plexus, the anterior septal vein, and the thalamostriate vein (Fig. 30.2A). The endoscope is then advanced into the third ventricle, and the floor of the third ventricle is confirmed in the midline, anterior to the mammillary bodies and posterior to the infundibular recess (Fig. 30.2B). The floor of the third ventricle was subsequently fenestrated in a standard fashion, often with balloon dilation through the endoscope.

Ventricular Shunt Placement

A thorough review of preoperative imaging should precede any ventricular shunt placement or revision given the potential for abnormal anatomic variations in patients with hydrocephalus. Careful note should be made of ventricular size and configuration, patient history including any prior incisions, and aberrant anatomy such as distorted venous sinus locations.

Frontal and occipital entry points are most often employed for ventricular shunt placement, with typical termination in the frontal horn. The impact of entry site selection on risk of shunt malfunction is controversial within the literature, with systematic review not demonstrating clear evidence in favor of either location.[1] Positioning the catheter within a defined CSF space, away from ventricular walls and choroid plexus, may lower shunt malfunction risk.[2] It is important to always include a reservoir in the shunt system to tap the shunt in an emergency or to evaluate for infection.

The peritoneal space is the most frequent distal terminus for ventricular shunts. Other considerations include the pleural space and the right atrium of the heart, though these are primarily chosen in cases where the peritoneal space is contraindicated. A pleural shunt is often not tolerated in a child less than 2 years of age due to poor absorption from the pleural space. An atrial shunt may need to be revised in a young child due to growth, since the catheter would migrate out of the right atrium and into the subclavian vein and thrombose. In patients with significant prior abdominal surgical history or with less common distal terminus sites, surgical assistance from specialists trained in accessing these anatomic areas safely and minimally invasively is often appropriate.

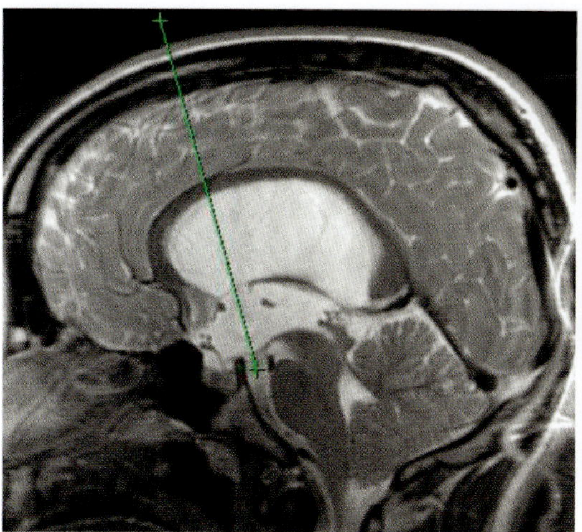
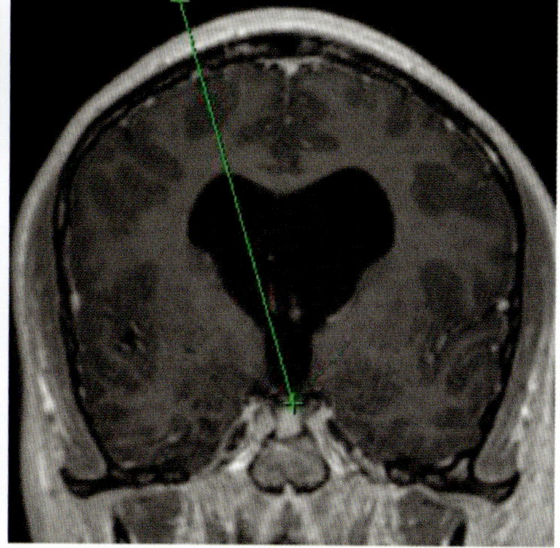

• **Fig. 30.1** An appropriate trajectory and entry point for endoscopic third ventriculostomy can be determined by extending a straight line from the floor of the third ventricle through the foramen of Monro. Neuronavigation may be helpful in cases with challenging ventricular anatomy.

RED FLAGS

- Patients with lower chances of ETV success can be identified preoperatively using the ETV Success Score.[3]
- Risk of shunt infection is highest directly after external ventricular drainage, especially if this was in the setting of a recent infection.[4]
- Age less than 6 months, cardiac comorbidities, and use of an endoscope for ventricular catheter placement are factors that have been statistically correlated with higher risk of shunt malfunction in a large multiinstitutional analysis.[5]

Prevention

Good surgical outcomes start with appropriate patient and procedure selection. Determining which patients would most benefit from ETV or shunting requires familiarity with not only the respective procedures but also the best available data to guide clinical decisions.

Endoscopic Third Ventriculostomy Complications

Preoperatively, the chances of successfully treating hydrocephalus with an ETV should be considered and discussed with patients and their families. The ETV Success Score is a validated measure that allows calculation of this potential risk.[3] Patient age is the largest determinant of this score, followed by the etiology of hydrocephalus and history of prior shunting (Table 30.1).

TABLE 30.1 ETV Success Score, With the Sum of Scores in Three Categories Approximating the Probability of Successful Hydrocephalus Management With an ETV Alone

Score	Patient Age	Hydrocephalus Etiology	History of Prior CSF Shunt
0	<1 month	Postinfectious	Yes
10	1–6 months		No
20		Myelomeningocele, intraventricular hemorrhage, nontectal brain tumor	
30	6–12 months	Aqueductal stenosis, tectal tumor, other	
40	1–10 years		
50	>10 years		

CSF, Cerebrospinal fluid; *ETV*, endoscopic third ventriculostomy.

Bleeding is a risk of any intraventricular procedure. Hemorrhage risk is mitigated by careful avoidance of the vascular choroid plexus, except in cases where choroid plexus cauterization is added to decrease CSF production. Minimizing nonaxial endoscope movement limits the risk of ependymal bleeding; this is much easier with careful preoperative incision planning, aided by neuronavigation in more challenging cases and using a peel-away sheath in the brain. Most recently, robotic assistance has been used to ensure precise navigation and steady endoscope positioning.[6,7] The most dreaded complication of ETV, however, is injury to the critical basilar and pontine vessels immediately subjacent to the floor of the third ventricle. Injury to these vessels can be avoided by confirming an adequate prepontine space on preoperative imaging, by a good understanding of the anatomy of the third ventricular floor, by identifying the clivus through the floor utilizing tactile feedback, and by aborting the procedure in favor of other treatment options in cases where the endoscopic anatomy is not clear enough to proceed safely. If an injury to the basilar or posterior cerebral arteries occurs intraoperatively, it is important not to pull back the endoscope but instead to use the endoscope to hold pressure on the artery and to irrigate for several minutes to stop the bleeding. Consider direct transfer to the angio suite for a neurointerventional procedure to coil the vessel if needed. If the endoscope is pulled back, which can be a natural reflex at the moment, the blood will quickly fill the ventricles, and visualization will be lost.

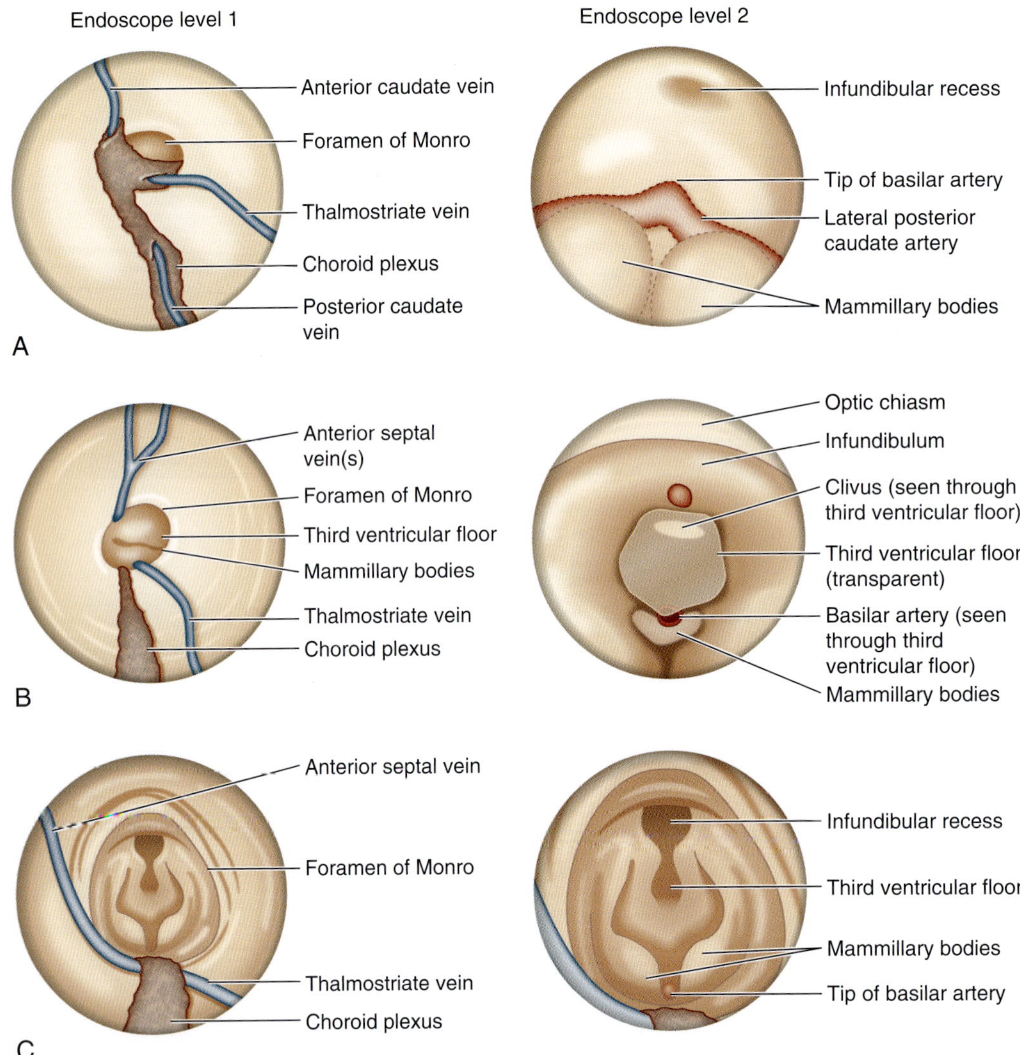

• **Fig. 30.2** The endoscopic anatomy encountered while performing an endoscopic third ventriculostomy (A) at the foramen of Monro, and (B) within the third ventricle.

Other complications of ETV include CSF leak or pseudomeningocele, wound infection, meningitis, new neurologic deficits, endocrinopathies, and perioperative seizure.[8] Occlusion of the epidural opening before closure and meticulous wound management may mitigate these risks. The fornix is at highest risk within the brain, with injury noted in up to 16.6% of cases and thus potential permanent short-term memory loss[8]; as with hemorrhage, this risk is lowered by minimizing nonaxial endoscope movement and torque applied at the level of the foramen of Monro. Other complications, such as third nerve injury or hypothalamic disturbances, may be similarly avoided.

Shunt Complications

Shunt Infection

Shunt infections present a challenge given the requisite foreign bodies and direct communication with the central nervous system. Infection is reported in 4% to 30% of cases, varying according to patient history, presence of external drainage, and history of recent infection.[4,9–11] The latency between surgery and presentation for infection ranges from 15 days to 12 months, with a bimodal distribution weighted toward early presentation.[11] Gram-positive organisms cause most shunt infections, with coagulase-negative staphylococci reported in 17% to 78% of cases and *Staphylococcus aureus* found in 4% to 30%.[11,12] Risk factors for shunt infection are numerous and include prematurity and low birth weight, relative immunosuppression, repeat shunt revisions or aspirations, and lack of compliance with established infection-control protocols both in the operating room and perioperative setting.[4,11,13,14]

Operative protocols have demonstrated success in reducing shunt infection rates, and currently most institutions have established perioperative management plans regarding antibiotics, skin sterilization, handling of shunt components, and flow of operating room personnel.[4,13,15–17] Antibiotic-impregnated catheters may have some benefit, though conclusive data for this is limited.[18] As with any procedure, infection rates are likely improved with careful and meticulous surgical technique, copious irrigation, and adherence to wound-healing principles with the incisions and closure.

Mechanical Shunt Failure

Shunt failure can take many clinical forms and often is patient-specific in presentation. Frustratingly to the surgeon, there are no absolute ways of preventing shunt failures. The highest risk of failure is in the early postoperative period after insertion or revision, though in practice, examples of late failures are easily produced as well.[5,19] The largest prospective cohort studying risk factors for shunt failure identified three risk factors associated with reduced shunt survival: age less than 6 months, a cardiac comorbidity, and use of an endoscope for ventricular catheter placement.[5] Of these, use of an endoscope is the only modifiable risk factor, so an endoscope is generally not recommended for routine ventricular catheter placement.[5,20,21]

Shunt occlusion can occur at the proximal catheter, valve, or distal system. As described above, the choice of frontal or occipital entry site does not appear to affect shunt survival, though maintaining an open CSF space around the catheter, away from the ventricular walls and choroid plexus, may reduce shunt malfunction.[1,2] Selection of valve design does not change the risk of shunt malfunction.[5,22–24] Laparoscopic placement may reduce the risk of distal catheter occlusion in ventriculoperitoneal shunts.[25,26]

Shunts may disconnect, fracture, or migrate. The risk of disconnection may be mitigated by securing the shunt system tightly with nondissolvable suture and limiting the number of connections when possible. Placement of the valve and connections over the skull, where these connections are not subjected to repetitive movement at the neck, is also encouraged. Shunt fracture is typically seen in older, calcified catheters and does not require a history of significant trauma. Early shunt migrations are avoided by securing the ventricular catheter and valve to the pericranium or skull as possible, avoiding unnecessary subgaleal dissection, and closing the abdominal wall layers securely around the distal catheter. Late migration of the shunt catheters, including the ventricular catheter into the brain parenchyma and the distal catheter out of the abdomen or other terminus, may be seen as a result of relative growth of the child; this late migration can be minimized when the shunt is inserted by accounting for the child's anticipated growth.

Overdrainage

Multiple longer-term risks of CSF diversion are related to CSF overdrainage. Creation of subdural hematomas or hygromas, slit ventricle syndrome, shunt-induced craniosynostosis, low-pressure headaches, and ventricular collapse with loculations are all complications of shunt overdrainage. Valve selection, including the setting of programmable valves, may help avoid some of these complications, though predicting CSF hydrodynamics is imperfect and incompletely studied. Patients are routinely followed clinically and radiographically, with intervention as needed, to avoid these concerns and their sequelae as possible.

Long-Term Shunt Complications

There are many complications related to CSF shunts that deserve recognition by patient care teams, especially as general health maintenance of these patients is challenged by comorbidities and paucity of multidisciplinary transitional clinics. These findings should be periodically screened, with referral to appropriate experts as needed to prevent significant progression.

Shunted patients may have endocrine disturbances. Growth hormone abnormalities can be seen as a result of intracranial hypertension or can be related to tumor treatment when applicable.[27] Early puberty and infertility are related concerns.[28,29] Diabetes insipidus is an uncommon complication after ETV. Obesity is a significant problem in the shunted population, with the higher risk related to both associated neurologic deficits and potential contributions from hypothalamic dysfunction.[30]

In addition to findings related to their underlying pathology, shunted patients may present with long-term neurologic complications. Headaches unrelated to shunt function are common, reported in up to 44% of patients with shunts.[31] Epilepsy is found in 30% of patients with nontumoral hydrocephalus.[32] Neuropsychologic and cognitive sequelae of chronic shunting are understudied and undertreated.

There is always a question as to whether a patient will remain shunt dependent years after the shunt placement. It is most likely that, if the shunt was placed early in life, the patient is still dependent on the shunt. If a patient presents with a shunt disconnection and is asymptomatic, CSF may still be draining via the previously established tract. To confirm shunt independence, a shunt may be surgically ligated with the patient carefully observed in the hospital, or the shunt can be externalized with the external ventricular drain (EVD) clamped to monitor intracranial pressure over 3 to 5 days. A patient with a history of a meningomyelocele is usually shunt dependent for life.

Management

Intraoperative Complication Management

Intraoperative complications must be identified and managed in accordance with the surgeon's best clinical judgment. Difficulty accessing the ventricle, for either ETV or shunt placement, can be eased with neuronavigation or intraoperative ultrasonography. For shunt placement in patients with significant prior abdominal surgeries or less familiar distal terminus locations, assistance from other surgical specialists may be helpful.

Intraventricular hemorrhage in endoscopic cases presents a surgical challenge. Traditional methods of hemostasis used in open surgical cases, such as hemostatic gelatin sponges and matrices or direct isolation and coagulation of vessels, are not available to the surgeon. Compounding this difficulty is the obscuration of the endoscopic field by blood clouding the ventricular fluid. Bleeding is often best managed by gentle yet persistent irrigation of the ventricle, and copious amounts of irrigant and patience may be needed.[33] If a focal source of bleeding is identified, bipolar electrocautery may also be applied. Though fortunately rare, injury to critical vessels may warrant angiographic studies and treatment.

External ventricular drainage is an important consideration in cases with unexpected challenges intraoperatively, and this possibility should be discussed with patients and families preoperatively. In cases with significant bleeding intraoperatively, complications with the distal terminus while placing a shunt, questionable infection or contamination, patient instability, or other intraoperative concerns, external drainage allows for intracranial pressure monitoring and patient stabilization while further evaluation is completed. When safe, the patient can then be definitively treated in a controlled surgical fashion.

Investigation and Management of Potential Shunt Infection

Shunt infection should be suspected in any shunted patient with an apparent wound infection, meningitis/ventriculitis, or peritonitis. Patients may have fever, leukocytosis, or signs and symptoms of shunt malfunction. Positive blood cultures or findings of a pleural empyema may be seen in patients with infected ventriculoatrial or ventriculopleural shunts, respectively.

CSF sampling is often helpful in the evaluation of a potential shunt infection. When the CSF profile is concerning for infection or when the cultures of this fluid demonstrate infection, the most common management involves removal of any implants that are reasonably presumed to be infected and subsequent treatment of the infection before reimplantation.[11,13,34] Conservative management of shunt infections is less common, though it has been successful in select cases with prolonged systemic antibiotics for up to 6 weeks for gram-positive infections.[13] Some patients present with erythema or swelling around the shunt. This patient likely needs externalization; a shunt tap may risk contaminating the CSF if the infection is outside of the shunt, called an external shunt infection.

Although abdominal pseudocysts often present secondary to mechanical outflow obstruction of the distal shunt system, it is important to recognize the potential for infection. Up to half of patients with shunt-related abdominal pseudocysts demonstrate positive cultures on presentation, a finding even more common in younger children.[35,36] Pseudocyst formation should be suspected particularly in patients with a history of abdominal pain or abdominal surgeries. Diagnosis is confirmed with either ultrasound or cross-sectional imaging. In patients with a pseudocyst, partial removal or externalization of the shunt, drainage and culturing of the abdominal fluid, and empiric treatment of a presumed infection may help expedite resolution of the pseudocyst before reimplantation in either the peritoneal space or other distal terminus as indicated.

Investigation and Management of Potential Shunt Malfunction

Identification of shunt malfunction starts with patient and family education regarding concerning signs and symptoms of shunt malfunction. Symptoms may be subtle and identified only by the patient's closest family members or caregivers. Suspicion is raised by different findings in progressive age groups: Whereas infants may show irritability and a bulging fontanelle, an older child or adult may have findings of headache, nausea, vomiting, or lethargy. The clinical picture is typically consistent overall with progressively increased intracranial pressure, however. Dictated by the specific clinical scenario, the standard investigation of potential shunt malfunction includes clinical history and physical examination, cross-sectional cranial imaging, and potentially plain radiographs of the shunt system or abdominal imaging depending on these findings. Additional evaluation, such as with shunt aspiration, radionuclide shuntography, or contrast-enhanced shunt series, may have additional benefit in the proper clinical context.[37–39] Ultimately, however, determination of shunt malfunction is based on a multitude of patient-specific clinical and radiographic correlates, with no perfectly sensitive or specific testing.[40] It is important to keep in mind that some patients have slit ventricles or do not dilate their ventricles with a shunt malfunction. These patients can be very challenging to manage given the absence of standard changes on imaging. However, these patients are also high risk to be sent home from the emergency room and die if left untreated.

When malfunction is suspected, prompt shunt exploration and revision are recommended. The proximal ventricular system is routinely explored first, with manometry for evaluation of intracranial pressure and confirmation of the valve and distal system function. All shunt components are tested as needed to confirm appropriate function, with revision of any nonfunctioning elements. In challenging cases or situations of uncertainty, external ventricular drainage may be used to stabilize a patient while further evaluation is completed and a controlled operative plan is developed. The old saying not to let the sun set on a patient with a proximal shunt malfunction refers to the urgency of repairing the shunt to avoid sudden neurologic deterioration.

SURGICAL REWIND

My Worst Case

A 15 year-old young man was admitted with progressive headaches after a concussion. He had a long-standing history of headaches, but they escalated in severity and frequency after his concussion. His magnetic resonance imaging scan showed obstructive hydrocephalus, and ophthalmologic examination confirmed papilledema. We recommended an ETV. The patient was placed supine, and we proceeded with a right frontal ETV. As soon as we fenestrated the floor of the third ventricle, we visualized the basilar and perforating arteries beautifully. At that moment, the patient coughed, and the screen turned bright red. The endoscope was pulled back to the lateral ventricles, and we irrigated for over 30 minutes. We could no longer visualize any appreciable ventricular anatomy and left an external ventricular drain behind. Ultimately, we converted the EVD into a shunt, which got infected and required another EVD and eventual shunt replacement on the opposite side. He suffered a brainstem stroke and developed a severe injury to both fornices, resulting in severe short-term memory dysfunction. The moral of the story is to be sure the patient is paralyzed during the ETV!

NEUROSURGICAL SELFIE MOMENT

CSF diversion, whether accomplished via ETV or ventricular shunt placement, is an important approach for many conditions, having a direct impact on patient quantity and quality of life. Complications related to these procedures take a variety of forms, including hemorrhage, ventriculostomy failure, infection, mechanical failure of the shunt, and long-term issues related to the CSF diversion. Careful preoperative evaluation and perioperative management may help avoid many complications. When complications of CSF diversion are suspected, thorough evaluation is warranted, with treatment as needed to improve patient outcomes. The planning of the first shunt is the most critical due to the likely need for revisions in the future. If the shunt does not look "perfect" before closure and is not dripping spontaneously before distal insertion, it will come back to haunt the surgeon.

References

1. Kemp J, Flannery AM, Tamber MS, Duhaime AC, Pediatric Hydrocephalus Systematic R, Evidence-Based Guidelines Task F. Pediatric hydrocephalus: systematic literature review and evidence-based guidelines. Part 9: effect of ventricular catheter entry point and position. *J Neurosurg Pediatr*. 2014;14(suppl 1):72–76.
2. Tuli S, O'Hayon B, Drake J, Clarke M, Kestle J. Change in ventricular size and effect of ventricular catheter placement in pediatric patients with shunted hydrocephalus. *Neurosurgery*. 1999;45(6):1329–1333, discussion 33-5.
3. Kulkarni AV, Drake JM, Kestle JR, et al. Predicting who will benefit from endoscopic third ventriculostomy compared with shunt insertion in childhood hydrocephalus using the ETV Success Score. *J Neurosurg Pediatr*. 2010;6(4):310–315.

4. Kestle JR, Holubkov R, Douglas Cochrane D, et al. A new Hydrocephalus Clinical Research Network protocol to reduce cerebrospinal fluid shunt infection. *J Neurosurg Pediatr*. 2016;17(4):391–396.
5. Riva-Cambrin J, Kestle JR, Holubkov R, et al. Risk factors for shunt malfunction in pediatric hydrocephalus: a multicenter prospective cohort study. *J Neurosurg Pediatr*. 2016;17(4):382–390.
6. Hoshide R, Calayag M, Meltzer H, Levy ML, Gonda D. Robot-assisted endoscopic third ventriculostomy: institutional experience in 9 patients. *J Neurosurg Pediatr*. 2017;20.125-133.
7. De Benedictis A, Trezza A, Carai A, et al. Robot-assisted procedures in pediatric neurosurgery. *Neurosurg Focus*. 2017;42(5):E7.
8. Kulkarni AV, Riva-Cambrin J, Holubkov R, et al. Endoscopic third ventriculostomy in children: prospective, multicenter results from the Hydrocephalus Clinical Research Network. *J Neurosurg Pediatr*. 2016;18(4):423–429.
9. Guzelbag E, Ersahin Y, Mutluer S. Cerebrospinal fluid shunt complications. *Turk J Pediatr*. 1997;39(3):363–371.
10. Shapiro S, Boaz J, Kleiman M, Kalsbeck J, Mealey J. Origin of organisms infecting ventricular shunts. *Neurosurgery*. 1988;22(5):868–872.
11. Prusseit J, Simon M, von der Brelie C, et al. Epidemiology, prevention and management of ventriculoperitoneal shunt infections in children. *Pediatr Neurosurg*. 2009;45(5):325–336.
12. Lee JK, Seok JY, Lee JH, et al. Incidence and risk factors of ventriculoperitoneal shunt infections in children: a study of 333 consecutive shunts in 6 years. *J Korean Med Sci*. 2012;27(12):1563–1568.
13. Tamber MS, Klimo P Jr, Mazzola CA, Flannery AM, Pediatric Hydrocephalus Systematic R, Evidence-Based Guidelines Task F. Pediatric hydrocephalus: systematic literature review and evidence-based guidelines. Part 8: management of cerebrospinal fluid shunt infection. *J Neurosurg Pediatr*. 2014;14(suppl 1):60–71.
14. Kulkarni AV, Rabin D, Lamberti-Pasculli M, Drake JM. Repeat cerebrospinal fluid shunt infection in children. *Pediatr Neurosurg*. 2001;35(2):66–71.
15. Kulkarni AV, Riva-Cambrin J, Butler J, et al. Outcomes of CSF shunting in children: comparison of Hydrocephalus Clinical Research Network cohort with historical controls: clinical article. *J Neurosurg Pediatr*. 2013;12(4):334–338.
16. Klimo P Jr, Van Poppel M, Thompson CJ, et al. Pediatric hydrocephalus: systematic literature review and evidence-based guidelines. Part 6: preoperative antibiotics for shunt surgery in children with hydrocephalus: a systematic review and meta-analysis. *J Neurosurg Pediatr*. 2014;14(suppl 1):44–52.
17. Hommelstad J, Madso A, Eide PK. Significant reduction of shunt infection rate in children below 1 year of age after implementation of a perioperative protocol. *Acta Neurochir (Wien)*. 2013;155(3):523–531.
18. Klimo P Jr, Thompson CJ, Baird LC, Flannery AM, Pediatric Hydrocephalus Systematic R, Evidence-Based Guidelines Task F. Pediatric hydrocephalus: systematic literature review and evidence-based guidelines. Part 7: antibiotic-impregnated shunt systems versus conventional shunts in children: a systematic review and meta-analysis. *J Neurosurg Pediatr*. 2014;14(suppl 1):53–59.
19. Drake JM, Sainte-Rose C. *The Shunt Book*. Cambridge, MA: Blackwell Science; 1995:xii, 228.
20. Flannery AM, Duhaime AC, Tamber MS, Kemp J, Pediatric Hydrocephalus Systematic R, Evidence-Based Guidelines Task F. Pediatric hydrocephalus: systematic literature review and evidence-based guidelines. Part 3: endoscopic computer-assisted electromagnetic navigation and ultrasonography as technical adjuvants for shunt placement. *J Neurosurg Pediatr*. 2014;14(suppl 1):24–29.
21. Kestle JR, Drake JM, Cochrane DD, et al. Lack of benefit of endoscopic ventriculoperitoneal shunt insertion: a multicenter randomized trial. *J Neurosurg*. 2003;98(2):284–290.
22. Baird LC, Mazzola CA, Auguste KI, et al. Pediatric hydrocephalus: systematic literature review and evidence-based guidelines. Part 5: effect of valve type on cerebrospinal fluid shunt efficacy. *J Neurosurg Pediatr*. 2014;14(suppl 1):35–43.
23. Drake JM, Kestle JR, Milner R, et al. Randomized trial of cerebrospinal fluid shunt valve design in pediatric hydrocephalus. *Neurosurgery*. 1998;43(2):294–303, discussion 303–305.
24. Warf BC. Comparison of 1-year outcomes for the Chhabra and Codman-Hakim Micro Precision shunt systems in Uganda: a prospective study in 195 children. *J Neurosurg*. 2005;102(4 suppl): 358–362.
25. He M, Ouyang L, Wang S, Zheng M, Liu A. Laparoscopy versus mini-laparotomy peritoneal catheter insertion of ventriculoperitoneal shunts: a systematic review and meta-analysis. *Neurosurg Focus*. 2016;41(3):E7.
26. Schucht P, Banz V, Trochsler M, et al. Laparoscopically assisted ventriculoperitoneal shunt placement: a prospective randomized controlled trial. *J Neurosurg*. 2015;122(5):1058–1067.
27. Cholley F, Trivin C, Sainte-Rose C, Souberbielle JC, Cinalli G, Brauner R. Disorders of growth and puberty in children with non-tumoral hydrocephalus. *J Pediatr Endocrinol Metab*. 2001;14(3): 319–327.
28. Proos LA, Tuvemo T, Ahlsten G, Gustafsson J, Dahl M. Increased perinatal intracranial pressure and brainstem dysfunction predict early puberty in boys with myelomeningocele. *Acta Paediatr*. 2011;100(10):1368–1372.
29. Proos LA, Dahl M, Ahlsten G, Tuvemo T, Gustafsson J. Increased perinatal intracranial pressure and prediction of early puberty in girls with myelomeningocele. *Arch Dis Child*. 1996;75(1):42–45.
30. Vinchon M, Dhellemmes P. The transition from child to adult in neurosurgery. *Adv Tech Stand Neurosurg*. 2007;32:3–24.
31. Rekate HL, Kranz D. Headaches in patients with shunts. *Semin Pediatr Neurol*. 2009;16(1):27–30.
32. Bourgeois M, Sainte-Rose C, Cinalli G, et al. Epilepsy in children with shunted hydrocephalus. *J Neurosurg*. 1999;90(2):274–281.
33. Amelot A. Letter: Washing and irrigation: faithful allies of the neurosurgeon for endoscopy hemostasis. *Neurosurgery*. 2017;81(4): E48–E49.
34. Simon TD, Kronman MP, Whitlock KB, et al. Variability in management of first cerebrospinal fluid shunt infection: a prospective multi-institutional observational cohort study. *J Pediatr*. 2016;179: 185–191.e2.
35. Dabdoub CB, Dabdoub CF, Chavez M, et al. Abdominal cerebrospinal fluid pseudocyst: a comparative analysis between children and adults. *Childs Nerv Syst*. 2014;30(4):579–589.
36. Baird C, O'Connor D, Pittman T. Late shunt infections. *Pediatr Neurosurg*. 1999;31(5):269–273.
37. Tsai SY, Wang SY, Shiau YC, Yang LH, Wu YW. Clinical value of radionuclide shuntography by qualitative methods in hydrocephalic adult patients with suspected ventriculoperitoneal shunt malfunction. *Medicine (Baltimore)*. 2017;96(17):e6767.
38. Rocque BG, Lapsiwala S, Iskandar BJ. Ventricular shunt tap as a predictor of proximal shunt malfunction in children: a prospective study. *J Neurosurg Pediatr*. 2008;1(6):439–443.
39. von Eckardstein KL, Kallenberg K, Psychogios MN, et al. Contrast-enhanced shunt series ("shuntography") compare favorably to other shunt imaging modalities in detecting shunt occlusion. *Acta Neurochir (Wien)*. 2017;159(1):63–70.
40. Nikas DC, Post AF, Choudhri AF, et al. Pediatric hydrocephalus: systematic literature review and evidence-based guidelines. Part 10: change in ventricle size as a measurement of effective treatment of hydrocephalus. *J Neurosurg Pediatr*. 2014;14(suppl 1):77–81.

31

Complications After Myelomeningocele Repair: CSF Leak and Retethering

IRENE KIM, W. JERRY OAKES

HIGHLIGHTS

- Cerebrospinal fluid leak and retethering are two of the more common complications after myelomeningocele repair.
- Watertight dural closure and adequate cerebrospinal fluid diversion are important in preventing and managing cerebrospinal fluid leak.
- Imbrication of the neural placode not only may help prevent retethering, but also may make untethering at a later date, when indicated, easier to perform.
- Retethering typically is caused by scarring of the neural placode or imbrication suture line to the dorsal dura.
- Other causes of tethering are inclusion dermoids or unrecognized concomitant lesions, such as split cord malformation (hemimyelia).

"Le mieux est l'ennemi du bien."
("The best is the enemy of the good.")

—VOLTAIRE

Background

In the post–folic acid fortification era, an estimated 1500 children in the United States are born with spina bifida every year.[1] The vast majority of patients with myelomeningocele undergo surgical closure within 48 hours after birth.[2,3] Complications that occur shortly after surgery include worsened neurologic function or level, cerebrospinal fluid (CSF) leak, wound dehiscence, meningitis, and wound infection.[4] Unfortunately, some of these complications may occur concomitantly. Complications that occur in a delayed fashion include symptomatic Chiari II malformation, which can occur within weeks to months of birth, and retethering, which typically occurs years to decades later.[4]

Anatomic Insights

Understanding the anatomy is critical to successful myelomeningocele repair (Fig. 31.1). The neural placode is a flattened, open embryologic form of the caudal aspect of the spinal cord. The dorsal surface corresponds to the unclosed interior of the neural tube. The central canal of the normal, closed spinal cord above is in direct continuity with the primitive neural groove down the midline of the placode.[5] The ventral surface corresponds to the entire exterior pial-lined surface of what should have formed into a closed neural tube. Thus, both the ventral and dorsal nerve roots arise from the ventral surface of the placode, with the dorsal sensory roots lateral to the ventral motor roots.[3,4]

Surrounding the edge of the placode is the arachnoid membrane, which extends laterally to fuse with the edge of normal skin. Ventral to the placode is an intact subarachnoid space. Although the ventral dura develops normally, rather than fusing in the dorsal midline, the dura fuses with the free edges of the surrounding soft tissue, including the paraspinal musculature, lumbodorsal fascia, and/or periosteum of the incomplete neural arch.[4] What would have been the dorsal dura therefore lies laterally just beneath the surface of the skin.

Due to the incomplete formation of the posterior neural arch, the dorsal paraspinal musculature and lumbodorsal fascia are displaced ventrolaterally and may be attenuated. The underlying vertebral bodies typically are flattened and widened. The pedicles are usually everted, which, in combination with wider vertebral bodies, results in an increased interpedicular distance. The laminae remnants typically are hypoplastic and may also be everted. The spinous processes are absent.

To identify all of the important structures, closure of the myelomeningocele begins with a circumference incision around the myelomeningocele at the junction of the arachnoid and the advancing edge of epithelium. Attention is then turned toward dissection of the neural placode. The nerve roots are dissected free from the arachnoid. The arachnoid and remaining epithelium are then sharply divided away from the neural placode, allowing it to move freely within the CSF.[3–5] The superior and, to a lesser degree, inferior poles of the placode are technically the most challenging to separate. Although there is some debate about it, the neural placode likely contains residual functional neural elements with a reflex arc especially important for rectal sphincter tone, so it should be handled with care to minimize injury.[2,3,6] It is also important to ensure that no epithelium is retained within the neural placode, because it can result in an inclusion dermoid, which not only enlarges over time, but also can cause arachnoiditis and enhance the tethering process.[5,6]

This idealized description may seem moot when one is faced with significant variation from the individualized patient. Although the goal is the maintenance of neurologic integrity and the exclusion of all dermal elements in the closure of the neural placode, in practice this can prove technically challenging.[7]

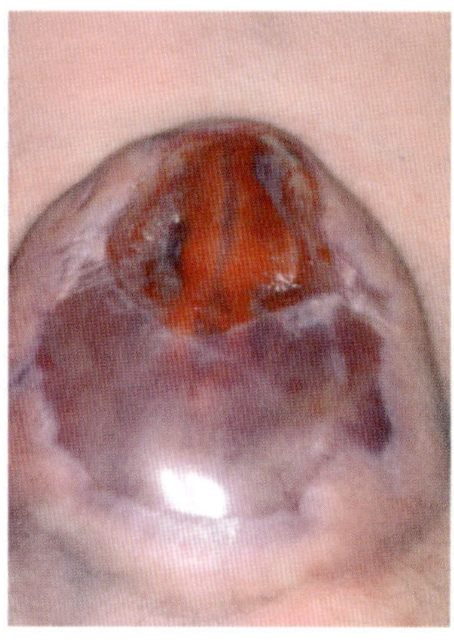

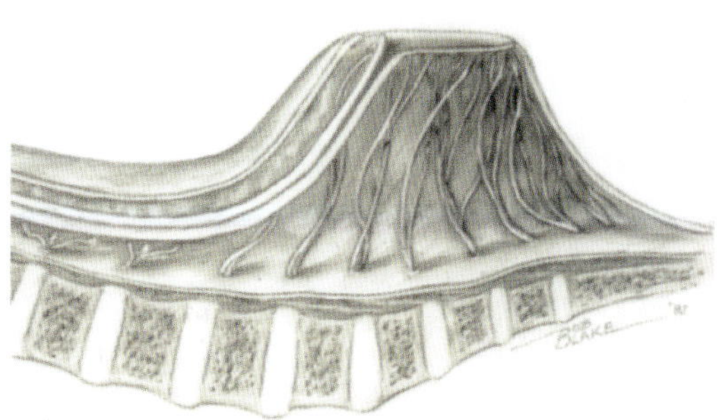

• **Fig. 31.1** Photograph of myelomeningocele on left. Illustration of anatomy of myelomeningocele on right.

RED FLAGS

Cerebrospinal Fluid Leak

- Large, wide epithelial deficiency for skin closure
- Hydrocephalus
- Kyphotic deformity
- Lesions involving deficient sacral skin

Retethering

- No imbrication of placode at time of initial myelomeningocele closure
- Shallow spinal canal
- Inclusion dermoid
- Thickened filum terminale
- Split cord malformation (hemimyelia)

Prevention

Cerebrospinal Fluid Leak

A meticulous watertight primary dural closure is important to the prevention of a CSF leak.[3,4] We prefer to use a 6-0 polydioxanone (PDS) suture with a small tapered needle in a running fashion. If care is taken to identify the extreme lateral aspect of the dura, there is almost always adequate material for primary closure without tension. After the dural closure is completed, Valsalva maneuvers should be performed to evaluate the integrity of the closure.[2–4]

After the primary dural closure, it is desirable to perform a strong, multilayered wound closure. Mobilizing paraspinal musculature and fascia for soft-tissue coverage over the midline can help tamponade and contain small CSF pseudomeningoceles and may help prevent CSF leakage through the skin.[3,4,6] With wide areas of absent skin, these tissues may not be available to assist in the closure, leaving only the skin. If the lesion is especially large, it may be prudent to consider requesting assistance from plastic surgery colleagues with the skin closure.

Although dural closure is the surgeon's primary defense against CSF leak, this must be balanced against tight soft-tissue compression of the neural elements, particularly when they are positioned proud of the skin surface, which can compromise the blood supply to the neural placode.[3]

Postoperatively, keeping the patient prone and relatively flat may also help prevent CSF leak. This decreases pressures within the lumbar thecal sac, allowing any small tears or holes within the dura to heal. At our institution, the more precarious the wound closure, the longer we tend to keep the patient flat. However, this must be balanced with the upright nurturing of the patient by the mother.

Finally, it should be emphasized that CSF leaks cannot be avoided if intracranial pressure (ICP) is elevated and hydrocephalus is not appropriately treated.[4] For lesions with large skin defects and limited soft-tissue coverage that require complex skin closures, an external ventricular drain (EVD) for temporary CSF diversion to allow for better wound healing may be a consideration. Even if it is not present at birth, progressive hydrocephalus may develop over time, especially after closure of a leaking myelomeningocele. Prompt treatment of hydrocephalus with a ventriculoperitoneal (VP) shunt or endoscopic third ventriculostomy (ETV) is important for prevention of CSF leaks and meningitis.[4]

Retethering

Preventing retethering remains a significant neurosurgical challenge. Unfortunately, there are no infallible methods for avoiding retethering, but the stage should be set to minimize this problem during the initial myelomeningocele repair.

Imbrication of the placode, that is, reapproximation of the pial edges of the placode into a tubular structure, may help because it decreases the exposed raw surface area available for retethering. It also makes untethering at a later date easier because the anatomy can be more readily identified.[3–6] We prefer to use interrupted 7-0 nylon sutures in an inverted fashion to imbricate the placode to minimize the exposed suture line, which is the most common site of tethering after myelomeningocele repair.

After imbrication of the placode, it is important to inspect for the presence of other concomitant tethering lesions. Occasionally, there is a thickened filum terminale that should be sectioned if present.[3] In our institution, the last intact spinal lamina is cut during the initial myelomeningocele repair to inspect for evidence of a split spinal cord malformation, which is present in 6% of patients.[8] Hemimyelia is the presence of a terminal split cord

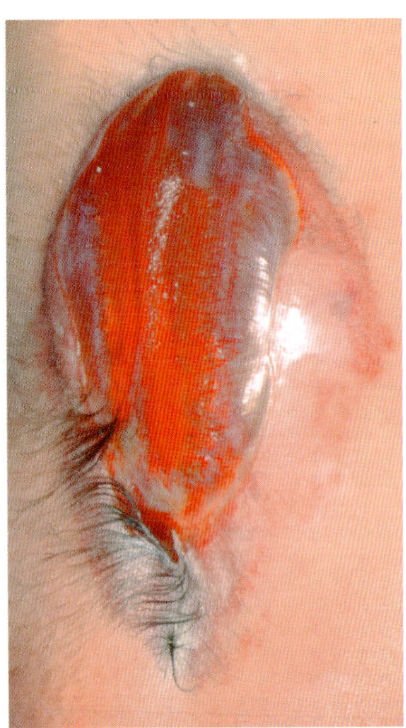

• **Fig. 31.2** Myelomeningocele with focal hirsutism on left side due to split cord malformation with hemimyelia (myelomeningocele on only one hemicord).

malformation with a myelomeningocele involving only one of the hemicords (Fig. 31.2). These patients often present with asymmetry in lower-extremity neurologic examination, with greater distal dysfunction ipsilateral to hemicord with myelomeningocele. Although these lesions per se do not technically cause retethering, if unrecognized and untreated during the initial repair, they can cause progressive loss of neurologic function over time.

Management

Cerebrospinal Fluid Leak

If a patient develops a CSF leak, he or she is also at risk of developing meningitis, wound dehiscence, and/or wound infection. The patient should be started on broad-spectrum empiric antibiotics with meningitis coverage, and attempts should be made to minimize ICP, add reinforcing skin sutures, and avoid stool contamination of the wound.

CSF diversion is essential to the management of CSF leaks.[4] If not already in place, an EVD may be placed to divert CSF away from the wound to allow it to heal. The height of the EVD can then be adjusted accordingly until there is no further egress of CSF from the wound. After adequate wound healing, the EVD can be raised in an attempt to wean it. It should be noted that with a single CSF leak, some surgeons may prefer to proceed with VP shunt placement rather than a temporary EVD.

If CSF leaks persist despite adequate CSF diversion, or if they recur after the EVD is raised, wound exploration may be helpful.[4] At the time of surgery, a dural defect can often be identified, which should be repaired primarily. The EVD should be kept in place postoperatively for additional CSF diversion to allow the fresh wound to heal before another attempt is made to wean the EVD.

Retethering

After repair of the myelomeningocele, nearly all patients will have radiographic evidence of spinal cord tethering or fixation.[9] Symptomatic tethering, when it occurs, is delayed for years to decades and rarely occurs within the first five years of life. If symptoms develop early, other causes of neurologic dysfunction are much more common, such as a second expression of neural tube defect (i.e., split cord malformation, second skin-covered lesion, etc.). The brain and entire spine should be imaged.

The diagnosis of symptomatic tethered cord is based on clinical symptoms.[9] The most common symptoms include progressive motor dysfunction, worsening urologic dysfunction, deteriorating gait, scoliosis and, rarely, spasticity and/or pain.[9–11] It is our experience that by 10 years of age, approximately half of ambulatory patients will have some clinical evidence of neurologic decline. The decision regarding whether this deterioration crosses the risks vs. benefits threshold for untethering depends on the severity of these symptoms. Before proceeding with tethered cord release, it is important to ensure that hydrocephalus is adequately treated and that symptoms are not secondary to worsening syringomyclia.

To perform a tethered cord release, the patient's existing incision is used. Although not strictly required, it is often necessary to reopen the entire incision due to extensive tethering. The incision should be extended cranially to expose the inferiormost intact lamina to identify normal anatomic landmarks.[11]

A laminectomy of the inferiormost intact lamina may be necessary to identify a safe place to open the dura and enter the subarachnoid space above the point of tethering. The dural opening is extended inferiorly toward the site of tethering, which most commonly occurs in the midline along the suture line of the imbrication.[11] When the dorsal surface of the neural elements is densely adherent to the overlying dura, it is safest to open just lateral to the point of fixation.

After the dura is opened and the subarachnoid space is identified, it is ideal to keep the arachnoid intact and to work in the subdural, extraarachnoidal space for as long as possible. We prefer to use the blunt nerve hook to sweep under the dura from lateral to medial toward the point of tethering, that is, the junction of the dura with scar and neural elements. The dura is then incised sharply just lateral to the nerve hook. This minimizes the risk of injury to the functional sensory roots exiting the placode but adherent to the undersurface of the dura. We use this technique to open the dura laterally around the point of dorsal fixation, working from cephalad to caudad, until the dura is opened circumferentially around the scar, allowing the cord to fall ventrally back into its normal position within the spinal canal.

Attention can then be directed to the scar fixed to the dorsal surface of the cord. This maneuver should be performed last, only after all of the nerve roots have been identified and dissected free. This is the point of maximum risk of injury to the underlying cord. This dorsal nonneural mass should then be separated sharply and removed. Once the neural placode is completely free and untethered, the wound should be carefully inspected for any other abnormalities before attention is turned toward the closure. As with the initial repair, a watertight dural closure is important. A dural graft is sometimes required to achieve a primary dural closure.

SURGICAL REWIND

My Worst Cases

Cerebrospinal Fluid Leak

A full-term infant male was born with a wide upper lumbar myelomeningocele that was significantly elevated relative to the level of the surrounding skin (Fig. 31.3). Preoperative workup including scoliosis x-rays confirmed a significant kyphotic deformity (Fig. 31.4). The patient was taken to the operating room (OR) for myelomeningocele repair. The placode was imbricated and the dura mobilized and closed primarily without difficulty. However, due to the kyphotic deformity, the neural elements and dural sac remained significantly proud relative to the level of the skin. Kerrison punches and rongeurs were used to remove the remaining hypoplastic, splayed lamina and pedicles bilaterally, resulting in a shallow spinal canal. Due to the wide defect, the paraspinal musculature was attenuated and could not be mobilized without significantly compressing the neural elements.

Despite adequate dural closure and partially because of the attenuated skin closure, a CSF leak was seen on the third postoperative day. EVD was placed to allow wound healing of the attenuated soft-tissue closure. The patient did not require return to the OR for wound revision, but he did undergo placement of VP shunt after the wound was appropriately healed.

Retethering

A 12-year-old male child who had undergone myelomeningocele repair shortly after birth at an outside institution presented to our spina bifida clinic with progressive lower-extremity weakness and worsening gait. Neurologic examination was notable for asymmetric lower-extremity function with intact toe flexion and extension on the right but only iliopsoas and quadriceps function on the left. Physical examination was notable for a well-healed midline incision with hypertrichosis (Fig. 31.5). Computed tomographic myelogram demonstrated a complex split cord with the myelomeningocele occurring on the left hemicord and the right hemicord folded under but with recognizable neural anatomy (Fig. 31.6).

Patient was taken to the OR for exploration and tethered cord release. Intraoperative findings confirmed imaging findings of hemimyelia. The bony median septum was rotated, making its excision difficult. The dural sleeve between the two hemicords was removed down to the level of the ventral dural floor. A thickened filum terminale was identified and sectioned on the left hemicord.

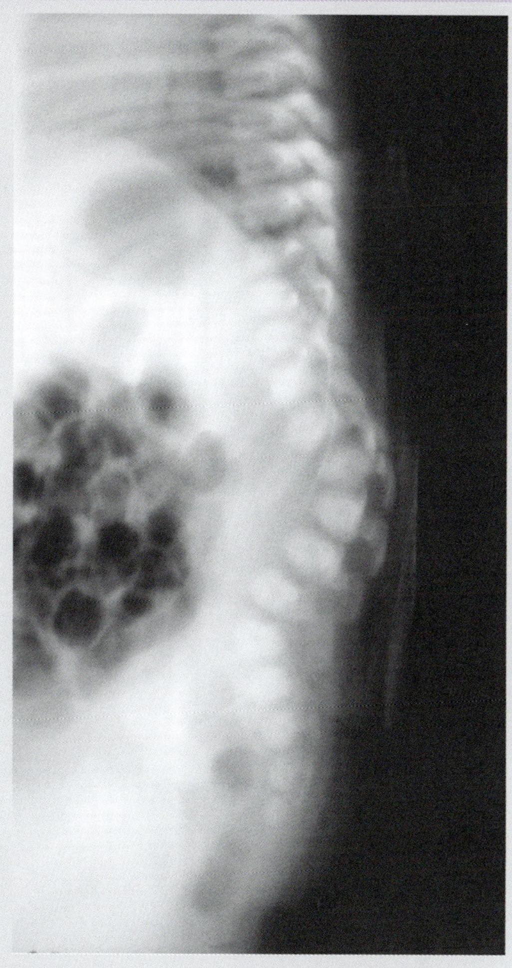

• **Fig. 31.4** Lateral x-ray demonstrating kyphotic deformity in patient with myelomeningocele.

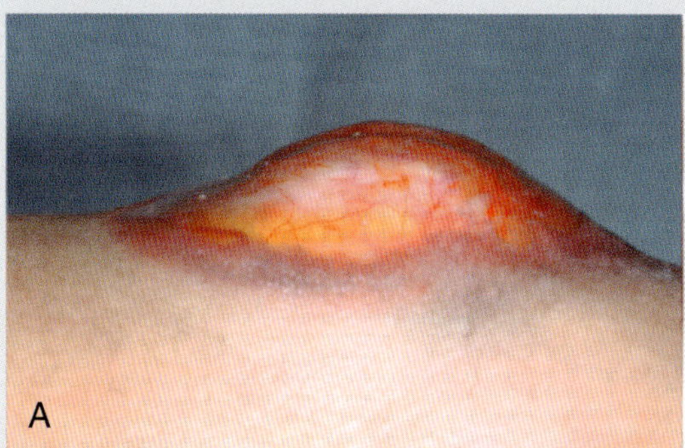

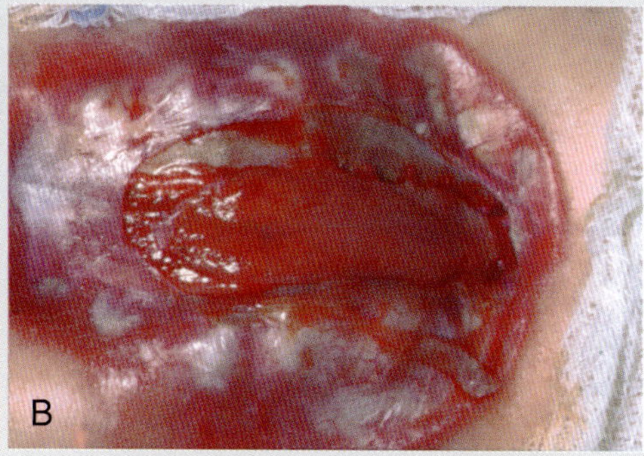

• **Fig. 31.3** Lateral view (A), and overhead view (B), of myelomeningocele with significant kyphotic deformity.

Continued

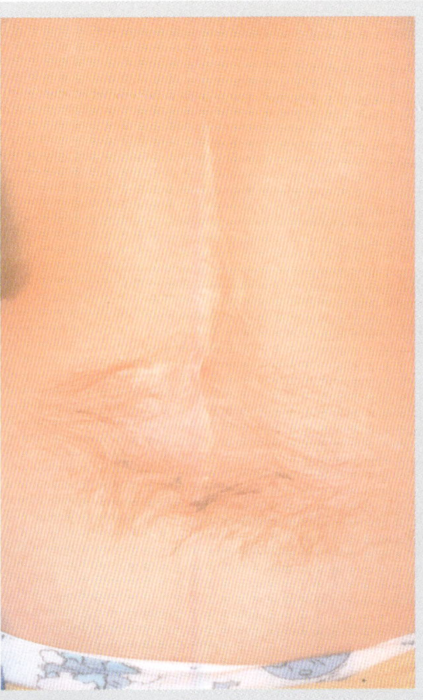

• **Fig. 31.5** 12-year-old male who had undergone myelomeningocele repair at birth at outside institution who presents with neurologic deterioration. Focal hirsutism suggests presence of split cord malformation (hemimyelia).

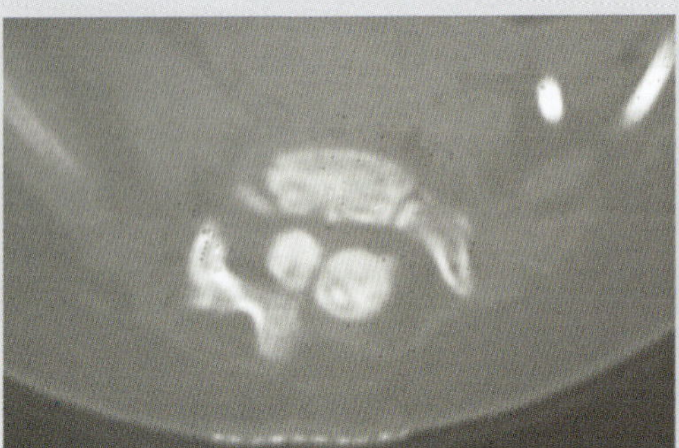

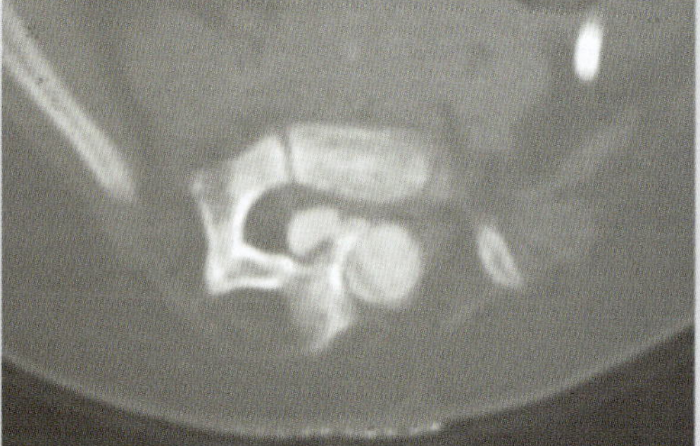

• **Fig. 31.6** Computed tomographic myelogram demonstrating split cord malformation with two hemicords and hemimyelia on the left side. The bony septum is deviated to the left, resulting in the right hemicord being slightly more ventral to the left hemicord within the spinal canal. This slight rotation can make it very difficult to identify a split cord malformation intraoperatively.

NEUROSURGICAL SELFIE MOMENT

CSF leaks and retethering are among the more common complications after myelomeningocele repair. Care taken during the initial repair can help minimize complications as well as make future operations less challenging. CSF diversion is the key to management of CSF leaks. Treatment of secondary tethering is indicated if clinical symptoms are significant enough that benefits outweigh risks of tethered cord release.

References

1. Parker SE, Mai CT, Canfield MA, et al. Updated national birth prevalence estimates for selected birth defects in the United States, 2004–2006. *Birth Defects Res A Clin Mol Teratol.* 2010;88(12):1008–1016.
2. Mattogno PP, Massimi L, Tamburrini G, et al. Myelomeningocele repair: surgical management based on a 30-year experience. *Acta Neurochir Suppl.* 2017;124:143–148.
3. Caldarelli M, Rocco CD. Myelomeningocele primary repair surgical technique. In: Özek MM, Cinalli G, Maixner WJ, eds. *The Spina Bifida: Management and Outcome.* Milano: Springer Milan; 2008: 143–155.
4. Pang D. Surgical complications of open spinal dysraphism. *Neurosurg Clin N Am.* 1995;6(2):243–257.
5. Akalan N. Myelomeningocele (open spina bifida) - surgical management. *Adv Tech Stand Neurosurg.* 2011;37:113–141.
6. McLone DG, Dias MS. Complications of myelomeningocele closure. *Pediatr Neurosurg.* 1991;17(5):267–273.
7. Danzer E, Adzick NS, Rintoul NE, et al. Intradural inclusion cysts following in utero closure of myelomeningocele: clinical implications and follow-up findings. *J Neurosurg Pediatr.* 2008;2(6): 406–413.

8. Iskandar BJ, McLaughlin C, Oakes WJ. Split cord malformations in myelomeningocele patients. *Br J Neurosurg*. 2000;14(3):200–203.
9. Mehta VA, Bettegowda C, Ahmadi SA, et al. Spinal cord tethering following myelomeningocele repair. *J Neurosurg Pediatr*. 2010;6(5): 498–505.
10. Herman JM, McLone DG, Storrs BB, et al. Analysis of 153 patients with myelomeningocele or spinal lipoma reoperated upon for a tethered cord. Presentation, management and outcome. *Pediatr Neurosurg*. 1993;19(5):243–249.
11. Caldarelli M, Boscarelli A, Massimi L. Recurrent tethered cord: radiological investigation and management. *Childs Nerv Syst*. 2013;29(9):1601–1609.

32 Complications of Various Treatment Options for Trigeminal Neuralgia

ANIL NANDA, DEVI PRASAD PATRA

HIGHLIGHTS

- Complications after treatment of trigeminal neuralgias are rare, but they are debilitating when they occur.
- Facial numbness and masseter weakness are common complications after all treatment modalities.
- Stereotactic radiosurgery is least invasive and is associated with fewer complications but with higher recurrence rates.
- Microvascular decompression is invasive but is associated with fewer complications and higher success rates.

Introduction

Trigeminal neuralgia (TN) is a chronic debilitating disease characterized by paroxysmal lancinating pain along the distribution of trigeminal nerve. Compression at the root entry zone (REZ) of the trigeminal nerve is the most common proposed pathogenesis, but a definite compression may not be found in a large subset of patients. Historically, section of the nerve at the extracranial location was the most commonly practiced method to alleviate the pain, but it was associated with complete loss of nerve function. Over the years, multiple treatment methods have evolved, including various percutaneous ablation methods [retrogasserian glycerol rhizotomy (RGR), balloon compression rhizotomy (BCR), radiofrequency rhizotomy (RFR)], stereotactic radiosurgery (SRS), and microvascular decompression (MVD). All the treatment methods have been compared with one another and have their own merits and demerits. Ablation methods are less invasive, but the overall efficacy depends on the size of the lesion created during the ablation procedure; therefore adequate pain relief is associated with a greater degree of facial numbness and keratitis. SRS is least invasive but requires a longer time for pain relief and is associated with a higher recurrence rate. MVD relieves the compression at the REZ and hence is associated with immediate pain relief; therefore it is considered the most effective and gold standard modality. However, it requires a craniotomy and general anesthesia with the associated risks and complications. Recently, less invasive methods have been developed, including endoscope-assisted MVD, which requires a small burr hole for the whole procedure; however, it is still associated with the complications related to microsurgery itself.

Complications After Treatment of Trigeminal Neuralgia

The complication profiles for each procedure are different and are related to the approach and technical details. However, few complications are common for each procedure and are better discussed collectively and comparatively.

Complications Common to Each Treatment Method

The trigeminal nerve is a mixed nerve carrying both sensory and motor nerve fibers. The sensory nerve fibers include pathways carrying pain as well as touch and proprioception. The mechanism of pain relief in all the treatment modalities except MVD involves the manipulation of the nerve conduction by producing lesions to ablate the pain pathway using different methods. Therefore all these methods are expected to produce some degree of nerve dysfunction that involves not only pain pathway but also other sensory and motor function. MVD essentially relieves the compression at the REZ by separating the offending artery or vein from the trigeminal nerve. Direct manipulation of the nerve is usually avoided, though many surgeons prefer some degree of nerve massaging for optimal pain relief. Therefore the incidence of nerve dysfunction is much less with MVD.

Sensory Dysfunction

The rates of postoperative dysesthesia are mostly comparable among the three percutaneous ablation methods. The rate of dysesthesia after BCR ranges from 1.5% to 19% and is related to the compression time.[1–5] Similar rates have been reported after RFR (1%–15.2%).[1,6–11] Facial numbness is considered as a predictor of pain relief after RGR, and some degree of sensory loss is always expected for an adequate pain relief. Most of the series have reported dysesthesia in the range of 1% to 11.7%[1,12]; however, a few series have reported much higher rates (49%–53%).[13,14] Corneal hypoesthesia is a common complication after RFR because the V1 segment is mostly targeted during the ablation. Corneal complications can occur in 1% to 20% of patients after RFR.[1,6–8] Though similar rates are observed after RGR (0%–16%), this complication is particularly rare after BCR (nearly 0%).[10] This is due to the observation that balloon compression selectively spares the small fibers carrying the corneal reflex. Pain over the area of numbness, also called anesthesia dolorosa, is fairly common after RFR. In a series of 1600 patients of TN treated by RFR by Kanpolat et al., this was the most common complication encountered, occurring in as many as 12% of cases.[8] However, anesthesia dolorosa is rare after RGR (0%–5%) and BCR (0%–0.6%).

Sensory dysfunction is the most common complication after SRS and is related to the radiation dose and location of the isocenter. The rates of sensory dysfunction range from 6% to 42% among most of the series.[15–23] A higher radiation dose is thought to be associated with higher rates of sensory dysfunction. In a study by Pollock et al., sensory dysfunction was noted in more than half of the patients who received 90 Gy, which dropped to 15% in patients receiving 70 Gy.[19] Similarly, facial numbness is more common when the target is closer to the brainstem. In a study by Xu et al., the rate of facial numbness in patients with a proximal target was significantly higher (53%) than in those with distal targets (25%).[24] Postoperative anesthesia dolorosa is rare after SRS and reported only in less than 1% of cases.[18,23,25] MVD is associated with the least incidence of facial numbness.[20,26] In the largest series of 1204 patients by Barker et al., only 11 (0.01%) patients developed severe facial numbness after first surgery[27]; however, there was an increase in rate to 0.08% (11 of 132 patients) in patients undergoing reoperation. In a recent study, Theodros et al. reported facial numbness in up to 1% of their surgically treated patients.[28]

Motor Dysfunction

The most common motor dysfunctions after treatment of TNs are diplopia and masseter weakness. Diplopia occurs in 0% to 3% of patients after BCR, which is a little higher than for RFR (0%–0.8%). Similarly, the rates of masseter weakness are higher after BCR and RFR, ranging from 3% to 29% and 6.2% to 33%, respectively. In a prospective study of 105 patients, the rate of mandibular weakness was as high as 50% after BCR.[29] RGR is thought to be associated with less motor nerve dysfunction, with rates of diplopia and masseter nerve dysfunction being 0% to 0.2% and 0% to 4%, respectively.[1,12,30,31] Motor weakness after SRS or MVD is extremely rare and has been reported in less than 1% of cases.[27,28,32]

Complications Specific to Each Treatment Method

Percutaneous Ablation Procedures

The percutaneous procedures are associated with complications inherent to their techniques. The usual site of access in all three type of percutaneous procedures is the foramen ovale, which is surrounded by important neurovascular structures. All the access methods are landmark based and are relatively blind; therefore they can be associated with disastrous complications. Puncture of the internal carotid artery in the neck or in the skull base can lead to neck hematoma or internal carotid artery dissection. Similarly, inadvertent puncture of the jugular foramen, which lies just posterolateral to foramen ovale, can lead to venous bleeding and cranial nerve palsies. Other possible complications are reactivation of herpes labialis, subdural hematoma (venous injury), occlusion of cavernous sinus, ocular motor nerve palsies (cannulation of superior orbital fissure or nerve injury at the ganglion), optic nerve injury leading to blindness,[33] and brainstem injury.[34] Sudden cardiac arrest may occur during engagement of foramen ovale and has been reported in two patients.[3] Meningitis is another serious complication after percutaneous accesses and has been reported in up to 6% of cases in some series.[35] Mortality during the procedure is rare and has been reported in only two cases of BCR.[36,37] One patient developed hemorrhage after puncture of the arteriovenous fistula, and the other developed brainstem hematoma.

Stereotactic Radiosurgery

SRS is one of the safest treatment options for TN. Acute complications apart from frame-related complications are rare and mostly due to the immediate effect of radiation on the brainstem. Higher doses on the brainstem may produce brainstem edema, which may be prevented in some cases with the use of steroids. Delayed parenchymal changes applicable to any radiosurgery, including postradiation malignancy and vascular occlusion, are also potential complications.

Microvascular Decompression

MVD is one of the safest, albeit invasive, procedures in microneurosurgery. Complications after MVD have been dramatically reduced over the years, with the lowest rates reported in high-volume centers.[38] Specific complications may include cranial nerve dysfunctions during manipulation of the nerves in the cerebellopontine angle. Some degree of hearing loss is not infrequent after MVD; in most cases it is due to conductive impairment secondary to fluid ingression into the middle ear cavity through the mastoid bone.[26] This hearing problem is transient and improves over 2 to 3 weeks. Sensory neural hearing loss is troublesome and should call for more attention. It is the possible result of retraction injury of the cochlear nerve or may be secondary to vasospasm of the anterior inferior cerebellar artery (AICA) during separation of the vessel. Facial nerve paresis, tinnitus, and vertigo are the other few reported cranial nerve complications.[27] Another important complication during surgery is venous bleeding while coagulating the petrosal vein or venous loop over the trigeminal nerve. Though not frequent, the bleeding can sometimes be troublesome and can lead to postoperative cerebellar or brainstem edema. Injury to the transverse or sigmoid sinus during craniotomy and cerebellar contusion during retraction are some important avoidable intraoperative complications. Postoperative complications include cerebrospinal fluid (CSF) leak, wound infection, and CSF rhinorrhea.

RED FLAGS

- Percutaneous treatment: indistinct radiologic landmarks, skull base anomalies, abnormal curvature of extracranial internal carotid artery
- SRS: no specific risk factors; short cisternal segment of trigeminal nerve may pose problem in appropriate fixing of target
- Microvascular surgery: previous radiosurgery, previous MVD, vascular malformation in the cerebellopontine angle
- Previous medical therapy (especially prolonged dopamine agonist therapy)
- Lesions invading the cavernous sinus

Prevention

Most complications during the treatment of TN can be easily prevented.

Percutaneous Procedures

Proper identification of the landmarks is essential for safe percutaneous approaches. High-quality multiplanar fluoroscopy aids in identification of right trajectory. In BCR, the most important factors that affect the complication profile are the compression pressure and compression time. Brown et al. in their study have defined the ideal compression pressure to be 750 to 1250 mm Hg for 1.15 minutes.[35] A compression time of less than 1 minute is usually advised to decrease complications with adequate pain relief. Similarly, the complication profile in RFR depends on the area of target; therefore accurate mapping should decrease the complication rate. Karol and Karol have developed a quadripolar electrode that improves the accuracy of somatotropic mapping and thereby reduces the lesion size to 1.5 × 3 mm.[39] Such an effort translated into an improved patient outcome with a significant decrease in complications. In RGR, both pain relief and postoperative numbness depend on the volume of the glycerol injected, so accurate volume calculation is helpful in producing desired pain relief in a specific trigeminal division.

Stereotactic Radiosurgery

As already discussed, a precise treatment plan with a target at the REZ is necessary for adequate pain relief after SRS. Utilizing the optimal dose plan with rapid dose falloff at the brainstem is another prerequisite to prevent unnecessary complications. Most of the centers use 70 to 85 Gy in a single isocenter using a 4-mm collimator. A larger target volume or increased radiation time does not appear to benefit in terms of pain relief but may have definite adverse effects.

Microvascular Decompression

MVD is mostly a straightforward surgery and should not give rise to complications if done meticulously using standard precautions. Adequate CSF release after craniotomy should provide adequate relaxation of the cerebellum, so a very gentle retraction is all that is needed to get the view of the cerebellopontine angle. Sharp arachnoid dissection usually makes the separation of the offending vessel easier. Care should be taken to avoid unnecessary manipulation of the arteries and coagulation of the cerebellar veins. Venous bleedings can usually be controlled with minimal pressure over cottonoids. In the presence of obvious compression, the trigeminal nerve should not be manipulated unnecessarily, and only separation of the vessel and placement of Teflon balls is required. In the absence of the definite compression, some degree of nerve massage may be tried. Finally, appropriate obliteration of the mastoid air cells with bone wax and meticulous wound closure is essential to prevent postoperative wound complications and CSF rhinorrhea.

SURGICAL REWIND

My Worst Cases

Case 1 (Fig. 32.1)

A 70-year-old female patient with a prior history of MVD and SRS for TN presented with recurrent pain. Repeat MVD was planned, and the patient was operated through the previous craniotomy. Intraoperatively, there was some fibrosis of the arachnoid because of the previous surgery and radiation, and the dissection was difficult. The petrosal vein was adhered to the trigeminal nerve, and attempted release of the vein led to avulsion of the vein from the base, resulting in troublesome bleeding. However, we could control the bleeding with pressure application using cottonoids over shredded cellulose and Teflon. Postoperatively, the patient did well and had no complication related to the event.

Case 2 (Fig. 32.2)

A 68-year-old male patient with a prior history of SRS underwent MVD because of recurrent pain. Postoperatively, the patient had a CSF leak from the wound, which subsided after a lumbar drain was put in. However, on the follow-up office visit, he had fluctuant swelling over the incision site suggestive of pseudomeningocele. A lumboperitoneal shunt was subsequently placed, and there was resolution of the swelling with symptomatic relief.

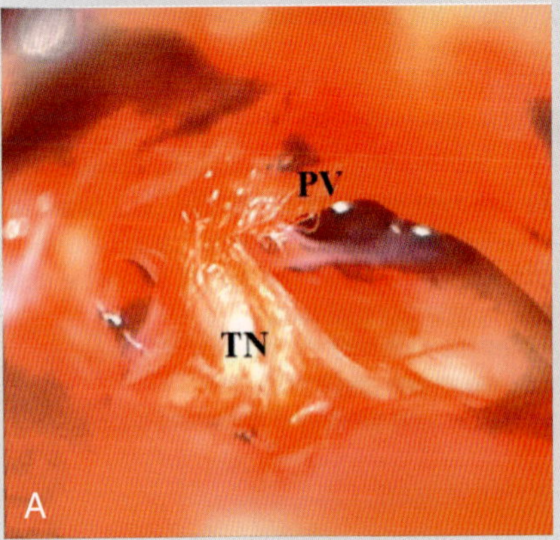

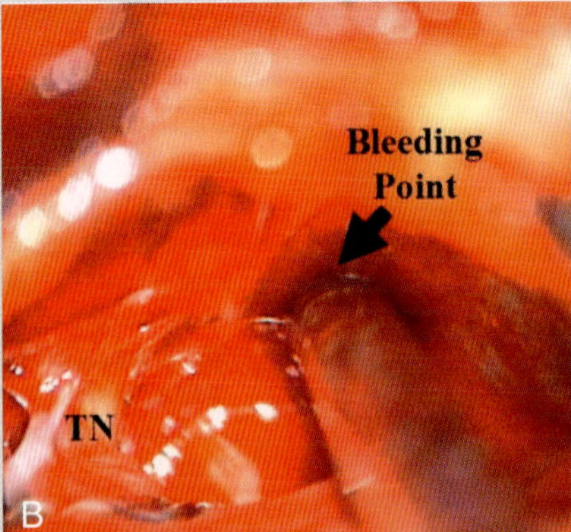

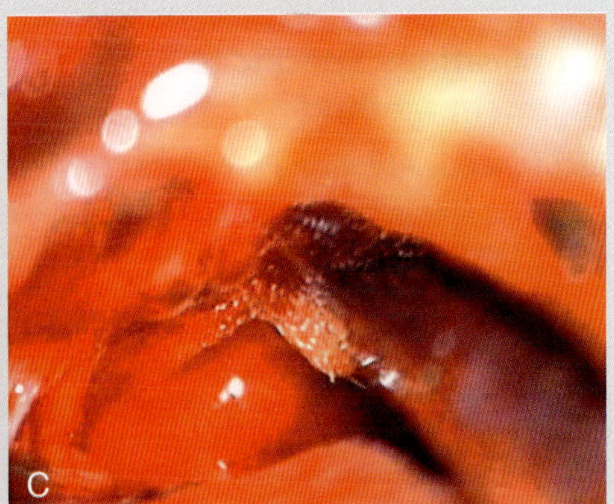

• **Fig. 32.1** Intraoperative picture showing (A) the trigeminal nerve and the petrosal vein in relation to it. Note the thickened arachnoid and adhesions. (B) Bleeding from the petrosal vein at its attachment to the petrous bone. (C) Bleeding is being controlled with pressure over a cottonoid and oxidized cellulose balls. *TN,* Trigeminal nerve; *PV,* petrosal vein.

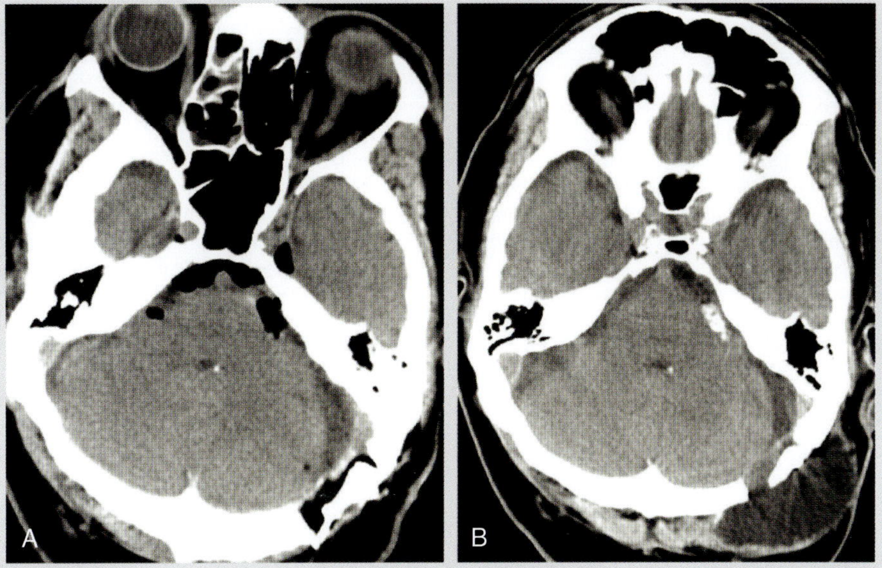

• **Fig. 32.2** Computed tomography scans: (A) Immediate postoperative scan showing the craniotomy defect and the bone flap in situ. (B) Follow-up scan showing fluid collection under the skin flap suggestive of pseudomeningocele.

NEUROSURGICAL SELFIE MOMENT

Complications after treatment of TNs are not infrequent and should be carefully discussed with the patient during treatment planning. A few complications like facial numbness and weakness are common but can be decreased to a significant extent. Many of the serious complications specific to each procedure are avoidable. MVD and SRS, the most common procedures performed, should be carefully selected for individual patients because of their different complication profiles.

References

1. Fraioli B, Esposito V, Guidetti B, Cruccu G, Manfredi M. Treatment of trigeminal neuralgia by thermocoagulation, glycerolization, and percutaneous compression of the gasserian ganglion and/or retrogasserian rootlets: long-term results and therapeutic protocol. *Neurosurgery*. 1989;24(2):239–245.
2. Lobato RD, Rivas JJ, Sarabia R, Lamas E. Percutaneous microcompression of the gasserian ganglion for trigeminal neuralgia. *J Neurosurg*. 1990;72(4):546–553.
3. Skirving DJ, Dan NG. A 20-year review of percutaneous balloon compression of the trigeminal ganglion. *J Neurosurg*. 2001;94(6):913–917.
4. Chen JF, Tu PH, Lee ST. Long-term follow-up of patients treated with percutaneous balloon compression for trigeminal neuralgia in Taiwan. *World Neurosurg*. 2011;76(6):586–591.
5. Abdennebi B, Guenane L. Technical considerations and outcome assessment in retrogasserian balloon compression for treatment of trigeminal neuralgia. Series of 901 patients. *Surg Neurol Int*. 2014;5:118.
6. Frank F, Fabrizi AP. Percutaneous surgical treatment of trigeminal neuralgia. *Acta Neurochir (Wien)*. 1989;97(3–4):128–130.
7. Broggi G, Franzini A, Lasio G, Giorgi C, Servello D. Long-term results of percutaneous retrogasserian thermorhizotomy for "essential" trigeminal neuralgia: considerations in 1000 consecutive patients. *Neurosurgery*. 1990;26(5):783–786, discussion 786-787.
8. Kanpolat Y, Savas A, Bekar A, Berk C. Percutaneous controlled radiofrequency trigeminal rhizotomy for the treatment of idiopathic trigeminal neuralgia: 25-year experience with 1,600 patients. *Neurosurgery*. 2001;48(3):524–532, discussion 532-524.
9. Cheng JS, Lim DA, Chang EF, Barbaro NM. A review of percutaneous treatments for trigeminal neuralgia. *Neurosurgery*. 2014;10(suppl 1):25–33, discussion 33.
10. Wang JY, Bender MT, Bettegowda C. Percutaneous procedures for the treatment of trigeminal neuralgia. *Neurosurg Clin N Am*. 2016;27(3):277–295.
11. Ko AL, Burchiel KJ. Percutaneous procedures for trigeminal neuralgia. In: Winn HR, ed. *Youmans and Winn Neurological Surgery*. Vol. 2. 7th ed. Philadelphia, PA: Elsevier, Inc; 2017:5463–5476.
12. Saini SS. Reterogasserian anhydrous glycerol injection therapy in trigeminal neuralgia: observations in 552 patients. *J Neurol Neurosurg Psychiatry*. 1987;50(11):1536–1538.
13. Pollock BE. Percutaneous retrogasserian glycerol rhizotomy for patients with idiopathic trigeminal neuralgia: a prospective analysis of factors related to pain relief. *J Neurosurg*. 2005;102(2):223–228.
14. Blomstedt PC, Bergenheim AT. Technical difficulties and perioperative complications of retrogasserian glycerol rhizotomy for trigeminal neuralgia. *Stereotact Funct Neurosurg*. 2002;79(3–4):168–181.
15. Regis J, Tuleasca C, Resseguier N, et al. Long-term safety and efficacy of Gamma Knife surgery in classical trigeminal neuralgia: a 497-patient historical cohort study. *J Neurosurg*. 2016;124(4):1079–1087.
16. Lucas JT Jr, Nida AM, Isom S, et al. Predictive nomogram for the durability of pain relief from Gamma Knife radiation surgery in the treatment of trigeminal neuralgia. *Int J Radiat Oncol Biol Phys*. 2014;89(1):120–126.
17. Marshall K, Chan MD, McCoy TP, et al. Predictive variables for the successful treatment of trigeminal neuralgia with Gamma Knife radiosurgery. *Neurosurgery*. 2012;70(3):566–572, discussion 572-563.
18. Verheul JB, Hanssens PE, Lie ST, Leenstra S, Piersma H, Beute GN. Gamma Knife surgery for trigeminal neuralgia: a review of 450 consecutive cases. *J Neurosurg*. 2010;113(suppl):160–167.
19. Pollock BE, Phuong LK, Foote RL, Stafford SL, Gorman DA. High-dose trigeminal neuralgia radiosurgery associated with increased risk of trigeminal nerve dysfunction. *Neurosurgery*. 2001;49(1):58–62, discussion 62-54.

20. Nanda A, Javalkar V, Zhang S, Ahmed O. Long term efficacy and patient satisfaction of microvascular decompression and Gamma Knife radiosurgery for trigeminal neuralgia. *J Clin Neurosci.* 2015; 22(5):818–822.
21. Jawahar A, Wadhwa R, Berk C, et al. Assessment of pain control, quality of life, and predictors of success after Gamma Knife surgery for the treatment of trigeminal neuralgia. *Neurosurg Focus.* 2005;18(5):E8.
22. Shaya M, Jawahar A, Caldito G, Sin A, Willis BK, Nanda A. Gamma Knife radiosurgery for trigeminal neuralgia: a study of predictors of success, efficacy, safety, and outcome at LSUHSC. *Surg Neurol.* 2004;61(6):529–534, discussion 534–525.
23. Xu Z, Sheehan JP. Stereotactic radiosurgery for trigeminal neuralgia. In: Winn HR, ed. *Youmans and Winn Neurological Surgery.* Vol. 2. 7th ed. Philadelphia, PA: Elsevier, Inc; 2017:5486–5498.
24. Xu Z, Schlesinger D, Moldovan K, et al. Impact of target location on the response of trigeminal neuralgia to stereotactic radiosurgery. *J Neurosurg.* 2014;120(3):716–724.
25. Kondziolka D, Zorro O, Lobato-Polo J, et al. Gamma Knife stereotactic radiosurgery for idiopathic trigeminal neuralgia. *J Neurosurg.* 2010;112(4):758–765.
26. Miller JP, Burchiel KJ. Microvascular decompression for trigeminal neuralgia. In: Winn HR, ed. *Youmans and Winn Neurological Surgery.* Vol. 2. 7th ed. Philadelphia, PA: Elsevier, Inc; 2017:5506–5518.
27. Barker FG 2nd, Jannetta PJ, Bissonette DJ, Larkins MV, Jho HD. The long-term outcome of microvascular decompression for trigeminal neuralgia. *N Engl J Med.* 1996;334(17):1077–1083.
28. Theodros D, Rory Goodwin C, Bender MT, et al. Efficacy of primary microvascular decompression versus subsequent microvascular decompression for trigeminal neuralgia. *J Neurosurg.* 2017;126(5):1691–1697.
29. de Siqueira SR, da Nobrega JC, de Siqueira JT, Teixeira MJ. Frequency of postoperative complications after balloon compression for idiopathic trigeminal neuralgia: prospective study. *Oral Surg Oral Med Oral Pathol Oral Radiol Endod.* 2006;102(5):e39–e45.
30. Bender M, Pradilla G, Batra S, et al. Effectiveness of repeat glycerol rhizotomy in treating recurrent trigeminal neuralgia. *Neurosurgery.* 2012;70(5):1125–1133, discussion 1133–1124.
31. Steiger HJ. Prognostic factors in the treatment of trigeminal neuralgia. Analysis of a differential therapeutic approach. *Acta Neurochir (Wien).* 1991;113(1–2):11–17.
32. Wolf A, Kondziolka D. Gamma Knife Surgery in trigeminal neuralgia. *Neurosurg Clin N Am.* 2016;27(3):297–304.
33. Agazzi S, Chang S, Drucker MD, Youssef AS, Van Loveren HR. Sudden blindness as a complication of percutaneous trigeminal procedures: mechanism analysis and prevention. *J Neurosurg.* 2009;110(4):638–641.
34. Bergenheim AT, Asplund P, Linderoth B. Percutaneous retrogasserian balloon compression for trigeminal neuralgia: review of critical technical details and outcomes. *World Neurosurg.* 2013;79(2):359–368.
35. Brown JA, McDaniel MD, Weaver MT. Percutaneous trigeminal nerve compression for treatment of trigeminal neuralgia: results in 50 patients. *Neurosurgery.* 1993;32(4):570–573.
36. Abdennebi B, Mahfouf L, Nedjahi T. Long-term results of percutaneous compression of the gasserian ganglion in trigeminal neuralgia (series of 200 patients). *Stereotact Funct Neurosurg.* 1997;68(1–4 Pt 1):190–195.
37. Brown JA, Pilitsis JG. Percutaneous balloon compression for the treatment of trigeminal neuralgia: results in 56 patients based on balloon compression pressure monitoring. *Neurosurg Focus.* 2005;18(5):E10.
38. Kalkanis SN, Eskandar EN, Carter BS, Barker FG 2nd. Microvascular decompression surgery in the United States, 1996 to 2000: mortality rates, morbidity rates, and the effects of hospital and surgeon volumes. *Neurosurgery.* 2003;52(6):1251–1261, discussion 1261–1252.
39. Karol EA, Karol MN. A multiarray electrode mapping method for percutaneous thermocoagulation as treatment of trigeminal neuralgia. Technical note on a series of 178 consecutive procedures. *Surg Neurol.* 2009;71(1):11–17, discussion 17-18.

33 Complications of Deep Brain Stimulation (DBS)

PHILIPPE MAGOWN, KIM J. BURCHIEL

Case Report

A 63-year-old man presented on referral from a neurologist specializing in movement disorders, with medically intractable Parkinson disease (PD). The patient had levodopa-induced dyskinesias, rigidity, bradykinesia, freezing, and some rest tremor bilaterally. After neuropsychological, speech and swallowing, and on/off levodopa testing, the patient was considered an appropriate candidate for bilateral deep brain stimulation (DBS) electrode implantation. The target chosen by the neurologist was the subthalamic nucleus (STN). The patient underwent this image-guided procedure in two stages, both under general anesthesia, the first stage being the implantation of the electrodes, and the second stage, the implantation of the internal pulse generator (IPG). The patient did well after these procedures and 3 weeks postoperatively started stimulation with the goal to optimize his DBS system and drug management of his PD symptoms.

His initial response to DBS was encouraging, with resolution of his dyskinesias, more consistent "on time," and a significant reduction in his dosage of Sinemet. However, at approximately 4 months postoperatively, the patient began to develop uncontrolled flailing movements of his left arm. This was concerning for hemiballismus, and the patient underwent high-resolution 1.5T magnetic resonance imaging (MRI) with contrast. This showed what appeared to be a small ring-enhancing lesion around his right STN electrode, with some minimal enhancement around the left STN electrode. Both distal electrodes also appeared to have a much wider surrounding area of T2 hyperintensity, interpreted as "edema." At this time, the patient showed no systemic signs of infection. One week after the development of his hemiballismus, his entire DBS system, including the generator and extension leads, was removed. The patient was initially placed on broad-spectrum cerebrospinal fluid (CSF) penetrating antibiotics, but when the culture from the right electrode tip yielded *Propionibacterium acnes*, the regimen was simplified to just vancomycin. He was treated with a 3-week course of parenteral vancomycin and then observed off antibiotics for 6 weeks. His hemiballismus stabilized but did not improve, and he developed no additional neurologic deficits. Two months after the explant of his DBS system, his entire system was replaced, this time using a globus pallidus internus (GPI) target bilaterally. GPI DBS alleviated his left arm hemiballismus as well as his dyskinesias and other cardinal symptoms of PD. Over the course of two years, he has done well with DBS at this location and has had neither recurrence of his hemiballismus nor signs of recurring infection.

Discussion of the Case Report

This case is illustrative in several ways. First, it highlights what is an uncommon, but serious, complication of DBS implantation, namely infection. Most infections become apparent at the generator site, but rarely, the initial presentation may be at the brain electrode site, with attendant neurologic problems. MRI scanning is the definitive test in these cases because systemic or laboratory signs of infection are insensitive. As discussed below, the treatment for this complication is partial or complete removal of the system, parenteral antibiotics, followed by a short course of oral antibiotics. In this instance, GPI DBS was effectively used to treat a complication of STN damage from the infection: hemiballismus.

Complications of DBS

DBS has become an important therapy for a variety of neurologic conditions, including movement disorders,[1–3] epilepsy,[4] and potentially psychiatric conditions (reviewed by Holtzheimer and Mayberg[5]). For movement disorders in particular, DBS has been proven to be more effective than the best medical therapy at the highest level of evidence.[6,7] Remarkably, complications of DBS surgery have diminished steadily over the past 25 years, yet the classification of DBS complications remains unstandardized. Most of the morbidity of DBS falls into three categories: procedure-related, hardware-related, and stimulation-related complications (adverse events). Surgical complications include intraoperative events and those arising within 30 days of the procedure: cerebrovascular events (strokes), postsurgical edema, seizures, electrode malposition, and miscellaneous complications associated with any surgery. Infections are best classified as hardware-related complications considering that the incidence of infections generally increases with implanted foreign bodies. As such, hardware-related complications include infections and erosions, lead migration, hardware fracture, and electrical malfunction. Stimulation-related complications revolve mainly around so-called "off-target" effects.

Utilizing the following categorization, this chapter will review the current evidence with regard to each of these complications and discuss best practices to avoid these complications. This chapter intentionally leaves aside patient selection and target selection, despite both being fundamentally important in the success of DBS therapy.[8]

1. **Procedure-related complications:**
   a. Stroke
      i. Intracerebral hemorrhage (ICH)
      ii. Nonhemorrhagic transient or permanent neurologic deficit
         1. Ischemic infarction
         2. Venous infarction
         3. Postsurgical edema
         4. Seizures
   b. Electrode malposition
2. **Hardware-related complications:**
   a. Infection and skin erosion
   b. Lead migration, lead fracture, and electrical malfunction
3. **Stimulation-related complications:**
   a. Off-target effects

Procedure-Related Complications

Stroke

Intracerebral Hemorrhage

Perhaps the most devastating complication of DBS electrode implantation is ICH resulting in permanent neurologic deficit(s). Fortunately, the incidence of symptomatic ICH is low, ranging from 0.7% to 3.9% per lead with a permanent neurologic morbidity of up to 1.1%[9,10] and a very low mortality risk of 0.4% or less.[11–13]

Systematic reviews of surgical risk for DBS have reported ICH rates of 3.2% to 5%.[12–14] The risk of ICH is related to the use of microelectrode recording (MER), the number of MER penetrations, and a sulcal or transventricular course of the electrodes.[15] The bulk of the evidence indicates that making multiple instrumented passes into the brain with a microelectrode for recording contributes to the risk of ICH, with the per-trajectory ICH rate estimated at 1.6%.[16] Hypertension further increases the ICH risk by 2.5-fold.[17–21]

ICH related to DBS further divides equally between asymptomatic and symptomatic, 1.9% and 2.1%, respectively. Hemorrhages resulting in permanent deficit or death are estimated at 1.1%.[14] The incidence of hemorrhage in studies adopting an image-guided and image-verified approach without MER was significantly lower than reported with other operative techniques for total number of hemorrhages, asymptomatic and symptomatic hemorrhages, and hemorrhage leading to permanent deficit.[14,22] Although the risk of MER-guided versus image-guided DBS implantation has not been subjected to a randomized controlled trial, multiple studies have shown that there is an associated risk of MER mapping.[14,18,20,23–28] It is also worth emphasizing that MER guidance has *never* been demonstrated to be more effective at target localization than image guidance. Whether MER guidance adds substantively to the efficacy of DBS electrode localization and clinical outcome, to an extent that would justify the risk, remains an unanswered question.[29]

Best Practice

Keeping the number of MER penetrations to a clinically indicated minimum and avoiding sulcal or transventricular electrode trajectories can mitigate the risk of ICH and intraventricular hemorrhage during DBS electrode implantation. Intraoperative hypertension (≥160 mm Hg systolic) has been associated with ICH,[18] so blood pressure must be carefully monitored, particularly in procedures performed under local anesthetic. Postoperative computed tomography (CT) or MRI imaging may be warranted if the patient experiences an unexpected neurologic deficit after implantation.

Full anticoagulation must be reversed (international normalized ratio [INR] ≤1.4) before surgery.[30] Although our practice has been to aim for an INR ≤1.2 for neurosurgical procedures, there is a lack of evidence to support this.[31] Bridge anticoagulant treatment is often not required but may be appropriate in very high risk patients with thromboembolic disorders.[32] So-called "bridging" is usually performed with low-molecular-weight heparin up to 24 hours before the DBS procedure. The timing of the discontinuance of oral anticoagulants must be appropriate to the therapeutic half-life of the drug, typically 4 to 5 days before the surgery. However, each individual case should be carefully assessed for proper timing of discontinuation.[33] Importantly, before DBS implantation, aspirin (ASA) must be discontinued a minimum of 7 to 10 days before surgery.[30,34] However, many institutions, including our own, still prefer to discontinue ASA and other antiplatelet agents 2 weeks before surgery.[35] NSAIDs should be discontinued 3 to 4 days before DBS surgery.[36]

Nonhemorrhagic Transient or Permanent Neurologic Deficit

Probably the most common reason for a postoperative neurologic deficit is ICH. However, some patients do experience temporary or permanent neurologic deterioration, either from cortical or subcortical ischemia, cortical venous infarct, or perielectrode "edema." Ischemic infarcts are rarely reported, ranging from 0.3% to 0.9%.[9,37,38] Cortical venous infarcts can occur in 1.3% of cases, usually becoming symptomatic only during postoperative day 1. A full recovery can be expected in nearly all cases. Most are avoidable by planning the electrode trajectory away from veins and cortical sulci visible on preoperative enhanced MRI.[39]

Most neurologic deficits appear to be due to "edema" along the electrode trajectory or at the DBS target site.[38] The origin(s) of this "edema," revealed in some cases by T2 or FLAIR MRI, is not clear. Symptoms usually occur 1 to 2 days postoperatively, whereas the edema might take on average 1 month to resolve.[40] The incidence of MRI signal changes along the electrode trajectory has been estimated around 6.3%, with the majority of cases being asymptomatic.[41] Possibilities include mechanical tissue disruption from passing the insertion cannula(s), DBS electrodes, or microelectrodes. Rarely, this swelling can be indicative of cerebritis, or deep infection, although this complication is rare.[42] Furthermore, if a patient exhibits a neurologic deficit in the immediate perioperative interval and no ICH can be demonstrated, it is highly unlikely that the deficit relates to an infectious etiology.

Seizures can happen around the time of electrode implantation. A metaanalysis has reported a rate of 2.4% occurring acutely within 24 to 48 hours and 0.5% chronically.[43] An abnormal postoperative imaging study demonstrating a hemorrhage, ischemia, or edema increases the risk of seizures by 30- to 50-fold.[44]

Best Practice

Cortical veins should be avoided especially if visualized during planning on preoperative MRI. In the face of limited understanding regarding the trajectory of swelling and infarction, it is difficult to recommend a best practice. Given the relative infrequency of unexpected neurologic deficits not related to ICH, it is tempting to argue that this problem is related to some intrinsic property of the patient's brain, such as microvascular disease, gliosis, plaque formation, or amyloid angiopathy. It is certainly conceivable that preoperative corticosteroid administration might mitigate symptomatic edema, but this would need to be confirmed with a prospective study. Again, minimizing the number of penetrations may also minimize this complication, but this remains unproven. Clearly, further investigations of this phenomenon are imperative.

Malposition of Electrodes

The fundamental goal of DBS surgery is to accurately implant each electrode precisely at the desired target. In practice there is a fair degree of variance with regard to the "best target" for STN, GPI, and ventral intermediate nucleus (VIM). In the final analysis, the best electrode location is defined by the patient's clinical outcome and tolerance for off-target effects.

Malpositioned electrodes are infrequently reported. Even a previous literature review encompassing large trials in PD revealed only a 1.6% rate of misplaced electrodes.[12,37,45] Many factors can lead to electrode malposition: a misaligned stereotactic frame, instability of the frame, incorrect interpretation of MER, or intracranial air with intraoperative brain shift. Perhaps an underappreciated cause of lead misplacement is lead "deflection," possibly due to variations in tissue density along the planned path of the electrode, the coronal angle of the trajectory, or superficial collision of the insertion cannula with either the burr hole edges or the dura. It is interesting that larger numbers of patients are being referred to specialized centers for second opinions after poor clinical DBS effects.[46] Consequently, malposition rates may, in fact, be systematically underestimated in the literature. Indeed, a recent review of both CMS (Centers for Medicare & Medicaid Services), and NSQIP (National Surgical Quality Improvement Program) data revealed that somewhere between 15.2% and 34% of DBS electrode placements are removed or revised.[47] The authors estimated that up to 48.5% of revisions may have been due to improper targeting, or to lack of therapeutic effect. Similar findings have also been shown on multiple occasions by another group.[8,46] Together, these reports make the point that we need to understand the true prevalence and nature of such failures as they occur in the wider surgical community. If these statistics are representative of the degree to which electrodes are malpositioned, this complication *alone* dwarfs all others combined, by an order of magnitude.

Best Practice

The variance in target selection for DBS seems to be inherent in the field at present. No studies have convincingly demonstrated that minor variations in electrode position within a given nucleus result in a clinically significant difference, and opinions continue to dominate discussions. Proprietary targeting seems to be the norm. Electrodes that are clearly outside the target structure are suspect, although targeting the margin of a nucleus may exploit the fact that DBS recruits *axons*, not *neurons*, directly. Off-target effects also limit therapy, and the incidence of these phenomena is not consistently described in the literature.

Once a target has been planned, "off-target" can be defined as greater than a 1- to 2-mm malposition. By comparison, DBS electrodes measure 1.24 mm in diameter. If the average accuracy of DBS electrode placement is within this range, the method for placement can probably be considered "accurate." In a recent study of image-guided DBS electrode placement, we determined the accuracy of placement was "past target" by 1.66 ± 0.76 mm, and "off plan" by 1.44 ± 0.73 mm,[22] which we consider to be within the "acceptable" range of accuracy. Other authors have reached similar conclusions regarding accuracy.[48,49] Whether image guidance or MER guidance offers superior placement accuracy is still being debated, although the value of intraoperative imaging and accurate DBS electrode placement verification before leaving the operating room (OR) seems increasingly to be recognized. In all instances, postimplant imaging confirmation of DBS electrode locations should be performed and correlated with improvement on clinical rating scales.[8]

Hardware-Related Complications

Infection

An infection is the most pernicious of all complications after DBS system implantation. Reported infection rates with DBS range from 0% to 15%,[9,37,38,50] which effectively eclipses all other reported postoperative adverse outcomes. It is difficult to determine an average infection rate that could be considered "standard of care." Nevertheless, the largest available evidence comes from a random effects meta-analysis pooling 3550 patients from 35 studies, averaging 134 patients per study, published between 1997 and 2009[50]; it reports a mean infection rate of 4.7% with a large prediction interval ranging from 0.9% to 22%. In comparison, the largest published population reported an infection rate of 0.4% within 30 days of implantation.[11]

It is unlikely that a "true" infection rate, which could be used as standard of care, will ever be determined. With a binomial distribution, more than 1000 patients treated identically would be required to demonstrate that the "true" infection rate could be around 4.7% ± 1.2%, but the required sample size enlarges as the "true" infection rate decreases. With an infection rate of 0.4%, the sample size would be above 15,000. Similarly, with an average of 134 patients per study, the 95% confidence interval for a "true" infection rate spans from 1.7% to 10.5%, representing the reported infection rate for the majority of published studies and leaving the neurosurgical community with uncertainty as to the "true" infection rate.

Alternatively, an acceptable infection rate could be derived from literature in other specialties where similar devices are implanted. Orthopedic surgery is heavily involved with hardware implantation, and the rates of surgical site infections (SSIs) after hip or knee arthroplasties are around 2.18%.[51] The rate of infections after primary implant for implantable cardiac electronic devices ranges from 0.5% to 0.8%, and 1% to 4% for revisions.[52] One would expect that DBS infection rates closer to these should be achievable.

There is a somewhat artificial distinction being established in the neurosurgical literature regarding "infection" based on the timing of the infection. What is reported as an "infection" presents early (<6 months) with the classic signs and symptoms of SSI: erythema, warmth, pain, with or without purulence or drainage. Later surgical site complications (>6 months) are reported as "erosions" irrespective of a proven primary infection.[53] Erosions are thought to be due to skin breakdown, typically over a prominent generator or connector in an elderly patient with thin and fragile skin. By the time these erosions present clinically, hardware is already exposed and there is *de facto* colonization of the underlying hardware by skin flora. These definitions are somewhat arbitrary. As such, we suggest that we recapitulate the definitions of SSI from the CDC[51,54] and the American College of Surgeons,[55] while incorporating the extensive neurosurgical experience with ventriculoperitoneal (VP) shunts.

The CDC National Healthcare Safety Network classifies SSI based on the depth of the infection and timing of onset.[51,54] Depth is divided into superficial, deep, or involving an organ space. Timing of infection is used as a surrogate to the virulence of the infectious organisms and is divided into early (<3 months), delayed (3–24 months), and late (>24 months). However, these time frames do not fully represent the trend found in neurosurgical implants such as VP shunts. Two thirds of VP shunt infections occur within 30 days, and nearly all infections occur by 12 months.[56] In fact, shunt failures secondary to infection plateau by 3 months, and that plateau remains stable up to 6 months, the latest time point reported.[57] With this in mind, we would suggest that early surgical site complications be composed of superficial infections occurring within 1 month and deep infections occurring within 3 months of surgery. Delayed surgical site complications involve the deep skin tissues and can occur between 3 and 12 months after surgery. Late surgical site complications occur beyond 12 months and are the result of either hematogenous spread of infectious organisms, trauma, or noninfectious erosion. Of note, the American College of Surgeons defines SSI specifically for implants as any infection involving the implanted hardware for the 12 months after implantation,[55] a concept not consistently applied for neurosurgical implants.

Incision dehiscence is obligatorily deep and infected, and these commonly occur within 30 days. Pocket hematomas, which are fortunately rare, fall along an early deep surgical site complication and substantially raise the rate of infection.[58] Erosion without a priori signs of infection are infrequent at 0.48% and most common at the connector site, followed by the pulse generator pocket, and occasionally at the skull-anchoring device.[59]

This classification could provide guidance in managing surgical site complications. In superficial SSI, which occurs only within 30 days of surgery, hardware could be salvaged with an aggressive antibiotic regimen.[50,60] Deep SSIs, early or delayed, require hardware explantation followed by an aggressive antibiotic regimen to salvage the distant hardware left in situ. Late complications, beyond 12 months, may not always be infectious. Certainly, many individuals who are implanted with DBS are older, often with thin and fragile skin along the scalp and chest wall, and many have lost subcutaneous fat. These patients may be prone to simple failure of the skin overlying the implants due to ischemia, pressure, or abrasion. However, once these later erosions present clinically, the distinction is moot because the wound and underlying hardware are now contaminated with skin flora.

Most DBS hardware infections occur at the pocket site, involving the pulse generator in one-third of cases or the lead extensions.[59,61] Luckily, intracranial lead infections with possible intracerebral abscess formation are rare.[42,62] Rates of infection with pulse generator replacement or revision have been reported to be increased by some[63] but not others.[64]

Best Practice

Implantation of DBS electrodes, extensions, and a generator can be performed in one or more stages. The infection risk does not increase with temporary externalized wires.[65–67] The procedure should be performed after screening the patient for nasal methicillin-resistant *Staphylococcus aureus* (MRSA) and completing a decolonization, if timely possible.[55] We recommend an antibacterial shower or cleansing the night before surgery, despite a possible lack of effect on SSI rates.[68] All patients receive a dose of parenteral antibiotics within an hour before skin incision, at each stage.[51,55] We remove hair with a clipper for technical and postoperative hygienic convenience. There is no statistical evidence that hair increases the infection rate, although no study has been specifically done for hardware implantation.[69,70] Surgical sites should be prepped with an alcohol-based chlorhexidine or iodine solution.[71] Although not proven, reopening a recent incision for wire connection is best avoided to reduce the infection rate. The use of water- based or alcohol-based surgical hand antiseptics does not affect the rate of infections.[72] Double-gloving is done for all procedures.[73] Iodinated-adhesive drapes are used only for stage one procedures to cover the fiducials, which get contaminated during the nonsterile registration. There is otherwise no evidence for the use of adhesive drapes.[74]

Irrigation with bacitracin at 10,000 U/L is used to copiously irrigate the wound before closure. A mixture of 200,000 units of polymyxin B and 40 mg of neomycin diluted in saline 1 : 10 (v/v) is distributed in surgical sites after the deep sutures are tied and the wounds are watertight.[75] No antibiotics are administered after surgery in concordance with the lack of evidence supporting a prolonged postoperative antibiotic administration.[51,55]

Topical antibiotics are applied to incisions; the risk to benefit ratio is valuable in our opinion, despite the low level of evidence supporting a number needed to treat of 50.[76] Occlusive dressings are placed over the incisions and not removed for at least 24 hours after surgery,[77] although we prefer to keep the dressing on for 2 days. After this period, the principle of "clean and dry" is followed. We advise our patients to cover the incisions with a waterproof dressing while showering for 2 weeks postimplantation and to wait 4 weeks before submerging the surgical sites.

If the infection or erosion occurs over the generator site, often the DBS leads can be salvaged by first dividing the extensions just distal to the connectors, closing that wound completely, isolating that part of the field (usually behind the ear), and then removing the generator and extension lead segment. Cultures are performed at both the retroauricular connector and chest generator sites. If the retroauricular wound shows growth on culture, the DBS leads, skull anchors, and connectors are subsequently removed. If the culture at the retroauricular connector site shows no growth, the patient is treated with 4 to 6 weeks of parenteral antibiotic based on the bacterial sensitivities obtained from the chest wound. The patient is observed and monitored for recurrent infection for a month post cessation of antibiotics. The patient is then placed on a 10-day course of doxycycline 100 mg per oral twice a day starting on the day of reimplantation of new hardware. The same protocol is observed if the entire system is removed, replacing the entire DBS system only after the treatment regimen and a period of observation.

Lead Migration, Lead Fracture, and Electrical Malfunction

As long as hardware is being implanted, some will eventually break or malfunction. This is to be expected because hardware can be subjected to repetitive movements, stretching, and even trauma. A rough estimate would be 8% per lead-year,[12] keeping in mind that most data has been retrieved from older hardware models and that this rate should substantially reduce with technologic advancements. Lead fractures have been estimated around 1.8% per lead.[9,10,59] The majority of lead fractures are associated with the implantation of connectors at or below the mastoid, allowing the extensions to track down toward the chest and pull the leads along the way.[78,79] Lead extensions can also occasionally become tethered (0.12%), leading to a phenomenon described as "bowstringing."[59,80,81]

Electrode migrations are very uncommon now with the advent of reliable skull-anchoring devices. Despite this, reported rates, irrespective of anchoring technology, average around 4.4% per lead.[10] With improvement of skull-anchoring devices, rates of lead migration should plummet. Again, intraoperative imaging is of utmost assistance in confirming lead proper positioning until the lead is secured in place. Rare occurrence of "twiddling" syndrome has been linked to lead migration, mostly in children, and raises the necessity to anchor the pulse generator when there is a possibility of its moving in the pocket.[82]

Electrical malfunctions, mainly short or open circuits, are intrinsic to DBS implantation, ranging between 0.9% and 9.9%.[10] Most of the time, programming can be done around malfunctioning contacts, avoiding revising electrodes or extensions. With sturdier connector and electrode designs, these rates should also decrease over time. Pulse generator malfunctions are now uncommon, and these devices are highly reliable. MRI-compatible models have been designed to be free of magnetic interferences. At most, malfunctions are no more than 1%.[59]

Best Practice

Lead fractures from migration of the lead extensions can be prevented by implanting the connectors posterior and superior to the ear. We implant our DBS systems in two stages, and during the first stage we bring the lead caps over the parietal convexity, above the ear, in the subgaleal space. This means that the DBS lead caps are sitting at the border of the temporalis muscle. During the second stage, the lead extension connectors are implanted above the upper third of the pinna, positioning the connectors above the nuchal fascia attachment to the skull. This prevents downward migration of the extensions.

"Bowstringing" extensions require opening the posterior auricular incision and the pocket incision and readjusting the extensions to release the tethering. Generally, extensions are replaced with new ones, keeping in mind a minimal risk of damaging the DBS leads when manipulating the connectors. Finally, pulse generators should be anchored to the fascia unless the pocket is well established and tight enough to prevent rotation or flipping of the generator. Rechargeable generators should always be anchored to the pocket wall.

Stimulation-Related Complications

Off-Target Effects

As discussed above, the incidence of off-target effects as a limitation of DBS therapy for movement disorders has not been quantitatively described in the literature. The best available systematic reviews on management and recommendations for off-target effects bring into focus the low level of evidences available in the literature.[83,84] These effects do seem to be a major limitation of DBS therapy due to patient intolerance of these side effects. DBS electrode placement accuracy may mitigate this complication, and the advent of "steerable" fields in the newest generation of DBS leads may help reduce the incidence of untoward effects.

Stimulation off-target effects can be divided between stimulation-independent versus stimulation-dependent effects. That is, stimulation-dependent effects should resolve after turning the stimulation off. This distinction is not always clearly established among publications.[12] Most off-target effects are target dependent and have been extensively reviewed.[12,38,85] A few side effects are worth discussing. Postsurgical suicide rates are higher after DBS therapy, reaching up to 4.3%,[86] and could be preventable. There is an overall higher incidence of cognitive adverse events after STN DBS compared with GPI DBS. Behavioral changes, including hypomania and depression, have been reported with stimulation of the STN. Gait disturbance seems to occur more commonly after STN DBS compared with GPI DBS.[87–90] Nonreversible speech disturbances are also more common after STN DBS, whereas reversible effects may be more prominent with GPI stimulation.[87] Gait and speech disturbances are well recognized both as reversible and nonreversible side effects of VIM DBS.[87]

Best Practice

Accurate placement of DBS leads, confirmation of lead placement before leaving the OR, "steerable" leads, and maintenance of the lowest possible therapeutic current density at the active DBS contacts should all help minimize off-target effects. Again, this is an area in which a consensus approach would be advantageous and a standardized workup more efficient.[83–85]

Summary

Overall, with current practice, the procedure to implant DBS electrodes and generators is remarkably complication free. There are still questions about the morbidity of MER and whether this guidance technique adds more value than risk. Malposition of electrodes does seem to be the overwhelming complication of DBS implantation surgery, but the magnitude of this problem is only just now being recognized. If recent data is to be accepted, the complication of electrode malposition is by far the most common adverse event associated with DBS surgery. This issue should be addressed promptly by consensus and eventually by prospective trials. Other complications seem to be well mitigated by existing protocols, which can always be improved.

If DBS as a therapy, for movement disorders and other conditions, is to be accessible and appealing to the majority of candidates for the procedure, its attendant complications must be minimized. Clearly more work will be required before we can accomplish that goal.

References

1. Larson PS. Deep brain stimulation for movement disorders. *Neurother.* 2014;11(3):465–474.
2. Flora ED, Perera CL, Cameron AL, Maddern GJ. Deep brain stimulation for essential tremor: a systematic review. *Mov Disord.* 2010; 25(11):1550–1559.
3. Ostrem JL, Starr PA. Treatment of dystonia with deep brain stimulation. *Neurother.* 2008;5(2):320–330.
4. Sprengers M, Vonck K, Carrette E. *Deep brain and cortical stimulation for epilepsy. Cochrane Database Syst Rev.* 2017;7:CD008497.
5. Holtzheimer PE, Mayberg HS. Deep brain stimulation for psychiatric disorders. *Annu Rev Neurosci.* 2011;34(1):289–307.
6. Weaver FM, Follett K, Stern M, et al. Bilateral deep brain stimulation vs best medical therapy for patients with advanced Parkinson disease: a randomized controlled trial. *JAMA.* 2009;301(1):63–73.
7. Weaver FM, Follett KA, Stern M, et al. Randomized trial of deep brain stimulation for Parkinson disease: thirty-six-month outcomes. *Neurology.* 2012;79(1):55–65.
8. Okun MS, Tagliati M, Pourfar M, et al. Management of referred deep brain stimulation failures: a retrospective analysis from 2 movement disorders centers. *Arch Neurol.* 2005;62(8):1250–1255.
9. Falowski SM, Ooi YC, Bakay RAE. Long-term evaluation of changes in operative technique and hardware-related complications with deep brain stimulation. *Neuromodulation.* 2015;18(8):670–677.
10. Bakay R, Smith A. Deep brain stimulation: complications and attempts at avoiding them. *Open Neurosurg J.* 2011;4:42–52.
11. Voges J, Hilker R, Bötzel K, et al. Thirty days complication rate following surgery performed for deep-brain-stimulation. *Mov Disord.* 2007;22(10):1486–1489.
12. Videnovic A, Metman LV. Deep brain stimulation for Parkinson's disease: prevalence of adverse events and need for standardized reporting. *Mov Disord.* 2008;23(3):343–349.

13. Kleiner-Fisman G, Herzog J, Fisman DN, et al. Subthalamic nucleus deep brain stimulation: summary and meta-analysis of outcomes. *Mov Disord.* 2006;21(suppl 14):S290–S304.
14. Zrinzo L, Foltynie T, Limousin P, Hariz MI. Reducing hemorrhagic complications in functional neurosurgery: a large case series and systematic literature review. *J Neurosurg.* 2012;116(1):84–94.
15. Ben-Haim S, Asaad WF, Gale JT, Eskandar EN. Risk factors for hemorrhage during microelectrode-guided deep brain stimulation and the introduction of an improved microelectrode design. *Neurosurgery.* 2009;64(4):754–762, discussion 762–763.
16. Kimmelman J, Duckworth K, Ramsay T, Voss T, Ravina B, Emborg ME. Risk of surgical delivery to deep nuclei: a meta-analysis. *Mov Disord.* 2011;26(8):1415–1421.
17. Hu X, Jiang X, Zhou X, et al. Avoidance and management of surgical and hardware-related complications of deep brain stimulation. *Stereotact Funct Neurosurg.* 2010;88(5):296–303.
18. Gorgulho A, De Salles AAF, Frighetto L, Behnke E. Incidence of hemorrhage associated with electrophysiological studies performed using macroelectrodes and microelectrodes in functional neurosurgery. *J Neurosurg.* 2005;102(5):888–896.
19. Elias WJ, Sansur CA, Frysinger RC. Sulcal and ventricular trajectories in stereotactic surgery. *J Neurosurg.* 2009;110(2):201–207.
20. Higuchi Y, Iacono RP. Surgical complications in patients with Parkinson's disease after posteroventral pallidotomy. *Neurosurgery.* 2003;52(3):558–571, discussion 568–571.
21. Sansur CA, Frysinger RC, Pouratian N, et al. Incidence of symptomatic hemorrhage after stereotactic electrode placement. *J Neurosurg.* 2007;107(5):998–1003.
22. Burchiel KJ, McCartney S, Lee A, Raslan AM. Accuracy of deep brain stimulation electrode placement using intraoperative computed tomography without microelectrode recording. *J Neurosurg.* 2013;119(2):301–306.
23. Alkhani A, Lozano AM. Pallidotomy for Parkinson disease: a review of contemporary literature. *J Neurosurg.* 2001;94(1):43–49.
24. Palur RS, Berk C, Schulzer M, Honey CR. A metaanalysis comparing the results of pallidotomy performed using microelectrode recording or macroelectrode stimulation. *J Neurosurg.* 2002;96(6):1058–1062.
25. de Bie RMA, de Haan RJ, Schuurman PR, Esselink RAJ, Bosch DA, Speelman JD. Morbidity and mortality following pallidotomy in Parkinson's disease: a systematic review. *Neurology.* 2002;58(7):1008–1012.
26. Hariz MI. Safety and risk of microelectrode recording in surgery for movement disorders. *Stereotact Funct Neurosurg.* 2002;78(3–4):146–157.
27. Deep-Brain Stimulation for Parkinson's Disease Study Group, Obeso JA, Olanow CW, et al. Deep-brain stimulation of the subthalamic nucleus or the pars interna of the globus pallidus in Parkinson's disease. *NEJM.* 2001;345(13):956–963.
28. Binder DK, Rau GM, Starr PA. Risk factors for hemorrhage during microelectrode-guided deep brain stimulator implantation for movement disorders. *Neurosurgery.* 2005;56(4):722–732, discussion 722–732.
29. Kocabicak E, Alptekin O, Ackermans L, et al. Is there still need for microelectrode recording now the subthalamic nucleus can be well visualized with high field and ultrahigh MR imaging? *Front Integr Neurosci.* 2015;9(876):46.
30. Douketis JD, Spyropoulos AC, Spencer FA, et al. Perioperative management of antithrombotic therapy: antithrombotic therapy and prevention of thrombosis, 9th ed: American College of Chest Physicians Evidence-Based Clinical Practice Guidelines. *Chest.* 2012;141 (2 suppl):e326S–e350S.
31. Bauer DF, McGwin G, Melton SM, George RL, Markert JM. The relationship between INR and development of hemorrhage with placement of ventriculostomy. *J Trauma.* 2011;70(5):1112–1117.
32. Beyer-Westendorf J, Gelbricht V, Förster K, et al. Peri-interventional management of novel oral anticoagulants in daily care: results from the prospective Dresden NOAC registry. *Eur Heart J.* 2014; 35(28):1888–1896.
33. Albaladejo P, Bonhomme F, Blais N, et al. Management of direct oral anticoagulants in patients undergoing elective surgeries and invasive procedures: updated guidelines from the French Working Group on Perioperative Hemostasis (GIHP) - September 2015. *Anaesth Crit Care Pain Med.* 2017;36:73–76.
34. Oprea AD, Popescu WM. Perioperative management of antiplatelet therapy. *Br J Anaesth.* 2013;111(suppl 1):i3–i17.
35. Palmer JD, Sparrow OC, Iannotti F. Postoperative hematoma: a 5-year survey and identification of avoidable risk factors. *Neurosurgery.* 1994;35(6):1061–1064, discussion 1064–1065.
36. Schafer AI. Effects of nonsteroidal antiinflammatory drugs on platelet function and systemic hemostasis. *J Clin Pharmacol.* 1995; 35(3):209–219.
37. Fenoy AJ, Simpson RK. Risks of common complications in deep brain stimulation surgery: management and avoidance. *J Neurosurg.* 2014;120(1):132–139.
38. Tong F, Ramirez-Zamora A, Gee L, Pilitsis J. Unusual complications of deep brain stimulation. *Neurosurg Rev.* 2015;38(2):245–252, discussion 252.
39. Morishita T, Okun MS, Burdick A, Jacobson CE, Foote KD. Cerebral venous infarction: a potentially avoidable complication of deep brain stimulation surgery. *Neuromodulation.* 2013;16(5):407–413, discussion 413.
40. Deogaonkar M, Nazzaro JM, Machado A, Rezai A. Transient, symptomatic, post-operative, non-infectious hypodensity around the deep brain stimulation (DBS) electrode. *J Clin Neurosci.* 2011; 18(7):910–915.
41. Englot DJ, Glastonbury CM, Larson PS. Abnormal T2-weighted MRI signal surrounding leads in a subset of deep brain stimulation patients. *Stereotact Funct Neurosurg.* 2011;89(5):311–317.
42. Merello M, Cammarota A, Leiguarda R, Pikielny R. Delayed intracerebral electrode infection after bilateral STN implantation for Parkinson's disease. Case report. *Mov Disord.* 2001;16(1):168–170.
43. Coley E, Farhadi R, Lewis S, Whittle IR. The incidence of seizures following deep brain stimulating electrode implantation for movement disorders, pain and psychiatric conditions. *Br J Neurosurg.* 2009; 23(2):179–183.
44. Pouratian N, Reames DL, Frysinger R, Elias WJ. Comprehensive analysis of risk factors for seizures after deep brain stimulation surgery. Clinical article. *J Neurosurg.* 2011;115(2):310–315.
45. Ellis T-M, Foote KD, Fernandez HH, et al. Reoperation for suboptimal outcomes after deep brain stimulation surgery. *Neurosurgery.* 2008;63(4):754–760, discussion 760–761.
46. Kluger BM, Foote KD, Jacobson CE, Okun MS. Lessons learned from a large single center cohort of patients referred for DBS management. *Parkinsonism Relat Disord.* 2011;17(4):236–239.
47. Rolston JD, Englot DJ, Starr PA, Larson PS. An unexpectedly high rate of revisions and removals in deep brain stimulation surgery: Analysis of multiple databases. *Parkinsonism Relat Disord.* 2016;33:72–77.
48. Shahlaie K, Larson PS, Starr PA. Intraoperative computed tomography for deep brain stimulation surgery: technique and accuracy assessment. *Neurosurgery.* 2011;68(1 Suppl Operative):114–124, discussion 124.
49. Starr PA, Martin AJ, Ostrem JL, Talke P, Levesque N, Larson PS. Subthalamic nucleus deep brain stimulator placement using high-field interventional magnetic resonance imaging and a skull-mounted aiming device: technique and application accuracy. *J Neurosurg.* 2010;112(3):479–490.
50. Bhatia R, Dalton A, Richards M, Hopkins C, Aziz T, Nandi D. The incidence of deep brain stimulator hardware infection: the effect of change in antibiotic prophylaxis regimen and review of the literature. *Br J Neurosurg.* 2011;25(5):625–631.
51. Berríos-Torres SI, Umscheid CA, Bratzler DW, et al. Centers for Disease Control and Prevention guideline for the prevention of surgical site infection, 2017. *JAMA Surg.* 2017;152(8):784–791.
52. Sandoe JAT, Barlow G, Chambers JB, et al. Guidelines for the diagnosis, prevention and management of implantable cardiac electronic device infection. Report of a joint Working Party project on behalf of the British Society for Antimicrobial Chemotherapy (BSAC, host organization), British Heart Rhythm Society (BHRS), British Cardiovascular Society (BCS), British Heart Valve Society

(BHVS) and British Society for Echocardiography (BSE). *J Antimicrob Chemother*. 2014;70(2):325–359.
53. Sillay KA, Larson PS, Starr PA. Deep brain stimulator hardware-related infections: incidence and management in a large series. *Neurosurgery*. 2008;62(2):360–366, discussion 366–367.
54. Mangram A, Horan T, Pearson M, et al. Guideline for Prevention of Surgical Site Infection, 1999. Centers for Disease Control and Prevention (CDC) Hospital Infection Control Practices Advisory Committee. *Am J Infect Control*. 1999;27(2):97–132.
55. Ban KA, Minei JP, Laronga C, et al. American College of Surgeons and Surgical Infection Society: surgical site infection guidelines, 2016 update. *J Am Coll Surg*. 2017;224(1):59–74.
56. Gutiérrez-González R, Boto GR, Pérez-Zamarrón A. Cerebrospinal fluid diversion devices and infection. A comprehensive review. *Eur J Clin Microbiol Infect Dis*. 2012;31(6):889–897.
57. Kulkarni AV, Drake JM, Lamberti-Pasculli M. Cerebrospinal fluid shunt infection: a prospective study of risk factors. *J Neurosurg*. 2001;94(2):195–201.
58. Polyzos KA, Konstantelias AA, Falagas ME. Risk factors for cardiac implantable electronic device infection: a systematic review and meta-analysis. *Europace*. 2015;17(5):767–777.
59. Jitkritsadakul O, Bhidayasiri R, Kalia SK, Hodaie M, Lozano AM, Fasano A. Systematic review of hardware-related complications of deep brain stimulation: Do new indications pose an increased risk? *Brain Stimul*. 2017;10(5):967–976.
60. Fenoy AJ, Simpson RKJ. Management of device-related wound complications in deep brain stimulation surgery. *J Neurosurg*. 2012; 116(6):1324–1332.
61. Hamani C, Lozano AM. Hardware-related complications of deep brain stimulation: a review of the published literature. *Stereotact Funct Neurosurg*. 2006;84(5–6):248–251.
62. Blomstedt P, Bjartmarz H. Intracerebral infections as a complication of deep brain stimulation. *Stereotact Funct Neurosurg*. 2012;90(2): 92–96.
63. Pepper J, Zrinzo L, Mirza B, Foltynie T, Limousin P, Hariz M. The risk of hardware infection in deep brain stimulation surgery is greater at impulse generator replacement than at the primary procedure. *Stereotact Funct Neurosurg*. 2013;91(1):56–65.
64. Frizon LA, Hogue O, Wathen C, et al. Subsequent pulse generator replacement surgery does not increase the infection rate in patients with deep brain stimulator systems: a review of 1537 unique implants at a single center. *Neuromodulation*. 2017;349:1925.
65. Rosa M, Scelzo E, Locatelli M, et al. Risk of infection after local field potential recording from externalized deep brain stimulation leads in Parkinson's disease. *World Neurosurg*. 2017;97:64–69.
66. Sixel-Döring F, Trenkwalder C, Kappus C, Hellwig D. Skin complications in deep brain stimulation for Parkinson's disease: frequency, time course, and risk factors. *Acta Neurochir (Wien)*. 2010;152(2): 195–200.
67. Oh MY, Abosch A, Kim SH, Lang AE, Lozano AM. Long-term hardware-related complications of deep brain stimulation. *Neurosurgery*. 2002;50(6):1268–1274, discussion 1274–1276.
68. Webster J, Osborne S. Preoperative bathing or showering with skin antiseptics to prevent surgical site infection. *Cochrane Database Syst Rev*. 2015;(2):CD004985.
69. Tanner J, Norrie P, Melen K. Preoperative hair removal to reduce surgical site infection. *Cochrane Database Syst Rev*. 2011;(11):CD004122.
70. Lefebvre A, Saliou P, Lucet JC, et al. Preoperative hair removal and surgical site infections: network meta-analysis of randomized controlled trials. *J Hosp Infect*. 2015;91(2):100–108.
71. Darouiche RO, Wall MJ, Itani KMF, et al. Chlorhexidine-alcohol versus povidone-iodine for surgical-site antisepsis. *N Engl J Med*. 2010;362(1):18–26.
72. Tanner J, Dumville JC, Norman G, Fortnam M. Surgical hand antisepsis to reduce surgical site infection. *Cochrane Database Syst Rev*. 2016;(1):CD004288.
73. Tanner J, Parkinson H. Double gloving to reduce surgical cross-infection. *Cochrane Database Syst Rev*. 2006;(3):CD003087.
74. Webster J, Alghamdi A. Use of plastic adhesive drapes during surgery for preventing surgical site infection. *Cochrane Database Syst Rev*. 2015;(4):CD006353.
75. Miller JP, Acar F, Burchiel KJ. Significant reduction in stereotactic and functional neurosurgical hardware infection after local neomycin/polymyxin application. *J Neurosurg*. 2009;110(2):247–250.
76. Heal CF, Banks JL, Lepper PD, Kontopantelis E, van Driel ML. Topical antibiotics for preventing surgical site infection in wounds healing by primary intention. *Cochrane Database Syst Rev*. 2016;(11): CD011426.
77. Dumville JC, Gray TA, Walter CJ, et al. Dressings for the prevention of surgical site infection. *Cochrane Database Syst Rev*. 2016;(12): CD003091.
78. Schwalb JM, Riina HA, Skolnick B, Jaggi JL, Simuni T, Baltuch GH. Revision of deep brain stimulator for tremor. Technical note. *J Neurosurg*. 2001;94(6):1010–1012.
79. Hariz MI. Complications of deep brain stimulation surgery. *Mov Disord*. 2002;17(suppl 3):S162–S166.
80. Miller PM, Gross RE. Wire tethering or "bowstringing" as a long-term hardware-related complication of deep brain stimulation. *Stereotact Funct Neurosurg*. 2009;87(6):353–359.
81. Janson C, Maxwell R, Gupte AA, Abosch A. Bowstringing as a complication of deep brain stimulation: case report. *Neurosurgery*. 2010;66(6):E1205, discussion E1205.
82. Geissinger G, Neal JH. Spontaneous twiddler's syndrome in a patient with a deep brain stimulator. *Surg Neurol*. 2007;68(4):454–456, discussion 456.
83. Picillo M, Lozano AM, Kou N, Munhoz RP, Fasano A. Programming deep brain stimulation for tremor and dystonia: The Toronto Western Hospital Algorithms. *Brain Stimul*. 2016;9(3):438–452.
84. Picillo M, Lozano AM, Kou N, Puppi Munhoz R, Fasano A. Programming deep brain stimulation for Parkinson's disease: The Toronto Western Hospital Algorithms. *Brain Stimul*. 2016;9(3):425–437.
85. Deuschl G, Herzog J, Kleiner-Fisman G, et al. Deep brain stimulation: postoperative issues. *Mov Disord*. 2006;21 Suppl 14:S219–S237.
86. Burkhard PR, Vingerhoets FJG, Berney A, Bogousslavsky J, Villemure JG, Ghika J. Suicide after successful deep brain stimulation for movement disorders. *Neurology*. 2004;63(11):2170–2172.
87. Buhmann C, Huckhagel T, Engel K, et al. Adverse events in deep brain stimulation: A retrospective long-term analysis of neurological, psychiatric and other occurrences. *PLoS ONE*. 2017;12(7):e0178984.
88. Rocchi L, Carlson-Kuhta P, Chiari L, Burchiel KJ, Hogarth P, Horak FB. Effects of deep brain stimulation in the subthalamic nucleus or globus pallidus internus on step initiation in Parkinson disease: laboratory investigation. *J Neurosurg*. 2012;117(6):1141–1149.
89. St George RJ, Carlson-Kuhta P, King LA, Burchiel KJ, Horak FB. Compensatory stepping in Parkinson's disease is still a problem after deep brain stimulation randomized to STN or GPi. *J Neurophysiol*. 2015;114(3):1417–1423.
90. St George RJ, Nutt JG, Burchiel KJ, Horak FB. A meta-regression of the long-term effects of deep brain stimulation on balance and gait in PD. *Neurology*. 2010;75(14):1292–1299.

34

Complications After Epilepsy Surgery

KEVIN MANSFIELD, PIYUSH KALAKOTI, HAI SUN, ANDY REKITO, FABIO GRASSIA, JEFF OJEMANN, KIM J. BURCHIEL

HIGHLIGHTS

- The safety and efficacy of epilepsy surgery have been demonstrated in several randomized trials; however, it is critical to reiterate potential complications arising from epilepsy surgery to ensure best practices of care.
- The association of vascular injury, particularly with the anterior choroidal artery during medial temporal resections, the most commonly performed epilepsy surgery, can have deleterious effects ranging from clinically silent infarctions to hemiplegia, hemianopsia, and more.
- Visual deficits from direct injury to the Meyer loop are potentially avoidable.
- Prevention of injury through adequate visualization, aided by the surgeon's anatomic knowledge and neuronavigation, is a key to successful surgery.

Introduction

Epilepsy is a well-known chronic neurologic disorder affecting an estimated 1% of the general population.[1,2] Despite advancement in therapeutic management, approximately one-third of cases are refractory to medical therapy alone. Patients with drug-resistant epilepsies (DRE) are at increased propensity for developing serious morbidities including cognitive disorders, depression, and sudden death in epilepsy.[3] In selective patients with DRE, including adults and the pediatric population, epilepsy surgery is widely regarded as a gold standard therapeutic modality for seizure remission, thereby increasing quality of life. Patient selection is critical because not all patients with DRE are surgical candidates. The safety and efficacy of epilepsy surgery compared with medical therapy alone in patients with temporal lobe epilepsy has been demonstrated in several randomized controlled trials.[1,4,5] Temporal lobe epilepsy emanating from a focal lesion with a unilateral onset is the most common diagnosis associated with surgical resectability. Despite the utility of surgical therapy in treating DRE, it is often underutilized, with a meager 3.6% of temporal lobe DRE undergoing surgical management.[6] In patients with mesial temporal sclerosis or other focal temporal lobe epilepsies, the response rates range from 67% to 82%.[5,7]

With improvements in surgical technique including preoperative planning, neuronavigation and, most importantly, appropriate patient selection, algorithms have dramatically reduced the rates of morbidity and mortality from this therapy over the years. A study comparing adverse events across various epilepsy surgeries between 1980–1996 and 1996–2012 noted a pronounced decline in neurologic complications from 42% to 5%, whereas permanent neurologic deficits decreased from 10% to 1%.[8] Although rare, these permanent complications are of sufficient impact to outweigh much, if not all, of the benefit that even Engel class 1A seizure control would provide; as such, all efforts to avoid these rare but potentially devastating complications should be made. In this chapter we provide a comprehensive overview of the surgical modalities available for epilepsy, discussing anatomic insights and considerations and the potential complications associated with surgical epilepsy procedures.

Epilepsy Surgery: Anatomic Considerations

Most complications after epilepsy surgery occur as a direct result of severance to the local vasculature, particularly the anterior choroidal artery (AChA), and the visual pathways. Anatomic insights on these pertinent structures can help mitigate life-threatening complications; hence a review of these critical structures is necessary.

The AChA, the terminal branch of the internal carotid artery before bifurcation into the middle and anterior cerebral arteries, courses posteriorly between the lateral diencephalic and medial telencephalic structures. Intraoperative severance to the AChA can cause symptomatology related to the affected structures supplied by the artery, such as the anterior perforated substance, optic tract and optic radiations, uncus, cerebral peduncle, temporal horn, choroid plexus of the temporal horn, lateral geniculate body, posterior two-thirds of the posterior limb of the internal capsule, and globus pallidus. Rarely, the head of the caudate, the pyriform cortex, posteromedial amygdala, substantia nigra, subthalamic nucleus, red nucleus, caudate tail, the hypothalamus, and the superficial part of the ventrolateral nucleus of the thalamus can also be supplied by the AChA.[3] It is interesting to note the developmental equilibrium between the posterior communicating artery (PComm) and the AChA; a robust PComm results in a diminished field for the AChA, whereas a diminutive PComm is associated with a greater territory for the AChA. Overlap with the areas supplied by the posterior choroidal artery and the posterior cerebral artery occurs with a similar balance, and often there are anastomoses between the AChA and these posterior circulation vessels.[9–12] Interruption of the AChA supply to these various components can be predicted to potentially produce visual loss, speech deficits, and sensory and motor deficits described in the epilepsy surgery literature, and it is commonly associated with injury to the AChA itself.

The visual system's importance to our day-to-day function is underscored by its extensive and highly organized network of white matter tracts and gray matter connections. The Meyer loop, a white matter tract, carries visual information about the contralateral superior quadrant from the lateral geniculate body to the inferior primary visual cortex. As it leaves the lateral geniculate body, it passes through the temporal stem and sweeps forward over the lateral roof of the temporal horn, eventually turning back toward the inferior occipital pole and visual cortex. Its anterior extent is on average less than a centimeter posterior to the tip of the temporal horn, with the left side often slightly more anterior than the right.[13,14] The fibers have a visuotopic arrangement, with anterior fibers corresponding to the medial visual field, whereas the posterior fibers carry the lateral field. However, there exists significant variability from patient to patient; additionally, inability to distinguish these fibers from other white matter intraoperatively can likely account for high estimated injury risk to visual pathways.

Epilepsy Surgery: Indications and Complications

Surgical intervention for epilepsy is often age independent. Patients with persistent, frequent seizures that adversely impact quality of life, including those with impaired cognition and psychosocial development despite being on a dose-adjusted medical regimen, are ideal candidates. However, the choice of surgical selection is often tailored based upon a comprehensive epilepsy evaluation including tracing of the epileptogenic focus, determination of the extent of resection needed, seizure semiology, and frequency and severity as well as patient tolerance to surgery.[1] Components of presurgical evaluation usually include clinical examination, neuropsychological testing, scalp and video electroencephalography (EEG), high-resolution magnetic resonance imaging (MRI), and other magnetic resonance techniques including assessment of functional and structural integrity, and positron emission tomography/single-photon emission computed tomography (PET/SPECT) scans as needed. Routinely performed surgical procedures (Table 34.1) for seizure remission are as follows:

Temporal Lobe Surgery

Temporal lobectomy, the most common "resective" surgery or lesionectomy, is a highly successful seizure control procedure where the epileptogenic focus is known to be localized from a distinct area of the brain (temporal lobe). The rationale is simply to remove a portion of the lesion (defect), such as a tumor or malformed vessel, known to induce seizure. It involves removal of a portion of the lobe, usually the size of a golf ball. In most cases, complete remission is achieved while the risk of permanent brain damage is mitigated.

Permanent deficits include contralateral superior quadrantanopsia (most common), hemianopsia, hemiparesis (more common in extratemporal resections), stroke/cerebrovascular accident, and aphasia.[15,16] Although on the face of things these varied complications may seem to be unrelated, there is a common thread connecting

TABLE 34.1 Overview of Surgical Epilepsy Procedures and Associated Complications

Epilepsy Surgery	Indications	Common Complications
1. Temporal lobectomy and/or selective amygdalohippocampectomy (SAH)	Hippocampal sclerosis Lesional focus Nonlesional	• Injury to brain stem, cranial nerve III • Issues related to cognition, speech abnormalities, language, visual impairments (double vision, reduced visual field) • Vascular injury, especially to the anterior choroidal artery • Hemiparesis • Infections
2. Extratemporal lobe resections including hemispherectomy, functional surgeries (corpus callosectomy, multiple subpial transection)	Lesional Nonlesional	• Behavioral changes including motivation, attention or concentration, mood changes, impulsivity • Postoperative hydrocephalus • Infections • Complications involving anterior skull base including infarction of the basal ganglia, internal capsule and ventricular striae vessels, middle cerebral artery/anterior cerebral artery infarction
3. Stereotactic procedures including laser ablation of mesial temporal structures, grid placement (depth electrodes)		• Relatively new procedure, less invasive than SAH • Associated with psychiatric symptoms • Postoperative hematoma • Infections • Bone flap out
4. Vagus nerve stimulator		• Technical issues related to vagus nerve stimulation implantation (electrode fracture, dislocation and generator malfunction)[28] • Surgical-related complications are relatively low and include infections, hoarseness or temporary vocal cord paralysis due to recurrent laryngeal nerve palsy, dysphagia, facial hypoesthesia, neck hematoma.[48] • Delayed complications include scarring, vagus nerve stimulation becoming less effective over time
5. Neurostimulatory procedures (deep brain stimulation, transcranial magnetic stimulation, cranial nerve V stimulation)	Refractory epilepsy	• Depression • Impaired cognition • Hemorrhage • Implant site infections

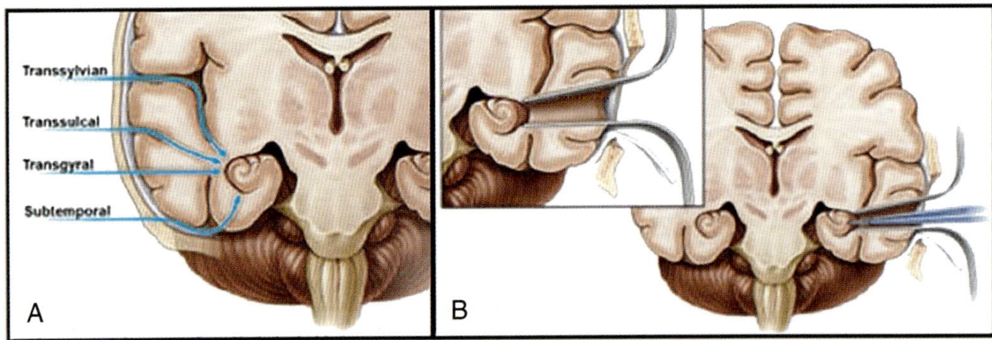

• **Fig. 34.1** Selective Amygdalohippocampectomy (SAH). (A) Commonly utilized approaches for SAH (coronal view). Note that a very anterior entry must be used in a transsylvian approach to avoid injury to the temporal stem. (B) A small craniotomy allows a 1- to 2-cm corridor of access to the ventricle and mesial structures in a transcortical SAH.

them all: the AChA. The reported incidence of quadrantanopsia varies substantially, but reasonable estimates suggest rates between 18% and 26% for anterior temporal lobectomy (ATL).[15,16] Quadrantanopsia is frequently unnoticed by the patient unless it is severe, and it is markedly underreported.[17] To distinguish partial or full quadrantanopsia from hemianopsia, injury localization is valuable. AChA injury causes hemianopsia by ischemic damage to the optic tract, whereas superior quadrantanopsia is produced as a resultant direct injury to the Meyer loop.

Selective Amygdalohippocampectomy

As an alternative to ATL, selective amygdalohippocampectomy has emerged as a viable option for surgical seizure control. In contrast to the traditional temporal lobectomy that involves en bloc resection of approximately 3 to 6 cm of the temporal neocortex to ensure permissible access to the mesial structures, SAH is a more targeted approach for mesial temporal resections that spares the temporal lobe neocortex. Commonly employed approaches for SAH include transsylvian, transsucal, transgyral, and subtemporal corridors (Fig. 34.1A). A small craniotomy is adequate for a 1- to 2-cm permissible corridor to provide access to mesial structures (Fig. 34.1B). However, consideration of patient selection is critical for SAH. Patients with well-defined mesial temporal onset seizures, including bitemporal onset seizures, are at increased risk for memory impairment and thus should be excluded.[18] Likewise, patients with a dominant seizure focus in the temporal lobe are at risk for postsurgical functional decline, including speech abnormalities. Patients with extratemporal focal epilepsy or with seizure focus in the temporal neocortex, along with those with primary idiopathic generalized epilepsies and those with psychogenic nonepileptic seizures (PNES), are not suitable candidates for SAH. Potential surgical complications include, but are not limited to, hemorrhage, infarction (lacunar strokes), infections, incomplete resection, neurocognitive impairments including speech disorders and memory loss, and mood disorders.

Whether performing an SAH to remove only the mesial structures or carrying out a full ATL, the key element of the surgery is maximal safe resection of the hippocampus, uncus, and parahippocampus.[15,19,20] Relevant knowledge of the AChA course can minimize morbidity. The course of the AChA carries it directly into the field of resection during temporal lobe epilepsy resection. After passing through the crural cistern, the AChA pierces the choroidal fissure superior to the uncus, usually around the posterior half of the uncus, and enters the temporal horn of the lateral ventricle to supply the choroid plexus. The choroid plexus of the temporal horn lies immediately superior and medial to the hippocampus and its fimbria.

Extratemporal Lobe Resection

Hemispherectomy

Considered a radical surgical approach for epilepsy, hemispherectomy involves complete removal of the outer layer of one-half of the brain. The rationale is to mechanically sever the functional connectivity across the two cerebral hemispheres. Common indications of hemispherectomy include cortical dysplasias (36%), large ischemic infarcts (34%), Rasmussen encephalitis (19%), and other pathologies including Sturge-Weber syndrome, hemiconvulsion-hemiplegia-epilepsy, and trauma.[21] It usually is performed in infants born with brain damage and in children with severe seizure disorders. Common complications after hemispherectomy include hydrocephalus (9%–81%) and those relating to any major intracranial complication including, but not limited to, infections, aseptic meningitis, neurologic deficits, strokes, and even mortality.[21] With the morbidity rates and possible marked alteration of brain composition associated with hemispherectomy, along with the inherent risks, the procedure is rarely indicated. Functional hemispherectomies are more commonly performed as compared with anatomic (mechanical) hemispherectomy.

Functional Epilepsy Surgeries

Functional hemispherectomy, popularly known as corpus callosectomy, is widely gaining momentum in most centers. Its utility is being explored in children with disabling "drop" attacks where the epileptogenic focus emanates from one hemisphere and spreads to the contralateral hemisphere. The rationale for surgery is severing the white matter connection between the two hemispheres, i.e., functional discontinuation, and surgery is often performed in a staged manner. The first surgery is aimed at resecting the anterior two-thirds of the corpus callosum while leaving the remainder intact.[22] In cases with inadequate seizure control, the remainder of the viable portion of the corpus callosum is removed.[22] Common application is in atonic patients with Lennox-Gastaut syndrome who incur repeated falls.[23] Significant reduction in seizure severity and frequency is achieved.

SURGICAL REWIND

My Worst Case

A 40-year-old woman presented with a long history of drug-resistant complex partial seizures. An EEG localized the epileptic focus to the left temporal region. MRI shows mesial temporal sclerosis in the ipsilateral hippocampus. Neuropsychological testing reveals a full-scale intelligence quotient (FSIQ) of 95 with specific verbal memory deficits and minimal visual perceptual deficits. The patient underwent left-side selective microsurgical amygdalohippocampectomy without intraoperative complication. While in the recovery room, the patient was noted to have right hemiparesis and a left homonymous hemianopsia. MRI shows a diffusion-weighted imaging (DWI) 2-cm irregular defect in the left anterior internal capsule and the region of the left optic tract (Fig. 34.2). After transfer to inpatient rehabilitation, a slow improvement in hemiparesis over the course of 6 weeks and a reduction of her visual field deficit to a right superior quadrantanopsia were noted. Five years after surgery, she remains Engel class I on a single anticonvulsant. Mild right-hand weakness and a right superior quadrantanopsia persist.

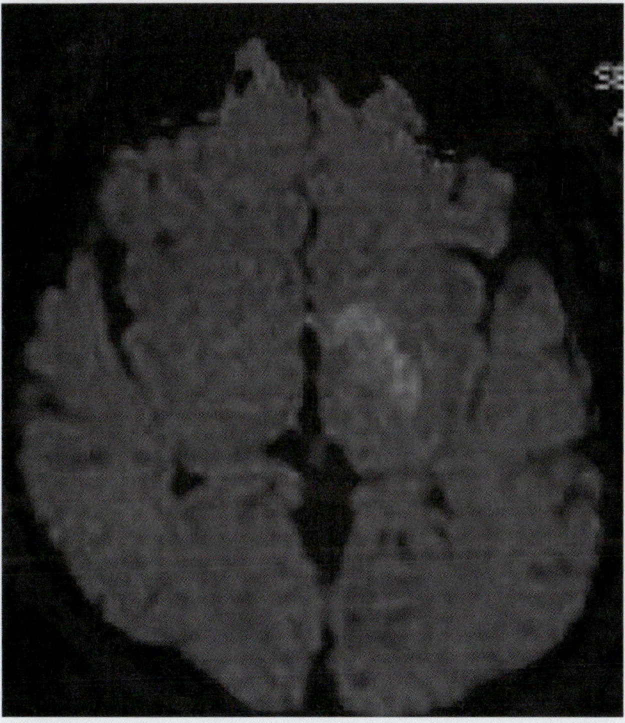

• **Fig. 34.2** Diffusion-weighted magnetic resonance imaging obtained postoperative day 1 after transcortical selective amygdalohippocampectomy. Hyperintensity in the area of the left internal capsule and globus pallidus can be visualized.

Multiple subpial transection (MST), an alternate functional procedure, is useful for seizures emanating from eloquent areas that are too vital to remove. The procedure involves a series of shallow cuts in the brain parenchyma, called "transections," that aim to disrupt the flow of abnormal seizure impulses without disturbing normal brain activity. Although rarely performed, MST may be more effective than resective surgery for diffuse seizures not originating from the same focus.

Grid Placement (Depth Electrodes)

Stereoelectroencephalography (SEEG) was primitively developed for invasive mapping of refractory focal epilepsy and includes implanting deep electrodes. Compared with grid placements, SEEG is less invasive and offers precise recordings from cortical and subcortical structures without using large craniotomies. Postoperative complications are rare and include hemorrhage (subdural, epidural, and intraparenchymal). Postoperative hematoma, usually seen as an immediate complication within 24 to 48 hours after surgery, often requires return to the operating room for evacuation to prevent complications from mass effect. Other potential complications include infections or wound-related problems, often necessitating readmission within 2 weeks after surgery. Cerebrospinal fluid (CSF) leaks are common, as are electrodes that malposition or surface to the scalp. To prevent displaced bone flap, osteoclast craniotomy is recommended. This includes moving intact temporalis muscle away from the bone flap, ensuring patent blood supply to the bony flap, and minimizing changes of wound infections.

Radio-Frequency Ablation

Radio-frequency ablation for temporal lobe epilepsy has expanded over the years with improvements in targeting and imaging technologies.[24] Laser ablation of mesial temporal structures is a relatively new surgical technique. Although less invasive than amygdalohippocampectomy, it is associated with a faster recovery and less postsurgical cognitive verbal deficits.[25]

Vagus Nerve Stimulation (VNS)

VNS implantation is an approved neuromodulatory adjunct treatment of drug-resistant partial-onset seizures. VNS is usually implanted in children with DRE who are not eligible candidates for resective epilepsy surgery. An estimated 30% to 40% of patients achieve over 50% reduction in their seizure rates.[26,27] Although deleterious events are seldom encountered with VNS implantation, common complications include those related to hardware failure, including electrode fracture or dislocation and generator malfunctions.[28] *Staphylococcal aureus* infection of subcutaneous pocket holding the VNS generator occurs in 2% to 7% of cases and can be managed by prophylactic antibiotics and wound debridement. Other potential complications include voice hoarseness (37%), throat pain (11%), persistent cough (7%), and shortness of breath (6%).[26] Horner syndrome, although rare, has been reported in some isolated cases implanted with VNS due to intraoperative manipulation of the sympathetic fibers.[29]

Neurostimulatory Procedures

Certain groups of patients with DRE are not likely candidates for resective epilepsy surgery. Neurostimulatory procedures such as deep brain stimulation, transcranial magnetic stimulation (TMS), and trigeminal nerve stimulation have shown promising results. The utility of neuromodulation and subcortical stimulation to the thalamus, caudate, hippocampus and the cerebellum in several open-label and small-series blinded trials has unveiled its potential use in controlling refractory seizure in patients who are not ideal for resective surgery.[30–35] In a recent randomized clinical trial (SANTE trial) involving 110 DRE patients, subcortical stimulation of the thalamic anterior nuclei was associated with seizure reduction by nearly one-third at 3 months compared with sham stimulation.

Over half the cohort had seizure remission by 50% at 2 years.[36] Beneficial effect was observed in patients with seizure semiology consistent with complex partial types. Likely complications witnessed in the stimulated group were depression (15% vs 2%) and issues related to cognition (13% vs 2%). Other complications included hemorrhages (5%) and implant site infections (13%). However, the long-term follow reported rates of depression, suicidal ideations, and sudden unexpected death in epilepsy (SUDEP) comparable to those in general patients with DRE.[37] Although the device is approved in Europe, Canada, and Australia, its approval by the U.S. Food and Drug Administration is pending.

Use of low-frequency TMS in reducing cortical excitability has been shown in isolated reports and small trials,[38–41] albeit with mixed results and low level of evidence. Similarly, low-frequency external stimulation of the trigeminal nerve has shown promising results in seizure and mood control in patients with DRE.[42,43] However, the device is currently being investigated for use in the United States.

Prevention and Complication Avoidance

Vascular Injury

Most technical descriptions involve entering and emptying the parahippocampal gyrus via the collateral sulcus first, to allow the hippocampus to be rolled laterally/inferiorly away from the choroid plexus and AChA. This highlights the unifying feature of the various approaches to the surgery: obtaining proper visualization and orientation intraoperatively. When an ATL is performed, this is accomplished by first resecting the cortex lateral to the ventricle so that direct visual inspection of the ependymal surface and mesial structures is easily accomplished. Fig. 34.1A shows the various surgical approaches to SAH. The various approaches to SAH allow a more limited view and thus require greater familiarity with the anatomy involved.

The transcortical technique for SAH (Fig. 34.1B), used in our index case, is attractive in that it allows the most minimally invasive approach. A small craniotomy centered over the middle temporal gyrus (or, less commonly, the superior temporal gyrus) of the anterior temporal lobe provides adequate exposure for a 1- to 2-cm corticectomy. This provides the corridor to the ventricle; inspection of the ependyma and identification of the choroid plexus, hippocampus, parahippocampus, and collateral eminence/sulcus then follow under direct visualization. As in the ATL, mobilization of the hippocampus away from the choroid ultimately occurs in a plane roughly orthogonal to the direction of view. Visualization of the choroid plexus and the hippocampal feeding arteries from the AChA is usually straightforward, presuming an appropriate approach trajectory was utilized from the outset.

The subtemporal approach was developed to produce even less impact on the lateral cortical structures during an SAH. A slightly larger exposure and craniotomy are required, but by entering the parahippocampal gyrus via the adjacent collateral sulcus, the only neural structures directly injured are those that are resected. An elegant approach, this trajectory requires the resection of the parahippocampal gyrus before the hippocampus can even be visualized; the hippocampus is then rolled toward the surgeon, revealing the vascular structures behind. Variations in anatomy may make visualization of the vasculature difficult; strict adherence to subpial dissection technique and resection of the hippocampus from lateral to medial may allow for better visualization of the vessels as the operation progresses.

The transsylvian approach, which aims to completely spare the lateral temporal cortex and utilizes a familiar approach from aneurysm surgery,[44] poses a different challenge. A larger craniotomy is required, and the sylvian fissure must be opened. A successful approach yields visualization of the optic tract, carotid siphon, middle cerebral artery, PComm, and AChA as they pass through the cisterns medial to the temporal lobe. The uncus is incised and resected, leading the operator to the anterior temporal horn. The subpial dissection is then continued posteriorly along the medial border of the ventricle. Visualization of the AChA (and the other surrounding vessels and nerves) is achieved here even before the resection targets are visualized. Care must be taken to avoid injuring these structures throughout the case; the course of the AChA superior and posterior to the uncus as it transitions from its cisternal to its plexal portion may lie directly over the resection area. Even without direct vascular injury, vasospasm can produce significant downstream injury and is most likely to occur from a transsylvian approach.[44–46]

In all cases, a clear and accurate understanding of the anatomy of each patient is crucial to establish an appropriate trajectory and to ensure a safe resection. One of the most useful methods of preventing complications is stereotactic image guidance. Although arguably less valuable in those approaches with larger exposures, it can provide valuable information about distant relevant anatomy. Selection of the precise location of the craniotomy in a transcortical SAH, or confirmation of the location of the collateral sulcus in the subtemporal SAH, helps to maximize the minimally invasive potential these approaches offer. Identification of the central sulcus, temporal pole, tectum, and temporal stem allows precise guidance for the extent of resection in these approaches, without the need for extensive craniotomy. Use of intraoperative navigation has been shown to reduce rates of complications and submaximal resection,[47] and is utilized routinely in our practice.

Separation of the hippocampus and fimbria from their arterial supply should be done with gentle microdissection. Care should be taken to avoid opening the choroidal fissure, and for much of the dissection, the neural tissue can be carefully peeled away from the vessels. When direct cauterization of vessels is required, this should be done as close to the surface of the hippocampus as possible to sacrifice only the terminal branches feeding the hippocampus and to avoid the *en passage* vessels. Careless traction/dissection of the neural structures may tear the main feeding branch of the AChA or create bleeding from a terminal vessel that is difficult to stop without also cauterizing the AChA branch. Indirect injury can even induce arterial spasm or thermal injury from cautery spread. Optimal visualization of the vascular interface of the hippocampus and fimbria is key to avoiding problems here; this in turn is predicated on an optimal approach trajectory. As stated before, emptying the parahippocampal gyrus before attacking the hippocampus allows easier mobilization and visualization of the hippocampus, reducing the chance for this type of error. The choroid plexus can be carefully swept upward and covered with a cotton patty to prevent inadvertent trauma and bleeding during the dissection as well; it should not be coagulated.

Visual Pathway Injury

Avoidance of the temporal stem and the Meyer loop during resection is the best way to prevent injury to the optic radiations. This is most challenging in ATL because the lateral cortical and white matter lesions of the anterior temporal lobe are removed as part of the surgery. However, during the SAH procedures, it is easy to inadvertently continue resection of the mesial temporal lobe into the temporal stem unless careful attention is paid to intraoperative landmarks.

The most common location of injury to the Meyer loop is at its anterior limit where it lies superior and lateral to the anterior temporal horn. If careful attention to technique is maintained, this area can be completely avoided via the transsylvian and subtemporal approaches. The transcortical approach may transgress this area unless an approach trajectory inferior to the fiber tract is used. Thus a superior temporal gyrus entry is more likely than a middle temporal gyrus entry to injure the Meyer loop. Also, a more anterior entry site is less likely to cause injury than a posterior entry site.

If there is major preoperative concern about the consequences of even a partial quadrantanopsia, preoperative imaging can be obtained to locate the fibers of the Meyer loop. Diffusion tensor imaging (DTI) and tractography are now available in many facilities; these images can be fused with the anatomic scans used for intraoperative neuronavigation. Such advanced imaging techniques facilitate virtual visualization of the Meyer loop for planning the trajectory and extent of resection to minimize injury to the fibers.

Complication Avoidance

Vascular Injury

In the event of vascular injury, overaggressive cauterization to regain control should be avoided. Instead, adopting standard microvascular surgical techniques—including gentle pressure to the suspected area of bleed using cotton patties, and warm irrigation to optimize view—may yield adequate control. Careful inspection is required to identify the precise source of bleeding and to control it as close to the terminal end as possible. In this way, sometimes, an indelicate injury can be kept from becoming a parent vessel sacrifice.

In the event of a major injury to the AChA at any point along its course, there are currently no alternatives but to sacrifice the vessel to stop the bleeding. Endovascular repair with stenting or other methods is not possible due to the very small caliber of the vessel, and most approaches do not provide the proper access to perform a direct or indirect repair or bypass of the vessel. Therefore before sacrifice, all efforts must be taken to confirm that it is in fact the parent branch of the AChA that is bleeding, not a terminal side branch that can be more easily controlled.

If the AChA is taken during the procedure, some degree of postoperative infarction is expected. The size of the ischemic field depends on the degree of anastomosis of the AChA with the posterior choroidal, posterior cerebral, and PComm arteries. Postoperative management should balance the typical concerns after resective brain surgery (i.e., hemorrhage into the resection cavity) with those of acute ischemic stroke management (i.e., maintaining adequate perfusion pressure to allow optimal blood flow in watershed areas). Meticulous hemostasis during the remainder of the procedure and closure will allow for more permissive blood pressure control. Postoperative imaging to evaluate for stroke is not necessary unless there is clinical indication of deficit that is worsening over time; this may help guide medical management to help reduce further ischemic sequelae.

Visual Pathway Injury

Inadvertent injury to the optic radiations will likely go undetected intraoperatively unless advanced imaging with tractography is utilized with intraoperative neuronavigation. Regardless, once the fibers are injured, there is no remedy. Patients should be counseled preoperatively about the potential for visual field defect. Postoperatively, visual field testing can detect the extent of any deficit; in cases where there is significant visual field deficit, and especially in cases where it is noticeable to the patient, occupational therapy and other types of rehabilitation can help the patient compensate for the deficit.

NEUROSURGICAL SELFIE MOMENT

Epilepsy surgery in appropriately selected patients is safe and effective and provides significant improvements in quality of life. The described procedures for seizure control are often tailored based upon clinical symptomatology, including patient presentation, seizure severity and frequency, and impact on quality of life. Although underutilized in clinical practice, epilepsy surgery is associated with low mortality and morbidity rates. Major intraoperative complications include vascular injury, particularly to the AChA, that may predispose to postsurgical sequelae based on the territory involved. Anatomic consideration with regard to the course of the AChA is essential for complication prevention. Common complications include cognitive impairments and visual field deficits. Preservation of the superior visual fields, although not always possible, should also be a goal of surgical planning. Appropriate surgical approach should include patient-specific needs (e.g., cortical resection needed) as well as the surgeon's comfort and familiarity with a given approach. Correct trajectory to the temporal horn of the lateral ventricle and adequate visualization of each of the key structures are mandatory to prevent inadvertent injury to the AChA and the Meyer loop. Utilization of stereotactic neuronavigation to confirm key landmark sites can be a valuable adjunct to the procedure. Lastly, meticulous dissection techniques and disconnection of the hippocampal blood supply at the entrance of the terminal branches to the neural tissue minimize the risk to the parent artery.

RED FLAGS

- During transcortical SAH, difficulty accessing the temporal horn of the lateral ventricle suggests an incorrect trajectory. This may result in abnormally difficult or impossible visualization of the vascular structures medial to the hippocampus.
- Breach of the pia-arachnoid layer into the medial cisternal spaces during resection exposes the vasculature, cranial nerves, diencephalon, and midbrain to injury. Sudden influx of CSF into the operative field (except during transsylvian approaches) may indicate inadvertent transgression into the cistern and should prompt extreme caution. Every effort to reestablish the pia-arachnoid border medial to the resection should be taken.
- Inability to visualize the entrance of terminal arterial branches into the hippocampus suggests inadequate resection of the parahippocampal gyrus and increases the risk of AChA injury during devascularization of the hippocampus.
- Considering the proximity of AChA, the resection of the pes hippocampi, amygdala, and uncus should be undertaken carefully while respecting the regional anatomy.
- Entering the lateral ventricle from a superior trajectory or damage to the temporal stem can increase the chance of injury to the Meyer loop, resulting in contralateral superior quadrantanopsia.
- Procedures related to the opercular-insular region, disruption to the perforating arterial segments branching off the M2–M3 and M2–M3 junction, especially those supplying the superior part of the posterior short gyrus and the superior limiting sulcus, may lead to severe neurologic deficits.

References

1. Wiebe S, Blume WT, Girvin JP, et al. A randomized, controlled trial of surgery for temporal-lobe epilepsy. *N Engl J Med.* 2001;345(5):311–318.
2. Georgiadis I, Kapsalaki EZ, Fountas KN. Temporal lobe resective surgery for medically intractable epilepsy: a review of complications and side effects. *Epilepsy Res Treat.* 2013;2013:752195.
3. Kwan P, Brodie MJ. Early identification of refractory epilepsy. *N Engl J Med.* 2000;342(5):314–319.
4. Dwivedi R, Ramanujam B, Chandra PS, et al. Surgery for drug-resistant epilepsy in children. *N Engl J Med.* 2017;377(17):1639–1647.
5. Engel J Jr, McDermott MP, Wiebe S, et al. Early surgical therapy for drug-resistant temporal lobe epilepsy: a randomized trial. *JAMA.* 2012;307(9):922–930.
6. Sharma K, Kalakoti P, Henry M, et al. Revisiting racial disparities in access to surgical management of drug-resistant temporal lobe epilepsy post implementation of Affordable Care Act. *Clin Neurol Neurosurg.* 2017;158:82–89.
7. Acar G, Acar F, Miller J, et al. Seizure outcome following transcortical selective amygdalohippocampectomy in mesial temporal lobe epilepsy. *Stereotact Funct Neurosurg.* 2008;86(5):314–319.
8. Tebo CC, Evins AI, Christos PJ, et al. Evolution of cranial epilepsy surgery complication rates: a 32-year systematic review and meta-analysis. *J Neurosurg.* 2014;120(6):1415–1427.
9. Abbie AA. The blood supply of the lateral geniculate body, with a note on the morphology of the choroidal arteries. *J Anat.* 1933;67(Pt 4):491–521.
10. Rhoton AL. The anterior choroidal artery. In: Rhoton A, ed. *Cranial anatomy and surgical approaches.* Philadelphia, PA: Lippincott Williams & Wilkins; 2003:89–96.
11. Uflacker R. Arteries of the head and neck. In: Uflacker R, ed. *Atlas of vascular anatomy: an angiographic approach.* Philadelphia, PA: Lippincott Williams & Wilkins; 1997:9–10.
12. Abbie AA. The clinical significance of the anterior choroidal artery. *J Nerv Ment Dis.* 1934;80(1):90.
13. Borius PY, Roux FE, Valton L, et al. Can DTI fiber tracking of the optic radiations predict visual deficit after surgery? *Clin Neurol Neurosurg.* 2014;122:87–91.
14. James JS, Radhakrishnan A, Thomas B, et al. Diffusion tensor imaging tractography of Meyer's loop in planning resective surgery for drug-resistant temporal lobe epilepsy. *Epilepsy Res.* 2015;110:95–104.
15. Attiah MA, Paulo DL, Danish SF, et al. Anterior temporal lobectomy compared with laser thermal hippocampectomy for mesial temporal epilepsy: a threshold analysis study. *Epilepsy Res.* 2015;115:1–7.
16. Hader WJ, Tellez-Zenteno J, Metcalfe A, et al. Complications of epilepsy surgery: a systematic review of focal surgical resections and invasive EEG monitoring. *Epilepsia.* 2013;54(5):840–847.
17. Yeni SN, Tanriover N, Uyanik O, et al. Visual field defects in selective amygdalohippocampectomy for hippocampal sclerosis: the fate of Meyer's loop during the transsylvian approach to the temporal horn. *Neurosurgery.* 2008;63(3):507–513, discussion 513–5.
18. Abosch A, Bernasconi N, Boling W, et al. Factors predictive of suboptimal seizure control following selective amygdalohippocampectomy. *J Neurosurg.* 2002;97(5):1142–1151.
19. Tonini C, Beghi E, Berg AT, et al. Predictors of epilepsy surgery outcome: a meta-analysis. *Epilepsy Res.* 2004;62(1):75–87.
20. Wyler AR, Hermann BP, Somes G. Extent of medial temporal resection on outcome from anterior temporal lobectomy: a randomized prospective study. *Neurosurgery.* 1995;37(5):982–990, discussion 990–991.
21. Lew SM. Hemispherectomy in the treatment of seizures: a review. *Transl Pediatr.* 2014;3(3):208–217.
22. Graham D, Tisdall MM, Gill D. Corpus callosotomy outcomes in pediatric patients: a systematic review. *Epilepsia.* 2016;57(7):1053–1068.
23. Asadi-Pooya AA, Sharan A, Nei M, et al. Corpus callosotomy. *Epilepsy Behav.* 2008;13(2):271–278.
24. Blume WT, Parrent AG, Kaibara M. Stereotactic amygdalohippocampotomy and mesial temporal spikes. *Epilepsia.* 1997;38(8):930–936.
25. Kanner A, Ribot R, Serrano E, et al. Laser ablation of mesial temporal structures: a new treatment for epilepsy surgery (P6.231). *Neurology.* 2017;88(16 suppl):P6–P231.
26. A randomized controlled trial of chronic vagus nerve stimulation for treatment of medically intractable seizures. The vagus nerve stimulation study group. *Neurology.* 1995;45(2):224–230.
27. DeGiorgio CM, Schachter SC, Handforth A, et al. Prospective long-term study of vagus nerve stimulation for the treatment of refractory seizures. *Epilepsia.* 2000;41(9):1195–1200.
28. Spuck S, Tronnier V, Orosz I, et al. Operative and technical complications of vagus nerve stimulator implantation. *Neurosurgery.* 2010;67 (2 Suppl Operative):489–494.
29. Kim W, Clancy RR, Liu GT. Horner syndrome associated with implantation of a vagus nerve stimulator. *Am J Ophthalmol.* 2001;131(3):383–384.
30. Cohen-Gadol AA, Britton JW, Wetjen NM, et al. Neurostimulation therapy for epilepsy: current modalities and future directions. *Mayo Clin Proc.* 2003;78(2):238–248.
31. Theodore WH, Fisher RS. Brain stimulation for epilepsy. *Lancet Neurol.* 2004;3(2):111–118.
32. Andrade DM, Zumsteg D, Hamani C, et al. Long-term follow-up of patients with thalamic deep brain stimulation for epilepsy. *Neurology.* 2006;66(10):1571–1573.
33. Cukiert A, Cukiert CM, Burattini JA, et al. Seizure outcome after hippocampal deep brain stimulation in patients with refractory temporal lobe epilepsy: a prospective, controlled, randomized, double-blind study. *Epilepsia.* 2017;58(10):1728–1733.
34. Sprengers M, Vonck K, Carrette E, et al. Deep brain and cortical stimulation for epilepsy. *Cochrane Database Syst Rev.* 2017;(7):CD008497.
35. Velasco F, Velasco M, Jiménez F, et al. Predictors in the treatment of difficult-to-control seizures by electrical stimulation of the centromedian thalamic nucleus. *Neurosurgery.* 2000;47(2):295–304, discussion 304–5.
36. Fisher R, Salanova V, Witt T, et al. Electrical stimulation of the anterior nucleus of thalamus for treatment of refractory epilepsy. *Epilepsia.* 2010;51(5):899–908.
37. Salanova V, Witt T, Worth R, et al. Long-term efficacy and safety of thalamic stimulation for drug-resistant partial epilepsy. *Neurology.* 2015;84(10):1017–1025.
38. Chen R, Spencer DC, Weston J, et al. Transcranial magnetic stimulation for the treatment of epilepsy. *Cochrane Database Syst Rev.* 2016;(8):CD011025.
39. Fregni F, Otachi PT, Do Valle A, et al. A randomized clinical trial of repetitive transcranial magnetic stimulation in patients with refractory epilepsy. *Ann Neurol.* 2006;60(4):447–455.
40. Seynaeve L, Devroye A, Dupont P, et al. Randomized crossover sham-controlled clinical trial of targeted low-frequency transcranial magnetic stimulation comparing a figure-8 and a round coil to treat refractory neocortical epilepsy. *Epilepsia.* 2016;57(1):141–150.
41. Theodore WH, Hunter K, Chen R, et al. Transcranial magnetic stimulation for the treatment of seizures: a controlled study. *Neurology.* 2002;59(4):560–562.
42. DeGiorgio CM, Soss J, Cook IA, et al. Randomized controlled trial of trigeminal nerve stimulation for drug-resistant epilepsy. *Neurology.* 2013;80(9):786–791.
43. Soss J, Heck C, Murray D, et al. A prospective long-term study of external trigeminal nerve stimulation for drug-resistant epilepsy. *Epilepsy Behav.* 2015;42:44–47.
44. Martens T, Merkel M, Holst B, et al. Vascular events after transsylvian selective amygdalohippocampectomy and impact on epilepsy outcome. *Epilepsia.* 2014;55(5):763–769.
45. Hoyt AT, Smith KA. Selective amygdalohippocampectomy. *Neurosurg Clin N Am.* 2016;27(1):1–17.
46. Schaller C, Jung A, Clusmann H, et al. Rate of vasospasm following the transsylvian versus transcortical approach for selective amygdalohippocampectomy. *Neurol Res.* 2004;26(6):666–670.
47. Oertel J, Gaab MR, Runge U, et al. Neuronavigation and complication rate in epilepsy surgery. *Neurosurg Rev.* 2004;27(3):214–217.
48. Kahlow H, Olivecrona M. Complications of vagal nerve stimulation for drug-resistant epilepsy: a single center longitudinal study of 143 patients. *Seizure.* 2013;22(10):827–833.

35 Complications After Stereotactic Radiosurgery

BRUCE E. POLLOCK

HIGHLIGHTS

- Complications after stereotactic radiosurgery relate primarily to either temporary or permanent radiation injury to the structures adjacent to the irradiated target.
- Risk factors are history of prior irradiation, lesion size, lesion location, nonconformal dose planning, and radiation dose.
- Reversible imaging changes (areas of increased signal on T2-weighted magnetic resonance imaging) are common and generally occur in the first 6 to 12 months after stereotactic radiosurgery. Most are asymptomatic and resolve without treatment, whereas patients with symptomatic reversible imaging changes can usually be managed with corticosteroid therapy.
- Radiation necrosis (persistent areas of enhancement with adjacent edema) is much less common and represents permanent vascular damage with resultant immune response. Treatment of symptomatic patients can include corticosteroids, bevacizumab, hyperbaric oxygen therapy, or surgical resection.
- Late adverse radiation effects develop 5 or more years after stereotactic radiosurgery and are characterized by perilesional edema or cyst formation. Symptomatic late adverse radiation effects frequently require surgical removal to improve the patient's neurologic condition.

Introduction

The concept of stereotactic radiosurgery (SRS) was developed by Lars Leksell from the Karolinska Institute in Stockholm, Sweden in 1951.[1,2] SRS utilizes the principles of stereotactic localization combined with the precise delivery of radiation to an imaging-defined target. In the past 40 years, SRS has experienced exponential growth and has become an integral part of both neurosurgery and radiation oncology. Advances in neuroimaging and dose-planning software, together with the accumulated clinical experience of more than 1,000,000 treated patients to date, have made SRS safer and more effective for a wide variety of clinical indications.[3–5] Whereas once SRS was available in only a few academic centers, now SRS is available to patients at both academic and community medical centers around the world.

The goal of SRS is to deliver a clinically effective radiation dose to an imaging-defined target. At first, SRS was a single-fraction technique limited to the brain. Now SRS is defined as stereotactically delivered radiation in 1 to 5 fractions to both intracranial and extracranial targets. As with any radiation treatment, SRS aims to damage the target more than the adjacent normal tissues. Two primary approaches are used to increase the therapeutic ratio in different types of radiation treatment. One, dose fractionation, exploits the differential radiosensitivity of normal and abnormal tissues. Typically, normal tissues are better able to repair sublethal DNA damage than tumors because of aberrant cell cycle control mechanisms in tumors. This is the rationale behind external beam radiation therapy (EBRT), whereby multiple small doses of radiation are delivered to the target and the adjacent normal tissue. Two, and in contrast to EBRT, single-fraction SRS achieves its therapeutic effect by minimizing the radiation delivered to the nearby normal structures by using highly conformal dose plans. Within several millimeters of the edge of the target, the radiation dose drops from a therapeutic level (10–25 Gy) to doses that approximate a single fraction of EBRT (2 Gy). Multisession SRS (2–5 fractions) theoretically takes advantage of both of these approaches by using conformal dose planning delivered in a small number of sessions.

Types of Radiation Complications

Parenchymal Injury

Imaging changes noted after SRS are common and can be divided into three categories. First, reversible imaging changes (RIC) (areas of increased signal on T2-weighted magnetic resonance imaging [MRI]) generally occur in the first 6 to 12 months after SRS (Fig. 35.1).[6–8] Most are asymptomatic and resolve without treatment. Second, radiation necrosis (persistent areas of enhancement with adjacent edema) is much less common and represents permanent vascular damage with resultant immune response. Distinguishing between RIC, radiation necrosis, and tumor growth after SRS is important, and no imaging technique is perfect at guiding clinical decision-making.[9] For small areas in asymptomatic patients, observation with repeat imaging is preferred. Comparison of the area on gadolinium-enhanced T1-weighted and T2-weighted MRI is commonly used after brain metastases SRS.[10,11] Third, late adverse radiation effects (ARE) develop 5 or more years after SRS and are characterized by perilesional edema or cyst formation.[12,13]

Cranial Neuropathy

Cranial nerve deficits after SRS of skull base lesions are uncommon.[14–21] Most occur within the first year after SRS, but delayed injury can occur. Special somatic sensory nerves (optic,

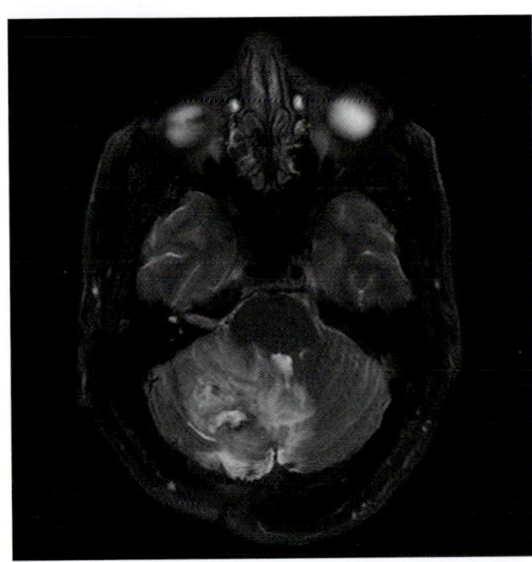

• **Fig. 35.1** Axial T2-weighted magnetic resonance imaging (MRI) of a 58-year-old man who developed mild headaches 7 months after SRS of a recurrent posterior fossa pilocytic astrocytoma. The MRI showed edema throughout the right cerebellar hemisphere and mild mass effect on the fourth ventricle. The patient was started on corticosteroid therapy with resolution of his symptoms.

vestibulo-cochlear) are the most radiation sensitive, followed by the general somatic sensory nerves (trigeminal). The motor nerves are particularly radiation resistant.

Vascular

Large vessel injury is uncommon after SRS, although cases of internal carotid artery occlusion and stroke have been reported after SRS of cavernous sinus meningiomas,[19] and focal morphologic changes and aneurysm formation have been seen in the superior cerebellar artery in patients after trigeminal neuralgia SRS.[22,23]

Secondary Tumor Formation

The most significant complication of any radiation-based procedure is the development of secondary tumors caused by irradiation. Cahan et al. reported 11 cases of bone sarcomas that arose after radiation treatment and outlined four criteria that are required before a secondary tumor could be deemed radiation induced.[24] First, the second tumor must arise within the prior radiation field. Second, there must be an adequate latency between the radiation exposure and the development of the second tumor. Third, the secondary tumor must be histologically different from the original tumor. Fourth, the patient must not have a genetic predisposition for tumor development. Often it is difficult to separate cases that are more likely coincidental than radiation induced.[25,26] The risk of radiation-induced tumors after SRS has been reported between 0% and 2.6% at 15 years and should not be used as a justification for choosing other treatment approaches over SRS for appropriate patients.[27–29]

Risk Factors for Radiation Complications

The primary risk factors for ARE after SRS are a history of prior irradiation, large treatment volume, target location, poor (nonconformal) dose planning, and higher radiation doses. Numerous studies have correlated the chance of RIC after SRS with some measure of the radiation dose to the surrounding tissue and the location of the target.[6,7,30] The most commonly cited parameter is the 12-Gy volume that is the total volume in the treatment field that receives a radiation dose of 12 Gy or more.[6] Patients with lesions in deep parenchymal locations (thalamus, basal ganglia, and brainstem) are more likely to develop neurologic deficits secondary to imaging changes noted on MRI. Advances in SRS technique including improved neuroimaging, better dose-planning software, and more precise radiation delivery devices have all contributed to a reduction in the incidence of ARE after SRS.[3–5] In addition, medical knowledge based on the last 40 years has been instrumental in guiding clinical decision-making and proper patient selection for SRS. Patients with large lesions with symptomatic mass effect are rarely good candidates for SRS.

One area that has received a great deal of attention is the risk of radiation-induced optic neuropathy (RION) after single-fraction SRS in the parasellar region. Early studies concluded that the risk of RION was increased if the radiation dose to the anterior visual pathways (optic nerves or chiasm) exceeded 8 Gy.[31] However, more recent studies have shown that radiation doses of 10 to 14 Gy are well tolerated and have a low risk of RION (Fig. 35.2).[15,17,18] Acceptance of this higher dose threshold for the anterior visual pathways increases the applicability and likely the effectiveness of single-fraction SRS for patients with lesions in the parasellar region.

Volume-staged SRS (VS-SRS) is another approach that has reduced the risk of ARE in arteriovenous malformation (AVM) SRS. Although SRS is an accepted treatment option for patients with small- to moderate-sized intracranial AVM, SRS is generally recommended only for AVM with a diameter of 3 cm or less (approximately 14 cm^3). Over the past 20 years, a number of centers have performed VS-SRS for patients with large-volume AVM.[32–35] Volume staging of large AVM into multiple radiosurgical sessions permits a higher radiation dose to be delivered to the entire AVM volume while reducing the radiation exposure to the adjacent brain. Early papers have shown that VS-SRS permits large-volume intracranial AVM to be treated with a low rate of ARE. More work on escalating dose and decreasing the treatment volume per stage is needed to determine whether this will increase the rate of obliteration with this technique.

Treatment of Radiation Complications

In neurologically stable patients, follow-up after SRS consists of periodic clinical examination and MRI. For patients with metastatic brain disease or primary brain tumors, this is usually performed every 3 months for the first year, then less frequently thereafter. Patients with AVM and most benign tumors (meningiomas, vestibular schwannoma, pituitary adenoma, glomus tumor) now undergo MRI between 6 and 12 months after SRS, then every 1 to 2 years. MRI review consists of lesion response, determination of RIC, and new tumor formation.

In asymptomatic patients, areas of increased signal on T2-weighted MRI adjacent to the treated lesion are followed, and further imaging is recommended. Most resolve without treatment, but patients with symptomatic RIC can usually be managed with corticosteroid therapy. Patients with symptomatic radiation necrosis can also be managed most times with corticosteroid therapy, but sometimes they cannot be successfully weaned off steroids, and other treatments are required. Treatment of persistent radiation necrosis can include bevacizumab, hyperbaric oxygen therapy, or surgical resection.[9,36–38] For patients with late ARE, again observation with serial imaging is recommended if they are asymptomatic.[12,13] Patients with symptomatic late ARE frequently require surgical removal to improve the patient's neurologic condition.

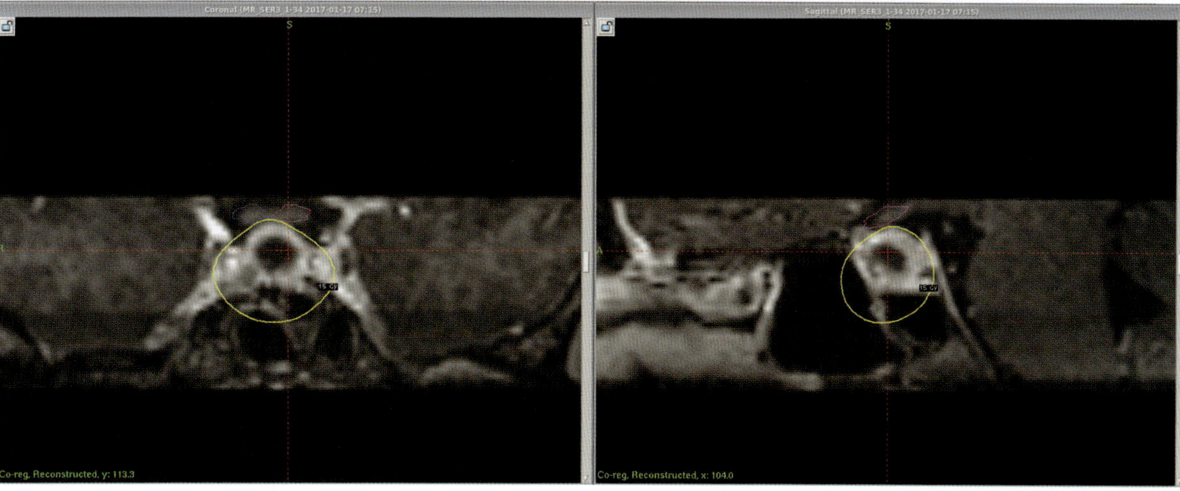

• **Fig. 35.2** Dose plan for a 52-year-old woman with a recurrent nonfunctioning pituitary adenoma after two prior transsphenoidal resections. The tumor margin dose was 15 Gy. The maximum dose to the right and left optic nerves was 13.2 and 13.4 Gy, respectively.

SURGICAL REWIND

My Worst Case

The patient was a 51-year-old man who had undergone complete resection of a left-sided 6-cm parasagittal fronto-parietal WHO grade II meningioma (Fig. 35.3). Postoperatively he did well but continued to have intermittent partial motor seizures. Follow-up MRI performed 7 months after surgery showed a tumor recurrence measuring 28 mm in greatest dimension. After discussing the options of repeat resection, EBRT, or SRS, the patient decided to proceed with SRS. Gamma Knife SRS was performed using 17 isocenters of radiation to cover a volume of 10.2 cm^3. The tumor margin dose was 16 Gy. Three months after SRS, he began to have more frequent seizures, and MRI showed slight tumor enlargement and adjacent edema. His anticonvulsant medications were increased, and he was placed on corticosteroid therapy. Over the next 5 months, he was not able to discontinue corticosteroid therapy without worsening headaches and more seizure activity. In addition, he developed steroid-induced diabetes mellitus and had a pulmonary embolus. He was started on bevacizumab therapy with improvement in the vasogenic edema. The bevacizumab therapy was stopped after 3 doses, and he was tapered off corticosteroids. Within several weeks, he started having more seizures again, and MRI showed the tumor to be larger with significant edema and mass effect. The patient underwent repeat tumor resection 15 months after SRS. A near-complete tumor resection was achieved, but he had a right-sided hemiparesis that required inpatient rehabilitation therapy. Within several weeks, his strength improved to normal, he was able to discontinue corticosteroid therapy, and he had no further seizure activity. One month after his second resection, he was treated with EBRT (59.4 Gy/33 fractions).

The decisions in this patient's management that contributed to his difficult course relate primarily to the timing and use of EBRT and SRS. It could be argued that EBRT given after his initial surgery may have prevented tumor recurrence and the need for SRS. However, the patient was not operated on at our center, and the usefulness of postoperative EBRT after complete removal of WHO grade II meningiomas remains controversial. In my opinion, the greater error was proceeding with SRS for a tumor >10 cm^3 in a location that is very high risk for ARE.[39,40] In retrospect, repeat surgical resection would have been a better option than SRS for this rapidly enlarging tumor. The lesson to learn is that poor patient selection cannot be overcome by advances in SRS technique.

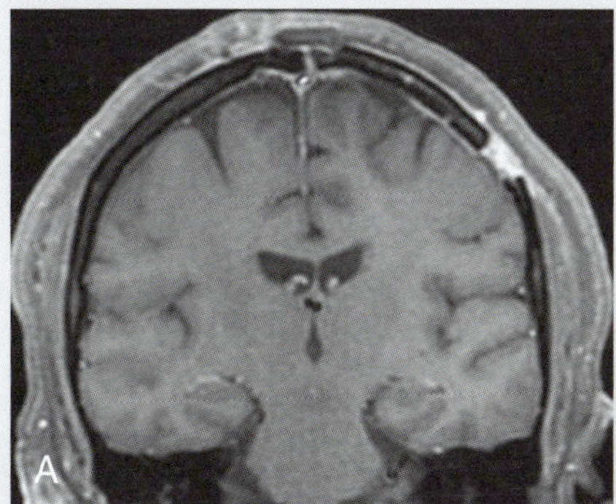

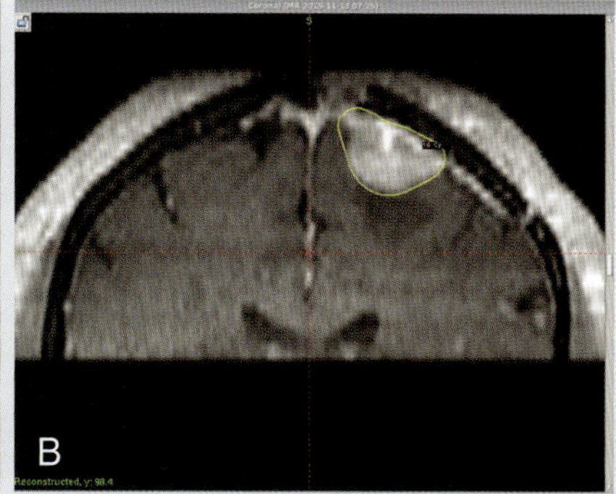

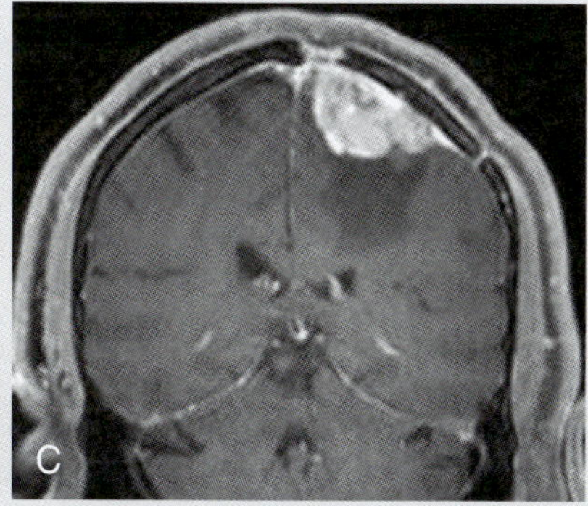

• **Fig. 35.3** Coronal postgadolinium magnetic resonance imaging (MRI) and dose plan of a 51-year-old man who underwent SRS for a recurrent WHO grade II meningioma. (A) MRI 3 months after initial resection showing no gross evidence of tumor. (B) Dose plan at the time of SRS 7 months after initial resection. (C) MRI 15 months after SRS shows the tumor to be increased in size with adjacent edema and mass effect.

NEUROSURGICAL SELFIE MOMENT

Major complications after contemporary SRS are uncommon, and most can be well managed by experienced physicians. The risks of ARE are greater in patients with a history of prior radiation treatment, large treatment volumes, and nonconformal dose plans. Late ARE can occur after both AVM and benign tumor SRS, emphasizing the need for ongoing MRI follow-up many years after SRS. The risk of radiation-induced tumors after single-fraction SRS is very low and should not be used as a reason to choose alternative treatment strategies for appropriate patients.

References

1. Leksell L. The stereotactic method and radiosurgery of the brain. *Acta Chir Scand*. 1951;102:316–319.
2. Leksell L. Stereotactic radiosurgery. *J Neurol Neurosurg Psychiatry*. 1983;46:797–803.
3. Flickinger JC, Kondziolka D, Pollock BE, et al. Evolution in technique for vestibular schwannoma radiosurgery and effect on outcome. *Int J Radiat Oncol Biol Phys*. 1996;36:275–280.
4. Nagy G, Rowe JG, Radatz MWR, et al. A historical analysis of single-staged Gamma Knife radiosurgical treatment for large arteriovenous malformations: evolution and outcomes. *Acta Neurochir*. 2012;154:383–394.
5. Pollock BE, Link MJ, Stafford SL, et al. Stereotactic radiosurgery for arteriovenous malformations: the effect of treatment period on patient outcomes. *Neurosurgery*. 2016;78:499–509.
6. Flickinger JC, Kondziolka D, Lunsford LD, et al. Development of a model to predict permanent symptomatic post-radiosurgery injury for arteriovenous malformation patients. *Int J Radiat Oncol Biol Phys*. 2000;46:1143–1148.
7. Kano H, Flickinger JC, Tonetti D, et al. Estimating the risks of adverse radiation effects after Gamma Knife radiosurgery for arteriovenous malformations. *Stroke*. 2017;48:84–90.
8. Yen CP, Matsumoto JA, Wintermark M, et al. Radiation-induced imaging changes following Gamma Knife surgery for cerebral arteriovenous malformations. *J Neurosurg*. 2013;118:63–73.
9. Chao ST, Ahluwalia MS, Barnett GH, et al. Challenges with the diagnosis and treatment of cerebral radiation necrosis. *Int J Radiat Oncol Biol Phys*. 2013;87:449–457.
10. Dequesada IM, Quisling RG, Yachnis A, et al. Can standard magnetic resonance imaging reliably distinguish recurrent tumor from radiation necrosis after radiosurgery for brain metastases? A radiographic-pathologic study. *Neurosurgery*. 2008;63:898–904.
11. Kano H, Kondziolka D, Lobato-Polo J, et al. T1/T2 matching to differentiate tumor growth from radiation effects after stereotactic radiosurgery. *Neurosurgery*. 2010;66:486–492.
12. Pan H, Sheehan J, Stroila M, et al. Late cyst formation following Gamma Knife surgery of arteriovenous malformations. *J Neurosurg*. 2005;102(suppl):124–127.
13. Pollock BE, Link MJ, Branda ME, et al. Incidence and management of late adverse radiation effects after arteriovenous malformation radiosurgery. *Neurosurgery*. 2017;81(6):928–934.
14. Carlson ML, Jacob JT, Pollock BE, et al. Long-term hearing outcomes following low-dose stereotactic radiosurgery for vestibular schwannoma: patterns of hearing loss and variables influencing audiometric decline. *J Neurosurg*. 2013;118:579–587.
15. Hasegawa T, Kobayashi T, Kida Y. Tolerance of the optic apparatus in single-fraction irradiation using stereotactic radiosurgery: evaluation in 100 patients with craniopharyngioma. *Neurosurgery*. 2010;66:688–695.
16. Kano H, Park KJ, Kondziolka D, et al. Does prior microsurgery improve or worsen the outcomes of stereotactic radiosurgery for cavernous sinus meningiomas? *Neurosurgery*. 2013;73:401–410.
17. Leavitt JA, Stafford SL, Link MJ, et al. Long-term evaluation of radiation-induced optic neuropathy after single-fraction stereotactic radiosurgery. *Int J Radiat Oncol Biol Phys*. 2013;87:524–527.
18. Pollock BE, Link MJ, Leavitt JL, et al. Dose-volume analysis of radiation-induced optic neuropathy after single-fraction stereotactic radiosurgery. *Neurosurgery*. 2014;75:456–460.
19. Pollock BE, Stafford SL, Link MJ, et al. Single-fraction radiosurgery of benign cavernous sinus meningiomas. *J Neurosurg*. 2013;119:675–682.
20. Sheehan JP, Starke RM, Mathieu D, et al. Gamma Knife radiosurgery for the management of nonfunctioning pituitary adenomas: a multicenter study. *J Neurosurg*. 2013;119:446–456.
21. Skeie BS, Enger PO, Skeie GO, et al. Gamma Knife surgery of meningiomas involving the cavernous sinus: long-term follow-up of 100 patients. *Neurosurgery*. 2010;66:661–669.
22. Chen JC, Chao K, Rahimian J. De novo superior cerebellar artery aneurysm following radiosurgery for trigeminal neuralgia. *J Clin Neurosci*. 2017;38:87–90.
23. Maher CO, Pollock BE. Radiation induced vascular injury after stereotactic radiosurgery for trigeminal neuralgia. *Surg Neurol*. 2000;54:189–193.
24. Cahan WG, Woodard HQ, Higonbotham NL, et al. Sarcoma arising in irradiated bone. Report of 11 cases. *Cancer*. 1948;1:3–29.
25. Carlson ML, Glasgow AE, Jacob JT, et al. The short- and intermediate-term risk of second neoplasms after diagnosis and treatment of unilateral vestibular schwannoma: analysis of 9,460 cases. *Int J Radiat Oncol Biol Phys*. 2016;95(4):1149–1157.
26. Rowe J, Grainger A, Walton L, et al. Risk of malignancy after Gamma Knife stereotactic radiosurgery. *Neurosurgery*. 2007;60:60–66.
27. Patel TR, Chiang VL. Secondary neoplasms after stereotactic radiosurgery. *World Neurosurg*. 2014;81:594–599.
28. Pollock BE, Link MJ, Stafford SL, et al. The risk of radiation-induced tumors or malignant transformation after single-fraction intracranial radiosurgery: results based on a 25-year experience. *Int J Radiat Oncol Biol Phys*. 2017;97(5):919–923.
29. Starke RM, Yen CP, Chen CJ, et al. An updated assessment of the risk of radiation-induced neoplasia after radiosurgery of arteriovenous malformations. *World Neurosurg*. 2014;82:395–401.
30. Voges J, Treuer H, Lehrke R, et al. Risk analysis of LINAC radiosurgery in patients with arterio-venous malformations (AVM). *Acta Neurochir*. 1997;68:118–123.
31. Tishler RB, Loeffler JS, Lunsford LD, et al. Tolerance of cranial nerves of the cavernous sinus to radiosurgery. *Int J Radiat Oncol Biol Phys*. 1993;27:215–221.
32. Kano H, Kondziolka D, Flickinger JC, et al. Stereotactic radiosurgery for arteriovenous malformations, part 6: multistaged volumetric management of large arteriovenous malformations. *J Neurosurg*. 2012;116:54–65.
33. Nagy G, Grainger A, Hodgson T, et al. Staged volume radiosurgery of large arteriovenous malformations improves outcome by reducing the rate of adverse radiation effects. *Neurosurgery*. 2017;80:180–192.
34. Pollock BE, Link MJ, Stafford SL, et al. Volume-staged stereotactic radiosurgery for intracranial arteriovenous malformations: outcomes based on an 18-year experience. *Neurosurgery*. 2017;80(4):543–550.
35. Seymour ZA, Sneed PK, Gupta N, et al. Volume-staged radiosurgery for large arteriovenous malformations: an evolving paradigm. *J Neurosurg*. 2016;124:163–174.
36. Boothe D, Young R, Yamada Y, et al. Bevacizumab as a treatment for radiation necrosis of brain metastases post stereotactic radiosurgery. *Neuro Oncol*. 2013;15:1257–1263.
37. Kohshi K, Imada H, Nomoto S, et al. Successful treatment of radiation-induced brain necrosis by hyperbaric oxygen therapy. *J Neurol Sci*. 2003;209:115–117.
38. Levin VA, Bidaut L, Hou P, et al. Randomized double-blind placebo-controlled trial of bevacizumab therapy for radiation necrosis of the central nervous system. *Int J Radiat Oncol Biol Phys*. 2011;79:1487–1495.
39. Bledsoe JM, Link MJ, Stafford SL, et al. Radiosurgery for large volume (>10 cc) benign meningiomas. *J Neurosurg*. 2010;112:951–956.
40. Pollock BE, Stafford SL, Link MJ, et al. Single-fraction radiosurgery of benign intracranial meningiomas. *Neurosurgery*. 2012;71:604–613.

36

Complications of Endoscopic Endonasal Skull Base Surgery

PAUL A. GARDNER, CARL H. SNYDERMAN, ERIC W. WANG, JUAN C. FERNANDEZ-MIRANDA

HIGHLIGHTS

- Cerebrospinal fluid leak remains the most common complication of endoscopic endonasal skull base surgery, but this has decreased dramatically with the use of vascularized nasoseptal flaps.
- Lumbar drains have been shown to decrease the risk of cerebrospinal fluid leak after endonasal skull base surgery, primarily for larger anterior and posterior fossa defects.
- Major vascular injury can be controlled during endoscopic ESBS, but it often requires immediate endovascular evaluation and/or treatment.
- Nasal instrumentation should be avoided in the postoperative period unless under direct endoscopic visualization.
- There is a significant learning curve with endonasal skull base surgery that should be respected to keep complication rates low.

Background

Endoscopic endonasal skull base surgery (ESBS) has seen a dramatic increase in adoption since its introduction and development over the last two decades. Initially used only for pituitary tumors,[1,2] the approach has expanded significantly to include the entire ventral skull base.[3–6] However, multiple articles have demonstrated that there is a significant learning curve with these approaches,[7–9] with improved resection and decreased complication rates such as cerebrospinal fluid (CSF) leak over time. In addition, the introduction of vascularized flaps such as the nasoseptal flap[10] has significantly improved the reconstruction of the skull base after these approaches.

With all skull base approaches, nerve and vascular injury make up the remainder of the majority of complications.[11] In general, endonasal approaches were developed to allow wide and well-visualized anterior access for tumors that originate in the midline or paramedian skull base and displace involved neurovascular structures laterally. Respecting this concept in approach selection, as well as the learning curve, helps minimize neurovascular complications.

Anatomic Insights

The anterior cranial base slopes inferiorly from anterior to posterior with varying degree. During exposure, care should be taken not to violate the skull base during anterior to posterior dissection, especially during maneuvers such as middle turbinate resection. Excessive head extension during positioning may alter the trajectory and predispose to anterior skull base injury during exposure.

A thorough understanding of vascular and neural anatomy is critical for navigating the skull base. The internal carotid artery (ICA) is a key anatomic landmark for orientation and classification of endonasal approaches (Fig. 36.1). Endonasal landmarks include:

- The Eustachian tube lies medial to the parapharyngeal ICA as it enters the skull base.
- The vidian nerve is located just inferior and lateral to the foramen lacerum ICA, and it crosses over the horizontal petrous ICA to connect with the greater superficial petrosal nerve (GSPN).
- The pterygoid process marks the medial plane of the foramen lacerum and the pterygo-sphenoidal fissure (between pterygoid process and sphenoid sinus floor) and attaches posteriorly to the foramen lacerum ICA.
- The middle clinoid process, when present, is located between the cavernous ICA and the clinoidal ICA.[12]
- The "medial optic-carotid recess (OCR)" is a landmark for the clinoidal segment of the ICA and dural ring.
- The lateral OCR is located laterally between the clinoidal ICA and optic canal.

Sphenopalatine artery anatomy (Fig. 36.2) is critical to understand for a multitude of reasons. It can be a source of postoperative epistaxis after pituitary surgery, is the key supply for the nasoseptal (posterior nasal artery) and other posteriorly based flaps, and must be dissected and managed to access the pterygoid canal and base of the pterygoid for transpterygoid approaches.[13]

Limitations for the endoscopic endonasal approach (EEA) are largely laterally located or displaced nerves and/or arteries. Crossing the plane of nerves defeats the main advantage of an endoscopic endonasal corridor, which is avoidance of neurovascular manipulation. Understanding these limitations and the

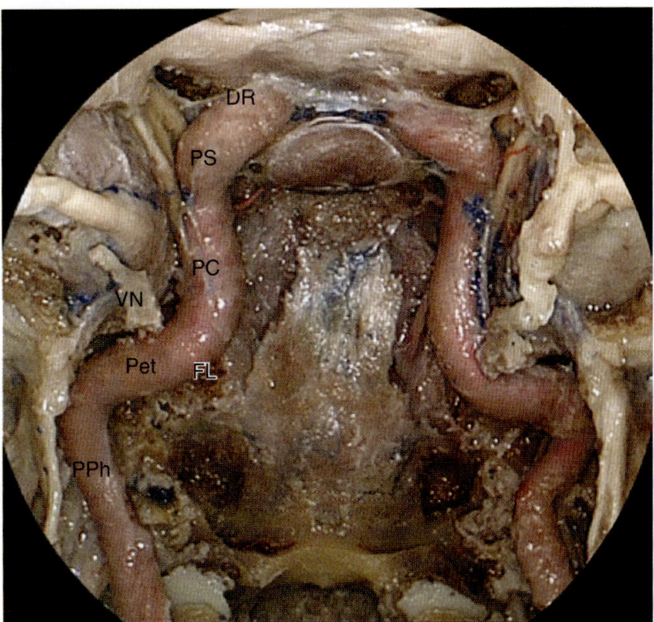

• **Fig. 36.1** Endoscopic endonasal view of a cadaver dissection showing the segments of the internal carotid artery (ICA) that create the lateral limit of many endonasal approaches. *DR,* Dural ring confluence; *FL,* foramen lacerum; *PC,* paraclival ICA; *Pet,* horizontal petrous ICA; *PPh,* Parapharyngeal ICA; *PS,* parasellar ICA; *VN,* vidian nerve.

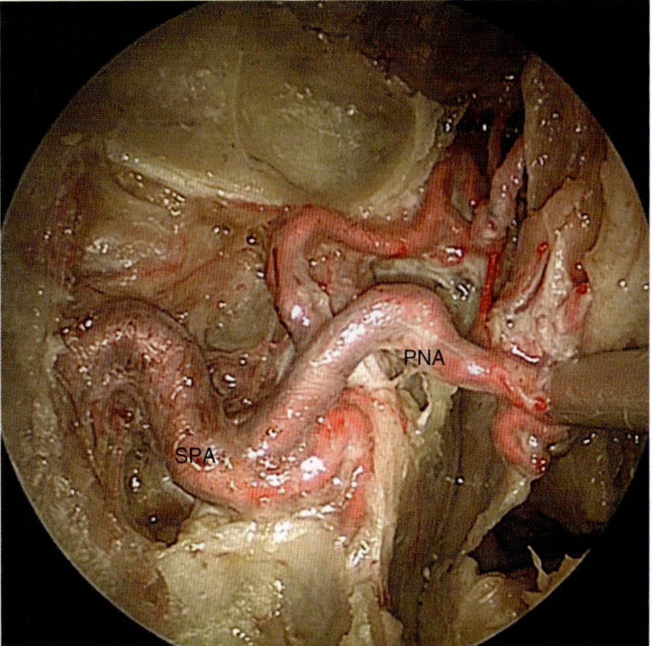

• **Fig. 36.2** Endoscopic endonasal view of the right pterygopalatine fossa showing the sphenopalatine artery (SPA) and key posterior nasal artery (PNA) branch. The latter provides blood supply to the vascularized nasoseptal flap and can also be a source of postoperative epistaxis when sacrificed.

anatomy of the cranial nerves in these key locations is critical for avoiding injury.

In the suprasellar space, the optic nerves enter the dural sheath of the optic canal at the medial aspect of the optic strut/lateral OCR. The canal can be widely decompressed by carefully drilling all bone overlying the medial canal. A suprasellar dural opening can be extended laterally to the medial falciform ligament above the optic nerve, to avoid injury to the ophthalmic artery, which often originates on the medial supraclinoidal ICA or loops medially before travelling to its usual position, just inferior to the optic nerve, until it crosses superiorly more distally.

The sella is limited laterally by the ICA, but tumors can be dissected from the various compartments of the cavernous sinus, named based on their relationship to the genu of the cavernous ICA.[14] The superior compartment (where most medially originating tumors extend) is related to the third cranial nerve, whereas the posterior and inferior compartments only have segments of the abducens nerve (CN VI). The lateral compartment contains segments of all cavernous cranial nerves (III, IV, V1, and VI). Though III and IV are generally ensheathed in the lateral cavernous wall dura, entrance into this compartment is generally reserved for aggressive tumors or those with symptoms indicative of oculomotor nerve involvement.

The midclivus is bounded laterally by the petrous apex, Dorello's canal, and the abducens nerve. This nerve is most likely to be injured during any transclival approach, so understanding its anatomy is essential. CN VI exits the brainstem at the vertebrobasilar junction and runs obliquely up to Dorello's canal, which runs behind the upper half of the paraclival ICA. There is a venous channel, the inferior petrosal sinus, immediately below the nerve, which can be a conduit for tumor growth. "Gardner's triangle" is a medial anatomic triangle providing access to the petrous apex. It is bounded superiorly by the abducens nerve, anteriorly by the paraclival ICA, and inferiorly by the petroclival synchondrosis.

The lateral limitation in the lower clivus, below the foramen lacerum, is the hypoglossal canal and nerve. Extending exposure to this landmark increases access by 50%.[15,16] Immediately above the canal lies the medial jugular tubercle and below it, the medial occipital condyle. Inferior extension of dissection beyond the tip of the odontoid process may cause craniocervical instability, especially if the anterior ring of C1 is disrupted.

RED FLAGS

- Prior endonasal surgery increases risk of nasoseptal flap necrosis.
- Chondroid tumors (chordoma and chondrosarcoma) have the highest risk of ICA injury.
- Growth hormone–secreting tumors are associated with ICA ectasia and increased risk of injury.
- Recurrent tumors, especially after radiation therapy, have an increased risk of both neural and vascular injury.
- Nonadenomas invading the cavernous sinus are at much higher risk than adenomas for nerve and artery injury during cavernous sinus dissection.
- Coronal plane (paramedian) approaches have an increased risk of complications, especially ICA injury.

Prevention

Important aspects of prevention of complications during ESBS include preoperative preparation; a careful understanding of the normal anatomy from an endonasal perspective; proper imaging (computed tomography [CT] angiography) to assess the circle of Willis; evaluation of nasal structures if the patient has had prior

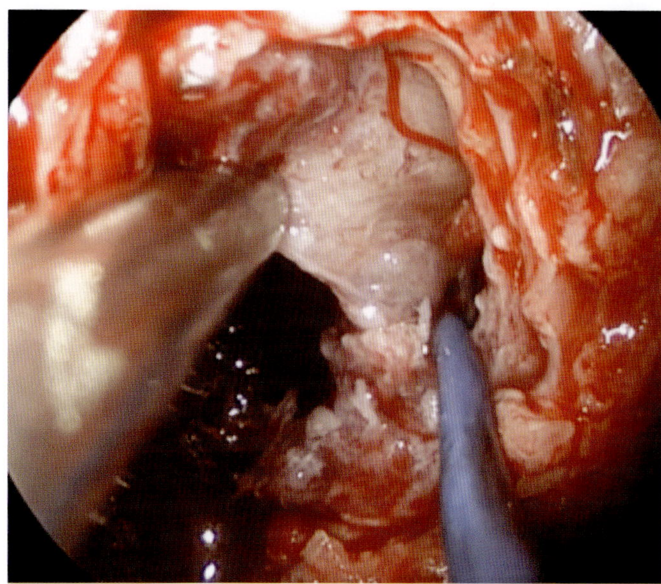

• **Fig. 36.3** Intraoperative endoscopic endonasal view showing a Kartush stimulator being used to dissect the abducens nerve from a petroclival meningioma. Identification and verification of cranial nerves with stimulating dissectors can decrease the risk of injury.

endonasal surgery; and full evaluation of hormonal and ophthalmologic function preoperatively.

Intraoperatively, the use of image guidance and Doppler probes provides accurate localization of the ICA to avoid injury. Electromyography (EMG) (both free-running and stimulated) can help identify motor cranial nerves and is associated with lower risk of postoperative loss of function (Fig. 36.3). In addition, team surgery (two surgeons, 3–4 hands) has significant advantages with respect to visualization, dynamic endoscopy, and microsurgical dissection, as well as avoidance and management of complications. A second surgeon will often notice impending complications when the other does not. Two surgeons (especially from different specialties) will often focus on different aspects, thereby increasing the likelihood of complication avoidance.

Postoperatively, close follow-up by both otolaryngological and neurosurgical teams will help avoid respective complications. Lumbar drainage has been shown to reduce postoperative CSF leak risk in patients with large anterior or posterior fossa dural defects.[17] If CSF leak is suspected, early re-exploration is key to preventing subsequent complications such as meningitis.

Frequent screening for deep venous thrombosis in the lower extremities with Doppler sonography is important in patients with prolonged procedures or hospital stays.

Management

Nerve Injury

In general, there is little that can be done for a nerve injury. Limited suturing ability combined with common sites of injury adjacent to or intimate with the ICA makes reapproximation difficult or impossible. If there is still a detectable EMG threshold across the nerve, no further measures are needed, although corticosteroids are often used intraoperatively and for a period of days postoperatively, depending on the severity of weakness and balanced with the impact of steroids on healing. There is some data on facial nerve injury suggesting that calcium channel blockers may aid recovery, but this has never been widely accepted or studied in other cranial nerves.[18–20] If the two ends of the nerve can be placed into contact with each other, covering them with fibrin glue is a means of both re-approximation and protection against further injury.

In general, vision loss after EEA is rare and seems to be less severe than with open approaches.[8,21–23] Patients with greater severity of vision loss preoperatively may have a higher risk of worsening postoperatively. This may be a reflection of degree of compression or compromise of perfusion. If patients are worse on awakening, they should be closely monitored with a mean arterial blood pressure (MAP) floor of 80 or more, even if pressors are required, and high-dose steroids. Unless the source of injury is known, imaging with CT scan should be performed to look for early hematoma or overpacking with fat graft. Intradural fat graft in the suprasellar region due to the latter risk is generally avoided at our center. Delayed worsening should generally be treated in the same manner, though hematoma becomes a more likely scenario. If visual status is unclear, bedside ophthalmologic examination and urgent magnetic resonance imaging (MRI) can be used to determine need for reoperation. If there is any concern for mass effect associated with vision loss, reoperation to evacuate the source should be done as efficiently as possible. In the absence of compression, microvascular vasospasm of the superior hypophyseal branches and other optic apparatus perforators is the presumed cause. This is managed with hypertension, as described, and by considering the addition of calcium channel blockers such as nimodipine.

Vascular Injury

Injury to the ICA or other intracranial vasculature is one of the most feared complications in any cranial base surgery, but especially during ESBS. The first step with any injury is control of the bleeding. This requires localization of the site of injury and maintenance of visualization. The former is obtained by using a large-bore suction to follow the bleeding while introducing a cottonoid to cover and contain it. If this cannot be achieved, other maneuvers should be used: adenosine (0.3 mg/kg) can give a 10- to 20-second cardiac pause; for ICA injury, firm percutaneous compression of the cervical ICA can provide a degree of proximal control.

Hypotension can aid in initial control, but once compression is applied and/or the artery is occluded, it should be avoided in favor of perfusion. Small holes in an artery or avulsion of a perforator can be effectively controlled with careful, fine bipolar electrocautery on a lower setting with saline irrigation by the co-surgeon. Bipolar electrocautery can be an effective means of hemostasis while maintaining vessel patency, depending on the caliber. Other options such as aneurysm clips placed with a single shaft applier are possible, but the most reliable solution for a large vessel injury is packing with muscle, either from the abdominal rectus or temporalis muscle (if prepped), or from the nasopharyngeal capitis muscle, which can be harvested in-field once bleeding is controlled. Ideally, packing will be tight enough to control bleeding, but not so tight that it occludes the vessel. Doppler sonography can be critical to confirm maintenance of flow, and intraoperative neurophysiologic monitoring with somatosensory evoked potentials (SSEP) is an important adjunct to detect ischemia.

The muscle graft (or cotton if used) ideally is covered with a tissue flap before placement of additional packing. This separates the site of injury from the sinus to prevent future contamination.

An algorithm to this effect has been previously published.[24] If control of the injury requires excessive or repeated manipulation of the artery, intraoperative anticoagulation should be considered, though this is often counterintuitive at a time of uncontrolled bleeding. However, once the vessel is controlled, the thrombus formation from endothelial injury can lead to complete occlusion or embolus.

Immediate postoperative angiography (digital subtraction angiography [DSA] or CT angiography [CTA]) is critical in the setting of any vascular injury. Unless an injury is minor and easily controlled, minimal tumor resection should proceed, because vessel stenosis and/or manipulation can lead to unforeseen complications, such as thromboembolism, that can result in devastating but avoidable consequences. "Emergent" bypass is not pragmatic. The majority of patients will tolerate ICA sacrifice, and those who do not typically will infarct rapidly, much sooner than the 4+ hours it would take even the most skilled surgeons to complete a high-flow bypass. Therefore endovascular salvage remains the main reasonable option.

The advantage of DSA is the ability to treat any active issue such as extravasation, stenosis, or pseudoaneurysm. Newer flow-diversion devices have improved coverage and can provide a good solution for all three of these. However, if this is not possible due to tortuosity of the carotid siphon, a large defect, or lack of technical expertise, coiling and even ICA sacrifice should be considered, assuming neurophysiologic parameters are stable.

Delayed vascular imaging is also important, because vascular injuries will often result in pseudoaneurysm formation. Follow-up vascular imaging (CTA or DSA is preferred, but MR angiography is an option) typically is performed around 1 week, 1 month, and 3 to 6 months postoperatively in the setting of arterial injury without sacrifice.

Postoperative Cerebrospinal Fluid Leak

CSF leak is the most common complication after ESBS.[7–8,25] Early detection and treatment of leak are critical to prevent further sequelae. The introduction and widespread usage of the vascularized nasoseptal flap have led to a dramatic decrease in the risk of postoperative leak, and the flap is recommended in any high-flow leak setting.[26,27] Proper healing requires removal of any intervening tissue (mucosa, blood clot) or foreign body (bone wax) between the flap and native bone or dura surrounding the defect. This maximizes contact between vascularized tissues. A multilayer reconstruction with an auto- or allograft onlay deep to the flap is sometimes necessary if the flap is not adequate to cover the defect with overlap. It is important to ensure that the flap is in contact with a demucosalized surface along its entire length, including the pedicle. Any part of the flap that is stretched across an air space will retract and cause shift of the flap in the postoperative period. Tissue glues play an unclear role but are used routinely. Nasal packing is important to hold the flap in place and counteract CSF pulsations exacerbated by the patient's activities.

There are also clear patient factors that contribute to CSF leak.[28] Foremost among these is increased body mass index (BMI), a setting in which CSF leak rates were most significantly reduced with use of a nasoseptal flap. Posterior fossa tumor location has also been shown repeatedly to be associated with higher pressures and therefore higher leak rates.

Also likely related to increased posterior fossa pressures is pontine encephalocele, a radiographic finding, typically without clinical sequelae, noted after wide bony and dural transclival resection.[29] The pons can slowly herniate into the defect during the period of healing (Fig. 36.4). This complication can severely limit postoperative radiation fields and could create problems for repeat surgery.

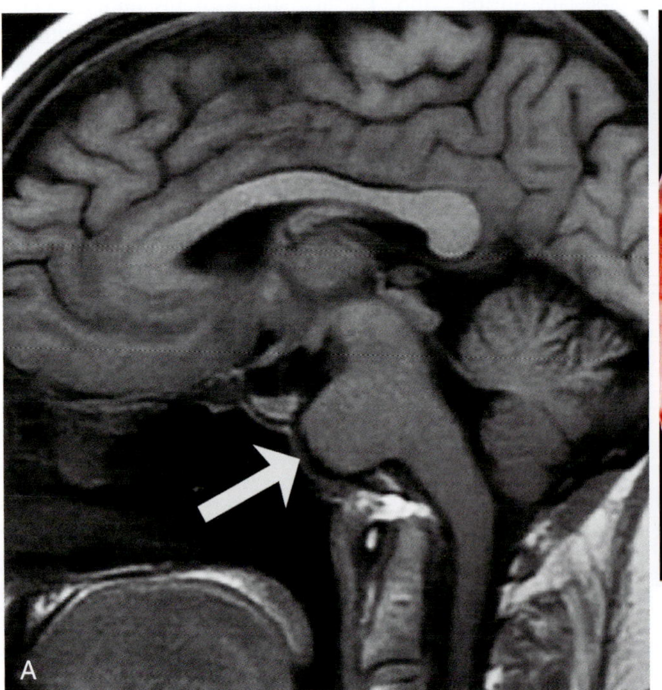

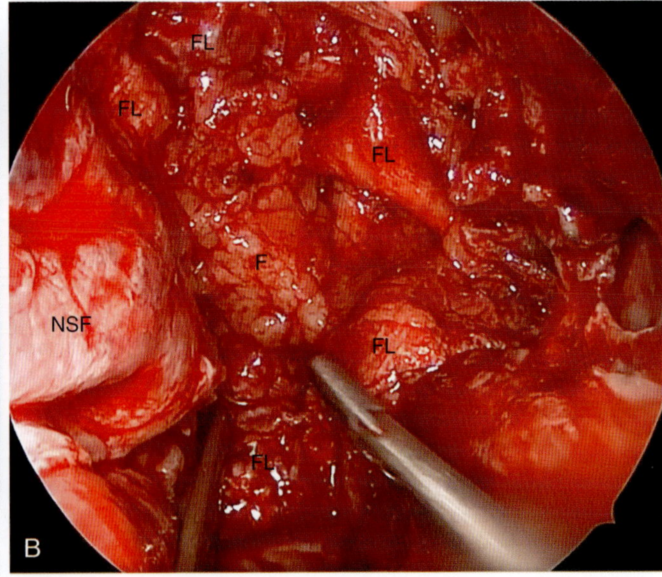

• **Fig. 36.4** (A) Sagittal T1-weighted magnetic resonance imaging showing bulging of the ventral pons (arrow) into a large clival defect after endoscopic endonasal surgery (EES). (B) Intraoperative endoscopic endonasal view showing abdominal fat-graft as part of a multilayered reconstruction of a large clival defect, which lowers risk of pontine encephalocele. *F*, Fat-graft; *FL*, fascia lata autograft covering the entire bony and dural defect; *NSF*, nasoseptal flap.

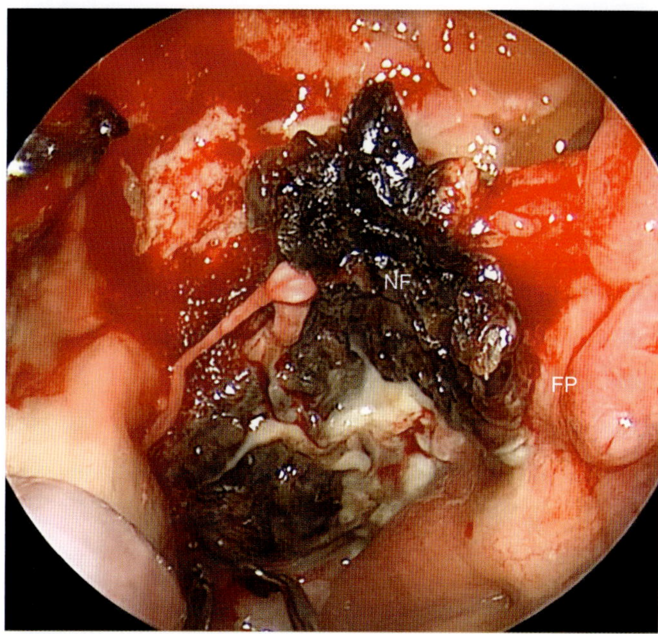

• **Fig. 36.5** Intraoperative endoscopic endonasal view showing a necrotic flap in a patient who presented with meningitis but no cerebrospinal fluid leak. *FP,* Flap pedicle; *NF,* necrotic flap.

Meningitis and young age increase this complication, whereas use of a fat graft as part of multilayer reconstruction (typically in between a deep allo- or autograft and the vascularized nasoseptal flap) lowered the risk by 91%.

Another rare complication is nasoseptal flap necrosis (Fig. 36.5). Occurring in 1.2% of patients,[30] it typically presents with signs of meningitis. Patients with prior nasal surgery are at higher risk, likely due to compromised vascularity of the flap pedicle or mucosa. Doppler sonography or ICG fluorescence endoscopy can be used to assess flap viability intraoperatively. Taking care to avoid narrowing the flap pedicle during harvest and protecting the pedicle during drilling and dissection are critical to avoid damage to the blood supply. A viable flap should enhance brightly on MRI. Failure to do so should lead to increased vigilance for necrosis and can be used to diagnose necrosis if the patient presents with meningismus or other signs of infection. Patients may also have a vaguely necrotic odor or halitosis.

If symptomatic flap necrosis is suspected, MRI can confirm the diagnosis, and a lumbar puncture should be performed if there is any concern for superinfection. It is treated by endonasal exploration with debridement of the necrotic tissue and replacement with vascularized tissue whenever possible (inferior turbinate/lateral nasal wall flap is the first option). A lumbar drain can be placed, especially if there is evidence of increased intracranial pressure as a result of meningitis.

SURGICAL REWIND

My Worst Case (Video 36.1)

A 39-year-old woman presented with florid acromegaly. Imaging showed an invasive adenoma with circumferential involvement of the right ICA (Knosp grade 4). Intraoperatively, the tumor was very fibrous and required sharp dissection and debridement. During the last portion of the surgery, an attempt at dissection of the ICA, which could not be visualized or accurately localized with Doppler sonography, resulted in torrential bleeding from the medial aspect of the cavernous ICA. Attempts at bipolar coagulation were unsuccessful. A cottonoid was placed over the bleeding site and compression held with a suction. Distal control with an aneurysm clip could be obtained at the paraclinoidal cavernous segment, but proximal control was unsuccessful due to tumor involvement, and neck compression did not slow the bleeding. A muscle patch was harvested from the rectus abdominal muscle while compression was once again held with a cottonoid. The muscle patch was placed at the site of bleeding and reinforced with multiple cottonoids. Mean arterial pressures were then increased as SSEPs began to decrease. The patient was taken immediately to the endovascular suite, where the ICA was seen to be completely occluded with no evidence of contralateral cross-fill. Fortunately, deployment of a stent across the area of occlusion was adequate to reopen the artery. The patient was placed on aspirin and Plavix. Postoperative MRI showed a near-complete tumor removal and only minor, scattered watershed infarcts.

The patient returned to the operating room more than a week later for removal of packing. Attempts at removal of the last cottonoid over the area of injury resulted in bleeding. This cottonoid was left in place but was covered with a vascularized nasoseptal flap to separate it from the nasal cavity. Repeat angiography showed that this resulted in a pseudoaneurysm that was treated with a flow diverter inside the previously deployed stent. Follow-up angiography showed resolution of the pseudoaneurysm. The patient was asymptomatic at this point and in biochemical remission. Later, she developed expected recurrence in the cavernous sinus, which was successfully treated with Gamma knife radiosurgery.

NEUROSURGICAL SELFIE MOMENT

Complications of endoscopic ESBS generally fall into three categories: neural injury, vascular injury, and failure of reconstruction. Avoidance of all three requires a complete understanding of the relevant anatomy and respect for the learning curve associated with these approaches. Careful case selection, guided by the principle of minimizing neurovascular manipulation and the concept of team surgery, provides for the safe application of the EEA to the skull base.

References

1. Jho HD, Carrau RL. Endoscopic endonasal transsphenoidal surgery: experience with 50 patients. *J Neurosurg.* 1997;87(1):44–51.
2. Cappabianca P, Alfieri A, de Divitiis E. Endoscopic endonasal transsphenoidal approach to the sella: towards functional endoscopic pituitary surgery (FEPS). *Minim Invasive Neurosurg.* 1998;41(2):66–73.
3. Kassam A, Snyderman CH, Mintz A, Gardner P, Carrau RL. Expanded endonasal approach: the rostrocaudal axis. Part I. Crista galli to the sella turcica. *Neurosurg Focus.* 2005;19(1):E3.

4. Kassam A, Snyderman CH, Mintz A, Gardner P, Carrau RL. Expanded endonasal approach: the rostrocaudal axis. Part II. Posterior clinoids to the foramen magnum. *Neurosurg Focus.* 2005;19(1):E4.
5. Cavallo LM, Messina A, Gardner P, et al. Extended endoscopic endonasal approach to the pterygopalatine fossa: anatomical study and clinical considerations. *Neurosurg Focus.* 2005;19(1):E5.
6. Kassam AB, Gardner P, Snyderman C, Mintz A, Carrau R. Expanded endonasal approach: fully endoscopic, completely transnasal approach to the middle third of the clivus, petrous bone, middle cranial fossa, and infratemporal fossa. *Neurosurg Focus.* 2005;19(1):E6.
7. Koutourousiou M, Gardner PA, Tormenti MJ, et al. Endoscopic endonasal approach for resection of skull base chordomas: outcomes and learning curve. *Neurosurgery.* 2012;71(3):614–625.
8. Koutourousiou M, Fernandez-Miranda JC, Stefko ST, Wang EW, Snyderman CH, Gardner PA. Endoscopic endonasal surgery for suprasellar meningiomas: experience with 75 patients. *J Neurosurg.* 2014;120(6):1326–1339.
9. Koutourousiou M, Fernandez-Miranda JC, Wang EW, Snyderman CH, Gardner PA. Endoscopic endonasal surgery for olfactory groove meningiomas: outcomes and limitations in 50 patients. *Neurosurg Focus.* 2014;37(4):E8.
10. Hadad G, Bassagasteguy L, Carrau RL, et al. A novel reconstructive technique after endoscopic expanded endonasal approaches: vascular pedicle nasoseptal flap. *Laryngoscope.* 2006;116(10):1882–1886.
11. Kassam AB, Prevedello DM, Carrau RL, et al. Endoscopic endonasal skull base surgery: analysis of complications in the authors' initial 800 patients. *J Neurosurg.* 2011;114(6):1544–1568.
12. Fernandez-Miranda JC, Tormenti M, Latorre F, Gardner P, Snyderman C. Endoscopic endonasal middle clinoidectomy: anatomical, radiological, and technical note. *Neurosurgery.* 2012;71(2 Suppl Operative): ons233–ons239.
13. Zhang X, Wang EW, Wei H, et al. Anatomy of the posterior septal artery with surgical implications on the vascularized pedicled nasoseptal flap. *Head Neck.* 2015;37(10):1470–1476.
14. Fernandez-Miranda JC, Zwagerman NT, Abhinav K, et al. Cavernous sinus compartments from the endonasal endoscopic approach: anatomical considerations and surgical relevance to adenoma surgery. *J Neurosurg.* 2018;129(2):430–441.
15. Morera VA, Fernandez-Miranda JC, Prevedello DM, et al. "Far-medial" expanded endonasal approach to the inferior third of the clivus: the transcondylar and transjugular tubercle approaches. *Neurosurgery.* 2010;66(6 Suppl Operative):211–219, discussion 219–220.
16. Wang WH, Abhinav K, Wang E, Snyderman C, Gardner PA, Fernandez-Miranda JC. Endoscopic endonasal transclival transcondylar approach for foramen magnum meningiomas: surgical anatomy and technical note. *Oper Neurosurg.* 2016;12(2):153–162.
17. Zwagerman NT, Wang EW, Shin S, et al. Does lumbar drainage reduce postoperative cerebrospinal fluid leak after endoscopic endonasal skull base surgery? A prospective, randomized controlled trial. *J Neurosurg*, submitted for publication. 2017;October.
18. Scheller C, Wienke A, Tatagiba M, et al. Prophylactic nimodipine treatment for cochlear and facial nerve preservation after vestibular schwannoma surgery: a randomized multicenter Phase III trial. *J Neurosurg.* 2016;124(3):657–664.
19. Scheller K, Scheller C. Nimodipine promotes regeneration of peripheral facial nerve function after traumatic injury following maxillofacial surgery: an off-label pilot study. *J Craniomaxillofac Surg.* 2012;40(5):427–434.
20. Lindsay RW, Heaton JT, Edwards C, Smitson C, Hadlock TA. Nimodipine and acceleration of functional recovery of the facial nerve after crush injury. *Arch Facial Plast Surg.* 2010;12(1):49–52.
21. Bander ED, Singh H, Ogilvie CB, et al. Endoscopic endonasal versus transcranial approach to tuberculum sellae and planum sphenoidale meningiomas in a similar cohort of patients. *J Neurosurg.* 2018;128(1):40–44.
22. Clark AJ, Jahangiri A, Garcia RM, et al. Endoscopic surgery for tuberculum sellae meningiomas: a systematic review and meta-analysis. *Neurosurg Rev.* 2013;36(3):349–359.
23. Stefko ST, Snyderman C, Fernandez-Miranda J, et al. Visual outcomes after endoscopic endonasal approach for craniopharyngioma: the Pittsburgh experience. *J Neurol Surg B.* 2016;77(4):326–332.
24. Gardner PA, Tormenti MJ, Pant H, Fernandez-Miranda JC, Snyderman CH, Horowitz MB. Carotid artery injury during endoscopic endonasal skull base surgery: incidence and outcomes. *Neurosurgery.* 2013;73 (2 Suppl Operative):ons261–ons270.
25. Koutourousiou M, Gardner PA, Fernandez-Miranda JC, Tyler-Kabara EC, Wang EW, Snyderman CH. Endoscopic endonasal surgery for craniopharyngiomas: surgical outcome in 64 patients. *J Neurosurg.* 2013;1119(5):1194–1207.
26. Zanation AM, Carrau RL, Snyderman CH, et al. Nasoseptal flap reconstruction of high flow intraoperative cerebral spinal fluid leaks during endoscopic skull base surgery. *Am J Rhinol Allergy.* 2009; 23(5):518–521.
27. Harvey RJ, Parmar P, Sacks R, Zanation AM. Endoscopic skull base reconstruction of large dural defects: a systematic review of published evidence. *Laryngoscope.* 2012;122(2):452–459.
28. Fraser S, Gardner PA, Koutourousiou M, et al. Risk factors associated with postoperative cerebrospinal fluid leak after endoscopic endonasal skull base surgery. *J Neurosurg.* 2018;128(4):1066–1071.
29. Koutourousiou M, Vaz Guimaraes Filho F, Costacou T, et al. Pontine encephalocele and abnormalities of the posterior fossa following transclival endoscopic endonasal surgery. *J Neurosurg.* 2014; 121(2):359–366.
30. Chabot JD, Patel C, Hughes M, et al. Nasoseptal flap necrosis: a rare complication of endoscopic endonasal surgery. *J Neurosurg.* 2018;128(5):1463–1472.

37

Vascular Injuries During Transsphenoidal Surgery

ANIL NANDA, TANMOY KUMAR MAITI, DEVI PRASAD PATRA

HIGHLIGHTS

- Sphenopalatine artery, internal carotid artery, and intercavernous sinus are the most common vessels susceptible to inadvertent injury during the transsphenoidal approach.
- Endovascular treatment is preferred to surgical intervention to confront the resultant bleeding or pseudoaneurysm.
- Sacrificing the internal carotid artery should be considered as salvage therapy or a last resort treatment, but it is the most practiced method in an acute setting.

Introduction

The transsphenoidal approach is an excellent portal to the pituitary gland, yet it is more vulnerable to vascular injuries owing to the anatomic proximity to major vessels, especially the internal carotid artery (ICA). Intraoperative carotid injury is well reported, often with catastrophic sequelae that can range from (1) hemorrhage, (2) spasm, (3) thrombosis of ICA or cavernous sinus, (4) embolism, and (5) pseudoaneurysm formation to delayed complications like ICA stenosis. Incidence of ICA injury during transsphenoidal surgery varies from 0.2% to 2% in large series.[1,2] A recent study using the National Inpatient Sample (NIS) database suggested that transsphenoidal surgery was followed by endovascular intervention in 0.1% cases, which did not differ much in a high-volume center when compared with a low-volume center.[3] Injury to sphenopalatine artery is another complication discussed, though it is minor and easily manageable. However, serious epistaxis is not uncommon (3.4%).[4]

Anatomic Insights

Arterial

Internal Carotid Artery

The most important vessel that is related to the transsphenoidal approach is the ICA. The cavernous ICA is the most common segment that is encountered during routine transsphenoidal surgery. However, with the advent of endoscopy, more extended transsphenoidal approaches are being done where other segments of ICA, starting from the petrous ICA to the supraclinoid ICA, are exposed. Fig. 37.1A illustrates a standard view of transsphenoidal surgery, showing the anatomy of the ICA in relation to sella. Intercarotid distance (ICD) between cavernous carotid arteries (CCAs) is 15 to 17 mm on MR coronal images in healthy individuals.[5] This distance increases to 20 to 22 mm for patients with pituitary adenomas.[5–7] Anterior and posterior parts of the CCAs are usually closer to the midline sagittal plane in comparison with the middle part of the CCAs.[7] The anterior horizontal segment of the CCA was close to the pituitary gland in most of the specimens in an anatomic study.[7] Renn and Rhoton[8] found the shortest distance between the two carotid arteries in the supraclinoid area in 82% of cases, in the cavernous sinus along the side of the sella in 14%, and in the sphenoid sinus in 4%. In 10% of cases, CCAs were within 4 mm of the midline.[8] Ectasia of cavernous ICA or kissing carotid artery can pose a significant challenge and may force the surgeon to access a different route.[9] This dolichoectasia may be seen in pituitary fossa, sphenoid bone or sinus, and it is more common in acromegalic patients. Protrusion of ICA into sphenoid sinus occurs in 25% to 30% of cases. The dehiscence of the bony sphenoidal wall of the ICA occurred in about 10% of cases.[10] Bilateral involvement may be seen in 1% of cases. The anatomic differences must be noted especially in acromegalic patients where the ICD is significantly smaller than in nonacromegalic patients. Interestingly, cavernous sinus invasion of adenoma was found to be independently associated with ICD contraction >2 mm ($P = 0.027$) in postoperative images. But a pituitary adenoma encasing ICA rarely causes compression of the artery (only 1.7%).[11]

Arterial bleeding may also arise from the branches of ICA, such as the inferior hypophyseal artery or a small capsular artery.[12,13] With the increasing use of the endoscope, an injury to the A1–A2 complex with its perforating vessels or basilar or posterior cerebral arteries is possible while approaching suprasellar and retrosellar pathologies.[14]

Association of intracranial aneurysm and pituitary adenoma has been discussed in the literature. Though this rare occurrence does not merit any added workup, the possibility should be kept in mind in the context of an anticipated torrential bleeding.[1]

Sphenopalatine Artery

This is the second most commonly observed vessel that is encountered during the nasal phase of the transsphenoidal surgery. The sphenopalatine artery is the terminal branch of the maxillary artery and enters the nasal cavity through the sphenopalatine foramen, which is located behind the end of the middle turbinate corresponding to the inferolateral corner of the sphenoidal sinus (Fig. 37.1B). Next, it splits into two branches: (A) nasopalatine artery, coursing medially above the choana, leading to the nasal septum, and (B)

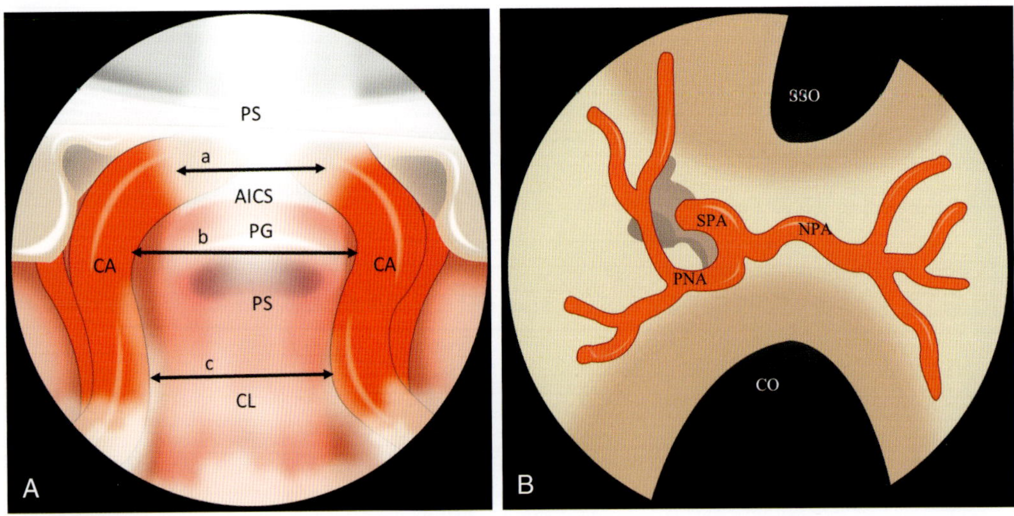

• **Fig. 37.1** Illustrations showing endoscopic anatomy of the sellar region (A) and the sphenopalatine artery (B); (a) intercarotid distance (ICD) at anterior aspect of sella near planum sphenoidate; (b) ICD at the middle part of sella; (c) ICD at posterior aspect of sella near clivus. *AICS,* Anterior intercavernous sinus; *CA,* carotid artery; *CL,* clivus; *CO,* choanae; *CS,* cavernous sinus; *NPA,* nasopalatine artery; *PG,* pituitary gland; *PICS,* posterior intercavernous sinus; *PNA,* posterior nasal artery; *PS,* planum sphenoidate; *SPA,* sphenopalatine artery; *SSO,* sphenoid sinus osteum. Note: Anterior and posterior intercavernous sinuses are observed as two blue lines during pituitary surgery and guide the limit of the dural opening.

posterior nasal artery passing laterally, reaching the lateral wall of the nasal cavity. The chance of arterial injury is higher with the endoscopic endonasal approach than with the microscopic approach because of a more lateral route. Entering the anterior wall of the sphenoid sinus 1.5 cm above the upper border of the choana is a safer trajectory. Sphenoidotomy may be restricted at the inferolateral corner.

Venous

Intercavernous sinuses are seen as two blue lines in the anterior and posterior part of the pituitary gland, which guides the anterior and posterior limit of the dural opening, respectively. The variation in the anatomy of the intercavernous sinus must be emphasized while planning dural opening.[15] In case of microadenoma, especially in a case of Cushing's disease, the entire sellar dura may be covered by a venous channel, and torrential bleeding may initiate as soon as the incision is placed on the dura.[14]

RED FLAGS

- Large invasive adenoma
- Previous transsphenoidal surgery
- Previous radiation therapy
- Previous medical therapy (especially prolonged dopamine agonist therapy)
- Lesions invading the cavernous sinus

Prevention

Appropriate imaging of the ICA and use of an intraoperative neuronavigation system and micro-Doppler ultrasonography are essential to avoid ICA injury at surgery, especially in revision surgeries when there has been cavernous sinus invasion before the primary surgery.[16]

Management of Internal Carotid Artery Injury

Steps to Control Torrential Bleeding[14,17,18]

It is preferable that two surgeons be engaged, allowing one surgeon to control the bloodstream, directing it away from the endoscope, while the other obtains visualization to attempt hemostasis. The packing of sella and/or of the sphenoid sinus should be performed by moving the endoscope back to the level of the head of the middle turbinate and inserting the hemostatic substances under endoscopic control. Two large-bore (10F) suction devices and a lens cleaning system for the endoscope will be helpful in this scenario. An endoscope equipped with an irrigating system enables continuous cleaning of the distal lens. The primary surgeon may place the endoscope down the contralateral side, using the posterior septal edge as a shield from the blood flow. Also he must try to clear blood ahead of the endoscope using the second suction device. A pedicled septal flap should also be cleared and pushed into the nasopharynx. At the same time, the second surgeon uses suction downside the nose with predominant bleeding to direct flow away from the other side. The second surgeon is then free to "hover" the suction device directly over the site of injury to help gain visualization for the primary surgeon. Nevertheless, neurosurgeons with less training on the endoscope must be prepared to swap the endoscope for the speculum and the microscope to avoid delay in endoscopic control of bleeding.

Hemostasis: Maneuvers and Materials

Several maneuvers have been discussed in the literature to aid the control of bleeding. The efficacy of head elevation and controlled hypotension, a common practice, is doubtful.[17] Ipsilateral common carotid artery compression can allow time for adequate nasal packing.[19] Weidenbecher et al. advocated bilateral carotid artery compression in the neck with concurrent surgical widening of the sphenoid sinus ostium to facilitate nasal pack placement.[20] It is also widely recommended that normotension be maintained through resuscitative measures to preserve adequate cerebral perfusion.[19] Several packing agents have been described in the literature. These include Teflon (Medox Medical, Oakland, NJ) and methyl methacrylate patch, fibrin glue, Gelfoam (Pfizer, New York City, NY), oxidized cellulose packing thrombin-gelatin matrix, oxygel, and glue and muslin gauze.[19,21] Muscle patch from fascia lata, sternocleidomastoid, or quadriceps may be used, along with oxidized cellulose and fibrin glue. Despite numerous options, gauze was most frequently used due to its availability and ease of use.[19] Packing is not without its own complications. Overpacking can contribute to ICA occlusion/stenosis leading to increased morbidity and mortality.[22]

Open and Endovascular Treatment Options

A direct suture repair or a Sundt-type clip graft has been described.[23,24] A U-clip anastomotic device or T2 aneurysm clip (Mizuho, Tokyo, Japan) may be useful as well.[17,25] Electrocauterization is often performed to gain rapid hemostasis, but this can potentially lead to carotid occlusion or delayed secondary hemorrhage and therefore cannot be recommended. However, bleeding from intercavernous sinus may be successfully controlled with electrocautery, if two layers of dura can be approximated together.[14]

Endovascular options have become frontline choices in present days. However, treatment options may vary according to type of injury and time of identification. Though ICA preservation is always the goal, sacrificing ICA remains the definitive treatment in acute uncontrollable bleeding. Balloon occlusion test (BOT) or some form of angiographic assessment of collateral circulation should be performed before sacrifice of ICA because permanent neurologic complication occurs in approximately one-fifth of them.[2] A covered stent may be considered as a valuable option in active bleeding or Carotico-Cavernous fistula (CCF) (JoStent: Jomed International and Symbiot self-expanding stent). However, the rigidity of a covered stent can be a concern because negotiation into tortuous cavernous ICA may be difficult and occlusion of branching arteries is not uncommon.[2] Vasospasm and in-stent thrombosis are other potential complications.[26,27] Kim et al. have advised use of abciximab to treat in-stent thrombosis.[26]

Patients with pseudoaneurysm should be started with dual antiplatelet therapy whenever possible. A covered stent is a reasonable option here as well. A stent-assisted coiling (Enterprise and Neuroform) is useful for wide-necked and traumatic pseudoaneurysms. Pipeline embolization device, the first flow-diverting device approved by US Food and Drug Administration for intracranial use, can successfully lead to complete exclusion of a pseudoaneurysm in 2 weeks to 6 months.[28,29] Coil embolization without stent placement should be considered in pseudoaneurysms with poor collateral circulation. This strategy obviates the need for dual antiplatelet therapy. Luo et al. expressed doubt over use of coils alone for treatment of acute traumatic carotid aneurysms, citing inherent fragility, wide neck, and indistinct anatomy of these aneurysms.[30] But it can certainly be considered as a bridge therapy. Onyx embolization may be another good treatment option.[31]

What a Neurosurgeon Can Offer

Sacrifice of ICA with endovascular coiling should be considered strongly in cases of acute, uncontrolled bleeding. BTO may be considered to assess the collateral circulation before ICA sacrifice. It is difficult to perform any concrete test when the patient is already under general anesthesia, and neurologic deficit may be unavoidable. With increasing realm of endovascular surgery, ICA sacrifice may be discarded only as a last resort/salvage therapy. A high-flow extracranial-intracranial (EC-IC) bypass can be considered for patients with inadequate collaterals where vessel preservation is deemed difficult or proved a failure.[32] A bypass surgery may be especially useful where the collateral is not adequate and a tortuous course of cavernous ICA prevents the implant of a stent.

Medical Treatment

Dual antiplatelet therapy is advised after stent graft or flow diverter placement to minimize the risk of stent thrombosis and distal emboli.[2] However, the timing to start the treatment is controversial because the benefit must be weighed against the risk of increased perioperative hemorrhage. An active bleeding, a large pseudoaneurysm, and a significant mechanism of injury warrant immediate start of this therapy.[2] The presence of a residual tumor could be a contraindication for initiation of dual antiplatelet therapy considering the increased risk of bleeding from healing vasculature within the tumor.[29]

Management of Sphenopalatine Artery Injuries

Detachment of mucosa from the rostrum sphenoidale followed by coagulation of the bleeding vessel may be the most effective treatment to control the bleeding of sphenopalatine artery or one of its branches. However, a proximal bleeding point may be difficult to control as the artery tends to withdraw toward the sphenopalatine foramen. In that scenario, an incision may be placed at approximately one centimeter anterior to the end of the middle turbinate in the lateral wall of the nasal cavity. Next, dissection is performed toward the sphenopalatine foramen above the terminal portion of the middle turbinate until the artery is isolated and hemostasis is achieved.[14] Reoperation and clipping of a bleeding sphenopalatine after transsphenoidal surgery have also been described.[22] Delayed postoperative bleeding from the sphenopalatine artery requires an anterior and/or posterior nasal packing.[14] Embolization of distal internal maxillary artery or sphenopalatine artery, often both, is required to control the bleeding. During embolization, branches of the internal maxillary artery around the sphenopalatine artery, which anastomoses to the meningeal branches of the carotid artery supplying the trigeminal nerve, must be preserved.

Management of Intercavernous Sinus Injury

Intercavernous sinuses are low-flow channels, so are easily controlled with compression and topical hemostatic agents. Rarely, there can be troublesome bleeding where controlled bipolar cauterization or the application of a miniclip may be required.

SURGICAL REWIND

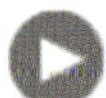

My Worst Case (Fig. 37.2 and Video 37.1)

A 46-year-old gentleman was diagnosed with nonfunctioning pituitary adenoma. In view of worsening vision and failure of conservative therapy, the patient was scheduled for a microscopic transnasal transsphenoidal approach. The tumor was calcific and difficult to remove. Sudden, torrential bleeding followed the removal of tumor from the left upper part of the operative field. A carotid tear was anticipated, but about 2 L of bleeding occurred in no time; finally, hemostasis was achieved with packing. The patient was shifted to neuro ICU for stabilization. On postoperative day 2, the patient underwent angiogram. It revealed a medially directed pseudoaneurysm of ICA, distal to the ophthalmic artery. There was narrowing of the C7 segment with distal filling of MCA. The perfusion to the left hemisphere was through the anterior communicating artery and left posterior communicating artery. The left vertebral artery injection did not fill the pseudoaneurysm. An attempt to place a wingspan stent across the stenotic segment failed. An angioplasty balloon was exchanged for the stent. When several attempts to place the stent past the stenotic segment failed, the carotid artery was sacrificed at C6 and C5 segment. Postocclusion digital subtraction angiography showed impaired perfusion to the distal territory of the left MCA. Massive cerebral edema resulted, and the left hemisphere developed a massive infarct. The patient died 5 days after the intervention, 8 days after the original surgery.

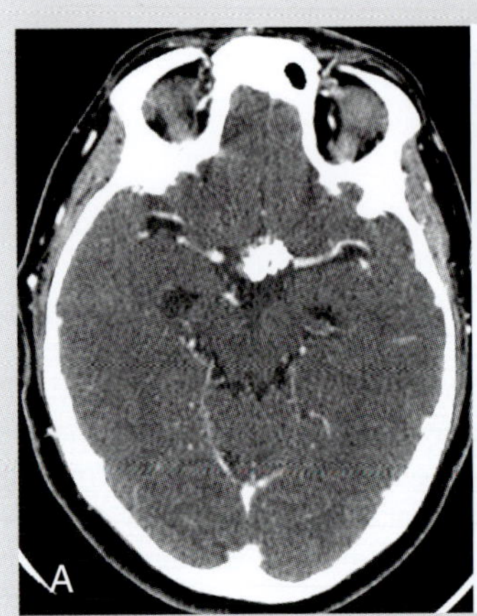

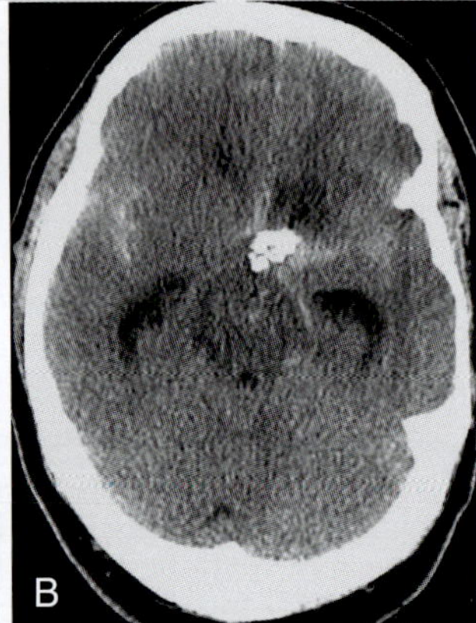

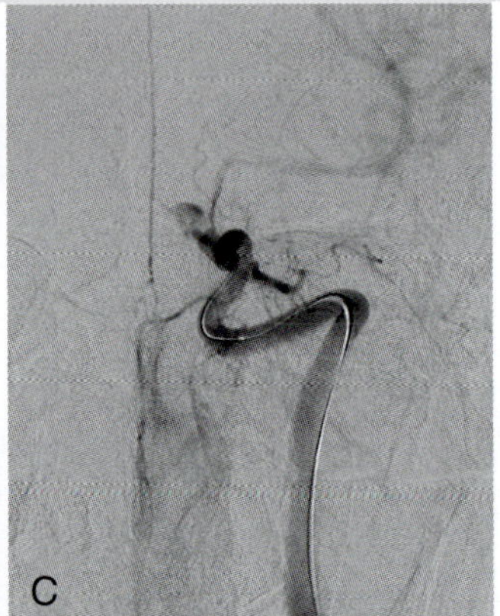

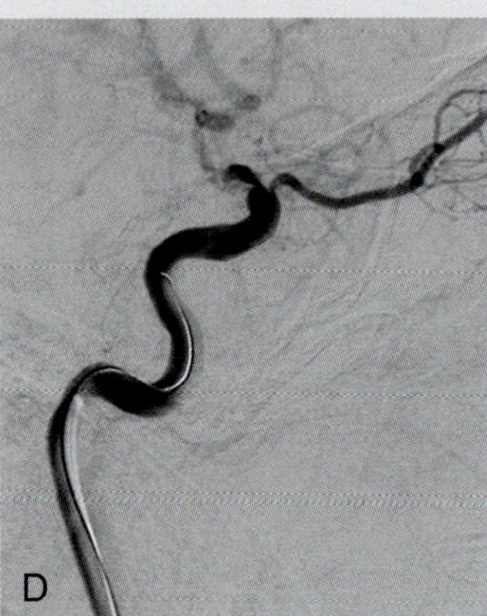

• **Fig. 37.2** Preoperative computed tomography (CT) (A) suggest a calcified pituitary adenoma. Postoperative CT showed subarachnoid hemorrhage and diffuse edema (B). Postoperative angiogram AP (C) and lateral (D) suggested formation of pseudoaneurysm with hypoperfusion of the distal segment.

NEUROSURGICAL SELFIE MOMENT

Vascular injury during transsphenoidal surgery can have dreadful consequences. The common injuries involve sphenopalatine arteries, but carotid injuries are associated with catastrophic sequelae. Venous injuries may be especially troublesome for microadenomas and potentially compel the surgeon to abandon the procedure. Endovascular approaches increasingly are adopted for immediate control and for delayed complications of ICA injury. However, the choice must be tailored to the individual type of injury and the time of intervention. A multidisciplinary approach is essential for safe and optimum treatment.

References

1. Berker M, Aghayev K, Saatci I, Palaoglu S, Onerci M. Overview of vascular complications of pituitary surgery with special emphasis on unexpected abnormality. *Pituitary*. 2010;13:160–167.
2. Sylvester PT, Moran CJ, Derdeyn CP, et al. Endovascular management of internal carotid artery injuries secondary to endonasal surgery: case series and review of the literature. *J Neurosurg*. 2016;125(5):1256–1276.
3. Brinjikji W, Lanzino G, Cloft HJ. Cerebrovascular complications and utilization of endovascular techniques following transsphenoidal resection of pituitary adenomas: a study of the Nationwide Inpatient Sample 2001–2010. *Pituitary*. 2014;17:430–435.
4. Ciric I, Ragin A, Baumgartner C, Pierce D. Complications of transsphenoidal surgery: results of a national survey, review of the literature, and personal experience. *Neurosurgery*. 1997;40:225–236, discussion 236-227.
5. Scotti G, Yu CY, Dillon WP, et al. MR imaging of cavernous sinus involvement by pituitary adenomas. *AJR Am J Roentgenol*. 1988;151:799–806.
6. Sasagawa Y, Tachibana O, Doai M, Akai T, Tonami H, Iizuka H. Internal carotid arterial shift after transsphenoidal surgery in pituitary adenomas with cavernous sinus invasion. *Pituitary*. 2013;16:465–470.
7. Yilmazlar S, Kocaeli H, Eyigor O, Hakyemez B, Korfali E. Clinical importance of the basal cavernous sinuses and cavernous carotid arteries relative to the pituitary gland and macroadenomas: quantitative analysis of the complete anatomy. *Surg Neurol*. 2008;70:165–174, discussion 174–175.
8. Renn WH, Rhoton AL Jr. Microsurgical anatomy of the sellar region. *J Neurosurg*. 1975;43:288–298.
9. Pereira Filho Ade A, Gobbato PL, Pereira Filho Gde A, Silva SB, Kraemer JL. Intracranial intrasellar kissing carotid arteries: case report. *Arq Neuropsiquiatr*. 2007;65:355–357.
10. Hewaidi G, Omami G. Anatomic Variation of sphenoid sinus and related structures in Libyan population: CT scan study. *Libyan J Med*. 2008;3:128–133.
11. Molitch ME, Cowen L, Stadiem R, Uihlein A, Naidich M, Russell E. Tumors invading the cavernous sinus that cause internal carotid artery compression are rarely pituitary adenomas. *Pituitary*. 2012;15:598–600.
12. Isolan GR, de Aguiar PH, Laws ER, Strapasson AC, Piltcher O. The implications of microsurgical anatomy for surgical approaches to the sellar region. *Pituitary*. 2009;12:360–367.

13. Laws ER Jr, Kern EB. Complications of trans-sphenoidal surgery. *Clin Neurosurg*. 1976;23:401–416.
14. Cavallo LM, Briganti F, Cappabianca P, et al. Hemorrhagic vascular complications of endoscopic transsphenoidal surgery. *Minim Invasive Neurosurg*. 2004;47:145–150.
15. Deng X, Chen S, Bai Y, et al. Vascular complications of intercavernous sinuses during transsphenoidal surgery: an anatomical analysis based on autopsy and magnetic resonance venography. *PLoS ONE*. 2015; 10:e0144771.
16. Dusick JR, Esposito F, Malkasian D, Kelly DF. Avoidance of carotid artery injuries in transsphenoidal surgery with the Doppler probe and micro-hook blades. *Neurosurgery*. 2007;60:322–328, discussion 328-329.
17. Padhye V, Valentine R, Wormald PJ. Management of carotid artery injury in endonasal surgery. *Int Arch Otorhinolaryngol*. 2014; 18:S173–S178.
18. Valentine R, Wormald PJ. Controlling the surgical field during a large endoscopic vascular injury. *Laryngoscope*. 2011;121:562–566.
19. Valentine R, Wormald PJ. Carotid artery injury after endonasal surgery. *Otolaryngol Clin North Am*. 2011;44:1059–1079.
20. Weidenbecher M, Huk WJ, Iro H. Internal carotid artery injury during functional endoscopic sinus surgery and its management. *Eur Arch Otorhinolaryngol*. 2005;262:640–645.
21. Inamasu J, Guiot BH. Iatrogenic carotid artery injury in neurosurgery. *Neurosurg Rev*. 2005;28:239–247, discussion 248.
22. Raymond J, Hardy J, Czepko R, Roy D. Arterial injuries in transsphenoidal surgery for pituitary adenoma; the role of angiography and endovascular treatment. *AJNR Am J Neuroradiol*. 1997;18:655–665.
23. Laws ER Jr. Vascular complications of transsphenoidal surgery. *Pituitary*. 1999;2:163–170.
24. Solares CA, Ong YK, Carrau RL, et al. Prevention and management of vascular injuries in endoscopic surgery of the sinonasal tract and skull base. *Otolaryngol Clin North Am*. 2010;43:817–825.
25. Valentine R, Boase S, Jervis-Bardy J, Dones Cabral JD, Robinson S, Wormald PJ. The efficacy of hemostatic techniques in the sheep model of carotid artery injury. *Int Forum Allergy Rhinol*. 2011;1:118–122.
26. Kim BM, Jeon P, Kim DJ, Kim DI, Suh SH, Park KY. Jostent covered stent placement for emergency reconstruction of a ruptured internal carotid artery during or after transsphenoidal surgery. *J Neurosurg*. 2015;122:1223–1228.
27. Kocer N, Kizilkilic O, Albayram S, Adaletli I, Kantarci F, Islak C. Treatment of iatrogenic internal carotid artery laceration and carotid cavernous fistula with endovascular stent-graft placement. *AJNR Am J Neuroradiol*. 2002;23:442–446.
28. Amenta PS, Starke RM, Jabbour PM, et al. Successful treatment of a traumatic carotid pseudoaneurysm with the Pipeline stent: case report and review of the literature. *Surg Neurol Int*. 2012;3:160.
29. Nerva JD, Morton RP, Levitt MR, et al. Pipeline Embolization Device as primary treatment for blister aneurysms and iatrogenic pseudoaneurysms of the internal carotid artery. *J Neurointerv Surg*. 2015;7:210–216.
30. Luo CB, Teng MM, Chang FC, Lirng JF, Chang CY. Endovascular management of the traumatic cerebral aneurysms associated with traumatic carotid cavernous fistulas. *AJNR Am J Neuroradiol*. 2004;25:501–505.
31. Medel R, Crowley RW, Hamilton DK, Dumont AS. Endovascular obliteration of an intracranial pseudoaneurysm: the utility of Onyx. *J Neurosurg Pediatr*. 2009;4:445–448.
32. Rangel-Castilla L, McDougall CG, Spetzler RF, Nakaji P. Urgent cerebral revascularization bypass surgery for iatrogenic skull base internal carotid artery injury. *Neurosurgery*. 2014;10(suppl 4):640–647, discussion 647-648.

38

Complications of Ventricular Endoscopy

ROBERTA REHDER, ALAN R. COHEN

HIGHLIGHTS

- Complications in ventricular endoscopy are best managed by prevention.
- Comprehensive knowledge of intraventricular anatomy is essential for safe endoscopic navigation, not because the anatomy is difficult but because one sees only a small part of it at any given time.
- The endoscope has no rear-view mirror, so structures can be injured outside the endoscopic field of vision.
- In the event of intraventricular bleeding:
  - *Keep the endoscope focused on the site where the bleeding occurred, even if the field is obscured.*
  - *Irrigate with a warmed solution of Ringer's lactate.*
  - *Be sure to keep an exit port open.*
  - *Use an endoscopic bipolar device to coagulate a bleeding vessel when feasible.*
  - *Leave an external ventricular drain if the bleeding cannot be controlled.*
  - *Obtain a vascular study if there is concern about a significant arterial injury.*

Background

In recent decades, advances in optics, illumination, miniaturization, and computer technology have provided a means for neurosurgeons to approach selected conditions with reduced parenchymal exposure, manipulation, and trauma.[1] There has been an increasing interest in the performance of endoscopic ventricular surgery to treat selected disorders such as hydrocephalus, cysts, and neoplasms.[2–5] Ventricular endoscopy can be both diagnostic and therapeutic, in that the procedure is performed with minimal invasiveness.[6]

Although ventricular endoscopy is a minimally invasive procedure, it is not risk free, and associated complications can be significant. Among the reported complications are intraventricular hemorrhage, subdural hygroma, thalamic contusions, cerebrospinal fluid (CSF) leak, and technical failures.[7] In most cases, unexpected events can be prevented by understanding the underlying causes of the pathologies. Overall, many complications can be avoided by selecting the right candidate for the procedure, having the most appropriate instrumentation, and having a thorough knowledge of the anatomy and pathology.

Two minimally invasive procedures commonly performed using endoscopic techniques are fenestration of the third ventricular floor, known as endoscopic third ventriculostomy (ETV), and endoscopic resection of colloid cysts of the third ventricle. ETV is a powerful method for treating selected cases of noncommunicating hydrocephalus without the need for implanted shunts (Fig. 38.1). Endoscopic resection of colloid cysts, when feasible, eliminates the need for brain manipulation and retraction that occur with open craniotomy.

Anatomic Insights

The ventricular endoscope is introduced into the ventricle either blindly or with the aid of image guidance. Once the endoscope is in the lateral ventricle, anatomic landmarks can be identified, including the choroid plexus, anterior septal and thalamostriate veins, and fornix. These constant landmarks guide the surgeon to the foramen of Monro, a paired structure that connects the lateral and the third ventricles. The operator can identify the mammillary bodies, tuber cinereum, and infundibular recess located on the floor of the third ventricle. In dilated ventricles, the tuber cinereum, a translucent membrane, runs from the mammillary bodies to the dorsum sellae. The surgeon can visualize the basilar apex in the interpeduncular cistern below (Fig. 38.2).

RED FLAGS

- For ETV, one should use a precoronal burr hole, which should be a bit more medial in location than the conventional midpupillary line. This enables the operator to have easier access to the midline third ventricular floor using a rigid endoscope.
- For ETV, one can identify the basilar apex directly underneath the translucent floor of the third ventricle.
- For ETV, thermal energy sources should be avoided along the third ventricular floor to prevent transmitted injury to the underlying basilar artery.
- In case of massive intraventricular bleeding, the endoscopic procedure should be aborted; an emergency angiography is recommended to find the bleeding source.
- For endoscopic colloid cyst resection, the precoronal burr hole should be more anterior and lateral than that for ETV. This provides the operator with a better view of the mass at the foramen of Monro. Image guidance can be helpful for this approach.
- If problems are encountered during endoscopic colloid cyst resection, the procedure can be easily converted to a microsurgical approach.

Risk Factors

Ventricular endoscopy can be challenging in patients presenting distorted ventricular anatomy.[8] For instance, anatomic variations are commonly seen in patients with hydrocephalus and myelomeningocele, including a vertically oriented third ventricular floor, thickened massa intermedia, and hindbrain descent.[9–11] Therefore careful analysis of the preoperative magnetic resonance imaging (MRI) study is helpful in planning the surgical procedure.

Stereotactic guidance should be considered for patients with small ventricles and distorted anatomy. It improves the accuracy of the surgical approach and minimizes trauma.[12] Frameless stereotactic localization can be useful for planning the surgical trajectory precisely, from the entry point to the target site, thus minimizing the risk of injury to the superior sagittal sinus and emissary veins.

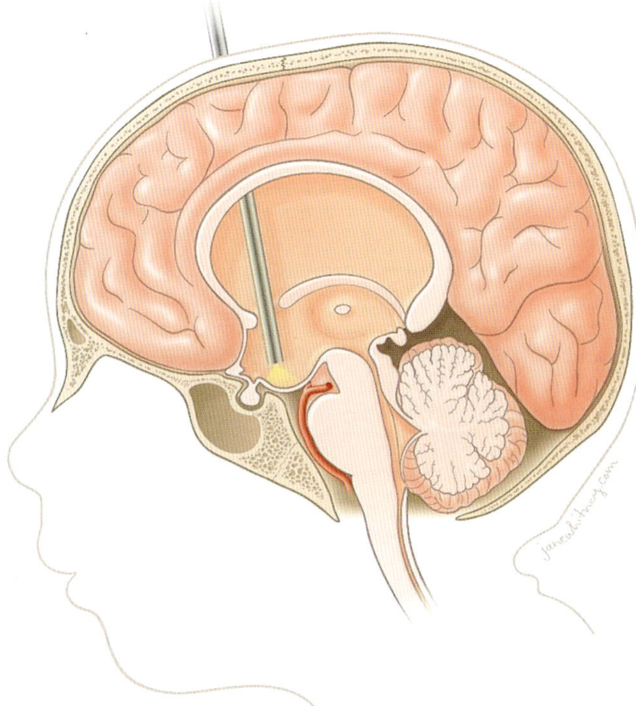

• **Fig. 38.1** Illustration showing the trajectory of the rigid endoscope during the performance of endoscopic third ventriculostomy.

Such a maneuver can potentially reduce the risk of neural and vascular injuries during ventricular endoscopy.[13,14]

Poor intraoperative visibility is an important risk factor for ventricular endoscopy complications. It can be caused by a murky CSF or bleeding. In cases of massive bleeding from injury of major vessels, the procedure must be interrupted; an emergency angiographic study is recommended to find the bleeding source.

Prevention of Complications

Complications in ventricular endoscopy can be avoided by identifying preventable adverse events such as distorted intraventricular anatomy and inadequate endoscopic instruments. Surgical complications may result in increased morbidity, length of hospital stay, and hospital costs for the patient. Here we describe how to prevent adverse events during the performance of ventricular endoscopy.

Preoperative Prevention

Instrumentation

In neurosurgery, there are two types of endoscopes: the flexible fiber-optic and the rigid rod-lens scope. The flexible scope has the advantage of steerability and maneuverability, although the imaging quality is not as clear as that provided by the rigid scope.[15,16] The operator should properly synchronize the endoscope with the camera so that the true anatomic orientation correlates with the orientation seen on the screen. Rarely, a piece of the endoscope lens can break off into the ventricle and may need to be retrieved.[4,17–20] The use of thermal energy sources, such as laser instruments, should be avoided on the floor of the third ventricle due to the risk of basilar artery injury.

Perioperative Prevention

Vascular Injury

Intraventricular bleeding from small subependymal vessels is the most frequent hemorrhagic complication in ventricular endoscopy. It is usually caused by the endoscopic instrumentation and can be

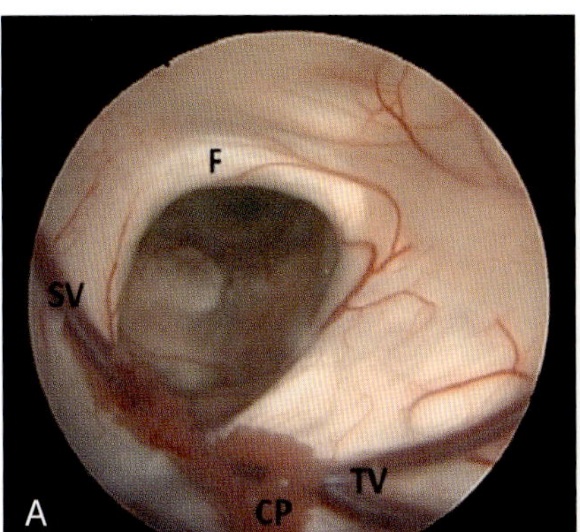

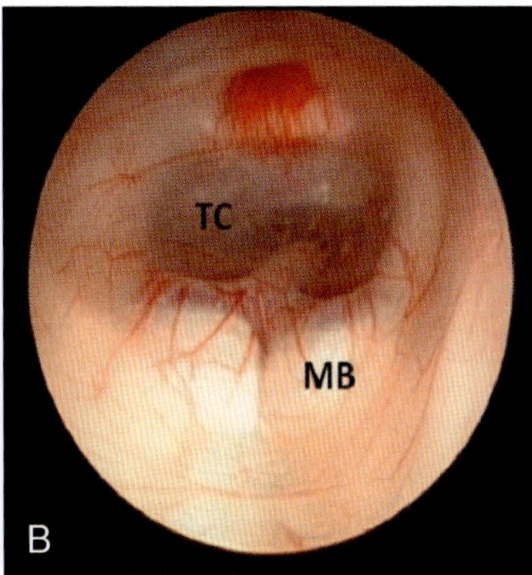

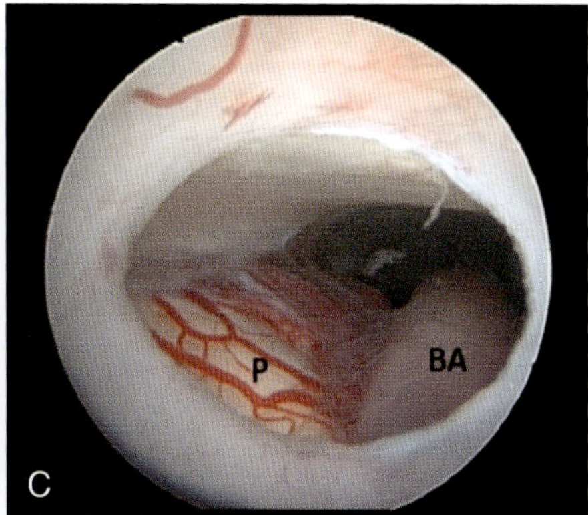

• **Fig. 38.2** Endoscopic view of the intraventricular structures using a 0-degree rigid scope. (A) Visualization of the foramen of Monro and identification of the choroid plexus and septal and thalamostriate veins. (B) Endoscopic view of the floor of the third ventricle and identification of the mammillary bodies and tuber cinereum. Note the basilar artery underneath the translucent membrane of the floor of the third ventricle. (C) Visualization of the interpeduncular cistern, basilar artery, and pons after the fenestration of the floor of the third ventricle. *BA,* Basilar artery; *CP,* choroid plexus; *F,* fornix; *MB,* mammillary bodies; *P,* pons; *SV,* septal vein; *TC,* tuber cinereum; *TV,* thalamostriate vein.

easily managed by gentle irrigation or coagulation of the bleeding source using the endoscopic bipolar device.

On the other hand, hemorrhage from larger vessels can significantly impair operative visibility. Generous irrigation with Ringer's lactate solution should be attempted.[7] In that case, one should be certain that an exit port in the endoscope sheath is open, thus preventing the increase of intracranial pressure. In severe cases of hemorrhage, one may need to leave an external ventricular drain in place.[21] Angiography may be necessary to identify a pseudoaneurysm, which may require endovascular repair.[22–25]

For ETV procedures, minimal bleeding may arise around the edges of the ventriculostomy after deflation of the balloon catheter. Often this injury can be controlled by tamponade after reinflating the balloon.[26] The most fearful complication in ETV is injury of the basilar artery or its perforators, a life-threatening injury. Its prevalence is reported to be about 1% of cases.[23] One tries to avoid basilar artery injury by fenestrating the floor of the third ventricle anteriorly, as close to the dorsum sellae as possible. Injuries to the anterior cerebral or pericallosal arteries have been reported infrequently during ETV.[27,28]

Neural Injury

Neural injury can occur anywhere along the endoscope trajectory. Investigators report the overall rate of neural injury between 3% and 4%.[23,29] Most serious injuries occur in the deep structures surrounding the ventricles, including contusions of the fornices, mammillary bodies, hypothalamus, thalamus, brainstem, and cranial nerves.[7,25,30] The risk of these lesions increases in cases of structural anomalies, such as a small foramen of Monro.[25]

Investigators have reported intraocular hemorrhage secondary to an acute increase of intracranial pressure (ICP) due to obstruction of the outflow channel by debris, blood clot, or kinking of the tubes.[31,32] Such acute increase of ICP results in bradycardia and tachycardia during intraventricular irrigation.[32–35] Cardiac instability can cease if the inciting factors are corrected, such as by releasing the irrigation fluid. Other described neurologic complications after ventricular endoscopy include hemiparesis, transient third and sixth cranial nerve palsies, speech delay, and transient personality changes.[23,25,29,36]

For endoscopic treatment of arachnoid cysts, the most common complication is bleeding obscuring the endoscopic view. Therefore one should coagulate the arachnoid vessels in the entry zone of the endoscope to prevent bleeding. For anatomic orientation, the middle cerebral artery is the main landmark in arachnoid cysts of the sylvian fissure. In this case, the cystocisternostomy should be performed between the carotid artery and the oculomotor nerve. There is an increased risk of injury of the oculomotor nerve and posterior communicating and anterior choroidal arteries.[37]

For the resection of colloid cysts, the removal of the cyst capsule from the roof of the third ventricle can be challenging (Fig. 38.3). If the cyst wall is firmly adherent to the roof, there is an increased risk of venous bleeding when the removal of the cyst capsule is attempted. In those cases, cyst wall remnants should be coagulated using bipolar coagulation devices and left in place.

Technical Failure

In some cases, procedural interruption may be necessary to avoid life-threatening injuries. The incidence of aborted procedures ranges between 2% and 7%.[23] Among the causes of aborted procedure are hemorrhages, unfavorable anatomy, CSF features (murky fluid), and those related to the instrumentation, such as dislodged lens and broken endoscope. Procedural interruption may be necessary to avoid complications or life-threatening injuries.[38]

Conclusion

Minimally invasive neurosurgery plays an important role in the treatment of various neurosurgical pathologies, including hydrocephalus, ventricular cysts, tumor biopsy, and tumor resection. Although the complication rates of ventricular endoscopy are low, they should not be negligible. As the field of ventricular endoscopy continues to evolve, novel techniques will be introduced to facilitate the performance of the procedure and to minimize the risks of related complications. The incidence of preventable complications can be reduced by selecting the right candidate for the procedure, having the optimal instruments available, and recognizing the potential pitfalls in advance.

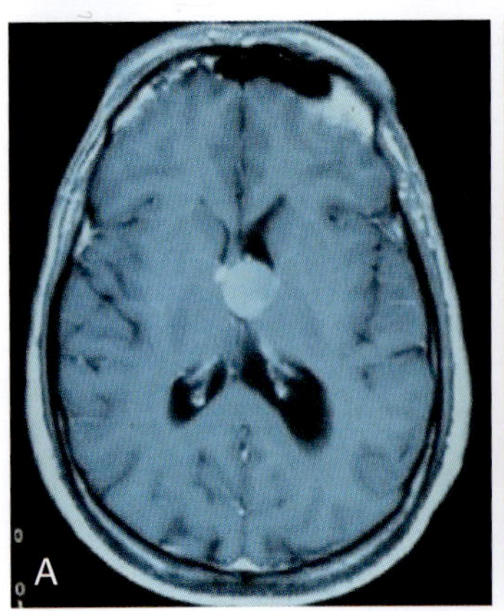

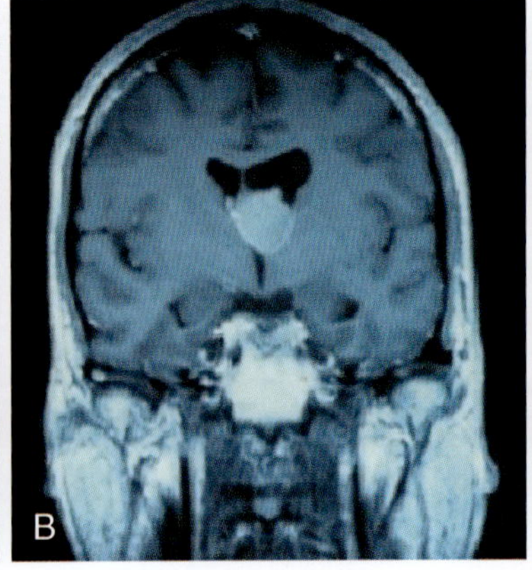

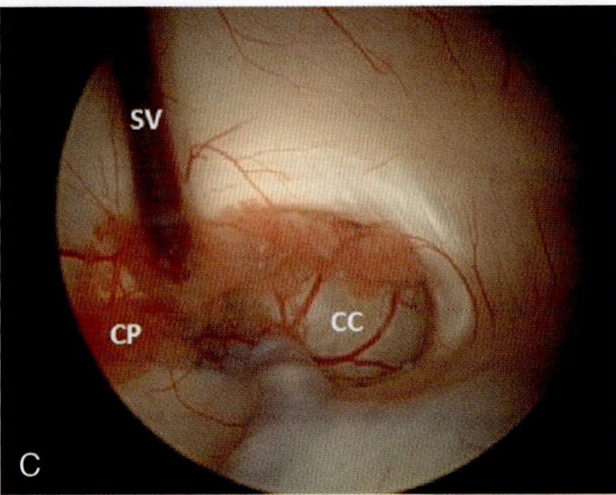

• **Fig. 38.3** Colloid cyst is a benign lesion commonly located in the rostral portion of the third ventricle. (A) Axial contrast-enhanced magnetic resonance imaging (MRI) study showing colloid cyst in the third ventricle. (B) Coronal contrast-enhanced MRI study. (C) Endoscopic visualization of the colloid cyst obstructing the foramen of Monro. *CC*, Colloid cyst; *CP*, choroid plexus; *SV*, septal vein.

SURGICAL REWIND

My Worst Case

Presentation

A 9-year-old left-handed girl was admitted to the hospital emergently with progressive headache, vomiting, and ataxia over 3 weeks. A cranial computed tomography scan showed an enhancing fourth ventricular brain tumor with hydrocephalus and multiple small enhancing masses along the walls of the lateral ventricles (Fig. 38.4). She was obtunded on admission and was brought urgently to the operating room.

Treatment

Because she had significant hydrocephalus, we elected to place an external ventricular drain before opening the posterior fossa. Because of the ependymal seeding, we chose to place the drain endoscopically in the left frontal horn and to biopsy the supratentorial ependymal tumor at the same time, using a rigid endoscope system with a solid rod lens. We attempted to remove a small portion of the tumor that was adherent to the ependymal wall of the frontal horn of the left lateral ventricle. A small biopsy forceps was inserted through a working channel in the endoscope sheath (Fig. 38.5).

Complication

The tumor was soft. As we began to lift it off of the ependyma, we encountered brisk arterial bleeding from the tumor. The operative field rapidly turned red, and we lost all visualization within seconds (Fig. 38.6).

Management

We held the endoscope in the original position, even though we had lost all anatomic landmarks. The biopsy forceps was removed. We gently irrigated

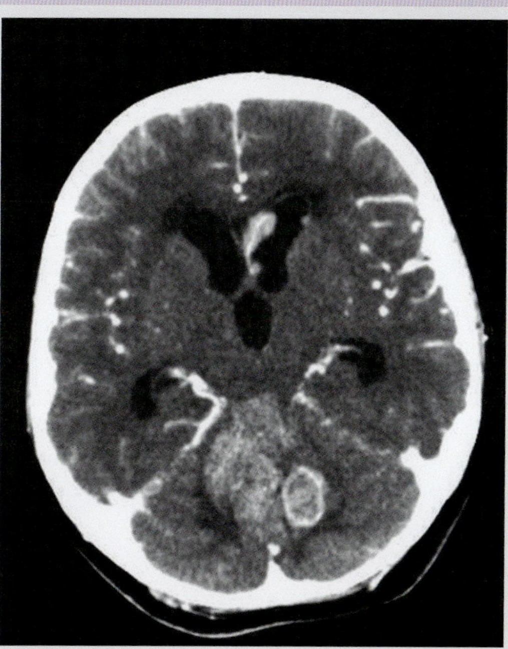

• **Fig. 38.4** Preoperative cranial computed tomography scan showing a large enhancing tumor filling the fourth ventricle. There is hydrocephalus with nodular masses lining the ependyma of the frontal horn of the left lateral ventricle and diffuse enhancement of the subarachnoid space.

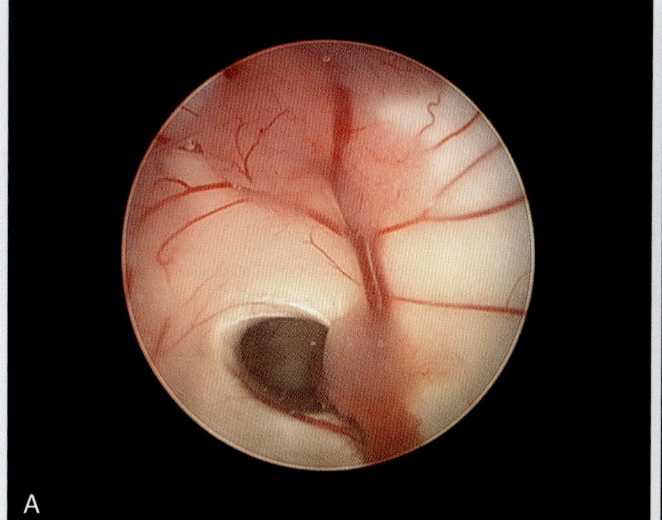

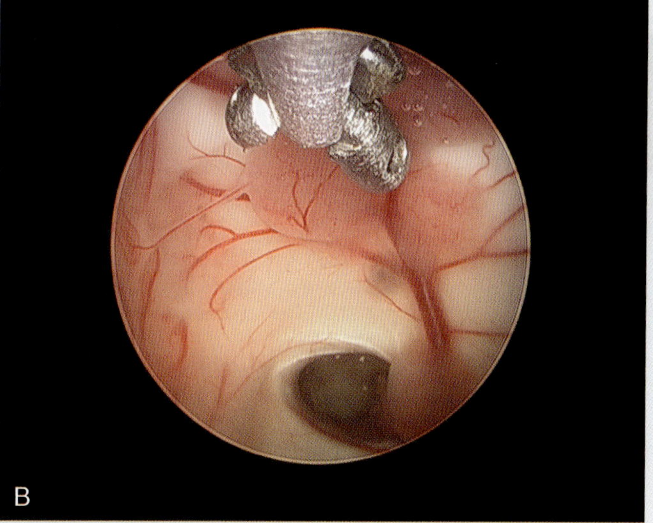

• **Fig. 38.5** Endoscopic cannulation of the frontal horn of the left lateral ventricle. 0-degree solid rod lens. (A) The patent foramen of Monro is seen inferiorly at about 7 o'clock. The septum pellucidum is to the right. The anterior septal vein is seen running vertically, just to the right of the foramen. Note the multiple pink ependymal-based tumor nodules adjacent to the course of the anterior septal vein. (B) A small tumor biopsy forceps has been introduced through a working channel in the endoscope sheath.

Continued

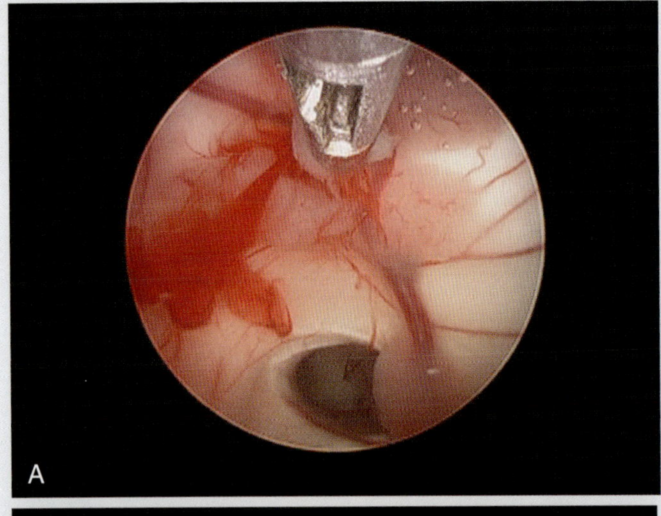

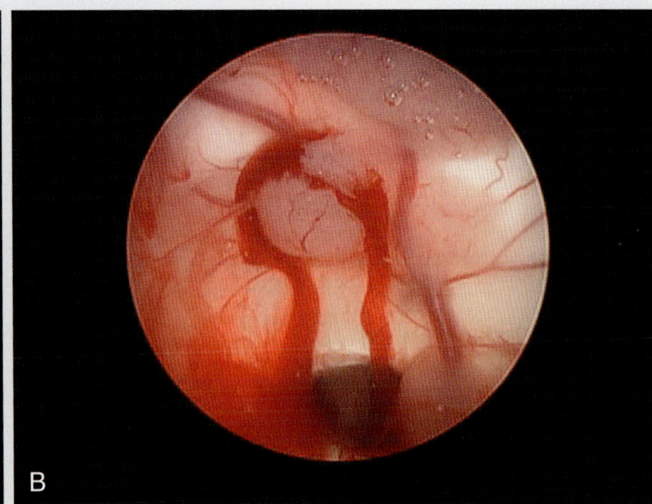

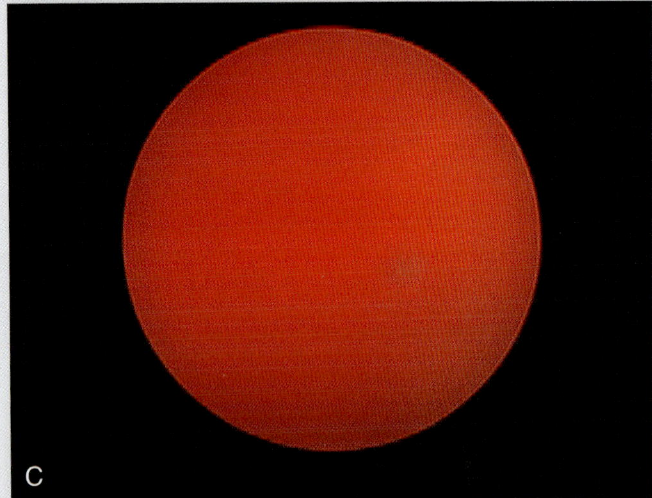

• **Fig. 38.6** Endoscopic tumor biopsy. (A) A small piece of tumor was grasped by the jaws of the biopsy forceps, and the forceps was twisted 180 degrees. Note the jet of arterial blood coming from the left side of the tumor. (B) The tumor was immediately released, and the forceps was removed. Within seconds the bleeding increased and now can be seen coming from both sides of the tumor. Small air bubbles are seen as a result of irrigation with warm Ringer's lactate solution. (C) Several seconds later the entire endoscopic field turned red, and all anatomic landmarks have been lost. The endoscope is held in its original position while ventricular irrigation is continued.

the ventricles with a warmed solution of Ringer's lactate for 7 minutes, instilled continuously through a working channel in the endoscope sheath. The bleeding site was deep to the tumor, and we were unable to reach it or see it to attempt coagulation with an endoscopic bipolar forceps. Another working channel in the endoscope sheath was left open as an exit port for the irrigation fluid. Ultimately, the bleeding stopped. The endoscope was removed, and we left a tunneled external ventricular drain at the same site.

The patient was then turned prone, and we removed the fourth ventricular tumor through a midline posterior fossa craniotomy under microscopic magnification. The tumor arose from the inferior medullary velum and was soft, purplish, and vascular. A gross total resection was achieved. Pathology was medulloblastoma.

Outcome

The patient was lethargic for 48 hours but made a smooth recovery. The external ventricular drain was removed on postoperative day 5. Neuraxis MRI confirmed the presence of the small tumor nodules studding the ependymal walls of the lateral ventricles. No enhancement was seen in the postoperative bed in the fourth ventricle. There was no enhancement in the spine.

The patient underwent treatment with craniospinal radiation. She received adjuvant chemotherapy for 1 year. At the time of this writing, 7 years after surgery, she is doing remarkably well as a junior in high school, on the honor roll and active in sports. She did not require ventricular shunting. She has hearing loss in the left ear and mild truncal ataxia. She takes Synthroid but is on no other medications. Her MR imaging 7 years after surgery shows no evaluable disease.

NEUROSURGICAL SELFIE MOMENT

Advances in optics, miniaturization, and computer technology have enabled surgeons to operate in the depths of the brain, within the cerebral ventricles, with minimal invasiveness. Minimally invasive techniques can be highly effective, but they are not risk free. The same factors that make minimally invasive neuroendoscopy so effective also make it difficult for the surgeon to deal with complications, should they occur.

The most feared complications of endoscopic ventricular surgery are bleeding and injury to neural structures. Endoscopic complications are best managed by prevention, with thorough knowledge of the regional anatomy and meticulous operative technique. Great care is taken to prevent bleeding. One tries to avoid significant movements of the endoscope sheath so as not to injure vessels such as subependymal veins that are outside the field of view. The endoscope has no rear-view mirror.

Should bleeding occur, it often looks worse than it really is, because the endoscope brings the surgeon so close to the anatomy and pathology. It is important not to panic. Every effort is made to keep the endoscope positioned in its original orientation, even when all anatomic landmarks are obscured by blood. Gentle, continuous irrigation with warmed Ringer's lactate solution will often clear the operative field and let the bleeding vessel come into view. Venous bleeding can sometimes be controlled with an endoscopic bipolar inserted through a working channel in the endoscope sheath. Some arterial bleeding will stop with irrigation. Basilar artery injury is an especially feared complication of endoscopic third ventriculostomy. We recommend avoiding the use of coagulating devices along the floor of the third ventricle to avert transmitting a heat injury to the basilar. In selected cases of arterial injury, external ventricular drainage and angiography may be indicated.

In this particular case the bleeding stopped with ventricular lavage, and the patient made a nice recovery with no ill effects. However, intraventricular bleeding can be catastrophic during neuroendoscopic procedures. With the wisdom of retrospective analysis, were we to do this case again, we would not have biopsied the intraventricular tumor.

References

1. Grunert P, Charalampaki P, Hopf N, Filippi R. The role of third ventriculostomy in the management of obstructive hydrocephalus. *Minim Invasive Neurosurg.* 2003;46(1):16–21.
2. Bilginer B, Oguz KK, Akalan N. Endoscopic third ventriculostomy for malfunction in previously shunted infants. *Childs Nerv Syst.* 2009;25(6):683–688.
3. Sgaramella E, Sotgiu S, Crotti FM. Neuroendoscopy: one year of experience–personal results, observations and limits. *Minim Invasive Neurosurg.* 2003;46(4):215–219.
4. Vogel TW, Bahuleyan B, Robinson S, Cohen AR. The role of endoscopic third ventriculostomy in the treatment of hydrocephalus. *J Neurosurg Pediatr.* 2013;12(1):54–61.
5. Kamikawa S, Inui A, Kobayashi N, et al. Endoscopic treatment of hydrocephalus in children: a controlled study using newly developed Yamadori-type ventriculoscopes. *Minim Invasive Neurosurg.* 2001;44(1):25–30.
6. Cohen AR. Images in clinical medicine. Endoscopic laser third ventriculostomy. *N Engl J Med.* 1993;328(8):552.
7. Cinalli G, Spennato P, Ruggiero C, et al. Complications following endoscopic intracranial procedures in children. *Childs Nerv Syst.* 2007;23(6):633–644.
8. Tamburrini G, Frassanito P, Iakovaki K, et al. Myelomeningocele: the management of the associated hydrocephalus. *Childs Nerv Syst.* 2013;29(9):1569–1579.
9. Hopf NJ, Grunert P, Fries G, Resch KD, Perneczky A. Endoscopic third ventriculostomy: outcome analysis of 100 consecutive procedures. *Neurosurgery.* 1999;44(4):795–804, discussion 804–805.
10. Jones RF, Kwok BC, Stening WA, Vonau M. Third ventriculostomy for hydrocephalus associated with spinal dysraphism: indications and contraindications. *Eur J Pediatr Surg.* 1996;6(suppl 1):5–6.
11. Teo C, Jones R. Management of hydrocephalus by endoscopic third ventriculostomy in patients with myelomeningocele. *Pediatr Neurosurg.* 1996;25(2):57–63, discussion 63.
12. Schroeder HW, Wagner W, Tschiltschke W, Gaab MR. Frameless neuronavigation in intracranial endoscopic neurosurgery. *J Neurosurg.* 2001;94(1):72–79.
13. Kadri H, Mawla AA. Variations of endoscopic ventricular anatomy in children suffering from hydrocephalus associated with myelomeningocele. *Minim Invasive Neurosurg.* 2004;47(6):339–341.
14. Pavez A, Salazar C, Rivera R, et al. Description of endoscopic ventricular anatomy in myelomeningocele. *Minim Invasive Neurosurg.* 2006;49(3):161–167.
15. Kehler U, Regelsberger J, Gliemroth J. Pro and cons of different designs of rigid endoscopes. *Minim Invasive Neurosurg.* 2003;46(4):205–207.
16. Kehler U, Regelsberger J, Gliemroth J. The mechanism of fornix lesions in 3rd ventriculostomy. *Minim Invasive Neurosurg.* 2003;46(4):202–204.
17. Chowdhry SA, Cohen AR. Intraventricular neuroendoscopy: complication avoidance and management. *World Neurosurg.* 2013;79(2):S15, e1-0.
18. McLaughlin MR, Wahlig JB, Kaufmann AM, Albright AL. Traumatic basilar aneurysm after endoscopic third ventriculostomy: case report. *Neurosurgery.* 1997;41(6):1400–1403, discussion 1403–1404.
19. Peretta P, Ragazzi P, Galarza M, et al. Complications and pitfalls of neuroendoscopic surgery in children. *J Neurosurg.* 2006;105(3 suppl): 187–193.
20. Vandertop WP, Verdaasdonk RM, van Swol CF. Laser-assisted neuroendoscopy using a neodymium-yttrium aluminum garnet or diode contact laser with pretreated fiber tips. *J Neurosurg.* 1998;88(1):82–92.
21. Navarro R, Gil-Parra R, Reitman AJ, Olavarria G, Grant JA, Tomita T. Endoscopic third ventriculostomy in children: early and late complications and their avoidance. *Childs Nerv Syst.* 2006;22(5):506–513.
22. Abtin K, Thompson BG, Walker ML. Basilar artery perforation as a complication of endoscopic third ventriculostomy. *Pediatr Neurosurg.* 1998;28(1):35–41.
23. Schroeder HW, Oertel J, Gaab MR. Incidence of complications in neuroendoscopic surgery. *Childs Nerv Syst.* 2004;20(11–12):878–883.
24. Schroeder HW, Warzok RW, Assaf JA, Gaab MR. Fatal subarachnoid hemorrhage after endoscopic third ventriculostomy. Case report. *J Neurosurg.* 1999;90(1):153–155.
25. Di Rocco C, Massimi L, Tamburrini G. Shunts vs endoscopic third ventriculostomy in infants: are there different types and/or rates of complications? A review. *Childs Nerv Syst.* 2006;22(12):1573–1589.
26. Schroeder HW, Niendorf WR, Gaab MR. Complications of endoscopic third ventriculostomy. *J Neurosurg.* 2002;96:1032–1040.
27. Cohen AR. Endoscopic ventricular surgery. *Pediatr Neurosurg.* 1993;19(3):127–134.
28. Buxton N, Punt J. Cerebral infarction after neuroendoscopic third ventriculostomy: case report. *Neurosurgery.* 2000;46(4):999–1001, discussion 1001–1002.
29. Beems T, Grotenhuis JA. Long-term complications and definition of failure of neuroendoscopic procedures. *Childs Nerv Syst.* 2004; 20(11–12):868–877.
30. Dusick JR, McArthur DL, Bergsneider M. Success and complication rates of endoscopic third ventriculostomy for adult hydrocephalus: a series of 108 patients. *Surg Neurol.* 2008;69(1):5–15.
31. Grand W, Leonardo J, Chamczuk AJ, Korus AJ. Endoscopic Third ventriculostomy in 250 adults with hydrocephalus: patient selection, outcomes, and complications. *Neurosurgery.* 2016;78(1):109–119.
32. Hoving EW, Rahmani M, Los LI, Renardel de Lavalette VW. Bilateral retinal hemorrhage after endoscopic third ventriculostomy: iatrogenic Terson syndrome. *J Neurosurg.* 2009;110(5):858–860.
33. Handler MH, Abbott R, Lee M. A near-fatal complication of endoscopic third ventriculostomy: case report. *Neurosurgery.* 1994;35(3):525–527, discussion 527–528.
34. Boogaarts H, Grotenhuis A. Terson's syndrome after endoscopic colloid cyst removal: case report and a review of reported complications. *Minim Invasive Neurosurg.* 2008;51(5):303–305.
35. Kalmar AF, Van Aken J, Struys MM. Exceptional clinical observation: total brain ischemia during normal intracranial pressure readings caused by obstruction of the outflow of a neuroendoscope. *J Neurosurg Anesthesiol.* 2005;17(3):175–176.
36. Drake JM. The surgical management of pediatric hydrocephalus. *Neurosurgery.* 2008;62(suppl 2):633–640, discussion 640–642.
37. Schroeder HW, Gaab MR. Endoscopic management of intracranial arachnoid cysts. In: Hellwig D, Bauer BL, eds. *Minimally invasive techniques for neurosurgery: current status and future perspectives.* Berlin/ Heidelberg: 1998:101–105.
38. Kulkarni A, Warf B, Drake J, Mallucci C, Sgouros S, Constantini S. Surgery for hydrocephalus in sub-Saharan Africa versus developed nations: a risk-adjusted comparison of outcome. *Childs Nerv Syst.* 2010;26(12):1711–1717.

39

Access-Related Complications in Endovascular Neurosurgery

MITHUN G. SATTUR, MATTHEW E. WELZ, BERNARD R. BENDOK

HIGHLIGHTS

- Obtaining, maintaining, and exiting the vascular portal of entry in a safe and efficient manner are essential to achieve the goal of diagnosis and treatment of cranial, spinal, and head-neck neurovascular diseases.
- Transfemoral/groin access represents the most common route for endovascular access in vascular neurosurgery.
- Access-related complications are categorized as bleeding, pseudoaneurysm, infection, and other arterial abnormalities.
- A standard regimental approach to complication avoidance is the secret to successful outcome.

Introduction

The field of vascular neurosurgery has been enriched by significant advances in endovascular technology and techniques. Despite rapid evolution, certain basic tenets remain sacrosanct. Chief among them is the art and science of safe vascular access. Obtaining, maintaining, and exiting the vascular portal of entry in a safe and efficient manner are essential to achieve the goal of diagnosis and treatment of cranial, spinal, and head-neck neurovascular diseases. Catastrophic complications can arise, and access-related complications should never be underestimated or viewed with hubris. The present chapter provides a concise overview of the nuances for safe access for each of the various endovascular access routes.

Access-Related Complications

Access-related complications (ARC) should be considered if related to any of the following:

1. Injury at access site:
   a. Femoral
   b. Radial
   c. Brachial
   d. Carotid
   e. Vertebral
   f. Transorbital
   g. Transcranial access
2. Device navigation along vascular roadmap to the lesion
   a. Thoracoabdominal aortic
   b. Arch of aorta
   c. Carotid arteries
   d. Vertebral arteries
   e. Intracranial arteries and veins
3. Intracranial target lesion access
   a. Access to aneurysm
   b. Access to arteriovenous malformation/dural fistula
   c. Tumor access
4. Contrast-induced nephropathy

Femoral Access

Transfemoral/groin access represents the most common route for endovascular access in vascular neurosurgery. The large size of the artery that allows placement of large devices in co-axial fashion for a stable construct, location over the femoral head that allows compressibility, situation away from the fluoroscopy arms, and a long history of operator familiarity are main factors for this preference. Most devices available for intervention are configured and optimized for femoral access. Spinal angiography and intervention are almost always carried out via the transfemoral route. Complications from femoral access have been documented to occur in 1.6% to 6.0% of patients in the literature but can be minimized with proper precautions. Complications are categorized as follows:

1. Bleeding
   Groin hematoma
   Retroperitoneal hematoma
2. Pseudoaneurysm (PA)
3. Other arterial abnormalities (arteriovenous fistula, acute thrombosis, dissection, distal embolism)
4. Infection

Bleeding

Minor hematomas at the puncture site are common and do not necessarily represent complications. Major hematomas may occur either in the groin or retroperitoneum and represent difficulty with hemostasis. Risk factors for hematoma formation are:

a. Obesity
b. Puncture above inguinal ligament (high puncture)
c. Advanced atherosclerotic disease
d. Dual antiplatelet therapy (DAPT)
e. Anticoagulation
f. Uncontrolled hypertension
g. Large sheath
h. Rough catheterization of circumflex branch (and rupture)
i. Backwall puncture
j. Inability to deploy closure device
k. Inadequate rest before ambulation

A major hematoma manifests with increasing local pain, swelling, and bruising, along with declining hematocrit in the few hours post-procedure. However, a retroperitoneal hematoma is more treacherous because there is no external swelling. The only external sign sometimes is ipsilateral flank bruising. Typically with retroperitoneal hematoma, there is an initial transient episode of hypotension that improves with a fluid bolus; if left undiagnosed, it can lead to dangerous and rapid hemodynamic collapse.

Diagnosis

A high index of suspicion is needed to diagnose a retroperitoneal hematoma. Close attention to clinical examination and prompt serial hematocrit estimations are important. Ultrasound is helpful with a thigh hematoma in ruling out expanding PA. Definitive diagnosis of retroperitoneal hematoma requires computed tomography (CT) imaging.

Management

Many hematomas may not require surgical evacuation. Maintaining stable blood pressure and adequate circulatory status is paramount. Serial hematocrit estimation guides transfusion, and packed red cells should readily be available. It is prudent to obtain early vascular surgery consultation if a patient is being admitted for hematoma management. With active extravasation (which sometimes can be seen on contrast-enhanced CT) and impending cardiovascular collapse, vascular surgical intervention is indicated. Anticoagulated patients and those on DAPT pose a unique dilemma. Procedural anticoagulation usually reverses spontaneously in few hours. Reversal of chronic anticoagulation depends on the primary diagnosis for which this is indicated and should be undertaken on a case-by-case basis. DAPT patients tend to be more problematic due to difficulty in reversing platelet dysfunction and, more importantly, the fact that DAPT is indicated for recent intracranial or coronary (or other intravascular) stent. Placement of a covered stent across the site of leakage is an endovascular option in select cases.

Prevention

Though theoretically longer durations of bed rest might reduce bleeding, clinical studies have proven that a 2-hour bed rest period post sheath removal is adequate. One study used manual compression for hemostasis after use of 5 Fr sheaths in the majority of the 295 patients evaluated.[1] Close attention to steps involved in femoral access is mandatory to prevent complications (see "Complication avoidance").

Pseudoaneurysms

A hematoma that occurs in the vessel wall and is in communication with the arterial lumen can become PA. Clinical presentation is with an enlarging firm mass that is pulsatile and may have a bruit on auscultation. Some degree of pain/discomfort may be seen. PA typically becomes evident after 48 hours. Some authors describe simple (one lobe) and complex (more than one lobe) PA.[2] Whether use of a closure device in lieu of manual compression increases PA risk is debatable based on recent metaanalyses versus those from a decade ago.[3,4] Other risk factors include high puncture, large sheath, and puncture below bifurcation in superficial femoral artery.

Diagnosis

Duplex ultrasound (US) is the imaging modality of choice. PA neck, lobe(s), dimensions, and parent artery lumen communication are clearly visualized.

Management

Small PAs frequently do not require treatment, but occasional lesions progressively enlarge. Treatment modalities are delineated in Table 39.1.

The most common technique (including at our center) is thrombin injection because it is quick, highly effective, a bedside procedure, and largely safe.[2] It may be prudent to repeat a US in 1 to 2 weeks to rule out recurrence.

Other Femoral Artery Complications

Arterial thrombosis, dissection, and distal embolism are rare complications that present with pain, paresthesias, and diminished or absent pedal pulses. Thrombosis risk is strongly correlated with leaving the sheath in for prolonged duration post procedure. Risk factors include puncture below bifurcation of common femoral artery, large sheath placement, inadequate flush of heparinized saline, severe atherosclerosis, and rough technique. Arteriovenous fistula

TABLE 39.1 Various Treatment Modalities and Their Advantages/Concerns

Treatment	Advantages	Concerns
Ultrasound-guided manual compression	Simple, bedside Inexpensive No risk to parent artery lumen	Patient discomfort Vasovagal symptoms
Ultrasound-guided thrombin injection	Excellent success rates (over 90%) Minimal patient discomfort	Parent artery reflux Distal embolism Systemic effects Recurrence
Covered stent	Endovascular option in larger neck Indicated for failure of ultrasound-guided techniques	Antiplatelet therapy Cost
Open surgical repair	Effective for large/giant PA Indicated for rupture/infection	Major surgical procedure

is recognized by characteristic thrill and bruit and usually presents in a delayed fashion. US guidance to avoid the femoral vein and tributaries during arterial puncture and avoiding a simultaneous femoral vein puncture (when required) on the same side may help avoid this complication. It is imperative to recognize these potentially limb-threatening complications early and involve vascular surgery expeditiously for open or endovascular intervention. The imaging modality of choice to document these complications is duplex US. Early recognition and management leads to good outcomes.

Complication Avoidance

At our institution, all diagnostic angiography–related access is treated with a "nuclear launch code" protocol. Fluoroscopic confirmation of femoral head location is performed with a localizer (hemostat), and puncture occurs over this site (Fig. 39.1A–C). We use ultrasound to mark the bifurcation of the common femoral artery (into superficial femoral and profunda femoris artery), and we puncture above this point but still over the femoral head (Fig. 39.2D–G). Continuous heparinized saline flush is run through the sheath for the duration of the procedure. Invariably we endeavor to remove the femoral sheath on the table after the conclusion of the procedure. Femoral arteriography is performed before sheath removal. Particular attention is paid to puncture site vis-a-vis the bifurcation, location of puncture site (= sheath entry site) with respect to the femoral head, dissection, or thrombosis. Decision regarding closure device deployment proceeds as described later, after ensuring that the puncture is above the bifurcation.

Closure Device Use

Vascular closure devices are approved for femoral access closure and are currently available under various categories:

i. Collagen plug–based (Angio-Seal, Terumo, Somerset, NJ)
ii. Suture based (Perclose Abbott, Abbott Park, IL)
iii. Clip based (StarClose Abbott, Abbott Park, IL)

The advantages and disadvantages of using a closure device for femoral access are described in Table 39.2.

Closure device deployment also follows a strict set of rules:

i. Confirm location of puncture above common femoral artery bifurcation (Fig. 39.3)
ii. Repeat prep and draping of groin site
iii. Change of gloves by team
iv. Prophylactic antibiotics before insertion
v. Confirmation of intravascular placement
vi. Avoidance of closure device deployment in certain situations:
   a. Puncture at/below bifurcation (higher risk of dissection)
   b. Severe calcified atherosclerotic disease
   c. Small artery size
   d. Immunocompromised patient (infection risk)
   e. Access through bypass graft

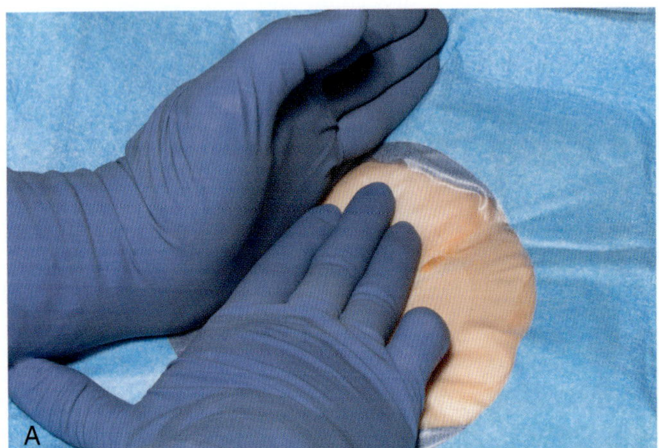

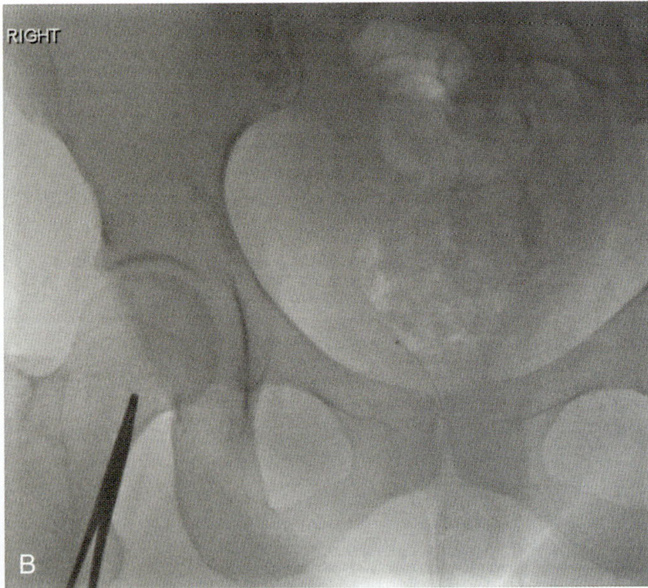

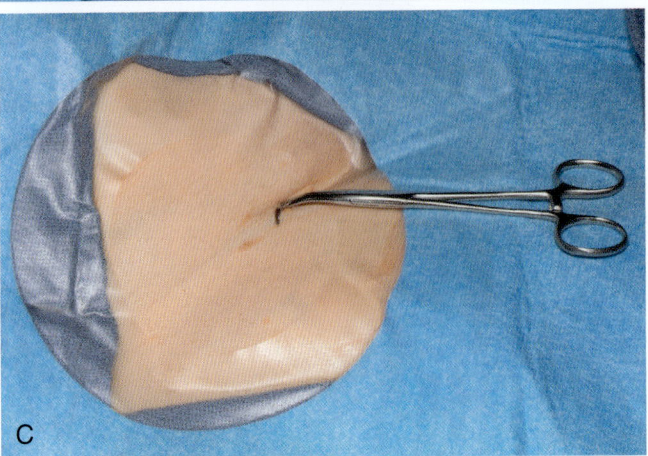

• **Fig. 39.1** Anatomic (A) and fluoroscopic (B and C) landmarks for groin puncture (shown here on right side). A good approximation of the femoral pulse is a site 3 finger-breadths below a line joining the anterior superior iliac spine and the pubic symphysis (A). A localizer is placed at this site and X-ray is obtained to confirm position over the femoral head (B). This site in turn is marked (C). (Used with permission of Mayo Foundation for Medical Education and Research, all rights reserved.)

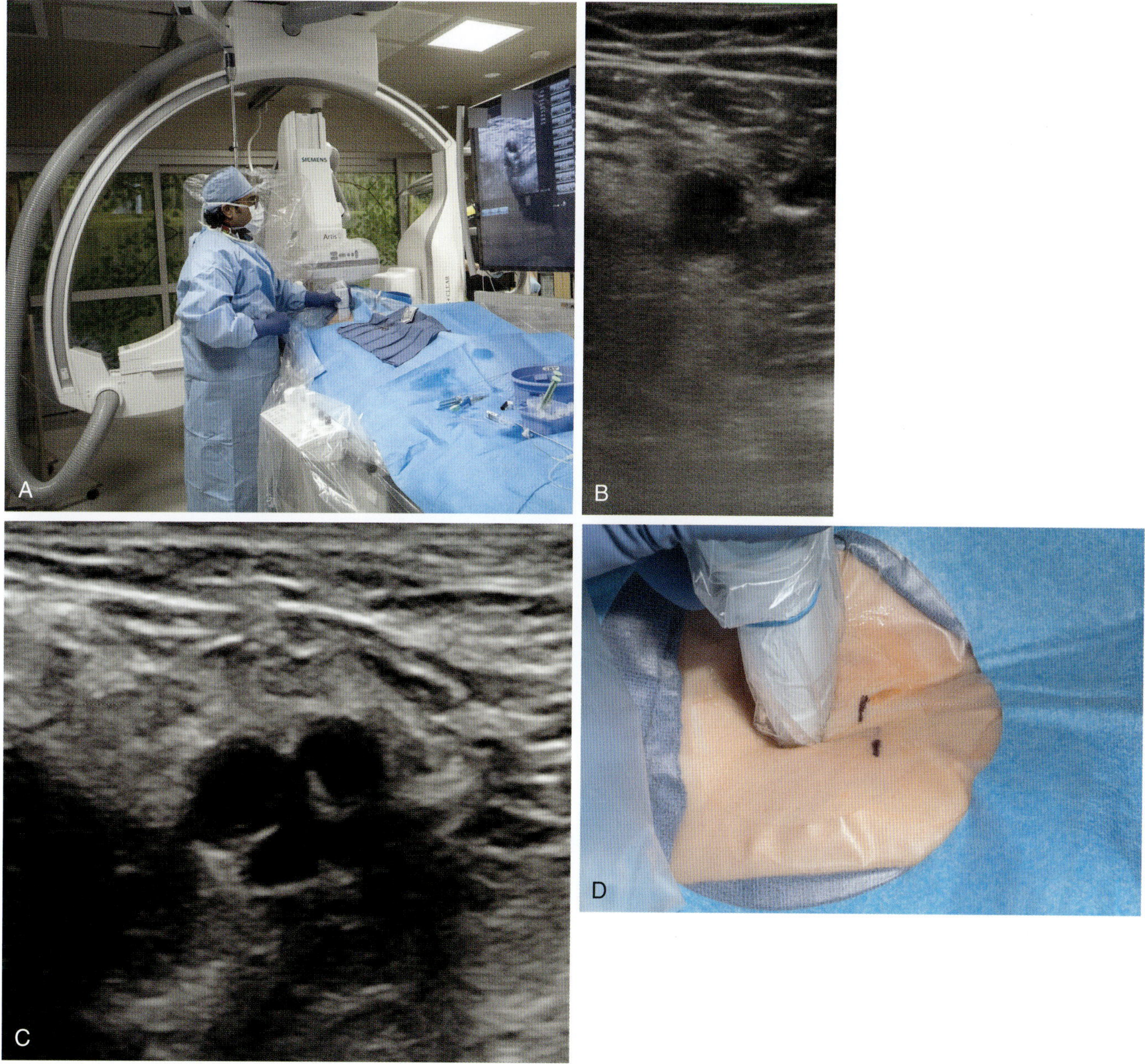

• **Fig. 39.2** Strategic use of ultrasound for safe femoral puncture (A). Ultrasound is used to visualize the common femoral artery (B) and the bifurcation (C). The bifurcation is marked on the groin (D) and puncture is above this yet over the femoral head. (Used with permission of Mayo Foundation for Medical Education and Research, all rights reserved.)

TABLE 39.2 Advantages and Disadvantages of Using a Closure Device for Femoral Access

Advantages	Disadvantages
Shortens bed rest	Potential vessel occlusion/ thrombosis
Less intense physician/nurse involvement	Dissection/PA risk may be greater
Cost benefit by reducing stay and personnel requirement	Infection
Potentially less incidence of hematoma formation	Cost

Infection of a closure device can be a severe complication and most commonly occurs in immunocompromised populations. It can potentially lead to vessel rupture in addition to bacteremia and sepsis. Treatment often involves open surgical resection and grafting and prolonged IV antibiotic therapy, but outcomes may not be satisfactory.

Transfemoral Venous Access

The principle of ensuring puncture over the femoral head is most important and probably more so than with arterial access, since typically closure devices cannot be deployed. Adequate manual compression is the key to achieving adequate hemostasis.

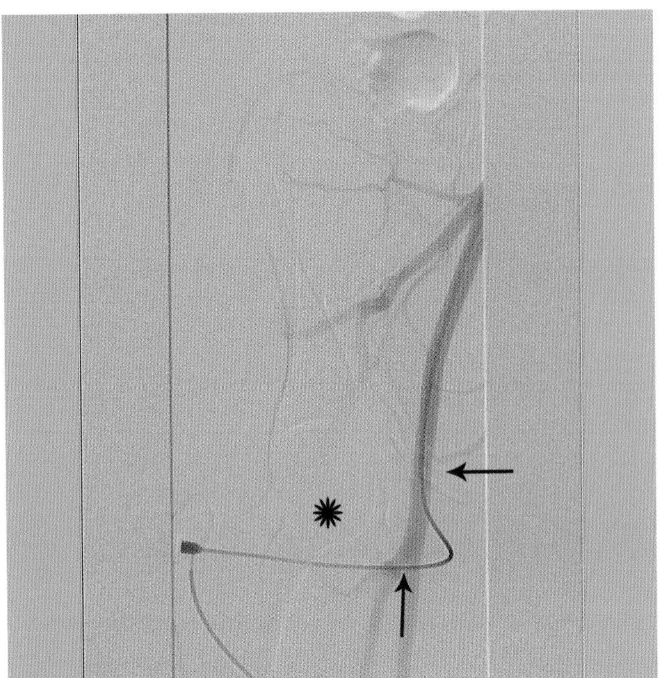

• **Fig. 39.3** Ideal puncture site (horizontal arrow) is over the femoral head (asterisk) and above the bifurcation (vertical arrow) for deployment of closure device. (Used with permission of Mayo Foundation for Medical Education and Research, all rights reserved.)

Radial Access

Traditional transfemoral access may not be feasible in patients with severe aortoiliac or iliofemoral atherosclerosis. Severe obesity not only makes puncture challenging, but applying manual compression after sheath removal is also very difficult in situations where a closure device cannot be employed. In such cases, radial artery access is very attractive. The superficial location of radial artery, radial-ulnar collaterals to hand, and unrestricted ambulation have encouraged increasing use of radial access for vascular, both extracranial and intracranial vascular neurosurgery indications.[5,6] For carotid stenting, radial artery access is attractive because of the ease of navigating a type III aortic arch and accessing a bovine carotid take-off.[6,7] Radial access on the right side avoids aortic arch navigation; catheter manipulation in the aortic arch has been postulated as a mechanism of periprocedural stroke in patients who undergo carotid artery stenting.[8] Based on success with cervical intervention, we have previously reported on the successful and effective application of the transradial approach for intracranial intervention[9] (Fig. 39.4). The radial arteries, however, are prone to spasm easily and require administration of nitroglycerine and verapamil along with heparin in the form of a vasodilatory "cocktail."[5] Thrombosis is documented in about 5% of transradial interventions, but in general it is well tolerated due to collaterals from ulnar territory. An Allen's test is performed before radial catheterization (Fig. 39.5). Immediate sheath removal and nonocclusive compression technique reduces the risk of occlusion Fig. 39.6). The size of the artery limits the size of devices that may be used for intervention, and usually it is difficult to insert devices larger than 6 Fr. Cross-over to femoral approach was documented to occur in 4.9% of patients who underwent carotid stenting, according to one large Italian study.[10–12]

Brachial Access

The attraction of brachial access lies in the fact that atherosclerotic disease and tortuosity is rare at this location and that a device of somewhat larger size than at a radial access site (7 Fr sheath, for example) can be used. A unique scenario where we have used the brachial approach is documented in a patient with severe coarctation of aorta.[13] Thrombosis and PA are potential complications. In a study of 214 patients who underwent transradial or transbrachial approach for carotid stenting, 4 had to be treated for acute thrombosis or PA of brachial artery (of 60 patients), and 6 had radial artery occlusion (of 154).[14] Thrombosis usually requires surgical thrombectomy by a vascular surgeon. Occurrence of PA after brachial access is more frequent than femoral access and may be treated with US-guided manual compression or injection of fibrin, but eventually surgical intervention may be required. Hematoma at the access site has the potential to cause compartment syndrome if very large, but most cases do not require surgical evacuation. Cross-over to a femoral approach occurs in about 1% to 7%.

Transorbital Access

This specific access route is unique to management of cavernous sinus dural arteriovenous fistulas (CS-DAVF). In well-selected cases, transvenous embolization of DAVFs can be accomplished via direct transorbital puncture of the superior or inferior ophthalmic vein, which is frequently arterialized and prominent.[15,16] Potential complications include orbital hematoma, infection, and puncture of the globe, vitreous leakage, and damage to the optic nerve and/or ocular motor nerves. Prevention of complications starts with appropriate case selection. Clear visualization of the arterialized ophthalmic vein on angiography is necessary. Meticulous technique and optimal use of angiographic working views are paramount. Three-dimensional rotational angiography can be helpful in selecting appropriate working views.

Carotid Access

Severe tortuosity of the aortic arch introduces a significant technical impediment in catheterizing arch vessels, especially the left common carotid artery. Transradial and transbrachial access is the next natural step in attempting access, but even these may prove unsuccessful. In such instances, direct carotid puncture remains an option.[17,18] Sheaths from 4 Fr to 8 Fr may be inserted. Complications may be severe and include carotid dissection, embolism of plaque fragments and, most importantly, neck hematoma. The latter is important given that most situations are complicated with anticoagulation and antiplatelet therapy. Sheath removal is usually followed by manual compression, but closure devices have also been used.[19] There has been recent resurgence in direct carotid access with the introduction of the ENROUTE transcarotid neuroprotection system (Silk Road Medical Inc., Sunnyvale, CA).[20]

Transcranial Access for Endovascular Therapy

Rare instances may dictate direct microsurgical access to treat an intracranial vascular lesion. Examples have included access to arterialized and dilated middle cerebral vein or middle meningeal artery or the cavernous sinus.[21] This situation is usually encountered with certain DAVFs where endovascular transarterial and/or transvenous access is not feasible and the only approach is via an arterialized vein accessible microsurgically. An apt example is

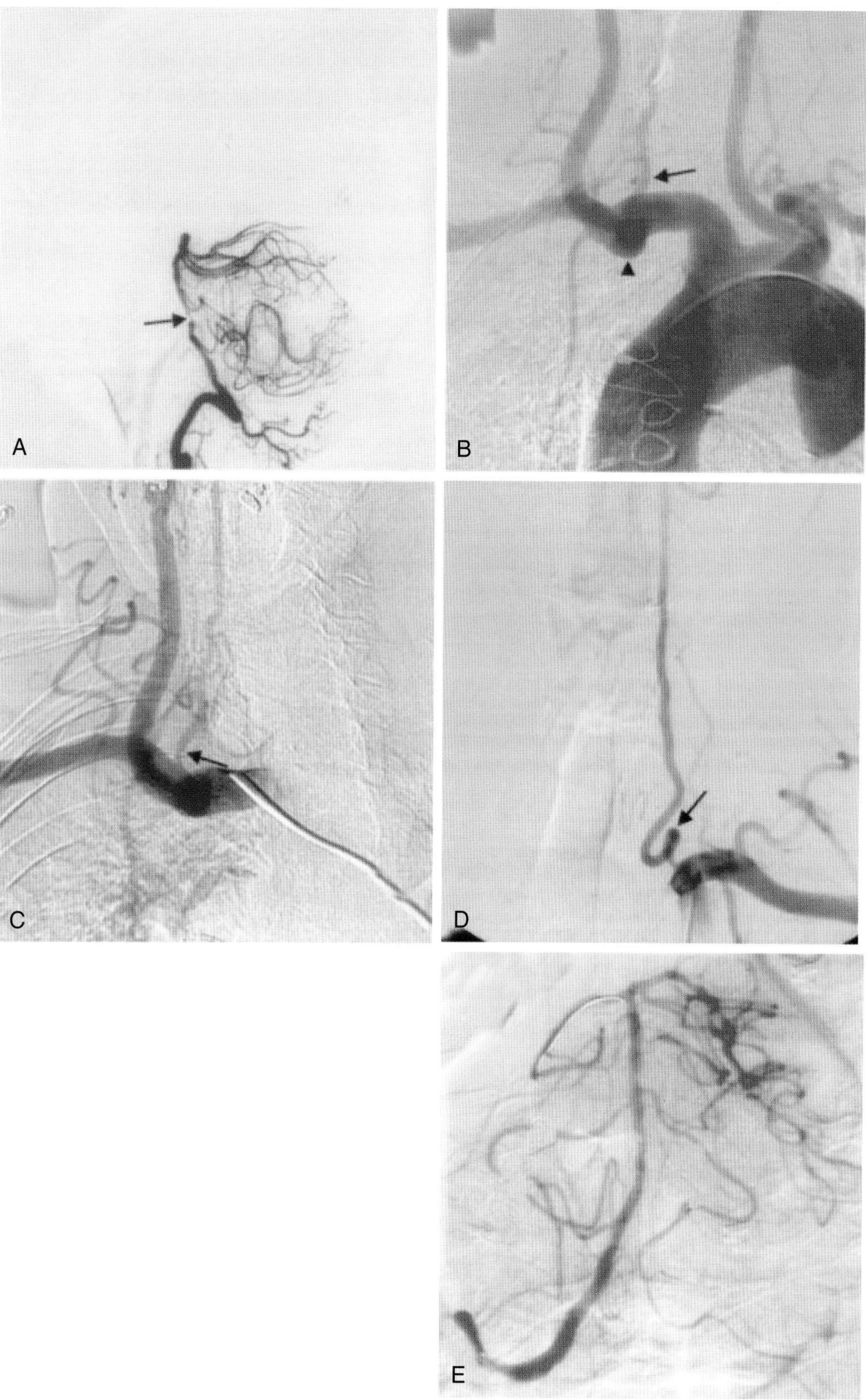

• **Fig. 39.4** Approach to basilar artery stenosis (A) via the radial approach because of severe tortuosity of the innominate artery (B) and left vertebral artery (D) for transfemoral access. The favorable angle of right vertebral artery off the right subclavian (C) enabled effective stent placement across the stenosis (E). (Adapted with permission Bendok BR, Przybylo JH, Parkinson R, Hu Y, Awad IA, Batjer HH. Neuroendovascular interventions for intracranial posterior circulation disease via the transradial approach: technical case report. *Neurosurgery.* 2005;56(3):E626)

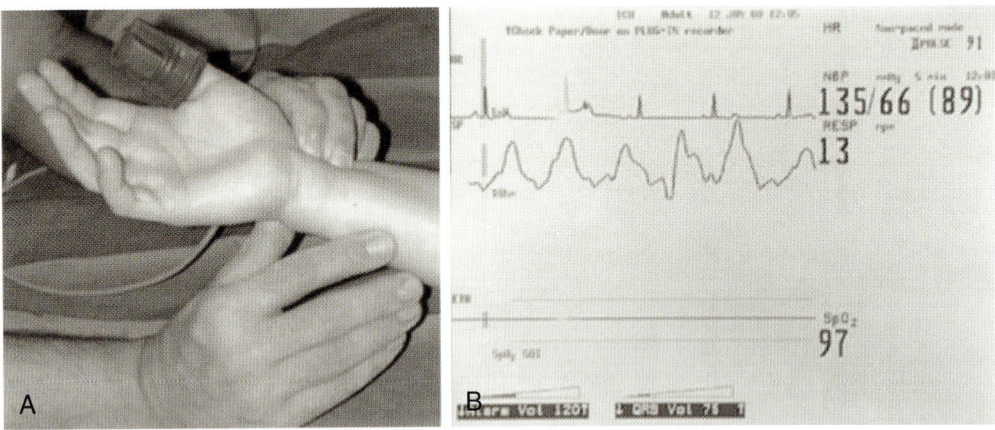

• **Fig. 39.5** Allen's test. Following simultaneous ulnar and radial artery compression till thumb oximeter saturation is no longer picked up, pressure over the ulnar artery is released. In the presence of adequate collateral circulation, the oxygen saturation rises to normal. (Adapted with permission Levy EI, Boulos AS, Fessler RD, et al. Transradial cerebral angiography: an alternative route. *Neurosurgery.* 2002;51(2): 335–340.)

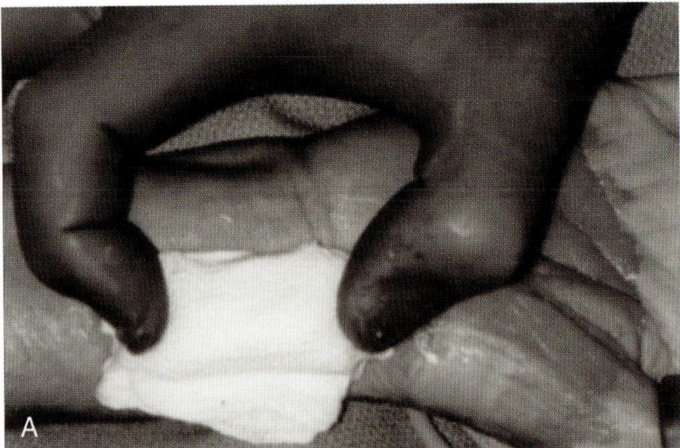

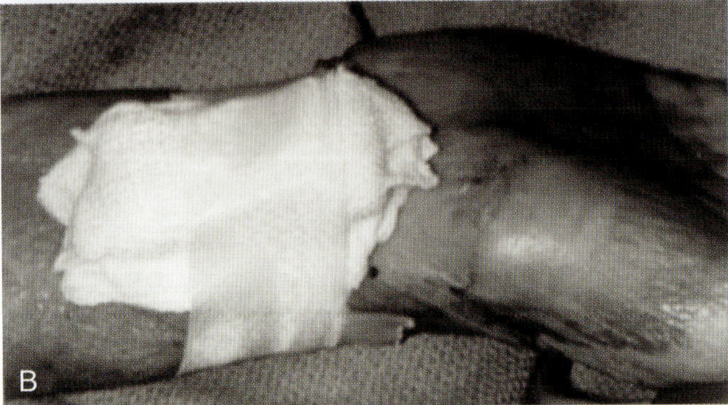

• **Fig. 39.6** Non-occlusive radial artery compression for hemostasis reduces risk of thrombosis. (Adapted with permission Levy EI, Boulos AS, Fessler RD, et al. Transradial cerebral angiography: an alternative route. *Neurosurgery.* 2002;51(2):335–340)

illustrated in the case of a challenging cavernous sinus DAVF that we treated via a strategic "hybrid" approach (Fig. 39.7i–v).[21]

Thromboembolic Complications From Intravascular Device Navigation in Large Vessels

After diagnostic and interventional cerebral angiography, there is clear evidence that patients experience increased hyperintense signals on diffusion-weighted magnetic resonance imaging (DWI) that represent microemboli.[22-30]

Ischemic thromboembolic events arise from following mechanisms:

i. Dislodged atheromatous debris mainly in the region of the aortic arch and carotid bifurcation
ii. Inherent thrombogenicity of an intravascular device
iii. Exogenous air/debris in the catheter system

The descending thoracic aorta and the distal aortic arch are the most common sites of atheromatous plaque in the aorta.[31] Catheter navigation with increasing age carries increasing risk and requires smooth maneuvers while in the tortuous arch. Risk factors for thromboembolic complications can be divided as described in Table 39.3.

The incidence of DWI "hits" ranges from about 11% to 22% in diagnostic angiography, to 20% to 60% in stent-assisted coiling of aneurysms, to as high as 86% with flow diverter placement. Most DWI signals interestingly spare deep perforator territories.[25] On follow-up, most of the small (<2 mm) signals disappear.[32] Not all signals correspond with clinical ischemic symptoms, but risk of neurologic adverse events can be as high as 3% with diagnostic cerebral angiography.[33] Clinical stroke rate with flow diversion may be as high as 6% to 13%.[22,34] The clinical stroke rate in carotid stenting ranges from 2% to 6.8% with far greater (>70%) new DWI lesions.[28,35] Nearly 25% of those with diffusion abnormalities will have contralateral lesions also.

Complication Avoidance

Table 39.4 outlines the steps that are rigorously followed at our institution to reduce the risk of thromboembolic events.

Extracranial Internal Carotid Artery/Vertebral Artery Spasm and Dissection

Catheter manipulation inside of the internal carotid artery (ICA) or vertebral artery can lead to spasm and on occasion lead to dissection. In diagnostic angiography, this has been noted to occur in about 1.2% of cases, according to a single-center study that reviewed 597 angiograms in 494 patients.[38] The vertebral artery tends to be more prone to dissection because of its smaller size

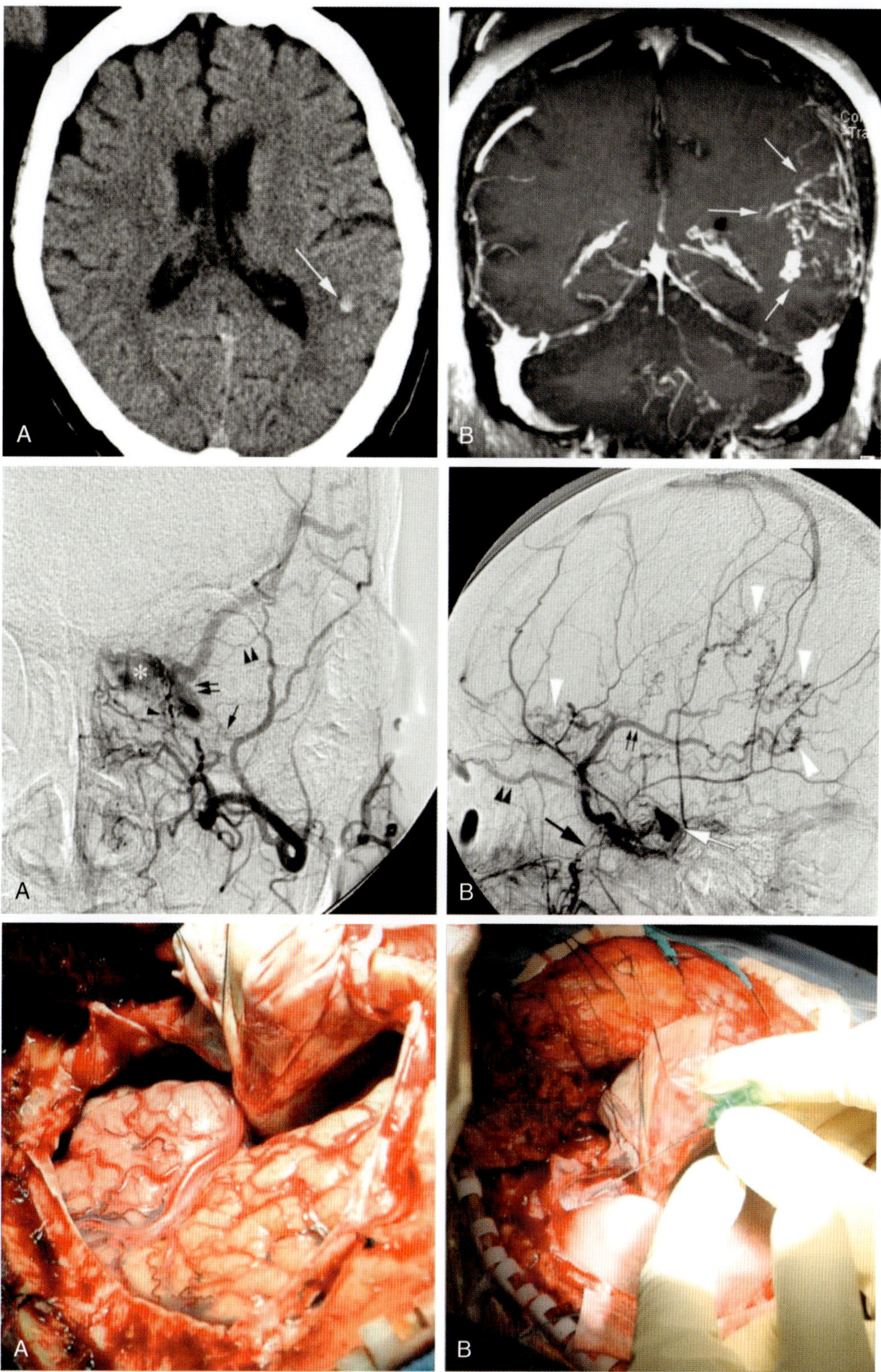

• **Fig. 39.7** Illustration of transcranial microsurgical 'hybrid' access. Left posterior temporal hematoma (i) due to venous hypertension from a high grade left cavernous sinus DAVF (ii) with a prominent arterialized superficial middle cerebral vein (SMCV). Endovascular direct access was not feasible since venous outflow was exclusively through cortical veins. While the initial angiogram showed a small superior ophthalmic vein, this was noted to be spontaneously thrombosed during the subsequent angiogram after 72 hours of the initial study. Left frontotemporal craniotomy with zygomatic osteotomy for microsurgical exposure of the SCMV (iii A). Micropuncture (iii B) and insertion of sheath in middle fossa floor at entrance of SMCV into dura (iv A and B) for coil embolization of the arterialized cavernous sinus (v A). Complete elimination of fistula was successfully achieved (v B). (Adapted with permission Hurley MC, Rahme RJ, Fishman AJ, Batjer HH, Bendok BR. Combined surgical and endovascular access of the superficial middle cerebral vein to occlude a high-grade cavernous dural arteriovenous fistula: case report. *Neurosurgery.* 2011;69(2):E475–E482.)

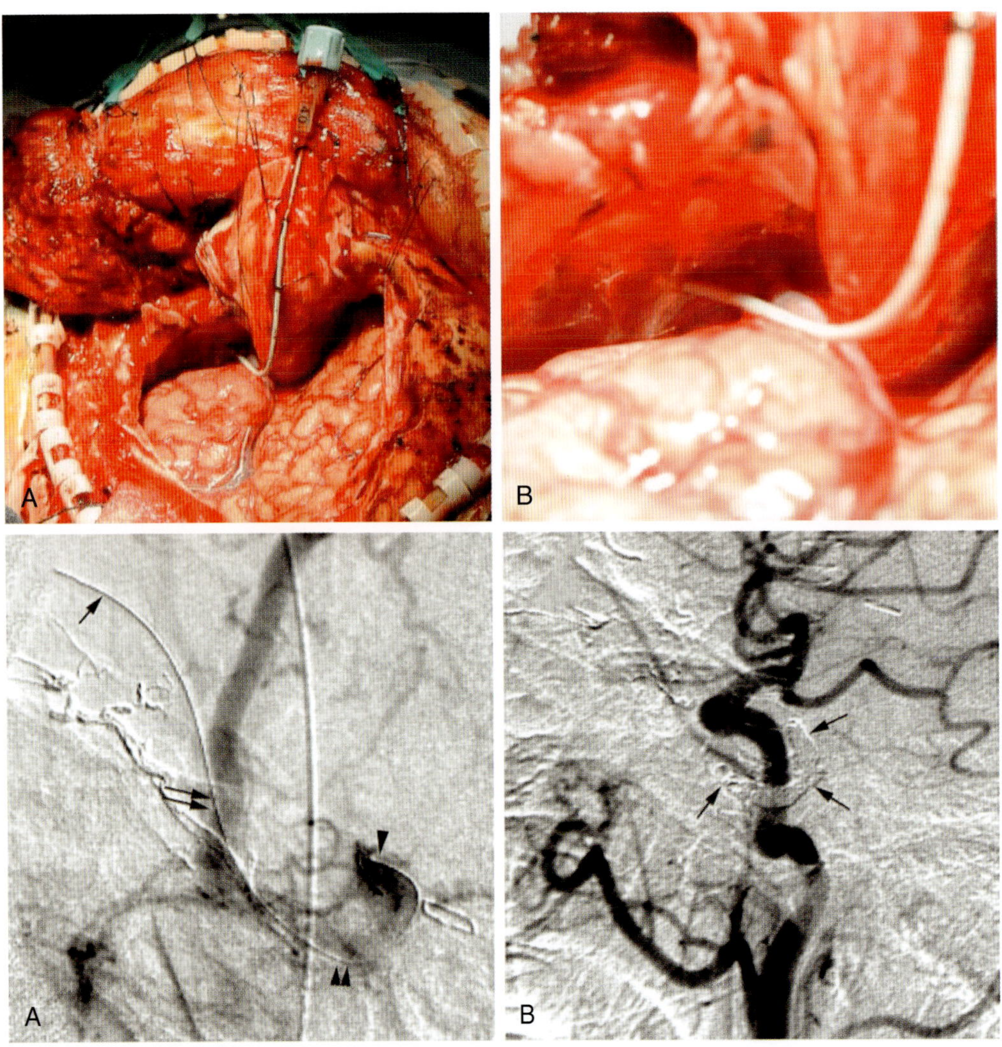

• **Fig. 39.7, cont'd**

TABLE 39.3 Risk Factors for Thromboembolic Complications

Patient Factors	Pharmacology	Procedural Factors
Increased age and atherosclerosis Tortuous arch anatomy Hypercoagulable state Unstable carotid plaque Tight carotid stenosis Contralateral carotid stenosis >50% Large, wide-neck aneurysm Resistance to antiplatelet agents Fibromuscular dysplasia Connective tissue diseases	Inadequate heparinization Inadequate platelet inhibition	Increased fluoroscopy time Increased contrast use Operator inexperience Complex intervention Flow diversion Inconsistent use of heparin flush with/without in-line filters Failure to use distal protection device

and the rigid nature of transverse foramina in its V2 segment. Complex interventions and operator technique are main risk factors, in addition to vessel wall abnormalities as in fibro muscular dysplasia.

Management

Spasm is usually relieved promptly with catheter withdrawal, time, and intraarterial verapamil or nitroglycerine. With ICA dissections the intimal flap is usually in the direction of flow (cranial), and this carries the risk of progression. At the same time, small dissections tend to heal excellently with medium-term antiplatelet or anticoagulant therapy. Hence decision-making has to occur on a case-by-case basis.

i. ***Subintimal dissection:*** this type carries the risk of stenosis and occlusion along with thromboembolic events. The initial therapy of choice is heparinization for 24 to 48 hours, followed by 1 to 3 months of Coumadin therapy. Milder degrees of stenosis may be alternatively treated with antiplatelet therapy such as aspirin for 3 to 6 months. Close follow-up with US is

TABLE 39.4 Steps to Reduce Thrombotic Events

Patient preparation	Anticipation of thromboembolic (TE) risk in elderly patients and atherosclerotic population Prophylactic aspirin for 5–7 days before planned diagnostic angiography[30] Adequate dual antiplatelet inhibition for stent placement procedures MR for carotid plaque imaging to risk-stratify unstable plaque[36] Noninvasive assessment (CTA or MRA) of arch and carotid/vertebral anatomy and atherosclerosis Radial or brachial access in case of prohibitive arch anatomy Consider microsurgical therapy
Pharmacology	Platelet inhibition testing
Technical steps	Meticulous "purging" of all flush lines of air, including line from power injector (Fig. 39.8) Keep field free of gauze fragments that may form embolizable debris during manipulation (Fig. 39.9) Heparin in flush lines and periodic check of pressure and content of bags to ensure continuous flush[37] Include above technical points in pre/post briefing and timeout Administration of IV heparin after access sheath in place (in endovascular procedures: full dose 60–80 IU/kg body weight; in diagnostic angiograms: half dose) Separate bowl of heparinized saline for cleaning gloves of blood and contrast material Frequent activated clotting time (ACT) checks (every 30–60 minutes) and bolus heparin doses as needed Hermetic technique during contrast injection Smooth and efficient technique: ALWAYS lead by wire Spend minimum necessary time intravascularly
Postoperative period	Continue antiplatelet agents as indicated Consider avoiding active heparin reversal Minimize neck manipulation with carotid stent

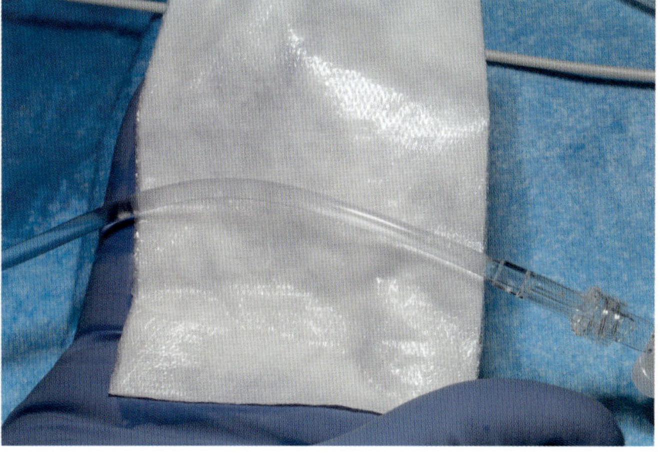

• **Fig. 39.8** Meticulous purging of flush lines of air at beginning of procedure and continual vigilance. (Used with permission of Mayo Foundation for Medical Education and Research, all rights reserved.)

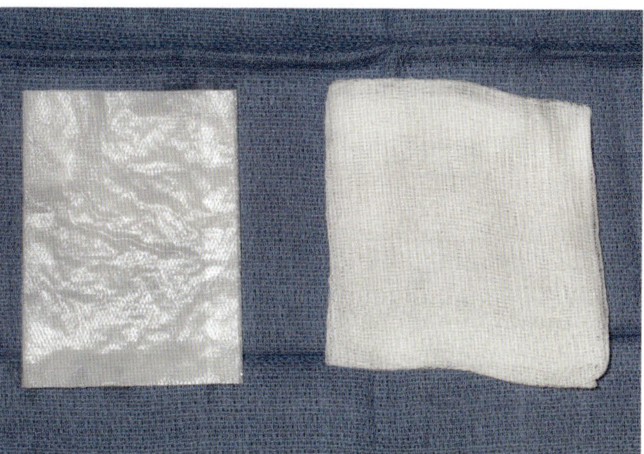

• **Fig. 39.9** Avoidance of material (such as gauze, on right) that can produce embolizable debris and preferential use of material such as Telfa (American Surgical Company, Salem, MA). (Used with permission of Mayo Foundation for Medical Education and Research, all rights reserved.)

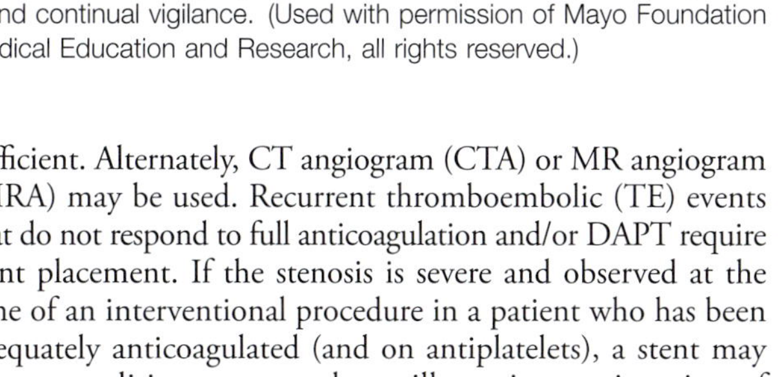

sufficient. Alternately, CT angiogram (CTA) or MR angiogram (MRA) may be used. Recurrent thromboembolic (TE) events that do not respond to full anticoagulation and/or DAPT require stent placement. If the stenosis is severe and observed at the time of an interventional procedure in a patient who has been adequately anticoagulated (and on antiplatelets), a stent may be an expeditious measure but will require continuation of DAPT.

ii. ***Subadventitial dissection:*** This type carries the risk of PA formation. Again, the first-line treatment is either anticoagulation or antiplatelet therapy to avoid thromboembolic events and to promote healing. An additional concern is periodic monitoring for PA enlargement, which can be accomplished with US or MRA or CTA. Progressive PA enlargement or recurrent TE events may require stent placement.

Complications Related to Target Lesion Access

These complications usually relate to microcatheter and microwire access and include:

i. Rupture of arterial feeder during transarterial embolization
ii. Aneurysm perforation and rupture
iii. Arteriovenous malformation rupture
iv. Rupture of draining vein during transvenous embolization

Avoidance of the above complications requires compulsive attention to technique and constant review of the position of the guide catheter and distal access catheter, especially with tortuous anatomy. Forcing wires through vessels such as the middle meningeal artery is absolutely prohibited. In aneurysm coiling, adequate sizing of the initial ("framing") coil and subsequent packing should be done carefully after a thorough assessment with rotational angiography.

Contrast Nephropathy

Contrast-induced nephropathy is defined as the rise in serum creatinine concentration in the 24 to 48 hours after contrast administration. Typically it remains asymptomatic other than a laboratory abnormality, and oliguria is surprisingly rare. The pathology is acute tubular necrosis. The risk factors identified are:

i. preexisting renal insufficiency, especially in combination with diabetes mellitus
ii. hemodynamic instability and hypovolemia with reduced renal perfusion
iii. arterial versus venous administration (such as CTA)
iv. interventional versus diagnostic angiography (related to volume of contrast)
v. use of nonionic hypo-osmolal agents such as iohexol or iopamidol.[39]

Complication Avoidance

Avoidance of renal dysfunction or exacerbation post angiography requires proper identification of high-risk patients. Steps that are taken to mitigate contrast-induced nephropathy are:

1. Hydration: Pre-, intra- and postprocedure hydration with isotonic normal saline reduces risk of kidney damage. Typically we prefer administration of about 0.5 to 1.0 L for diagnostic angiography and ensure ongoing hydration for more complex and lengthy interventions. Fluid overload should be avoided.
2. Acetylcysteine: Some evidence suggests benefit in the oral form given twice a day beginning the day before surgery and on the day of the procedure.[40]
3. Bicarbonate: Intravenous solution of bicarbonate has been compared with saline as a nephroprotectant with conflicting results, but most authorities consider it to be useful.[40] Our preference is saline hydration.
4. Contrast agent selection: The nonionic iso-osmolal agent iodixanol (Visipaque) is our preferred choice in high-risk patients and when frequent repeated examinations are necessary, such as in vasospasm. The other safer agents are iopamidol (Isovue) and loversol (Optiray), both of which are nonionic hypo-osmolal. The high-osmolal nonionic agent iohexol (Omnipaque) should be avoided.
5. Dose of contrast agent: Whichever agent is selected, it is important to limit volume administered to the absolute essential. Intelligent use of angiographic equipment and deliberate thought about the steps involved are important. Diluted contrast may be used conveniently without sacrificing image quality. We have used 20% diluted contrast with excellent imaging results in very high risk patients.

Management

As mentioned earlier, the incidence of oliguria is surprisingly low, and large studies have shown that the necessity of dialysis exists in less than 1%.[41] The elevated creatinine levels tend to drop back to baseline toward the end of the week after angiography.

SURGICAL REWIND

My Worst Case

Retroperitoneal Hematoma

A 72-year-old lady underwent a second stage of stent-assisted coiling for a residual unruptured basilar apex aneurysm (Fig. 39.10). Approach was via the right transfemoral route. The previous treatment session was also via a right transfemoral approach about 3 months prior and was uneventful with regard to groin hemostasis and follow-up. Groin access for the index procedure was achieved with an 8 Fr sheath, and after the procedure, an 8 Fr Angio-Seal closure device was deployed uneventfully (Fig. 39.11). Complete heparinization had been achieved, and no reversal was undertaken (she was also on dual antiplatelet therapy). The next morning she developed acute severe groin pain and hypotension with tenderness over and around the puncture site. Hemoglobin dropped from 10.1 to 6.5 g/dL, and packed cells were transfused. Coagulation profile was normal. CT scan/CTA of the abdomen and pelvis revealed a massive retroperitoneal hematoma with a small site of contrast extravasation (Fig. 39.12A–C). Emergent pigtail aortogram (Fig. 39.13A) and right iliofemoral angiography (Fig. 39.13B) from left-sided femoral access did not show active site of leak or PA. One day later she developed atrial fibrillation with rapid ventricular response from the acute hemodynamic insult and discontinuation of metoprolol; this settled readily with rate control using diltiazem. She was managed with bed rest for 48 hours, close hemodynamic monitoring, and gradual mobilization and was discharged on day 7 in stable condition. Follow-up at 6 weeks was unremarkable, and hemoglobin was 13.1 g/dL.

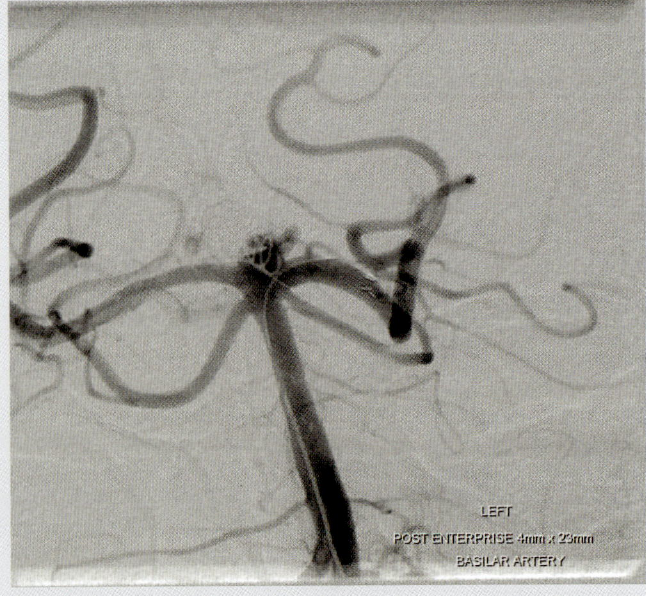

• **Fig. 39.10** Residual basilar apex aneurysm.

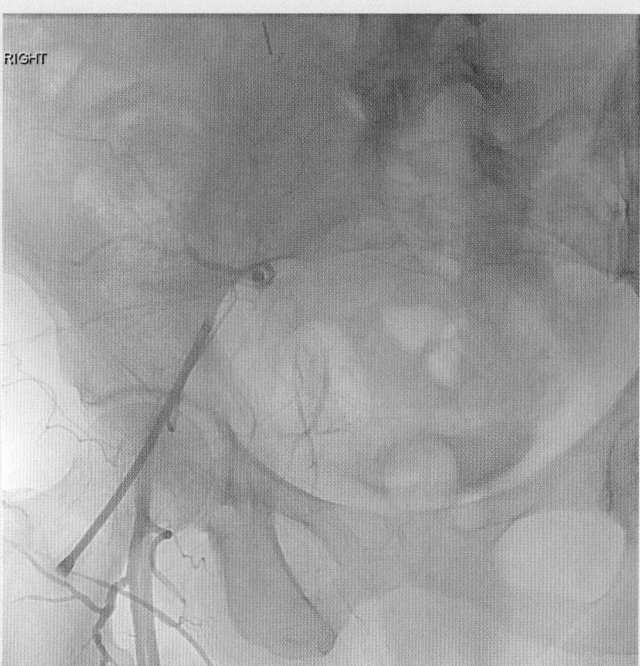

• **Fig. 39.11** Groin puncture site towards uppermost aspect of femoral head. This would constitute a 'high' puncture though it appears to be over the femoral head. Strategic obliquity with the sheath pulled away can often demonstrate exact puncture site (not done in this case). (Used with permission of Mayo Foundation for Medical Education and Research, all rights reserved.)

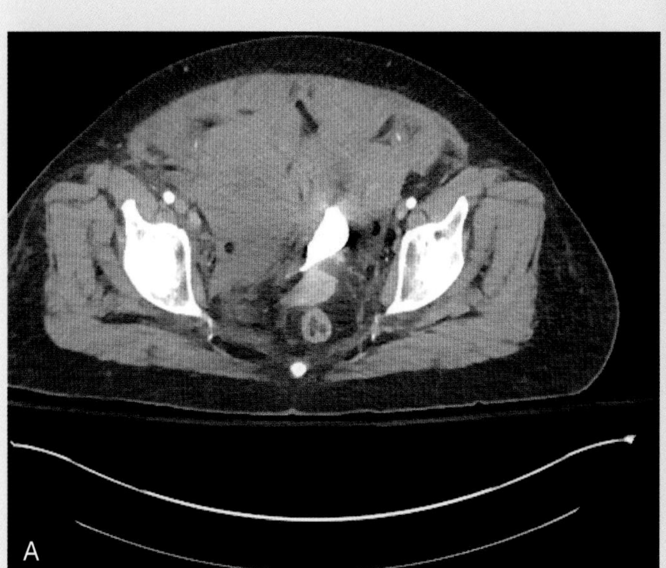

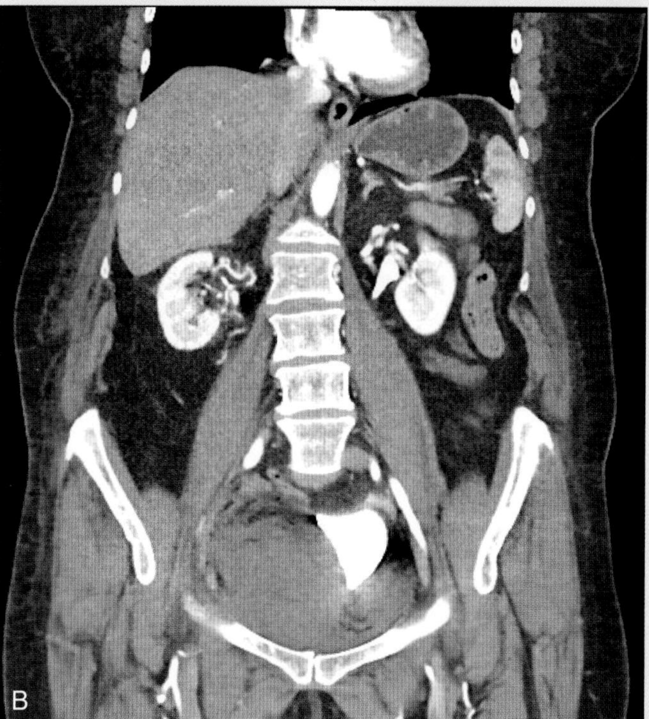

• **Fig. 39.12** Axial (A), coronal (B) and CT angiogram (C) images of abdomen and pelvis. A large retroperitoneal hematoma is evident (3A) that displaces the urinary bladder to the contralateral side and compresses it (3B, arrow). There is a site of contrast extravasation in the clot (3C, arrow). No pseudoaneurysm was evident. (Used with permission of Mayo Foundation for Medical Education and Research, all rights reserved.)

Continued

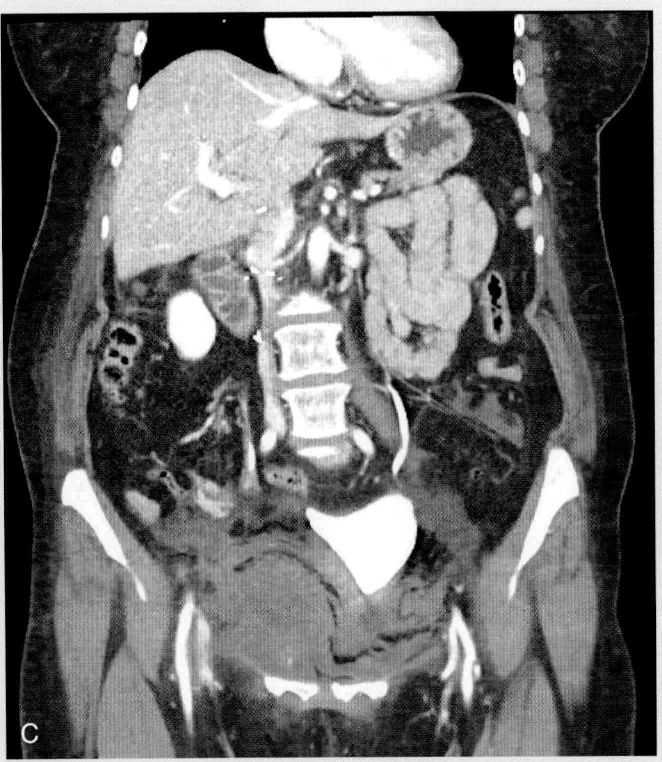

• **Fig. 39.12, cont'd**

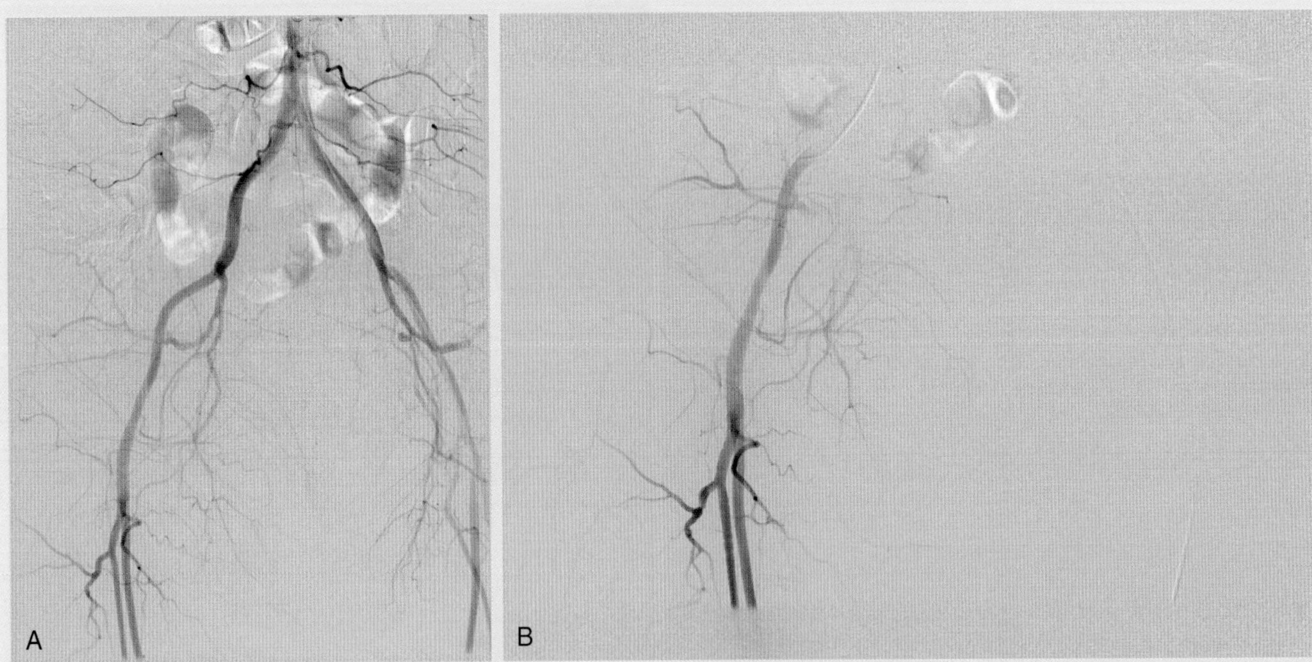

• **Fig. 39.13** Pigtail aortogram (A) and right iliofemoral run (B) via left femoral approach does not show pseudoaneurysm or active dye extravasation. (Used with permission of Mayo Foundation for Medical Education and Research, all rights reserved.)

NEUROSURGICAL SELFIE MOMENT

Access-related complications are not unusual in day-to-day endovascular neurosurgical practice. A standard regimental approach to complication avoidance is the secret to successful outcomes. Knowing your patient and patient-specific anatomy, identification of high-risk patients, brutal honesty about complications, minimizing procedural time, constant refinement of technique, and smooth techniques will help minimize the complications.

References

1. Wagenbach A, Saladino A, Daugherty WP, Cloft HJ, Kallmes DF, Lanzino G. Safety of early ambulation after diagnostic and therapeutic neuroendovascular procedures without use of closure devices. *Neurosurgery*. 2010;66(3):493–496, discussion 496–497.
2. Krueger K, Zaehringer M, Strohe D, Stuetzer H, Boecker J, Lackner K. Postcatheterization pseudoaneurysm: results of US-guided percutaneous thrombin injection in 240 patients. *Radiology*. 2005;236(3):1104–1110.
3. Robertson L, Andras A, Colgan F, Jackson R. Vascular closure devices for femoral arterial puncture site haemostasis. *Cochrane Database Syst Rev*. 2016;(3):CD009541.
4. Koreny M, Riedmuller E, Nikfardjam M, Siostrzonek P, Mullner M. Arterial puncture closing devices compared with standard manual compression after cardiac catheterization: systematic review and meta-analysis. *JAMA*. 2004;291(3):350–357.
5. Levy EI, Boulos AS, Fessler RD, et al. Transradial cerebral angiography: an alternative route. *Neurosurgery*. 2002;51(2):335–340, discussion 340–332.
6. Levy EI, Kim SH, Bendok BR, Qureshi AI, Guterman LR, Hopkins LN. Transradial stenting of the cervical internal carotid artery: technical case report. *Neurosurgery*. 2003;53(2):448–451, discussion 451–442.
7. Kedev S, Mann T. Skin to skin: transradial carotid angiography and stenting. *Intervent Cardiol Clin*. 2014;3(1):21–35.
8. Hill MD, Brooks W, Mackey A, et al. Stroke after carotid stenting and endarterectomy in the Carotid Revascularization Endarterectomy versus Stenting Trial (CREST). *Circulation*. 2012;126(25):3054–3061.
9. Bendok BR, Przybylo JH, Parkinson R, Hu Y, Awad IA, Batjer HH. Neuroendovascular interventions for intracranial posterior circulation disease via the transradial approach: technical case report. *Neurosurgery*. 2005;56(3):E626, discussion E626.
10. Mendiz OA, Fava C, Lev G, Caponi G, Valdivieso L. Transradial versus transfemoral carotid artery stenting: a 16-year single-center experience. *J Interv Cardiol*. 2016;29(6):588–593.
11. Faggioli G, Ferri M, Rapezzi C, Tonon C, Manzoli L, Stella A. Atherosclerotic aortic lesions increase the risk of cerebral embolism during carotid stenting in patients with complex aortic arch anatomy. *J Vasc Surg*. 2009;49(1):80–85.
12. Faggioli G, Ferri M, Gargiulo M, et al. Measurement and impact of proximal and distal tortuosity in carotid stenting procedures. *J Vasc Surg*. 2007;46(6):1119–1124.
13. Aoun SG, Bendok BR, Batjer HH. Acute management of ruptured arteriovenous malformations and dural arteriovenous fistulas. *Neurosurg Clin N Am*. 2012;23(1):87–103.
14. Montorsi P, Galli S, Ravagnani PM, et al. Carotid artery stenting with proximal embolic protection via a transradial or transbrachial approach: pushing the boundaries of the technique while maintaining safety and efficacy. *J Endovasc Ther*. 2016;23(4):549–560.
15. Dashti SR, Fiorella D, Spetzler RF, Albuquerque FC, McDougall CG. Transorbital endovascular embolization of dural carotid-cavernous fistula: access to cavernous sinus through direct puncture: case examples and technical report. *Neurosurgery*. 2011;68(1 Suppl Operative):75–83, discussion 83.
16. White JB, Layton KF, Evans AJ, et al. Transorbital puncture for the treatment of cavernous sinus dural arteriovenous fistulas. *AJNR Am J Neuroradiol*. 2007;28(7):1415–1417.
17. Blanc R, Piotin M, Mounayer C, Spelle L, Moret J. Direct cervical arterial access for intracranial endovascular treatment. *Neuroradiology*. 2006;48(12):925–929.
18. Mokin M, Snyder KV, Levy EI, Hopkins LN, Siddiqui AH. Direct carotid artery puncture access for endovascular treatment of acute ischemic stroke: technical aspects, advantages, and limitations. *J Neurointerv Surg*. 2015;7(2):108–113.
19. Blanc R, Mounayer C, Piotin M, Sadik J-C, Spelle L, Moret J. Hemostatic closure device after carotid puncture for stent and coil placement in an intracranial aneurysm: technical note. *AJNR Am J Neuroradiol*. 2002;23(6):978–981.
20. Kwolek CJ, Jaff MR, Leal JI, et al. Results of the ROADSTER multicenter trial of transcarotid stenting with dynamic flow reversal. *J Vasc Surg*. 2015;62(5):1227–1234.
21. Hurley MC, Rahme RJ, Fishman AJ, Batjer HH, Bendok BR. Combined surgical and endovascular access of the superficial middle cerebral vein to occlude a high-grade cavernous dural arteriovenous fistula: case report. *Neurosurgery*. 2011;69(2):E475–E482.
22. Iosif C, Camilleri Y, Saleme S, et al. Diffusion-weighted imaging-detected ischemic lesions associated with flow-diverting stents in intracranial aneurysms: safety, potential mechanisms, clinical outcome, and concerns. *J Neurosurg*. 2015;122(3):627–636.
23. Heller RS, Dandamudi V, Calnan D, Malek AM. Neuroform intracranial stenting for aneurysms using simple and multi-stent technique is associated with low risk of magnetic resonance diffusion-weighted imaging lesions. *Neurosurgery*. 2013;73(4):582–590, discussion 590–591.
24. Park JC, Lee DH, Kim JK, et al. Microembolism after endovascular coiling of unruptured cerebral aneurysms: incidence and risk factors. *J Neurosurg*. 2016;124(3):777–783.
25. Park KY, Chung PW, Kim YB, Moon HS, Suh BC, Yoon WT. Post-interventional microembolism: cortical border zone is a preferential site for ischemia. *Cerebrovasc Dis*. 2011;32(3):269–275.
26. Biondi A, Oppenheim C, Vivas E, et al. Cerebral aneurysms treated by Guglielmi detachable coils: evaluation with diffusion-weighted MR imaging. *AJNR Am J Neuroradiol*. 2000;21(5):957–963.
27. Albayram S, Selcuk H, Kara B, et al. Thromboembolic events associated with balloon-assisted coil embolization: evaluation with diffusion-weighted MR imaging. *AJNR Am J Neuroradiol*. 2004;25(10):1768–1777.
28. Bijuklic K, Wandler A, Varnakov Y, Tuebler T, Schofer J. Risk factors for cerebral embolization after carotid artery stenting with embolic protection: a diffusion-weighted magnetic resonance imaging study in 837 consecutive patients. *Circ Cardiovasc Interv*. 2013;6(3):311–316.
29. Bendszus M, Koltzenburg M, Burger R, Warmuth-Metz M, Hofmann E, Solymosi L. Silent embolism in diagnostic cerebral angiography and neurointerventional procedures: a prospective study. *Lancet*. 1999;354(9190):1594–1597.
30. Brockmann C, Hoefer T, Diepers M, et al. Abciximab does not prevent ischemic lesions related to cerebral angiography: a randomized placebo-controlled trial. *Cerebrovasc Dis*. 2011;31(4):353–357.
31. Meissner I, Whisnant JP, Khandheria BK, et al. Prevalence of potential risk factors for stroke assessed by transesophageal echocardiography and carotid ultrasonography: the SPARC study. Stroke Prevention: Assessment of Risk in a Community. *Mayo Clin Proc*. 1999;74(9):862–869.
32. Iosif C, Lecomte JC, Pedrolo-Silveira E, et al. Evaluation of ischemic lesion prevalence after endovascular treatment of intracranial aneurysms, as documented by 3-T diffusion-weighted imaging: a 2-year, single-center cohort study. *J Neurosurg*. 2018;128(4):982–991.
33. Dion JE, Gates PC, Fox AJ, Barnett HJ, Blom RJ. Clinical events following neuroangiography: a prospective study. *Stroke*. 1987;18(6):997–1004.
34. Brinjikji W, Kallmes DF, Cloft HJ, Lanzino G. Age-related outcomes following intracranial aneurysm treatment with the Pipeline Embolization Device: a subgroup analysis of the IntrePED registry. *J Neurosurg*. 2016;124(6):1726–1730.

35. Brott TG, Hobson RWI, Howard G, et al. Stenting versus endarterectomy for treatment of carotid-artery stenosis. *NEJM*. 2010; 363(1):11–23.
36. Akutsu N, Hosoda K, Fujita A, Kohmura E. A preliminary prediction model with MR plaque imaging to estimate risk for new ischemic brain lesions on diffusion-weighted imaging after endarterectomy or stenting in patients with carotid stenosis. *AJNR Am J Neuroradiol*. 2012;33(8):1557–1564.
37. Bendszus M, Koltzenburg M, Bartsch AJ, et al. Heparin and air filters reduce embolic events caused by intra-arterial cerebral angiography: a prospective, randomized trial. *Circulation*. 2004;110(15):2210–2215.
38. Le Roux PD, Elliott JP, Eskridge JM, Cohen W, Winn HR. Risks and benefits of diagnostic angiography after aneurysm surgery: a retrospective analysis of 597 studies. *Neurosurgery*. 1998;42(6):1248–1254, discussion 1254–1245.
39. Eng J, Wilson RF, Subramaniam RM, et al. Comparative effect of contrast media type on the incidence of contrast-induced nephropathy: a systematic review and meta-analysis. *Ann Intern Med*. 2016;164(6):417–424.
40. Gonzales DA, Norsworthy KJ, Kern SJ, et al. A meta-analysis of N-acetylcysteine in contrast-induced nephrotoxicity: unsupervised clustering to resolve heterogeneity. *BMC Med*. 2007; 5(1):32.
41. Rudnick MR, Goldfarb S, Wexler L, et al. Nephrotoxicity of ionic and nonionic contrast media in 1196 patients: a randomized trial. *Kidney Int*. 1995;47(1):254–261.

40

Procedure-Related Complications of Aneurysm Treatment: Intraprocedural Rupture, Thromboembolic Events, Coil Migration or Prolapse Into Parent Artery, and Recurrent Aneurysm Management

JACOB F. BARANOSKI, BRUNO C. FLORES, FELIPE C. ALBUQUERQUE

HIGHLIGHTS

- Endovascular techniques continue to evolve and are increasingly applied to more complex aneurysms.
- Potential devastating complications include intraprocedural rupture and rerupture, thromboembolic events, coil prolapse and migration, and aneurysm recurrence.
- Certain aneurysms are associated with higher rates of complications because of specific aneurysm characteristics and anatomy.
- Patient outcomes are improved by knowing how to help prevent complications, how to recognize them immediately when they occur, and how to utilize salvage techniques.

Background

The prevalence of intracranial aneurysms is about 3%, with the incidence of aneurysm subarachnoid hemorrhage (SAH) estimated to range from 10 to 15 cases per 100,000 people.[1] Both surgical and endovascular techniques are available for aneurysm treatment. Factors that should be considered when selecting an intervention include patient presentation (e.g., ruptured vs unruptured aneurysm, patient age, comorbidities), anatomic considerations (e.g., aneurysm size, location, morphology), and surgeon expertise. Studies have demonstrated clinical equipoise regarding endovascular coiling and open surgery for treatment of intracranial aneurysms.[2] However, as endovascular interventions continue to evolve, they are increasingly used for more complex aneurysms and have provided neurointerventionalists with an ever-expanding repertoire of technologies and techniques.

With the broader use of endovascular interventions has come an increased potential for devastating complications. We discuss the most common complications, their risk factors, and complication management strategies.

Potential Complications

The most common and clinically significant complications of coil embolization of intracranial aneurysms are hemorrhage from intraprocedural rupture and rerupture, ischemia from thromboembolic events, coil migration and prolapse of coils into the parent vessel, and aneurysm recanalization. A 2016 metaanalysis found a 12% overall complication rate for the coiling of intracranial aneurysms.[3]

Intraprocedural Rupture and Rerupture

Intraprocedural rupture and rerupture are serious and potentially devastating complications that result in a substantial increase in overall morbidity and mortality. In the Analysis of Treatment by Endovascular Approach of Nonruptured Aneurysms (ATENA) study, the rate of intraprocedural rupture for unruptured aneurysms was 2.6% (18 of 700 procedures).[4] The intraprocedural rate for ruptured aneurysms was somewhat higher in the Clinical and Anatomic Results in the Treatment of Ruptured Intracranial Aneurysms (CLARITY) study, which found the risk to be 3.7% (15 of 405 patients).[5] Rates of intraprocedural rupture are likely higher in patients with ruptured aneurysms because of a preexisting decrease in aneurysm wall strength and because of aggressive coiling of ruptured aneurysms in an attempt to achieve tighter coil packing.

With the increasing use of newer endovascular techniques, including balloon-assisted coiling (BAC) and stent-assisted coiling (SAC), intraprocedural rupture remains a potentially catastrophic complication. Although Sluzewski et al.[6] demonstrated a higher rate of intraprocedural rupture with BAC (4%; 3 of 71) than with coiling alone (0.8%; 6 of 756) in their 2006 study, Pierot et al.[7] later demonstrated in 2011 that intraprocedural rupture rates are similar for BAC (4.4%; 7 of 160) and conventional coil embolization (4.6%; 28 of 608). Likewise, there appears to be no significant difference in intraprocedural rupture risk between SAC and traditional coil embolization.[8,9] An important consideration is that SAC has been reserved primarily for patients who have not had a rupture because of the required use of antiplatelet therapy after stent deployment; the use of antiplatelet therapy can complicate the management of intracranial aneurysms when there is an intraprocedural rupture.

Thromboembolic Events

As with an intraprocedural rupture, ischemia from a thromboembolic event can be a potentially catastrophic event. The rates of ischemic events resulting from the endovascular treatment of unruptured and ruptured aneurysms were 7.3% (29 of 398) in the ATENA study and 13.3% (54 of 405) in the CLARITY study.[4,5] The use of the SAC technique and the use of flow diverters are associated with a higher risk of ischemic events than the use of traditional coil embolization.[3,8,9] This increased risk is likely a result of the permanent placement of a foreign object in the parent vessel. Although there is an obvious need for antiplatelet therapy upon the deployment of these devices, the optimal timing, regimen, and generalized standard of care have not been well established. Fortunately, many of the patients who experience thromboembolic events are generally asymptomatic or have only transient neurologic deficits; however, others have significant neurologic complications, and these ischemic events are associated with an overall increased morbidity and mortality.[10]

Coil Migration and Prolapse Into Parent Vessel

One of the many advantages of modern coils and delivery systems is that they allow the delivery, repositioning, and evaluation of the placement of coils in the aneurysm before detachment. In most cases, a suboptimally placed coil can be removed or repositioned before final deployment. However, these coils can still protrude from the aneurysm sac into the parent vessel after deployment, and they can become intertwined with other coils or stents. The attempted removal of such coils can result in the coil stretching, unraveling, and breaking. The consequences of coil migration or prolapse range from asymptomatic flow alterations in the parent artery to devastating thromboembolic occlusion of major intracranial vessels and subsequent large territory infarcts. Depending on the site of coil breakage, pieces of coil may be carried into distal cerebral or even systemic blood vessels, creating a potentially dangerous thrombogenic mass.[11] Data from a meta-analysis examining multiple series indicate that the incidence of cases with coil migration ranges from 2% to 6%.[12] Another potential consequence of coil migration is the need for long-term systemic antiplatelet medication to reduce the risk of thromboembolism, which carries its own inherent risks, particularly in cases of ruptured aneurysms.

Aneurysm Recanalization

With the continued establishment of endovascular techniques as the first-line treatment for intracranial aneurysms, one of the greatest concerns is the observed rate of aneurysm recanalization after treatment. Recanalization may result in aneurysm rupture or rerupture. A recent meta-analysis reported a recanalization incidence of 8% to 33.6% after endovascular treatment,[3] and another study reported a retreatment rate of 10.3% (572 of 5582) of all aneurysms because of recanalization.[13] Although numerous small case series studies have attempted to elucidate factors associated with aneurysm recanalization, no definitive conclusions have emerged. A prospective trial designed to help determine predictive factors associated with aneurysm recanalization recently completed patient enrollment (ARETA; NCT01942512).[14]

Anatomic Insights

A key component of preoperative and intraoperative decision-making and treatment execution for cerebral aneurysms is the careful study of the anatomic characteristics of the aneurysm and its relationship to the parent vessel. Certain characteristics (e.g., neck size, dome size, location, parent vessel angle, and rupture status) have been demonstrated to correlate with rates of complications after endovascular intervention (Fig. 40.1).

Wide-Neck Aneurysms

Numerous studies have identified wide-neck aneurysms, which are typically defined as aneurysms with a neck diameter >4 mm, as having an increased risk of complications when treated by endovascular techniques.[4,9,15–17] These complications include thromboembolic events and intraoperative rupture.

In addition to the absolute size of the aneurysm neck, the relative size of the neck is also an important anatomic characteristic of the aneurysm. A relatively wide neck, as calculated by the aneurysm dome-to-neck ratio (i.e., dome width to neck width) and by the aspect ratio (i.e., dome height to neck width), correlates with the need for adjunctive techniques during endovascular treatment.[18]

Aneurysm Dome Size

The size of the aneurysm dome has also been associated with adverse effects of endovascular treatment; however, its relationship to complication rates is complex. Some studies have demonstrated that, unlike smaller lesions, large aneurysms (>10 mm) carry a higher risk of treatment-related thromboembolic events and overall greater rates of periprocedural morbidity and mortality.[4,9,16] Aneurysms >10 mm have also been associated with an increased risk of revascularization and the need for retreatment.[13,19] However, other studies have demonstrated that small aneurysms (<4 mm) carry a greater risk of procedural rupture or rerupture.[4,17]

Aneurysm Location

Aneurysm location may be associated with the risk of complications after endovascular interventions; however, this relationship has not been fully elucidated. Some authors have reported higher rates of complications, including thromboembolic events and intraprocedural rupture, with middle cerebral artery aneurysms than with aneurysms in other locations.[9,16] Other authors have demonstrated that posterior circulation aneurysms carry an increased risk of retreatment[13] or that there is no correlation between location and risk.[15]

Parent Vessel Angle

Fan et al.[17] reported that a small parent vessel angle (<60 degrees) is associated with thromboembolic complications. They postulated that these complications may result from increased microcatheter

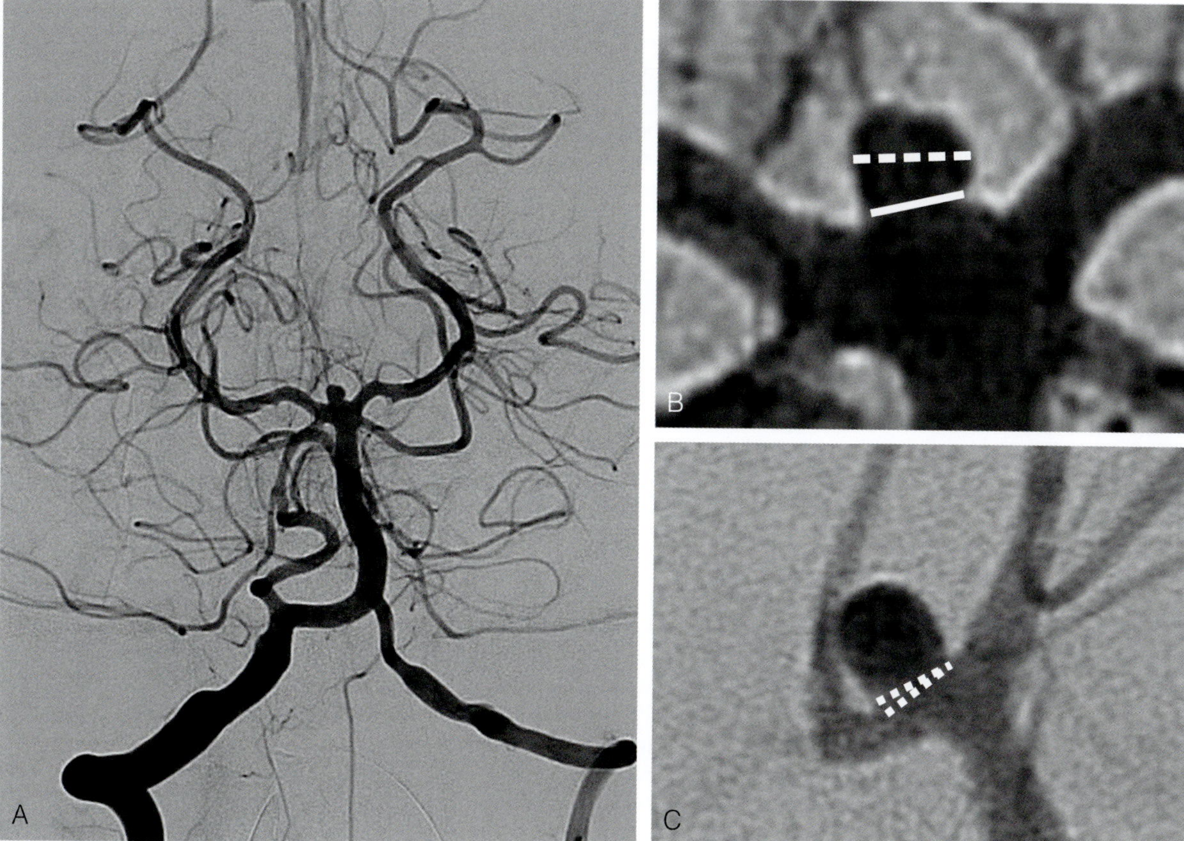

• **Fig. 40.1** Angiograms highlighting key aspects of aneurysm anatomy. (A) Anteroposterior angiogram demonstrating a basilar tip aneurysm. (B) A magnified view of the basilar tip aneurysm illustrating the size of its neck (solid line) and the size of its dome (dashed line). The high neck-to-dome size ratio correlates with an increased risk for complications, and it highlights the need for balloon-assisted coiling or stent-assisted coiling techniques for adequate treatment. (C) Magnified working-angle view of an anterior communicating artery aneurysm depicting a measurement of the parent vessel angle (dotted lines). Small parent vessel angles (<60 degrees), as shown in this example, are associated with an increased risk of complications. (Used with permission from Barrow Neurological Institute, Phoenix, Arizona.)

instability and that repeat catheterization may cause endothelial injury and thrombi.

Ruptured Aneurysms

Aneurysms treated after rupture and SAH are associated with higher complication rates than those for unruptured lesions or aneurysms treated electively.[20] Complications include intraprocedural rerupture,[4,5,21] recanalization,[19] thromboembolism,[22] and procedural morbidity and mortality.[23] Two possible reasons for higher rates of intraprocedural rerupture are decreased aneurysm wall strength and aggressive coiling of ruptured aneurysms to achieve tighter coil packing.

RED FLAGS

- Unfavorable aneurysm characteristics or anatomy (e.g., wide neck, very large or small dome, middle cerebral artery location, small parent vessel angle)
- Unfamiliarity with indicated technique
- Insufficient medical management of SAH sequelae
- Multiple medical comorbidities and challenging aneurysm anatomy for elective cases

Prevention

Prevention remains the most effective strategy for management of endovascular complications. It requires appropriate preoperative care, selection of the patient and technique, understanding and acknowledgment of device and personal capabilities and limitations, and meticulous study of anatomic information from both preprocedural and intraprocedural imaging studies.

Preoperative Care

For ruptured aneurysms, preprocedural stabilization with appropriate resuscitation, blood pressure and comorbidity management, neurologic monitoring, and possible external ventricular drain placement with intracranial pressure monitoring can improve both periprocedural and overall morbidity and mortality.[24] Patients with aneurysmal SAH treated by experienced and multidisciplinary medical staff have improved overall outcomes.[25]

Patient Selection

Nearly all patients with aneurysmal SAH should be considered for intervention, and patients with unruptured aneurysms who opt for elective intervention should be counseled on their risks based on patient-specific factors, such as family history and comorbidities.[1] Certain comorbidities, such as smoking and hypertension, increase the likelihood of complications during endovascular surgery.[16,17] Older age of patients undergoing endovascular treatment for cerebral aneurysms does not significantly increase the risk of complications[9,15,16,26]; however, some authors have reported a higher rate of complications in the elderly.[27]

Intervention Selection

Like appropriate patient selection, optimal intervention selection based on the natural history of the disease and aneurysm anatomy must be considered. Doing so helps decrease complication rates and helps improve overall outcomes.

In elective treatment of wide-neck aneurysms or in other cases requiring the use of SAC or a flow diverter, initiation of antiplatelet therapy before the procedure may help reduce the likelihood of periprocedural thromboembolic events.[28] Antiplatelet therapy regimens differ among institutions. We typically initiate dual antiplatelet therapy with clopidogrel and aspirin 10 to 15 days before the procedure and then assess the patient for platelet inhibition during preoperative testing. If patients were not pretreated but required dual antiplatelet coverage, we successfully used intraoperative intravenous and intra-arterial administration of abciximab, followed by postoperative aspirin and clopidogrel. Our group recently showed that this strategy was not associated with an increased risk of perioperative thromboembolic complications.[29] Both SAC and BAC have been demonstrated to be safe and effective techniques for technically challenging wide-neck aneurysms, resulting in improved obliteration and decreased recurrence or progression.[3,7–9] SAC has also been used for ruptured aneurysms with encouraging results.[30] The optimal antiplatelet therapy strategy for these challenging cases and the implications for traditional SAH treatments (e.g., timing of external ventricular drain placement) remain to be fully elucidated.

Flushing catheters with heparinized saline to prevent formation of microthrombi that can subsequently embolize helps reduce the rates of thromboembolism. For unruptured lesions, we systemically heparinize all patients for the duration of the procedure, with no protamine sulfate reversal unless bleeding complications occur. Ruptured lesions are systemically heparinized just before intracranial microcatheterization, with protamine readily available in the angiography suite for rapid reversal in case of intraoperative rupture. This practice is not universal, and some surgeons prefer to hold systemic anticoagulation until partial dome protection is achieved.

Operator Ability

Microsurgical or endovascular treatment options are available for most intracranial aneurysms. Selecting the right treatment, for the right aneurysm, for the right patient is the first step in minimizing complications and improving outcomes. Complication rates have been associated with advanced endovascular techniques, and improved outcomes have been strongly correlated with experience, reflecting a learning-curve effect.[31] As with all aspects of neurosurgery, understanding one's own limitations and feeling comfortable with specific pathologies and techniques are crucial to providing appropriate patient care, especially for elective cases. For neurointerventionalists, this treatment selection process includes recognizing that open clipping will sometimes be the superior choice.

Management

Recognizing Complications

The most important factor in managing procedure-related complications is arguably their immediate recognition. For intraprocedural rupture and coil migration, recognition includes observing active contrast extravasation, coil protrusion, or both from the aneurysm into the extravascular space or into the parent vessel. Timely recognition requires vigilant awareness of the location of the coils and conceptualization of the three-dimensional anatomy of the lesion, parent vessel, and coil mass. For thromboembolic events, such recognition involves inspecting the distal vasculature and paying attention to alterations in stent and parent vessel diameter. In addition to operative and angiographic findings, clinical and neurophysiologic monitoring data can help identify complications. Obtaining these data requires good communication with the anesthesiologist and close monitoring of vital signs, intracranial pressure, and external ventricular drain output. Neurophysiologic monitoring of changes in regional cerebral blood flow during endovascular treatment is also proving useful, particularly when neurologic examination is not possible (e.g., the patient is under general anesthesia or obtunded).[32]

Intraoperative Techniques

After a complication has been identified, its successful resolution depends largely on the familiarity of the surgeon with salvage and adjuvant techniques for complication management. Some of the intraoperative techniques that all endovascular surgeons should know include balloon deployment, stent deployment, use of thrombolytic agents, snare and coil retrieval techniques, and treatment strategies for recurrent or residual aneurysms.

Intraprocedural Rupture

The microcatheter, guidewire, and coils can all be sources of potential aneurysm wall perforation.[21] Therefore, one should minimize guidewire and microcatheter contact with the aneurysm wall. When an intraprocedural rupture occurs, immediate recognition and action are required. Heparinization should be emergently reversed using protamine. If the now-ruptured or reruptured dome can be secured by quickly completing the coiling, doing so should result in aneurysm obliteration and prevention of further SAH. Temporary intraluminal balloon vessel occlusion may also limit arterial hemorrhage from the ruptured dome and facilitate rapid coiling. The use of a balloon occlusion catheter in patients who experience intraprocedural rupture may improve outcomes.[33] If a ruptured aneurysm cannot be adequately coiled, emergent surgical clipping or parent vessel sacrifice should be considered. Throughout this scenario, good communication with the anesthesiologist and other team members is essential.

Thrombolysis of Intraprocedural Thrombus

Thromboembolic events can occur distally as embolic occlusions of smaller-caliber arteries or arterioles, focally at the parent vessel–aneurysm interface, or within the deployed stent or flow diverter. Immediate recognition of thromboembolic events is critical.

In patients with unruptured aneurysms, immediate thrombolysis should be performed when a clot is identified. Thrombolysis is typically performed with the use of focal intra-arterial infusion of a glycoprotein IIb (GpIIb)/IIIa inhibitor, such as abciximab or tirofiban.[34] In their 2015 meta-analysis, Brinjikji et al.[34] found GpIIb/IIIa inhibitors to be superior to fibrinolytics. In a 2017 case review and meta-analysis, Kansagra et al.[35] demonstrated the superiority of intra-arterial versus intravenous abciximab for thrombolysis during endovascular coiling. Although the use of abciximab for thrombolysis in patients with unruptured aneurysms is relatively safe, intracranial hemorrhages may follow such treatment.[34]

In patients with ruptured aneurysms, thrombolysis can result in aneurysm rerupture.[36] This risk appears to be decreased by securing the aneurysm before administration of a GpIIb/IIIa inhibitor.[37] If a thrombus is identified before the aneurysm is obliterated, the decision about how to proceed must be decided on a case-by-case basis: (1) complete the coiling and then address the thrombus; (2) treat the thrombus and then resume coiling; or (3) treat the thrombus only.

As an adjunct to medical management, a clot-retrieval device can be used in patients with large thrombi. Although many surgeons advocate for postprocedural antiplatelet or anticoagulation treatment in patients who have experienced a thromboembolic event, these regimens are not standardized across institutions.

Coil Migration and Prolapse Into Parent Vessel

Prolapsed and migrated coils can result in parent vessel stenosis, can disrupt laminar flow, or can become a source for thrombus formation. If coil prolapse is noted after detachment of the coil, inflating a balloon or deploying a stent across the neck of the aneurysm may allow the coil to be pushed back into and secured within the aneurysm. These strategies may also permit the deployment of additional securing coils or stent placement to provide a permanent barrier across the neck.[38] Alternatively, coil removal can be attempted with a retrieval device.[11] If the prolapsed coil cannot be safely reinserted into the aneurysm or removed, and it continues to protrude into the lumen of the parent vessel, initiation of antiplatelet therapy should be considered to decrease the risk of thromboembolic events.

Coil unraveling and migration are estimated to occur in 2% to 6% of cases.[12] Retrieval of migrated and unraveled coils can be difficult and hazardous. As with any complication, immediate recognition is paramount. Various techniques have been used for retrieval of migrated and unraveled coils, including the use of retrieval devices, stent retrievers, microwires, and snares.[12] One technique involves running the retrieval device over the coil-delivering microcatheter to facilely reach the unraveled portion of the coil for safe removal.[11] Prompt retrieval of unraveling coils is critical before breakage occurs, because broken coil pieces may be carried into distal cerebral or systemic blood vessels.

Treatment of Recurrent Aneurysm

Aneurysm recurrence after coiling is increasingly recognized as a potential delayed complication of endovascular intervention.[2,14] Recurrent and residual ruptured aneurysms carry an increased risk of rerupture and therefore often warrant additional intervention.[39] The optimal treatment strategy for a recurrent aneurysm must be determined individually, and both open and endovascular options should be considered. In general, for recurrent aneurysms, better rates of obliteration can be achieved with SAC and flow diverters than with primary coiling alone.[40]

SURGICAL REWIND

My Worst Case

An 83-year-old woman was diagnosed with an unruptured right superior hypophyseal artery aneurysm during a workup for a transient ischemic attack. Her anxiety about her aneurysm interfered with her daily activities, and she adamantly requested treatment. She was taken to the angiography suite with plans for possible BAC. A diagnostic angiogram was performed with the patient under general anesthesia with systemic heparinization via transfemoral access with a 6 French short sheath. The angiogram demonstrated a right superior hypophyseal artery aneurysm with dysplastic features and several daughter sacs (Fig. 40.2A).

In light of the identified high-risk features of the aneurysm, a decision was made to proceed with BAC. A Benchmark-95 catheter (Penumbra, Inc., Alameda, CA) was positioned in the right internal carotid artery. A HyperGlide balloon (Medtronic, plc, Dublin, Ireland) was placed across the neck of the aneurysm. The aneurysm was catheterized with an Excelsior SL-10 microcatheter and a Synchro2 microwire (both Stryker Corp., Kalamazoo, MI) without issue, and the balloon was inflated. We next attempted to place a framing coil (Target 360 Soft, 5×20; Stryker Corp.), but the dome of the aneurysm ruptured, and active extravasation and coil herniation were noted. Protamine was emergently administered for reversal of heparinization, and systolic blood pressure was kept below 100 mm Hg. The balloon remained inflated, and the aneurysm was quickly coiled with 12 additional coils of various types. During coiling, additional coil herniations and active extravasation were observed (Fig. 40.2B and 40.2C). After coiling, the aneurysm was angiographically obliterated, and no further extravasation was identified (Fig. 40.2D). However, a parent thrombus was noted without any distal vessel flow alteration (Fig. 40.2E). Because of the proximity of the thrombus to the rupture site and its non–flow-limiting nature, and because of the potential risk for rerupture with thrombolysis, we opted to observe the thrombus. CT demonstrated significant SAH and hydrocephalus (Fig. 40.2F). An external ventricular drain was emergently placed. Repeat angiograms demonstrated stable appearance of the coiled aneurysm, parent vessel thrombus, and distal vasculature. We again opted not to attempt thrombolysis because of the risk of rerupture or embolic shower. Unfortunately, the patient never recovered from this devastating complication and died on post-angiogram day 5.

Continued

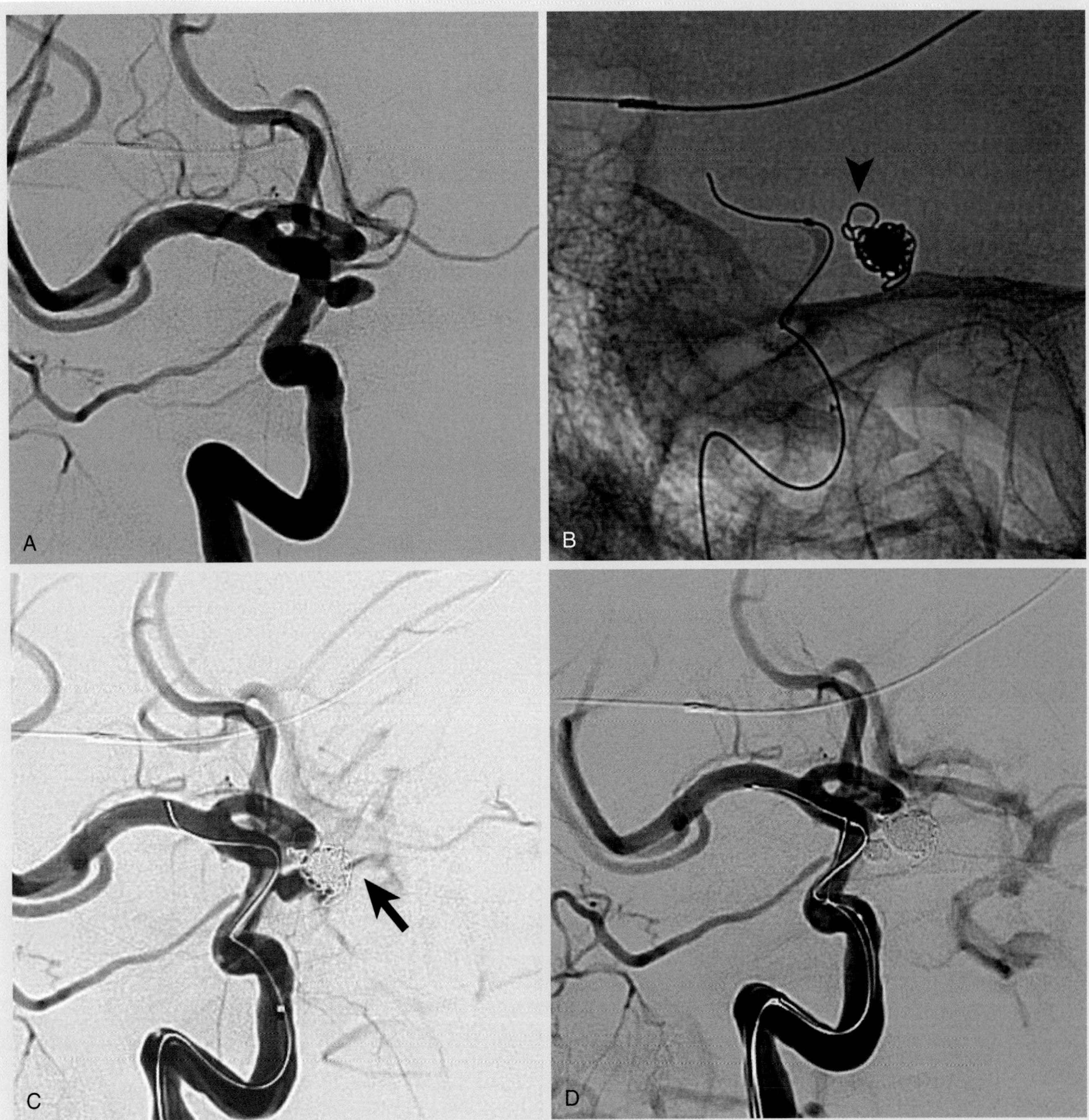

• **Fig. 40.2** (A) Working-angle view of a right superior hypophyseal artery aneurysm with dysplastic features and several daughter sacs. (B and C) Angiographic evidence of intraprocedural rupture with coil herniation (B, arrowhead) and active contrast extravasation (C, arrow). (D) Angiographic obliteration of the aneurysm after multiple rounds of additional coil deployment.

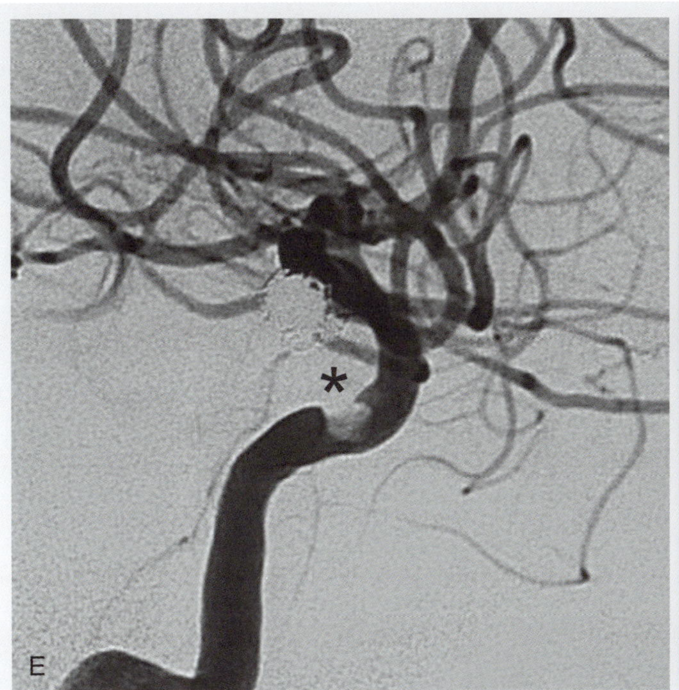

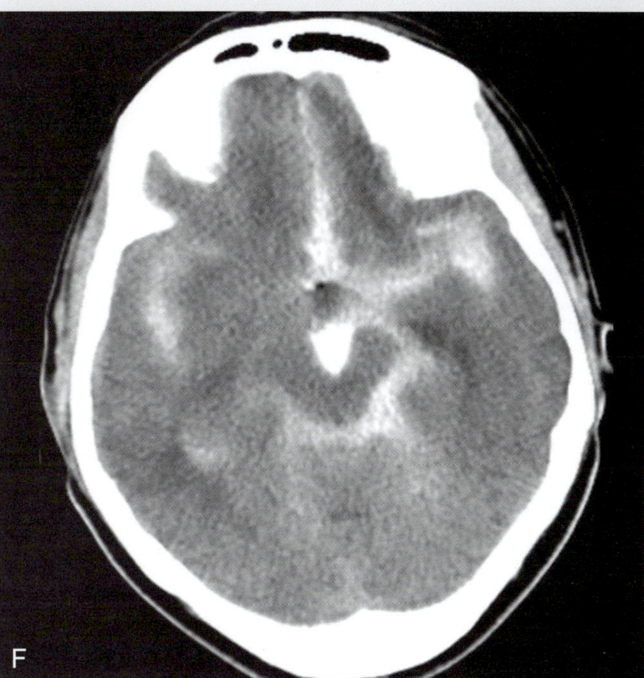

• **Fig. 40.2, cont'd** (E) Identification of proximal parent vessel thrombus (*) without distal flow alteration. (F) Intraprocedural three-dimensional rotational computed tomogram demonstrating diffuse subarachnoid hemorrhage. (Used with permission from Barrow Neurological Institute, Phoenix, Arizona.)

NEUROSURGICAL SELFIE MOMENT

Endovascular techniques are evolving and being applied to increasingly more complex aneurysms. As their use increases, so does the potential for devastating complications. The most common and significant complications of coil embolization of intracranial aneurysm are hemorrhage from intraprocedural rupture or rerupture, ischemia from thromboembolic events, coil migration or prolapse into the parent vessel, and aneurysm recanalization. Certain aneurysm characteristics (e.g., neck size, dome size, aneurysm location, parent vessel angle, rupture status) correlate with rates of procedural complications. The most effective management strategy for potentially catastrophic complications is prevention. When complications occur, their immediate recognition and one's familiarity with salvage techniques aid improved patient outcomes.

References

1. Rinkel GJ, Djibuti M, Algra A, van Gijn J. Prevalence and risk of rupture of intracranial aneurysms: a systematic review. *Stroke.* 1998;29(1):251–256.
2. Spetzler RF, McDougall CG, Zabramski JM, et al. The Barrow Ruptured Aneurysm Trial: 6-year results. *J Neurosurg.* 2015;123(3):609–617.
3. Phan K, Huo YR, Jia F, et al. Meta-analysis of stent-assisted coiling versus coiling-only for the treatment of intracranial aneurysms. *J Clin Neurosci.* 2016;31:15–22.
4. Pierot L, Spelle L, Vitry F, ATENA Investigators. Immediate clinical outcome of patients harboring unruptured intracranial aneurysms treated by endovascular approach: results of the ATENA study. *Stroke.* 2008;39(9):2497–2504.
5. Cognard C, Pierot L, Anxionnat R, Ricolfi F, Clarity Study Group. Results of embolization used as the first treatment choice in a consecutive nonselected population of ruptured aneurysms: clinical results of the CLARITY GDC study. *Neurosurgery.* 2011;69(4):837–841, discussion 842.
6. Sluzewski M, van Rooij WJ, Beute GN, Nijssen PC. Balloon-assisted coil embolization of intracranial aneurysms: incidence, complications, and angiography results. *J Neurosurg.* 2006;105(3):396–399.
7. Pierot L, Cognard C, Anxionnat R, Ricolfi F, CLARITY Investigators. Remodeling technique for endovascular treatment of ruptured intracranial aneurysms had a higher rate of adequate postoperative occlusion than did conventional coil embolization with comparable safety. *Radiology.* 2011;258(2):546–553.
8. Hetts SW, Turk A, English JD, et al. Stent-assisted coiling versus coiling alone in unruptured intracranial aneurysms in the Matrix and Platinum Science Trial: safety, efficacy, and mid-term outcomes. *AJNR Am J Neuroradiol.* 2014;35(4):698–705.
9. Nishido H, Piotin M, Bartolini B, Pistocchi S, Redjem H, Blanc R. Analysis of complications and recurrences of aneurysm coiling with special emphasis on the stent-assisted technique. *AJNR Am J Neuroradiol.* 2014;35(2):339–344.
10. Kang DH, Kim BM, Kim DJ, et al. MR-DWI–positive lesions and symptomatic ischemic complications after coiling of unruptured intracranial aneurysms. *Stroke.* 2013;44(3):789–791.
11. Fiorella D, Albuquerque FC, Deshmukh VR, McDougall CG. Monorail snare technique for the recovery of stretched platinum coils: technical case report. *Neurosurgery.* 2005;57(1 suppl):E210, discussion E210.
12. Ding D, Liu KC. Management strategies for intraprocedural coil migration during endovascular treatment of intracranial aneurysms. *J Neurointerv Surg.* 2014;6(6):428–431.
13. Ferns SP, Sprengers ME, van Rooij WJ, et al. Coiling of intracranial aneurysms: a systematic review on initial occlusion and reopening and retreatment rates. *Stroke.* 2009;40(8):e523–e529.
14. Benaissa A, Barbe C, Pierot L. Analysis of recanalization after endovascular treatment of intracranial aneurysm (ARETA trial): presentation of a prospective multicenter study. *J Neuroradiol.* 2015;42(2):80–85.

15. van Rooij WJ, Sluzewski M, Beute GN, Nijssen PC. Procedural complications of coiling of ruptured intracranial aneurysms: incidence and risk factors in a consecutive series of 681 patients. *AJNR Am J Neuroradiol.* 2006;27(7):1498–1501.
16. Pierot L, Cognard C, Anxionnat R, Ricolfi F. Ruptured intracranial aneurysms: factors affecting the rate and outcome of endovascular treatment complications in a series of 782 patients (CLARITY study). *Radiology.* 2010;256(3):916–923.
17. Fan L, Lin B, Xu T, et al. Predicting intraprocedural rupture and thrombus formation during coiling of ruptured anterior communicating artery aneurysms. *J Neurointerv Surg.* 2017;9(4):370–375.
18. Brinjikji W, Cloft HJ, Kallmes DF. Difficult aneurysms for endovascular treatment: overwide or undertall? *AJNR Am J Neuroradiol.* 2009;30(8):1513–1517.
19. Nguyen TN, Hoh BL, Amin-Hanjani S, Pryor JC, Ogilvy CS. Comparison of ruptured vs unruptured aneurysms in recanalization after coil embolization. *Surg Neurol.* 2007;68(1):19–23.
20. Mocco J, Snyder KV, Albuquerque FC, et al. Treatment of intracranial aneurysms with the Enterprise stent: a multicenter registry. *J Neurosurg.* 2009;110(1):35–39.
21. Cloft HJ, Kallmes DF. Cerebral aneurysm perforations complicating therapy with Guglielmi detachable coils: a meta-analysis. *AJNR Am J Neuroradiol.* 2002;23(10):1706–1709.
22. Ishibashi T, Murayama Y, Saguchi T, et al. Thromboembolic events during endovascular coil embolization of cerebral aneurysms. *Interv Neuroradiol.* 2006;12(suppl 1):112–116.
23. Park HK, Horowitz M, Jungreis C, et al. Periprocedural morbidity and mortality associated with endovascular treatment of intracranial aneurysms. *AJNR Am J Neuroradiol.* 2005;26(3):506–514.
24. Connolly ES Jr, Rabinstein AA, Carhuapoma JR, et al. Guidelines for the management of aneurysmal subarachnoid hemorrhage: a guideline for healthcare professionals from the American Heart Association/American Stroke Association. *Stroke.* 2012;43(6):1711–1737.
25. McNeill L, English SW, Borg N, Matta BF, Menon DK. Effects of institutional caseload of subarachnoid hemorrhage on mortality: a secondary analysis of administrative data. *Stroke.* 2013;44(3):647–652.
26. Stiefel MF, Park MS, McDougall CG, Albuquerque FC. Endovascular treatment of unruptured intracranial aneurysms in the elderly: analysis of procedure related complications. *J Neurointerv Surg.* 2010;2(1):11–15.
27. Sturiale CL, Brinjikji W, Murad MH, Lanzino G. Endovascular treatment of intracranial aneurysms in elderly patients: a systematic review and meta-analysis. *Stroke.* 2013;44(7):1897–1902.
28. Hwang G, Jung C, Park SQ, et al. Thromboembolic complications of elective coil embolization of unruptured aneurysms: the effect of oral antiplatelet preparation on periprocedural thromboembolic complication. *Neurosurgery.* 2010;67(3):743–748, discussion 748.
29. Levitt MR, Moon K, Albuquerque FC, Mulholland CB, Kalani MY, McDougall CG. Intraprocedural abciximab bolus versus pretreatment oral dual antiplatelet medication for endovascular stenting of unruptured intracranial aneurysms. *J Neurointerv Surg.* 2016;8(9):909–912.
30. Yang H, Sun Y, Jiang Y, et al. Comparison of stent-assisted coiling vs coiling alone in 563 intracranial aneurysms: safety and efficacy at a high-volume center. *Neurosurgery.* 2015;77(2):241–247, discussion 247.
31. Shapiro M, Becske T, Sahlein D, Babb J, Nelson PK. Stent-supported aneurysm coiling: a literature survey of treatment and follow-up. *AJNR Am J Neuroradiol.* 2012;33(1):159–163.
32. Chen L, Spetzler RF, McDougall CG, Albuquerque FC, Xu B. Detection of ischemia in endovascular therapy of cerebral aneurysms: a perspective in the era of neurophysiological monitoring. *Neurosurg Rev.* 2011;34(1):69–75.
33. Santillan A, Gobin YP, Greenberg ED, et al. Intraprocedural aneurysmal rupture during coil embolization of brain aneurysms: role of balloon-assisted coiling. *AJNR Am J Neuroradiol.* 2012;33(10):2017–2021.
34. Brinjikji W, Morales-Valero SF, Murad MH, Cloft HJ, Kallmes DF. Rescue treatment of thromboembolic complications during endovascular treatment of cerebral aneurysms: a meta-analysis. *AJNR Am J Neuroradiol.* 2015;36(1):121–125.
35. Kansagra AP, McEachern JD, Madaelil TP, et al. Intra-arterial versus intravenous abciximab therapy for thromboembolic complications of neuroendovascular procedures: case review and meta-analysis. *J Neurointerv Surg.* 2017;9(2):131–136.
36. Park JH, Kim JE, Sheen SH, et al. Intraarterial abciximab for treatment of thromboembolism during coil embolization of intracranial aneurysms: outcome and fatal hemorrhagic complications. *J Neurosurg.* 2008;108(3):450–457.
37. Gentric JC, Brisson J, Batista AL, et al. Safety of abciximab injection during endovascular treatment of ruptured aneurysms. *Interv Neuroradiol.* 2015;21(3):332–336.
38. Lavine SD, Larsen DW, Giannotta SL, Teitelbaum GP. Parent vessel Guglielmi detachable coil herniation during wide-necked aneurysm embolization: treatment with intracranial stent placement: two technical case reports. *Neurosurgery.* 2000;46(4):1013–1017.
39. Johnston SC, Dowd CF, Higashida RT, et al. Predictors of rehemorrhage after treatment of ruptured intracranial aneurysms: the Cerebral Aneurysm Rerupture After Treatment (CARAT) study. *Stroke.* 2008;39(1):120–125.
40. Mascitelli JR, Oermann EK, Mocco J, et al. Predictors of success following endovascular retreatment of intracranial aneurysms. *Interv Neuroradiol.* 2015;21(4):426–432.

41 Procedure-Related Complications: AVMs

BRIAN M. CORLISS, BRIAN L. HOH

HIGHLIGHTS

- Endovascular therapy for brain arteriovenous malformations is one piece of a multidisciplinary therapeutic approach.
- Neurologic complications from AVM embolization are often devastating and only occasionally can be managed endovascularly.
- Complication management must be focused on prevention.

Background

Cerebral arteriovenous malformations (AVMs) are rare lesions that are best addressed using a combination of complementary technologies and medical subspecialists, including neurosurgeons, neurologists, radiologists, and radiation therapy specialists, such as radiation oncologists or surgeons with specialized training in stereotactic radiosurgery. These lesions harbor a significant risk of rupture—in general, about 2% to 3% per year—with high rates of resultant neurologic disability or death.[1,2] The ARUBA (A Randomized Trial of Unruptured Brain Arteriovenous Malformation) study raised important questions about the safety and necessity of therapies undertaken to prevent morbidity and mortality associated with these lesions.[3] Endovascular approaches have evolved over several decades and now represent powerful adjunctive therapies aiding in the surgical treatment of AVMs; in some cases, endovascular therapies can serve as stand-alone cures.[4–13]

Many specialized catheters and embolization agents have been developed since the inception of endovascular AVM embolization, but the most frequently encountered complications remain the same. The most common complication resulting from AVM embolization is hemorrhage—either from inadvertent vessel perforation, venous hypertension after venous outflow occlusion, or normal perfusion pressure breakthrough after extensive or complete embolizations.[11,12,14] Ischemic complications are similarly common, resulting from either reflux into or direct embolization of vessels supplying normal brain tissue.[15] Complications directly attributable to catheter technologies and malfunctions are also more commonly seen as endovascular interventions gain widespread implementation. In this chapter, we will review the sources of these complications and discuss strategies for their avoidance.

Anatomic Considerations

Cerebral AVMs are an anatomically diverse group of lesions. In general, a brain AVM consists of one or more feeding arteries that drain directly into one or more draining veins without any intervening capillary bed (Fig. 41.1). Unlike most arteriovenous fistulae, in an AVM there is a complex nidus of small arteries and arterialized veins at the site of the arteriovenous communication. There may be varying amounts of brain matter insinuated between vessels within the nidus, but this brain is invariably gliotic due to vascular steal away from normal capillary beds. There may be loss of cerebral vascular autoregulation globally in the affected brain region, which predisposes to hemorrhagic complications and edema after treatment, as we will discuss later.[16]

In terms of natural history risk of hemorrhage, it appears that deep venous drainage pattern increases the 5-year risk of rupture for all-comers with the diagnosis of brain AVM from 21% to 34% and increases the 20-year risk from 39% to 52%.[1] Size >5 cm increases the 20-year risk of rupture to 52% as well. Other anatomic considerations that impact the risk associated with brain AVM include the presence of prenidal or intranidal aneurysms, infratentorial location, and previous rupture.[1,17]

The most commonly used classification schema for characterizing the surgical risk of AVMs is the Spetzler-Martin (SM) grading scale.[18] This scale assigns points on the basis of AVM nidus diameter (1 point for <3 cm, 2 points for 3–6 cm, and 3 points for >6 cm), eloquence of the brain surrounding the lesion (0 points for noneloquent, 1 point for eloquent), and pattern of venous drainage (0 points for cortical/superficial, 1 point for deep venous drainage). Spetzler's own case series, presented with the description of his eponymous classification system, demonstrated dramatically increased surgical morbidity and mortality when attempting to surgically excise high-grade brain AVMs.[18,19] Unfortunately, SM grade, although an established predictor of surgical risk, fails to predict the likelihood of complications related to endovascular embolization.[8,15]

Alternative grading scales have been developed to attempt to quantify the risks undertaken during endovascular embolization of AVMs. In 2010, the AVM neurovascular grade was developed from a review of the literature on embolization-related complications using either Onyx or n-butyl cyanoacrylate glue.[20] This schema scores an AVM on the number of feeding vessels (1 point for <3, 2 points for 3–6, and 3 points for >6), the eloquence of the surrounding brain (similar to SM system), and the presence of an arteriovenous fistula (0 points if absent, 1 point if present). Fistulae can be defined according to the criteria of Yuki et al.[21] as the direct communication of a feeding artery to draining vein without intervening nidus, or as abnormal dilatation to twofold or greater

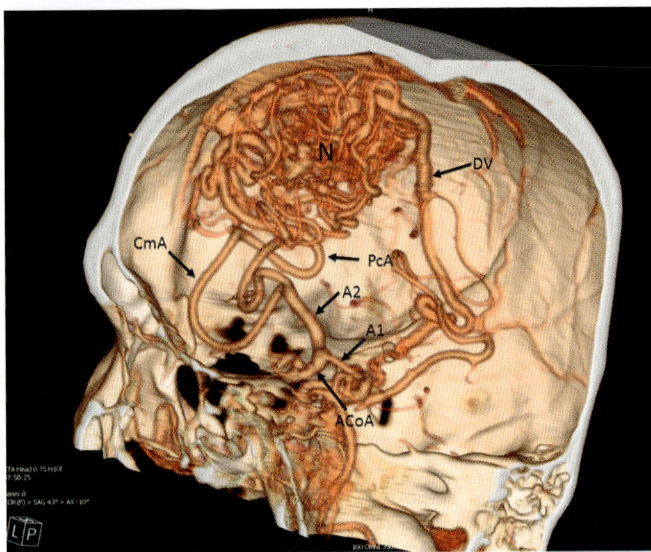

• **Fig. 41.1** Anatomy of a Spetzler-Martin grade 2 arteriovenous malformation of the right frontal lobe fed by branches of the left anterior cerebral artery (ACA), draining via an enlarged cortical vein. Note the enlarged ACA branches feeding the nidus, consistent with a fistula according to the criteria of Yuki. *A1,* First segment, right anterior cerebral artery; *A2,* second segment, right anterior cerebral artery; *ACoA,* anterior communicating artery; *CmA,* callosomarginal artery; *DV,* draining vein; *N,* nidus; *PcA,* pericallosal artery.

enlargement of the feeding artery compared with a comparable vessel (e.g., in the same territory as the feeding vessel, or compared with the contralateral side). A retrospective validation study[5] of 127 patients demonstrated good interrater reliability and significant differences in scores for patients who were cured with endovascular techniques (median score = 2), patients who required multimodal therapy (median score = 3), and patients who suffered complications attributed to embolization (median score = 4).

In 2015, the Buffalo score was described.[22] This score is determined by the number of arterial pedicles feeding the AVM (1 point for 1 or 2, 2 points for 3 or 4, and 3 points for 5 or more), the diameter of the arterial pedicles (0 points for most >1 mm, 1 point for most <1 mm), and the nidus location (similar to the SM system). In their initial retrospective application of this scale to 50 patients, the Buffalo group demonstrated correlation between their score and complication risk, with >50% risk of complications after embolization for patients with scores of 4 or 5. More recently, however, neither the SM scale, nor the AVM neurovascular grade, nor the Buffalo score was seen to be predictive of complications when retrospectively applied to a group of patients undergoing 55 embolization procedures.[8] The small sample size and low numbers of grade 4 (<10%) or 5 (0%) lesions contribute to this result, however.

RED FLAGS

- Many small feeder vessels
- Close proximity of nidus to circle of Willis
- Deep venous drainage through single draining vein
- Marked hypertrophy of feeding artery
- Significant perilesional edema or gliosis
- Prenidal aneurysms

AVM Hemorrhage and Hemorrhagic Complications

Hemorrhage continues to be the primary mode of symptom presentation in surgical series of patients with previously undiagnosed AVM,[4,7,11,17,23] although increasingly, unruptured AVMs are being identified incidentally due to high sensitivity and availability of modern noninvasive imaging modalities. Hemorrhage is also the most common and most devastating complication after endovascular embolization. Hemorrhagic complications can generally be thought of in two categories: those resulting from technical issues, such as vessel perforation or rupture, or those that occur spontaneously and are unrelated to inadvertent vessel rupture. We will discuss these categories separately.

Spontaneous Postembolization Hemorrhage

Spontaneous postembolization hemorrhage is among the most vexing and devastating complications of AVM embolization. There are multiple theories of spontaneous AVM hemorrhage before treatment, and it is believed that these factors contribute to hemorrhage after embolization as well, usually due to changes in transmural vessel pressures or blood flow patterns. The most important concept to be discussed in this regard is that of normal perfusion pressure breakthrough.[16,18]

The normal perfusion pressure breakthrough hypothesis was posited in 1978 by Spetzler as a mechanism to explain postoperative hemorrhage seen in the brain after complete excision of a high-flow AVM. In normal brain parenchyma, perfusion pressures are maintained within a narrow window by vessel caliber regulation through means that are both extrinsic and intrinsic to the vessels themselves. Cerebral capillary perfusion pressures can be regulated over a wide range of arterial blood pressures as a result. Although extrinsic sympathetic regulation of vascular tone does play a role in the central nervous system, it is primarily through intrinsic smooth muscle autoregulation that capillary perfusion is maintained. Importantly, arterioles appear to have a greater ability to dilate in response to hypotension than they do to constrict in response to hypertension.

In the brain of a patient harboring an AVM, there is an area of low vascular resistance due to the loss of the capillary bed and enlargement of feeding arterial and draining venous calibers. Parallel vascular beds are therefore subjected to relative hypotension with respect to perfusion pressures. The AVM essentially presents a short circuit through which blood will preferentially flow. As a result, vessels irrigating normal brain near the AVM will become chronically dilated in a constant effort to maintain flow to these relatively ischemic regions of the brain. These vessels may either lose their autoregulation abilities, or their autoregulatory set points may be dramatically shifted to remain dilated even in the face of relatively high capillary perfusion pressures. Chronically low tissue oxygen tension may also result in effusive neovascularization with frail, "leaky" capillaries.

The result of these phenomena is a vascular system in which feeding arteries are chronically dilated with reduced capacity to respond appropriately to changes in perfusion pressure heads, and with downstream capillary beds that are prone to rupture. Embolization of an AVM results in decreased flow across the fistula and a compensatory increase in flow through these fragile systems. It would be expected, therefore, that postembolization hemorrhage would be common—and it is.

Several recent studies have evaluated hemorrhage risk after endovascular embolization. Asadi et al.[4] reported post- or intraprocedural hemorrhages in 57 of 199 patients (29%) treated with endovascular embolization, 47% of which occurred spontaneously at a site remote from the embolization after uncomplicated completion of the embolization procedure. This hemorrhage rate is relatively high compared with other series, probably because the majority of patients in this series presented with hemorrhage from the AVM; in addition, almost all patients underwent multiple embolizations (i.e., the risk of complications from an individual embolization procedure is a fraction of these numbers), and an aggressive strategy of endovascular therapy was pursued, with 45% of patients achieving cure of the AVM without supplemental radiosurgery or open microsurgical resection.

Baharvahdat et al.[23] reported post- or intraprocedural hemorrhages after endovascular embolization—again with the goal of complete obliteration of the lesion—in 92 of 408 patients (23% of patients, 11% of embolization procedures). Fifty-two percent of these complications were felt to be related to spontaneous hemorrhage unrelated to inadvertent vessel rupture or perforation during the procedure. Eighty-one percent of these occurred just hours or days after the procedure was complete, with a mean of 34 hours postprocedure. Once again, this study is remarkable for the fact that endovascular embolization was utilized as the sole therapeutic modality in 91% of cases. Spontaneous hemorrhages resulted in 37 patients suffering an acquired neurologic deficit, 58% of which resulted in permanent disability and 10% in death. Types of hemorrhages encountered included intracerebral, intraventricular, and subarachnoid hemorrhage; 71% of spontaneous hemorrhages were intraparenchymal. Importantly, the authors of this study identified premature embolization of the draining vein as a contributing factor in delayed hemorrhage, with 17% of hemorrhages occurring in this context, although other authors have reported successful transvenous embolization strategies in small patient samples.[9]

In neurosurgical series using embolization as an adjunctive therapeutic modality followed by either microsurgical resection or stereotactic radiosurgery, hemorrhagic complications appear to be less common. Crowley et al.[7] reported permanent neurologic morbidity from all causes in 9.6% of patients with only 1 death out of 327 patients treated. Six of 153 patients (4%) suffered unexpected postprocedural neurologic deficits secondary to hemorrhagic complications in an earlier, smaller series published by the same group.[15] Only 13% and 2.3% of procedures in the smaller and larger series, respectively, were curative, whereas 70% and 79%, respectively, were performed before microsurgical resection of the lesion, thus highlighting differences in treatment strategies employed around the world and by different subspecialists. One should bear this in mind when comparing studies, because the surgical complications after craniotomy may not be included in the reported data. In an older surgical series, Taylor et al.[14] reported permanent neurologic deficits after embolization in 18 of 201 patients (9%) and death in 4 patients (2%). Again, in this series embolization was used primarily as an adjunct to surgical resection.

In summary, periprocedural intracerebral hemorrhage after endovascular embolization of is most common in patients in whom: (1) complete embolization of the lesion is attempted in one session, (2) when embolic material enters the draining veins during subtotal embolization, and (3) when high-risk features (e.g., intranidal aneurysms) are left untreated.[24] Hemorrhage in these situations is caused either by worsening of venous or intraaneurysmal hypertension or by normal perfusion pressure breakthrough. Avoidance of hemorrhage may therefore be accomplished by staging attempts at embolization, targeting high-risk features of the lesion early in treatment, and maintaining strict blood pressure control after embolization. The risks of hemorrhage from attempted endovascular cure of the AVM should be weighed against the risks of microsurgical resection, which are patient- specific but may be accurately predicted by the SM grading scheme.

At our institution, all cerebral AVMs are treated by neurosurgeons with training in both open surgical and endovascular treatment modalities, and with access to state-of-the-art radiosurgical therapy. Embolizations are generally staged with no more than 30% to 50% of the lesion embolized in a single session, except in very small lesions fed by a single artery, when cure may be achieved in a single sitting and partial embolization is not possible. Postoperatively, systolic blood pressures are controlled to <120 mm Hg, frequently requiring intravenous infusions of nicardipine. Labetalol is a second-line agent that is also used as a continuous infusion or, more commonly, on an as-needed basis for breakthrough hypertension. Postembolization, all patients are monitored in the neurosurgical intensive care unit at least overnight. Neurologic deterioration from delayed postembolization hemorrhage generally prompts immediate evacuation of the hematoma and resection of the AVM.

Iatrogenic Complications

Iatrogenic complications resulting from the endovascular treatment of AVMs include those common to all endovascular procedures, including access vessel injury and vessel dissection, as well as complications related to microcatheterization and embolization that are specific to AVM therapy. Later we will consider those unique to AVM therapy.

Iatrogenic Hemorrhage

As discussed above, some hemorrhages after AVM embolization may be related to factors that are under the control of the treating interventionalist. Specifically, these factors include large (>40%–50%) or complete AVM embolizations undertaken in a single sitting, or embolization of the draining vein(s) during a subtotal embolization. Intraprocedural hemorrhage, however, is usually unintentional and iatrogenic owing to vessel perforation.

The walls of nidal vessels in cerebral AVMs are histopathologically abnormal, which may account for their fragility. This fragility is likely related to increased proportions of collagen type 1 compared with type 3, abnormal polymerization of collagen 1 fibrils, and resultant vessel wall rigidity and relative loss of elasticity.[25] Smooth muscle hypertrophy and mural hyalinization also contribute to vessel stiffness and risk of rupture. During embolization, the treatment microcatheter must be positioned as close to the AVM nidus as possible for embolization of the nidus itself. Vessel walls are increasingly fragile, however, as the nidus is approached, making vessel wall perforation a significant concern. Vessel perforation is not uniformly reported in the literature, but likely occurs in 1% to 5% of cases, many of which result in little or no morbidity.[10–12,26–28] A similar rate is seen in pediatric series.[29,30] Vessel perforation may be increasing in the Onyx era, a phenomenon that may be related to the properties of Onyx-compatible catheters. This is not well established, however.

Avoidance of vessel perforation requires careful microcatheter manipulation, selection of soft microwires, or avoidance of microwire manipulation by utilization of flow-directed catheters. In general, the softest, most steerable wire should be used in conjunction with the most flexible microcatheter that is compatible with the embolic agent being employed. If vessel perforation is encountered in the small feeding arteries near the AVM being treated, vessel sacrifice is often the most expedient solution to halt extravasation with relatively low risk of neurologic deficits induced by cerebral ischemia. Liquid embolic agents have the advantage of being useful for hemorrhage control without necessarily losing the necessary access for embolization of the nidus. If more proximal vessel perforation is encountered, balloon tamponade and reversal of anticoagulation (if administered) may be employed to attempt to preserve parent vessel patency.

Retained Catheters

Embolizations performed using liquid embolic agents/glues carry the risk of unintentional catheter retention. This complication can be seen with Onyx. The incidence of catheter retention after Onyx embolization appears to be on the order of 3% to 5%.[8,31–33]

Management of glued-in catheters frequently involves cutting the retained microcatheter at the point of skin penetration. These catheters may be removed subsequently at the time of surgery if the AVM is ultimately resected.[34] Although retained catheters may eventually become incorporated into the wall of cervicocerebral vessels, thereby limiting the long-term probability of thromboembolic complications,[35] other complications, including access vessel (e.g., femoral) pseudoaneurysm, may result from this practice.[36] Other techniques have been described, including the coaxial placement of a distal access catheter (DAC) over the microcatheter after cutting the hub end off.[33] The DAC may be advanced up to the Onyx plug and used to apply countertraction so that the necessary force can be applied to the microcatheter without avulsing the feeding vascular pedicle when attempting to remove it.

Avoidance of gluing in a catheter can be accomplished by avoiding reflux of the liquid embolic agent, or by avoiding liquid embolic agents altogether. Newer detachable tip catheters have been developed recently that demonstrate efficacy in published studies.[37,38] These catheters have a short tip that can break away (Fig. 41.3) from the main microcatheter shaft if enough tension is applied, thereby allowing for removal of the majority of the catheter if the tip does become glued in place. If a detachable tip catheter is used, the embolic agent should not be allowed to reflux more proximal than the proximal radiopaque tip marker.

Ischemic Complications

All central nervous system embolization procedures harbor a risk of inadvertent embolization of normal tissue, with resultant neurologic deficits that are commensurate with the extent of embolization and the eloquence of the tissue embolized. Microcatheters should be checked for defects before use. Selective microcatheter contrast injection of any target pedicle should be performed before embolization. Given the sensitivity of cerebral microcatheter injection for detection of normal brain perfusion, we do not routinely use neuromonitoring for cerebral AVM embolization, though this has been described.[39] If concerns about the safety of embolization of a particular target exist, strong consideration should be given to open microsurgical obliteration or stereotactic radiosurgery without embolization. When a safe target has been identified, navigation of the microcatheter as close to the nidus as possible, and careful control of reflux of any liquid embolic agents, should prevent inadvertent embolization of normal brain (Fig. 41.4). After an individual pedicle has been embolized, we routinely remove and exchange the microcatheter—and often the guiding catheter—before repeat contrast injections.

Neuromonitoring in the form of motor and somatosensory evoked potentials (MEP/SSEP) may be of use for spinal cord embolizations. Provocative testing using intraarterial administration of 2 to 5 mg of methohexital[40] to anesthetize spinal cord gray matter, followed by up to 40 mg of preservative-free 2% lidocaine[41,42] to anesthetize spinal white matter, can produce detectable changes in monitored potentials if the target pedicle provides blood supply to the spinal cord that is below the visible resolution of the microcatheter injection. If changes are observed in monitored potentials, open surgical ligation of the target fistula may be advisable. It should be noted that methohexital and lidocaine are not compatible drugs and should not be admixed, because this can result in precipitation of the constituent medications. Catheters should be thoroughly flushed between medication doses.

SURGICAL REWIND

My Worst Case

A 59-year-old man was referred for neurosurgical consultation regarding a large right frontal AVM (SM grade 2) discovered incidentally on imaging workup for persistent otitis media (Fig. 41.2). He had no history of seizures or other neurologic complaints, and formal neurologic examination was normal. Given his young age and the AVM size, he was recommended to undergo staged Onyx embolization followed by microsurgical resection on an elective basis. He was admitted and underwent uncomplicated Onyx embolization of about 50% of the AVM on hospital day 0. He underwent stage 2 embolization on hospital day 2. Angiography at the completion of stage 2 of the embolization demonstrated occlusion of about 80% of the AVM. Several hours later, while eating dinner in the recovery room, the patient experienced sudden onset of headache, left hemiplegia, anisocoria, and depressed mental status. He was emergently intubated, and mannitol was bolused IV. A STAT head computed tomography demonstrated a 9.5 × 7-cm right frontal intracerebral hemorrhage. The patient was taken emergently to the operating room for right frontal craniotomy, evacuation of the hematoma, and resection of the AVM. Postoperatively, he was monitored in the neurosurgical intensive care unit, where he ultimately was able to be weaned from the ventilator. He did eventually require a gastrostomy tube, but was discharged to rehab in fair condition with left hemiplegia on hospital day 41. At 3-year follow-up, he was ambulatory with a walker and had residual 4/5 left hemiparesis.

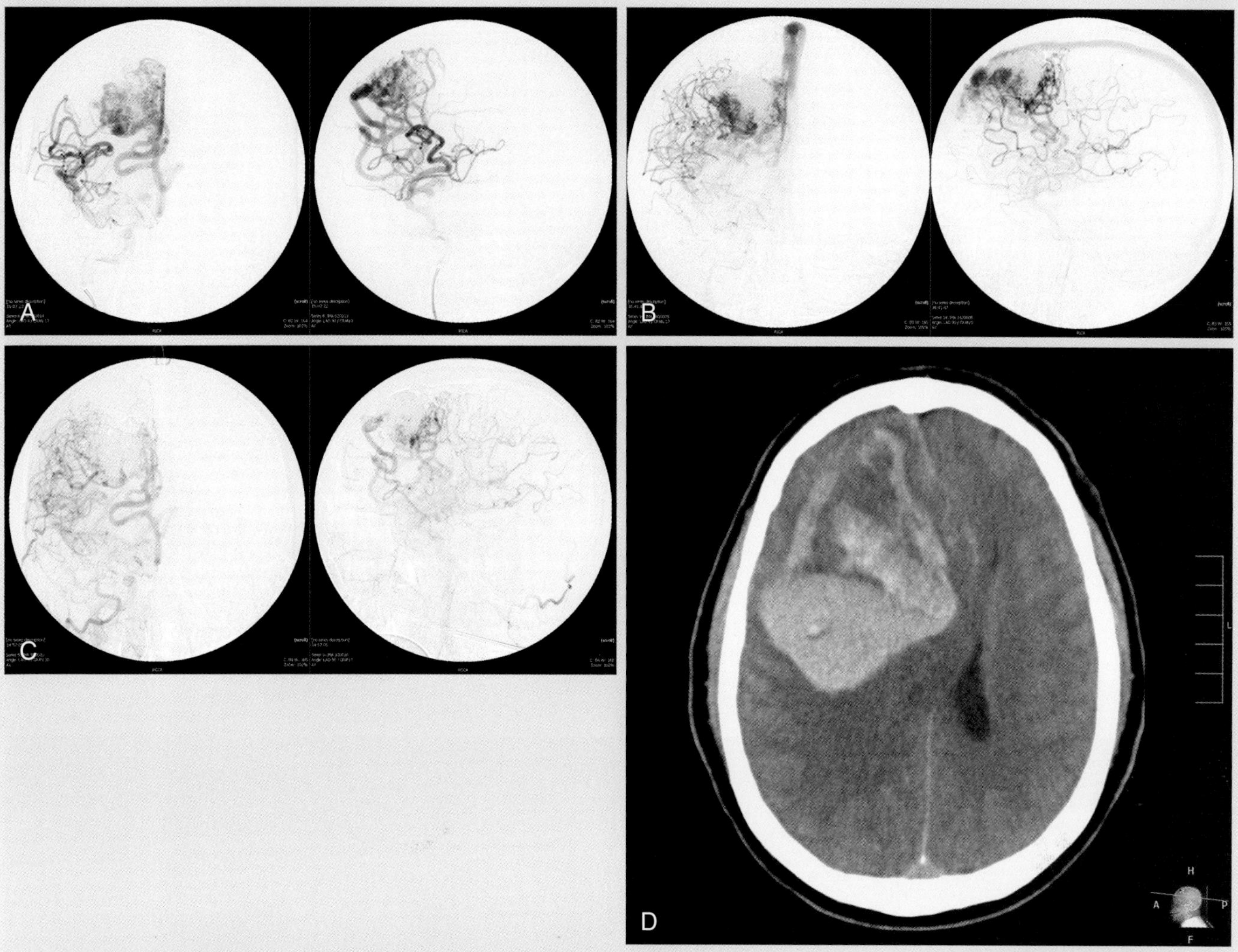

• **Fig. 41.2** 59-year-old male with incidentally discovered right frontal arteriovenous malformation (AVM). Mid-arterial pre-embolization (A) internal carotid artery angiogram demonstrating a 5 cm right frontal arteriovenous malformation with superficial drainage to the superior sagittal sinus fed from right anterior cerebral artery branches. After stage 1 embolization (B), the rate of flow through AVM is reduced and an Onyx cast can be seen occupying approximately 50% of the original nidus volume. After stage 2 embolization (C) 80% of the AVM nidus has been embolized. (D) Postembolization head computed tomography demonstrating large right frontal hemorrhage.

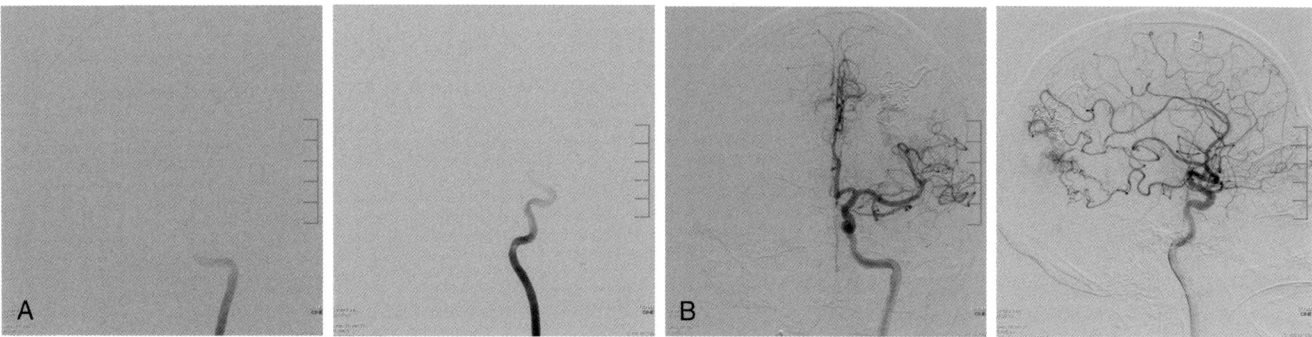

• **Fig. 41.3** 59-year-old man with left parieto-occipital arteriovenous malformation (AVM) presenting with seizures, cognitive dysfunction, and seizures. Staged embolization was planned before surgical resection. Stage 1 embolization was performed with a detachable tip microcatheter. Postembolization early (A) and mid (B) arterial phase internal carotid artery angiograms demonstrated a retained catheter tip within the cavernous left internal carotid segment. The detached tip had either migrated after removal of the microcatheter or sheared off as the microcatheter was withdrawn into the guiding catheter.

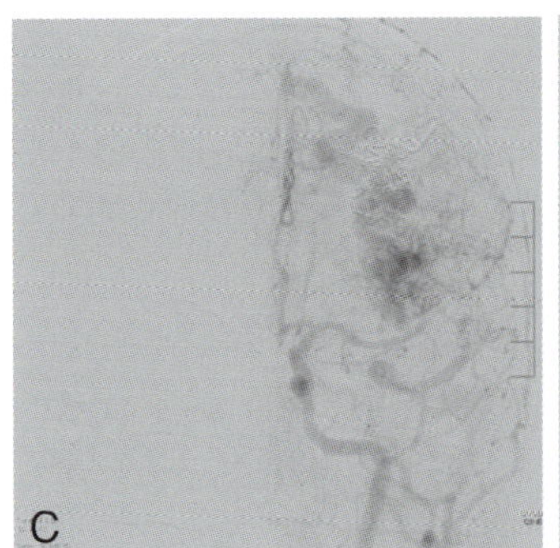
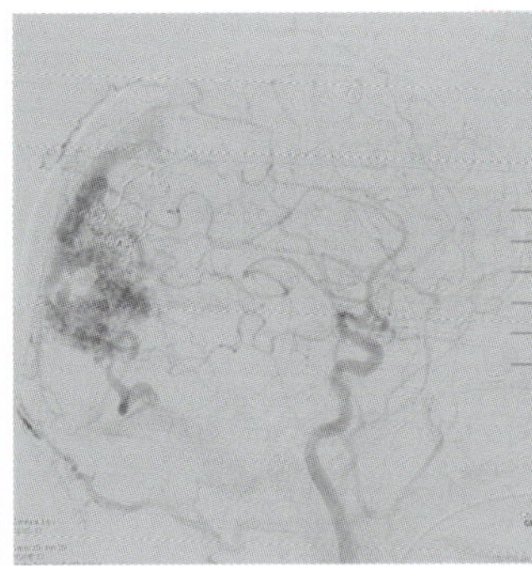
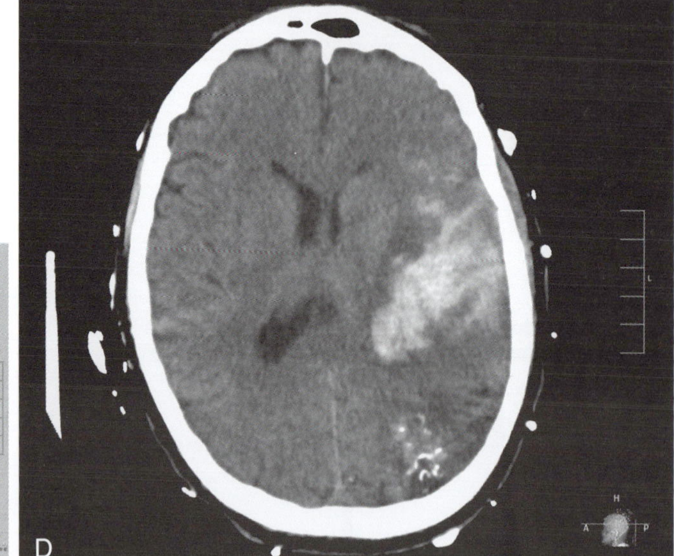

• **Fig. 41.3, cont'd** (C) Mid-arterial common carotid artery angiogram after retrieval of the retained tip using a combination of suction/aspiration and a stent-retriever device. (D) Postembolization computed tomography demonstrating intracerebral and subarachnoid hemorrhage remote from the embolization site. No extravasation was noted during the procedure.

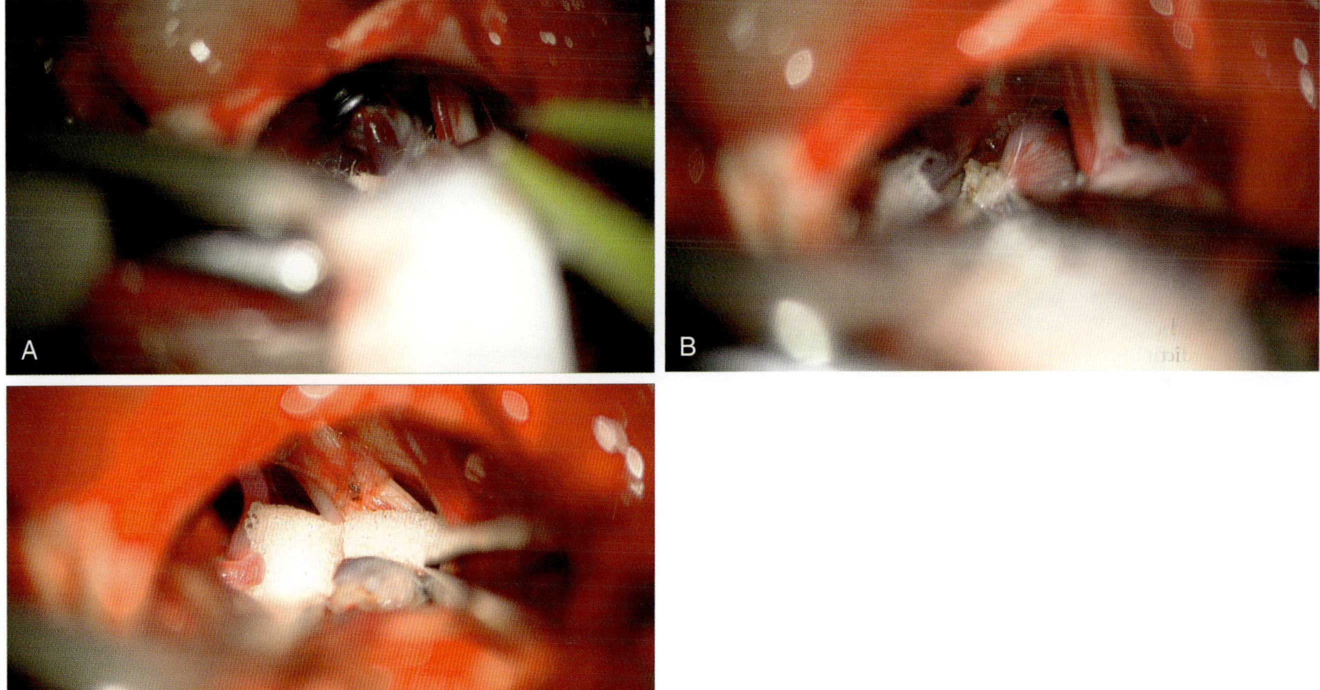

• **Fig. 41.4** 50-year-old man presenting with a posterior fossa Borden type-3 dural arteriovenous fistula presenting with symptoms of trigeminal neuralgia. Embolization of the fistula was planned. First, trans-arterial embolization was attempted without successful obliteration of the fistula. The patient returned for a second attempt at trans-venous embolization. On injection of Onyx, the agent migrated from the fistula into the straight sinus (Videos 41.1 and 41.2). Due to high treatment radiation exposure, further attempts at embolization were abandoned, and the fistula was successfully clip-ligated (A). At the time of surgery, a large venous aneurysm (B) was noted compressing the trigeminal nerve. This was coagulated and the trigeminal nerve was padded with a polyvinyl acetal sponge (C) before closure. His trigeminal neuralgia was completely relieved after surgical decompression.

NEUROSURGICAL SELFIE MOMENT

AVM embolization can be an important adjunct to make AVM surgery safer. Although the anatomy of every AVM is unique, certain high-risk features appear repeatedly; if they are recognized early, strategies can be employed to help prevent complications. Ultimately the risks and utility of AVM therapy must be weighed on a patient-by-patient basis, and the benefit of endovascular embolization should be considered within the fuller context of a multidisciplinary approach to therapy.

References

1. Hernesniemi JA, Dashti R, Juvela S, Vaart K, Niemela M, Laakso A. Natural history of brain arteriovenous malformations: a long-term follow-up study of risk of hemorrhage in 238 patients. *Neurosurgery*. 2008;63(5):823–831.
2. Brown RD, Wiebers DO, Forbes G, et al. The natural history of unruptured intracranial arteriovenous malformations. *J Neurosurg*. 1988;68:352–357.
3. Mohr JP, Parides MK, Stapf C, et al. Medical therapy with or without interventional therapy for unruptured brain arteriovenous malformations (ARUBA): a multicentre, non-blinded, randomised trial. *Lancet*. 2014;383:614–621.
4. Asadi H, Kok HK, Looby S, Brennan P, O'Hare A, Thornton J. Outcomes and complications after endovascular treatment of brain arteriovenous malformations: a prognostication attempt using artificial intelligence. *World Neurosurg*. 2016;96:562–569.
5. Bell DL, Leslie-Mazwi TM, Yoo AJ, et al. Application of a novel brain arteriovenous malformation endovascular grading scale for transarterial embolization. *AJNR Am J Neuroradiol*. 2015;36:1303–1309.
6. Castro-Afonso LH, Nakiri GS, Oliveira RS, et al. Curative embolization of pediatric intracranial arteriovenous malformations using Onyx: the role of new embolization techniques on patient outcomes. *Neuroradiology*. 2016;58:585–594.
7. Crowley RW, Ducruet AF, Kalani YS, Kim LJ, Albuquerque FC, McDougall CG. Neurological morbidity and mortality associated with endovascular treatment of cerebral arteriovenous malformations before and during the Onyx era. *J Neurosurg*. 2015;122:1492–1497.
8. Gupta R, Adeeb N, Moore JM, et al. Validity assessment of grading scales predicting complications from embolization of cerebral arteriovenous malformations. *Clin Neurol Neurosurg*. 2016;151:102–107.
9. Iosif C, Mendes GAC, Saleme S, et al. Endovascular transvenous cure for ruptured brain arteriovenous malformations in complex cases with high Spetzler-Martin grades. *J Neurosurg*. 2015;122:1229–1238.
10. Katsaridis V, Papagiannaki C, Aimar E. Curative embolization of cerebral arteriovenous malformations (AVMs) with Onyx in 101 patients. *Neuroradiology*. 2008;50:589–597.
11. Pierot L, Cognard C, Herbreteau D, et al. Endovascular treatment of brain arteriovenous malformations using a liquid embolic agent: results of a prospective, multicentre study (BRAVO). *Eur Radiol*. 2013;23:2838–2845.
12. Strauss I, Frolov V, Buchbut D, Gonen L, Maimon S. Critical appraisal of endovascular treatment of brain arteriovenous malformations using Onyx in a series of 92 consecutive patients. *Acta Neurochir*. 2013;155:611–617.
13. Yu SCH, Chan MSY, Lam JMK, Tam PHT, Poon WS. Complete obliteration of intracranial arteriovenous malformation with endovascular cyanoacrylate embolization: initial success and rate of permanent cure. *AJNR Am J Neuroradiol*. 2004;25:1139–1143.
14. Taylor CL, Dutton K, Rappard G, et al. Complications of preoperative embolization of cerebral arteriovenous malformations. *J Neurosurg*. 2004;100:810–812.
15. Kim LJ, Albuquerque FC, Spetzler RF, McDougall CG. Postembolization neurological deficits in cerebral arteriovenous malformations: stratification by arteriovenous malformation grade. *Neurosurgery*. 2006;58(7):53–58.
16. Rangel-Castilla L, Spetzler RF, Nakaji P. Normal perfusion pressure breakthrough theory: a reappraisal after 35 years. *Neurosurg Rev*. 2015;38:399–405.
17. Platz J, Berkefeld J, Singer OC, et al. Frequency, risk of hemorrhage, and treatment considerations for cerebral arteriovenous malformations with associated aneurysms. *Acta Neurochir*. 2014;156:2025–2034.
18. Spetzler RF, Martin NA. A proposed grading system for arteriovenous malformations. *J Neurosurg*. 1986;65:476–483.
19. Hamilton MG, Spetzler RF. The prospective application of a grading system for arteriovenous malformations. *Neurosurgery*. 1994;34(1):2–6.
20. Feliciano CE, Leon-Berra R, Hernandez-Gaitan MS, Rodriguez-Mercado R. A proposal for a new arteriovenous malformation grading scale for neuroendovascular procedures and literature review. *P R Health Sci J*. 2010;29(2):117–120.
21. Yuki I, Kim RH, Duckwiler G, et al. Treatment of brain arteriovenous malformations with high-flow arteriovenous fistulas: risk and complications associated with endovascular embolization in multimodality treatment. Clinical Article. *J Neurosurg*. 2010;113(4):715–722.
22. Dumont TM, Kan P, Snyder KV, Hopkins LN, Siddiqui AH, Levy EI. A proposed grading system for endovascular treatment of cerebral arteriovenous malformations: Buffalo Score. *Surg Neurol Int*. 2015;6:3.
23. Baharvahdat H, Blanc R, Termechi R, et al. Hemorrhagic complications after endovascular treatment of cerebral arteriovenous malformations. *AJNR Am J Neuroradiol*. 2014;35:978–983.
24. Jordan JA, Llibre JC, Vazquez F, Rodriguez R, Prince JA, Ugarte JC. Predictors of hemorrhagic complications from endovascular treatment of cerebral arteriovenous malformations. *Interv Neuroradiol*. 2014;20:74–82.
25. Zhang R, Zhu W, Su H. Vascular integrity in the pathogenesis of brain arteriovenous malformation. *Acta Neurochir Suppl*. 2016;121:29–35.
26. Sugiu K, Tokunaga K, Sasahara W, et al. Complications of embolization for cerebral arteriovenous malformations. *Interv Neuroradiol*. 2004;10(suppl 2):59–61.
27. Halbach VV, Higashida RT, Dowd CF, Barnwell SL, Hieshima GB. Management of vascular perforations that occur during neurointerventional procedures. *AJNR Am J Neuroradiol*. 1991;12(2):319–327.
28. Weber W, Kis B, Siekmann R, Kuehne D. Endovascular treatment of intracranial arteriovenous malformations with Onyx: technical aspects. *AJNR Am J Neuroradiol*. 2007;28:371–377.
29. Ashour R, Aziz-Sultan MA, Soltanolkotabi M, et al. Safety and efficacy of Onyx embolization for pediatric cranial and spinal vascular lesions and tumors. *Neurosurgery*. 2012;71(4):773–784.
30. Lin N, Smith ER, Scott RM, Orbach DB. Safety of neuroangiography and embolization in children: complication analysis of 697 consecutive procedures in 394 patients. *J Neurosurg Pediatr*. 2015;16:432–438.
31. van Rooij WJ, Sluzewski M, Beute GN. Brian AVM embolization with Onyx. *AJNR Am J Neuroradiol*. 2007;28:172–177.
32. Mounayer C, Hammami N, Piotin M, et al. Nidal embolization of brain arteriovenous malformations using Onyx in 94 patients. *AJNR Am J Neuroradiol*. 2007;28:518–523.
33. Newman CB, Park MS, Kerber CW, Levy ML, Barr JD, Pakbaz RS. Over-the-catheter retrieval of a retained microcatheter following Onyx embolization: a technical report. *J Neurointervent Surg*. 2012;4:e13.
34. Pandey P, Shetty R, Sabharwal P, Aravinda HR. Retrieval of a microcatheter from arteriovenous malformation after hemorrhage following Onyx embolization. *Neurol India*. 2013;61:523–525.
35. Zoarski GH, Lilly MP, Sperling JS, Mathis JM. Surgically confirmed incorporation of a chronically retained neurointerventional microcatheter in the carotid artery. *AJNR Am J Neuroradiol*. 1999;20:177–178.
36. Bingol H, Sirin G, Akay HT, Iyem H, Demirkilic U, Tatar H. Management of a retained catheter in an arteriovenous malformation. *J Neurosurg*. 2007;106:481–483.
37. Altschul D, Paramasivam S, Ortega-Gutierrez S, Fifi JT, Berenstein A. Safety and efficacy of using a detachable tip microcatheter in the

embolization of pediatric arteriovenous malformations. *Childs Nerv Syst*. 2014;30:1099–1107.
38. Herial NA, Khan AA, Sherr GT, Qureshi MH, Suri MFK, Qureshi AI. Detachable tip microcatheters for liquid embolization of brain arteriovenous malformations and fistulas: a United States single-center experience. *Neurosurgery*. 2015;11(3):404–411.
39. Peters K, Quisling RG, Gilmore R, Mickle P, Kuperus JH. Intraarterial use of sodium methohexital for provocative testing during brain embolotherapy. *AJNR Am J Neuroradiol*. 1993;14:171–174.
40. Glasser R, Masson R, Mickle JP, Peters KR. Embolization of a dural arteriovenous fistula of the ventral cervical spinal canal in a nine-year-old boy. *Neurosurgery*. 1993;33(6):1089–1093.
41. Niimi Y, Deletis V, Berenstein A. Provocative testing for embolization of spinal cord AVMs. *Interv Neuroradiol*. 2000;6(suppl 1):191–194.
42. Niimi Y, Sala F, Deletis V, Setton A, Bueno de Camargo A, Berenstein A. Neurophysiologic monitoring and pharmacologic provocative testing for embolization of spinal cord arteriovenous malformations. *AJNR Am J Neuroradiol*. 2004;25:1131–1138.

42

Procedure-Related Complications: Stroke

HIRAD S. HEDAYAT, YASIR AL-KHALILI, MANDY J. BINNING, EROL VEZNEDAROGLU

HIGHLIGHTS

- Post-thrombectomy symptomatic hemorrhage and hemorrhage requiring craniectomy are potentially devastating complications after successful endovascular intervention.
- Vessel perforation from catheter manipulation carries significant morbidity and mortality with it.
- Postprocedural intensive care monitoring and aggressive control of blood pressure help diminish the risk of post-reperfusion hemorrhagic complications.

Background

Each year approximately 795,000 patients will experience a new or recurrent stroke with approximately 610,000 of these as first occurrences.[1] In compiled assessments 87% were ischemic, 10% intracerebral hemorrhages, and 3% subarachnoid hemorrhages (SAHs).[2] The main goal in treating ischemic stroke patients is to restore cerebral perfusion as fast and safely as possible given that roughly 2 million neurons die per minute after vessel occlusion without recanalization.[3] Intravenous tissue plasminogen activator (IV tPA) may successfully recanalize about 30% of occlusions but has only a 10% to 15% efficacy in large vessel occlusions, namely those involving the internal carotid artery (ICA), proximal middle cerebral artery (MCA), or basilar artery (BA).[4] IV tPA has not demonstrated efficacy in thrombus lengths above 8 mm,[5] and reocclusions of the involved vascular segment may also occur.[6,7] The recent multicenter MR CLEAN, ESCAPE, and EXTEND IA trials[8–10] demonstrated that for large vessel occlusions, mechanical thrombectomy with stent retrievers had the highest recanalization rates in the anterior circulation and were superior to medical management with IV tPA. Additionally, good neurologic outcomes (mRS ≤2 at 90 days) were demonstrated in 40% to 60% of patients according to the TREVO trial.[11] However, these benefits come with the potentially devastating complication of intracranial hemorrhage.[12]

Endovascular Thrombectomy Complications

Although the total rate of complications is below 5%,[13] endovascular treatments carry risks related to vascular access at the groin site,[14] along with device- or procedure-related complications such as stent retriever detachment, arterial dissection, carotid-cavernous fistula, or vessel perforation.[15–19] Additional complications may be related to arterial-related infarct or ischemic complications such as reocclusion, vessel vasospasm, or reperfusion injuries[20] that may progress to devastating parenchymal hemorrhages. Rare medical complications of the procedure include contrast-induced nephropathy at a rate of 1.5%.[21]

Hemorrhagic Complications

The risk of hemorrhagic transformation of an acute ischemic stroke without any intervention is nearly 0.6%, whereas intraarterial pharmacologic treatments and mechanical interventions increase this risk to 15.4% and 10%, respectively.[22] After revascularization of an occluded vessel, the vasculature distal to the occlusion may show dilations or "luxury perfusion" that can be visualized on angiograms because the vessel has been maximally dilated to maintain cerebral perfusion secondary to autoregulation. It has been postulated that these dilated vessels in the salvageable ischemic penumbra are less tolerant of higher pressures, suggesting a higher vulnerability for damage and resultant hemorrhage.[22] It has been noted when using intraoperative transcranial Doppler[23] that increased blood flow and decreased pulsatility distal to the stent retriever device were seen. Given this knowledge, transient aggressive postoperative blood pressure control could help prevent hemorrhage after mechanical thrombectomy with a blood pressure reduction of 25% to 30% from preoperative baseline.[23]

The majority of patients with intracranial hemorrhage after thrombectomy remain asymptomatic with a 2% to 15% reported rate of symptomatic hemorrhages.[24,25] Decompressive craniectomy for hemorrhage or malignant cerebral edema has also been reported in up to 15% of patients after thrombectomy, and both symptomatic hemorrhage and need for craniectomy were associated with poor outcome.[25]

Subarachnoid Hemorrhagic Complications

The occurrence of peri-interventional subarachnoid hemorrhage has been reported in 5% to 16% of cases,[26] whereas angiographically detectable vessel perforations were reported at a rate of 0% to 3%, meaning that the majority of peri-interventional SAH is likely due to angiographically occult perforations.[27] The majority of these perithrombectomy SAH cases are asymptomatic but were found to have a higher chance of developing asymptomatic intraparenchymal hemorrhage within the first 24 hours after recanalization, according to a retrospective case control study (57% vs 0%, $P = 0.018$).[11]

SURGICAL REWIND

My Worst Case

A 58-year-old man presented with National Institutes of Health (NIH) Stroke Scale 19 and an occlusion of the left M2 superior division on computed tomography (CT) angiography. CT perfusion suggested salvageable penumbra in the distribution of the occlusion. He received IV tPA without improvement in his neurologic examination and subsequently underwent uneventful and successful thrombectomy with a thrombolysis in cerebral infarction (TICI) 3 recanalization. While in the ICU he had elevated blood pressures postprocedurally and had a significant neurologic decline. CT head demonstrated a devastating intraparenchymal reperfusion hemorrhage. After a discussion with his family, they elected to withdraw care.

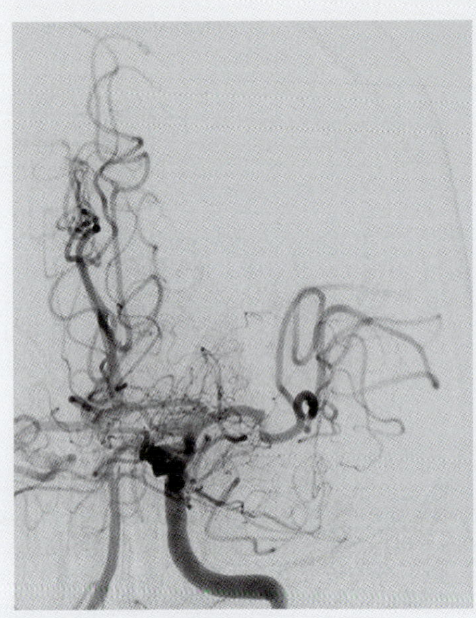

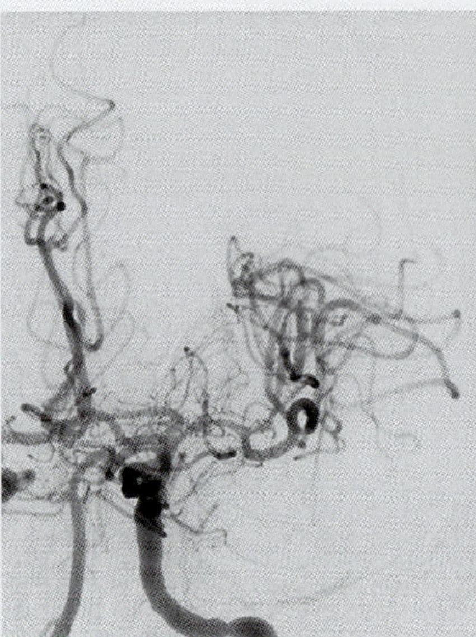

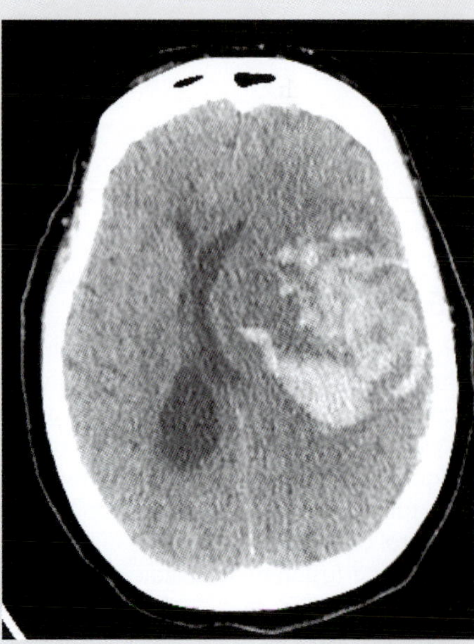

Apart from true SAH, sulcal hyperdensities that resemble SAH may be seen on postinterventional CTs in 3.5% to 16.2% of stroke interventions[28] secondary to either small vessel perforation or, more commonly, mechanical destruction of the endothelial integrity during thrombectomy and seepage of contrast. The chances of developing SAH increase with a longer time interval between clinical onset and recanalization, an extensive procedure time, and a higher number of recanalization attempts.[28]

RED FLAGS

- Tortuous vascular anatomy
- Vessel wall calcifications
- Difficulty navigating microwires or microcatheters past thrombus
- tPA administration before thrombectomy
- Poorly controlled blood pressure peri- and postintervention
- Stasis or nonfilling of distal vasculature

Intracranial Vascular Perforation

Perforation of a vessel is a rare occurrence during thrombectomy, although its mechanisms, risk factors, outcomes, and rescue approaches have not been well described in the literature. It is usually related to micro-guidewire manipulation making a 29- to 30-gauge hole (about 0.014 in. or 0.09 mm[24]), which is usually self-sealing if it occurs in a nondiseased vessel. The sequela of this will depend on the location of the perforation in the vessel (subarachnoid space vs intraparenchymal), duration of bleeding, and rate of bleeding. Most of the time, the microwire perforation will be identified by extravasation seen on microcatheter injection beyond the vessel occlusion before the stent retriever is inserted. When this occurs, it is typically wise to forgo thrombectomy so that the occluded vessel will prevent hemorrhage from the small vessel perforation. When this is not possible, or if extravasation persists, treatment may require occlusion of the vessel over the hole or just proximal to it with a small coil or the use of Onyx embolization material.[29] Intraprocedural vessel perforation during stent retriever thrombectomy cases occurred in 1.0% with most perforations occurring at distal locations.[30] Mortality during hospitalization and at 3 months were 56% and 63%, respectively, whereas 25% of patients achieved good functional outcome at 90 days postprocedure.[30]

Vasospasm

Vasospasm of both intracranial and cervical vessels happens secondary to intraluminal manipulation with catheters and guidewires at a reported rate of up to 23% of patients with approximately 0.5% being symptomatic.[31] Vasospasm during interventions is mostly self-resolving. In the setting of severe, nonresolving, flow-limiting vasospasm, infusion of intraarterial Nimodipine, Verapamil, or Diltiazem may be necessary for treatment.[20] Balloon angioplasty is less likely required for catheter spasm because it is not recurring as seen with subarachnoid hemorrhage–associated vasospasm; therefore the results from intraarterial calcium channel blockers tend to be durable. The best preventive method to avoid vasospasm is to avoid inducing it via careful, efficient manipulation of catheters and guidewire to minimize intraluminal intimal irritation of the vessels. When vasospasm occurs, withdrawing or removing the offending item and waiting while acquiring serial angiographic runs will demonstrate resolution.

Arterial Dissection

Arterial dissection related to mechanical thrombectomy is typically related to the guide-catheter dissecting the ICA either during initial placement or during clot retrieval when the guide moves distally due to pulling back on a well-integrated, hard clot. Typically, small dissection flaps can be seen that are not flow-limiting and that can be treated with an antiplatelet agent. If thrombus formation is identified on a dissection flap, anticoagulation is typically warranted. When a dissection is flow-limiting or occlusive, the dissection can often be opened by finding the true lumen of the carotid with the wire and placing the guide (if petrous or proximal) beyond the occlusion. If the occlusion is distal to the petrous ICA, an intermediate catheter or microcatheter can be placed distal to the occlusion. An angiographic run after this maneuver will often show that the flow has been restored. In cases in which this does not restore flow, stenting may be required to tack down the dissection flap and restore the true lumen.

Carotid-Cavernous Fistula

A direct carotid-cavernous fistula (CCF) usually occurs from trauma or aneurysmal rupture and is rarely iatrogenic. CCF is reported to occur in 0.8% of all endovascular procedures, including stroke interventions.[32] CCFs occurred significantly more often in women, suggesting a sex difference in vascular weakness.[32] When a CCF occurs, one option is not to proceed with further passes with the stent retriever if revascularization is not complete. If revascularization is complete with TICI 3 flow, the CCF can be treated in a delayed or staged fashion if it becomes symptomatic.

Stent Retriever Detachment/Device Malfunction

With the continued evolution of technical advances in endovascular technologies, the rate of stent retriever device detachment or malfunction is quite rare. Arterial stenoses, tortuosity, and wall calcifications cause luminal surface irregularities that may cause detachment of the stent during withdrawal.[33] The number of stent passes is also thought to contribute to detachment because the stent attachment site weakens with repetitive thrombectomies.[33] Most of the reported cases have shown poor outcomes along with the unsuccessful retrieval of the detached devices. Removal of the detached stent with another thrombectomy stent may serve as an alternative option that can produce favorable outcomes.[32] However, in cases of stent detachment in the parent vessel with resultant patency, it is best to leave the stent retriever in place and place the patient on dual-antiplatelet agents as one would for any intracranial stent. One must remember that all is not lost, especially if the result is a patent vessel.

Reperfusion Injury

Chronically decreased perfusion pressures are found in patients with occlusive atherosclerotic disease, and when normal pressure is restored after vessel recanalization, there may be resultant edema or frank hemorrhage because these areas have little to no cerebrovascular reserve.[34] The arterioles lose their normal pressure sensitivity such that when normal pressure is restored, suddenly there is vascular disruption, leakage of blood contents, edema, or hemorrhage. When this occurs, the aggressive use of antihypertensives is indicated to reduce the high flow of blood into these areas after revascularization occurred.

Conclusion

Endovascular thrombectomy has become the standard of care in large vessel occlusive stroke management for patients who fit the appropriate criteria for intervention. Randomized trials have revealed significant improvement in neurologic outcomes with this therapy. As these interventions become more commonplace throughout hospitals caring for stroke patients, the role of experienced, efficient, and careful practitioners who may face cases with challenging anatomy and pathology that increase the complication rate is crucial. Postprocedural management of these patients in an intensive care setting with specially trained nurses who maintain aggressive blood pressure control and close neurologic monitoring are as crucial to good outcomes as are procedural-related factors.

Reference

1. Go AS, Mozaffarian D, Roger VL, et al. Heart disease and stroke statistics–2014 update: a report from the American Heart Association. *Circulation*. 2014;129:282–292.
2. Serrone J, Jimenez L, Ringer A. The role of endovascular therapy in the treatment of acute ischemic stroke. *Neurosurgery*. 2014;74:133–141.
3. Saver JL. Time is brain—quantified. *Stroke*. 2006;37:263–266.
4. Behrens L, Mohlenbruch M, Stampfl S, et al. Effect of thrombus size on recanalization by bridging intravenous thrombolysis. *Eur J Neurol*. 2014;21:1406–1410.
5. Riedel CH, Zimmermann P, Jensen-Kondering U, et al. The importance of size: successful recanalization by intravenous thrombolysis in acute anterior stroke depends on thrombus length. *Stroke*. 2011;42:1775–1777.
6. del Zoppo GJ, Higashida RT, Furlan AJ, et al. PROACT: a phase II randomized trial of recombinant pro-urokinase by direct arterial delivery in acute middle cerebral artery stroke. PROACT Investigators. Prolyse in Acute Cerebral Thromboembolism. *Stroke*. 1998;29: 4–11.
7. Dorado L, Castallano C, Mill M. Hemorrhagic risk of emergent endovascular treatment plus stenting in patients with acute ischemic stroke. *J Stroke Cerebrovasc Dis*. 2013;22:1326–1331.
8. Berkhemer OA, Fransen PS, Beumer D, et al. A randomized trial of intraarterial treatment for acute ischemic stroke. *NEJM*. 2015;372:11–20.
9. Demchuk AM, Goyal M, Menon BK, et al. Endovascular treatment for Small Core and Anterior circulation Proximal occlusion with Emphasis on minimizing CT to recanalization times (ESCAPE) trial: methodology. *Int J Stroke*. 2015;10:429–438.
10. Campbell BCV, Mitchell P, Kleinig T. Endovascular therapy for ischemic stroke with perfusion-imaging selection. *N Engl J Med*. 2015;372:1009–1018.
11. Yilmaz U, Walter S, Körner H, et al. Peri-interventional subarachnoid hemorrhage during mechanical thrombectomy with stent retrievers in acute stroke: a retrospective case-control study. *Clin Neuroradiol*. 2015;25:173–176.
12. Ansari S, Rahman M, McConnell DJ, et al. Recanalization therapy for acute ischemic stroke, part 2: mechanical intra-arterial technologies. *Neurosurg Rev*. 2011;34:11–20.
13. Bösel J. Intensive care management of the endovascular stroke patient. *Semin Neurol*. 2016;36:520–530.

14. Schickel S, Cronin SN, Mize A, et al. Removal of femoral sheaths by registered nurses: issues and outcomes. *Crit Care Nurse.* 1996;16:32–36.
15. Lawson MF, Velat GJ, Fargen KM, et al. Interventional neurovascular disease: avoidance and management of complications and review of the current literature. *J Neurosurg Sci.* 2011;55:233–242.
16. Kaufmann TJ, Huston J 3rd, Mandrekar JN, et al. Complications of diagnostic cerebral angiography: evaluation of 19,826 consecutive patients. *Radiology.* 2007;243:812–819.
17. Gill HL, Siracuse JJ, Parrack IK, et al. Complications of the endovascular management of acute ischemic stroke. *Vasc Health Risk Manag.* 2014;10:675–681.
18. Akins PT, Amar AP, Pakbaz RS, Fields JD, SWIFT Investigators. Complications of endovascular treatment for acute stroke in the SWIFT trial with solitaire and AJNR. *AJNR Am J Neuroradiol.* 2014;35:524–528.
19. Kwon HJ, Chueh JY, Puri AS, et al. Early detachment of the Solitaire stent during thrombectomy retrieval: an in vitro investigation. *J Neurointerv Surg.* 2014;2:114–117.
20. Akpinar SH, Yilmaz G. Periprocedural complications in endovascular stroke treatment. *Br J Radiol.* 2016;89:1057.
21. Pereira VM, Gralla J, Davalos A. Prospective, multicenter, single-arm study of mechanical thrombectomy using Solitaire Flow Restoration in acute ischemic stroke. *Stroke.* 2013;44:2802–2807.
22. Vollman AT, Bruno CA Jr, Dumeer S. Angiographic warning of hemorrhagic transformation after stent retriever thrombectomy procedure. *J Neurointerv Surg.* 2014;6(1):e6.
23. Brus-Ramer M, Starke RM, Komotar RJ, et al. Radiographic evidence of cerebral hyperperfusion and reversal following angioplasty and stenting of intracranial carotid and middle cerebral artery stenosis: case report and review of the literature. *J Neuroimaging.* 2010;20:280–283.
24. Nogueira RG, Yoo AJ, Buonanno FS, et al. Endovascular approaches to acute stroke, part 2: a comprehensive review of studies and trials. *AJNR Am J Neuroradiol.* 2009;30:859–875.
25. Cappelen-Smith C, Cordato D, Calic Z, et al. Endovascular thrombectomy for acute ischaemic stroke: a real-world experience. *Intern Med J.* 2016;46:1038–1043.
26. Hong H, Zeng J-S, Kreulen DL, et al. Atorvastatin protects against cerebral infarction via inhibition of NADPH oxidase-derived superoxide in ischemic stroke. *Am J Physiol Heart Circ Physiol.* 2006; 291:2210–2215.
27. Dorn F, Stehle S, Lockau H, et al. Endovascular treatment of acute intracerebral artery occlusions with the Solitaire stent: single-centre experience with 108 recanalization procedures. *Cerebrovasc Dis.* 2012;34:70–77.
28. Nikoubashman O, Reich A, Pjontek R, et al. Postinterventional subarachnoid haemorrhage after endovascular stroke treatment with stent retrievers. *Neuroradiology.* 2014;56:1087–1096.
29. Kostov D, Kanaan H, Lin R, et al. Review of intracranial vessel perforation with Onyx-18 using an exovascular retreating catheter technique. *J Neurointerv Surg.* 2012;4:121–124.
30. Mokin M, Fargen KM, Primiani CT, et al. Vessel perforation during stent retriever thrombectomy for acute ischemic stroke: technical details and clinical outcomes. *J Neurointerv Surg.* 2016;10:1136–1141.
31. Shi ZS, Liebeskind D, Loh Y. Predictors of subarachnoid hemorrhage in acute ischemic stroke with endovascular therapy. *Stroke.* 2010;41:2775–2781.
32. Ono K, Oishi H, Tanouse S, et al. Direct carotid-cavernous fistulas occurring during neurointerventional procedures. *J Neurointerv Surg.* 2016;22:91–96.
33. Akpinar S, Yilmaz G. Spontaneous Solitaire™ AB thrombectomy stent detachment during stroke treatment. *Cardiovasc Intervent Radiol.* 2015;38:475–478.
34. Samaniego EA, Dabus G, Linfante I. Avoiding complications in neurosurgical interventional procedures. *J Neurosurg Sci.* 2011;55: 71–80.

43

Complications in Endovascular Management of Carotid-Cavernous and Dural Arteriovenous Fistulas

MICHAEL J. LANG, M. REID GOOCH, ROBERT H. ROSENWASSER

HIGHLIGHTS

- The vast majority of dural arteriovenous fistulas and carotid-cavernous fistulas should be treated with an endovascular-first strategy.
- Major complications include unintended embolic migration, cranial neuropathy, and occlusion of normal venous drainage.
- Most complications can be avoided by understanding the relevant cerebral vascular anatomy before any embolization procedure.

Background

Carotid-cavernous fistulas (CCF) and dural arteriovenous fistulas (dAVF) are abnormal communications between the branches of the internal carotid artery (ICA) or external carotid artery (ECA) and the dural venous structures of the head. They vary in clinical presentation, severity, natural history, and indications for treatment largely on the basis of their neurovascular anatomic features. Regardless of location and type, clinical manifestations are the result of venous hypertension. Furthermore, while open surgical interruption of dAVFs is a primary treatment in certain locations, endovascular embolization has become the mainstay of treatment for the vast majority of CCFs and dAVFs. As such, a thorough knowledge of arterial and venous anatomy is essential for the safe endovascular treatment of these lesions, particularly insofar as the dangerous anastomoses responsible for many complications are not always visible on angiography.

CCFs were classified by Barrow et al. into four types based on arterial supply (Table 43.1).[1] Type A fistulas are high-flow fistulas resulting from a direct connection between the ICA and the cavernous sinus (CS). Types B, C, and D fistulas are all low-flow lesions from dural vessels supplying the wall of the CS and originating from the ICA, ECA, or both, respectively. The presenting symptoms are not always the classic triad of exophthalmos, vision loss, and chemosis, and these lesions are often found to present with orbital bruit or cranial neuropathy as well.[2] In general, Type A fistulas tend to present acutely, with more significant clinical manifestations. Direct fistulas have been reported to account for up to 80% of all CCFs, and they are most frequently the result of craniofacial trauma. Spontaneous direct CCFs can occur in the setting of cavernous ICA aneurysm rupture or connective tissue disease, such as Ehlers-Danlos type IV or pseudoxanthoma elasticum. In 2% to 3% of cases, direct fistulas can present up to several weeks after the initial trauma as severe, potentially life-threatening epistaxis.[3] Indirect fistulas, conversely, tend to be more indolent, and spontaneous resolution is common. Presentation varies with the location of the fistulous point within the CS (discussed below). In both direct and indirect fistulas, intracerebral or subarachnoid hemorrhage is a rare finding (less than 5% of patients) but can occur in patients with cortical venous reflux (CVR).[4] Evidence of large varices of the CS or thrombosis of major venous outflow tracts can also predispose to hemorrhagic presentation, and it should lead to emergent evaluation and treatment of the fistula.

Dural arteriovenous fistulas are supplied by the dural branches of the ECA, ICA, and vertebral arteries (VAs). These fistulas are named and classified on the venous drainage location and pattern. The Borden classification divides dAVFs into three categories. Drainage of Type I fistulas is anterograde into a dural sinus, Type II fistulas anterograde into a dural sinus and retrograde into cortical veins, and Type III fistulas exhibit isolated retrograde drainage.[5] The Cognard classification follows a similar pattern, but differentiates Type II into IIa and IIb subtypes such that Type IIa fistulas drain anterograde and retrograde into a sinus/sinuses and Type IIb drain anterograde into the main sinus but with retrograde venous reflux.[6] Cognard also added Type IV to denote ectasia of the cortical draining veins (highest risk of hemorrhage), as well as Type V to denote drainage into the perimedullary venous plexus (which can mimic spinal dAVF presentation, particularly for fistulas located near the foramen magnum). CVR has been shown to confer a 10% annual risk of hemorrhage, and Cognard reported that Type III and Type IV lesions were found to be hemorrhagic at presentation in 40% and 65% of patients, respectively.[7] Nonhemorrhagic presentation is most common for low-grade lesions, and can include pulsatile tinnitus, bruit over the fistulous point, and headaches. Encephalopathy can occur from diffuse venous hypertension, and seizures and focal neurologic deficits can be present depending on location.[8]

In both CCFs and dAVFs the urgency of evaluation depends on the acuity and severity of symptoms at presentation. Initial workup with noninvasive imaging, including noninvasive vascular imaging, may suggest an underlying fistula when evidence of an

TABLE 43.1 Classification of Carotid-Cavernous and Dural Arteriovenous Fistulas

CAROTID-CAVERNOUS FISTULAS		DURAL ARTERIOVENOUS FISTULA			
Barrow Classification		**Borden Classification**		**Cognard Classification**	
Type	Definition	Type	Definition	Type	Definition
A	Direct ICA to CS, high flow	I	Drainage into sinus with antegrade flow	I	Drainage into sinus with antergrade flow
B	Indirect ICA to CS, low flow	II	Drainage into sinus with retrograde flow and cortical venous reflux (CVR)	IIa	Drainage into sinus with retrograde flow and CVR
C	Indirect ECA to CS, low flow			IIb	Drainage into sinus with retrograde flow and CVR
D	Indirect ICA+ECA to CS, Low flow			IIa+b	Drainage into sinus with retrograde flow anf CVR
		III	Drainage into cortical vein (CVR only)	III	Drainage into cortical vein (CVR only)
				IV	Drainage into cortical vein with venous varix
				V	Drainage into spinal perimedullary veins

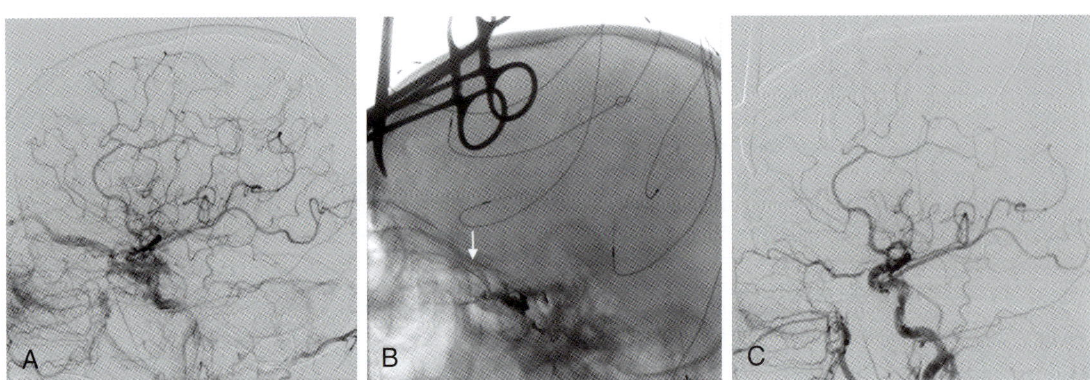

• **Fig. 43.1** Left common carotid artery (CCA) injection (A) demonstrates the presence of a Type D carotid-cavernous fistula (CCF) in a patient presenting with increased intraocular pressure, ophthalmoparesis, chemosis, and exophthalmos. After failure to catheterize the inferior petrosal sinus, transvenous embolization was performed through the superior ophthalmic vein, which was cannulated (arrow) by means of a transpalpebral cutdown (B). Postembolization CCA injection shows complete resolution of the fistula (C).

enlarged CS/superior ophthalmic vein (SOV), proptosis, sinus thrombosis, or diffuse engorgement of cerebral veins is seen. However, the gold standard for diagnosis of a CCF or dAVF remains catheter angiography, and endovascular approaches encompass the overwhelming majority of interventions for these lesions.

Anatomic Insights

Venous Anatomy

The cavernous sinus, first described by Jacobus Winslow in 1734, is a misnomer insofar as it is neither cavernous nor a sinus, as demonstrated by the pioneering work of Dwight Parkinson, who preferred *lateral sellar compartment* as the more anatomically correct term.[9] The reasoning for this designation is that the CS does not contain true cavernous tissue but instead is a plexiform arrangement of septated, compartmentalized venous channels. Furthermore, it is not a true sinus because it lies between the paired dural layers periosteum of the sphenoid bone (not between the two layers of dura). The CS has a number of venous tributaries and routes of egress, which include the superior and inferior ophthalmic veins (IOV), the sphenoparietal sinus, the pterygoid venous plexus via the foramen ovale, the superior and inferior petrosal sinuses (SPS and IPS), the anterior and posterior intercavernous sinuses (known collectively as the circular sinus), and the clival venous plexus. Anatomic variation is the rule in this region, resulting in substantial symptomatic heterogeneity.[10]

These venous pathways to the CS form the basis for the major transvenous embolization techniques. At our institution, indirect CCFs are generally addressed transvenously, proceeding in a stepwise progression from transfemoral access to the IPS, then transfemoral access via the common facial vein system into the SOV, and finally by transpalpebral exposure for direct SOV puncture (Fig. 43.1). Generally speaking, CCFs with fistulous points located anteriorly in the CS tend to present with more significant proptosis/chemosis due to reversal of flow within the SOV, whereas posteriorly positioned fistulas can present with bilateral or contralateral symptoms. Access via the IPS can be variable, based on embryologic development and position of the fistula, but it avoids the intraocular complications of trans-SOV access to the CS.[11,12] In the setting of long-standing venous hypertension, dilatation of the SOV can expand the veins of the common facial system, enabling transvenous access through this route, but in the absence of these findings, competent venous valves and tortuous pathways can complicate this approach to the SOV. Regardless of the route chosen, a thorough understanding of CS anatomy is essential to understand the unique properties of a given fistula and the likelihood of success with a given embolization strategy.

Dural AVFs vary in presenting symptoms and severity based on how likely a fistula at a given location is to give rise to CVR. Awad et al. reported that over 60% of all dAVFs in their series and metaanalysis were located at the sigmoid sinus and/or transverse sinus, but only one-fourth of these patients presented with aggressive clinical features.[13] Conversely, dAVFs of the tentorium and anterior cranial fossa (ethmoidal dAVFs) almost always present aggressive features and have high rates of hemorrhagic features due to the near-universal absence of direct sinus drainage of these fistulas. Superior sagittal sinus (SSS) dAVFs have a rate of aggressive presentation between these two extremes but often present with extensive bilateral feeding arteries, and torcular fistulas can be a particularly aggressive variant. Drainage patterns of dAVFs at the foramen magnum (including jugular bulb, marginal sinus, and hypoglossal canal) frequently present with myelopathy due to drainage into the perimedullary spinal venous plexus.

Arterial Anatomy

The relevant arterial microanatomy is complex, but certain common arterial anatomic features warrant particular attention because they can be the source of unintended injury to the brain or cranial nerves.[14] Lasjaunias et al., in their comprehensive study of the vascular anatomy of the head and neck, described three regions that serve as the major source of endogenous ECA-ICA anastomoses: the orbital region (via anastomoses with the ophthalmic artery [OphA]), the petrous-cavernous region (via anastomoses with the ICA), and the upper cervical region (via anastomoses with the VAs).[15]

The relevance of the extracranial-intracranial (EC-IC) anastomoses in the orbital region relates to risk of embolization of the central retinal artery (CRA), which arises as the first or second branch of the second segment of the OphA, resulting in blindness. The OphA can collateralize with the middle meningeal artery (MMA) via the anterior falcine artery and the anterior and posterior ethmoidal arteries, or by the meningo-orbital artery and superficial recurrent meningeal arteries that form anastomoses between the MMA and the lacrimal division of the OphA.[16]

Anastomoses in the cavernous-petrous region can result in distal embolization into the ICA via the inferolateral trunk (ILT), as injury to nearby cranial nerves. The cavernous branches of the MMA anastomose with the superior (tentorial) branch of the ILT, both of which anastomose with the petrous arcade supplying the geniculate ganglion through the fallopian hiatus.[17] The ILT also has connections with the superior recurrent meningeal artery to the MMA as well as to the internal maxillary artery (IMA) via the artery of the foramen rotundum (from the distal IMA) and the accessory meningeal artery (AMA) (passing through the foramen ovale or Vesalius to connect to the proximal IMA). Importantly, the ILT has perineural arterial divisions that supply the Gasserian ganglion as well as the cranial nerves running in the lateral wall of the CS. Anastomosis between the carotid canal branch of the ascending pharyngeal artery (APA) and the ILT is also common.

The upper cervical region harbors several anastomoses that are clinically relevant as well. The occipital artery (OA), being a remnant of the embryologic type I and II proatlantal arteries, still serves as an endogenous connection between the VA and the ECA, sending branches from its horizontal segment to the VA at the level of C1/C2. In some patients this embryologic origin is clearer, with shared origin of the distal OA from both the ECA and VA visible angiographically (Fig. 43.2). The neuromeningeal branches of the APA (jugular and hypoglossal) anastomose with the VA at the artery of the dens, and also form connections with the ILT and meningohypophyseal trunk (MHT) via their clival branches.

RED FLAGS

Avoidance of complications starts with patient selection. Patients with minimal or mild symptoms can be offered conservative management in the absence of any high-risk features. Temporizing medical therapy combined with intermittent cervical carotid artery compression with the contralateral hand has a 20% to 25% success rate for spontaneous resolution of low-flow CCFs.[18] The same rationale holds for grade I dAVFs, which have a high rate of spontaneous resolution.[19] Once a patient has been identified as warranting surgical intervention, a number of specific risk factors must be considered. The following is a discussion of some of the major considerations and risk factors to weigh when selecting an endovascular course of action for CCFs and dAVFs.

Selection of Approach

Techniques for embolization include coils, detachable balloons, and liquid embolic agents, such as *n*-Butyl cyanoacrylate (NBCA) and ethyl-vinyl alcohol (Onyx, Medtronic Inc., USA), which enable transarterial embolization across the fistulous point. The use of proximal Onyx plug formation, wedged microcatheter technique,

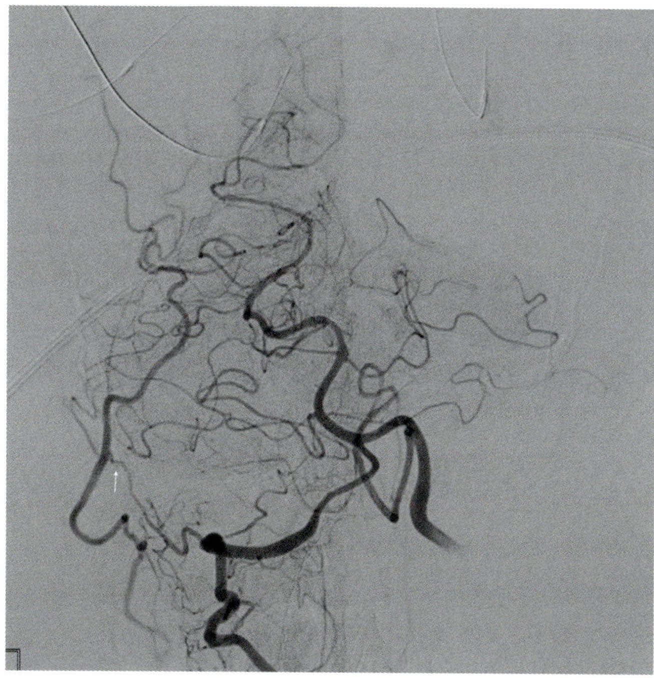

• **Fig. 43.2** Right vertebral artery (VA) injection demonstrates the presence of a persistent anastomosis between the VA and the occipital artery (arrow). Embolization through the occipital artery warrants particular attention to this anatomic variant, which may not be evident until flow is altered by treatment.

or proximal flow arrest with a separate balloon or a dual-lumen balloon catheter (such as the Scepter balloon [Microvention Inc., USA]) also enables more complete penetrance of arterial feeders with lower likelihood of proximal reflux.[20] For certain lesions, such as Barrow Type A CCFs, a transarterial approach is nearly always favored, and recent reports have also suggested a role for flow-diverting stents in these fistulas (despite concerns about dual-antiplatelet therapy in this patient population).[21] In other cases, the choice of approach is less clear. Fistulas that are fed by multiple small feeders or by arteries harboring dangerous anastomoses, or in which proximal reflux into a parent artery cannot be tolerated, may be better suited for transvenous treatment.[22] Conversely, transvenous therapies have higher cure rates for certain types of fistulas (type B-D CCFs, for example) and lower rates of cranial neuropathy in general compared with transarterial therapy, but several unique red flags must be considered. Thrombosis of the affected sinus may limit access to the draining vein (and may result in vessel perforation if attempted), and compartmentalization of sinus drainage may make it difficult to identify the true venous outflow.[23] Finally, in some cases, an endovascular approach should not be considered first-line, in lieu of open surgical disconnection. This is frequently the case with ethmoidal dAVFs, in which transarterial therapy carries significant risk of injury to the CRA (by embolysate reflux or retrograde thrombosis of the ophthalmic artery) and transvenous access via distal cortical veins can be difficult to achieve.[24]

Alteration of Flow Dynamics During Embolization

A central consideration, either by transvenous or transarterial approach, is that during the course of endovascular treatment, flow patterns seen on control or supraselective microcatheter angiograms may change during the course of embolization.[25] Decreasing capacitance of an embolized pedicle will occur during the course of injection, which can overcome the antireflux techniques. In this regard, the development of Onyx has been extremely useful because embolization can be halted, repeat angiography checked, and treatment continued or discontinued as indicated.[26] Venous approaches risk rapid redirection of flow into previously nonarterialized channels (with resultant venous infarction or hemorrhage) if the entire fistula outflow is not occluded. Normal venous drainage must also be respected. During transvenous treatment of CCFs, complete outflow obstruction of the CS, particularly with concomitant embolization into both the SOV and IOV, can result in rapid decrease in ocular venous outflow and rapid rise in intraocular pressure (IOP).

The Fistulous Point

Treatment failure and complication often arise from an inability to clearly visualize or reach the fistulous point. Increasing proximal support can improve distal access in tortuous vessels, as can the use of small flow-directed microcatheters (such as the Marathon catheter [Medtronic Inc., USA]). Direct puncture can mitigate access issues from traditional transfemoral routes. Visualization of the fistulous point throughout embolization is also essential. When using a blank road map technique during liquid embolic injection, reference angiograms should be displayed side-by-side so that the venous pouch can be clearly identified and injection halted before further migration into normal venous structures.

Numerous Feeding Arteries

Fistulas supplied by multiple large feeding arteries present a specific challenge to the interventionalist. In patients with extensive fistulas of the SSS, embolization of multiple, bilateral scalp arteries can cause significant scalp necrosis, even requiring free skin flap reconstruction.[27] Prolonged treatment times can result in radiation skin burns or alopecia. For fistulas of the skull base supplied bilaterally, transarterial embolization can risk potentially devastating bilateral cranial neuropathies.[28] This is particularly true when considering bilateral embolization of APA feeders and the inherent risk of lower cranial neuropathy. For this reason, we prefer staged intervention for these complex lesions.

High-Flow Fistulas

High flow through a CCF or dAVF can result in cardiopulmonary embolization as a result of treatment with liquid embolic agents. Treatment planning should include consideration of embolic formulations with higher viscosity and careful monitoring of embolysate flow during injection.

Equipment Considerations

Technical complications related to embolization with liquid embolic agents have been well documented in the literature. Catheters must be selected that are compatible with NBCA or DMSO. The potential for microcatheter retention has been shown to be higher with the use of NBCA as compared with Onyx.[26] If the catheter cannot be removed successfully, it must be cut at the groin access site. Detachable microcatheters, such as the Apollo catheter (Medtronic Inc., USA), have been developed to avoid this complication.

Management

As discussed above, the most important steps for avoiding complication in fistula embolization are the selection of appropriate patients, careful study of the relevant anatomy, selection of the optimal approach, and staged intervention when necessary. Intraoperatively, avoidance of unintended embolization can be managed by careful observation of embolic flow. With the use of Onyx, repeated angiography to assess degree of fistula/feeder occlusion followed by continuation of injection can be performed due to the so-called "lava-like" flow properties of Onyx.[29] In cases where embolic material has refluxed into critical parent arteries or migrated through critical anastomoses (such as into the vertebrobasilar system through the OA), the patient is maintained on a heparin infusion in the postoperative period. Depending on the severity, heparin can be converted to oral anticoagulant or antiplatelet therapy, or discontinued and the patient observed in-hospital until concern for ischemia lessens. Postoperative heparin therapy is also utilized in cases with potential impairment of normal venous drainage. Cranial neuropathies typically are managed with steroid tapers and expectant management, particularly in the transvenous treatment of CCFs, in which symptomatic neuropathies of the cranial nerves in the CS (CN III–VI) are common but generally resolve completely. In some cases of transvenous treatment of CCFs, particularly with transpalpebral direct cannulations of the SOV (as mentioned above), rapid, though invariably transient, increase of IOP often necessitates that an emergent canthotomy be performed at the bedside.

SURGICAL REWIND

My Worst Case

A 59-year-old male presented to our institution with 6-day history of progressive chemosis, exophthalmos, and subjective blurry vision of his left eye. Tonometry demonstrated elevation of IOP to 40 mm Hg in the affected eye, which was reduced to 26 mm Hg with medical therapy. Noninvasive imaging demonstrated a dilated SOV and proptosis, suggesting CCF. The following day, a diagnostic angiogram was performed, which demonstrated the presence of a fistula between the AMA and isolated drainage into the confluence of the SOV and IOV at the anterior extent of the CS, without posterior drainage into the rest of the CS. Given the presence of an easily accessible single feeding vessel, transarterial embolization was performed (Fig. 43.3). Using a 5F Berenstein guide catheter, a 0.017-in. microcatheter (Headway Duo, Microvention Inc., USA) was introduced into the AMA and into the venous sac. Embolization with 0.3 mL of Onyx 34 was performed, but subsequent ECA angiogram demonstrated persistence of the fistula. A second microcatheter was introduced, and another 0.3 mL of Onyx 34 was injected into the AMA, with occlusion of the arterial feeder to the level of the skull base.

The patient awoke from anesthesia without complication, but beginning 2 hours after embolization was found to have progressive ophthalmoparesis, facial anesthesia, and facial weakness, rapidly progressing to complete ophthalmoplegia, House-Brackmann grade 6 facial palsy, and dense hemianesthesia of V1 and V2 branches of the trigeminal nerve.

Post-procedures, a computed tomography scan was performed, which did not demonstrate any evidence of parenchymal infarct, but evidence of Onyx cast could be seen in the region of the ILT collaterals and petrous facial arcade. The patient was started on IV heparin and Decadron, and hypertension was induced with NeoSynephrine infusion. The patient was discharged with these symptoms unchanged, and with instructions for eye care in the setting of combined facial and trigeminal palsy and with a plan for early neurosurgical and ophthalmologic follow-up. In spite of these precautions, the patient developed a corneal ulcer, which required prolonged treatment with ophthalmic antibiotics and steroids, as well as tarsorrhaphy. At the 3-month follow-up, the patient had recovered a mild degree of extraocular muscle function and facial sensation, but with disabling House-Brackmann grade 5 facial palsy.

In retrospect, this disabling complication could potentially have been avoided by performing coil embolization of the venous pouch, given that we were able to directly access the venous outflow from the solitary arterial feeder, and potentially augmenting with a small amount of Onyx 34 into the coil mass, if necessary. Up-front use of such a strategy would have vastly decreased the risk of cranial neuropathy. Furthermore, after the initial Onyx injection, use of a dual-lumen balloon catheter could have aided in deposition of Onyx solely at the fistulous point while avoiding reflux down to the level of the skull base, where the dangerous anastomoses of the AMA are found.

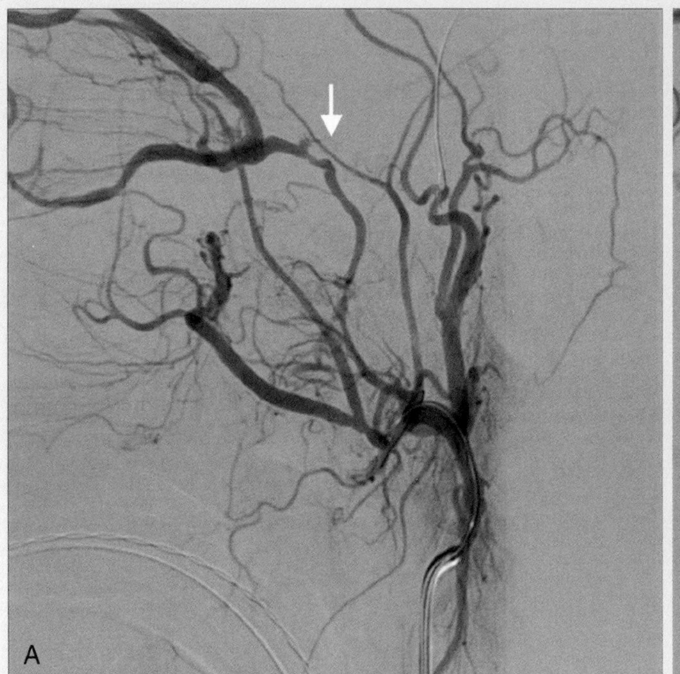

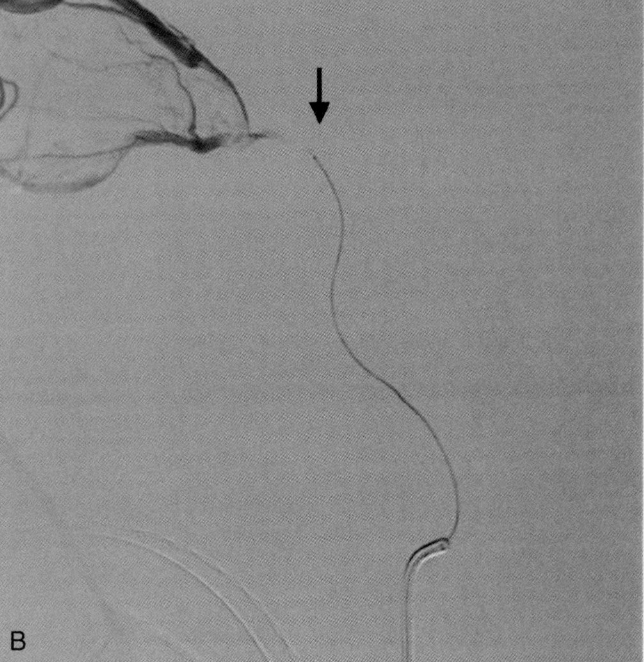

• **Fig. 43.3** Left external carotid artery (ECA) injection demonstrates a type C carotid-cavernous fistula (CCF) arising from a direct connection between the accessory meningeal artery and the anterior cavernous sinus (CS) at the junction of the superior ophthalmic vein (SOV) and inferior ophthalmic vein (IOV) (A, white arrow). There is no evidence of venous outflow posteriorly into the body of the CS. Supraselective injection demonstrates the navigation of the Duo microcatheter to the fistulous point (B, black arrow). After the injection of 0.3 mL of Onyx 34 into the venous sac, repeat ECA injection demonstrates persistent filling of the fistula with outflow via both the IOV and, to a lesser extent, the SOV (C, double black arrows). Subsequent injection of an additional 0.3 mL of Onyx 34 resulted in complete occlusion of the CCF, and the feeding accessory meningeal artery was occluded down to its entry at the foramen of Vesalius (D, double white arrows).

Continued

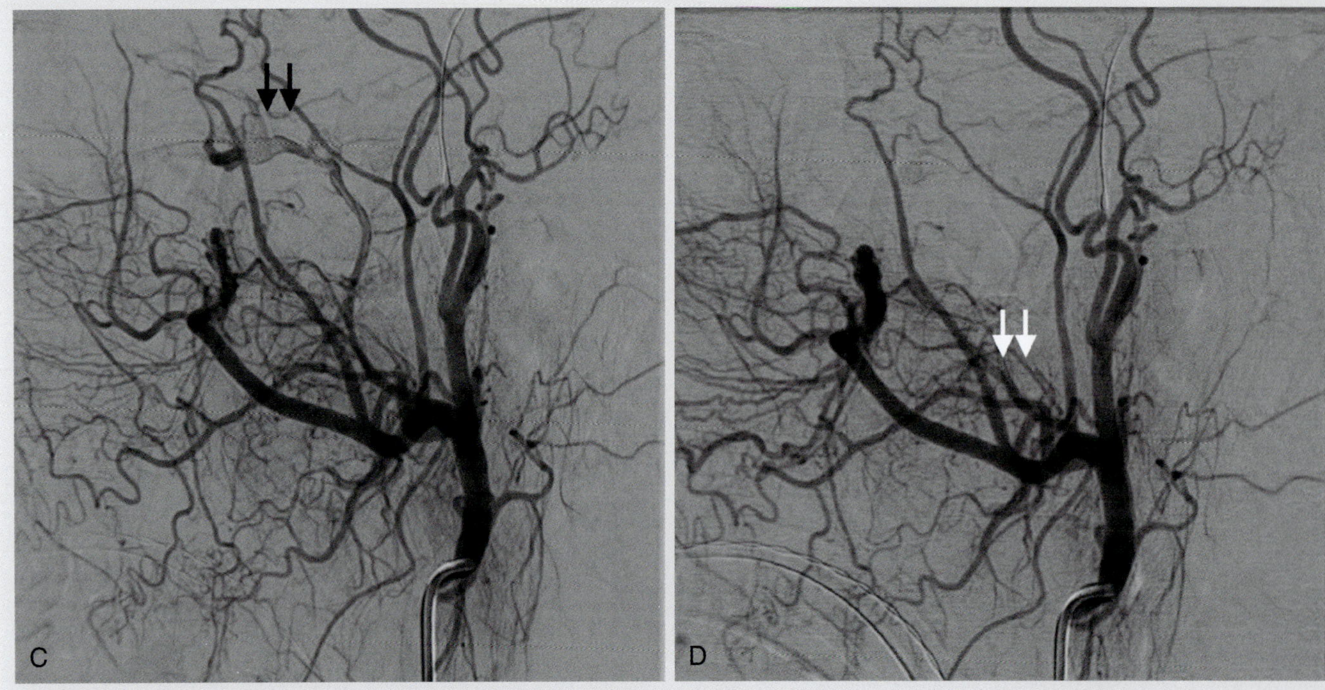

• Fig. 43.3, cont'd

NEUROSURGICAL SELFIE MOMENT

Endovascular approaches should be considered first-line for the vast majority of CCFs and dAVFs. Although technical advances have increased the safety and successful occlusion of both transvenous and transarterial approaches to these lesions, these advances are no substitute for a comprehensive knowledge of cerebrovascular anatomy, particularly dangerous anastomoses of feeding arteries and venous outflow of fistulas. This is particularly true because small-vessel anatomy may not be clearly evident angiographically, even with supraselective runs, and flow patterns may change drastically over the course of embolization.

References

1. Barrow DL, Spector RH, Braun IF, Landman JA, Tindall SC, Tindall GT. Classification and treatment of spontaneous carotid-cavernous sinus fistulas. *J Neurosurg*. 1985;62(2):248–256.
2. Ellis JA, Goldstein H, Connolly ES, Meyers PM. Carotid-cavernous fistulas. *Neurosurg Focus*. 2012;32(5):E9.
3. Wilson CB, Markesbery W. Traumatic carotid-cavernous fistula with fatal epistaxis. Report of a case. *J Neurosurg*. 1966;24(1):111–113.
4. Hiramatsu K, Utsumi S, Kyoi K, et al. Intracerebral hemorrhage in carotid-cavernous fistula. *Neuroradiology*. 1991;33(1):67–69.
5. Borden JA, Wu JK, Shucart WA. A proposed classification for spinal and cranial dural arteriovenous fistulous malformations and implications for treatment. *J Neurosurg*. 1995;82(2):166–179.
6. Cognard C, Gobin YP, Pierot L, et al. Cerebral dural arteriovenous fistulas: clinical and angiographic correlation with a revised classification of venous drainage. *Radiology*. 1995;194(3):671–680.
7. Rammos S, Bortolotti C, Lanzino G. Endovascular management of intracranial dural arteriovenous fistulae. *Neurosurg Clin N Am*. 2014;25(3):539–549.
8. McConnell KA, Tjoumakaris SI, Allen J, et al. Neuroendovascular management of dural arteriovenous malformations. *Neurosurg Clin N Am*. 2009;20(4):431–439.
9. Parkinson D. Lateral sellar compartment O.T. (cavernous sinus): history, anatomy, terminology. *Anat Rec*. 1998;251(4):486–490.
10. Sekhar LN, Biswas A, Hallam D, Kim LJ, Douglas J, Ghodke B. Neuroendovascular management of tumors and vascular malformations of the head and neck. *Neurosurg Clin N Am*. 2009;20(4):453–485.
11. Chan HHL, Asadi H, Dowling R, Hardy TG, Mitchell PJ. Facial nerve injury as a complication of endovascular treatment for cavernous dural arteriovenous fistula. *Orbit*. 2014;33(6):462–464.
12. Phan K, Xu J, Leung V, et al. Orbital approaches for treatment of carotid cavernous fistulas: a systematic review. *World Neurosurg*. 2016; 96(C):243–251.
13. Awad IA, Little JR, Akarawi WP, Ahl J. Intracranial dural arteriovenous malformations: factors predisposing to an aggressive neurological course. *J Neurosurg*. 1990;72(6):839–850.
14. Geibprasert S, Pongpech S, Armstrong D, Krings T. Dangerous extracranial-intracranial anastomoses and supply to the cranial nerves: vessels the neurointerventionalist needs to know. *AJNR Am J Neuroradiol*. 2009;30(8):1459–1468.
15. Lasjaunias P, Berenstein A, ter Brugge KG. *Clinical vascular anatomy and variations*. Berlin, Heidelberg: Springer; 2001.
16. Perrini P, Cardia A, Fraser K, Lanzino G. A microsurgical study of the anatomy and course of the ophthalmic artery and its possibly dangerous anastomoses. *J Neurosurg*. 2007;106(1):142–150.
17. Nyberg EM, Chaudry MI, Turk AS, Turner RD. Transient cranial neuropathies as sequelae of Onyx embolization of arteriovenous shunt lesions near the skull base: possible axonotmetic traction injuries. *J Neurointerv Surg*. 2013;5(4):e21.
18. Hu YC, Newman CB, Dashti SR, Albuquerque FC, McDougall CG. Cranial dural arteriovenous fistula: transarterial Onyx embolization experience and technical nuances. *J Neurointerv Surg*. 2011;3(1): 5–13.
19. Lv X, Jiang C, Zhang J, Li Y, Wu Z. Complications related to percutaneous transarterial embolization of intracranial dural arteriovenous fistulas in 40 patients. *AJNR Am J Neuroradiol*. 2009;30(3): 462–468.
20. de Castro-Afonso LH, Trivelato FP, Rezende MT, et al. Transvenous embolization of dural carotid cavernous fistulas: the role of liquid

embolic agents in association with coils on patient outcomes. *J Neurointerv Surg*. 2018;10(5):461–462.

21. Pradeep N, Nottingham R, Kam A, Gandhi D, Razack N. Treatment of post-traumatic carotid–cavernous fistulas using pipeline embolization device assistance. *BMJ Case Rep*. 2015;bcr2015011786.
22. Torok CM, Nogueira RG, Yoo AJ, et al. Transarterial venous sinus occlusion of dural arteriovenous fistulas using Onyx. *Interv Neuroradiol.* 2016;22(6):711–716.
23. Vanlandingham M, Fox B, Hoit D, Elijovich L, Arthur AS. Endovascular treatment of intracranial dural arteriovenous fistulas. *Neurosurgery*. 2014;74:S42–S49.
24. Lv X, Jiang C, Li Y, Liu L, Liu J, Wu Z. The limitations and risks of transarterial Onyx injections in the treatment of grade I and II DAVFs. *Eur J Radiol.* 2011;80(3):e385–e388.
25. Chandra RV, Leslie-Mazwi TM, Mehta BP, et al. Transarterial onyx embolization of cranial dural arteriovenous fistulas: long-term follow-up. *AJNR Am J Neuroradiol.* 2014;35(9):1793–1797.
26. Rabinov JD, Yoo AJ, Ogilvy CS, Carter BS, Hirsch JA. Onyx versus n-BCA for embolization of cranial dural arteriovenous fistulas. *J Neurointerv Surg*. 2013;5(4):306–310.
27. Watanabe J, Maruya J, Nishimaki K, Ito Y. Onyx removal after embolization of a superior sagittal sinus dural arteriovenous fistula involving scalp artery. *Surg Neurol Int*. 2016;7(15):410.
28. Gross BA, Albuquerque FC, Moon K, McDougall CG. The road less traveled: transarterial embolization of dural arteriovenous fistulas via the ascending pharyngeal artery. *J Neurointerv Surg*. 2016;9(1):97–101.
29. Zanaty M, Chalouhi N, Tjoumakaris SI, Hasan D, Rosenwasser RH, Jabbour P. Endovascular treatment of carotid-cavernous fistulas. *Neurosurg Clin N Am*. 2014;25(3):551–563.

44

Complications After Decompressive Craniectomy and Cranioplasty

JEFFREY V. ROSENFELD, JIN W. TEE

HIGHLIGHTS

- The common complications of decompressive craniectomy are acute postoperative hemorrhage (subgaleal, epidural, subdural), delayed subdural effusion, hydrocephalus, and syndrome of the trephined.
- The common complications of cranioplasty are resorption of cranial bone flap, subflap hematomas, and infection.
- The cranioplasty should be performed as early as possible after the brain swelling has subsided and before the late complications of decompressive craniectomy have developed. The management of decompressed patients with secondary hydrocephalus is challenging.
- An uncommon but serious complication of decompressive craniectomy is paradoxical herniation with brainstem compression, which is a life-threatening emergency.
- An uncommon but serious complication of cranioplasty is massive postoperative cerebral swelling with subsequent death.
- Careful surgical planning, meticulous surgical technique, and assiduous postoperative care will help prevent much of the morbidity associated with decompressive craniectomy and cranioplasty.
- The commonest error in surgical technique is to make the craniectomy too small, which results in inadequate relief of intracranial hypertension and results in brain herniation out of the defect and further secondary brain injury.

Background

Decompressive craniectomy (DC) and subsequent cranioplasty are common operations in neurosurgical practice. The purpose of DC is to control elevated intracranial pressure (ICP). The indications for DC are blunt or penetrating severe traumatic brain injury (TBI), malignant middle cerebral artery occlusion syndrome, acute cerebellar infarction, acute cerebellar hemorrhage, acute intra- or postoperative cerebral swelling/hematoma, and refractory nontraumatic intracranial hypertension in children due to infection, infarction, or Reye's syndrome.

The controversies surrounding the indications, timing, and selection of patients for DC are not discussed in this chapter. The surgical technique for unilateral hemicraniectomy and bilateral frontotemporo-parietal DC has been well described.[1,2] The size of the craniectomy is an important consideration because an inadequately sized craniectomy will not adequately control the intracranial hypertension and will result in a brain herniation out of the defect with secondary injury to this brain, particularly at the edges of the defect where veins are occluded. The herniated brain may be hemorrhagic and infarcted when re-explored.

The fourth edition of the Brain Trauma Foundation guidelines recommends that a unilateral frontotemporo-parietal DC in the civilian context be not less than 12 × 5 cm or 15 cm in diameter.[3] Bell et al., from their military experience with bomb blasts and penetrating TBI due to gunshot wounds, recommend that a hemicraniectomy for frontotemporo-parietal decompression have at a minimum dimensions of 14 cm anteroposterior by 12 cm superioinferior.[4]

The systematic review by Kurland et al. subtyped DC-associated complications into three main types: (1) hemorrhagic, (2) infection/inflammatory, and (3) disturbances of the cerebrospinal compartment. According to their analysis, one in 10 patients undergoing a DC suffers a complication necessitating additional medical or surgical intervention.[5] Individual studies have reported a high incidence of complications overall. In a series of 164 patients who had DC for TBI, 81 patients (55.5%) had at least one complication.[6] The occurrence of at least one complication was significantly associated with an increased risk of prolonged hospital or rehabilitation stay after adjusting for the predicted risk of unfavorable outcome from the TBI.[6] In a series of 108 patients with TBI, 50% developed complications related to the surgical decompression, and of these, 25.9% of patients developed more than one type of complication.[7] Older patients and those with more severe head trauma had a higher occurrence of complications. In a series of 12 children who had DC after severe TBI, the most frequent complications were hygroma formation (83%), aseptic bone resorption of the reimplanted bone (50%), hydrocephalus (42%), secondary infection or dysfunction of ventriculoperitoneal shunt (25%) or cranioplasty (33%), and epilepsy. 75% of the patients required reoperation in addition to the cranioplasty, with up to 8 interventions.[8]

The common complications after DC are acute postoperative hematoma, brain herniation through the bone defect, subdural effusion, expansion of hemorrhagic contusions, seizures, hydrocephalus, and syndrome of the trephined.[5,6] New contralateral or remote subdural or epidural hematomas may also occur, usually during the first week after DC.[5,7,9] Hemorrhagic transformation of ischemic infarction has been reported after DC.[5] Infectious complications include meningitis, ventriculitis, and wound infection (Figs 44.1–44.3).

The common complications of cranioplasty are new ipsilateral hematoma (usually epidural); infectious, inflammatory, and wound healing complications (superficial or deep, including abscess formation and osteomyelitis); meningitis and ventriculitis; cerebrospinal fluid (CSF) disturbance including subdural effusion/hygroma and CSF leak/fistula; bone flap aseptic necrosis and resorption and cosmetic defects; less commonly, seizures; and hydrocephalus.[5,10,11] A rare, fatal allergy to titanium bone replacement has been reported.[12] Zanaty et al. reported an overall complication rate of 31.3% and a mortality rate of 3.16% in a mixed series of 348 cranioplasties.[13]

Anatomic Insights

The scalp flaps for DC should be planned carefully. The scalp flaps are large, and the main blood supply for the hemicraniectomy flap is from the superficial temporal artery (STA). The STA and its accompanying draining veins should be preserved to avoid scalp flap ischemia and subsequent wound breakdown. The STA should be palpated and marked on the scalp so that the incision avoids it. The scalp flap can reach the midline, but the bone cuts must avoid the major venous sinuses (sagittal and transverse). Some neurosurgeons leave a central bone strut over the sagittal sinus to protect the sinus. It is helpful to mark out the position of the venous sinuses and the scalp incision before draping commences.

A flap design that lessens the risk of ischemia of large scalp flaps is the T-shaped incision that is favored by some military surgeons. A midline sagittal incision with a "T-bar" extension was described by Ludwig G. Kempe for hemispherectomy.[14] The midline incision extends from the hairline to the inion. The T-bar incision starts 1 to 2 cm anterior to the tragus at the root of the zygoma and extends superiorly to meet the midline incision just behind the coronal suture. This incision largely preserves the STA and occipital artery angiosomes.

Falx. The anterior falx is frequently divided along with the sagittal sinus during the bifrontal craniectomy. A bilateral horizontal fish-mouth opening in the dura including falx and sagittal sinus division was described by Polin et al.[15] This theoretically permits both cerebral hemispheres and the corpus callosum to expand forward without being tethered or injured by the falx. An alternative is to open the dura separately on each side without dividing the falx.

Frontal sinus. The lower bone cut for the bifrontal craniectomy may open the frontal sinus. The surgeon can avoid the sinus by steering the craniotome above it, but a small opening should be covered with pericranial flap. A larger opening requires "cranialization" of the sinus, including removal of the posterior wall of the sinus and the mucosa of the sinus. This will help prevent infection and late mucocele formation.

Air cells are present in the temporal and sphenoid bones. The hemicraniectomy may open these air cells. The surgeon should carefully examine the exposed bone edge for any air cells and occlude them with bone wax to prevent CSF leaks. Larger air cell openings will require a flap of pericranium to close them.

Cerebrospinal fluid pathways. CSF dynamics are disturbed after DC. CSF fistula between the subarachnoid space or ventricles could lead to subdural hygromas and pseudomeningoceles. Also,

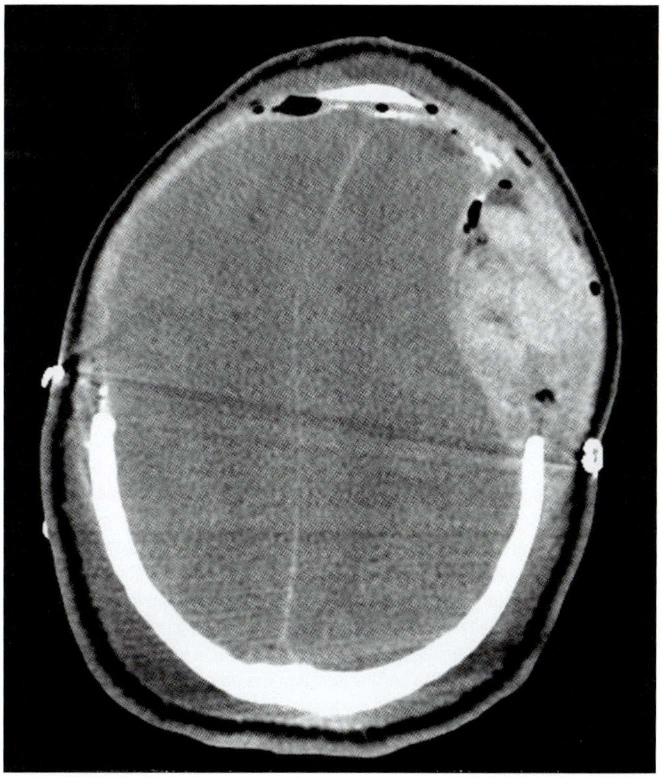

• **Fig. 44.1** Early postoperative computed tomography scan showing acute subgaleal and subdural hematoma in a patient with severe traumatic brain injury and coagulopathy who has had a decompressive craniectomy.

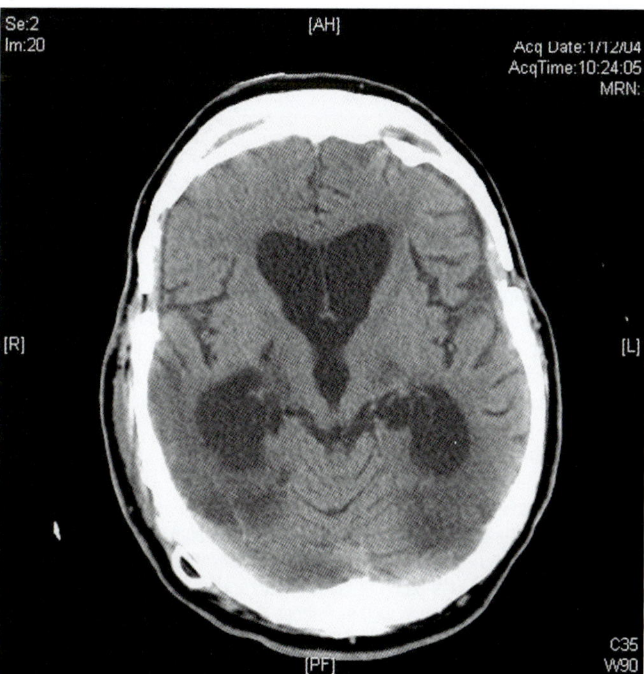

• **Fig. 44.2** Late computed tomography scan after bifrontal cranioplasty in a patient with severe traumatic brain injury. Gross communicating hydrocephalus developed, which required ventriculoperitoneal shunting.

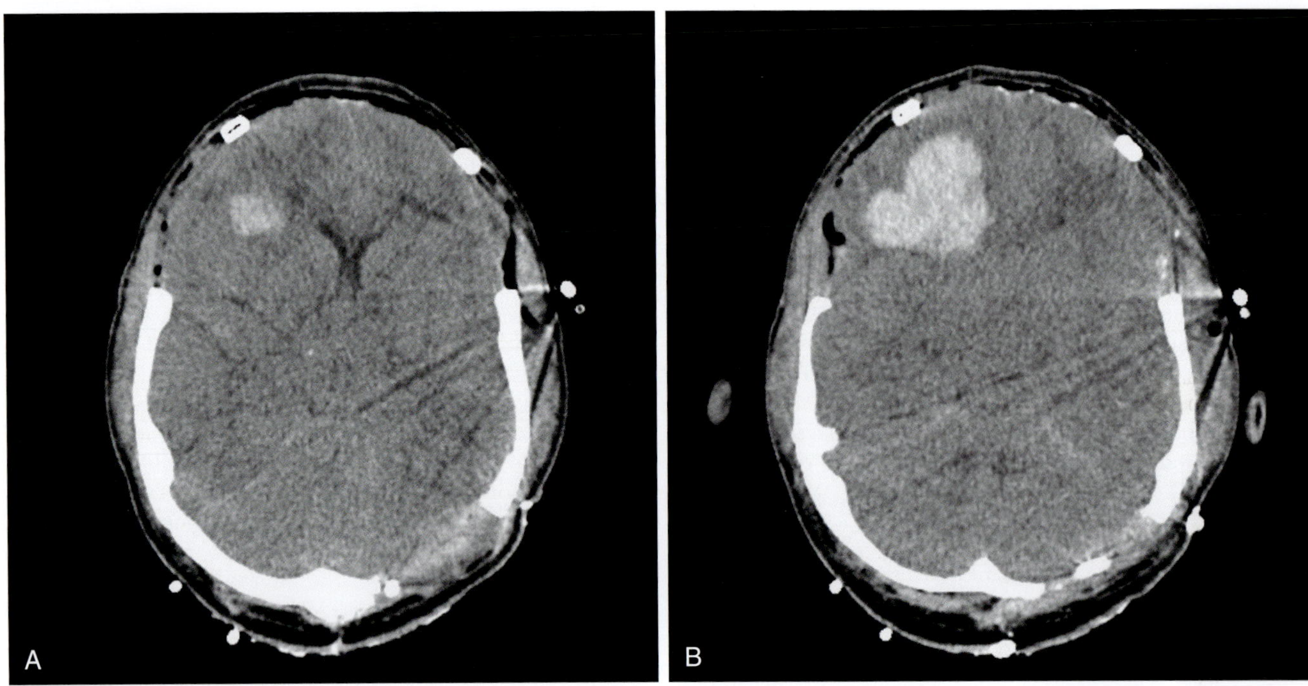

• **Fig. 44.3** (A) Early computed tomography (CT) scan after a bifrontal decompressive craniectomy for severe traumatic brain injury. Note the small right frontal intracerebral hematoma. A left parietal craniotomy was performed for an epidural collection. (B) CT scan 24 hours later showing enlargement of the intracerebral hematoma.

the entry of blood into the ventricular system could lead to communicating hydrocephalus. A further suggested mechanism is an increased venous outflow to the sagittal sinus after DC that results in an increase in extracellular fluid absorption, reduced brain parenchyma volume, and increased ventricular size.[16] The development of an interhemispheric hygroma that occurs within the first 9 days after DC is a predictive radiologic sign for hydrocephalus developing within the first 6 months in patients with severe TBI.[17]

RED FLAGS

Decompressive Craniectomy

Coagulopathy will increase the risk of hemorrhagic complications. Reversal of the coagulopathy should occur preoperatively or be continued intraoperatively in an emergency.

Hemorrhagic cerebral contusions frequently expand after DC. In a retrospective study of 40 consecutive patients, new or expanded hemorrhagic contusions ≥5 cc were observed in 48% of patients having a hemicraniectomy. Expanded hemorrhagic contusion volume >20 cc after hemicraniectomy was strongly associated with poor outcome and mortality.[18] The expansion of contusions may also occur in the absence of a DC. Particular attention should be directed to optimizing coagulation parameters in these patients.

Inadequate wound debridement in compound injuries to the cranium will increase the risk of wound breakdown and infection.

Dura left open. The dura should ideally be closed watertight after DC by duroplasty using a dural patch of fascia, pericranium, or dural substitute. This prevents CSF fistula as well as subflap and subgaleal collections and reduces the risk of infection.

Open frontal sinus will increase the risk of CSF rhinorrhea, infection, and mucocele.

One-layer scalp closure will increase the risk of poor scalp healing and CSF fistula and wound infection. The scalp should be closed in two layers.

Tense scalp closure will increase the risk of wound edge necrosis, wound dehiscence, CSF fistula, and infection.

Seizures may indicate progressive intracranial pathology such as postoperative hemorrhage, infection, and swelling and should be investigated.

Fever may indicate intracranial infection. Cranial infections typically do not manifest in the first five postoperative days and may be accompanied by fever, reddening of the wound site, and elevated white cell counts and C-reactive protein (CRP) values.

Deteriorating cognitive function or conscious state requires urgent imaging and further investigation.

CSF fistula (wound/nose/ear)

Chronic headaches, seizures, and cognitive decline may be signs of a low-grade infection that will need to be investigated with infection markers and imaging. If a collection is developing around the bone flap or substitute, re-exploration and removal of the flap may be required if infection is the likely cause.

Sunken scalp flap. The development of new focal neurologic deficits and cognitive decline raises the possibility of the *syndrome of the trephined* or sinking skin flap syndrome.[19] In this condition, the difference between atmospheric and intracranial pressure due to the absence of the cranium causes the scalp to be infolded, and mass effect to be exerted on the cerebral cortex, affecting cerebral perfusion and CSF flow dynamics. This syndrome occurs 5.1 ± 10.8 months after the DC for trauma. The presenting symptoms include unilateral motor deficits, cognitive deficits, language deficits, altered level of consciousness, headache, seizure, and cranial nerve deficits. Investigations include electroencephalography, computed tomography (CT) perfusion scan, and phase contrast magnetic resonance imaging. The neurologic deficits are usually recoverable in the ensuing days to months after the cranioplasty. In many cases improvement is seen within 24 hours of cranioplasty. Minimizing the time interval to cranioplasty will reduce the risk of this complication.[19] The bone should be replaced when the brain swelling has subsided and the patient is fit enough for surgery. This is usually at 4 to 6 weeks after the DC.

CSF drainage by lumbar puncture, ventriculostomy, lumbar drain on continuous drainage, or ventriculoperitoneal shunt exacerbates the pressure gradient of atmospheric pressure exceeding ICP, which may precipitate downward shift of the brain, tonsillar herniation, and death. This is called **paradoxical herniation (PH)** because it occurs in the presence of a sunken bone flap. This is a life-threatening emergency. PH occurred in 13/429 (3.03%) consecutive DCs, and all 13 patients were treated and survived beyond 6 months.[20] PH may also occur in the absence of CSF drainage.[21] Upright posture, mannitol, and hyperventilation may also be risk factors.[5] The patient is placed in the Trendelenburg position (15 degrees, head down) and hydrated intravenously, and CSF drainage is ceased.

Unprotected brain at the site of the craniectomy. The patient should be fitted with a custom-made plastic helmet (Fig. 44.1) to protect the exposed brain, and this should be worn even before the patient is mobilized. Direct trauma to the craniectomy site may have serious consequences or result in death (Fig. 44.4).[22]

Cranioplasty

Elevating the scalp flap overlying exposed cerebral cortex. If the dura has not been closed, the scalp adheres to the cortex with fibrous adhesions. At the cranioplasty, the neurosurgeon must be very careful not to injure the cortex when the scalp is reflected. These injuries to the cortex cause bleeding and further scarring and heighten the risk of epilepsy. These patients should receive prophylactic anticonvulsants.

Large defect and sunken scalp. The development of massive cerebral swelling with fixed dilated pupils is an uncommon event after cranioplasty but particularly affects young men who have had TBI and a DC with a large bony defect and significantly sunken craniotomy site. The negative pressure of subgaleal drains may have contributed.[23] This complication may also occur in patients who developed hydrocephalus post DC and required ventriculoperitoneal shunts.[24] The mechanism may relate to altered brain compliance and disturbed autoregulation. This disastrous complication should be included in the consent process. Suction drains should be avoided.

Titanium mesh. We have observed scalp thinning and eventual ulceration overlying titanium mesh. We have had to remove the titanium. The mesh seems to create a suction effect on the scalp. Covering the mesh with methyl methacrylate should prevent this complication.

Delayed cranioplasty. The scalp shrinks progressively when the bone is missing for months, and when the bone flap or bone substitute flap is replaced, the scalp has to be stretched over the restored curve of the skull, which creates tension on the wound. A rotation flap may be required to ease the tension, and a split skin graft is placed on the pericranium (not directly on bone) to cover the donor site. Tissue expanders with a temporary acrylic graft have also been used.[25]

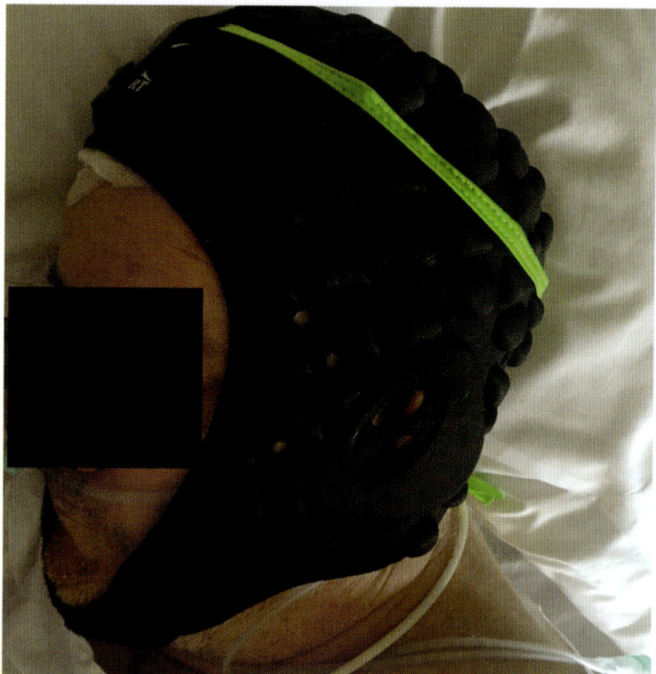

• **Fig. 44.4** A patient wearing a custom-made plastic helmet to protect the brain after decompressive craniectomy.

Risk Factors

The optimal timing of cranioplasty is uncertain. Malcolm et al. in a systematic review and metaanalysis reported that cranioplasty within 90 days after DC was associated with increased odds of hydrocephalus, but there was no difference in odds of developing other complications. In the trauma population, there were fewer extraaxial collections with earlier cranioplasty.[26] However, Huang et al. found no relation of neurologic outcome to timing of cranioplasty.[27] We recommend early cranioplasty with the aim of normalizing ICP and vascular dynamics after DC.

Perioperative risk factors for complications after cranioplasty were identified in a retrospective review of 348 patients. Predictors of complications were hypertension, hemorrhagic stroke, diabetes mellitus, seizures, bifrontal cranioplasty, and repeated surgery for hematoma evacuation. This provides the neurosurgeon with better information to assess risk, control risk factors, and treat complications at an early stage.[13]

The method of storage of bone flaps by cryopreservation or subcutaneous abdominal implantation does not seem to differ in terms of infection, resorption, or reoperation.[28] Bone flap resorption is associated with young age, bone flap fragmentation, long storage time, and Glasgow Outcome Scale at the time of cranioplasty.[29]

There is a lower rate of reoperation for cranioplasty in patients who have had bone substitute implants such as titanium compared with autologous bone replacement. This is because of resorption of autologous bone, particularly in patients <30 years of age and in older patients with fragmented flaps.[30,31] Complete resorption of autologous bone flaps was reported in 22% of patients in the randomized controlled trial (RCT) of Honeybul et al.[31] Takeuchi et al. reported only one patient out of 40 with mild bone resorption when the autologous bone flaps were cryopreserved with glycerol.[32] Lindner et al. performed an RCT comparing custom-made hydroxylapatite (HA) cranioplasty with titanium and found that there was a higher number of epidural hematomas in the HA group. Infection and reoperation rates were similar between the two groups.[33]

Wound dehiscence and the presence of a postoperative fluid collection are common factors associated with infections after cranioplasty.[34]

Prevention

Preoperative

The patient's medical fitness, nutritional status, coagulation profile, immune status, and electrolytes should be optimized before cranioplasty. This is not possible before the emergent DC.

Perioperative

Thorough cleansing of skin contamination is performed. Prophylactic antibiotics and antiepileptic drugs (AEDs) are administered.

The choice of antibiotics depends on the degree of contamination.[35] In a noncontaminated DC, the antibiotics are continued 24 hours; in a contaminated case, for 5 days. Prophylactic AEDs are continued for 7 days after DC and are recommenced if seizures occur.

Prevention of hydrocephalus. Waziri et al. found a strong correlation between prolonged time to replacement of bone flap and persistence of hydrocephalus,[36] although these findings were not replicated in a similar study.[37] Nevertheless, we aim for early cranioplasty, which may restore normal ICP dynamics and prevent persistent hydrocephalus and thus the need for permanent CSF diversion. De Bonis et al. studied 41 patients who underwent DC for closed head injury. The distance of the craniectomy from the midline was independently associated with the development of hydrocephalus. When the superior limit of the craniectomy was <25 mm from the midline, those patients had a markedly increased risk of developing hydrocephalus (OR = 17). Based on this evidence, the superior limit of the DC should be performed >25 mm from the midline to lessen the chance of hydrocephalus.[16] One additional step we have found helpful (if the wound is not compromised), is to place a piece of sterile plastic sheeting between the dura and the scalp. At the time of cranioplasty, there are no adhesions and the scalp can be elevated freely off the plastic.

Epidural fluid collections after cranioplasty may be reduced by attention to closure of the dura at the time of cranioplasty.[38] Dural hitching sutures should be used where the dura splits away from the skull edge to avoid epidural hematoma formation. The placement of a Poppen suture in the center of the dura at the time of cranioplasty may help prevent postoperative epidural collections.

Management of Complications

Some aspects of management have been discussed above. Patient deterioration or instability requires urgent reimaging. Epidural or subdural hematomas may require evacuation depending on size and mass effect. Persistent CSF fistula will require investigation for the source of the fistula and re-exploration and sealing of the dural opening either by re-exploring the craniectomy wound or performing an endoscopic transnasal skull base repair. Suspected infections after cranioplasty will usually require re-exploration and removal of the bone flap or bone substitute and extended periods of administration of intravenous antibiotic through a peripherally inserted central catheter (PICC) line. Bone flap resorption will require revision of the cranioplasty and replacement with acrylic titanium or HA.

Subdural effusions or hygromas or effusions are usually small, ipsilateral to the craniectomy, and resolve spontaneously. Application of an early pressure dressing with an elastic bandage over the scalp for 7 to 10 days after DC was found to reduce subdural effusions in a controlled trial of 169 patients. The control group had general wrapping of the scalp.[39] Contralateral subdural effusions are less common and may cause symptomatic cerebral compression and should be suspected in patients having delayed neurologic deterioration, particularly where the flap is bulging. They may also occur in those who have remained in a poor neurologic state. The probable cause of these contralateral effusions is an arachnoid tear. One treatment option is to place a subdural-peritoneal shunt and perform a simultaneous cranioplasty. This is effective in relieving the subdural collection and in improving alertness and motor deficit, but some patients will still develop hydrocephalus. They may require a ventriculoperitoneal shunt in addition to the subdural–peritoneal shunt.[40] An alternative is tapping the effusion and applying cranial strapping.[41]

Hydrocephalus

Symptomatic or progressive hydrocephalus will require CSF diversion. The timing of shunt placement in relation to the cranioplasty is not straightforward. Shunting without cranioplasty would worsen the sinking of the flap, promote further brain shift, and could precipitate paradoxical coning. The preferred options are to place a shunt at the same time as the cranioplasty, or alternatively, an external ventricular drain is placed at the same time as the cranioplasty. The ICP is monitored for 3 to 5 days, then the ventriculoperitoneal shunt is placed. Based on the results, the most appropriate opening pressure is chosen if a simple valve is available. However, the use of a programmable valve will allow for regular noninvasive revision of the pressure. In a series of 23 patients, Pachatouridis et al. found that the latter sequence had fewer complications.[42]

SURGICAL REWIND

My Worst Case

A 55-year-old man was involved in an interstate motor vehicle accident with fatality at the scene. He was found at the scene with a Glasgow Coma Scale (GCS) score of 3 and a dilated left pupil. Investigations at the regional trauma service revealed a large left-sided acute subdural hemorrhage causing significant midline shift and uncal herniation (Fig. 44.5A). Because there was no neurosurgical service in that remote setting, a general surgeon performed a lifesaving DC and hematoma evacuation (Fig. 44.5B). After stabilization of his other injuries (abdomen and chest), he was transferred to our state trauma service 4 weeks later (6 weeks after the accident).

On arrival at our Level 1 trauma center, he had a GCS of 5 with a right-sided hemiplegia. On removal of his head dressings, the skin flap edge was necrotic and a large tense pseudomeningocele was present. An urgent CT scan was performed (Fig. 44.5C) that showed gross hydrocephalus. A wound swab was also sent off, which returned florid growth of gram-positive cocci. There was no contrast enhancement beneath the scalp. He was started on intravenous meropenem and vancomycin while awaiting pathogen identification and antibiotic sensitivities. An external ventricular drain (EVD) was placed to treat the hydrocephalus. Two further EVDs were placed due to intraluminal blockages. The third blocked EVD was removed, and a lumbar drain was inserted. Two hours later, the patient dropped his GCS from 10 to 5 and was found to be bradycardic and hypertensive with bilateral dilated pupils. He had a generalized tonic-clonic seizure. An urgent CT brain showed a large-volume intracerebral and intraventricular hemorrhage with mass effect (Fig. 44.5D). The scan also showed transcalvarial herniation, leftward subfalcine, and right-sided uncal herniation. Based on the severity of his original injury, the complications, and the poor prognosis for meaningful recovery, further active management was thought to be futile, and he received palliative care and died.

The complications (aside from the TBI itself) followed a craniectomy that was too small, tense scalp flap with necrotic edge, wound infection, hydrocephalus requiring EVDs and spinal drainage, gross cerebral herniation, and hemorrhage after removal on an EVD.

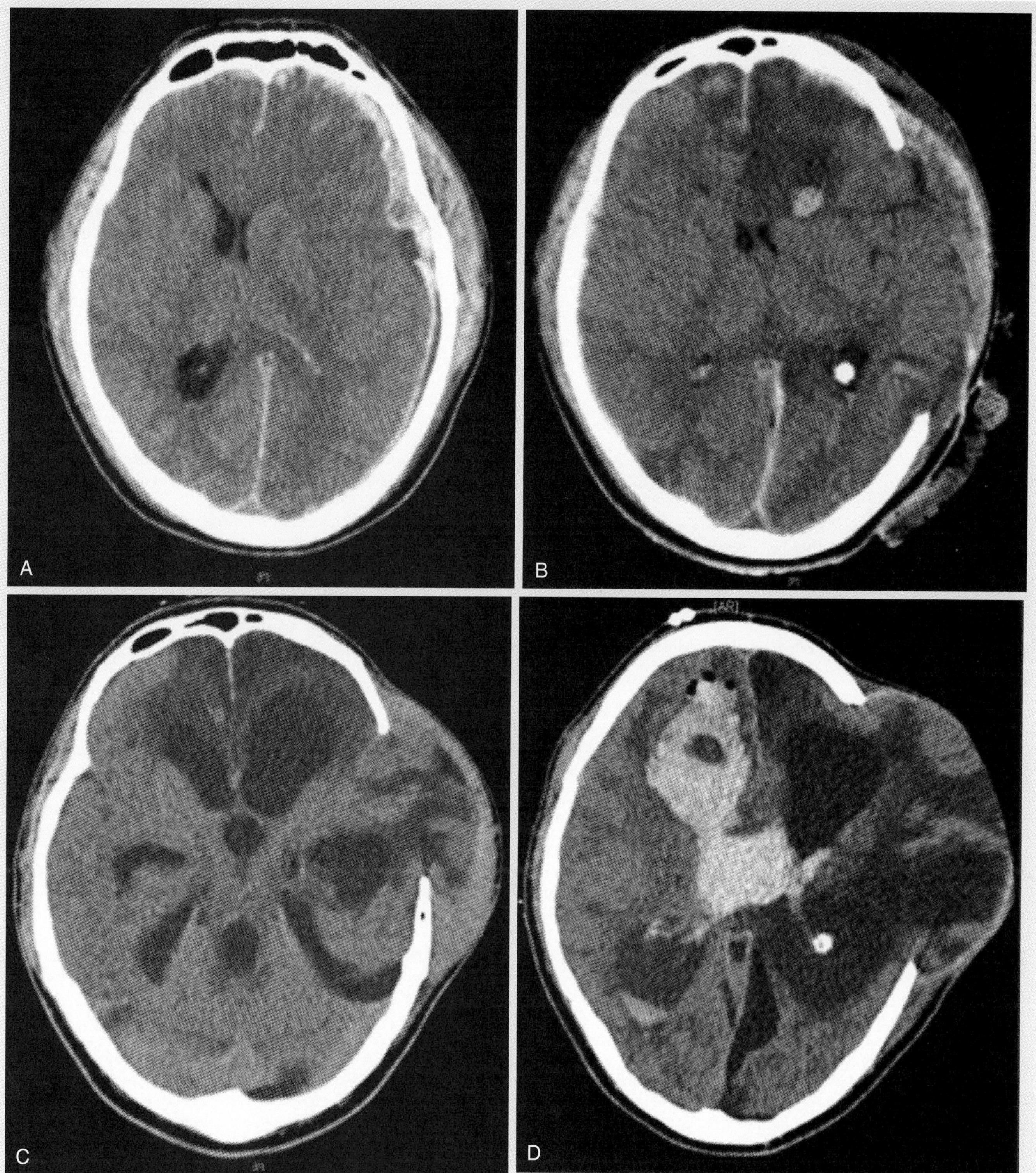

• **Fig. 44.5** (A) computed tomography (CT) scan showing an extensive right-sided acute subdural hemorrhage (SDH) with falcine hemorrhage, significant left hemisphere swelling, and gross midline shift in a 55-year-old male after a motor vehicle accident. Note also the bilateral scalp hematomas. (B) Postoperative CT scan showing the craniectomy and the evacuation of the acute SDH. The craniectomy size is inadequate. There is brain herniation with partial correction of the midline shift, a new deep left frontal intracerebral hematoma, and bifrontal edema. (C) CT brain showing severe generalized hydrocephalus and severe focal brain herniation through the craniectomy site. Note the bifrontal edema/infarction. (D) CT scan showing a large intracerebral and intraventricular hemorrhage with gross hydrocephalus, left frontal lobe infarction, posterior left parafalcine hygroma, and grotesque cerebral herniation through the skull defect.

NEUROSURGICAL SELFIE MOMENT

Complications after DC and cranioplasty are frequent and range from the minor to the most major life-threatening events, such as PH after DC and diffuse brain swelling and coning after cranioplasty. The neurosurgeon should carefully consider the risk-benefit ratio before proceeding with a DC, because the surgery is a major procedure with significant risks. As with all neurosurgery, avoidance of complications after DC and cranioplasty requires the patient to be in optimal medical condition, and it necessitates meticulous surgical technique and assiduous postoperative care of the patient. The neurosurgeon should have knowledge of all the potential complications and should use all the preventive strategies required to lessen these risks. DC and cranioplasty may seem to be straightforward procedures and are often relegated to the most junior member of the neurosurgery team, but this delegation will likely result in a higher incidence of complications. These operations are often challenging even for experienced neurosurgeons. They are great learning experiences for trainees, but adequate supervision is required to ensure optimal performance of this unforgiving surgery.

References

1. Ragel BT, Klimo P Jr, Martin JE, Teff RJ, Bakken HE, Armonda RA. Wartime decompressive craniectomy: technique and lessons learned. *Neurosurg*. 2010;28(5):E2.
2. Quinn TM, Taylor JJ, Magarik JA, Vought E, Kindy MS, Ellegala DB. Decompressive craniectomy: technical note. *Acta Neurol Scand*. 2011;123(4):239–244.
3. Carney N, Totten AM, O'Reilly C, et al. Guidelines for the management of severe traumatic brain injury, fourth edition. *Neurosurgery*. 2017;80(1):6–15.
4. Bell RS, Mossop CM, Dirks MS, et al. Early decompressive craniectomy for severe penetrating and closed head injury during wartime. *Neurosurg*. 2010;28(5):E1.
5. Kurland DB, Khaladj-Ghom A, Stokum JA, et al. Complications associated with decompressive craniectomy: a systematic review. *Neurocrit Care*. 2015;23(2):292–304.
6. Honeybul S, Ho KM. Long-term complications of decompressive craniectomy for head injury. *J Neurotrauma*. 2011;28(6):929–935.
7. Yang XF, Wen L, Shen F, et al. Surgical complications secondary to decompressive craniectomy in patients with a head injury: a series of 108 consecutive cases. *Acta Neurochir (Wien)*. 2008;150(12):1241–1247, discussion 1248.
8. Pechmann A, Anastasopoulos C, Korinthenberg R, van Velthoven-Wurster V, Kirschner J. Decompressive craniectomy after severe traumatic brain injury in children: complications and outcome. *Neuropediatrics*. 2015;46(1):5–12.
9. Stiver SI. Complications of decompressive craniectomy for traumatic brain injury. *Neurosurg Focus*. 2009;26(6):E7.
10. Sobani ZA, Shamim MS, Zafar SN, et al. Cranioplasty after decompressive craniectomy: an institutional audit and analysis of factors related to complications. *Surg Neurol Int*. 2011;2:123.
11. Gooch MR, Gin GE, Kenning TJ, German JW. Complications of cranioplasty following decompressive craniectomy: analysis of 62 cases. *Neurosurg Focus*. 2009;26(6):E9.
12. Hettige S, Norris JS. Mortality after local allergic response to titanium cranioplasty. *Acta Neurochir (Wien)*. 2012;154(9):1725–1726.
13. Zanaty M, Chalouhi N, Starke RM, et al. Complications following cranioplasty: incidence and predictors in 348 cases. *J Neurosurg*. 2015;123(1):182–188.
14. Kempe L. Hemispherectomy, in *Operative Neurosurgery*. New York, NY: Springer-Verlag; 1968, 180–189.
15. Polin RS, Shaffrey ME, Bogaev CA, et al. Decompressive bifrontal craniectomy in the treatment of severe refractory posttraumatic cerebral edema. *Neurosurgery*. 1997;41(1):84–92, discussion, 92–94.
16. De Bonis P, Pompucci A, Mangiola A, Rigante L, Anile C. Post-traumatic hydrocephalus after decompressive craniectomy: an underestimated risk factor. *J Neurotrauma*. 2010;27(11):1965–1970.
17. Kaen A, Jimenez-Roldan L, Alday R, et al. Interhemispheric hygroma after decompressive craniectomy: does it predict posttraumatic hydrocephalus? *J Neurosurg*. 2010;113(6):1287–1293.
18. Flint AC, Manley GT, Gean AD, Hemphill JC 3rd, Rosenthal G. Post-operative expansion of hemorrhagic contusions after unilateral decompressive hemicraniectomy in severe traumatic brain injury. *J Neurotrauma*. 2008;25(5):503–512.
19. Ashayeri K, MJ E, Huang J, Brem H, Gordon CR. Syndrome of the trephined: a systematic review. *Neurosurgery*. 2016;79(4):525–534.
20. Chen W, Guo J, Wu J, et al. Paradoxical herniation after unilateral decompressive craniectomy predicts better patient survival: a retrospective analysis of 429 cases. *Medicine (Baltimore)*. 2016;95(9): e2837.
21. Rahme R, Bojanowski MW. Overt cerebrospinal fluid drainage is not a sine qua non for paradoxical herniation after decompressive craniectomy: case report. *Neurosurgery*. 2010;67(1):214–215, discussion 215.
22. Honeybul S. Decompressive craniectomy: a new complication. *J Clin Neurosci*. 2009;16(5):727–729.
23. Sviri GE. Massive cerebral swelling immediately after cranioplasty, a fatal and unpredictable complication: report of 4 cases. *J Neurosurg*. 2015;123(5):1188–1193.
24. Honeybul S. Sudden death following cranioplasty: a complication of decompressive craniectomy for head injury. *Br J Neurosurg*. 2011;25(3):343–345.
25. Dos Santos Rubio EJ, Bos EM, Dammers R, Koudstaal MJ, Dumans AG. Two-stage cranioplasty: tissue expansion directly over the craniectomy defect prior to cranioplasty. *Craniomaxillofac Trauma Reconstr*. 2016;9(4):355–360.
26. Malcolm JG, Rindler RS, Chu JK, Grossberg JA, Pradilla G, Ahmad FU. Complications following cranioplasty and relationship to timing: a systematic review and meta-analysis. *J Clin Neurosci*. 2016;33:39–51.
27. Huang YH, Lee TC, Yang KY, Liao CC. Is timing of cranioplasty following posttraumatic craniectomy related to neurological outcome? *Int J Surg*. 2013;11(9):886–890.
28. Corliss B, Gooldy T, Vaziri S, Kubilis P, Murad G, Fargen K. Complications after in vivo and ex vivo autologous bone flap storage for cranioplasty: a comparative analysis of the literature. *World Neurosurg*. 2016;96:510–515.
29. Brommeland T, Rydning PN, Pripp AH, Helseth E. Cranioplasty complications and risk factors associated with bone flap resorption. *Scand J Trauma Resusc Emerg Med*. 2015;23:75.
30. Schwarz F, Dunisch P, Walter J, Sakr Y, Kalff R, Ewald C. Cranioplasty after decompressive craniectomy: is there a rationale for an initial artificial bone-substitute implant? A single-center experience after 631 procedures. *J Neurosurg*. 2016;124(3):710–715.
31. Honeybul S, Morrison DA, Ho KM, Lind CR, Geelhoed E. A randomized controlled trial comparing autologous cranioplasty with custom-made titanium cranioplasty. *J Neurosurg*. 2017;126(1):81–90.
32. Takeuchi H, Higashino Y, Hosoda T, et al. Long-term follow-up of cryopreservation with glycerol of autologous bone flaps for cranioplasty after decompressive craniectomy. *Acta Neurochir (Wien)*. 2016;158(3):571–575.
33. Lindner D, Schlothofer-Schumann K, Kern BC, Marx O, Muns A, Meixensberger J. Cranioplasty using custom-made hydroxyapatite versus titanium: a randomized clinical trial. *J Neurosurg*. 2017;126(1):175–183.
34. Riordan MA, Simpson VM, Hall WA. Analysis of factors contributing to infections after cranioplasty: a single-institution retrospective chart review. *World Neurosurg*. 2016;87:207–213.
35. Rosenfeld JV, Bell RS, Armonda R. Current concepts in penetrating and blast injury to the central nervous system. *World J Surg*. 2015;39(6):1352–1362.
36. Waziri A, Fusco D, Mayer SA, McKhann GM 2nd, Connolly ES Jr. Postoperative hydrocephalus in patients undergoing decompressive

hemicraniectomy for ischemic or hemorrhagic stroke. *Neurosurgery.* 2007;61(3):489–493, discussion 493–494.
37. Rahme R, Weil AG, Sabbagh M, Moumdjian R, Bouthillier A, Bojanowski MW. Decompressive craniectomy is not an independent risk factor for communicating hydrocephalus in patients with increased intracranial pressure. *Neurosurgery.* 2010;67(3):675–678, discussion 678.
38. Jeong SH, Wang US, Kim SW, Ha SW, Kim JK. Symptomatic epidural fluid collection following cranioplasty after decompressive craniectomy for traumatic brain injury. *Korean J Neurotrauma.* 2016;12(1):6–10.
39. Xu GZ, Li W, Liu KG, et al. Early pressure dressing for the prevention of subdural effusion secondary to decompressive craniectomy in patients with severe traumatic brain injury. *J Craniofac Surg.* 2014;25(5):1836–1839.
40. Lin MS, Chen TH, Kung WM, Chen ST. Simultaneous cranioplasty and subdural-peritoneal shunting for contralateral symptomatic subdural hygroma following decompressive craniectomy. *Scientific World Journal.* 2015;2015:518494.
41. Krishnan P, Roy Chowdhury S. Recurrent, symptomatic, late-onset, contralateral subdural effusion following decompressive craniectomy treated by cranial strapping. *Br J Neurosurg.* 2015;29(5):730–732.
42. Pachatouridis D, Alexiou GA, Zigouris A, et al. Management of hydrocephalus after decompressive craniectomy. *Turk Neurosurg.* 2014;24(6):855–858.

45

Complications After Surgery for Chronic Subdural Hematomas

EDOARDO VIAROLI, CORRADO IACCARINO, RODOLFO MADURI, ROY THOMAS DANIEL, FRANCO SERVADEI

Complications After Surgery for Chronic Subdural Hematomas

Chronic subdural hematoma (CSDH) (Fig. 45.1A–B) is an abnormal collection of liquefied blood degradation underneath the dura matter that may result in brain tissue compression and subsequent neurologic sequelae. Due to the aging population in developed countries, chronic subdural hematoma is becoming an increasingly common neurosurgical pathology that can reach up to 58.1 per 100,000 persons in the population over 65 years of age.[1,2] Toi et al.,[3] in a review of surgical databases on more than 63,000 cases, showed how the age of the patients has progressively increased in the last three decades. The high number of comorbidities at a higher age and the increasing number of surgeries for the evacuation of CSDH may lead to several complications due to a lack of evidence in the guidelines for the ideal management of this kind of hematoma.

Principal complication is a recurrence of the hematoma, which can reach a surprisingly high rate of 30% in some populations.[4]

Pathophysiological Insights

The physiopathology of chronic subdural hematoma still remains unclear. The most probable and cited hypothesis is that it starts as an acute subdural hematoma due to intermittent rupture of bridging veins in the subdural space. The persistence of blood in subdural space, often clinically asymptomatic due to cerebral atrophy of older people, enhances an inflammatory reaction; progressive involvement of fibroblasts leads to the formation of a cortical (or inner) and a dural (or outer) membrane. Inside this new "capsule," the clot of blood of ASDH is degraded by fibrinolytic enzymes and progressively liquefied; continuous proliferation of fibroblast may also lead to the formation of inner neomembranes. The increasing size of the newly formed hematoma is the result of the plasma effusion versus the liquid reabsorption; in most cases, this balance explains the differences in the timing of the appearance of clinical manifestations.[5]

SURGICAL MANAGEMENT

Surgical treatment of CSDH still lacks clear indications and guidelines; however, there are a few points that should be kept in mind to avoid complications:

- Before operation, coagulation parameters should be monitored and eventually reversed; surgical treatment should be avoided until internal normalized ratio (INR) is normalized or under 1,53.
- There are *no* guidelines about which type of anesthesia should be performed.
- There is *no* correlation between the outcome and recurrence of subdural hematoma in patients operated on with twist drill (<5 mm) or burr hole (1 cm)[1,6]; however, burr hole remains the most common procedure.[7]
- Systematic reviews have not found any difference in outcomes between one and two burr holes; however, two burr holes are recommended, especially if the operation is performed under general anesthesia.[8,9] The role of a single burr hole under local anesthesia should still be evaluated.
- Placement of a postoperative drainage improves neurologic outcome and decreases the rate of recurrence[1,6,10,11]; subdural drain is recommended according to the high-quality evidence found by Santarius et al.[10]

Complications

Recurrence

Recurrence (Fig. 45.1E-F) of the hematoma is the most common complication of CSDH, with an overall rate that varies between 2% and 87%.[4,7,12,13,14] Physiopathology of this complication is not fully understood but represents a significant problem due to the fact that around 20% of the patients require at least one reoperation.[13]

One of the most discussed explanations concerns the use and restarting of anticoagulant and/or antiplatelet therapy.

Due to the high number of comorbidities in patients with CSDH (e.g., FA, ischemic cardiopathy) there is an increasing interest in the management of anticoagulant therapy in this setting. Anticoagulant and antiplatelet therapies have been showed to be risk factors for the development and recurrence of hematoma by many groups[7,15,16]; however, the definition of the optimal management of these drugs is still lacking. Concerning anticoagulants, the therapy should be stopped at admission to the hospital, and the INR should be monitored to eventually normalize the level. In many patients, due to severe comorbidities or prolonged periods of immobilization, a prophylactic therapy (against deep vein thrombosis) should be started with heparin. These anticoagulant treatments, according to Kolias et al.[7] and

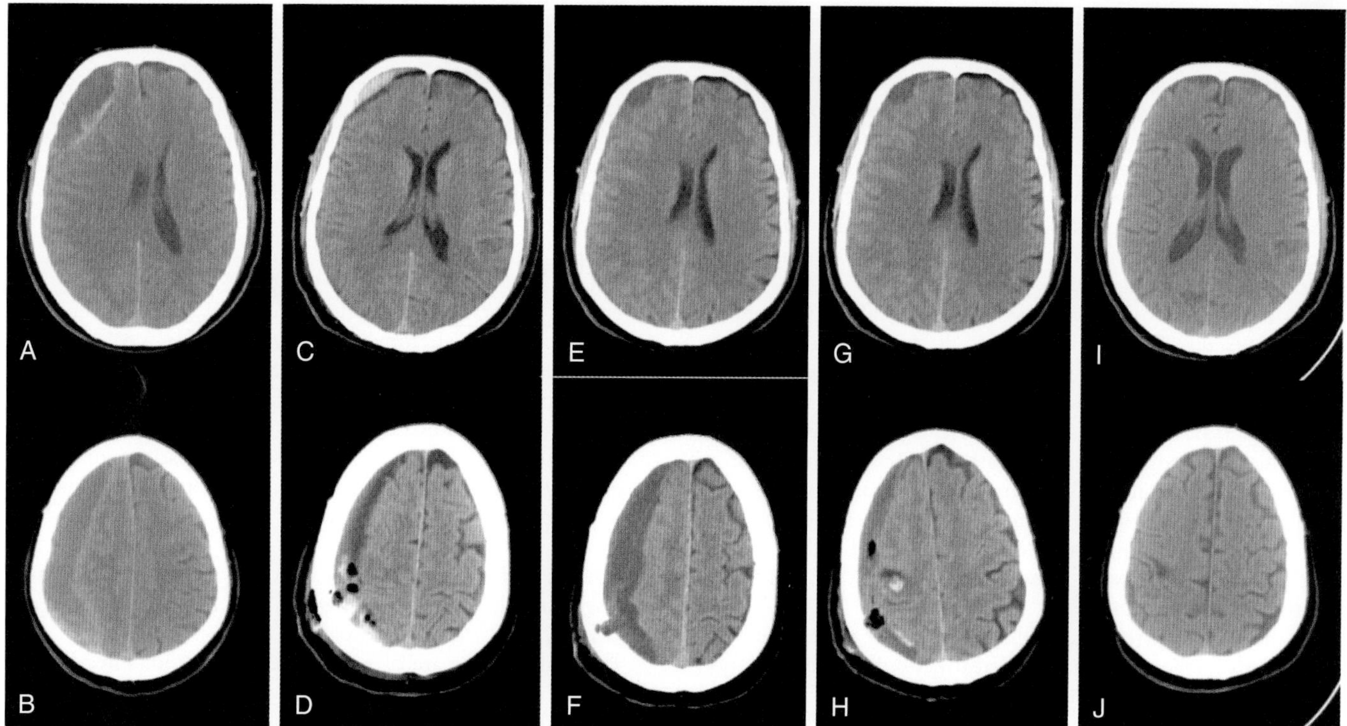

• **Fig. 45.1** (A and B) Admission computed tomography (CT) scan: presentation of a right chronic subdural hematoma (CSDH) in a 68-year-old male patient presenting with left motor hemisyndrome. (C and D) 24-hour postoperative CT scan: acute bleeding after surgical evacuation of right CSDH by parietal burr hole. After rebleeding, the patient was not reoperated due to the lack of neurologic symptoms. (E and F) 3 weeks postoperative CT scan: recurrence of the right CSDH after 3 weeks. (G and H) immediate postoperative (second surgery) CT scan: presence of a contusion in right motor cortex. Patient presenting with deficit of the left hand (M1). (I and J) 4 months postoperative (2nd surgery) CT scan: complete resorption of CSDH and contusion. Complete motor recuperation of the left hand.

Tahsim-Oglou et al.,[17] increase the risk of recurrence by 18.8%[7] and 32.1%[17], respectively; for these patients, a more strict surveillance should be performed. Another issue is represented by the timing of the restart of the anticoagulation. Is there an optimal range to minimize the risk? Several authors have tried to find an answer but without a clear result; at this moment the ideal timing to restart anticoagulant or antiplatelet therapy should be decided on an individual patient basis.[7,15,16,18] An objective method, that has been advised by Chari et al.,[19] that can be used for patients undergoing anticoagulant therapy for atrial fibrillation is to compare the CHA2DS2-VASc thromboembolism risk score with the HAS-BLED bleeding risk score. Although this method represents a good starting point to try to solve a significant problem, it has not yet been validated by sequent RCT. This field definitely needs further study, especially due to the introduction of new anticoagulants such as Rivaroxaban.

A second variable that should be considered is the type of hematoma the patient is experiencing; it has been shown that bilateral hematomas have a higher risk of recurrence after evacuation. In 2010 Kung et al.[20] tried to answer this question by reviewing computed tomography (CT) scans performed 14, and 30 days postoperatively. They concluded that the higher recurrence is probably related to a major shift produced by the higher volume of the lesion; this can lead to a stretch and new tearing of the bridging veins, which contributes to the reforming hematoma. This theory has not been validated by subsequent papers but still remains an interesting hypothesis.

Another possible explanation of recurrences deals with the organization of the hematoma: CSDH has a thicker outer membrane and a thinner inner membrane. These two enclose liquefied blood and often new vascularized membranes. In their randomized prospective trial, Unterhofer et al.[12] compared two groups of 28 patients; the first group underwent enlarged burr hole surgery with opening of the inner membrane, and the second group underwent enlarged burr hole surgery without opening. This study showed no difference in the need for of a revision surgery, size of residual hematoma during the follow-up, and outcome.

The problem of inner membranes has been discussed many times over the years, and it has been proven that it is statistically significant in the recurrence of CSDH.[13,21,22] Intraoperative opening of these septations is a common way to avoid the segregation of parts of the hematoma; however, in the case of thick or diffuse membranes, the opening could not be enough and a minicraniotomy would be required.

Another aspect to consider in the prevention of recurrency of the hematoma is the correct positioning of the patient.

Indications about the right placement of the head of the patient after surgery are not standardized. At the moment only two small randomized trials have been written about this topic with two opposite results: In 2010 Kurabe et al.[23] found a higher risk of recidivism in the patient with the head raised to 30 to 40 degrees, and Baouzari et al. in 2007[24] showed no difference between the two groups of patients. Further investigations are needed to clarify this point.

The need for a validated method to predict the recurrence of CSDH has led several authors to propose scores and scales. In a work published in 2015, Jack et al.[13] proposed a simple way to stratify the risk of recurrence; they attributed 0 or 1 point to age (<80 years = 0; >80 years = 1), CSDH volume (<160 mL = 0; >160 mL = 1) and presence of septations (absence = 0; presence = 1); the summary gives an estimation of risk of recurrence that ranges from 5% (total of 0) to >20% (total of 3). This paper represents a good starting point to stratify the risk, although more investigations are needed.

Recurrence of CSDH has not only been studied with respect to surgical factors. Schaumann et al.[4] in 2016 published the results of the RCT "COXIBRAIN": according to this paper the recurrence of CSDH is related to neoangiogenesis in the parietal membrane, which is VEGF-mediated. The aim of this study was to reduce the incidence of recurrence of operated CSDH by administering selective COX-2 inhibitors (Colecoxib). Unfortunately this study enrolled only 23 patients in 2 years and did not reach conclusions that can be used in clinical practice; on the other hand, it showed how 55% of patients were already treated by COX-2 inhibitors and they developed a relapse.

In the end, recurrence of CSDH is not fully understood and it still needs further investigations. Treatment of this complication is often surgical, but with a lack of high-quality evidence, it should be adapted on a case-by-case basis.

Steroid Treatment for Cdsh

The current role of steroids in the treatment of CSDH as substitute for or adjuvant to surgery has not been established. There are currently two ongoing RCTs, one promoted by the WHO (ICTRP) and the other promoted by the UK National Institute for Health Research.[25,26] At the moment the only recommendation is not to treat CSDH with steroids on a systematic manner but to use steroids in a case-by-case manner.

Acute Rebleeding and Focal Brain Injury

Acute rebleeding (Fig. 45.1C-D) after the evacuation of CSDH, with the development of ASDH, SAH or contusions, is an uncommon situation. SAH after evacuation of CSDH has been described by only two authors.[27,28] In the first case, Miyazaki et al. attributed the formation of this complication to hypertension and anticoagulation therapy taken by the patient; they also discussed, as mechanism of formation, the rapid shift of the brain after surgery with an overdrainage of subdural space and a hypoperfusion syndrome. This mechanism has also been discussed by Ogasawara et al.,[29] who attributed the formation of SAH to a loss of autoregulation of blood vessels with consequent hypertension and cortical hyperemia after reexpansion of the brain.

ICH as a complication of CSDH evacuation is a rare issue that has been described few times in the literature. This type of hematoma is usually ipsilateral to CSH; however, few cases of contralateral hematomas have been described.[27,30] Pathological explication of this complication remains unclear; several authors[27,30] believe that overdrainage of subdural fluid and CSF may lead to a rapid expansion of the brain and stretch of vessels with formation of acute hematomas.

This mechanism, even though not validated, could also explain another complication—namely, ASDH after evacuation of CSDH. This hematoma could also be related to a direct trauma during surgery or the ablation of subdural drain, but it remains rare and not very well explained. Spetzler et al.[31] have found a loss of regulation and loss of CO_2 reactivity in the brains of animals with CSDH; this mechanism, though not demonstrated in humans, could be another possible explanation for the formation of ASDH and ICH in patients with CSDH.

Even though the literature remains unclear about the management of postsurgical acute bleeding, treatment should be adapted to the individual patient. Many authors also recommend a slow brain decompression to prevent rapid intracranial changes.

Infections

Infections are a rare complication of chronic subdural hematoma that lead to subdural empyema (Figs 45.2 and 45.3). According to the latest review by Dabdoub et al.[32] there are only 46 cases described in the literature, and the real overall rate of this complication is less than 1% of cases of CSDH. There are no differences in the occurrence of this complication among patients of different sexes or ages; the only factors that seem related are the immunologic state of the patient and comorbidities like diabetes, chronic infections, and chronic hepatobiliary disorders. However, in the 50% of cases described, the source of infection remains unknown.[33,34] Pathogens involved usually belong to *E. Coli, Salmonella, Staphylococcus aureus,* and *Streptococcus* species.

Clinical features are often nonspecific, but an infection of a CSDH or evacuated CSDH should be suspected when the patient presents a decreased state of consciousness, which is seen in 81% of patients ($P = 0.020$, according to Dabdoub et al.[32]), and it should be investigated with a CT scan as first-line imaging. Injection of contrast should be useful to detect the membranes of the empyema. The role of magnetic resonance imaging (MRI) is progressively increasing due to its ability show convex fluid collection surrounded by a contrast-enhancing rim with a low signal on T1-weighted images and a relatively high signal on T2-weighted images. Narita et al.[34] emphasize that diffusion-weighted imaging may be useful to diagnose infected subdural hematoma and serial diffusion-weighted imaging evaluations may help monitor the therapeutic response in this condition.

As treatment, both burr hole washout and craniotomy with complete evacuation of the hematoma have been proposed as surgical adjuncts to antibiotic therapy. In 2007 Otsuka et al.[35] compared two groups of patients according to the treatment and

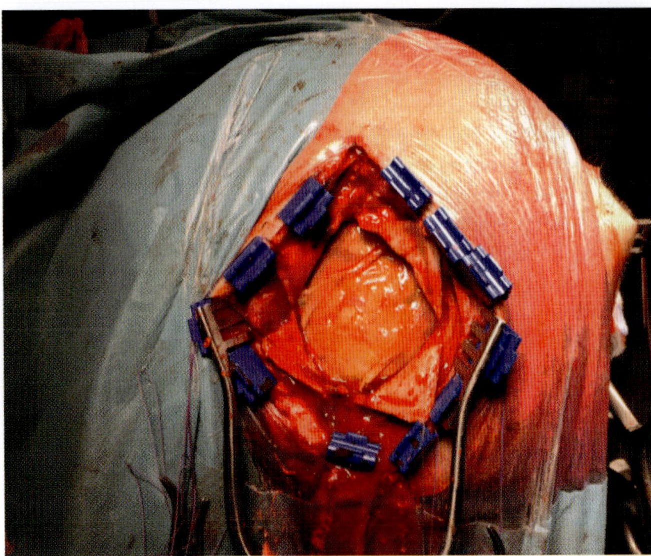

• **Fig. 45.2** Intraoperative photo showing the subdural empyema in the patient described in the previous image.

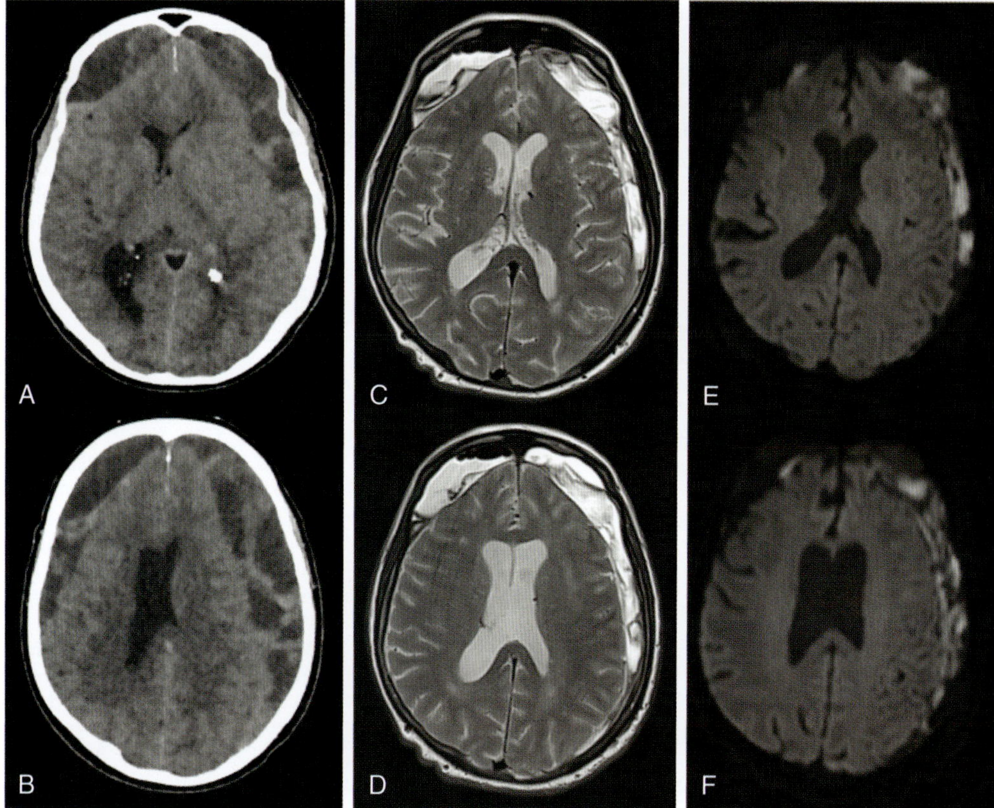

• **Fig. 45.3** (A and B) Admission computed tomography (CT) scan: presentation of a bilateral chronic subdural hematoma (CSDH) in a 72-year-old male patient presenting with cognitive impairment and gait instability. (C and D) 2 weeks post-operative MRI (T2): presence of a bilateral subdural collection. (E and F) 2 weeks post-operative MRI (DTI): presence of a subdural empyema on the left side and recurrence of the hematoma on the left side.

showed no difference in the outcome after either surgery. In the last review of 2015, Dabdoub et al. showed a high recurrence of the infection in patients treated by burr hole washout.[32] In conclusion, we recommend craniotomy as first-line surgical treatment associated with specific antibiotherapy.

Seizures and Epileptic Status

The development of seizures or status epilepticus after evacuation of CSDH is a complication with a global incidence that ranges from 1% to 23%.[36,37,38] The difference between these studies is probably related to the surgical technique adopted and the severity of the underlying condition.

In their paper, Hirakawa et al.[39] compared the outcomes of 309 patients and observed that patients undergoing burr hole treatment had a decreased incidence of seizures compared with patients who underwent craniotomy and opening of the membranes.

In the literature many risk factors, such as alcoholism (won),[38] previous stroke, change of mental status, mean GCS at discharge, and CT density, have been identified (di won)[30,35,38]; however, those studies do not differentiate between type of epilepsy, duration of epilepsy, and duration between surgery and inaugural seizure.[36]

SURGICAL REWIND

My Worst Cases

Case 1

A 68-year-old male patient presented with left-sided weakness. The CT scan showed left frontotemporoparietal chronic subdural hematoma. He underwent burr hole surgery and evacuation of hematoma. A postoperative CT scan taken at 24 hours showed a small bleed under the parietal burr hole. It was managed conservatively. At 3 weeks after surgery, there was a recurrence of chronic subdural hematoma with mass effect. Reexploration was done, and the hematoma was evacuated. Postoperatively he developed left upper hand weakness. A postoperative CT scan showed a small contusion of the motor cortex. At 4 months, there was complete resolution of CSDH and motor cortex contusion, and patient's hand function made a full recovery.

Case 2

A 72-year-old male patient presented with cognitive impairment and gait instability. A CT scan showed bilateral CSDH with significant mass effect. He underwent bilateral placement of burr holes and evacuation if subdural hematoma. The postoperative MRI at 2 weeks showed a recollection of hematoma. Diffusion tensor imaging indicated a possibility of subdural empyema. Reexploration was done and frank pus was noted in the subdural compartment. A craniotomy was performed, and subdural empyema was evacuated.

Management and prevention of this complication remains unclear: in a retrospective study[15] focused on operated CSDH, the use of phenytoin has showed a reduction of seizures, but neurologic outcome has not been described. In contrast, another retrospective paper showed no benefit in patients treated with antiepileptic drugs (AEDs) and no changes in neurologic outcome.

In conclusion, there is still no consensus about the use of AEDs in CSDH, and, as shown by the latest Cochrane Review of 2013,[40] there are no current RCTs that deal with the treatment of postoperative seizures. These studies clearly need to be performed.

NEUROSURGICAL SELFIE

In the last 30 years, the literature is replete with several studies concerning the clinical and surgical management of CSDH. However, there remain many obscure points regarding the complications of CSDH. By far, the best management remains surgical evacuation with burr-hole craniotomy and postoperative drainage as first-line treatment; however, further prospective studies are required to elucidate pitfalls of treatment with a view to avoid complications.

References

1. Almenawer SA, Farrokhyar F, Hong C, et al. Chronic subdural hematoma management: a systematic review and meta-analysis of 34,829 patients. *Ann Surg*. 2014;259(3):449–457.
2. Munoz-Bendix C, Pannewitz R, Remmel D, et al. Outcome following surgical treatment of chronic subdural hematoma in the oldest-old population. *Neurosurg Rev*. 2017;40(3):461–468.
3. Toi H, Kinoshita K, Hirai S, et al. Present epidemiology of chronic subdural hematoma in Japan: analysis of 63,358 cases recorded in a national administrative database. *J Neurosurg*. 2018;128(1):222–228.
4. Schaumann A, Klene W, Rosenstengel C, et al. COXIBRAIN: results of the prospective, randomised, phase II/III study for the selective COX-2 inhibition in chronic subdural haematoma patients. *Acta Neurochir (Wien)*. 2016;158(11):2039–2044.
5. Drapkin AJ. Chronic subdural hematoma: pathophysiological basis of treatment. *Br J Neurosurg*. 1991;5:467–473.
6. Liu W, Bakker NA, Groen RJ. Chronic subdural hematoma: a systematic review and meta-analysis of surgical procedures. *J Neurosurg*. 2014;121(3):665–673.
7. Kolias AG, Chari A, Santarius T, Hutchinson PJ. Chronic subdural haematoma: modern management and emerging therapies. *Nat Rev Neurol*. 2014;10(10):570–578.
8. Smith MD, Kishikova L, Norris JM. Surgical management of chronic subdural haematoma: one hole or two? *Int J Surg*. 2012;10:450–452.
9. Belkhair S, Pickett G. One versus double burr holes for treating chronic subdural hematoma meta-analysis. *Can J Neurol Sci*. 2013;40:56–60.
10. Santarius T, Kirkpatrick PJ, Ganesan D, et al. Use of drains versus no drains after burr-hole evacuation of chronic subdural haematoma: a randomised controlled trial. *Lancet*. 2009;374:1067–1073.
11. Ivamoto HS, Lemos HP Jr, Atallah AN. Surgical treatments for chronic subdural hematomas: a comprehensive systematic review. *World Neurosurg*. 2016;86:399–418.
12. Unterhofer C, Freyschlag CF, Thomé C, et al. Opening the internal hematoma membrane does not alter the recurrence rate of chronic subdural hematomas: a prospective randomized trial. *World Neurosurg*. 2016;92:31–36.
13. Jack A, O'Kelly C, McDougall C, Findlay JM. Predicting recurrence after chronic subdural haematoma drainage. *Can J Neurol Sci*. 2015;42(1):34–39.
14. Jang KM, Kwon JT, Hwang SN, et al. Comparison of the outcomes and recurrence with three surgical techniques for chronic subdural hematoma: single, double burr hole, and double burr hole drainage with irrigation. *Korean J Neurotrauma*. 2015;11(2):75–80.
15. De Bonis P, Trevisi G, de Waure C, et al. Antiplatelet/anticoagulant agents and chronic subdural hematoma in the elderly. *PLoS ONE*. 2013;8(7):e68732.
16. Gonugunta V, Buxton N. Warfarin and chronic subdural haematomas. *Br J Neurosurg*. 2001;15(6):514–517.
17. Tahsim-Oglou Y, Beseoglu K, Hanggi D, et al. Factors predicting recurrence of chronic subdural haematoma: the influence of intraoperative irrigation and low–molecular–weight heparin thromboprophylaxis. *Acta Neurochir (Wien)*. 2012;154:1063–1067.
18. Okano A, Oya S, Fujisawa N, et al. Analysis of risk factors for chronic subdural haematoma recurrence after burr hole surgery: optimal management of patients on antiplatelet therapy. *Br J Neurosurg*. 2014;28(2):204–208.
19. Chari A, Clemente Morgado T, Rigamonti D. Recommencement of anticoagulation in chronic subdural haematoma: a systematic review and meta-analysis. *Br J Neurosurg*. 2013;28:2–7.
20. Kung WM, Hung KS, Chiu WT, et al. Quantitative assessment of impaired postevacuation brain re-expansion in bilateral chronic subdural haematoma: possible mechanism of the higher recurrence rate. *Injury*. 2012;43(5):598–602.
21. Stanisic M, Lund-Johansen M, Mahesparan R. Treatment of chronic subdural hematoma by burr-hole craniostomy in adults: influence of some factors on postoperative recurrence. *Acta Neurochir (Wien)*. 2005;147:1249–1256, discussion 56–57.
22. Tanikawa M, Mase M, Yamada K, et al. Surgical treatment of chronic subdural hematoma based on intrahematomal membrane structure on MRI. *Acta Neurochir (Wien)*. 2001;143:613–618, discussion 618–619.
23. Kurabe S, Ozawa T, Watanabe T, Aiba T. Efficacy and safety of postoperative early mobilization for chronic subdural hematoma in elderly patients. *Acta Neurochir (Wien)*. 2010;152:1171–1174.
24. Abouzari M, Rashidi A, Rezaii J, et al. The role of postoperative patient posture in the recurrence of traumatic chronic subdural hematoma after burr-hole surgery. *Neurosurgery*. 2007;61:794–797.
25. International Clinical Trials Registry Platform (ICTRP). *WHO [online]*, 2014. http://www.who.int/ictrp/en/.
26. Emich S, Richling B, McCoy MR, et al. The efficacy of dexamethasone on reduction in the reoperation rate of chronic subdural hematoma—the DRESH study: straightforward study protocol for a randomized controlled trial. *Trials*. 2014;15:6.
27. Rusconi A, Sangiorgi S, Bifone L, Balbi S. Infrequent hemorrhagic complications following surgical drainage of chronic subdural hematomas. *J Korean Neurosurg Soc*. 2015;57(5):379–385.
28. Miyazaki T, Matsumoto Y, Ohta F, Daisu M, Moritake K. A case of unknown origin subarachnoid hemorrhage immediately following drainage for chronic subdural hematoma. *Kurume Med J*. 2004;51:163–167.
29. Ogasawara K, Ogawa A, Okuguchi T, Kobayashi M, Suzuki M, Yoshimoto T. Postoperative hyperperfusion syndrome in elderly patients with chronic subdural hematoma. *Surg Neurol*. 2000;54: 155–159.
30. Cohen-Gadol AA. Remote contralateral intraparenchymal hemorrhage after overdrainage of a chronic subdural hematoma. *Int J Surg Case Rep*. 2013;4:834–836.
31. Spetzler RF, Wilson CB, Weinstein P, Mehdorn M, Townsend J, Telles D. Normal perfusion pressure breakthrough theory. *Clin Neurosurg*. 1978;25:651–672.
32. Dabdoub CB, Adorno JO, Urbanp J, Silveira EN, Orlandi BMM. Review of the management of infected subdural hematoma. *World Neurosurg*. 2016;87:663.e1–663.e8.
33. Wagner FC, Preuss JM. Supratentorial epidural abscess and subdural empyema. In: Apuzzo MLJ, ed. *Brain Surgery*. vol. 2. New York: Churchill Livingstone; 1993:1401–1409.
34. Narita E, Maruya J, Nishimaki K, et al. Case of infected subdural hematoma diagnosed by diffusion-weighted imaging. *Brain Nerve*. 2009;61:319–323.
35. Otsuka T, Kato N, Kajiwara I, et al. A case of infected subdural hematoma. *No Shinkei Geka*. 2007;35:59–63.

36. Won SY, Konczalla J, Dubinski D, et al. A systematic review of epileptic seizures in adults with subdural haematomas. *Seizure*. 2017;45:28–35.
37. Ohno K, Maehara T, Ichimura K, et al. Low incidence of seizures in patients with chronic subdural haematoma. *J Neurol Neurosurg Psychiatry*. 1993;56:1231–1233.
38. Huang YH, Yang TM, Lin YJ, et al. Risk factors and outcome of seizures after chronic subdural hematoma. *Neurocrit Care*. 2011;14: 253–259.
39. Hirakawa K, Hashizume K, Fuchinoue T, et al. Statistical analysis of chronicsubdural hematoma in 309 adult cases. *Neurol Med Chir (Tokyo)*. 1972;12:71–83.
40. Ratilal BO, Pappamikail L, Costa J, et al. Anticonvulsants for preventing seizures in patients with chronic subdural haematoma. *Cochrane Database Syst Rev*. 2013;6(6):CD004893.

46

Overview of General and Degenerative Spine Surgery Complications

ANIL NANDA, MOHAMMED NASSER

Primum non nocere: First do no harm, the concept of nonmaleficence, holds true today more than ever before with the rapid technologic innovations in the field of spine surgery. It has become prudent to debate the use of an intervention that may carry a greater risk of harm than the presumed benefit. There is no such thing as a simple spine operation. The definition of the term *complication* in the spine literature and in the literature of the federal agencies is inconsistent.[1] A complication is defined as any clinical episode that may affect patient outcome or that may require intervention, further diagnostic tests, or monitoring. Added to this immediate complication are any long-term complications that develop long after the actual surgical procedure.

The prospective studies have shown higher rates of complications in spine surgeries than the retrospective studies.[2] In a review of 79,471 patients with 13,067 reported complications, the overall complication incidence was estimated to be 16.4% per patient.[2] It has been estimated that about 10% to 20% of patients undergoing spinal surgery may develop complications.[3] The overall complication incidence was highest for thoracolumbar surgery (17.8%) and for cervical spinal surgery (8.9%).[2] A study of 3475 patients from the database of the National Surgical Quality Improvement Program[4] found a complication rate of 7.6% and a mortality rate of 0.3%.[4] A study based on the Scoliosis Research Society Morbidity and Mortality's database of 22,857 patients, which includes 9409 cases of degenerative spine disorders, found a complication rate of 8.4%; the researchers also found that the patients with higher American Society of Anesthesiologists (ASA) grades undergoing spinal surgery had significantly higher rates of morbidity than those with lower ASA grades.[5] Increased patient age and contaminated or infected wounds were identified as independent predictors of mortality. Increased patient age, cardiac disease, preoperative neurologic abnormalities, prior wound infection, corticosteroid usage, history of sepsis, ASA classification of >2, and prolonged operative times were found to be independently associated with increased risk of complications.[4] In a large study by Hamilton et al.,[6] 108,419 spinal surgery patients were examined, and a 1.0% rate of new neurologic deficit was found in 1064 patients. Revision cases had a higher rate of deficits compared with primary cases. The pediatric cases had a higher rate of complications compared with the adult cases. The rate of new neurologic deficits for cases with implants was more than twice that for cases without implants.[6]

The complications during general and degenerative spine surgeries can be classified into general and specific causes. The general causes include infection, bleeding, deep vein thrombosis, pulmonary embolism, chest and urinary infection, complications related to positioning, wound hematoma, and bleeding and infection. The other complications are specific to the anatomic site and procedure used.

Dural tears are a familiar complication in spine surgery. Incidental dural tears have a wide range of clinical sequelae and are not always benign. Patients with incidental dural tears incur a longer hospital stay and greater incidence of perioperative complications.[7] The dural tears are an underreported adverse effect of spine surgery. A review of spine surgery cases has revealed that cerebrospinal fluid leaks after spinal surgery cost the US healthcare system an average incremental cost per patient of $6479 due to increased number of hospital stays, increased duration of hospital stays, and pharmacy costs.[8] The incidence of incidental dural tears in spine surgery is estimated to be between 1% and 17.4%[7,9,10] and is almost doubled in the revision cases (15.9%).[11] The problem of adjacent segment disease and pseudarthrosis after spinal fusion is unlikely to decline in the near future. The causation of adjacent level disease is still not clear. It has been widely debated as to whether the adjacent segment disease is a progression of the degenerative process or induced by the fusion process. The adjacent segment disease is found to have an incidence of 2.9% per year in the first 10 years after the cervical fusion.[12] It has been estimated that 25.6% of patients who had anterior arthrodesis would have adjacent level disease within 10 years of the operation.[12] A large review of lumbar surgeries has shown that about 23.6% of revision surgeries are done for pseudarthrosis.[13] Many risk factors have been found to be responsible for pseudarthrosis, such as smoking; osteoporosis; use of steroids, nonsteroidal antiinflammatory drugs, and antimetabolites; and use of allograft versus autograft.[14,15] The incidence of kyphosis after cervical laminectomy is estimated to be 20%.[16] The loss of posterior support leads to gradual development of kyphosis. This leads to constant contraction of extensor muscles, causing fatigue and neck pain.[17] Multilevel laminectomies are best avoided in younger patients.

Neurologic deterioration is the most feared consequence of any spine surgery. Acute neurologic deterioration due to postoperative epidural hematomas and compression from grafts and hardware needs to be addressed urgently and reexplored. Neurophysiologic monitoring during spinal surgery and use of navigational tools are essential to reduce the incidence of neurologic deterioration. Also to be considered is any comorbid medical illness that the patient may be having, which can give rise to spinal cord ischemia and neurologic deterioration. Injury to the vertebral artery is an uncommon yet feared complication of cervical spine surgery. The overall incidence of vertebral artery injury in cervical spine surgery is 0.14% to 1.4%.[18,19] The risk in instrumented posterior upper cervical surgeries is more than that involved in anterior subaxial spine surgery. The lateral dissection puts the vertebral artery under risk, and orientation of midline needs to be kept in mind throughout the surgery. The risk in instrumented posterior upper cervical surgeries (4%–8% incidence) is higher than that in anterior subaxial spine surgery (0.3%–0.5%).[20,21] Preoperative assessment of the course of the vertebral artery and the status of collateral circulation is important. The patient outcomes of vertebral artery injury can range from being clinically asymptomatic to experiencing infarcts, pseudoaneurysms, quadriparesis, sometimes coma, and even death.[18] The bleeding can be managed by tamponade, hemostatic agents, and blood transfusion. If repair is not possible and contralateral circulation is deemed adequate, endovascular coiling or primary ligation needs to be done.[22] Fortunately, 90% of vertebral artery injuries do not result in any permanent harm. Only 10% of cases end up with permanent neurologic injury.[23] Postinjury angiogram has to be done to rule out pseudoaneurysm or arteriovenous fistula formation. The use of intraoperative neuronavigation and a micro-Doppler probe is helpful to prevent this complication.[24]

Complications due to instrumentation can be avoided by careful perioperative workup. Cervical plate loosening is not a rare complication.[25] Osteoporosis, multilevel fusion, long lever arm imposed by the plate, and close proximity of screws to disc space are known to predispose the plate to loosening.[26,27] About two-thirds of loosening was associated with nonunions.[25] Multilevel cervical fusions have increased the complication rate of instrumentation failure and may need to be supplemented by posterior fusion. Most hardware failures are not symptomatic and can be treated conservatively.[27] Cervical lateral mass screws are associated with nerve root impingement by the screws. If the sagittal angulation is less than 15 degrees, there is a risk of nerve root impingement by the screws.[28] Exposure of the lumbar spine anteriorly can be associated with vascular injuries, with an incidence ranging from less than 1% to 15%.[29] Most injuries occur because of incorrect vessel dissection or identification, or lack of surgical control.[30] Venous lacerations are controlled by suture repair. Arterial injuries can have late presentation due to vessel thrombosis.

Minimally invasive spine surgery is gaining popularity, but with every new technique there is an associated learning curve. There is also the increased radiation exposure that is associated with doing minimally invasive procedures. The limited tactile feedback, the steep learning curve, the difficulty of depth perception, and the degree of manual dexterity required are the factors that one needs to keep in mind during minimally invasive spine surgery. Postoperative C5 palsy has an incidence of 3.4% after cervical laminectomy.[28] The C5 root has a short and direct course of exit and is subjected to traction with posterior displacement of the spinal cord after laminectomy.[28] Recovery may vary from weeks to several months.[31] The use of bone morphogenic protein in spine surgery has been shown to be associated with dysphagia, hematomas, seromas, osteolysis, increased neurologic deficits, and even cancer.[32]

This constantly evolving medical science is as yet imperfect, and complications will continue to occur. But it is important that the science of "complications" is understood and that a methodology is worked up to find solutions for these complications. The following chapters will address the complications that arise in general and degenerative spine surgery.

References

1. Dekutoski MB, Norvell DC, Dettori JR, et al. Surgeon perceptions and reported complications in spine surgery. *Spine*. 2010;35(suppl 9):S9–S21.
2. Nasser R, Yadla S, Maltenfort MG, et al. Complications in spine surgery. *J Neurosurg Spine*. 2010;13(2):144–157.
3. Deyo RA, Cherkin DC, Loeser JD, et al. Morbidity and mortality in association with operations on the lumbar spine. The influence of age, diagnosis, and procedure. *J Bone Joint Surg Am*. 1992;74(4):536–543.
4. Schoenfeld AJ, Ochoa LM, Bader JO, et al. Risk factors for immediate postoperative complications and mortality following spine surgery: a study of 3475 patients from the National Surgical Quality Improvement Program. *J Bone Joint Surg Am*. 2011;93(17):1577–1582.
5. Fu KM, Smith JS, Polly DW Jr, et al. Correlation of higher preoperative American Society of Anesthesiology grade and increased morbidity and mortality rates in patients undergoing spine surgery. *J Neurosurg Spine*. 2011;14(4):470–474.
6. Hamilton DK, Smith JS, Sansur CA, et al. Rates of new neurological deficit associated with spine surgery based on 108,419 procedures: a report of the scoliosis research society morbidity and mortality committee. *Spine*. 2011;36(15):1218–1228.
7. Cammisa FP Jr, Girardi FP, Sangani PK, et al. Incidental durotomy in spine surgery. *Spine*. 2000;25(20):2663–2667.
8. Jallo J, E.F., Minshall ME. The cost of cerebral spinal fluid leaks after spinal surgery in the USA. Abstract for presentation in *Congress of Neurological Surgeons*. 2009.
9. Bosacco SJ, Gardner MJ, Guille JT. Evaluation and treatment of dural tears in lumbar spine surgery: a review. *Clin Orthop Relat Res*. 2001;389:238–247.
10. Wang JC, Bohlman HH, Riew KD. Dural tears secondary to operations on the lumbar spine. Management and results after a two-year-minimum follow-up of eighty-eight patients. *J Bone Joint Surg Am*. 1998;80(12):1728–1732.
11. Khan MH, et al. Postoperative management protocol for incidental dural tears during degenerative lumbar spine surgery: a review of 3,183 consecutive degenerative lumbar cases. *Spine*. 2006;31(22):2609–2613.
12. Hilibrand AS, Carlson GD, Palumbo MA, et al. Radiculopathy and myelopathy at segments adjacent to the site of a previous anterior cervical arthrodesis. *J Bone Joint Surg Am*. 1999;81(4):519–528.
13. Martin BI, Mirza SK, Comstock BA, et al. Reoperation rates following lumbar spine surgery and the influence of spinal fusion procedures. *Spine*. 2007;32(3):382–387.
14. Phillips FM, Carlson G, Emery SE, et al. Anterior cervical pseudarthrosis. Natural history and treatment. *Spine*. 1997;22(14):1585–1589.
15. Hilibrand AS, Fye MA, Emery SE, et al. Impact of smoking on the outcome of anterior cervical arthrodesis with interbody or strut-grafting. *J Bone Joint Surg Am*. 2001;83-a(5):668–673.
16. Kaptain GJ, Simmons NE, Replogle RE, et al. Incidence and outcome of kyphotic deformity following laminectomy for cervical spondylotic myelopathy. *J Neurosurg*. 2000;93(suppl 2):199–204.
17. Cheung JPY, Luk KD-K. Complications of anterior and posterior cervical spine surgery. *Asian Spine J*. 2016;10(2):385–400.
18. Rampersaud YR, Moro ER, Neary MA, et al. Intraoperative adverse events and related postoperative complications in spine surgery: implications for enhancing patient safety founded on evidence-based protocols. *Spine*. 2006;31(13):1503–1510.

19. Neo M, Fujibayashi S, Miyata M, et al. Vertebral artery injury during cervical spine surgery: a survey of more than 5600 operations. *Spine.* 2008;33(7):779–785.
20. Madawi AA, Casey AT, Solanki GA, et al. Radiological and anatomical evaluation of the atlantoaxial transarticular screw fixation technique. *J Neurosurg.* 1997;86(6):961–968.
21. Wright NM, Lauryssen C. Vertebral artery injury in C1-2 transarticular screw fixation: results of a survey of the AANS/CNS section on disorders of the spine and peripheral nerves. American Association of Neurological Surgeons/Congress of Neurological Surgeons. *J Neurosurg.* 1998;88(4):634–640.
22. Devin CJ, Kang JD. Vertebral artery injury in cervical spine surgery. *Instr Course Lect.* 2009;58:717–728.
23. Lunardini DJ, et al. Vertebral artery injuries in cervical spine surgery. *Spine J.* 2014;14(8):1520–1525.
24. Peng CW, Chou BT, Bendo JA, et al. Vertebral artery injury in cervical spine surgery: anatomical considerations, management, and preventive measures. *Spine J.* 2009;9(1):70–76.
25. Sasso RC, Ruggiero RA Jr, Reilly TM, et al. Early reconstruction failures after multilevel cervical corpectomy. *Spine.* 2003;28(2):140–142.
26. Grubb MR, Currier BL, Shih JS, et al. Biomechanical evaluation of anterior cervical spine stabilization. *Spine.* 1998;23(8):886–892.
27. Ning X, Wen Y, Xiao-Jian Y, et al. Anterior cervical locking plate-related complications; prevention and treatment recommendations. *Int Orthop.* 2008;32(5):649–655.
28. Katonis P, Papadakis SA, Galanakos S, et al. Lateral mass screw complications: analysis of 1662 screws. *J Spinal Disord Tech.* 2011; 24(7):415–420.
29. Oskouian RJ Jr, Johnson JP. Vascular complications in anterior thoracolumbar spinal reconstruction. *J Neurosurg.* 2002;96(suppl 1): 1–5.
30. Hamdan AD, Malek JY, Schermerhorn ML, et al. Vascular injury during anterior exposure of the spine. *J Vasc Surg.* 2008;48(3): 650–654.
31. Satomi K, Nishu Y, Kohno T, et al. Long-term follow-up studies of open-door expansive laminoplasty for cervical stenotic myelopathy. *Spine.* 1994;19(5):507–510.
32. Epstein NE. Complications due to the use of BMP/INFUSE in spine surgery: The evidence continues to mount. *Surgical Neurology International.* 2013;4(suppl 5):S343–S352.

47

Adjacent Level Disc Degeneration and Pseudarthrosis

ANTHONY M. DIGIORGIO, ALEXANDER TENORIO, MICHAEL S. VIRK, PRAVEEN V. MUMMANENI

HIGHLIGHTS

- Adjacent segment disease occurs in up to 30% of patients 10 years after surgery.
- Pseudarthrosis rates for a one-, two-, and three-level anterior cervical fusion with allograft and a plate are approximately 4%, 9%, and 18%, respectively.
- Adjacent segment disease and pseudarthrosis rates can be reduced by surgical techniques.

Background

The use of fusion procedures to treat a variety of spinal pathologies in the United States is increasing as the population ages.[1,2] However, all spinal fusions carry a risk of pseudarthrosis and adjacent segment disease. Increased knowledge in spinal biomechanics, bone fusion biology, preoperative optimization, and spinal balance may help lower the rates of these problems.

Anterior cervical discectomy and fusion (ACDF) is one of the preferred treatments for degenerative cervical stenosis. The pseudarthrosis rate for this procedure ranges from 4% to 18%,[3,4] and the rates for adjacent segment disease have been reported at 3% to 30%, depending on the follow-up length.[5–7] Given the large volume of these cases done every year, neurosurgeons are likely to see these issues in their practices. We review the relevant literature on these issues in cervical spine surgery as well as their treatments here.

Anatomic Insights

Adjacent Level Disease

The pathophysiology of adjacent segment disease is still debated. The predominant theory postulates that when fusing previously mobile segments in the spine, forces that would have been absorbed by that segment are transmitted to the adjacent joints. This has been shown in cadaveric studies[8–10] and using fluoroscopy in patients.[10] However, some studies have failed to replicate these findings and instead postulate that adjacent segment disease is merely the progression of a preexisting spondylitic process.[11]

Regardless the cause of adjacent level disease, segments adjacent to a fusion often degenerate to the point of requiring repeat surgery. A study by Hilibrand et al. reviewed 374 patients and found a 2.9% annual incidence of adjacent level disease, with survivorship analysis estimating that 25% of patients will develop adjacent level disease within a decade.[5] Bydon et al. found a rate of 31% at 10 years and determined that the level or length of fusion did not change the incidence.[6] A study by Ishihara et al. found that adjacent level disease is more prevalent in levels that previously showed degeneration.[12]

Pseudarthrosis

Pseudarthrosis, or the failure to achieve bony fusion, can cause pain from continued motion at an arthritic joint. It can eventually lead to mechanical instability and hardware failure. The rates have declined with modern graft and plating technologies. The rates for a one-, two-, and three-level anterior cervical fusion with allograft and a plate are 4%, 9%, and 18%, respectively.[3,4] The pseudarthrosis rate of four-level anterior cervical discectomies and fusions remains unacceptably high, and those cases should probably be accompanied with posterior cervical fixation.

RED FLAGS

Adjacent Level Disease

- Preexisting multilevel spondylitic changes
- Global spinal imbalance or preexisting deformity
- Patient requiring a long fusion

Pseudarthrosis

- Smoking
- Nonsteroidal antiinflammatory drug (NSAID) use
- Steroid use
- Osteoporosis
- Poor nutrition
- Low vitamin D

Prevention

Adjacent Level Disease

A few studies have attempted to find interventions that decrease the rate of adjacent level disease. Hwang et al. found that, in cadavers, the amount of motion transmitted to adjacent segments was mitigated by the use of a larger lordotic cage.[13] Some surgeons advocate for matching the cage height to that of normal levels in the same patient. However, there are no large prospective trials to prove that this method works. The only intervention that has thus far been shown to decrease adjacent level disease in patients is the use of cervical arthroplasty. A review by Upadhyaya et al. examined the three cervical arthroplasty trials approved by the U.S. Food and Drug Administration (FDA) at the time. By combining the data from three FDA trials and using a fixed effects model, they found that the use of arthroplasty instead of fusion reduced the rate of adjacent level surgery, with a relative risk of 0.46.[14] Five-year follow-up data from one of those trials showed a reoperation rate of 11% in ACDF compared with 3% in arthroplasty.[15] This would favor the theory that adjacent level disease is at least partially caused by the fusion. Given these data, the authors typically counsel patients extensively about the possibility of accelerated spondylosis after cervical fusion.

The cervicothoracic junction (CTJ) deserves special mention because this level is especially prone to adjacent segment disease. Terminating a long segment cervical fusion at C7 creates a large lever arm that transmits force to the junction, theoretically accelerating degeneration there.[16] A study by Steinmetz et al. showed that fusions terminating at C7 trended toward more fusion failures in patients.[17] Yang et al. did not find that rod size had any effect on pseudarthrosis rate across the CTJ.[18]

Pseudarthrosis

It has long been known that smoking decreases fusion rates in the lumbar spine[19] and cervical spine.[20] Use of steroids has been shown to decrease fusion rates in rabbits.[21] Postoperative NSAID use has been shown to increase pseudarthrosis in the lumbar spine,[22] but these studies have not been performed in cervical fusion models. Postoperative infections impede wound healing and decrease fusion rates.[23] Lau et al. showed that two-level corpectomies and three-level ACDFs have equivalent pseudarthrosis rates.[24]

The risk of pseudarthrosis can be decreased with patient optimization. This can be done by counseling regarding tobacco cessation and NSAID avoidance. A multidisciplinary approach is needed if patients have comorbid conditions that are actively being treated with steroids because cessation of steroids is optimal but may not be possible. If osteoporosis is suspected, a preoperative dual-energy x-ray absorptiometry scan should be obtained. If low bone density is confirmed, teriparatide treatment has been shown to increase bone formation over bisphosphonates in spinal fusions.[25] Nutritional status should also be addressed. Although poor nutrition may not lead directly to a higher pseudarthrosis rate, it can adversely affect wound healing, which indirectly increases the pseudarthrosis rate. Decreased vitamin D levels have also been shown to impede bony fusion.[26] Levels should be measured and supplemented if needed. See Table 47.1 for a list of risk factors and how they can be addressed.

The use of autograft can decrease the pseudarthrosis rate.[27] For anterior cervical fusions, local osteophytes in a polyether ether ketone (PEEK) or allograft interbody along with a plate can be used in place of iliac autograft. For posterior procedures, local autograft is often mixed with iliac crest aspirate and a bone graft extender.

TABLE 47.1 List of Factors That Increase Pseudarthrosis Rate and Corrective Measures That Can Be Employed

Factors That Increase Pseudarthrosis Rate	Corrective Measures
Long segment fusion	Avoid fusing across four or more disc spaces with an anterior-only approach (supplement with posterior fixation)
Uninstrumented fusion	Use of cervical hardware increases fusion rates
Smoking/chewing tobacco	Patient counseling to cease tobacco products, preoperative testing
NSAID use	Patient counseling to avoid NSAID use 1–3 months postoperatively
Steroid use	Discussion with other physicians involved in care to see whether steroids can be weaned off
Infection	Meticulous sterile technique and patient nutritional optimization
Osteoporosis	Evaluate with preoperative DEXA scan and treat with teriparatide if needed
Vitamin D deficiency	Supplementation. Evaluate parathyroid hormone levels
Poor nutrition	Measure albumin/prealbumin levels. Optimize nutritional status.

DEXA, Dual-energy x-ray absorptiometry; *NSAID*, nonsteroidal antiinflammatory drug.

Management

Adjacent Level Disease

Adjacent segment disease can present with axial or radicular pain, often several years after the initial surgery. Gathering a careful history and physical examination is vital to assess the time of onset and to determine the distribution of the patient's symptoms. A patient who had a long period of symptom relief before experiencing a gradual onset of recurrent symptoms would be likely to have adjacent segment disease. Routine radiographic imaging will typically reveal the diagnosis.

If there are no symptoms of myelopathy, conservative management of adjacent level disease is an option. This can include epidural steroid injections and traction. Physical therapy and exercise can increase paraspinal muscle strength. Studies have reported varying levels of success using these nonoperative therapies, with between one-third and two-thirds going on to require surgery.[5,12] The surgical approach to adjacent segment disease will depend on the patient's extent and type of cervical pathology. Repeat anterior procedures are possible, although the complication rate is notable. Gok et al. found a complication rate of 27% in revision anterior cervical surgeries, with radiculopathy, dysphagia, and infection being the most common.[28] For patients requiring revision surgery who have prior anterior cervical plating and who have preoperative dysphagia or a history of radiation, assistance from otolaryngology may prove useful.

Pseudarthrosis

Pseudarthrosis can be asymptomatic. Patients may complain that their preoperative pain hasn't resolved, or they may have temporary resolution only to recur. One study described patients who had asymptomatic pseudarthrosis up to 2 years postoperatively, only to have symptoms recur after a traumatic event.[29]

Radiographic evaluation is used to confirm the diagnosis of pseudarthrosis. It is best evaluated with dynamic radiographs. Movement of the spinous processes by more than 2 mm with flexion and extension supports nonunion. Bone trabeculation on a computed tomography (CT) scan can be used as well. It has less sensitivity but a high positive predictive value.[30,31]

Once the patient is diagnosed, surgical revision of symptomatic pseudarthrosis is recommended. Revision surgeries have high rates of fusion, with recurrent pseudarthrosis rates from 0% to 14%.[28,32–34] Options for surgical revision include an additional anterior procedure with removal of the hardware and replacement of the interbody graft. Posterior approaches can also be used, with arthrodesis being performed using lateral mass screws or intrafacet allograft implants.[35,36] A metaanalysis on pseudarthrosis by McAnany et al. demonstrated that, although posterior approaches have a slightly higher fusion rate, clinical outcomes are equivalent for anterior and posterior approaches.[34] The use of recombinant bone morphogenic protein (BMP) in the cervical spine is off-label, and there is an FDA warning to avoid this product in the anterior cervical spine. Its use is controversial,[37] and it can increase seroma formation if used.[38,39] We do not typically use BMP in the cervical spine. Although revision surgery is typically successful in achieving arthrodesis, many patients will still continue to have pain.[40]

SURGICAL REWIND

My Worst Case

A 65-year-old man had a history of two prior cervical surgeries done at an outside institution, the most recent one 3 years prior (C5–6, 6–7 iliac crest autograft without a plate), and presented with a rapid progression of diffuse weakness, eventually requiring a wheelchair. He denied any bowel or bladder symptoms. He complained of recurrent neck pain since his last surgery that radiated into both upper extremities. On physical examination he had focal hand weakness with diminished leg strength as well. He was not hyperreflexic and had no Hoffman's or clonus.

Due to the rapid progression of his weakness, the patient was directly admitted to the hospital and underwent x-rays, CT, and magnetic resonance imaging (MRI) (see Figs 47.1–47.3 for his preoperative imaging). He was found to have a pseudarthrosis of his prior fusion and severe stenosis at C3–4. The patient underwent a posterior cervical decompression and fusion from C3–T1. He had lateral mass screws placed from C3–7 and pedicle screws at T1 with laminectomies, medial facetectomies, and bilateral foraminotomies performed from C3–T1 (see Fig. 47.4).

The patient had an uneventful postoperative course. He had excellent recovery of his strength and was able to ambulate with assistance. He was discharged to acute rehabilitation for further physical therapy and has done well since.

This case represents a delayed diagnosis of pseudarthrosis, becoming clinically relevant 3 years after his prior surgery. This was largely due to the symptoms he was experiencing secondary to his C3–4 stenosis. However, he did have a classic history of brief improvement of his neck and arm pain before recurrence. His preoperative x-rays showed >2 mm of movement between the spinous processes on flexion and extension. The CT scan clearly showed a nonunion, and his MRI revealed the C3–4 stenosis.

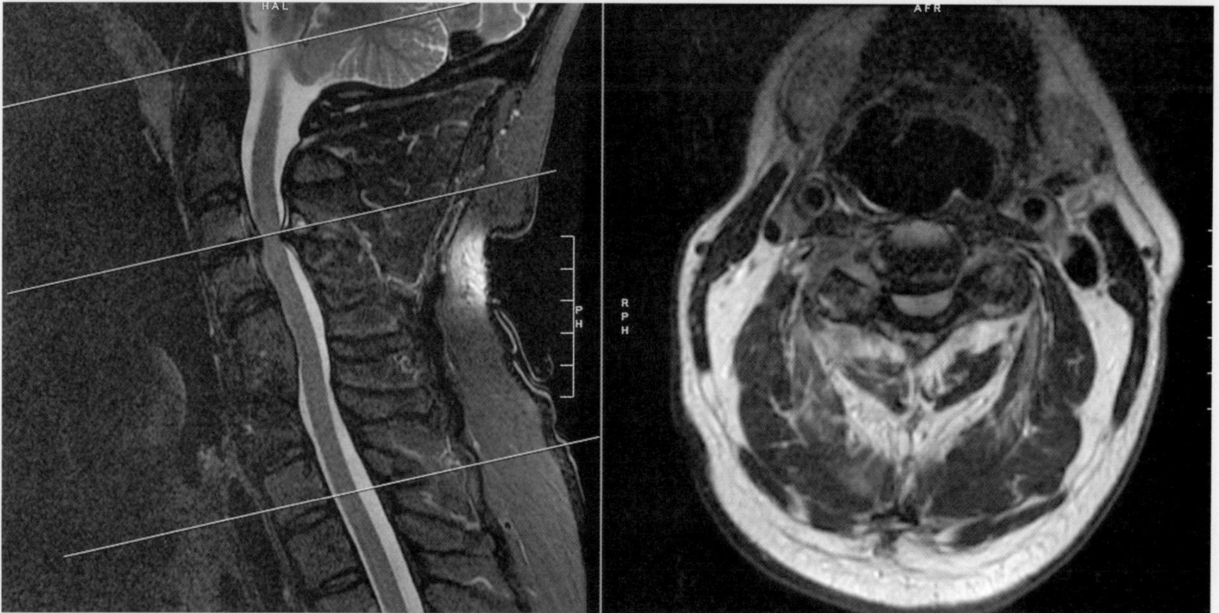

• **Fig. 47.1** Preoperative midline sagittal and axial T2-weighted magnetic resonance image showing severe stenosis and cord compression at C3–4.

Continued

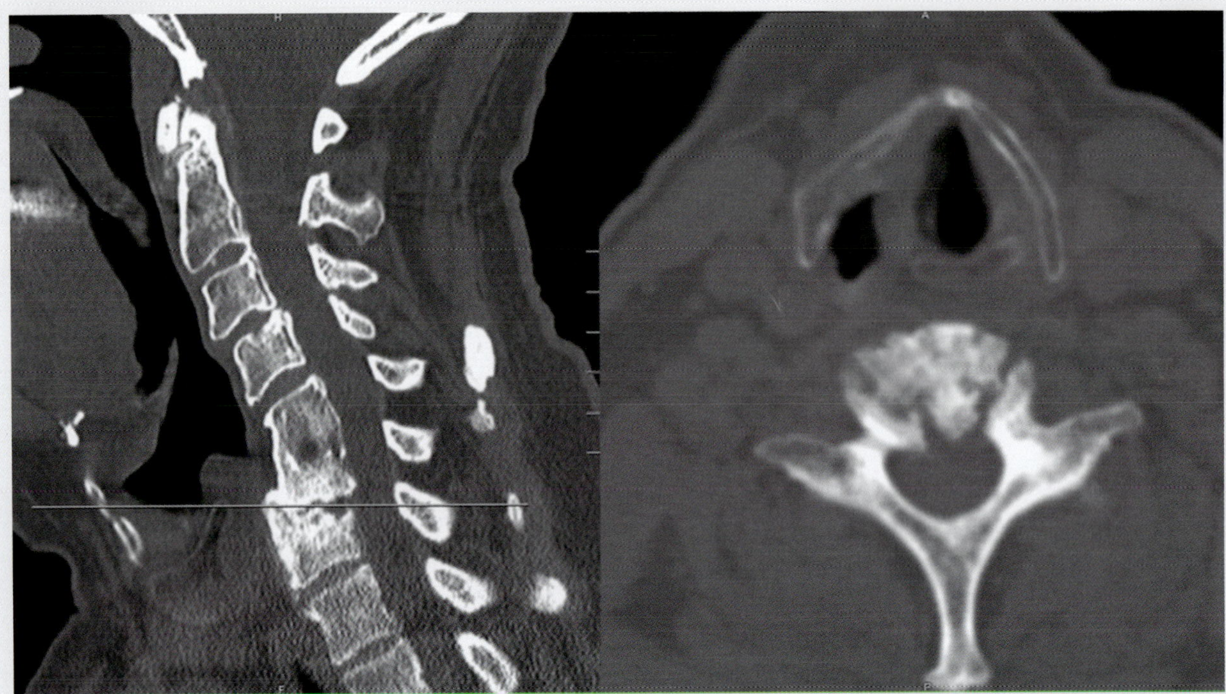

• **Fig. 47.2** Preoperative sagittal and axial computed tomography scan showing pseudarthrosis at C6–7 but a solid fusion at C5–6.

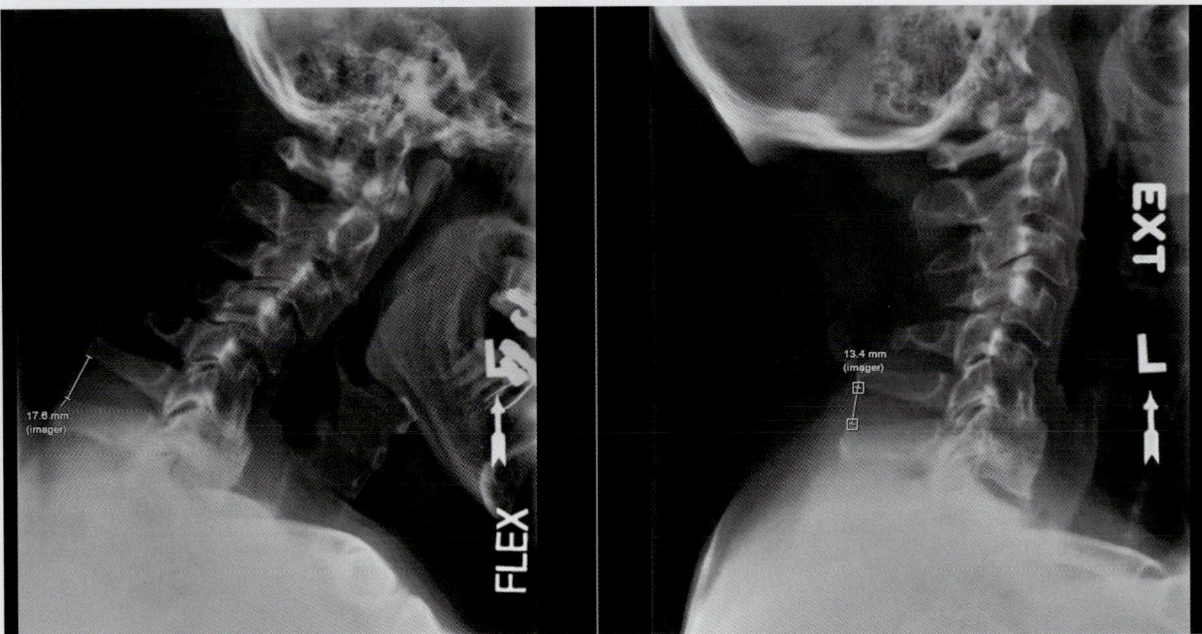

• **Fig. 47.3** Preoperative flexion/extension x-ray of the cervical spine. Note the change in C6–7 spinous process distance of over 4 mm, indicating pseudarthrosis at the prior fusion site.

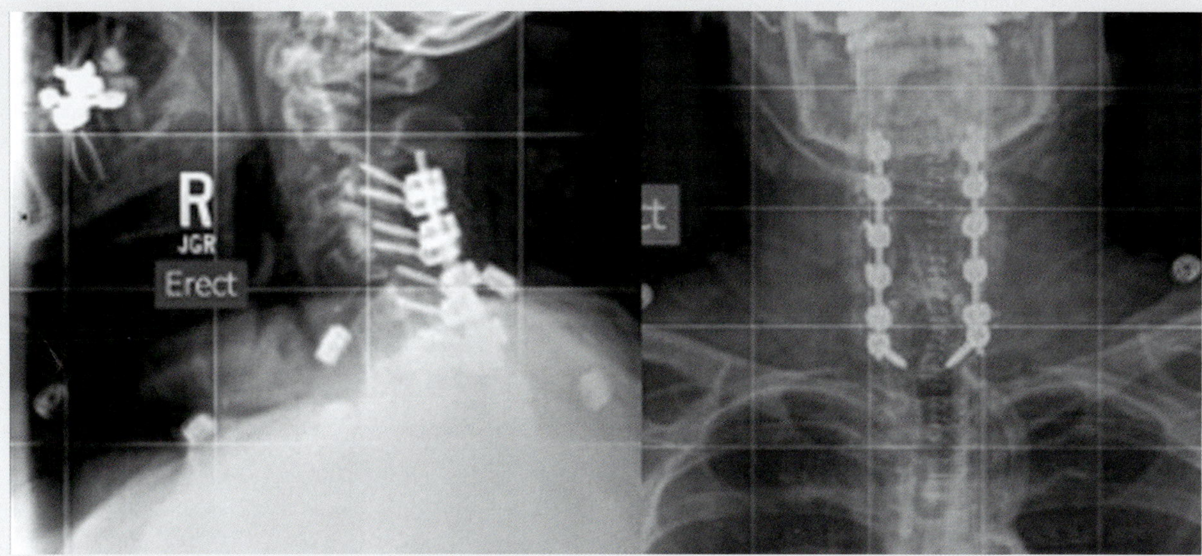

• **Fig. 47.4** Postoperative lateral and AP cervical spine x-rays showing posterior construct from C3–T1.

NEUROSURGICAL SELFIE MOMENT

With the increasing utilization of fusion techniques, more patients are suffering from the complications of adjacent level disease and pseudarthrosis. With current technologies and approaches, these sequelae unfortunately remain unavoidable. However, optimal surgical planning, patient counseling and optimization, and meticulous surgical technique can minimize their rates. When encountering these complications, revision surgeries often become necessary, but they can be performed with the techniques described here.

References

1. Lu Y, McAnany SJ, Hecht AC, Cho SK, Qureshi SA. Utilization trends of cervical artificial disc replacement after FDA approval compared with anterior cervical fusion: adoption of new technology. *Spine*. 2014;39(3):249–255.
2. Pannell WC, Savin DD, Scott TP, Wang JC, Daubs MD. Trends in the surgical treatment of lumbar spine disease in the United States. *Spine J*. 2015;15(8):1719–1727.
3. Wang JC, McDonough PW, Kanim LE, Endow KK, Delamarter RB. Increased fusion rates with cervical plating for three-level anterior cervical discectomy and fusion. *Spine*. 2001;26(6):643–646, discussion 646–647.
4. Kaiser MG, Haid RW Jr, Subach BR, Barnes B, Rodts GE Jr. Anterior cervical plating enhances arthrodesis after discectomy and fusion with cortical allograft. *Neurosurgery*. 2002;50(2):229–236, discussion 236–238.
5. Hilibrand AS, Carlson GD, Palumbo MA, Jones PK, Bohlman HH. Radiculopathy and myelopathy at segments adjacent to the site of a previous anterior cervical arthrodesis. *J Bone Joint Surg Am*. 1999;81(4):519–528.
6. Bydon M, Xu R, Macki M, et al. Adjacent segment disease after anterior cervical discectomy and fusion in a large series. *Neurosurgery*. 2014;74(2):139–146, discussion 146.
7. Mummaneni PV, Burkus JK, Haid RW, Traynelis VC, Zdeblick TA. Clinical and radiographic analysis of cervical disc arthroplasty compared with allograft fusion: a randomized controlled clinical trial. *J Neurosurg Spine*. 2007;6(3):198–209.
8. Eck JC, Humphreys SC, Lim TH, et al. Biomechanical study on the effect of cervical spine fusion on adjacent-level intradiscal pressure and segmental motion. *Spine*. 2002;27(22):2431–2434.
9. Maiman DJ, Kumaresan S, Yoganandan N, Pintar FA. Biomechanical effect of anterior cervical spine fusion on adjacent segments. *Biomed Mater Eng*. 1999;9(1):27–38.
10. Cheng JS, Liu F, Komistek RD, Mahfouz MR, Sharma A, Glaser D. Comparison of cervical spine kinematics using a fluoroscopic model for adjacent segment degeneration. Invited submission from the Joint Section on Disorders of the Spine and Peripheral Nerves, March 2007. *J Neurosurg Spine*. 2007;7(5):509–513.
11. Rao RD, Wang M, McGrady LM, Perlewitz TJ, David KS. Does anterior plating of the cervical spine predispose to adjacent segment changes? *Spine*. 2005;30(24):2788–2792, discussion 2793.
12. Ishihara H, Kanamori M, Kawaguchi Y, Nakamura H, Kimura T. Adjacent segment disease after anterior cervical interbody fusion. *Spine J*. 2004;4(6):624–628.
13. Hwang SH, Kayanja M, Milks RA, Benzel EC. Biomechanical comparison of adjacent segmental motion after ventral cervical fixation with varying angles of lordosis. *Spine J*. 2007;7(2):216–221.
14. Upadhyaya CD, Wu JC, Trost G, et al. Analysis of the three United States Food and Drug Administration investigational device exemption cervical arthroplasty trials. *J Neurosurg Spine*. 2012;16(3): 216–228.
15. Radcliff K, Coric D, Albert T. Five-year clinical results of cervical total disc replacement compared with anterior discectomy and fusion for treatment of 2-level symptomatic degenerative disc disease: a prospective, randomized, controlled, multicenter investigational device exemption clinical trial. *J Neurosurg Spine*. 2016;25(2):213–224.
16. Lapsiwala S, Benzel E. Surgical management of cervical myelopathy dealing with the cervical-thoracic junction. *Spine J*. 2006;6(6 suppl): 268S–273S.
17. Steinmetz MP, Miller J, Warbel A, Krishnaney AA, Bingaman W, Benzel EC. Regional instability following cervicothoracic junction surgery. *J Neurosurg Spine*. 2006;4(4):278–284.
18. Yang JS, Buchowski JM, Verma V. Construct type and risk factors for pseudarthrosis at the cervicothoracic junction. *Spine*. 2015;40(11): E613–E617.

19. Brown CW, Orme TJ, Richardson HD. The rate of pseudarthrosis (surgical nonunion) in patients who are smokers and patients who are nonsmokers: a comparison study. *Spine.* 1986;11(9): 942–943.
20. Lau D, Chou D, Ziewacz JE, Mummaneni PV. The effects of smoking on perioperative outcomes and pseudarthrosis following anterior cervical corpectomy: clinical article. *J Neurosurg Spine.* 2014;21(4):547–558.
21. Sawin PD, Dickman CA, Crawford NR, Melton MS, Bichard WD, Sonntag VK. The effects of dexamethasone on bone fusion in an experimental model of posterolateral lumbar spinal arthrodesis. *J Neurosurg.* 2001;94(1 suppl):76–81.
22. Glassman SD, Rose SM, Dimar JR, Puno RM, Campbell MJ, Johnson JR. The effect of postoperative nonsteroidal anti-inflammatory drug administration on spinal fusion. *Spine.* 1998;23(7):834–838.
23. Weiss LE, Vaccaro AR, Scuderi G, McGuire M, Garfin SR. Pseudarthrosis after postoperative wound infection in the lumbar spine. *J Spinal Disord.* 1997;10(6):482–487.
24. Lau D, Chou D, Mummaneni PV. Two-level corpectomy versus three-level discectomy for cervical spondylotic myelopathy: a comparison of perioperative, radiographic, and clinical outcomes. *J Neurosurg Spine.* 2015;23(3):280–289.
25. Ohtori S, Inoue G, Orita S, et al. Teriparatide accelerates lumbar posterolateral fusion in women with postmenopausal osteoporosis: prospective study. *Spine.* 2012;37(23):E1464–E1468.
26. Ravindra VM, Godzik J, Dailey AT, et al. Vitamin D levels and 1-year fusion outcomes in elective spine surgery: a prospective observational study. *Spine.* 2015;40(19):1536–1541.
27. Shriver MF, Lewis DJ, Kshettry VR, Rosenbaum BP, Benzel EC, Mroz TE. Pseudoarthrosis rates in anterior cervical discectomy and fusion: a meta-analysis. *Spine J.* 2015;15(9):2016–2027.
28. Gok B, Sciubba DM, McLoughlin GS, et al. Revision surgery for cervical spondylotic myelopathy: surgical results and outcome. *Neurosurgery.* 2008;63(2):292–298, discussion 298.
29. Phillips FM, Carlson G, Emery SE, Bohlman HH. Anterior cervical pseudarthrosis. Natural history and treatment. *Spine.* 1997;22(14): 1585–1589.
30. Kaiser MG, Mummaneni PV, Matz PG, et al. Radiographic assessment of cervical subaxial fusion. *J Neurosurg Spine.* 2009;11(2):221–227.
31. Ghiselli G, Wharton N, Hipp JA, Wong DA, Jatana S. Prospective analysis of imaging prediction of pseudarthrosis after anterior cervical discectomy and fusion: computed tomography versus flexion-extension motion analysis with intraoperative correlation. *Spine.* 2011;36(6):463–468.
32. Elder BD, Sankey EW, Theodros D, et al. Successful anterior fusion following posterior cervical fusion for revision of anterior cervical discectomy and fusion pseudarthrosis. *J Clin Neurosci.* 2016;24:57–62.
33. Kaiser MG, Mummaneni PV, Matz PG, et al. Management of anterior cervical pseudarthrosis. *J Neurosurg Spine.* 2009;11(2):228–237.
34. McAnany SJ, Baird EO, Overley SC, et al. A meta-analysis of the clinical and fusion results following treatment of symptomatic cervical pseudarthrosis. *Global Spine J.* 2015;5(2):148–155.
35. Mummaneni PV, Haid RW, Traynelis VC, et al. Posterior cervical fixation using a new polyaxial screw and rod system: technique and surgical results. *Neurosurg Focus.* 2002;12(1):E8.
36. Kasliwal MK, Corley JA, Traynelis VC. Posterior cervical fusion using cervical interfacet spacers in patients with symptomatic cervical pseudarthrosis. *Neurosurgery.* 2016;78(5):661–668.
37. Guppy KH, Harris J, Chen J, Paxton EW, Bernbeck JA. Reoperation rates for symptomatic nonunions in posterior cervicothoracic fusions with and without bone morphogenetic protein in a cohort of 450 patients. *J Neurosurg Spine.* 2016;25(3):309–317.
38. Hamilton DK, Smith JS, Reames DL, Williams BJ, Chernavvsky DR, Shaffrey CI. Safety, efficacy, and dosing of recombinant human bone morphogenetic protein-2 for posterior cervical and cervicothoracic instrumented fusion with a minimum 2-year follow-up. *Neurosurgery.* 2011;69(1):103–111, discussion 111.
39. Goode AP, Richardson WJ, Schectman RM, Carey TS. Complications, revision fusions, readmissions, and utilization over a 1-year period after bone morphogenetic protein use during primary cervical spine fusions. *Spine J.* 2014;14(9):2051–2059.
40. Kuhns CA, Geck MJ, Wang JC, Delamarter RB. An outcomes analysis of the treatment of cervical pseudarthrosis with posterior fusion. *Spine.* 2005;30(21):2424–2429.

48

Complications in Neurosurgery—Graft-Related Complications (Autograft, BMP, Synthetic)

WILLIAM J. KEMP, EDWARD C. BENZEL

HIGHLIGHTS

- Complications from bone grafting in the spine include poor bony fusion, pain at harvest sites, in addition to infection.
- Grafting in spine surgery includes autograft, allograft, bone morphogenetic protein, ceramics, and novel materials. Each graft type possesses benefits and drawbacks.
- New materials are intended to promote bony fusion while reducing further the possibility of complications.

Introduction

Neurosurgeons and orthopedic spine surgeons often utilize various forms of bone grafting to achieve successful spinal fusion. The process of achieving fusion with autograft, allograft, ceramic materials, or bone morphogenetic proteins (BMP) is not completely benign for the patient and presents the possibility for a variety of complications. This chapter details the complications with grafting for spinal fusion with various available materials, ranging from donor site pain, to infection, and to pseudarthrosis.

Spinal operations involving fusion are increasingly performed in the United States. To facilitate fusion, grafting has become requisite. Numerous factors influence whether a bone graft will achieve successful fusion or not. They include quality of preparation of the recipient site, the patient's history of radiation, the biomechanical stability of the graft complex, and the presence or absence of graft loading. Additionally, systemic patient factors such as general nutrition, history of smoking, osteoporosis, and presence of infection also affect the success of the bone graft and fusion.[1–3] If a patient has an unsuccessful fusion or pseudarthrosis, there is a greater likelihood of poor clinical outcome. Poor clinical outcome often leads to increased financial expenditure on the medical care of the patient, thus placing further burden on the health care system.

Bone grafting is associated with three requirements for successful spinal fusion: osteogenesis, osteoinduction, and osteoconduction. Osteogenesis refers to the provision of cells that can directly form bone. Osteoinduction describes the ability to induce differentiation of progenitor stem cells into osteoblasts for bone formation. Finally, osteoconduction is the provision of a sufficient scaffold to support bone formation. Autograft remains the most successful form of bone graft for spinal fusion since it involves all three requirements.[2–5] Unfortunately, utilizing autograft is associated with its own complications.

Autograft

Autograft is a very effective means for achieving successful fusion in anterior cervical discectomy and fusions. In 1952, Bailey and Badgley first performed an anterior cervical fusion, and in 1960 described a technique where a patient with instability due to neoplasm required onlay strut grafts harvested from the patient, thereby demonstrating the benefit of autograft. Autografts have a reported fusion rate of 83% to 99%.[2] The fusion rate decreases as the number of levels increases. After discectomy, an interbody potentially filled with structural bone can be utilized to avoid structural changes and maintain disc height.[1,2]

Autograft, usually in the form of corticocancellous bone, is harvested locally (Fig. 48.1) or with iliac crest bone graft (ICBG). This form of graft has been the most common and successful graft in spinal fusion, often referenced as the "gold standard."[3–5] In spine surgery, the bone harvested from a local site such as lamina or spinous process can be used later in the surgery for fusion. This cancellous autograft bone lacks possibility of disease transmission and has no risk of immunogenicity. Additionally, autograft is easily revascularized after removal from the donor site.[4]

ICBG, though effective at ensuring successful fusion, possesses inherent procedural potential for complications. Complicating factors include inadequate bone quantity, creation of another surgical incision, increased operative duration for harvesting, possibility of increased blood loss, and the potential need for transfusion.[2,3] Harvesting bone from the iliac crest can lead to pelvic fractures, vascular injuries, deep infection, and difficulty with ambulation due to pain. Minor complications include superficial infection and variable chronic donor site pain. Donor site pain can present as hyperesthesia or diminished sensitivity in the territory of the lateral femoral cutaneous nerve.[1–3,6] The incision should be made to avoid injury to the superior cluneal nerves and away from the sciatic notch to avoid injury to superior gluteal artery and nerve, the sciatic nerve, and the ureter.[5,7–9] Robertson and Wray performed a prospective analysis examining bone graft site donor morbidity for ICBG. Significant complications were low at 1.9% with donor

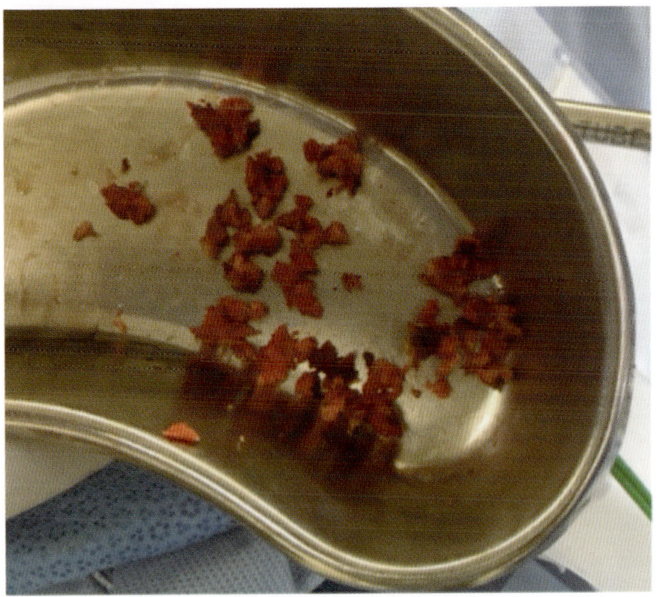

• **Fig. 48.1** Local autograft for posterior cervical fusion. (Intraoperative Photograph Cleveland Clinic Department of Neurosurgery 2018.)

site morbidity in 35% of patients. Patients reported donor site pain lasting up to 6 months that would significantly decrease by 12 months postoperatively.[7]

One case report describes a patient with non-Hodgkin's lymphoma on chemotherapy who experienced infection from a previous ICBG donor site 22 years prior for spinal arthrodesis. She was found to be infected with methicillin-resistant *Staphylococcus aureus* (MRSA) and underwent surgical debridement.[4] This case underscores the possibility of complications at the donor site, even decades after the initial surgery. Alternative sites of autograft also include the rib, fibula, and vertebral body when ICBG is deemed unsuitable.[5] The potential for complications associated with ICBG autograft has spurred spine surgeons to consider other options for bone grafting to achieve fusion.

Allograft

Serving as the most common substitute for autograft, cadaver allograft (Fig. 48.2), provides the benefits of fusion and spares the patient of a second surgical site.[3] Three types of allograft exist in the form of fresh frozen allograft, freeze-dried allograft, and demineralized bone matrix (DBM). Unfortunately, allografts possess minimal osteogenicity because cells do not survive the processing. Allograft advantages include immediate availability, storage ability, reduced blood loss, and decreased duration of surgery. Allograft is a reliable substitute in that the biomechanical stability is higher in allograft when compared with autograft.[10–12]

Fresh frozen allograft is the simplest of the allograft types. Typically, it is treated with antibiotic solution and stored at frozen temperature after harvesting. These allografts possess the greatest strength. Freeze-dried allograft is also treated with antibiotic and frozen, but the water is subsequently removed. This process can potentially decrease the mechanical stability and resistance to fracture.[5]

There are concerns that preservation via freezing or freeze-drying may negatively affect the osteoinductive and osteoconductive properties of the allograft, while also reducing its immunogenic properties.[5] Utilizing allograft also creates concern for donor to recipient disease transmission. This necessitates rigorous donor screening and sterilization to prevent bacterial and viral transmission.

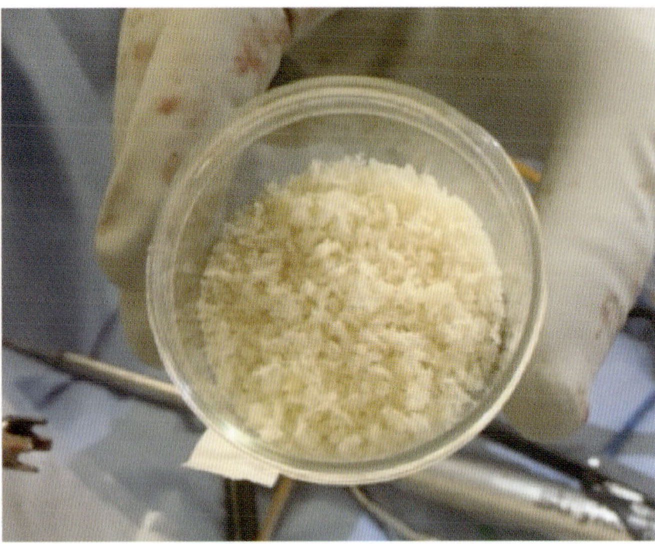

• **Fig. 48.2** Allograft cadaver bone for posterior cervical fusion. (Intraoperative Photograph Cleveland Clinic Department of Neurosurgery 2018.)

Though preservation effectively reduces immunogenicity, further sterilization may be needed with high-dose gamma irradiation or ethylene oxide gas. Unfortunately, these methods may further reduce osteoinductivity. Animal studies have shown that despite these sterilization procedures, viruses can survive, as in the case of feline leukemia virus, a retrovirus similar to the human immunodeficiency virus (HIV).[3,12] Additionally, there are long-term financial benefits associated with allogeneic bone graft, likely due to the increased costs of harvest site of morbidity.[2]

The third form of allograft is DBM. DBM has been acid treated for removal of the mineralized bone while keeping the organic scaffolding and growth factors.[5,11] DBM allograft has osteoconductive and variable osteoinductive properties without the structural strength of allograft. It has been shown that DBM products can act as a bone graft extender for posterior fusion in adults and adolescents with scoliosis.[5,6] One caveat noted in DBM animal studies is that it can be nephrotoxic.[6] DBM can also be used as a bone substitute for anterior lumbar body interbody fusion. Unfortunately, one study found that when allograft is combined with DBM, there is a higher rate of pseudarthrosis when compared with that of autograft.

The properties of the allograft are often variable due to lack of standardization among manufacturers and the heterogeneity of the donor population.[1,2] Human allograft has historically been available as mineralized or demineralized. Mineralized allograft is considered nonosteogenic, osteoinductive, and osteoconductive. DBM is osteoconductive and somewhat osteoinductive.

In addition to the risk of disease transmission, allografts can be associated with complications regarding malplacement and pseudarthrosis. Animal studies have shown that when compared with autograft in anterior and posterior spinal fusions, allograft is associated with a slower fusion rate, greater graft resorption, and increased infection rate.[3] Stand-alone impacted femoral ring allografts have been associated with pseudarthrosis and graft extrusion. Historically, use of autograft was more effective in achieving fusion when compared with allograft. Godzik et al. describe the case where they performed occipito-cervical fusion with allograft. They found the fusion in their series to be comparable to autograft when providing compressive forces.[8] To increase fusion rates, threaded allograft bone dowels were utilized in combination with recombinant human bone morphogenetic protein-2 (rhBMP-2).

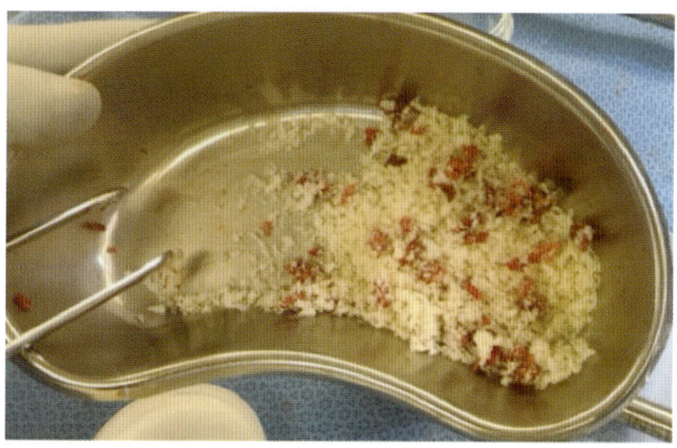

• **Fig. 48.3** Combined allograft and autograft for posterior cervical fusion. (Intraoperative Photograph Cleveland Clinic Department of Neurosurgery 2018.)

These threaded dowels were better able to resist expulsion and stabilize the implant.[10]

In 2000, a metaanalysis was performed on four studies comparing allograft and autograft in anterior cervical fusions. There was a significantly higher rate of bony union with a lower incidence of collapse with autograft versus allograft for one- and two-level fusions based on radiographic findings.[13] The authors did not report whether autograft was clinically superior to allograft. Ultimately, the decision to use autograft or allograft should be made by the surgeon to ensure the best clinical outcome.[13] Fig. 48.3 shows intraoperative combination of allograft and autograft to achieve fusion in the posterior cervical spine.

Ceramics

To avoid the donor site morbidity of autografts and the risk of infectious transmission, spine surgeons have also been looking to osteoconductive biodegradable materials such as ceramics.[3] Ceramic materials must possess biodegradability/biocompatibility with surrounding tissues in vivo, be capable of withstanding sterilization procedures, and be cost-effective in mass quantity. These materials are comprised of coralline hydroxyapatite, beta-tricalcium phosphate, silicate-substituted calcium phosphate, and calcium sulfate.[5,6,11] Unfortunately, these materials lack live cells, growth factors, and an organic matrix. Complications with ceramics involve their resorbability and mechanical strength. Lacking shear strength and fracture resistance, these materials do not have appropriate strength in the immediate postoperative period for lumbar surgery.[4,6] Tricalcium phosphates with a calcium phosphate molar ratio of 1.5 resorb too quickly for compressive requirements of cervical spine.[1] Hydroxyapatite with calcium phosphate ratio of 1.67 resorbs too slowly and shields bone from the mechanical stresses required for remodeling.[1] The utility of ceramics lies in their ability to be used as bone graft extenders in combination with local autograft.[11] With regard to ceramic materials, perhaps a happy medium in the future is needed to achieve successful fusion.

Bone Morphogenetic Protein

Surgeons are also utilizing adjuvant composite bone grafts and osteoconductive substrate.[3,4] In 1965, Urist discovered BMP after recognizing that bone growth could be achieved from animal DBM. Bone morphogenetic proteins, part of the transforming growth factor (TGF) receptor B family, help to facilitate intramembranous and endochondral bone formation. BMP stimulates mesenchymal cells to differentiate into osteoblasts and to produce bony matrix. Initially, BMP was considered to be too expensive. Today, recombinant human BMP (rhBMP) in forms of rhBMP-2 and rgBMP-7 (osteogenic protein 1 [OP-1]) can be produced for clinical use in unlimited quantity and without immunogenicity. The benefits provided by rhBMP include the ability to produce it in unlimited quantities and without immunogenic properties.[3,4] RhBMP was first used in anterior lumbar interbody fusion (ALIF) procedures, which remain the only FDA-approved indication for its use.[5] It often has been used off-label in posterior procedures.[5] The current literature has shown that the use of rhBMP is more effective in achieving posterior lumbar fusion when compared with iliac bone crest graft.

Though rhBMP has been utilized with efficacy, there have been complications regarding its use, especially in the cervical spine. There is a reported significant increase in swelling compared with those who did not receive the treatment. Other studies report complications of hematoma, dysphagia, hoarseness, and prolonged hospital stay.[14] Shields et al. discussed their retrospective results regarding the use of high-dose rhBMP-2 with an absorbable collagen sponge. The authors found that 23.2% of patients had complications, including hematoma that was distinguished from that obtained after anterior cervical interbody fusion (ACDF). The authors hypothesized that using the rhBMP-2 with the collagen sponge may cause an inflammatory reaction that can spread to the cervical area.[14] Additionally, there is a risk of ectopic bone formation possibly contributed by the formation of hematoma. Radiculitis also is a known complication after use of rhBMP. Vertebral osteolysis can also occur, typically associated with allograft resorption, cage migration, and subsidence. Park et al. hypothesized that this event may occur when there is violation of the end plate.[6]

Another complication discussed in the literature describes a phenomenon whereby rhBMP-2 causes aggressive resorption of an implanted graft, causing a resorption defect.[11] Nonetheless, animal studies have shown that when recombinant BMP is utilized, fusion rates are higher than with autograft alone. One long-term complication of rhBMP is the possibility of inducing cancer. As stated, BMP induces differentiation of pluripotent progenitor cells and stimulates osteogenesis. It is currently uncertain whether rhBMP-2 influences tumor formation or spread. There have been conflicting studies in vivo and in vitro regarding this significance. Currently, rhBMP-2 is contraindicated in patients with cancer.[15] In a systematic review, Devine et al. found that the cancer risk of rhBMP-2 may be dose dependent. Further studies are required to investigate this possible association.[16]

Autogenous Growth Factors

Autogenous growth factors have been utilized in patients who have recently undergone lumbar spine surgery. With these grafts, highly concentrated platelets are obtained from patient blood preoperatively. The platelets will include important growth factors such as platelet-derived growth factor (PDGF) and TGF that will enhance bone healing and formation. This graft can be utilized in combination with ICBG or allograft. Theoretical disadvantages are longer operative times and increased need for anesthesia. No specific complications are known at this time.[6,11]

Collagen-Based Matrices and Bone Marrow Aspirate

Collagen-based matrices describe a combination of bovine-based type 1 collagen and an osteoinductive agent such as an autograft. Possible disadvantages of these matrices include lack of structural strength and hypersensitivity to bovine collagen.[6] Bone marrow aspirate, both osteogenic and variably osteoinductive, is used with structural graft to enhance fusion rates in patients. Quality of the aspirate is variable based on the amount of osteoinductive factors in the harvested marrow.[6]

Conclusion

Bone graft via autograft, allograft, or other alternative means provides means of fusion. Although each is associated with benefits, these methods have individual risks that can result in complications for the patient. Ultimately, this can lead to poor patient outcomes and increased financial expenditure. The study of these products must be judiciously performed without bias. Industry is often involved in studies investigating various grafting products, potentially influencing conclusions regarding safety and efficacy. Because the ICBG has been time-tested and proven to work, researchers have had to justify the use of new materials.[5] Newer materials such as synthetic coralline hydroxyapatite are emerging into the field.[4,5] Perhaps new materials and techniques await to be achieved that will allow clinicians to minimize the risks of complications, enhance fusion rates, and improve patient outcomes.

SURGICAL REWIND

My Worst Case

Classic Complications Following Iliac Crest Bone Graft Harvest

Iliac crest bone graft harvesting is a known technique of obtaining autograft intraoperatively to aid in achieving bony spine fusion. Complications occur less often in current practice due to increased allograft availability thereby decreasing the need for iliac crest bone graft harvest. Nonetheless, it is important to understand the potential complications if this technique is employed.

Provided illustrations show normal anatomy with superior cluneal nerves exiting over the iliac crest as seen in Fig. 48.4. Fig. 48.5 shows these superior cluneal nerves passing in close proximity to iliac crest bone graft harvest site, placing them at risk for injury or irritation during the procedure. Patients may experience intense pain following the procedure that may be difficult to treat. Fig. 48.6 illustrates a pelvic fracture that may result following graft harvest at the iliac crest. Pelvis fracture secondary to this technique would ultimately require orthopaedic surgery consultation for repair. Additionally, another complication not illustrated includes infection of the harvest site.

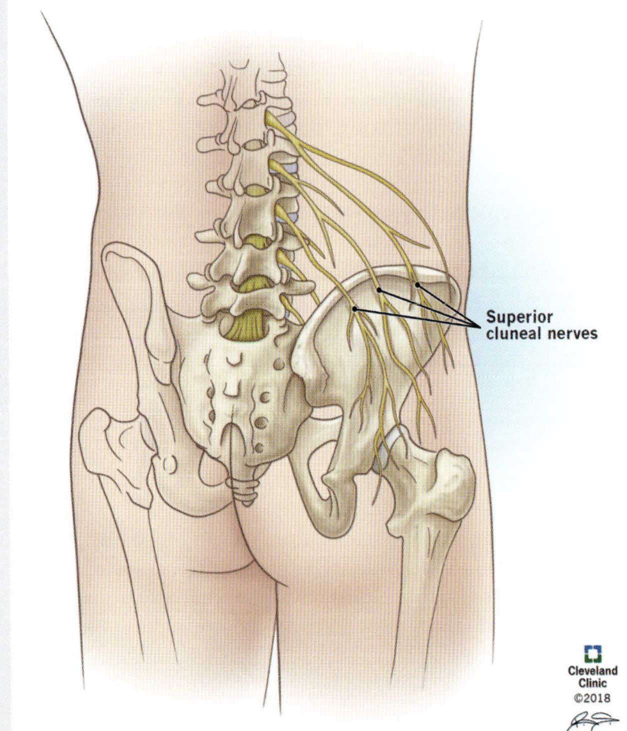

• **Fig. 48.4** Illustration of normal posterolateral lumbosacral anatomy with superior cluneal nerves traversing iliac crest. (Reprinted with permission, Cleveland Clinic Center for Medical Art & Photography © 2018. All Rights Reserved.)

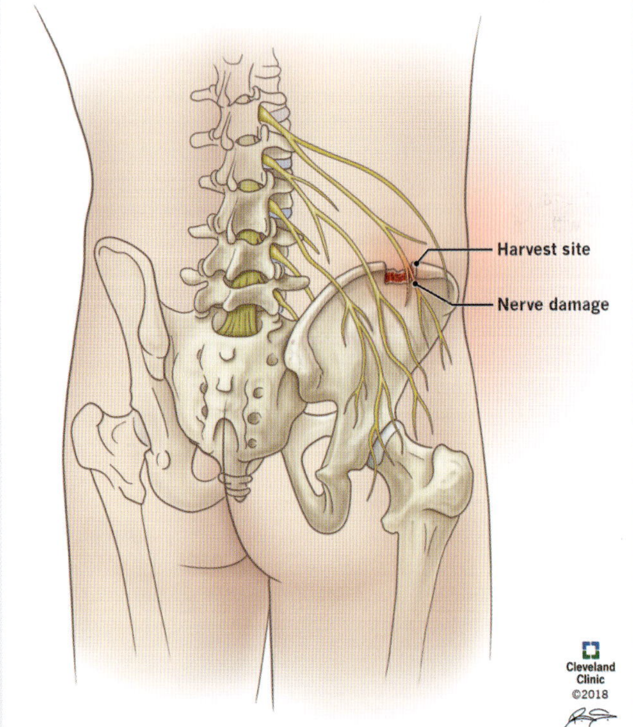

• **Fig. 48.5** Illustration of iliac crest bone graft harvest site with injured or irritated superior cluneal nerves traversing the donor site. (Reprinted with permission, Cleveland Clinic Center for Medical Art & Photography © 2018. All Rights Reserved.)

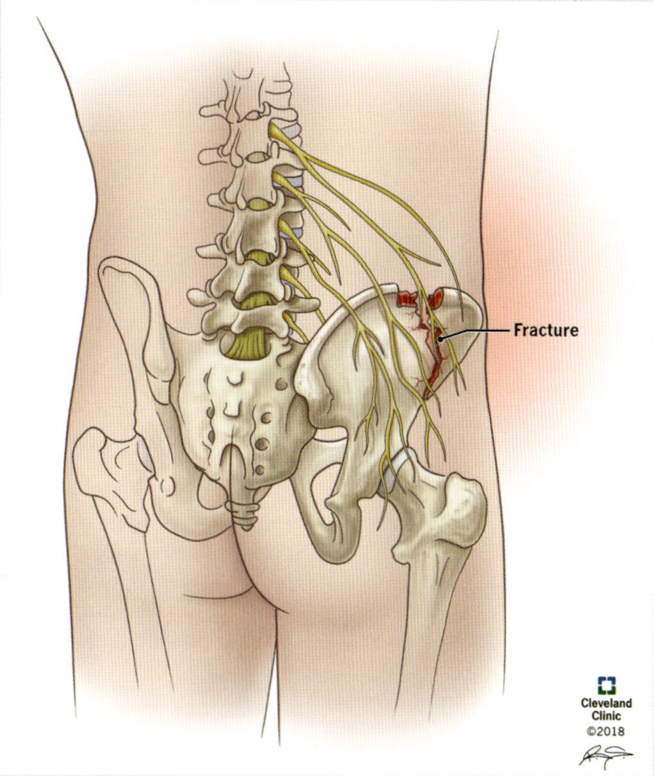

• **Fig. 48.6** Illustration of iliac crest bone graft harvest site with pelvic fracture. (Reprinted with permission, Cleveland Clinic Center for Medical Art & Photography © 2018. All Rights Reserved.)

NEUROSURGERY SELFIE MOMENT

When bony fusion of the spine is desired, the spine surgeon must decide which method of bone grafting is most appropriate for the patient. Whether it be utilization of autograft or allograft, use of BMP, or novel materials, all come with some risk of complication. These complications include poor bony fusion, increased operative time and anesthesia, pain to the patient, and potential for infection. Every bone grafting decision must be carefully tailored to the patient and the specific planned surgery coupled with the skill and experience of the surgeon.

References

1. Chau AMT, Mobbs RJ. Bone graft substitutes in anterior cervical discectomy and fusion. *Eur Spine J*. 2009;18:449–464.
2. Miller LE, Block JE. Safety and effectiveness of bone allografts in anterior cervical discectomy and fusion surgery. *Spine*. 2011;36:2045–2050.
3. Marchesi DG. Spinal fusions: bone and bone substitutes. *Eur Spine J*. 2000;9:372–378.
4. Babbi L, Barbanti-Brodano G, Gasbarrini A, Boriani S. Iliac crest bone graft: a 23-years history of infection at donor site in vertebral arthrodesis and a review of current bone substitutes. *Eur Rev Med Pharmacol Sci*. 2016;20(22):4670–4676.
5. Vaz K, Kushagra V, Protopsaltis T, Schwab F, Lonner B, Errico T. Bone grafting options for lumbar spine surgery: a review examining clinical efficacy and complications. *SAS J*. 2010;4(3):75–86.
6. Park JJ, Hershman SH, Kim YH. Updates in the use of bone grafts in the lumbar spine. *Bull Hosp Jt Dis (2013)*. 2013;71(1):39–48.
7. Robertson PA, Wray AC. Natural history of posterior iliac crest bone graft donation for spinal surgery. *Spine*. 2001;26(13):1473–1476.
8. Godzik J, Ravindra VM, Ray WZ, Schmidt MH, Bisson EF, Dailey AT. Comparison of structural allograft and traditional autograft technique in occipitocervical fusion: radiological and clinical outcomes from a single institution. *J Neurosurg Spine*. 2015;23:144–152.
9. Wetzel FT, Hoffman MA, Arcieri RR. Freeze-dried fibular allograft in anterior spinal surgery: cervical and lumbar applications. *Yale J Biol Med*. 1993;66:263–275.
10. Burkus JK, Harvinder SS, Gornet MF, Longley MC. Use of rhBMP-2 in combination with structural cortical allografts: clinical and radiographic outcomes in anterior lumbar spinal surgery. *J Bone Joint Surg Am*. 2005;87:1205–1212.
11. Miyazaki M, Tsmur H, Wang JC, Alanay A. An update on bone substitutes for spinal fusion. *Eur Spine J*. 2009;18:783–799.
12. Dodd CA, Fergusson CM, Freedman L, Houghton GR, Thomas D. Allograft versus autograft bone in scoliosis surgery. *J Bone Joint Surg Br*. 1988;70(3):431–434.
13. Floyd T, Ohnmeiss D. A meta-analysis of autograft versus allograft in anterior cervical fusion. *Eur Spine J*. 2000;9:398–403.
14. Shields LB, Raque GH, Glassman SD, et al. Adverse effects associated with high-dose recombinant human bone morphogenetic protein-2 use in anterior cervical spine fusion. *Spine*. 2006;31(5):542–547.
15. Thawani JP, Wayne AC, Than KD, Lin CY, La Marca F, Park P. Bone morphogenetic proteins and cancer: review of the literature. *Neurosurgery*. 2010;66:233–246.
16. Devine JG, Dettori JR, France JG, Brodt E, McGuire RA. The use of rhBMP in spine surgery: is there a cancer risk? *Evid Based Spine Care J*. 2012;3(2):35–41.

49

Procedure-Related Complications (Inadvertent Dural Tear, CSF Leak)

DARNELL T. JOSIAH, DANIEL K. RESNICK

HIGHLIGHTS

- Unintended durotomies are a known complication of spine surgery with the lowest incidence reported in the cervical spine and the highest in the thoracic spine for decompression of ossified posterior longitudinal ligament.
- Revision spine surgery, older age, and synovial cyst are significant risk factors for dural tears.
- Primary dural defect repair during the index procedure with augmentation has the highest success rate in the cervical and lumbar region, but the thoracic spine benefits from additional temporary cerebrospinal fluid diversion.

Background

Unintended durotomies and cerebrospinal fluid (CSF) leaks are a known complication of spine surgery with an incidence of 0.3% to 35% reported in the literature. CSF leaks after spine surgery have been estimated to increase the hospital stay cost on average by 50.4% with reimbursement increased only 21%, based on a prospective study from Germany.[1] Patients with CSF leak have been reported to cost the US healthcare system an additional $6479 compared with spine surgery patients who did not have any CSF leak complications.[2,3] Unintended durotomies may be complicated by postural headaches, pseudomeningoceles, meningitis, nerve rootlet entrapment, arachnoiditis, or postoperative wound dehiscence and infections. Older age, severe spinal stenosis, revision surgery, and synovial cysts are some of the risk factors for unintended durotomies. A prospective study of 1741 patients undergoing index lumbar spine fusion surgery assessed for the effects of inadvertent durotomy on patient-reported outcomes and postoperative complications. There was no significant difference found in postoperative infection, need for reoperation, or symptomatic neurologic damage in this population where the durotomy was recognized and addressed intraoperatively. Additionally, there was no difference in the final reported outcomes of back pain, leg pain, or functional disability.[4]

Anatomic Insights

In a retrospective study examining the pathologic anatomic variance that increased the risk for unintended durotomies, Takahashi et al. found that in discectomies, the durotomy usually occurred near the nerve root at the disc level. In degenerative spondylolisthesis, the durotomy often occurred at the medial facet or the rostral aspect of the inferior lamina, and in lumbar stenosis without spondylolisthesis, the durotomies occurred at the medial facet and the caudal aspect of the superior lamina. In those patients with synovial cysts, the dural tears occurred wherever the lesions made contact with the dura.[5]

RED FLAGS

- Signs of CSF egress are pulsatile clear fluid coming from a dry field or the swirl of lighter fluid with a bloodier border.
- Repeat bleeding from areas that previously were controlled should raise the concern that there has been CSF loss with thecal sac decompression or that an occult dural tear is possible.
- Postoperative postural headaches should be investigated as a sign of a CSF leak.
- A subfascial drain with consistently high output over several days with stable hemoglobin/hematocrit should prompt investigation for an asymptomatic CSF leak, and the fluid should be sent for Beta-2 transferrin.

Unintended Durotomies After Thoracic Decompression

CSF leaks after thoracic surgery for decompression are more frequently reported in the literature compared with after lumbar spine surgery, ranging from 20% to 30% with most cases attributed to ossified posterior longitudinal ligament (OPLL).[6,7] Dural violation may seem inevitable in patients with OPLL since the dura was found to be ossified in 25% of the cases reported by Sun et al.[8]

Incidence and Risk Factors

The overall reported incidence of unintended durotomies for all spine surgery is 3.1% with retrospective series reporting a 1% incidence for cervical surgeries, 7.6% incidence for index lumbar surgeries, and incidence for revision lumbar surgeries ranging from 8.1% to 15.9%.[9] As in the thoracic spine, OPLL is the biggest risk factor for dural tears in the cervical spine, and patients with OPLL are 13.7 times more likely to have a durotomy than patients without OPLL. Revision cervical surgery was the second most common risk factor for CSF leak in this series.[10] Synovial cyst adhesion is another leading cause, as is advanced patient age.[9] In a prospective study by Baker et al., multivariate analysis demonstrated that revision surgery patients were 2.21 times more likely to have an unintended durotomy than patients undergoing primary spine surgery.[11] Other mechanisms of unintended CSF leaks that can occur postoperatively include dural sac laceration or puncture from residual bone spicules or postoperative infection that may degrade a primarily repaired durotomy.

Prevention of Complication

Meticulous surgical technique and preoperative planning are the most effective means for mitigating unintended durotomies and CSF leaks. The use of high-speed drills, decompression of OPLL, and revision spine surgery increase the risk. Kerrison rongeurs must be used with great care, and less experienced surgeons should have the thecal sac protected while they use the instruments.[12]

Management for Lumbar Cerebrospinal Fluid Leak

Early detection of CSF leak is paramount and occurs either intraoperatively or postoperatively. An unintended durotomy occurring intraoperatively that is readily identified is the best-case scenario because it affords the surgeon a chance at primary repair and intraoperative testing through a Valsalva maneuver.

Direct primary suture repair is a widely accepted option for durotomies with the goal of obtaining a closure that is strong enough to withstand the intrathecal pressure during Valsalva maneuvers while the defect heals. The repair can be augmented with fibrin glue, muscle, fat-grafts, fascia, or gelatin sponges. There is evidence in the literature that primary dural repair may not always be necessary and that fibrin glue with gelatin sponges has been successful in selected cases in which direct repair is not possible (i.e., minimally invasive surgery cases).[2,12–14]

Postoperative detection of an unintended durotomy and CSF leak can be more problematic, and careful attention must be paid to patient symptoms (postural headaches) and subfascial fluid collection, persistent wound drainage, or wound infection, which may be clinical findings of an occult durotomy. Severe positional headache with neck stiffness, nausea, vomiting, or dizziness that improves when the patient is recumbent is a classic sign. CSF hypotension can be complicated by subdural hematoma or hygromas and cerebellar tonsillar herniation. Asymptomatic patients with CSF leaks may eventually present with a lumbar pseudomeningocele causing radiculopathy, the condition for which they initially underwent the index surgical procedure, which prompts repeat evaluation and imaging.[14]

The use of bedrest in the management after unintended durotomy continues to evolve and varies from no bedrest to a short period of bedrest of 24 to 48 hours. There is a trend of no bedrest with early mobilization if the durotomy is completely closed. In a study by Gautschi et al. surveying 175 neurosurgeons and orthopedic spine surgeons, 14.9% of surgeons never use bedrest, 35% use a 24-hour period, 28% use a 48-hour period of bedrest, and only 6.3% use a bedrest period of 72 hours.[15]

Management for Thoracic Cerebrospinal Fluid Leak

Suture repair of durotomies in the thoracic region is difficult compared with those in the cervical and lumbar areas, where the technical success rate is reported to be about 70%. Reported success rates in the thoracic region are closer to 30% because the dural tears in those procedures are usually irregularly shaped, often difficult to access, and often associated with defects related to ossification of the dura.[5,7,8,10,12,16,17] Suturing with the addition of fibrin glue, gelatin sponges, or tissue grafts increases the repair success rate. Sun et al. reported a success rate of only 23.5% with primary closure techniques in their series; operative and conservative modalities were used concurrently.[8] In dorsal wounds, a drain may be used for 2 to 3 days to eliminate the dead space and allow dural healing; to avoid a constant CSF flow through the dural defect, the drain is not placed on suction. Ventral tears, particularly if the chest cavity has been used to expose the spine, present a difficult dilemma and are discussed below.

There is controversy regarding bedrest for durotomies after primary dural repair in the thoracic spine. Sun et al. reported the use of 2 to 3 days of lateral or supine positioning for all patients; if there was persistent high output from the drain, those patients were placed prone for 5 to 7 days.[8] This is very difficult for many patients, and long periods of bedrest predispose patients to deep vein thrombosis and respiratory issues.[16,18]

Lumbar drains are another modality that reduces the flow and pressure across the dural defects, providing time for healing of the thecal sac. The recommended volume and duration are 120 to 360 mL/day for 4 to 5 days. This has been reported to resolve CSF leaks in 83% to 100% of cases.[6,16,17,19] When all else fails, exploration and repeat direct repair are warranted.

SURGICAL REWIND

My Worst Case (Fig. 49.1A)

A 54-year-old female presented to clinic with right-sided hemiparesis and pain and was found to have a large T8–9 herniated disc. She underwent a right-sided thoracotomy and partial corpectomies of T8–9 for removal of the large intradural calcified disc. There was an inevitable dural opening because the fragment was intradural; locally harvested muscle graft was used for the dural repair, augmented with DuraSeal and held in place by the bone graft. She was kept flat overnight with a right chest tube in place to water-seal. She did not have a lumbar drain in place. Her chest tube was eventually removed a few days later, and she was discharged home. She re-presented to the hospital 2 months postoperatively with positional headaches. Evaluation found a right pleural effusion with CSF leak from the operative site (Fig. 49.1B). She underwent re-exploration and repair with fascia lata graft and DuraSeal. She was kept flat and had a lumbar drain in place. Her headaches resolved, her drain was removed, and she was discharged home several days later. At her 4-month follow-up, she did not have any positional headaches or pleural effusions (Fig. 49.1C).

Continued

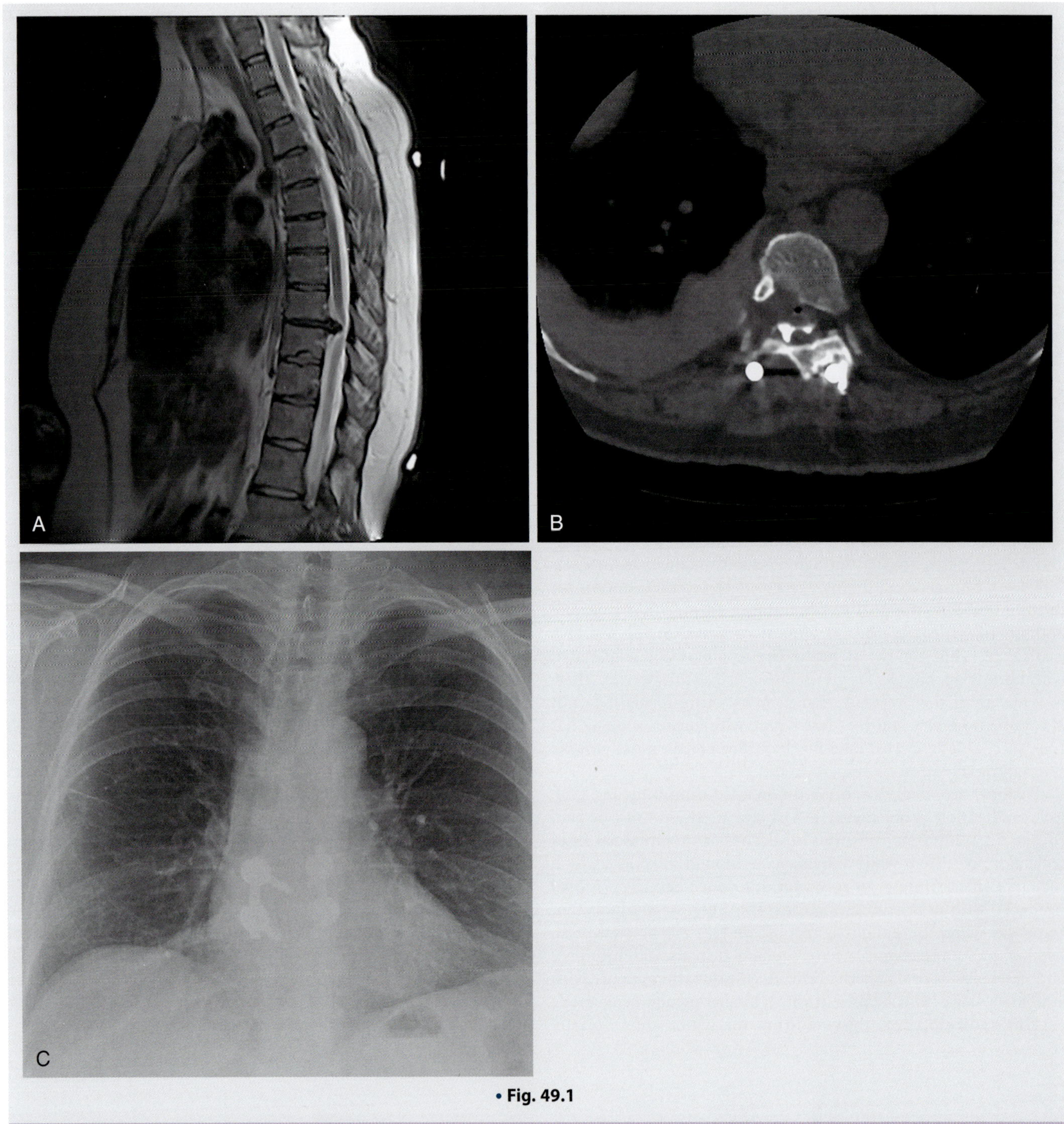

• **Fig. 49.1**

NEUROSURGICAL SELFIE MOMENT

Dural tears are a known complication of spine surgery, and prompt recognition and direct repair afford the best chance to avoid a CSF leak. Thoracic spine decompression for OPLL has an increased risk for CSF leaks; direct repair should be augmented, and the use of a lumbar drain for 2 to 3 days should be strongly considered.

References

1. Weber C, Piek J, Gunawan D. Health care costs of incidental durotomies and postoperative cerebrospinal fluid leaks after elective spinal surgery. *Eur Spine J*. 2015;24(9):2065–2068.
2. Menon SK, Onyia CU. A short review on a complication of lumbar spine surgery: CSF leak. *Clin Neurol Neurosurg*. 2015;139: 248–251.

3. Ghobrial GM, Theofanis T, Darden BV, Arnold P, Fehlings MG, Harrop JS. Unintended durotomy in lumbar degenerative spinal surgery: a 10-year systematic review of the literature. *Neurosurg Focus.* 2015;39(4):E8.
4. Adogwa O, Huang MI, Thompson PM, et al. No difference in postoperative complications, pain, and functional outcomes up to 2 years after incidental durotomy in lumbar spinal fusion: a prospective, multi-institutional, propensity-matched analysis of 1,741 patients. *Spine J.* 2014;14(9):1828–1834.
5. Takahashi Y, Sato T, Hyodo H, et al. Incidental durotomy during lumbar spine surgery: risk factors and anatomic locations: clinical article. *J Neurosurg Spine.* 2013;18(2):165–169.
6. Hu P, Yu M, Liu X, Liu Z, Jiang L. A circumferential decompression-based surgical strategy for multilevel ossification of thoracic posterior longitudinal ligament. *Spine J.* 2015;15(12):2484–2492.
7. Matsuyama Y, Yoshihara H, Tsuji T, et al. Surgical outcome of ossification of the posterior longitudinal ligament (OPLL) of the thoracic spine: implication of the type of ossification and surgical options. *J Spinal Disord Tech.* 2005;18(6):492–497; discussion 498.
8. Sun X, Sun C, Liu X, et al. The frequency and treatment of dural tears and cerebrospinal fluid leakage in 266 patients with thoracic myelopathy caused by ossification of the ligamentum flavum. *Spine.* 2012;37(12):E702–E707.
9. Espiritu MT, Rhyne A, Darden BV 2nd. Dural tears in spine surgery. *J Am Acad Orthop Surg.* 2010;18(9):537–545.
10. Hannallah D, Lee J, Khan M, Donaldson WF, Kang JD. Cerebrospinal fluid leaks following cervical spine surgery. *J Bone Joint Surg Am.* 2008;90(5):1101–1105.
11. Baker GA, Cizik AM, Bransford RJ, et al. Risk factors for unintended durotomy during spine surgery: a multivariate analysis. *Spine J.* 2012;12(2):121–126.
12. Guerin P, El Fegoun AB, Obeid I, et al. Incidental durotomy during spine surgery: incidence, management and complications. A retrospective review. *Injury.* 2012;43(4):397–401.
13. Dafford EE, Anderson PA. Comparison of dural repair techniques. *Spine J.* 2015;15(5):1099–1105.
14. Bosacco SJ, Gardner MJ, Guille JT. Evaluation and treatment of dural tears in lumbar spine surgery: a review. *Clin Orthop Relat Res.* 2001;389:238–247.
15. Gautschi OP, Stienen MN, Smoll NR, Corniola MV, Tessitore E, Schaller K. Incidental durotomy in lumbar spine surgery–a three-nation survey to evaluate its management. *Acta Neurochir (Wien).* 2014;156(9):1813–1820.
16. Hu PP, Liu XG, Yu M. Cerebrospinal fluid leakage after thoracic decompression. *Chin Med J.* 2016;129(16):1994–2000.
17. Mazur M, Jost GF, Schmidt MH, Bisson EF. Management of cerebrospinal fluid leaks after anterior decompression for ossification of the posterior longitudinal ligament: a review of the literature. *Neurosurg Focus.* 2011;30(3):E13.
18. Low JC, von Niederhausern B, Rutherford SA, King AT. Pilot study of perioperative accidental durotomy: does the period of postoperative bed rest reduce the incidence of complication? *Br J Neurosurg.* 2013;27(6):800–802.
19. Cho JY, Chan CK, Lee SH, Choi WC, Maeng DH, Lee HY. Management of cerebrospinal fluid leakage after anterior decompression for ossification of posterior longitudinal ligament in the thoracic spine: the utilization of a volume-controlled pseudomeningocele. *J Spinal Disord Tech.* 2012;25(4):E93–E102.

50 Complications of Surgery at the Craniocervical Junction

MARIO GANAU, MICHAEL G. FEHLINGS

HIGHLIGHTS

- The primary treatment goals for pathologies involving the craniocervical junction are the relief of bulbomedullary compression and the elimination of instability, if present. The choice of anterior or posterior approaches depends on the nature of the lesion, its natural history, and prognosis.
- A complete neuroradiologic workup, the use of neuronavigation (C-arm, O-arm, intraoperative computed tomography/magnetic resonance imaging), and neurophysiologic monitoring (somatosensory and motor evoked potentials) help reduce the risk of perioperative complications.
- Vertebral artery mobilization and occipital condyle resection may be needed depending on the extent and location of craniocervical junction tumors; in case of significant condylar resection, occipitocervical fixation is warranted.
- Although it is not ideal, the C2 ganglion can be sacrificed with minimal postoperative comorbidities, and in most cases, patients are asymptomatic from iatrogenic damage of the vertebral artery.
- Postoperatively, Halo immobilization or chemo-/proton-beam/ radiotherapy can be considered as adjuvant treatments, depending on the nature of the lesion.

Introduction

Like a cardan joint, the craniocervical junction (CCJ) allows simultaneous independent spatial movements around three axes; its primary role is in fact to ensure the maximal mobility of the head for visual and auditory exploration of space. These functional characteristics explain the complexity and fragility of this anatomic region. Over the years, many anterior, anterolateral, and posterior approaches to the CCJ (such as: transoral, transfacial, transmandibular, endoscopic transnasal, midline, or lateral or far lateral occipitocervical decompression coupled with instrumented fusion achievable by many techniques) have been developed to address the bulbomedullary compression caused by several degenerative, inflammatory, traumatic, congenital, and neoplastic spine pathologies[1–11] (Fig. 50.1). These include but are not limited to: (1) chronic inflammation of the CCJ osteoligament complex, mostly related to rheumatoid arthritis and metabolic disorders; (2) traumatic C1–C2 dislocations resulting in basilar invagination as well as unstable atlas and odontoid fractures; (3) congenital malformations causing instability and/or stenosis at the level of the CCJ, like those resulting from collagenopathies, osteogenesis imperfecta, Down's syndrome, and achondroplasia; and, (4) neoplastic (i.e., primary and secondary spinal tumors) and paraneoplastic (i.e., Paget's disease) lesions, usually affecting the body and dens of C2.

Anatomic Insights

The CCJ represents a transitional zone with a complex balance of different elements: osseous structures articulated with synovial joints, intrinsic ligaments, membranes, and muscles. From a biomechanical perspective, the CCJ can be thought of as a central pillar surrounded by two ringed structures: The first consists of clivus, anterior atlanto-occipital membrane (AAOM), odontoid process, and the vertebral body of C2, whereas the second includes the foramen magnum (FM) with the occipital condyles, the posterior atlanto-occipital membrane (PAOM), and the ring of C1 with its lateral masses and arches. Altogether those elements respond to seemingly opposed necessities: being at the same time loose enough to allow a great variety of movements yet strong enough to preserve the spinal cord and vertebral arteries. The anatomic structures more at risk of injury during surgical approaches to the CCJ are described below.

Brainstem, Spinal Cord, Cranial and Spinal Nerves

Among the structures passing behind the alar ligament that divides the posterior compartment of the FM from its anterior, osseoligamentous one are the lower end of the medulla oblongata (MO) with anterior and posterior spinal arteries, the spinal root of the accessory (XI) nerve and, occasionally, the lower aspect of the cerebellar tonsils. Pathologies causing bulbomedullary compression may result in concomitant involvement of the nuclei and ganglia of several cranial nerves arising from the MO: nucleus ambiguus of glossopharyngeal (IX) and vagus (X) nerves; dorsal nucleus, solitary nucleus, and inferior ganglion of X nerve; spinal accessory nucleus of IX nerve; and hypoglossal nucleus of the hypoglossal nerve (XII).[12] Pathologies eroding or infiltrating the occipital condyle and jugular foramen (JF) may result in a compression, stretching, or infiltration of IX nerve with its tympanic branch (for involvement of the pars nervosa of JF), X nerve with its auricular branch and XI nerve (for involvement of pars vascularis of JF).[13] Similarly, some upper cervical nerves may be affected by pathologies affecting the CCJ and extending caudally; those spinal nerves are: the suboccipital nerve (C1 root), the greater occipital nerve (C2 root) and,

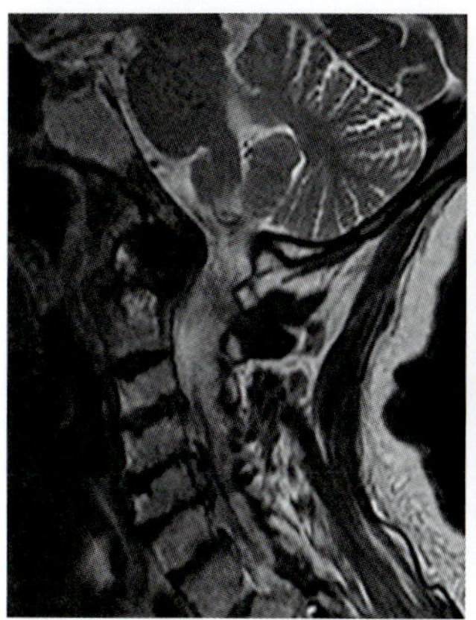
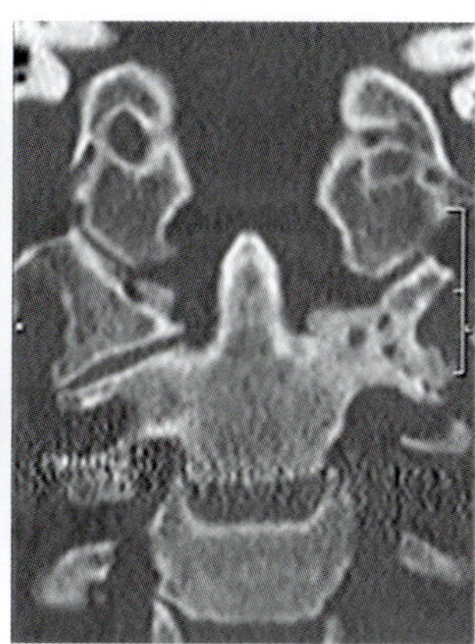
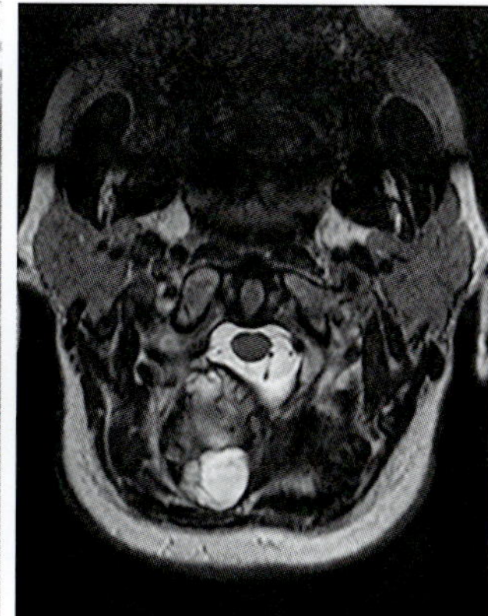
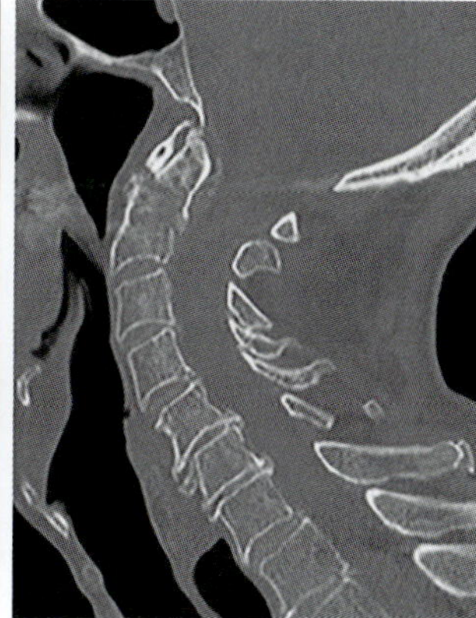

• **Fig. 50.1** From left to right, sagittal T2-weighted magnetic resonance imaging (MRI) scan showing periodontoid pseudotumor; coronal computed tomography (CT) scan showing seronegative osteoarthritis with geodic cavities and reabsorption of left C1–C2 joint; axial T2-weighted MRI scan showing a spindle cell tumor eroding the posterior arch of C2 and invading the craniocervical junction; sagittal CT scan showing a type II odontoid fracture.

rarely, the small occipital nerve (C3 root). Overall, the neurologic symptoms resulting from involvement of the neural elements cited above can range from dysphagia, dysarthria, and dysgeusia to neck pain and occipital neuralgia. Full neurologic examination with testing of gag reflex, light touch, and pinprick sensation in the territories of the upper spinal nerves is therefore recommended to identify subclinical signs.

Vertebral Artery

The vertebral artery (VA) provides segmental vertebral and spinal column blood supply; cranially, it continues with the basilar artery (BA), providing supply to the posterior fossa and the occipital lobes. Of the four segments of the VA, the two pertinent to the CCJ are the V3 and V4. The V3 segment emerges from the transverse process of C2, crosses the C2 root, and sweeps laterally to pass through the transverse foramen of C1 (vertical portion of V3).[14,15] From here it passes around the posterior border of the lateral mass of C1, keeping the C1 root on its medial side; it then lies in the groove on the upper surface of the posterior arch of C1 and enters the vertebral canal by passing beneath the PAOM, lateral to the cervicomedullary junction (horizontal portion of VA).[14,15] Finally, passing superomedially, it pierces the dura and the arachnoid to continue intracranially as the V4 segment of VA, which at the level of the FM is surrounded by a sympathetic plexus. The V4 segment inclines medially in front of the MO and is located between the XII nerve and the anterior root of the C1 nerve; at the lower border of the pons, it unites with its contralateral VA to form the BA.[12] In up to 18.8% of cases, a bony bridge called the arcuate foramen covers the VA groove on C1.[16] Asymmetry of VA may be due to hypoplasia or, more commonly, the presence of a dominant side: A statistically significant left dominance was found in ultrasonography and angiographic investigation testing several anatomic and functional parameters such as diameter, peak systolic velocity, end-diastolic velocity, time-averaged mean velocity, resistance index, and flow volume.[17–19] A strong correlation exists between the diameters of the transverse foramina and the blood flow of VA.[20] Anatomic variations of the V3 segment of VA include: fenestration, aberrant VA, and origin of posterior internal cerebral artery (PICA) at C2 or C1.[21] Damage to the VA is a concrete risk whenever performing an atlantoaxial fixation with Magerl technique, especially if the pars of C2 is narrow secondary to prominent looping of the VA into the pars.[22] The consequences of VA injury can be potentially catastrophic, leading to thrombosis, embolism, and cerebrovascular events, or causing iatrogenic pseudoaneurysm formation; usually, though, a unilateral injury has limited impact on the postoperative course, and most of the patients from the largest series are described as asymptomatic from unilateral arterial injury.[23]

Cervical Venous Plexus

Surgical techniques requiring careful exposure of the C1 lateral mass (e.g., C1–C2 screw-rod fixation with Goel or Harms techniques) have the advantage of reducing the risk of damage to the VA, but their complexity is increased by the venous plexus surrounding the C2 ganglion.[5,6] This venous plexus is part of an extensive sinusoidal network of posterior veins associated with the neural arches communicating with segmental veins forming the deep cervical vein complex. Of note, in correspondence to the C2 ganglion, this venous plexus may be quite extensive and further engorged due to the prone patient position required for these procedures.

Preoperative Workup

Prevention of complications starts with a careful preoperative workup. Regardless of the pathology and type of approach to the CCJ, every patient should undergo a magnetic resonance imaging study of the brain and cervical spine, coupled with a fine-cut

RED FLAGS

- Anatomic variations of VA course (fenestrated VA, aberrant VA, origin of PICA at C2 or C1)
- Thin squamous part of the occipital bone, small C1 lateral masses, small pedicles of C2/C3
- Poor-prognostic preoperative factors, such as: smoking habit, weight loss, osteopenia, prolonged steroid treatment, neurologic deficits, Ranawat Class IIIB, metastatic disease
- Risk of poor wound healing: anticipated blood loss exceeding 1000 mL, prolonged postoperative intubation/nasogastric feeding tube, need for adjuvant treatments (e.g., radiation therapy)
- Re-do of surgery for recurrence of disease (e.g., malignancies) or postoperative instability

computed tomography (CT) study of the CCJ and cervical spine. Appropriate imaging of the CCJ with CT angiography (CTA) or digital selective angiography (DSA) has to be considered for a careful study of the VA and its possible anatomic variations. The use of an intraoperative neuronavigation system and micro-Doppler ultrasonography can be advisable, depending on the pathology and the type of approach; intraoperative neurophysiologic monitoring with recording of somatosensory- and motor-evoked potentials is routinely recommended, with no exceptions. Patients with CCJ pathologies should always receive fiber-optic intubation; anterior approaches to the CCJ can require either nasotracheal or orotracheal intubation, depending on the use of a transoral or transnasal endoscopic approach.[24] In both cases, however, a triple-antibiotic prophylaxis covering for gram-positive and gram-negative cocci should be considered to reduce the risk of contamination, and a dose of steroids (dexamethasone 4 mg) should be administered preoperatively to prevent edema or swelling of the mucosae.[4,24] Patient positioning depends on the nature of the pathology addressed, the operative approach, and the surgeon's preference: transnasal endoscopic approaches are generally performed with the patient in supine, slight anti-Trendelenburg position (20 degrees); for lateral and far lateral approaches to the CCJ, options include prone, park bench, and sitting position; for occipitocervical fusion, our preference is to use the Jackson table with the head fixed in a Mayfield three-pins head holder.

Management of Cerebrospinal Fluid Leak

Cerebrospinal fluid (CSF) leak may occur with the use of a drill or rongeur during all sorts of anterior (endoscopic endonasal and transoral) or posterior approaches to CCJ. If the risk of dural breach can be anticipated preoperatively (e.g., with extradural tumors), a lumbar drain (LD) may be inserted before surgery and removed at the end of an uneventful procedure. If a dural leak occurs, the height of the LD should be adjusted to allow for a drainage of 10 to 15 mL of CSF hourly for 5 postoperative days to ensure dural and wound healing without tension. The management of dural tears depends on the location of the breach and the type of surgical exposure. As a general rule, if the surgeon has a direct visualization of the CSF leak, an attempt to close it through microsuture should be pursued; however, this may be technically challenging, especially in the case of ventrally or laterally located dural tears. Dural sutures in these areas increase the risk of making the tear even larger; in those instances, it is therefore better simply to use fibrin glue and perform a good two-layer waterproof closure; finally, a Valsalva maneuver should be carried out to confirm the good quality of the dural closure. Furthermore, the team should be aware of the risk of postoperative pneumocephalus, hydrocephalus, pseudomeningocele/seroma, meningitis, delayed CSF leak and, in rare cases, cerebral hypotension (Fig. 50.2).

Steps to Control Torrential Bleeding

The best way to reduce the risk of copious intraoperative bleeding, the need for transfusion, and the occurrence of possible neurovascular sequelae is understanding the mechanisms of injury to the VA and venous plexus. A few technical points must be highlighted: (1) intraoperative image-guided or stereotactic guidance may improve accuracy and significantly reduce the risk of vascular injury; (2) careful use of blunt instruments is recommended during the dissection and exposure of bone structures; (3) intraoperative systemic infusion of tranexamic acid should be considered to help reduce blood loss; (4) during the insertion of screws (especially at C1 and C2), the surgeon must be cautious with the use of probes or sounders meant to check the integrity of cortical bone. Once the desired screw trajectory is determined and prepared with the screwdriver and tapping instrument, it is advisable to proceed with the screw placement rather than to check the bone integrity, because this maneuver can result in inadvertent breach of the cortical wall and damage to neurovascular structures. The primary management of VA or venous plexus injury always includes the use of hemostatic agents followed by mechanical tamponade with a microsurgical cottonoid. Indulging in attempts to achieve hemostasis by coagulation with bipolar forceps is usually dangerous and useless. Of note, the need for direct surgical repair, ligation, and clipping of the VA during surgical approaches to the CCJ is extremely rare, with only a few cases reported during anterior C2 corpectomies.[25]

Instrumented Fusion: Tips and Tricks

The nature of the neural compression, the quality of the bone, and the patient's nutritional status play a large role in the decision-making process when considering anterior or posterior approaches to the CCJ; this said, approximately 70% of patients undergoing transoral decompression will also require subsequent occipitocervical fixation (OCF).[26] Occipital condyle resection may be needed,

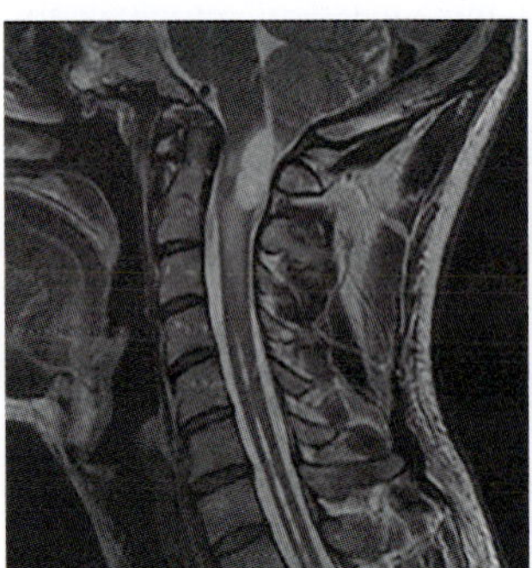
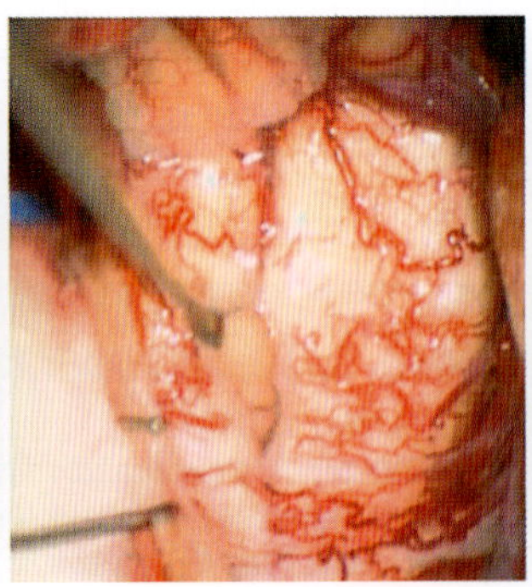
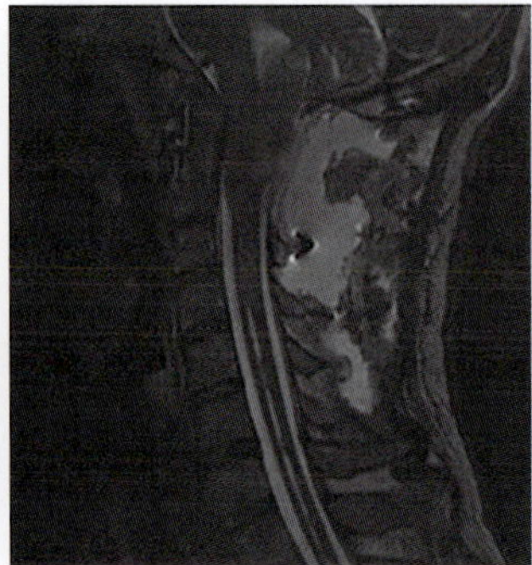
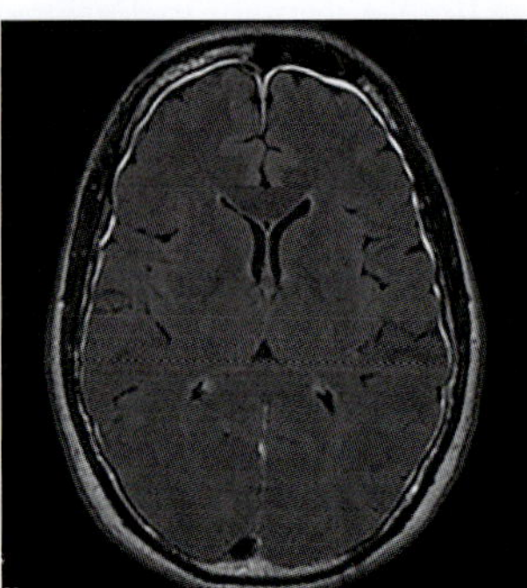

• **Fig. 50.2** From left to right, preoperative sagittal T2-weighted magnetic resonance imaging (MRI) scan showing a C1–C2 intramedullary cyst; intraoperative view showing the midline myelotomy to access the lesion (low-grade astrocytoma); postoperative sagittal T2-weighted MRI scan showing the complete resection with pseudomeningocele; postoperative T1-weighted MRI scan showing delayed intracranial hypotension.

depending on the extent and location of the CCJ tumors. In the case of significant condylar resection, OCF is warranted;[2,3,8] among patients with CCJ tumors, those with chordomas and metastases are more likely to require OCF.[10,27] Preoperative reduction/realignment can be considered in cases of severe deformity; these maneuvers ideally should be performed under sedation and neurophysiologic monitoring. Application of a Halo jacket before surgical decompression and fusion is a valuable option in selected cases, not only in the pediatric population. Transarticular screw fixation between C2 and C1 requires that the width of the pars interarticularis at C2 be satisfactory; the integrity of the lateral mass of C1 cannot be compromised by atrophy, compression, or significant osteoporosis.[28,29] Unfortunately, the VA groove may encroach on the pars articularis, and the risk of injury is high even in the most experienced hands; this situation can be identified as a potential problem on preoperative CT/CTA scans.[30] Immediate rigid fixation of the CCJ and a low rate of hardware failure are indispensable to achieving a high rate of fusion.[11] As a general rule, adding corticocancellous autografts obtained at the time of decompression and supplemented with bone morphogenic proteins, laterally to the instrumented fixation, is the best way to provide the four elements critical for successful bone healing: (a) an osteoconductive matrix, (b) osteoinductive factors, (c) viable osteogenic cells, and (d) structural support. Postoperative immobilization in a hard collar is usually not required, but in selected scenarios it can be considered for up to 3 months postoperatively.[9]

Wound Closure and Postoperative Care

After an accurate hemostasis, the surgical team must pay a great deal of attention to achieving satisfactory wound closure to avoid immediate or delayed wound breakdown. Posterior approaches to the CCJ are particularly at risk of wound dehiscence, which is favored by the absence of muscle layer over the occipital squama; dehiscence can become a dramatic complication whenever it is associated with the exposure of the hardware and its contamination. As such, early postoperative mobilization should be encouraged and nuchal decubitus avoided to prevent erosion of the skin, especially in patients with occipital plating after OCF. Besides the intraoperative risks highlighted above, patients undergoing surgery at the CCJ should be informed regarding the possible need for postoperative admission to the intensive care unit (ICU). In fact, surgery at the CCJ carries a high risk of delayed extubation, especially with long procedures or those requiring a combined anterior and posterior stage, or whenever the respiratory drive may be compromised, depending on the nature of the pathologic condition treated (brainstem and intramedullary lesions, high cervical cord injuries, etc.). Remote cerebellar hemorrhage after CCJ surgery is also infrequent but can complicate the immediate (24–48 hours) postoperative course. This type of bleeding is usually venous in nature and thought to occur secondary to VA occlusion or to sudden increases of transmural pressure gradient due to excessive intraoperative loss of CSF.[31]

SURGICAL REWIND

My Worst Case (Fig. 50.3)

A 63-year-old woman with a previous medical history of upper cervical fracture treated conservatively presented to our attention with clinical features of progressive cervical myelopathy and dysphagia. Imaging studies disclosed evidence of chronically nonunited odontoid fracture with significant cervical kyphosis and severe cord compression with T2 signal change. After Halo cervical traction with 15 pounds of weight to reduce the kyphotic

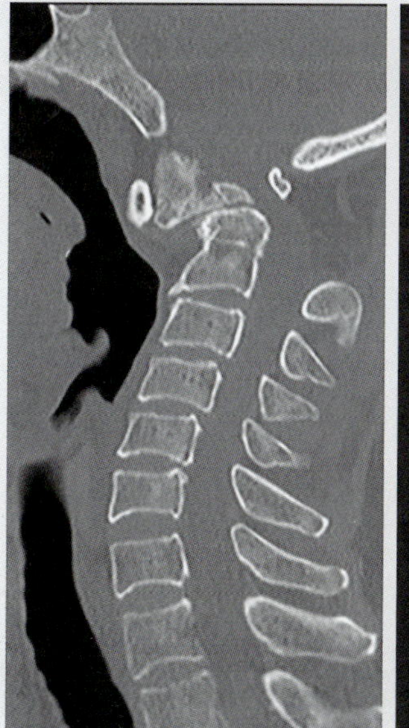
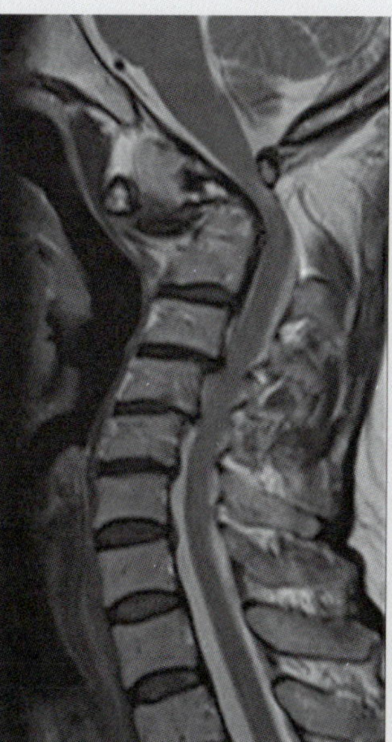
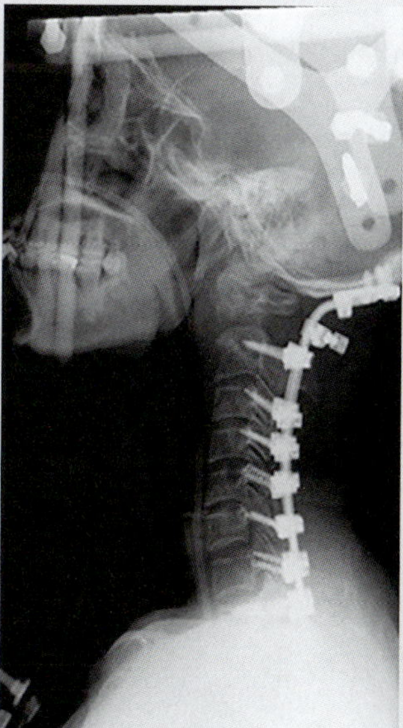
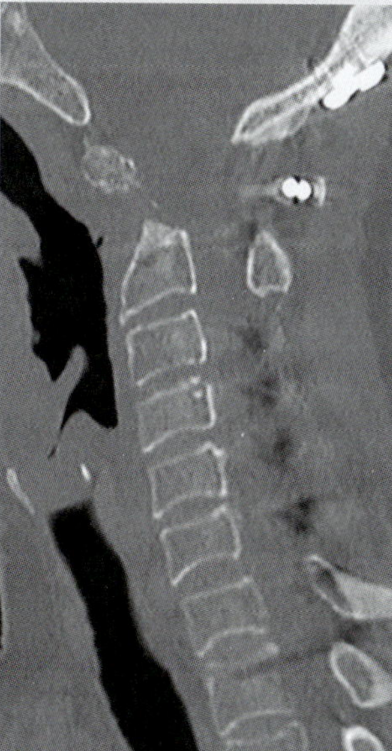

• **Fig. 50.3** From left to right, preoperative sagittal computed tomography (CT) and T2-weighted magnetic resonance imaging scans; note the T2 cord hyperintensity at the craniocervical junction and the subaxial cervical spondylosis. Postoperative x-ray and CT scan; note the satisfactory decompression and improvement of spinal alignment.

Continued

deformity, a transoral decompression was undertaken. A three-dimensional O-arm was used to obtain CT images of the skull base and upper cervical spine. The images were transferred to the stealth navigation system for intraoperative fiducially referenced stereotactic imaging. Baseline motor and somatosensory evoked potential were checked at the beginning of the procedure. A midline sharp incision of the pharyngeal wall was fashioned just above the arch of C1 and the base of the body of C2, and the odontoidectomy was performed with a high-speed drill and curettage until the tectorial membrane and posterior longitudinal ligament were exposed. A small dural breach was repaired with a multilayered complex duroplasty, followed by hemostasis and closure of the pharyngeal muscular layer. The patient was turned from the supine to prone position to undertake a lumbar drain insertion and then an occipito-cervico-thoracic fusion. Stereotactic guidance proved useful for cervical instrumentation, particularly for C2 pedicle screws; a C1 laminectomy was then performed, and the PAOM appeared completely disrupted by the osteoarthritic process. The occipital plate was placed, and so were the lateral mass screws at C3, C4, C5, C6, and C7 and the pedicle screws at T1. After placement of instrumentation, there were no changes in neurophysiologic status. The procedure was then completed with a C3–C7 laminectomy. A subfascial drain was positioned, and waterproof closure was sought. Patient was transferred to the ICU and was initially kept under nasotracheal ventilation. The lumbar drain was removed after 5 days, and the nasogastric feeding was discontinued after 1 week. The rest of the postoperative course was uneventful.

NEUROSURGICAL SELFIE MOMENT

Although the standard transoral approach provides a wide access to the CCJ, it requires a splitting of the soft palate and provides a wide but deep working channel; furthermore, it is affected by the risks of teeth traumatism, CSF leak, bacterial contamination, tongue swelling, and nasopharyngeal incompetence, often requiring prolonged intubation and nasogastric tube feeding. In summary, the more invasive the pathology, the longer the operative time and the riskier the extended procedure. The posterior approaches require a sound understanding of the biomechanics of the cervical spine; they also require the most appropriate choice of instrumented fixation technique to reduce the risks of neurovascular injuries and to achieve long-term fusion. As a general rule, the choice must be tailored to the specific type of pathology addressed, the patient's anatomic peculiarities, and the time of intervention. A thorough preoperative investigation is of paramount importance to achieve a satisfactory outcome; it must be borne in mind that the overall complication rate for surgery at the CCJ is 30%, whereas the reported infection rate for anterior and posterior approaches is 3.6% and 5%, respectively.[32,33] In the case of perioperative complications, a multidisciplinary approach is essential for safe and optimum management; despite that, the mortality rate of 1.7% for patients undergoing occipitocervical fixation clearly defines the relevant challenges of these procedures.[32]

References

1. Crockard HA, Pozo JL, Ransford AO, Stevens JM, Kendall BE, Essigman WK. Transoral decompression and posterior fusion for rheumatoid atlanto-axial subluxation. *J Bone Joint Surg Br*. 1986; 68:350–356.
2. Fehlings MG, David KS, Vialle L, Vialle E, Setzer M, Vrionis FD. Decision making in the surgical treatment of cervical spine metastases. *Spine*. 2009;34:S108–S117.
3. Fehlings MG, Errico T, Cooper P, Benjamin V, DiBartolo T. Occipitocervical fusion with a five-millimeter malleable rod and segmental fixation. *Neurosurgery*. 1993;32:198–208.
4. Fujii T, Platt A, Zada G. Endoscopic endonasal approaches to the craniovertebral junction: a systematic review of the literature. *J Neurol Surg B Skull Base*. 2015;76:480–488.
5. Goel A, Laheri V. Plate and screw fixation for atlanto-axial subluxation. *Acta Neurochir (Wien)*. 1994;129:47–53.
6. Harms J, Melcher RP. Posterior C1-C2 fusion with polyaxial screw and rod fixation. *Spine*. 2001;26:2467–2471.
7. Jeanneret B, Magerl F. Primary posterior fusion C1/2 in odontoid fractures: indications, technique, and results of transarticular screw fixation. *J Spinal Disord*. 1992;5:464–475.
8. Margalit NS, Lesser JB, Singer M, Sen C. Lateral approach to anterolateral tumors at the foramen magnum: factors determining surgical procedure. *Neurosurgery*. 2005;56:324–336.
9. Shiban E, Török E, Wostrack M, Meyer B, Lehmberg J. The far-lateral approach: destruction of the condyle does not necessarily result in clinically evident craniovertebral junction instability. *J Neurosurg*. 2016;125:196–201.
10. Shin H, Barrenechea IJ, Lesser J, Sen C, Perin NI. Occipitocervical fusion after resection of craniovertebral junction tumors. *J Neurosurg Spine*. 2006;4:137–144.
11. Singh SK, Rickards L, Apfelbaum RI, Hurlbert RJ, Maiman D, Fehlings MG. Occipitocervical reconstruction with the Ohio Medical Instruments Loop: results of a multicenter evaluation in 30 cases. *J Neurosurg*. 2003;98:239–246.
12. de Oliveira E, Rhoton AL Jr, Peace D. Microsurgical anatomy of the region of the foramen magnum. *Surg Neurol*. 1985;24:293–352.
13. Wen HT, Rhoton AL Jr, Katsuta T, de Oliveira E. Microsurgical anatomy of the transcondylar, supracondylar, and paracondylar extensions of the far-lateral approach. *J Neurosurg*. 1997;87:555–585.
14. Cacciola F, Phalke U, Goel A. Vertebral artery in relationship to C1-C2 vertebrae: an anatomical study. *Neurol India*. 2004;52:178–184.
15. Tubbs RS, Shah NA, Sullivan BP, Marchase ND, Cohen-Gadol AA. Surgical anatomy and quantitation of the branches of the V2 and V3 segments of the vertebral artery. Laboratory investigation. *J Neurosurg Spine*. 2009;11:84–87.
16. Elliott RE, Tanweer O. The prevalence of the ponticulus posticus (arcuate foramen) and its importance in the Goel-Harms procedure: meta-analysis and review of the literature. *World Neurosurg*. 2014;82:e335–e343.
17. Jeng JS, Yip PK. Evaluation of vertebral artery hypoplasia and asymmetry by color-coded duplex ultrasonography. *Ultrasound Med Biol*. 2004;30:605–609.
18. Sanelli PC, Tong S, Gonzalez RG, Eskey CJ. Normal variation of vertebral artery on CT angiography and its implications for diagnosis of acquired pathology. *J Comput Assist Tomogr*. 2002;26:462–470.
19. Trattnig S, Hübsch P, Schuster H, Pölzleitner D. Color-coded Doppler imaging of normal vertebral arteries. *Stroke*. 1990;21:1222–1225.
20. Kotil K, Kilincer C. Sizes of the transverse foramina correlate with blood flow and dominance of vertebral arteries. *Spine J*. 2014;14: 933–937.
21. Ivashchuk G, Fries FN, Loukas M, et al. Arterial variations around the atlas: a comprehensive review for avoiding neurosurgical complications. *Childs Nerv Syst*. 2016;32:1093–1100.
22. Sonntag VK. Beware of the arcuate foramen. *World Neurosurg*. 2014;82:e141–e142.
23. Casey AT, Madawi AA, Veres R, Crockard HA. Is the technique of posterior transarticular screw fixation suitable for rheumatoid atlanto-axial subluxation? *Br J Neurosurg*. 1997;11:508–519.
24. Marks RJ, Forrester PC, Calder I, Crockard HA. Anaesthesia for transoral craniocervical surgery. *Anaesthesia*. 1986;41:1049–1052.

25. Park HK, Jho HD. The management of vertebral artery injury in anterior cervical spine operation: a systematic review of published cases. *Eur Spine J*. 2012;21:2475–2485.
26. Dickman CA, Locantro J, Fessler RG. The influence of transoral odontoid resection on stability of the craniovertebral junction. *J Neurosurg*. 1992;77:525–530.
27. Colli B, Al-Mefty O. Chordomas of the craniocervical junction: follow-up review and prognostic factors. *J Neurosurg*. 2001;95:933–943.
28. Coyne TJ, Fehlings MG, Wallace MC, Bernstein M, Tator CH. C1-C2 posterior cervical fusion: long-term evaluation of results and efficacy. *Neurosurgery*. 1995;37:688–692.
29. Gunnarsson T, Massicotte EM, Govender PV, Raja Rampersaud Y, Fehlings MG. The use of C1 lateral mass screws in complex cervical spine surgery: indications, techniques, and outcome in a prospective consecutive series of 25 cases. *J Spinal Disord Tech*. 2007;20:308–316.
30. Paramore CG, Dickman CA, Sonntag VK. The anatomical suitability of the C1-2 complex for transarticular screw fixation. *J Neurosurg*. 1996;85:221–224.
31. Mikawa Y, Watanabe R, Hino Y, Ishii R, Hirano K. Cerebellar hemorrhage complicating cervical durotomy and revision C1-C2 fusion. *Spine*. 1994;19(10):1169–1171.
32. Deutsch H, Haid RW Jr, Rodts GE Jr, Mummaneni PV. Occipitocervical fixation: long-term results. *Spine*. 2005;30(5):530–535.
33. Shousha M, Mosafer A, Boehm H. Infection rate after transoral approach for the upper cervical spine. *Spine*. 2014;39(19):1578–1583.

51

Neurologic Deterioration After Spinal Surgery

ANDREW J. GROSSBACH, VINCENT C. TRAYNELIS

HIGHLIGHTS

- Postoperative neurologic decline includes a wide variety of etiologies.
- Care must be taken preoperatively to minimize neurologic risk to the patient.
- A swift, systematic approach should be taken to identify potential causes of postoperative neurologic decline.
- Once the etiology is identified, immediate action should be taken to remedy the situation and give the patient the best chance of neurologic recovery.

Background

Neurosurgery, at its very core, is a dangerous undertaking. When operating within and around vital neurologic structures, even with the utmost care and a deft touch, the risk of neurologic injury is always present. Care must always be taken to minimize the risk of neurologic injury to the patient. The causes of postoperative neurologic decline are numerous and varied. They include hemorrhagic and vascular etiologies and hardware/implant complications, or they could be secondary to systemic complications such as cardiovascular or respiratory issues. In this chapter we will discuss neurologic decline after spinal surgery, including what the potential risk factors are, how to minimize risk to the patient, how to work up a patient experiencing neurologic compromise after spine surgery, and how to manage these complications. Because of the wide variety of potential etiologies of postoperative neurologic decline, this chapter cannot be an all-encompassing text; however, we will attempt to point out the highlights of the aforementioned topics.

Anatomic Insights

The epidural venous plexus can be subdivided into two parts, the anterior venous plexus and the posterior venous plexus, the latter being larger and the most clinically significant because it is what is encountered during posterior approaches to the spine.[1] There is often an increased convolution of veins at the cervicothoracic junction.[1] This may put patients undergoing surgery in this region at a higher risk of epidural hematoma postoperatively, and therefore extra care should be taken to ensure adequate hemostasis. The epidural venous plexus is postulated to be the source for many postoperative epidural hematomas, although other etiologies may exist.[1]

The spinal cord receives blood flow mainly from one anterior spinal artery and two posterior spinal arteries.[2,3] The anterior spinal artery, which is formed by anterior spinal branches of the vertebral arteries at the level of the foramen magnum, lies over the anterior sulcus of the spinal cord and supplies the anterior two-thirds of the spinal cord.[2,3] Whether the anterior spinal artery is continuous or segmental is considered to be controversial.[3–5] The anterior spinal artery relies heavily on segmental feeders as it descends the spinal cord.[2–5] The posterior spinal arteries are formed by branches of the posterior inferior cerebellar arteries (PICA) and supply the posterior one-third of the spinal cord in the cervical region. As one moves more caudally, the segmental arteries assume a greater role in supplying blood to the anterior and posterior spinal cord.[2]

Paired radicular arteries originate from the thoracic aorta, enter the neuroforamina, penetrate the dura, and irrigate the spinal cord along with other local structures.[2,5] In the thoracic region, these arteries bifurcate into anterior and posterior branches that join the anterior spinal artery and posterior spinal arteries, respectively.[2] In the adult, many of these segmental arteries have become vestigial, with the cord being supplied by a few larger radicular arteries.[2] Although somewhat controversial, the largest radicular artery is known as the artery of Adamkiewicz, or the arteria radicularis magna. The artery of Adamkiewicz has been reported to originate from the left in 80% of the population,[2,4] from between T5–8 in 15%, T9–12 in 75%, and L1–2 in 10%.[2] Biglioli et al. in a 2000 cadaveric study reported that the artery of Adamkiewicz originated from the left in 68% of cases and from between T12–L3 in 84%.[3] This leaves areas prone to watershed infarcts around T1, T5, and T8–9.[2] Cheshire et al. reported a relative hypovascular zone from T4–T8.[5]

The neural structures of the spine are at risk from direct injury during spinal procedures, especially if instrumentation or hardware is used. Nerve roots pass medially and inferiorly to the pedicles in the spine and are at risk during pedicle screw placement, particularly in the thoracic spine due to relatively small pedicles.[6] In one cadaveric study, Ebraheim et al. found that inferiorly, the greatest distance between the pedicle and nerve root was at T6–T9 (3.1–3.7 mm) and that the smallest distance was at T1–T2 (1.7–1.8 mm).[6] They found no difference between the pedicle and thecal sac medially at any level.

When contemplating surgical intervention on patients with spinal deformity, care must be taken to appreciate all aspects of the deformity because the patient's spine may have aspects of coronal and sagittal as well as rotational deformity. Understanding these nuances could be a book in and of itself; therefore, we will touch only briefly on these topics in this chapter. Patients with scoliosis often have rotation of the spine toward the convexity of the deformity.[7] This leads to the pedicle screw on the concavity requiring a more medialized trajectory, and the opposite for the convexity. Furthermore, the neural elements will be shifted toward the concavity, leaving a relatively large free space lateral to the thecal sac at the convexity.[7] Patients with large coronal or sagittal deformities are at increased risk of neurologic compromise during corrective maneuvers,[8] and deformities in all planes must be measured out preoperatively for surgical planning and risk assessment.

RED FLAGS

Of the potential postoperative causes for neurologic decline after spinal surgery, postoperative epidural hematoma that compresses the spinal cord or cauda equina may be the most important to identify quickly and to intervene in surgically to restore a patient's neurologic function. However, this complication is fairly rare, occurring in 0.1% to 0.24% of spinal surgical cases.[9–11] Despite the relatively low number of symptomatic postoperative epidural hematomas, radiographic epidural hematomas have been reported in 33% to 100% of patients.[12] In a 2005 study, Awad et al. described several risk factors for postoperative epidural hematoma, including age >60 years old, the use of preoperative nonsteroidal antiinflammatories, Rh-positive blood group, hypertension, coagulopathy (hepatitis B, hepatitis C, liver cirrhosis, thrombocytopenia, history of easy bruising, pernicious anemia, and neoplasms), and tobacco use using univariate analysis.[13] When a logistic multivariate regression model was used, hypertension and medical coagulopathy proved not to be significant. When intraoperative variables were examined, risk factors for postoperative epidural hematoma included more than five operative levels, a hemoglobin <10 g/dL, and blood loss >1 L.[13] Postoperatively, the only risk factor for development of an epidural hematoma was an international normalized ratio (INR) >2.0 within 48 hours after surgery.[13] Sokolowski et al. reported in 2008 that age >60 years old, elevated preoperative INR, multilevel procedures, and higher levels of blood loss were associated with postoperative epidural hematomas.[12] In 2002, Kou et al. also discussed risk factors for the development of spinal epidural hematoma postoperatively. They identified undergoing a multilevel surgery as well as having a preoperative coagulopathy as increasing the risk of epidural hematoma.[14] Groen and Ponssen report larger exposures of the epidural space may increase the likelihood of bleeding from the venous plexus.[1]

In one series, Moufarrij reported an increased incidence of symptomatic postoperative epidural spinal hematomas after implantation of spinal cord stimulator paddle leads versus thoracic laminectomies without the implantation of leads (2.60% vs 0.84%).[15] None of these patients had identifiable risk factors for bleeding. Therefore, extra care should be taken when planning the placement of epidural paddle leads, and the patient should be counseled on this potential risk.

Patients with preexisting compressive lesions in the cervical or thoracic spine may be at significant risk for neurologic deterioration after a spinal surgery if the proximal lesion is not addressed first. Patients presenting with signs and/or symptoms of myelopathy should be further examined with MR imaging of the cervical and/or thoracic spine before surgery. Sensory abnormalities of the trunk may be a tip-off of thoracic pathology that can be masked in the setting of lumbar stenosis.[16] Therefore a careful neurologic examination and thorough documentation are a must for all patients undergoing planned spinal surgery.

Although postoperative urinary retention does not necessarily represent neurologic decline, it is a significant problem in spinal surgery patients. It has been reported in 8.8% of elective spine patients in a recent study.[17] Risk factors include posterior lumbar surgery, patients with preexisting benign prostatic hypertrophy, chronic constipation, prior history of urinary retention, long operative times, and the use of a patient-controlled analgesia pump postoperatively.[17]

Patients undergoing planned corrective procedures for spinal deformity may also be at an increased risk of postoperative neurologic decline, particularly in patients with sagittal imbalance.[18] Patients with >80 degrees of coronal or sagittal deformity are at significant risk of neurologic compromise during corrective procedures.[8,19] Lenke et al. report an incidence of new lower-extremity weakness of 22% in patients with coronal or sagittal deformities of >80 degrees.[19] They also report a relatively high risk for patients undergoing a 3-column osteotomy such as a vertebral column resection or a pedicle subtraction osteotomy.[19] The presence of preoperative motor deficits also significantly increased the risk of new postoperative deficits.[8,19] Patients with cardiopulmonary comorbidities may also be at higher risk, secondary to either systemic hypotension or to vascular injury causing ischemia of the spinal cord. There are several physiologic factors that determine perfusion of the spinal cord, including systemic blood pressure or mean arterial pressure, hemoglobin concentration of the blood, and intravascular volume.[18]

Prevention

Prevention of postoperative spinal epidural hematomas can best be achieved by limiting preoperative risk factors. Coagulopathies should be identified and corrected before surgery. Preoperative testing should include platelet count, prothrombin time/INR, and partial thromboplastin time. Patients should be counseled on when to stop medications such as anticoagulant, antiplatelet medication, and nonsteroidal antiinflammatory medications. Nonmodifiable risk factors such as advanced age, high anticipated blood loss, and a planned multilevel procedure should be acknowledged so the surgical team can maintain vigilance in the perioperative period. Postoperatively, intravenous anticoagulation use should be avoided for at least 12 hours.[9] Furthermore, INR should be maintained <2.0 for 48 hours postoperatively.[13]

Postoperative neurologic decline has also been associated with missed thoracic and/or cervical lesions.[16] Thorough neurologic examination and documentation—including sensory testing of the trunk because thoracic myelopathy may be masked in the face of lumbar stenosis—before any planned surgery is essential to identify any additional compressive lesions that may compromise neurologic functioning during or after a surgery. If there are any concerning signs or symptoms of a proximal compressive lesion causing myelopathy, magnetic resonance imaging (MRI) scans of the cervical and/or thoracic spine should be obtained before any planned surgeries.[16]

As spinal cord ischemia is another potential cause of postoperative neurologic decline, the patient should be optimized preoperatively to minimize the risk of spinal cord ischemia during surgery. Labs and vital signs should be noted to ensure adequate blood pressure, intravascular volume, and hemoglobin/hematocrit. Also, preparations should be made preoperatively so the surgical team is prepared in the case of excessive blood loss.

When planning a spinal surgery, intraoperative neuromonitoring (IONM) should be considered. Although IONM has not been shown to decrease neurologic complications in all types of spinal surgery, when performing a surgery to correct a spinal deformity, the use of multimodality monitoring has become commonplace.[20–24] The sensitivity and specificity values for detecting neurologic complications using multimodality IONM have been reported to be up to 100%.[20–25]

Although postoperative wound drains are common, either subfascial or suprafascial, several studies have shown no difference in the incidence of postoperative epidural hematoma between patients with postoperative wound drains versus no drains.[9,13,14,26–28]

There is one recent report, however, that showed less epidural hematomas on postoperative day 1 on MRI in patients with a subfascial drain.[29]

Management

When a patient awakens from spinal surgery with a new neurologic deficit, action must be taken swiftly to identify the cause of the deficit and, if possible, to remedy the situation.

Although evidence is lacking in the literature, adopting a policy to systematically address the patient should be considered, similarly to when there is a loss of IONM signals during surgery.[21] Systemic issues should be quickly assessed and remedied, including optimization of systemic blood pressure/mean arterial pressure (MAP), intravascular volume, hemoglobin/hematocrit, and respiratory status.[21]

An MRI of the surgical site should be obtained immediately.[10] A computed tomography (CT) scan should be obtained immediately if MRI is not available or there will be a delay obtaining the scan. It is often questioned whether a spinal epidural hematoma is the culprit in the development of a new deficit, because postoperative imaging often shows blood products at the surgical site.[9,10] Postoperative epidural hematomas may occur shortly after the operative procedure; however, delayed postoperative spinal epidural hematomas, occurring more than 3 days after surgery (average 5.3 days), have been described.[9] Yi et al. report that on MRI imaging, a postoperative spinal epidural hematoma will be isointense or hyperintense on T1-weighted imaging and heterogeneously hyperintense on T2-weighted imaging.[10] Uribe et al. report a hyperintense lesion on both T1- and T2-weighted images.[9] They also report a convex lens–shaped lesion on sagittal and parasagittal views.[9,10] The presentation of postoperative spinal epidural hematomas can vary, but a classic progression is sharp pain at the surgical site followed by radicular pain, then bowel/bladder dysfunction, motor weakness, and/or sensory loss.[9,10] Plain films or a CT scan should be obtained if there is hardware or instrumentation that is not able to be assessed on the MRI scan to ensure that it is not encroaching on the neural elements.

If a spinal epidural hematoma is identified, emergent reoperation for evacuation of the hematoma is warranted. Rapid decompression is associated with improved recovery.[10,11] Likewise, if spinal implants such as pedicle screws or interbody grafts have compromised neural structures, surgery should be undertaken immediately to revise or remove the offending instrumentation.

The differential diagnosis of patients with severe spinal pain and progressive neurologic deficit postoperatively includes intradural hemorrhage, spinal cord compression from hardware or instrumentation, infection, inflammatory conditions, spinal cord infarction, and other vascular processes.[9,30–32] Although this method is somewhat controversial, if a spinal cord infarction is suspected, oftentimes MAP is elevated to ensure optimal spinal cord perfusion, because this has been shown to be advantageous in the setting of spinal cord ischemia.[33] MAPs of >80 mm Hg to >90 mm Hg are frequently used.

If imaging does not reveal a compressive lesion at the site of surgery, a thorough neurologic examination and possible MR imaging should be performed to evaluate for proximal compressive lesions missed before surgery, such as cervical stenosis or a thoracic arachnoid cyst. If a lesion is detected, decompressive surgery should be performed on this lesion urgently because it has been reported to improve neurologic outcomes.[34]

SURGICAL REWIND

My Worst Case

A 44-year-old male with a history of prior C3–7 laminoplasty for cervical spondylotic myelopathy presented to the neurosurgery clinic with progressive symptoms of myelopathy. MR imaging and cervical x-rays revealed kyphotic deformity with continued compression of the cervical cord. He was taken to the operating room (OR) for a posterior cervical decompression from C3–7 with a C2–T2 posterior instrumentation and fusion (Fig. 51.1). He did well postoperatively and was discharged to a rehabilitation facility. On postoperative day 16 he developed acute worsening of his neck pain, followed shortly by progressive weakness in all four extremities as well as urinary retention. He was not on any antiplatelet agents or anticoagulation.

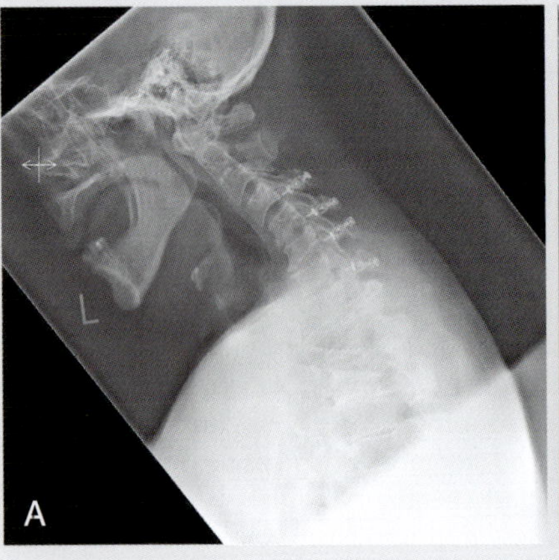

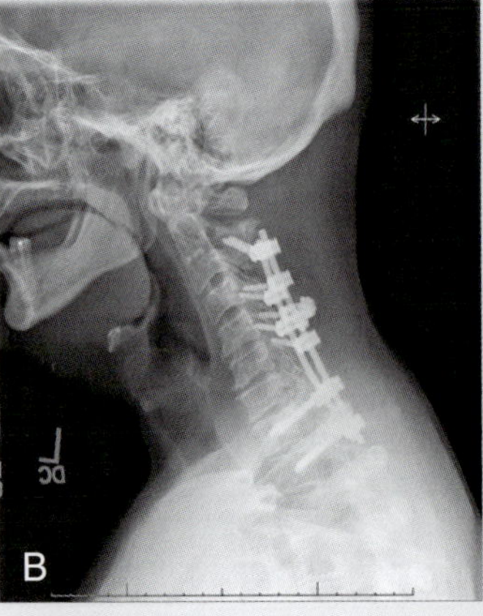

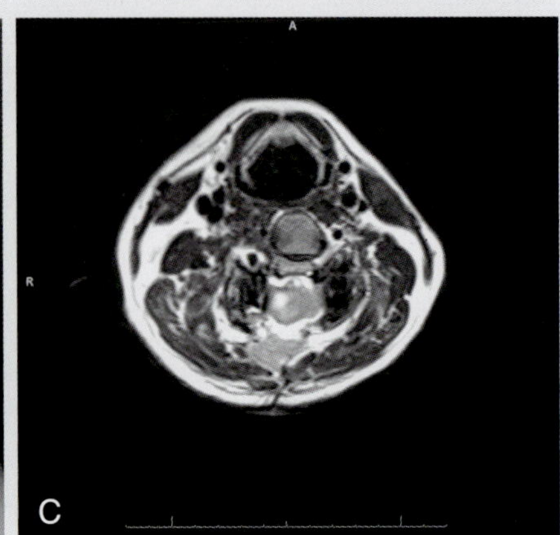

• **Fig. 51.1** (A) Preoperative lateral x-rays demonstrate prior laminoplasty with significant kyphotic deformity. (B) Postoperative x-rays demonstrate correction of kyphotic deformity. (C) Axial T2 magnetic resonance image (MRI) demonstrating posterior epidural hematoma with significant compression of the spinal cord.

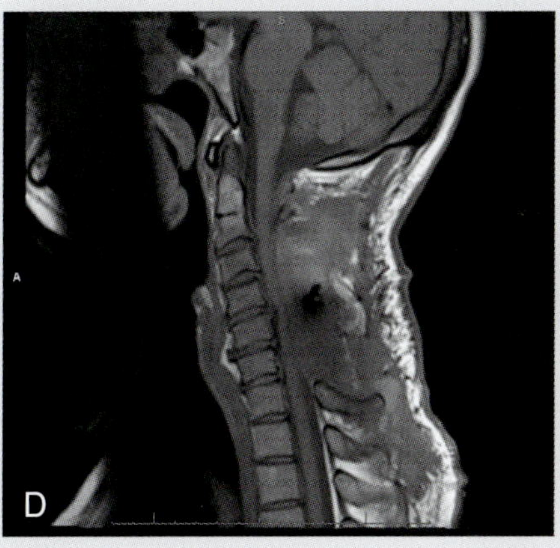

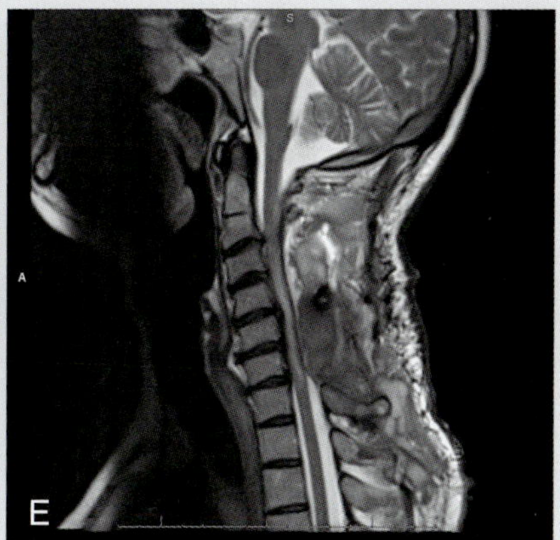

• **Fig. 51.1, cont'd** (D) Sagittal T1 MRI showing posterior epidural hematoma with significant compression of the spinal cord. (E) Sagittal T2 MRI showing posterior epidural hematoma with significant compression of the spinal cord.

He was transferred to the emergency room. He had 4/5 strength in the right upper and lower extremities, 2/5 strength in the left upper extremity, and 0/5 strength in the left lower extremity. A STAT MRI was obtained that showed an epidural hematoma extending from C3–7 with significant compression of the spinal cord and cord signal change. He was taken to the OR emergently for wound exploration and evacuation of the epidural hematoma. Upon opening the fascia, blood erupted from the epidural space under high pressure. The patient was again discharged to a rehabilitation facility 7 days later. At his 6-week follow-up, his strength had improved to 4+/5 in his bilateral upper extremities, 5/5 in the right lower extremity, and 4–/5 in his left lower extremity.

NEUROSURGICAL SELFIE MOMENT

Neurologic decline after spine surgery is every spine surgeon's worst fear. Although the etiologies may be varied, a rapid and thorough workup should be undertaken to identify potential causes that can be remedied. It is vital to maintain a cool head and to systematically work up the patient. If a remediable cause is identified, rapid intervention will ensure that the patient has the best chance to make a neurologic recovery.

References

1. Groen RJM, Ponssen H. The spontaneous spinal epidural hematoma. *J Neurol Sci*. 1990;98(2–3):121–138.
2. Shamji MF, Maziak DE, Shamji FM, Ginsberg RJ, Pon R. Circulation of the spinal cord: an important consideration for thoracic surgeons. *Ann Thorac Surg*. 2003;76(1):315–321.
3. Biglioli P, Spirito R, Roberto M, et al. The anterior spinal artery: the main arterial supply of the human spinal cord—a preliminary anatomic study. *J Thorac Cardiovasc Surg*. 2000;119(2):376–379.
4. Gharagozloo F, Neville RF Jr, Cox JL. Spinal cord protection during surgical procedures on the descending thoracic and thoracoabdominal aorta: a critical overview. *Semin Thorac Cardiovasc Surg*. 1998;10(1): 73–86.
5. Cheshire WP, Santos CC, Massey EW, Howard JF. Spinal cord infarction: etiology and outcome. *Neurology*. 1996; 47(2):321–330.
6. Ebraheim NA, Jabaly G, Xu R, Yeasting RA. Anatomic relations of the thoracic pedicle to the adjacent neural structures. *Spine*. 1997;22(14):1553–1556.
7. Suk SI, Kim WJ, Lee SM, Kim JH, Chung ER. Thoracic pedicle screw fixation in spinal deformities: are they really safe? *Spine*. 2001;26(18):2049–2057.
8. Iorio JA, Reid P, Kim HJ. Neurological complications in adult spinal deformity surgery. *Curr Rev Musculoskelet Med*. 2016;9(3):290–298.
9. Uribe J, Moza K, Jimenez O, Green B, Levi ADO. Delayed postoperative spinal epidural hematomas. *Spine J*. 2003;3(2):125–129.
10. Yi S, Yoon DH, Kim K-N, Kim SH, Shin HC. Postoperative spinal epidural hematoma: risk factor and clinical outcome. *Yonsei Med J*. 2006;47(3):326–332.
11. Scavarda D, Peruzzi P, Bazin A, et al. Postoperative spinal extradural hematomas. 14 cases. *Neurochirurgie*. 1997;43(4):220–227.
12. Sokolowski MJ, Garvey TA, Perl J, et al. Prospective study of postoperative lumbar epidural hematoma: incidence and risk factors. *Spine*. 2008;33(1):108–113.
13. Awad JN, Kebaish KM, Donigan J, Cohen DB, Kostuik JP. Analysis of the risk factors for the development of post-operative spinal epidural haematoma. *J Bone Joint Surg Br*. 2005;87(9):1248–1252.
14. Kou J, Fischgrund J, Biddinger A, Herkowitz H. Risk factors for spinal epidural hematoma after spinal surgery. *Spine*. 2002;27(15): 1670–1673.
15. Moufarrij NA. Epidural hematomas after the implantation of thoracic paddle spinal cord stimulators. *J Neurosurg*. 2016;125(4):982–985.
16. Takeuchi A, Miyamoto K, Hosoe H, Shimizu K. Thoracic paraplegia due to missed thoracic compressive lesions after lumbar spinal decompression surgery. Report of three cases. *J Neurosurg*. 2004;100 (Suppl 1):71–4.
17. Altschul D, Kobets A, Nakhla J, et al. Postoperative urinary retention in patients undergoing elective spinal surgery. *J Neurosurg Spine*. 2016;1–6.
18. Vitale MG, Moore DW, Matsumoto H, et al. Risk factors for spinal cord injury during surgery for spinal deformity. *J Bone Joint Surg Am*. 2010;92(1):64–71.
19. Lenke LG, Fehlings MG, Shaffrey CI, et al. Neurologic outcomes of complex adult spinal deformity surgery: results of the prospective, multicenter Scoli-RISK-1 study. *Spine*. 2016;41(3):204–212.
20. Pelosi L. Combined monitoring of motor and somatosensory evoked potentials in orthopaedic spinal surgery. *Clin Neurophysiol*. 2002;113(7):1082–1091.
21. Vitale MG, Skaggs DL, Pace GI, et al. Best practices in intraoperative neuromonitoring in spine deformity surgery: development of an

intraoperative checklist to optimize response. *Spine Deform.* 2014;2(5):333–339.

22. Sutter M, Eggspuehler A, Muller A, Dvorak J. Multimodal intraoperative monitoring: an overview and proposal of methodology based on 1,017 cases. *Eur Spine J.* 2007;16(2):153–161.
23. Quraishi NA, Lewis SJ, Kelleher MO, Sarjeant R. Intraoperative multimodality monitoring in adult spinal deformity: analysis of a prospective series of one hundred two cases with independent evaluation. *Spine.* 2009;34(14):1504–1512.
24. Thuet ED, Winscher JC, Padberg AM, Bridwell KH. Validity and reliability of intraoperative monitoring in pediatric spinal deformity surgery: a 23-year experience of 3436 surgical cases. *Spine.* 2010; 35(20):1880–1886.
25. Lall RR, Lall RR, Hauptman JS, et al. Intraoperative neurophysiological monitoring in spine surgery: indications, efficacy, and role of the preoperative checklist. *Neurosurg Focus.* 2012;33(5):E10.
26. Brown MD, Brookfield KFW. A randomized study of closed wound suction drainage for extensive lumbar spine surgery. *Spine.* 2004; 29(10):1066–1068.
27. Payne DH, Fischgrund JS, Herkowitz HN, Barry RL, Kurz LT, Montgomery DM. Efficacy of closed wound suction drainage after single-level lumbar laminectomy. *J Spinal Disord.* 1996;9(5):401–403.
28. Scuderi GJ, Brusovanik GV, Fitzhenry LN. Is wound drainage necessary after lumbar spinal fusion surgery? *Med Sci Monit.* 2005;11(2): CR64–CR66.
29. Mirzai H, Eminoglu M, Orguc S. Are drains useful for lumbar disc surgery? A prospective, randomized clinical study. *J Spinal Disord Tech.* 2006;19(3):171–177.
30. Boukobza M, Guichard JP, Boissonet M, et al. Spinal epidural haematoma: report of 11 cases and review of the literature. *Neuroradiology.* 1994;36(6):456–459.
31. Dickman CA, Shedd SA. Spinal epidural hematoma associated with epidural anesthesia: complications of systemic heparinization in patients receiving peripheral vascular thrombolytic therapy. *Anesthesiology.* 1990;72(5):947–950.
32. Müller H, Schramm J, Roggendorf W, Brock M. Vascular malformations as a cause of spontaneous spinal epidural haematoma. *Acta Neurochir (Wien).* 1982;62(3-4):297–305.
33. Ullery BW, Cheung AT, Fairman RM, et al. Risk factors, outcomes, and clinical manifestations of spinal cord ischemia following thoracic endovascular aortic repair. *J Vasc Surg.* 2011;54(3):677–684.
34. Takenaka S, Hosono N, Mukai Y, Tateishi K, Fuji T. Significant reduction in the incidence of C5 palsy after cervical laminoplasty using chilled irrigation water. *Bone Joint J.* 2016;98-B(1):117–124.

52

Vascular Injury During Approach to Lumbar Spine

ANIL NANDA, TANMOY KUMAR MAITI, DEVI PRASAD PATRA

HIGHLIGHTS

- Vascular injuries during lumbar spine surgery are underestimated in the present literature. The reported incidence of vascular injury is less than 1%.
- The sequelae may not be detected for years after the index surgery.
- Endovascular interventions are preferred over open surgery to encounter the sequelae of injury.

Background

Lumbar discectomy (with/without instrumentation) is one of the most common operations performed in spinal surgery practice. Vascular injury complications can be classified in two broad groups: (1) arterial bleeding from back muscles and epidural venous bleeding and (2) major vessel injury. Vascular injury to a major vessel is rare but is a life-threatening complication. The prevalence of vascular complications during lumbar disc surgery is reported to vary between 1 and 5 in every 10,000 disc operations.[1] About 300 cases with similar complications have been reported in the last 75 years. The offending vessels were abdominal aorta, inferior vena cava (IVC), common iliac arteries (CIAs) and/or common iliac veins (CIVs), and internal or external iliac artery. However, it may be an underestimation because complications often go unreported. Also, the complications may present in a delayed fashion.

Anatomic Insights (Fig. 52.1)

The most common vascular injury is related to L4–L5 and L5–S1 disc surgery.[2] The proximity of susceptible vessels varies according to the spinal level. Thus proximal (L2–L3 and L3–L4) level is associated with injuries predominantly to the aorta and the IVC, whereas iliac vessel injuries are seen mainly with L4–L5 and L5–S1 space surgery.[2,3] The course of the CIA begins at the distal portion of the abdominal aorta and extends inferolaterally for approximately 4 cm from the L4 vertebra to alongside the medial aspect of the psoas muscle, where it typically bifurcates anterior to the sacroiliac joint of the pelvis (Fig. 52.1). The left CIA is more susceptible to injury due to its medial course and close relation with the L4–L5 intervertebral disc.[4] Knowledge of common anomalies is also important. An aberrant iliac artery may impinge on the lumbar plexus, and a foraminal herniation at L4–L5 may pose difficulties in the transpsoas approach to an anterior lumbar interbody fusion (ALIF).[5] Although the occurrence is rare, there are examples of other vessels getting injured as well. Injury to L4 lumbar artery,[6] median sacral,[7] the inferior mesenteric,[8] and the superior rectal artery[9] have been described during the approach to the lumbar spine. Injuries to large veins have been documented in the literature. Injury to the left CIV is more common than to the right common iliac, right/left internal iliac, or IVC in one report.[10] Another report suggested that the left CIV was the vessel most commonly injured during an anterior approach to the lumbar spine.[11]

RED FLAGS

- In nearly all cases, the injury was caused by the pituitary rongeur pushed so far ventrally that it perforated the anterior vessels.[12]
- As the intervertebral disc is avascular, any unexpected bleeding from inside the disc should be considered suspicious. However, in more than half of the reported cases, bleeding is absent or mild.[13]
- Keep anesthesia involved: In very few reported cases, increase in heart rate and/or marked decrease in blood pressure occurred intraoperatively so as to lead to a suspicion of an abdominal vessel injury. Reduction in end-tidal CO_2 concentration may also be a clue on a few occasions.
- Surgeons may erroneously feel safe when an abnormal bleeding stops rapidly. The resulting annular flap might close the breach, acting like a valve, in a very short time interval. The elasticity of the annulus and ligament also plays a role.
- The iliac vessels, located laterally in the pelvis, may get compressed by the pads of the frame on which the patient was lying. Vessels may get compressed against lower lumbar vertebrae as well. This can lead to temporary hemostasis, which gets unmasked once the patient is back in the supine position.
- Any episode of intraoperative hypotension or bleeding should be carefully investigated. The abdomen should be auscultated before discharge. Emergency laparotomy should be considered in the unstable patient suspected of vascular injury. When patients with leg edema/ signs of cardiac insufficiency are examined, a history of previous discectomy should be sought to exclude an arteriovenous fistula (AVF).

Risk Factors

A number of factors may predispose to vascular injury during lumbar disc surgery. The common factors can be classified as congenital, acquired, and technical factors. These are summarized in Table 52.1.[13] Annulus fibrosis and degeneration of the anterior longitudinal ligament (ALL), advanced discopathy, vertebral anomalies (transitional lumbosacral vertebra), adhesion of intervertebral disc to the ALL, previous disc surgery, current or previous osteomyelitis or discogenic infection, aggressive exploration, and complex patient

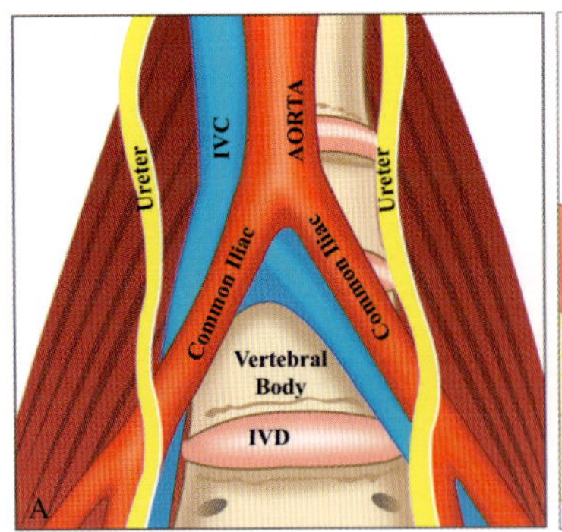

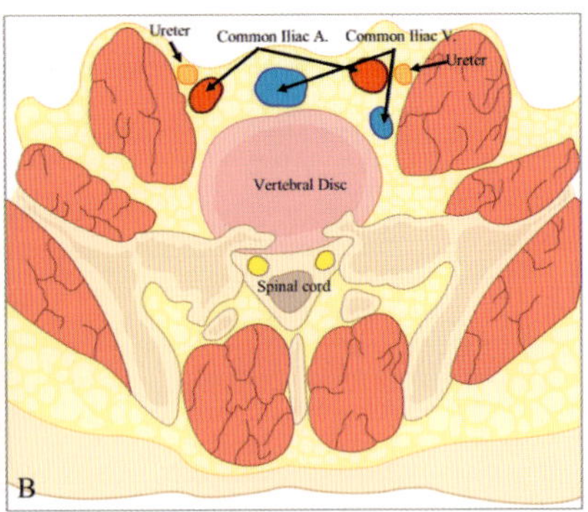

• **Fig. 52.1** (A) Relation of major vessel on posterior abdominal wall to fourth and fifth intervertebral disc. (B) Horizontal cross section at fifth lumbar disc showing vascualr relationship. *IVC,* Inferior vena cava; *IVD,* intervertebral disc.

TABLE 52.1 Risk Factors for Surgery-Related Vascular Complications

Congenital and Habitual

- Preexisting gaps and other defects of anterior annulus fibrosus (AAF) and anterior longitudinal ligament (ALL)
- Vertebral anomalies
- Variation in sagittal disc diameter
- Variation in and different configurations of the abdominal aorta and venous collectors and their branches

Acquired

- Degeneration of AAF and ALL
- Hypertrophic spurs
- Intraabdominal adhesion and fixation of the vessels due to previous abdominal surgery
- Previous disc surgery (reoperation)
- Preexisting peridiscal fibrosis with scarring of the vessels
- Previous radiotherapy
- Preexisting vascular disease (arteriosclerosis, arteriovenous malformation, arteriovenous fistula, aortic aneurysm)
- Pathologic weakness of the vascular wall due to degeneration or erosion of the ventral disc herniation or osteophytic spurs
- Patient's hiccup during surgery

Technical

- Improper or incorrect positioning of patient
- Different techniques
- Various (cutting and sucking, especially sharp) instruments: pituitary rongeur/forceps
- Using trephine to make an incision in hardened disc
- Lateral deviation of instruments
- Position of the jaws of the rongeur
- Plunge of the instruments
- Experience of the surgeon
- Unfamiliarity with microscope or erroneous depth perception with microscope
- Implant characteristics such as threaded cage

positioning are considered as important risk factors for vascular injury. Current or previous osteomyelitis or discogenic infection, spondylolisthesis, osteophyte formation, and anterior migration of interbody device point to an increased risk of vascular complication. Few studies have suggested that the exposure of L4–5 was associated with an increased chance of vascular injury during anterior approach.[14,15] Sasso et al. suggested that the use of threaded cage such as InterFix was associated with more vascular injury.[16] The incidence of vascular injury is more common with the anterior approach than the posterior approach.[10] The chance of injury is higher in the transperitoneal than in the retroperitoneal approach when performed anteriorly.[15] As expected, the incidence is higher in revision surgery than in primary surgery.[15,17]

Prevention of Complication

Preoperative Prevention

The image must be carefully evaluated with coronal and sagittal magnetic resonance imaging (MRI) to establish preexisting gaps and other defects of ALL. Vertebral anomalies, osteophytic spurs, and sagittal disc diameter must be noted with computed tomography (CT). The variation and different configurations of the abdominal aorta and IVC and their branches and preexisting vascular disease (arteriosclerosis, arteriovenous malformations, AVF, aortic aneurysm) must be documented with various CT and MRI techniques. Careful analysis of images is particularly useful in patients with previous abdominal surgery or radiotherapy. Ensuring the appropriate position is essential to avoid complications. The patient may be positioned in the park bench or other lateral position with an unsupported abdomen to reduce the venous pressure.

Perioperative Prevention

Use of "marked instruments" with safe depth (3 cm from the tip) that are painted in indelible blue or green (as a contrast to red) or use of instruments with adjustable mechanisms similar to those of an umbrella as a stopper (attachable and removable, depth regulator in respect to the patient's characteristics) to prevent an unexpected plunge can reduce complications to a great extent. A tactile sensation of the anterior border of the body and placement of the jaws of the rongeur in contact with the end plate before "biting" can be a protective measure. Use of instruments (pituitary rongeur/shaver) with an entirely rounded and smooth extremity reduces the chance of a tear on the annulus fibrosus or, if this does occur, a laceration of abdominal vessels. If the surgeon prefers to use a frame, the patient could be displaced out of the frame whenever a vascular injury is suspected, for a few minutes on one side and the other alternately, to decrease the compression on the iliac vessels, which are the most frequently injured vessels. Use of the lateral view of the x-ray in the C-arm would provide depth perception to the surgeon, and an AP view provides cautions about any lateral deviation of the instrument. Intraoperative discogram or saline/contrast injection is among the few widely practiced methods to demonstrate perforation of anterior annulus fibrosus (AAF) and anterior longitudinal ligament (ALL). Finally, in case of any suspected injury, intraoperative angiography must be sought without any hesitation. Surgeons must practice opening the jaws of the rongeur when it is introduced into the disc space because it is difficult for the instrument to pierce the ALL in this position.[8]

Sequelae of Vascular Injury

Depending on the trauma, the injury may be recognized immediately or may remain undetected for years. The detailed symptomatology after an injury has been discussed extensively in the literature.[18] Arterial lacerations present immediately and represent about one-third of vascular injuries.[19] Any delay in treatment of arterial lacerations is usually fatal.[20] AVF accounts for up to two-thirds of vascular injuries. Jarstfer and Rich reported that AVF symptoms may appear after a variable duration, at 24 h (9%), 24 h to 1 year (70%), and after 1 year (21%).[21] Pseudoaneurysms account for approximately 10% of sequelae of vascular injury.[2] Arterial thrombosis,[22] arterial vasospasm,[22] pulmonary embolism, and rhabdomyolysis[22] have been reported as concerning sequelae. All of these factors increase the length of hospital stay and hospital cost.

Management

Angiography is considered the gold standard in diagnosing iatrogenic vascular injury.[18] CT with CT angiography is a good first-line investigation. Ultrasonography is of value in confirming the presence of intraabdominal fluid when it is not appropriate to transfer the patient to a CT scanner.[23]

Treatment choice depends on the type and site of injury. Lacerations are repaired in acute settings to avoid rapid blood loss, whereas AVFs and pseudoaneurysms are suitable for repair in an elective setting.[18] The open approach to control acute bleeding has traditionally been described and recommended to repair lacerations.[24]

Open Vascular and Endovascular Intervention Techniques for Repair

Aorta and IVC lacerations can be repaired by lateral suturing.[2] This approach is sometimes difficult because the injury is located at the posterior wall. Therefore suturing from inside after an arteriotomy or graft interposition is an alternative procedure.[2,7] Large IVC injury is difficult to handle, even with the use of balloon catheters or sponge-stick compression. Ligation may sometimes be necessary and is preferred over a technically poor venous repair, which is likely to predispose to postoperative thrombosis and pulmonary embolism. However, IVC ligation may lead to chronic venous insufficiency with leg edema and recurrent cutaneous ulceration. In the case of aortocaval fistula, the procedure of choice is suturing from inside after arteriotomy or venotomy (in one case) or AVF division and lateral suturing.[2,25] Repair of late aortic pseudoaneurysm requires excision and primary suturing or interposition grafting or, alternatively, transluminal patching.[2,26] Iliac vessel lacerations can be sutured directly on most occasions. If suturing leads to arterial stenosis, development of thrombosis is impending, and graft interposition or patch angioplasty is the preferred alternative.[8] If a prosthetic graft is not available, extensive CIA damage could be repaired by means of an end-to-end anastomosis with the contralateral hypogastric artery.[27] In isolated lacerations of iliac veins, lateral suturing is widely used. If suturing leads to venous stenosis, venous patching with autologous saphenous vein patch is indicated because of the fear of impending deep vein thrombosis.[2,28] Ligation is reserved for severe vein damage.[9] For iliac AVFs (CIA-CIV or CIA-IVC), arteriotomy, along with suturing the lumen from inside and graft interposition, is preferred by vascular surgeons.[2] Alternatively, resection of the fistula with primary closure of the vein and reconstruction of the artery by graft interposition or end-to-end anastomosis can be performed. Division of the fistula and lateral suturing is the other technique practiced.[2] Simple ligation of the fistula is avoided to minimize recurrence.[2,29] Concomitant IVC and/or CIV ligation is usually well tolerated but sometimes may lead to transient leg edema. To avoid IVC ligation, venous patching is also used.[2,30] Rupture into an adherent jejunal segment at the suture line and sexual dysfunction are reported complications.[2,8] Stent-grafts have been used as well. The ureters should be inspected for integrity, because ureteral injuries coincident with vascular lacerations have, in the past, gone undetected.[2,26]

A major shift toward endovascular techniques (e.g., covered stents and coiling) has been observed over the past two decades for all types of vascular injury.[18] In acute settings, vascular access can be gained using either a percutaneous procedure or a cut-down. Once acute bleeding is suspected, balloon occlusion is an effective first step for management.[31] A balloon might be inflated right above the suspected level of injury to control the initial bleeding, stabilize the blood pressure, and allow time to identify the exact bleeding site. It is especially useful when the laceration flap goes the same direction as the blood flow. Risk of stenosis and embolism should be taken into account when performing endovascular repair. Endovascular therapy leads to promising results in the treatment of aortocaval fistulas associated with abdominal aortic aneurysms. Endovascular treatment with covered-stents has been effective for pseudoaneurysms.[32,33] A percutaneous or endoluminal stent graft has been deployed successfully for AVF.[34] A flexible stent graft such as Viabahn is better suited to negotiating tortuous iliac arteries.[35] The lacerations of internal iliac arteries could be managed by endovascular embolization. Coil embolization and glue injection may be required in some cases.

SURGICAL REWIND

My Worst Case (Fig. 52.2)

A 45-year-old man presented to the clinic with severe bilateral L5 radiculopathy. He underwent bilateral L4–L5 laminectomy and discectomy. During discectomy, considerable bleeding was encountered but was controlled with Gelfoam tamponade. The patient was hemodynamically stable, and bilateral L5 roots were decompressed. Postoperatively, he was neurologically intact. He moved his legs, but his hemoglobin kept dropping. On postoperative day 1, it dropped four points. The CT scan showed a retroperitoneal hematoma. The patient had an emergent arteriogram that showed a pseudoaneurysm in the iliac artery (Fig. 52.2A). He underwent stenting of the iliac artery without any adverse outcome (Fig. 52.2B and C). His radicular pain was relieved.

Continued

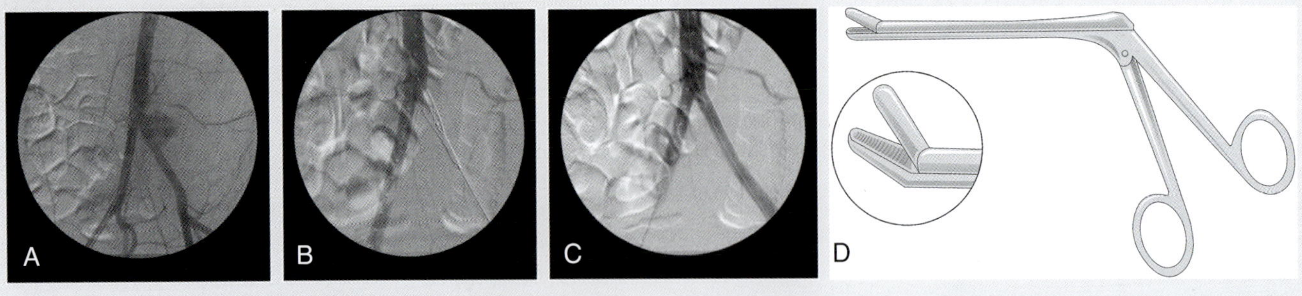

• **Fig. 52.2** Formation of iliac artery pseudoaneurysm after iatrogenic injury with rongeur.

NEUROSURGICAL SELFIE MOMENT

Surgery on the lumbar spine is an integral part of a neurosurgeon's practice. Detailed knowledge of the key anatomy involved in using different approaches is essential to avoiding complications. A high index of suspicion and careful evaluation are required to diagnose each complication in an appropriate time frame. Endovascular treatment options have been adopted over open surgical methods in the present era. However, treatment should be tailored to each site and mode of injury to ensure patient safety.

References

1. Ewah B, Calder I. Intraoperative death during lumbar discectomy. *Br J Anaesth*. 1991;66:721–723.
2. Papadoulas S, Konstantinou D, Kourea HP, Kritikos N, Haftouras N, Tsolakis JA. Vascular injury complicating lumbar disc surgery. A systematic review. *Eur J Vasc Endovasc Surg*. 2002;24:189–195.
3. Smith DW, Lawrence BD. Vascular complications of lumbar decompression laminectomy and foraminotomy. A unique case and review of the literature. *Spine*. 1991;16:387–390.
4. Bozok S, Ilhan G, Destan B, Gokalp O, Gunes T. Approach to the vascular complications of lumbar disc surgery. *Vascular*. 2013;21:79–82.
5. Delasotta LA, Radcliff K, Sonagli MA, Miller L. Aberrant iliac artery: far lateral lumbosacral surgical anatomy. *Orthopedics*. 2012;35:e294–e297.
6. Quigley TM, Stoney RJ. Arteriovenous fistulas following lumbar laminectomy: the anatomy defined. *J Vasc Surg*. 1985;2:828–833.
7. Szolar DH, Preidler KW, Steiner H, et al. Vascular complications in lumbar disk surgery: report of four cases. *Neuroradiology*. 1996;38:521–525.
8. Birkeland IW, Taylor TK. Major vascular injuries in lumbar disc surgery. *J Bone Joint Surg Br*. 1969;51:4–19.
9. Tsai YD, Yu PC, Lee TC, Chen HS, Wang SH, Kuo YL. Superior rectal artery injury following lumbar disc surgery. Case report. *J Neurosurg*. 2001;95:108–110.
10. Liu Y. Analysis of vascular injury in lumbar spine surgery. *Pak J Med Sci*. 2012;28:791–794.
11. Zahradnik V, Lubelski D, Abdullah KG, Kelso R, Mroz T, Kashyap VS. Vascular injuries during anterior exposure of the thoracolumbar spine. *Ann Vasc Surg*. 2013;27:306–313.
12. Erkut B, Unlu Y, Kaygin MA, Colak A, Erdem AF. Iatrogenic vascular injury during to lumbar disc surgery. *Acta Neurochir (Wien)*. 2007;149:511–515, discussion 516.
13. Dosoglu M, Is M, Pehlivan M, Yildiz KH. Nightmare of lumbar disc surgery: iliac artery injury. *Clin Neurol Neurosurg*. 2006;108:174–177.
14. Brau SA, Delamarter RB, Schiffman ML, Williams LA, Watkins RG. Vascular injury during anterior lumbar surgery. *Spine J*. 2004;4:409–412.
15. Wood KB, Devine J, Fischer D, Dettori JR, Janssen M. Vascular injury in elective anterior lumbosacral surgery. *Spine*. 2010;35:S66–S75.
16. Sasso RC, Kitchel SH, Dawson EG. A prospective, randomized controlled clinical trial of anterior lumbar interbody fusion using a titanium cylindrical threaded fusion device. *Spine*. 2004;29:113–122, discussion 121–122.
17. Nguyen HV, Akbarnia BA, van Dam BE, et al. Anterior exposure of the spine for removal of lumbar interbody devices and implants. *Spine*. 2006;31:2449–2453.
18. van Zitteren M, Fan B, Lohle PN, et al. A shift toward endovascular repair for vascular complications in lumbar disc surgery during the last decade. *Ann Vasc Surg*. 2013;27:810–819.
19. Skippage P, Raja J, McFarland R, Belli AM. Endovascular repair of iliac artery injury complicating lumbar disc surgery. *Eur Spine J*. 2008;17(suppl 2):S228–S231.
20. Nadstawek J, Wassmann HD, Boker DK, Schultheiss R, Hornchen U. Injuries to the large abdominal vessels during lumbar nucleotomy. *J Neurosurg Sci*. 1989;33:281–286.
21. Jarstfer BS, Rich NM. The challenge of arteriovenous fistula formation following disk surgery: a collective review. *J Trauma*. 1976;16:726–733.
22. Kulkarni SS, Lowery GL, Ross RE, Ravi Sankar K. Lykomitros V. Arterial complications following anterior lumbar interbody fusion: report of eight cases. *Eur Spine J*. 2003;12:48–54.
23. Nam TK, Park SW, Shim HJ, Hwang SN. Endovascular treatment for common iliac artery injury complicating lumbar disc surgery: limited usefulness of temporary balloon occlusion. *J Korean Neurosurg Soc*. 2009;46:261–264.
24. Inamasu J, Guiot BH. Vascular injury and complication in neurosurgical spine surgery. *Acta Neurochir (Wien)*. 2006;148:375–387.
25. Duque AC, Merlo I, Janeiro MJ, Madeira EN, Pinto-Ribeiro R. Postlaminectomy arteriovenous fistula: the Brazilian experience. *J Cardiovasc Surg (Torino)*. 1991;32:783–786.
26. Fruhwirth J, Koch G, Amann W, Hauser H, Flaschka G. Vascular complications of lumbar disc surgery. *Acta Neurochir (Wien)*. 1996;138:912–916.
27. Horacio. Alvarez J, Cazarez JC, Hernandez A. An alternative repair of major vascular injury inflicted during lumbar disk surgery. *Surgery*. 1987;101:505–507.
28. Baker JK, Reardon PR, Reardon MJ, Heggeness MH. Vascular injury in anterior lumbar surgery. *Spine*. 1993;18:2227–2230.
29. Anda S, Aakhus S, Skaanes KO, Sande E, Schrader H. Anterior perforations in lumbar discectomies. A report of four cases of vascular complications and a CT study of the prevertebral lumbar anatomy. *Spine*. 1991;16:54–60.
30. Franzini M, Altana P, Annessi V, Lodini V. Iatrogenic vascular injuries following lumbar disc surgery. Case report and review of the literature. *J Cardiovasc Surg (Torino)*. 1987;28:727–730.
31. Olcay A, Keskin K, Eren F. Iliac artery perforation and treatment during lumbar disc surgery by simple balloon tamponade. *Eur Spine J*. 2013;22(suppl 3):S350–S352.

32. Hong SJ, Oh JH, Yoon Y. Percutaneous endovascular stent-graft for iliac pseudoaneurysm following lumbar discectomy. *Cardiovasc Intervent Radiol.* 2000;23:475–477.
33. Luan JY, Li X. A misdiagnosed iliac pseudoaneurysm complicated lumbar disc surgery performed 13 years ago. *Spine.* 2012;37:E1594–E1597.
34. Hart JP, Wallis F, Kenny B, O'Sullivan B, Burke PE, Grace PA. Endovascular exclusion of iliac artery to iliac vein fistula after lumbar disk surgery. *J Vasc Surg.* 2003;37:1091–1093.
35. Canaud L, Hireche K, Joyeux F, et al. Endovascular repair of aorto-iliac artery injuries after lumbar-spine surgery. *Eur J Vasc Endovasc Surg.* 2011;42:167–171.

53

Vascular Complications in Cervical Spine Surgery (Anterior and Posterior Approach)

STEPHANIE A. DECARVALHO, MUHAMMAD M. ABD-EL-BARR, MICHAEL W. GROFF

HIGHLIGHTS

- Vertebral artery injury is the most common type of vascular complication in both anterior and posterior approaches to cervical spine surgery. Vertebral artery injury can occur during exposure, decompression, or instrumentation.
- Vertebral artery injury can result in catastrophic bleeding, permanent neurologic damage, and death.
- Direct tamponade is the most common method used in the management of vertebral artery injuries, but there are important immediate and delayed consequences of this type of management. Direct repair and endovascular techniques such as embolization and stenting are being used increasingly.
- It is imperative that the surgeon studies the preoperative films to avoid these types of injuries, is able to quickly assess when such an injury has occurred, and is able to quickly manage these injuries intraoperatively and the sequelae postoperatively.

Introduction

Cervical decompression and instrumentation are common in spinal surgery practice. Vascular complications can occur in both anterior and posterior approaches to cervical spine surgery. Vertebral artery injury (VAI) is the most common type of vascular complication in both approaches. Although rare, VAI can be a life-threatening complication. The incidence of VAI is reported to be 0.08% to 0.5%.[1–4] VAI can occur during exposure, decompression, or instrumentation of the cervical spine. The highest reported rates are associated with posterior instrumentation of the high cervical spine (such as C1–2 fusion) and anterior corpectomies.[1] As with other surgical complications, it is imperative that the surgeon studies the preoperative films to avoid these types of injuries, is able to quickly assess when such an injury has occurred, and is able to quickly manage these injuries intraoperatively and the consequences postoperatively.

Anatomic Insights

Understanding the anatomy of the vertebral artery is critical for the surgeon to avoid VAI injuries and to manage these injuries if they occur. It is critical to study the vertebral artery anatomy in all patients undergoing cervical spine surgeries. Traditional imaging for spine pathology such as magnetic resonance imaging (MRI) or computed tomography (CT) is usually sufficient, but dedicated vascular imaging in the form of MR, CT, or catheter angiography may be helpful in more complex procedures.

Normally, the vertebral artery branches off of the first part of the subclavian artery and divides into four segments as it ascends to provide circulation to the posterior fossa and brainstem (Fig. 53.1).[5] The first segment, known as V1, starts with the branching of the vertebral artery from the subclavian artery and travels anterior to the transverse foramen of C7 and enters the transverse foramen of C6. The V2 region determines a convergent course of the arteries as it passes through the transverse foramina from C6 to C1. The vertebral artery is typically at least 1.5 mm lateral to the uncovertebral joint.[6,7] It is important to note that the vertebral artery may enter the transverse foramen at a level other than C6 in almost 10% of cases.[8] The third segment, V3, includes the superior section of the arch of the atlas to the foramen magnum and can be encountered during posterior cervical approaches. It is important to note that as the vertebral artery exits the transverse foramen at C1, it runs medially on the vertebral artery groove (VAG), which is also known as the sulcus arteriosus, and then about 8 to 19 mm from midline and then turns abruptly upward toward the foramen magnum.[9] This is especially important during posterior approaches; as such, one should refrain from monopolar cautery when dissecting the ring of C1 laterally, especially along its superior border. The last segment, V4, extends from the foramen magnum to unite with contralateral vertebral artery. The vertebral arteries on either side join to form the basilar artery.

Understanding this anatomy should allow surgeons to avoid injuries to the vertebral arteries. In a multiinstitutional survey of spine surgeons, it was found that the most common procedures associated with VAIs are posterior instrumentation of the high (C1–2) spine (34%) and anterior corpectomies (23%), followed by posterior exposures more generally.[1] The relatively high rates of vertebral injuries during high cervical instrumentation can be understood by the fact that the vertebral artery has a winding course between C1 and C2, the course through C2 is highly variable, and that much of the instrumentation placed here runs very close to the normal course of the vertebral artery.

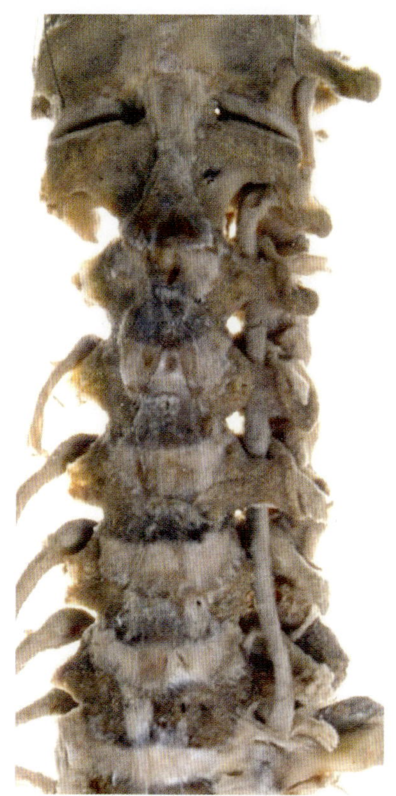

• **Fig. 53.1** Gross dissection of the cervical spine demonstrating typical anatomy of the left vertebral artery, including passage anterior to the transverse foramen at C7. The artery subsequently enters the C6 foramen and passes through each successive foramen to C1. (From Grabowski G, Cornett CA, Kang JD. Esophageal and vertebral artery injuries during complex cervical spine surgery–avoidance and management. *Orthop Clin North Am.* 2012;43[1]:63–74, viii with permission.)

Numerous methods are employed by surgeons for posterior C1–C2 fixation. The most common are Gallie-type fusion,[10] transarticular screw placement,[11] and C1 lateral mass with C2 pedicle screw (Harms fusion).[12] In both transarticular screw placement and C2 pedicle screw placement, the vertebral artery is at risk (Fig. 53.2A and B). Two characteristics that appear to be important in stratifying the risk of VAI during the placement of these screws is the size of the pedicle and the presence of a "high-riding" vertebral artery. The exact definition of a high-riding vertebral artery is somewhat vague but refers to the situation when the VAG is too medial and too high within the isthmus of the C2 pedicle to allow for the safe insertion of a C2 pedicle screw (Fig. 53.3).[11] It is crucial that the surgeon studies the course of the vertebral artery as it passes through C2 preoperatively for each individual patient before attempting to place C2 pedicle screws. If there is not a good trajectory for placement of a pedicle screw, it is our practice to place a shorter pars screw in C2, which most often provides more than adequate fixation. Several studies have shown that the vertebral artery is less susceptible to injury with C2 pedicle screws compared with transarticular screws,[11,13] and as such, we have limited our practice to only C2 pedicle or pars screws. A further benefit of C2 screws is that the trajectory can be modified to accommodate an aberrant course of the vertebral artery without the obligation to traverse the C1–2 joint.

Anatomic anomalies increase the likelihood of injury, especially if not appreciated preoperatively. Anomalies can be intraforaminal, extraforaminal, or arterial. Intraforaminal anomalies, also known as vertebral artery tortuosities, occur when the vertebral artery is located medial to the uncovertebral joint. This can cause erosion into the vertebral body, making the vertebral artery susceptible to injury, especially in corpectomy cases.[1,14] Extraforaminal anomalies are instances where the vertebral artery traverses anterior to the transverse foramen at levels between C6

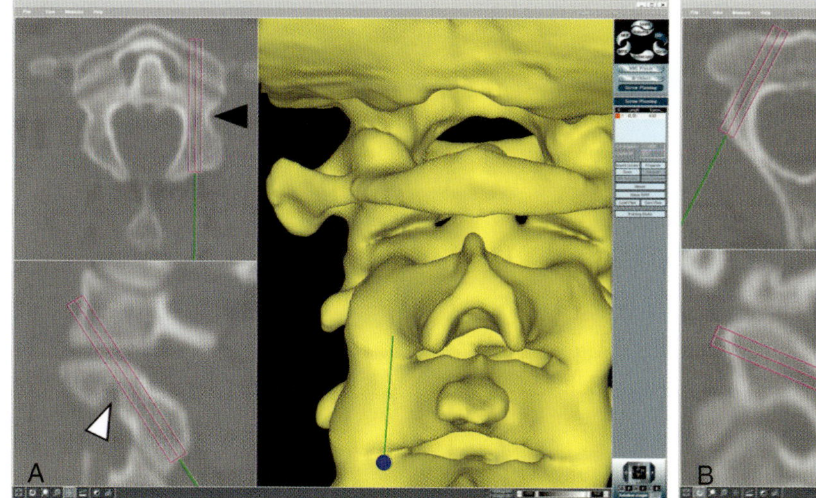

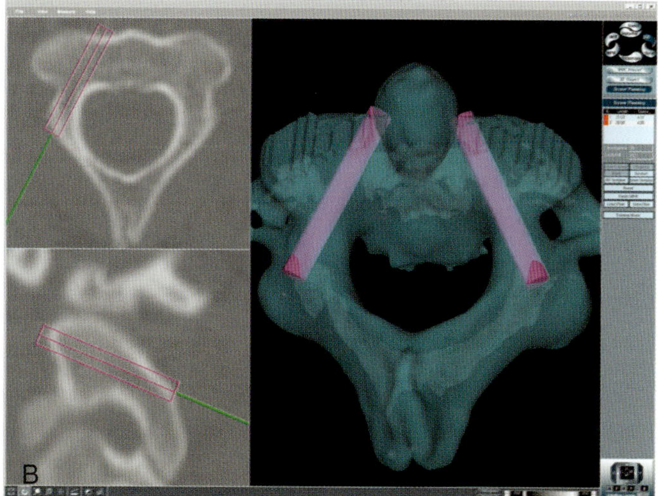

• **Fig. 53.2** (A) The trajectory of the transarticular screw is shown. The entry point is set at 3 mm above the C2–C3 joint line and as medial as possible without penetrating the lateral wall of the spinal canal at C2. The screw is angulated as dorsally as possible without perforating the dorsal cortical surface of C2. The vertebral artery groove of C2 is located lateral (black arrowhead) and anteroinferior (white arrowhead) to the screw. (B) The trajectory for the pedicle screw is shown. The entry point is set at the level of the upper end of the C2 lamina. Mediolaterally, it is located at a point that minimizes C2 vertebral artery groove violation, usually at the midportion of the pars interarticularis of C2. Medial and upward angulations are set at an angle that minimizes the groove violation. (From Yeom JS, Buchowski JM, Kim HJ, Chang BS, Lee CK, Riew KD. Risk of vertebral artery injury: comparison between C1-C2 transarticular and C2 pedicle screws. *Spine J.* 2013;13[7]:775–785 with permission.)

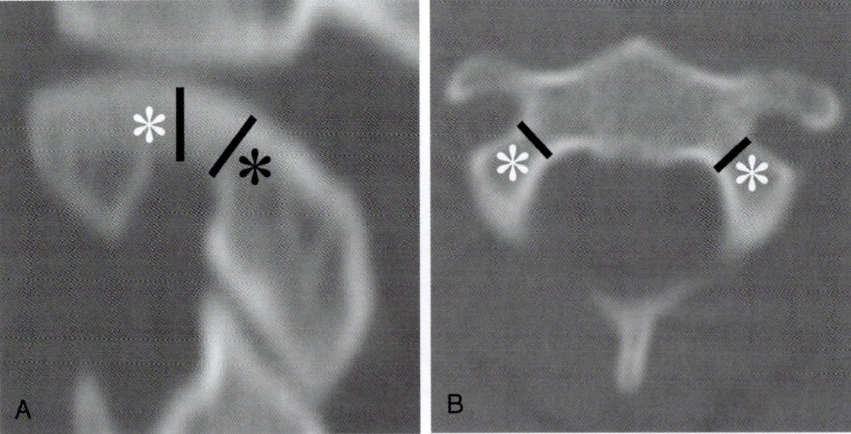

• **Fig. 53.3** (A) A high-riding vertebral artery is defined by an isthmus height (black asterisk) of 5 mm or less and/or an internal height (white asterisk) of 2 mm or less. (B) A narrow pedicle width is defined by a pedicle width of 4 mm or less (white asterisk). (From Yeom JS, Buchowski JM, Kim HJ, Chang BS, Lee CK, Riew KD. Risk of vertebral artery injury: comparison between C1-C2 transarticular and C2 pedicle screws. *Spine J.* 2013;13[7]:775–785 with permission.)

and C1. Arterial anomalies include dual-lumen and triple-lumen arteries or a hypoplastic vertebral artery. It is important to note a hypoplastic vertebral artery in the case of VAI because if the injury occurs on the dominant side, neurologic consequences may ensue if sacrifice of the artery is the only method available for management.

Carotid injuries during cervical spine surgery are extremely rare. Carotid injuries usually occur in anterior cervical spine surgery. In a retrospective, multicenter review of over 17,000 patients undergoing anterior cervical spine surgery in 21 centers, there were no cases of carotid artery injury (CAI) or cerebrovascular accidents (CVA).[15] In a review of the literature, these same authors were able to find only a few cases of carotid injury during anterior cervical procedures. Risk factors for carotid injury appeared to be extensive retraction on the carotid and long operative times.[15] Interestingly, in long anterior cervical procedures, it has been shown that the carotid artery may have up to an 80% decrease in its cross-sectional area,[16] leading to the suggestion that during long anterior cases, the surgeon should release the retraction on the carotid intermittently.

RED FLAGS

- Anomalous anatomy
- Copious bright red bleeding
- Drop in blood pressure/hemodynamically unstable

Risk Factors

- **Vertebral artery anomalies.** In a large multicenter review of VAIs that involved looking at over 16,000 surgical operations, it was noted that in 50% of VAIs, an anomalous vertebral artery was noted on preoperative imaging.[4] This underscores the importance of studying the vertebral artery anatomy preoperatively.
- **Abnormal bony anatomy.** Most surgeons use bony anatomy as landmarks during cervical spine surgery, and it is crucial to note cases where normal anatomy may be disrupted by degenerative processes, tumors, or other invasive properties.

Prevention

Preoperative Prevention

Identifying vertebral artery anomalies pre-operatively can reduce the likelihood of injury. Understanding vertebral artery anatomy with an awareness of potential anomalies allows surgeons to avoid injury. For posterior C1–2 fusions, it is critical to identify the presence of a high-riding vertebral artery. For anterior corpectomies a medial deviation of the vertebral artery needs to be accounted for.

Intraoperative Prevention

Care should be taken intraoperatively to avoid injury to the vertebral artery. For anterior approaches, it is important to find the midpoint between the longus colli muscles as a landmark for midline as well as the uncovertebral joints bilaterally. This will inform an accurate sense of midline and avoid injury to the laterally positioned vertebral artery during decompression. During foraminal decompression, one should limit the exposure to the uncovertebral joint because this will avoid the vertebral artery in most cases.[7] During corpectomies, one should limit the resection of the vertebral body to 16 mm because this will avoid injuring the vertebral artery.[17] Particular care should be taken when using a microscope not to create an oblique trajectory and resulting corpectomy trough that would place the contralateral vertebral artery at risk.[7]

During posterior cervical fusions, especially at C1, C2, the vertebral artery is at risk during both the exposure and the placement of instrumentation. During exposure, care must be taken at the superior side of the C1 ring. The venous plexus at C1–2 is particularly challenging, and if great care is not used in this area, profuse venous bleeding may ensue, complicating the establishment of the appropriate starting points for C1, C2 screws and thereby increasing the risk of VAI. As a useful adjunct, we have also used a micro-Doppler to find the carotid and vertebral arteries, especially in cases where normal anatomy is disrupted by tumors intimate with the vasculature.

Management

A VAI is usually detected at the time of injury due to bright, copious bleeding that is pressurized.[14] Once the VAI is identified, it is crucial for the surgeon to make fast decisions, because patients may lose tremendous amounts of blood in a short period of time. Even so, the dictate *primum non nocere* is paramount to ensure that the problem is not exacerbated. The first maneuver is to tamponade the bleed and the source with a cottonoid and then to remove as much blood as possible from the surgical field to allow for better visualization. The next maneuver is to try to identify where the injury to the artery has occurred. Due to the extensive bony anatomy around the vertebral artery, this is very difficult and may entail drilling off more bone in the face of copious bleeding. If a distinct hole or tear is found in the vertebral artery, direct repair may be attempted. However, this is often not possible. The use of hemostatic agents such as thrombin mixed with surgical patties may be helpful. However, even if tamponade is successful in decreasing bleeding, there is a greater awareness that this does not constitute a permanent solution, because there are reports of delayed hemorrhages, pseudoaneurysms, and fistulas that can occur with simple tamponade.[18–20] Before, during, or after local control has been established, it is important to communicate with the anesthesia members the graveness of the situation so that they may give fluids and blood products to resuscitate the patient. In a delayed fashion, arteriography can further define the injury. In a review of over 16,000 cervical spine cases, in which VAI occurred in only 0.08% of patients, only 23% of those patients required a transfusion, although the mean blood loss was significant at 770 mL.[4]

Arterial ligation is also an option but should not be done on dominant vertebral arteries, because significant neurologic consequences have been reported, and an overall mortality of 12% has been documented.[21] The canonical recommendation is to follow through with placement of the screw if the injury occurs during drilling of the screw trajectory or tapping. In this way the screw acts as a tamponading instrument. If this method is used, it is advisable not to instrument the contralateral side if it remains undone so as to avoid bilateral injuries to the vertebral arteries.

Endovascular techniques should be employed to diagnose the sequelae of the hemostatic and tamponading maneuvers as well as to provide definitive treatment. Even if tamponade is successful in stopping the torrid bleeding of an injury to the vertebral artery, it is advisable that patients who have this type of injury have a vessel angiogram postoperatively. Vessel sacrifice through embolic coils may be attempted if vessel injury is noted,[22,23] but again, this is not an option if this injury occurs to the dominant vertebral artery. It also should be noted that ligation or sacrifice of the artery should be done both proximally and distally to the injury site because delayed hemorrhages, fistulas, and pseudoaneurysms have been reported with only proximal ligation.[5,18,24] The use of newer stenting technologies is promising,[25,26] but these technologies require antiplatelet therapy, which has risks in the immediate perioperative period.

Remarkably, despite the high volumes of blood loss that are associated with VAI and the vital structures that the vertebral arteries supply, patients that are managed properly often do well. In a retrospective survey of cervical spine surgeons, they reported that almost 90% of patients that had suffered a VAI had no sequelae or only a temporary neurologic deficit. Five percent had a cerebellar infarct, and 5% mortality was reported.[1] In patients that have sustained a VAI, long-term follow-up is encouraged because delayed hemorrhages, pseudoaneurysms, and fistulas have been reported.[18,24,27]

SURGICAL REWIND

My Worst Case

A 50-year-old female was involved in a motor vehicle versus pedestrian accident. She suffered a traumatic subdural hematoma, pelvic fracture, right hip fracture, and a complicated C2 fracture. The C2 fracture was a combination of a Type III dens fracture, involving the body of C2 (Fig. 53.4A and B), and a hangman's fracture. On presentation, she was intoxicated but moving all four extremities. She was placed in a cervical orthosis for 4 weeks. Patient continued to have intractable neck pain.

Decision was made to undergo a posterior C1–C3 instrumented fusion. The C2 nerve roots were exposed and ligated bilaterally. During tapping of the right C2 pedicle screw, there was significant bleeding. This was tamponaded using Gelfoam (Pfizer Inc., New York, NY) and thrombin. Due to the small size of the right C2 pedicle, it was decided to place a shorter pars screw. Upon placement of the screw, bleeding subsided. Patient woke up neurologically intact. An immediate postoperative CT angiogram of the neck revealed a pseudoaneurysm adjacent to the C2 pedicle (Fig. 53.4C). Due to patient's good neurologic status, it was decided to start patient on aspirin (Bayer, Whippany, NJ). On postoperative day 3, patient complained of bilateral lower-extremity weakness and right arm weakness. STAT MRI revealed likely epidural hematoma with cord compression (Fig. 53.4D). Patient was taken to the operating room for evacuation of epidural hematoma and removal of rods. It was felt that some of the compression might be due to the persistent kyphotic deformity, so patient was placed in traction postoperatively. Her neurologic status improved, and a few days later she returned to the operating room for stabilization and replacement of the rods with an *in situ* fusion. Postoperative MRI revealed no residual cord compression (Fig. 53.4E). Patient was discharged a few days later.

Continued

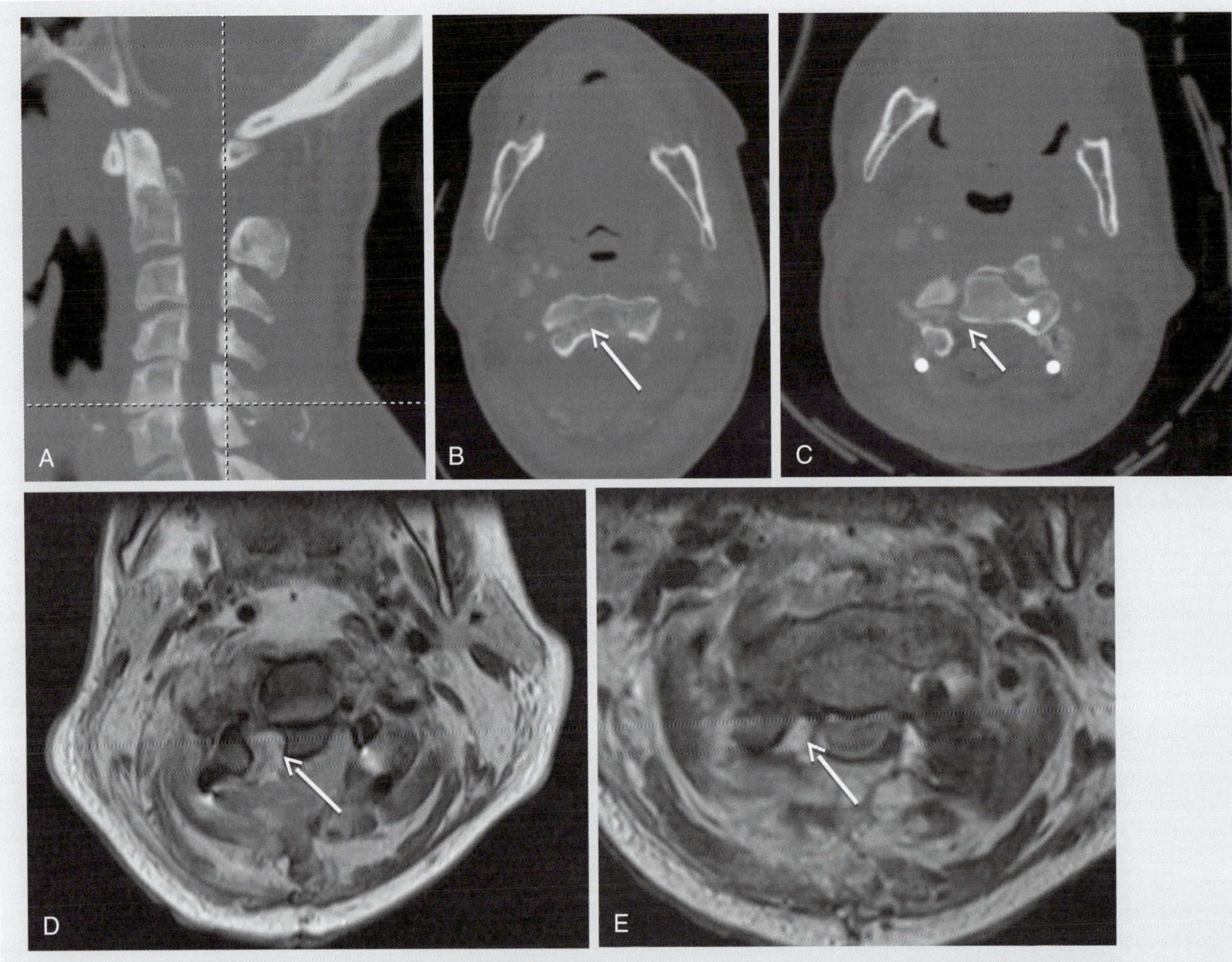

• **Fig. 53.4** (A and B) A 50-year-old female with complicated dens fracture, including a fracture through the body of the dens (white arrow). Patient underwent C1–3 posterior fusion. During tapping of right C2 pars, significant bleeding was noted that was treated with tamponade and placing of right C2 pars screw. (C) Postoperatively, patient underwent a computed tomography angiogram of the neck that revealed an outpouching of the right vertebral artery, likely representing a pseudoaneurysm (white arrow). Patient was started on aspirin. On postoperative day 3, patient was noted to be weak in the right arm and leg. (D) Magnetic resonance imaging (MRI) revealed cord compression due to kyphotic deformity and epidural hematoma. Patient was taken to the operating room for evacuation of epidural hematoma and removal of rods. Her neurologic status improved, and a few days later she returned to the operating room for replacement of the rods and *in situ* fusion. (E) Postoperative MRI revealed no residual cord compression (white arrow).

NEUROSURGICAL SELFIE MOMENT

Vascular complications during anterior and posterior cervical spine surgery can have drastic consequences. The most common injury is to the vertebral artery, due to its variable course and proximity to areas where instrumentation is placed. It is crucial for the surgeon to prevent these injuries from occurring by studying the preoperative imaging precisely, quickly ascertaining that such an injury has occurred, and managing the injury intraoperatively and monitoring for immediate and delayed sequelae.

References

1. Lunardini DJ, Eskander MS, Even JL, et al. Vertebral artery injuries in cervical spine surgery. *Spine J*. 2014;14(8):1520–1525.
2. Neo M, Fujibayashi S, Miyata M, Takemoto M, Nakamura T. Vertebral artery injury during cervical spine surgery: a survey of more than 5600 operations. *Spine*. 2008;33(7):779–785.
3. Wright NM, Lauryssen C. Vertebral artery injury in C1-2 transarticular screw fixation: results of a survey of the AANS/CNS section on disorders of the spine and peripheral nerves. American Association of Neurological Surgeons/Congress of Neurological Surgeons. *J Neurosurg*. 1998;88(4):634–640.

4. Hsu WK, Kannan A, Mai HT, et al. Epidemiology and outcomes of vertebral artery injury in 16 582 cervical spine surgery patients: an Aospine North America multicenter study. *Global Spine J.* 2017;7(1 suppl):21S–27S.
5. Peng CW, Chou BT, Bendo JA, Spivak JM. Vertebral artery injury in cervical spine surgery: anatomical considerations, management, and preventive measures. *Spine J.* 2009;9(1):70–76.
6. Bohlman HH. Cervical spondylosis and myelopathy. *Instr Course Lect.* 1995;44:81–97.
7. Grabowski G, Cornett CA, Kang JD. Esophageal and vertebral artery injuries during complex cervical spine surgery–avoidance and management. *Orthop Clin North Am.* 2012;43(1):63–74, viii.
8. Eskander MS, Drew JM, Aubin ME, et al. Vertebral artery anatomy: a review of two hundred fifty magnetic resonance imaging scans. *Spine.* 2010;35(23):2035–2040.
9. Ebraheim NA, Xu R, Ahmad M, Heck B. The quantitative anatomy of the vertebral artery groove of the atlas and its relation to the posterior atlantoaxial approach. *Spine.* 1998;23(3):320–323.
10. Farey ID, Nadkarni S, Smith N. Modified Gallie technique versus transarticular screw fixation in C1-C2 fusion. *Clin Orthop Relat Res.* 1999;359:126–135.
11. Yeom JS, Buchowski JM, Kim HJ, Chang BS, Lee CK, Riew KD. Risk of vertebral artery injury: comparison between C1-C2 transarticular and C2 pedicle screws. *Spine J.* 2013;13(7):775–785.
12. Harms J, Melcher RP. Posterior C1-C2 fusion with polyaxial screw and rod fixation. *Spine.* 2001;26(22):2467–2471.
13. Elliott RE, Tanweer O, Boah A, et al. Comparison of screw malposition and vertebral artery injury of C2 pedicle and transarticular screws: meta-analysis and review of the literature. *J Spinal Disord Tech.* 2014;27(6):305–315.
14. Maughan PH, Ducruet AF, Elhadi AM, et al. Multimodality management of vertebral artery injury sustained during cervical or craniocervical surgery. *Neurosurgery.* 2013;73(2 suppl Operative):ons271–ons281, discussion ons281–ons282.
15. Hartl R, Alimi M, Abdelatif Boukebir M, et al. Carotid artery injury in anterior cervical spine surgery: multicenter cohort study and literature review. *Global Spine J.* 2017;7(1 suppl):71S–75S.
16. Pollard ME, Little PW. Changes in carotid artery blood flow during anterior cervical spine surgery. *Spine.* 2002;27(2):152–155.
17. Smith MD, Emery SE, Dudley A, Murray KJ, Leventhal M. Vertebral artery injury during anterior decompression of the cervical spine. A retrospective review of ten patients. *J Bone Joint Surg Br.* 1993;75(3):410–415.
18. Cosgrove GR, Theron J. Vertebral arteriovenous fistula following anterior cervical spine surgery. Report of two cases. *J Neurosurg.* 1987;66(2):297–299.
19. de los Reyes RA, Moser FG, Sachs DP, Boehm FH. Direct repair of an extracranial vertebral artery pseudoaneurysm: case report and review of the literature. *Neurosurgery.* 1990;26(3):528–533.
20. Garcia Alzamora M, Rosahl SK, Lehmberg J, Klisch J. Life-threatening bleeding from a vertebral artery pseudoaneurysm after anterior cervical spine approach: endovascular repair by a triple stent-in-stent method. Case report. *Neuroradiology.* 2005;47(4):282–286.
21. Shintani A, Zervas NT. Consequence of ligation of the vertebral artery. *J Neurosurg.* 1972;36(4):447–450.
22. Choi JW, Lee JK, Moon KS, et al. Endovascular embolization of iatrogenic vertebral artery injury during anterior cervical spine surgery: report of two cases and review of the literature. *Spine.* 2006;31(23):E891–E894.
23. Jung HJ, Kim DM, Kim SW, Lee SM. Emergent endovascular embolization for iatrogenic vertebral artery injury during cervical discectomy and fusion. *J Korean Neurosurg Soc.* 2011;50(6):520–522.
24. Golfinos JG, Dickman CA, Zabramski JM, Sonntag VK, Spetzler RF. Repair of vertebral artery injury during anterior cervical decompression. *Spine.* 1994;19(22):2552–2556.
25. Ambekar S, Sharma M, Smith D, Cuellar H. Successful treatment of iatrogenic vertebral pseudoaneurysm using pipeline embolization device. *Case Rep Vasc Med.* 2014;2014:341748.
26. Obermuller T, Wostrack M, Shiban E, et al. Vertebral artery injury during foraminal decompression in "low-risk" cervical spine surgery: incidence and management. *Acta Neurochir (Wien).* 2015;157(11):1941–1945.
27. Diaz-Daza O, Arraiza FJ, Barkley JM, Whigham CJ. Endovascular therapy of traumatic vascular lesions of the head and neck. *Cardiovasc Intervent Radiol.* 2003;26(3):213–221.

54 Instrumentation-Related Complications

VICTOR SABOURIN, JOHN L. GILLICK, JAMES S. HARROP

HIGHLIGHTS

- During cervical instrumentation, one must be mindful of the location of the vertebral artery in relation to the cervical vertebrae or lateral mass being instrumented.
- For thoracic or lumbar pedicle screw placement, palpation of all four walls and floor of the bony channel is a critical portion of the procedure.
- The most important factor in preventing instrumentation-related complications is a thorough understanding of the relevant surgical anatomy.
- Furthermore, some method of intraoperative verification of hardware should be employed to avoid reoperation and to maximize accuracy.

Background

The treatment of traumatic spinal injuries in the written record dates back as far as the Edwin Smith Papyrus, which was transcribed in the 17th century BC and is theorized to be a copy of a more ancient record dating to sometime between 3000 and 2500 BC.[1,2] Spine surgery has evolved tremendously from ancient and medieval practices to the modern era, when advances have concentrated on spinal instrumentation and the techniques, trajectories, and locations in which spinal hardware can be placed.[1,3–5] In addition, because of the recognition of the significant cost of health care in the United States, the appropriate utilization and delivery of health care in the spine patient has come under thorough scrutiny.[6–9] Because spinal instrumentation is an integral component of the delivery of care in the modern-day spine patient, an understanding of the complications associated with spinal instrumentation is necessary to improve patient outcomes and reduce cost. This chapter will therefore focus on understanding the major complications associated with instrumenting the subaxial cervical, thoracic, lumbar, and sacral spine as well as the pelvis.

Although what follows will not be a definitive resource on all instrumentation-related complications, topics covered relate to common spinal instrumentation procedures, complications, and technique avoidance. Please note that complications related to the surgical exposure for instrumentation will not be discussed in this chapter as they are beyond its scope.

Anatomic Insights

Cervical Spine

Anatomy

The cervical spine consists of seven vertebrae and has a lordotic curvature that usually ranges from 16 to 25 degrees from C2 to T2. The vertebral bodies gradually increase in size from C2 to C7 and are usually 17 to 20 mm wide with uncovertebral joints defining the lateral margins. End plates make up the superior and inferior boundaries of the vertebral body and have intervertebral discs above and below, respectively. Lateral masses are connected to the vertebral body by pedicles and transverse processes with an intervening transverse foramen through which courses the vertebral artery. Vertebral arteries enter at C6 in approximately 90% of cases, with levels C3–5 and C7 receiving it in the other 10%. Lateral masses decrease in size traveling down the cervical spine, and the superior and inferior articulating processes of each cervical vertebra make up the superior and inferior borders of the lateral mass, respectively.[10]

Anterior Cervical Instrumentation

Anterior cervical instrumentation-related complications could include dysphagia, hoarseness, plate and screw loosening or fracture, end plate or posterior vertebral cortex disruption/fracture, plate migration, interbody graft migration, esophageal erosion/perforation, and nerve root injury.[11–14] Anterior cervical plates ideally sit at the midline of the vertebral body between each uncovertebral joint, with the cranial and caudal limits of the plate lying at the midpoint of the vertebral body. The plate should not overlap onto the adjacent disc space and ideally should be at least 5 mm away from the adjacent disc space to prevent the possibility of adjacent segment ossification.[15–17] Midline plate placement is important so as not to cause screws to be directed too far laterally and cause a neurovascular injury.[14] Screws should be angled 90 degrees to the plate and should be as long as possible, but not so long as to breach the posterior wall of the vertebral body.[14,18]

Posterior Cervical Instrumentation

Posterior cervical instrumentation complications can include vertebral artery injury, dural injury, nerve root injury, pedicle/lateral mass fracture, and screw/rod fracture or pullout.[10,19] Subaxial posterior cervical instrumentation is most often accomplished with lateral mass screws, with several techniques for screw placement available.[10] The Magerl technique is a common method that involves having a starting point of 1 mm medial and 1 to 2 mm superior from the center point of a cervical lateral mass and then directing the screw 25 degrees laterally and 30 degrees superiorly, or in parallel with the superior articulating process and that allows for bicortical bony purchase.[10,20] Pedicle screws carry a greater risk of neurovascular injury due to small cervical pedicles with vertebral arteries laterally and the spinal canal medially, but are used occasionally if lateral mass screws are not an option.[10]

Thoracic Spine

Anatomy

The thoracic spine consists of 12 vertebrae with associated rib articulation. The thoracic spine is naturally kyphotic due to the angulation of its vertebral bodies, with a normal kyphotic curvature ranging from 20 to 50 degrees.[10] Thoracic facets are coronally oriented in the upper levels and become progressively more sagittal in orientation caudally, down to T12. Thoracic spine pedicles become smaller from T1 to T4, with the smallest thoracic pedicles between T4 and T6, and then once again enlarge gradually down the thoracic spine to T12.[21] Pedicle angles also significantly vary in the thoracic spine with an angle of approximately 30 degrees at T1 to 5 degrees or perpendicular at T12.[21] The thoracic spine has two distinct transition zones: cervicothoracic and thoracolumbar. The cervicothoracic junction is a more abrupt transition zone than the thoracolumbar junction because of the relatively rigid upper thoracic spine and mobile cervical spine. In relation to the thoracic spine, important anatomic structures such as the esophagus, lungs, sympathetic chain, diaphragm, heart, thoracic duct, and great vessels sit in close proximity and bear significant consideration. An important artery to consider in lower thoracic spinal approaches is the artery of Adamkiewicz. This radicular artery most often enters from the left from T8 to L2, with T9 to T11 being the most likely location, and supplies the ventral spinal cord from the lower thoracic spinal cord to the conus.[10,21] Each of these structures poses a possible site of injury during posterior instrumentation.

Lateral/Anterior Thoracic Instrumentation

A detailed discussion on technique avoidance and complications of anterior and lateral thoracic instrumentation is outside the scope of this chapter. However, complications can include injury to closely related anatomic structures such as the heart, lungs, esophagus, great vessels, sympathetic plexus, and thoracic duct.[10,22]

Posterior Thoracic Instrumentation

Complications associated with thoracic pedicle instrumentation include spinal cord injury, dural tear, nerve root injury, pedicle breach/fracture, and injury to a major anatomic structure related to the thoracic spine as listed above.[10,21,23,24]

There are several approaches to the posterior thoracic spine for a variety of indications.[10] However, thoracic pedicle screws, which traverse the vertebral body, are the most commonly employed instrumentation technique. Thoracic pedicle screw starting points vary from T1 to T12 with upper thoracic levels being at the junction of the mid transverse process and lamina at the lateral pars, mid thoracic being at the junction of the proximal edge of the transverse process and lamina and lateral to the midpoint of the base of the superior articulating process, and at the junction of the bisected transverse process and lamina in the lower thoracic spine.[21,23] The axial trajectory of a thoracic pedicle screw is vital because if it is too medial, the spinal canal can be violated, resulting in spinal cord injury, whereas if it is too lateral, vital anatomic structures as listed above may be injured.[21] The appropriate angle at T1–2 should be approximately 30 degrees, whereas at T3–12 it should be approximately 20 degrees.[24] These angles should be appropriately contoured based on preoperative imaging and thoracic pedicle level with an understanding that there is a significant difference in angulation from T1 to T12. Pedicle breach is a known potential complication of all pedicle screws, and in the thoracic spine a medial breach is considered safe if less than 2 mm, probably safe between 2 and 4 mm, and questionably safe if there are no electrophysiologic changes in intraoperative monitoring between 4 and 8 mm of medial pedicle wall breach.[23] If the thoracic pedicle is breached laterally, up to 6 mm is considered acceptable; however, individual anatomy varies, and once again, it is important to consider proximally related structures as listed above. Sagittal angulation is also an important consideration with possible trajectories being more anatomic or straight on. The term *anatomic* refers to screws following the natural angle of the pedicle, which in the thoracic spine is posteriorly more rostral and anteriorly, more caudal. The term *straight on* refers to a screw trajectory that runs parallel to the surface of the superior end plate. One study comparing the two trajectories demonstrated that with straight-on screws, there is a 27% greater pullout strength and a 39% increase in maximum insertional torque when compared with anatomic screws.[25] Being able to find and clearly visualize thoracic spine transverse processes, laminae, and facets is critical when inserting thoracic pedicle screws to avoid complications.

Lumbar Spine

Anatomy

The lumbar spine classically consists of five vertebral bodies with an overall lordotic curvature of 20 to 65 degrees. Approximately 67% of lumbar lordosis occurs from L4 to the sacrum.[10] Lumbar vertebral bodies and pedicles increase in size from L1 to L5, and the facet joints are sagittally oriented and allow for significant resistance to rotational forces.[26] Relevant surgical anatomy associated with the lumbar spine includes the abdominal compartment as well as the retroperitoneum and their structures such as: bowel, aorta, inferior vena cava, kidneys, and ureters.[10] The lower lumbar spine can also occasionally contain transitional anatomy where the L5 vertebral body can display anatomic variations in degree of fusion to the sacrum. There is a prevalence of 4% to 30% of a lumbosacral transitional vertebrae and is important to recognize when counting vertebral levels for surgery.[27]

Anterior/Lateral Lumbar Instrumentation

As in the Thoracic Spine section, a detailed discussion on technique avoidance and complications of anterior and lateral lumbar instrumentation is outside the scope of this chapter. However, complications can include injury to closely related anatomic structures such as bowel, aorta, inferior vena cava, kidneys and ureters, pancreatitis, retrograde ejaculation, dural injury, and nerve root injury.[10,28]

Posterior Lumbar Instrumentation

The most common form of posterior lumbar instrumentation includes pedicle screws and rods.[10] The typical entry point for a lumbar pedicle screw is the junction of the pars interarticularis with the transverse process and mammillary process.[10,29] The most common trajectory of a lumbar pedicle screw is lateral to medial in the axis of the pedicle. However, another option is the cortical bone trajectory, which follows a medial to lateral and caudal to rostral pathway through the pedicle.[30] Complications associated with lumbar pedicle instrumentation can include pedicle breach/fracture, dural injury, nerve root injury, and vascular injury.[10] Although lumbar pedicles are robust, there still exists a risk of breach with resultant injury.[29] Therefore a thorough exposure of the posterior elements is necessary for safe access to the pedicle.

Sacrum/Pelvis

Anatomy

The sacrum consists of five vertebrae, which fuse together by the time a human reaches adulthood.[31] The sacrum articulates with four different bones: the lumbar spine rostrally, the coccyx caudally, and bilaterally with the ilium through the sacroiliac joint.[10] As in the lumbar spine, the sacrum can display transitional anatomy with a "lumbarized" sacral vertebral body.[27,31] An important anatomic consideration regarding instrumentation is the fact that S1 pedicles tend to be large and full of cancellous bone, which can limit screw purchase within pedicles.[32] Relevant posterior pelvic anatomy in relation to instrumentation includes: the posterior superior iliac spine, acetabulum, and sciatic notch, all of which contain the superior gluteal artery and sciatic nerve.[10]

Posterior Sacral/Pelvic Instrumentation

The sacrum is most commonly instrumented at S1 and S2.[33,34] Sacral screws can be directed through the pedicle into the sacral vertebral body and laterally into the sacral ala as well as through the sacral ala and into the iliac bone.[35] The S1 pedicle is the trajectory most commonly instrumented; however, because of its large cancellous bony component, screws are at risk for pullout. Therefore S1 screws are often placed in a way to engage as much cortical bone as possible, which can lead to anterior breach of the screw. The entry point for an S1 pedicle screw is the inferolateral margin of the L5/S1 facet and directed anteromedially through the pedicle and toward the sacral promontory.[32,34] However, complications related to S1 instrumentation are screw pullout and sacral fracture; to help prevent these complications, constructs are often extended to S2 and the ilium.[36] S2 screws are often directed laterally through the sacral ala and into the iliac bone (S2AI screw) to allow for a pelvic point of fixation, for instrumentation to remain in line and not require an offset connector. This also allows for less of a lateral dissection for exposure of the iliac screw start point.[35] The start point of an S2AI is 1 mm inferolateral to the S1 dorsal foramen. The screw is angulated toward the greater trochanter and ~30 degrees anterior to the floor.[35] One concern with the S2AI screw is the violation of the sacroiliac joint; however, it is still unknown whether this has a clinically significant adverse effect.[35] Finally, iliac screws are also an important consideration for helping to improve the caudal strength of a construct while fusion occurs by unloading the pressure off of S1 screws.[32] Potential complications associated with instrumenting the sacral spine include damaging the structures anterior and lateral to it, especially when considering that sacral screws are as long as possible to properly engage cortical bone and are liable to breach anteriorly. Potential structures at risk include the iliac veins and arteries, nerve roots, and rectum.[10,33] The pelvic screw start point correlates with the posterior superior iliac spine, and screws are directed to the cortical bone directly above the greater sciatic notch and toward the anterior inferior iliac spine. Potential complications while inserting pelvic screws include breaching cortical bone anteriorly or posteriorly, breaching the greater sciatic notch and causing injury to the superior gluteal artery or sciatic nerve, or breaching into the acetabulum.[10,32]

> **RED FLAGS**
>
> - During surgical planning for cervical instrumentation, knowledge of the vertebral artery anatomy and its course in the patient is of paramount importance. This anatomy is typically adequately visualized after a computed tomography (CT) scan and magnetic resonance imaging (MRI) of the cervical spine. Should the course or anatomy remain ambiguous after these images, a CT angiogram of the neck can be performed.
> - During preoperative planning of lumbosacral instrumentation, one must be mindful of segmentation anomalies: "lumbarized sacrum" or "sacralized L5 vertebrae." The presence of these anomalies can present a challenge regarding nomenclature, and it is up to the surgeon to ensure that the correct levels are addressed.
> - In today's environment, image guidance for instrumentation in some form must be employed. The modality used should be dictated by the surgeon's comfort level, hospital infrastructure, and complexity of the case. Certainly a single-level fusion can be safely performed with the use of the freehand technique. However, in cases of complex deformity, intraoperative CT scan may be more beneficial, especially in the hands of less experienced surgeons.
> - During instrumentation, hardware may be verified intraoperatively by several modalities. One may choose to use an intraoperative CT scan or simply anteroposterior and lateral x-rays. The goal of acquiring these images is to ensure that the patient leaves the operating room with hardware in optimal position.
> - Postoperatively, should the patient complain of symptoms that could possibly be attributed to hardware malposition, the initial workup would involve a repeat x-ray, followed by CT scan and, lastly, an MRI. The escalation of this algorithm depends on the detection of the etiology of the patient's symptoms. Should all of these studies be within normal limits, further workup may entail enlisting the help of nonsurgical specialists such as neurologists and physiatrists.

Prevention and Management

Above all else, a thorough understanding of anatomy and variants that may be present will prepare the surgeon adequately to avoid complications related to instrumentation placement. Regardless of the technique employed by the surgeon, should malposition be suspected, palpation remains a fundamental surgical step—that is, using a ball-tipped probe to detect the floor and all four walls of the pedicle. In addition, triggered electromyography (tEMG) has been a commonly utilized modality in which to further interrogate pedicle screw position in relation to the neural elements. A recent metaanalysis by Mikula et al. demonstrated that this modality has a specificity of 0.94 but a sensitivity of 0.78, extracted from the data of 2932 patients and 15,065 screws. The authors concluded that using a threshold of 10 to 12 mA and pulse duration of 300 μs provided the most accurate detection of misplaced screws.[37] The objective of each of these methods remains the same: to avoid screw malposition and decrease complications.

Over the years several other techniques of screw insertion have evolved with the goal of pedicle screw malposition avoidance. In a retrospective study of freehand thoracic pedicle screw placement by two senior spine surgeons, the authors found that in 577 screws there were 36 (6.2%) moderate cortical perforations (the central line of the pedicle screw lies outside the cortical wall of the pedicle) and 10 (1.7%) medial breaches. In addition, no screws were associated with neurologic, vascular, or visceral injuries.[23] However, these data represent only one sample from two senior spine surgeons.

In addition, as the trend toward outcome-based payments continues, accuracy of screw placement may become a metric that may eventually contribute to reimbursement. Therefore modalities of image guidance that may improve instrumentation accuracy to a level closer to 100% are gaining popularity, and are being employed more frequently.

The use of fluoroscopic guidance for the placement of pedicle screws represented an early effort to improve screw insertion accuracy. Overall, based on metaanalyses, the malposition rate for fluoroscopically guided pedicle screws has been published in the range of 10% to 15%.[38–42] However, some would view 85% to 90% accuracy as at best suboptimal and at worst unacceptable. New technologies in image guidance are beginning to demonstrate even more improved accuracy.

Currently, intraoperative CT scanning represents the most advanced form of image guidance. With systems such as the Iso-C (Siemens Healthcare USA, Malvern, PA) and the O-Arm (Medtronic Inc., Minneapolis, MN), surgeons can obtain intraoperative CT scans that can be transferred to a navigation platform and used for screw placement. This advance represents an improvement from navigation using preoperatively obtained CT scans. In a comparative study of patients undergoing pedicle screw placement using preoperative CT-based navigation versus intraoperative CT, Wood and Mannion found a 6.4% rate of screw malposition in the preoperative CT group versus 1.6% in the intraoperative CT group.[43] The accuracy of this technique was further demonstrated in a series of 599 consecutive patients by Bourgeois et al. who underwent placement of 2132 screws. The authors found a total of seven pedicle breaches, corresponding to a per-person breach rate of 1.15% (6/518) and a per-screw breach rate of 0.33% (7/2132).[38] Therefore with the advent of intraoperative CT-based navigation, improved accuracy can reduce the risk of pedicle screw malposition even further, thereby preventing instrumentation-related complications.

SURGICAL REWIND

My Worst Case

This is a 38-year-old male who presents with severe back and right leg pain and a grade 1 L4/5 spondylolisthesis who failed conservative therapy. He then underwent an L4/5 transforaminal lumbar interbody fusion (TLIF) from the right side. Screws were inserted under fluoroscopic guidance. During the procedure, the right L4 screw stimulated at 14 mA. The screw was removed, and four walls as well as the floor were palpated. The screw was then reinserted, and the patient was closed in the standard fashion. Immediately postoperatively, the patient was complaining of the same right leg pain he had preoperatively. Initially, this was felt to be secondary to retraction on the L4 nerve root. However, when his symptoms did not improve over the ensuing postoperative days, x-rays and a CT scan were performed (Fig. 54.1). These studies demonstrated not only a lateral breach of the left L4 screw, but also a possible breach into the foramen of the right L4 nerve root. The patient was managed conservatively for the next 2 to 3 weeks, but ultimately due to his persistent pain, he was taken back to operating room for screw revision.

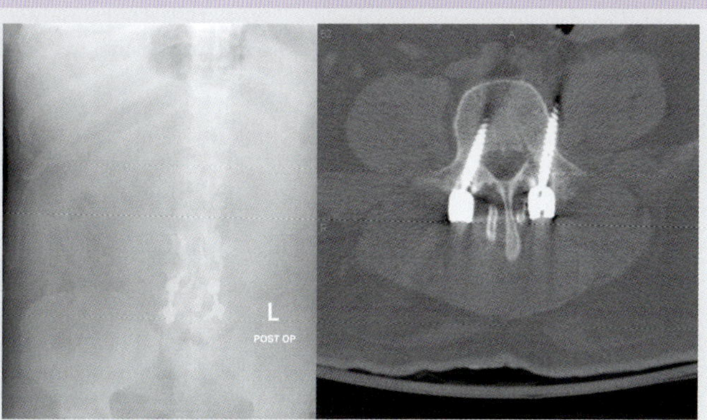

• **Fig. 54.1** Anteroposterior (AP) radiograph of patient with lateral breach of left L4 screw (left). Axial computed tomography scan demonstrating impingement of the right L4 screw on the foramen (right).

NEUROSURGICAL SELFIE MOMENT

Instrumentation-related complications regarding insertion can be avoided with the proper image guidance and intraoperative verification dependent on the comfort level of the surgeon and the complexity of the case. Furthermore, as the trend toward value-based payments continues, it stands to reason that instrumentation accuracy may eventually become a metric by which surgeons' skills are measured. Therefore ensuring the most optimal hardware placement through image guidance and intraoperative verification will result in excellent accuracy and avoidance of complications.

References

1. Goodrich JT. History of spine surgery in the ancient and medieval worlds. *Neurosurg Focus*. 2004;16(1):E2.
2. Breasted JH, New York hs. *The Edwin Smith surgical papyrus*. Chicago, IL: The University of Chicago press; 1930.
3. Kabins MB, James NW. The history of vertebral screw and pedicle screw fixation. *Iowa Ortho J*. 1991;11:127–136.
4. Jaikumar S, Kim DH, Kam AC. History of minimally invasive spine surgery. *Neurosurgery*. 2002;51(5 suppl):1.
5. Benzel EC, Francis TB. *Spine surgery: techniques, complication avoidance, and management*. Philadelphia, PA: Elsevier/Saunders; 2012.
6. Yadla S, Ghobrial GM, Campbell PG, et al. Identification of complications that have a significant effect on length of stay after spine surgery and predictive value of 90-day readmission rate. *J Neurosurg Spine*. 2015;23(6):807–811.
7. Lad SP, Babu R, Ugiliweneza B, Patil CG, Boakye M. Surgery for spinal stenosis: long-term reoperation rates, health care cost, and impact of instrumentation. *Spine*. 2014;39(12):978–987.
8. Alvin MD, Miller JA, Lubelski D, et al. Variations in cost calculations in spine surgery cost-effectiveness research. *Neurosurg Focus*. 2014; 36(6):E1.
9. Al-Khouja LT, Baron EM, Johnson JP, Kim TT, Drazin D. Cost-effectiveness analysis in minimally invasive spine surgery. *Neurosurg Focus*. 2014;36(6):E4.
10. Kim DH. *Surgical anatomy & techniques to the spine*. Philadelphia, PA: Saunders Elsevier; 2006.
11. Lu DC, Theodore P, Korn WM, Chou D. Esophageal erosion 9 years after anterior cervical plate implantation. *Surg Neurol*. 2008; 69(3):3.

12. Fountas KN, Kapsalaki EZ, Nikolakakos LG, et al. Anterior cervical discectomy and fusion associated complications. *Spine.* 2007;32(21):2310–2317.
13. Ning X, Wen Y, Xiao-Jian Y, et al. Anterior cervical locking plate-related complications; prevention and treatment recommendations. *Int Orthop.* 2008;32(5):649–655.
14. DiPaola CP, Jacobson JA, Awad H, Conrad BP, Rechtine GR. Screw pull-out force is dependent on screw orientation in an anterior cervical plate construct. *J Spinal Disord Tech.* 2007;20(5):369–373.
15. Herkowitz HN, Rothman RH, Simeone FA. *Rothman-Simeone: The spine.* 4th ed. Philadelphia, PA: W.B. Saunders; 1999.
16. Park JB, Cho YS, Riew KD. Development of adjacent-level ossification in patients with an anterior cervical plate. *J Bone Joint Surg Am.* 2005;87(3):558–563.
17. Kim HJ, Kelly MP, Ely CG, Dettori JR, Riew KD. The risk of adjacent-level ossification development after surgery in the cervical spine: are there factors that affect the risk? A systematic review. *Spine.* 2012;37(22 suppl):S65.
18. Park HG, Kang MS, Kim KH, Park JY, Kim KS, Kuh SU. A surgical method for determining proper screw length in ACDF. *Korean J Spine.* 2014;11(3):117–120.
19. Sekhon LH. Posterior cervical decompression and fusion for circumferential spondylotic cervical stenosis: review of 50 consecutive cases. *J Clin Neurosci.* 2006;13(1):23–30.
20. Jeanneret B, Magerl F, Ward EH, Ward JC. Posterior stabilization of the cervical spine with hook plates. *Spine.* 1991;16(3 suppl):56.
21. Kim YJ, Lenke LG. Thoracic pedicle screw placement: free-hand technique. *Neurol India.* 2005;53(4):512–519.
22. Ikard RW. Methods and complications of anterior exposure of the thoracic and lumbar spine. *Arch Surg.* 2006;141(10):1025–1034.
23. Kim YJ, Lenke LG, Bridwell KH, Cho YS, Riew KD. Free-hand pedicle screw placement in the thoracic spine: is it safe? *Spine.* 2004;29(3):42, discussion 342.
24. Avila MJ, Baaj AA. Freehand Thoracic pedicle screw placement: review of existing strategies and a step-by-step guide using uniform landmarks for all levels. *Cureus.* 2016;8(2):e501.
25. Lehman RA, Polly DW, Kuklo TR, Cunningham B, Kirk KL, Belmont PJ. Straight-forward versus anatomic trajectory technique of thoracic pedicle screw fixation: a biomechanical analysis. *Spine.* 2003;28(18): 2058–2065.
26. Benzel EC. *American Association of Neurological Surgeons. Biomechanics of spine stabilization.* Rolling Meadows, IL: American Association of Neurological Surgeons; 2001.
27. Konin GP, Walz DM. Lumbosacral transitional vertebrae: classification, imaging findings, and clinical relevance. *AJNR Am J Neuroradiol.* 2010;31(10):1778–1786.
28. Gumbs AA, Shah RV, Yue JJ, Sumpio B. The open anterior paramedian retroperitoneal approach for spine procedures. *Arch Surg.* 2005;140(4):339–343.
29. Parker SL, McGirt MJ, Farber SH, et al. Accuracy of free-hand pedicle screws in the thoracic and lumbar spine: analysis of 6816 consecutive screws. *Neurosurgery.* 2011;68(1):170–178, discussion 178.
30. Phan K, Hogan J, Maharaj M, Mobbs RJ. Cortical bone trajectory for lumbar pedicle screw placement: a review of published reports. *Orthop Surg.* 2015;7(3):213–221.
31. Cheng JS, Song JK. Anatomy of the sacrum. *Neurosurg Focus.* 2003;15(2):E3.
32. Tumialan LM, Mummaneni PV. Long-segment spinal fixation using pelvic screws. *Neurosurgery.* 2008;63(3 suppl):183–190.
33. Licht NJ, Rowe DE, Ross LM. Pitfalls of pedicle screw fixation in the sacrum. A cadaver model. *Spine.* 1992;17(8):892–896.
34. Arman C, Naderi S, Kiray A, et al. The human sacrum and safe approaches for screw placement. *J Clin Neurosci.* 2009;16(8):1046–1049.
35. Matteini LE, Kebaish KM, Volk WR, et al. An S-2 alar iliac pelvic fixation. Technical note. *Neurosurg Focus.* 2010;28(3):E13.
36. Kubaszewski L, Nowakowski A, Kaczmarczyk J. Evidence-based support for S1 transpedicular screw entry point modification. *J Orthop Surg Res.* 2014;9:22.
37. Mikula AL, Williams SK, Anderson PA. The use of intraoperative triggered electromyography to detect misplaced pedicle screws: a systematic review and meta-analysis. *J Neurosurg Spine.* 2016;24(4):624–638.
38. Bourgeois AC, Faulkner AR, Bradley YC, et al. Improved accuracy of minimally invasive transpedicular screw placement in the lumbar spine with 3-dimensional stereotactic image guidance: a comparative meta-analysis. *J Spinal Disord Tech.* 2015;28(9):324–329.
39. Bourgeois AC, Faulkner AR, Pasciak AS, Bradley YC. The evolution of image-guided lumbosacral spine surgery. *Ann Transl Med.* 2015;3(5):69.
40. Shin BJ, James AR, Njoku IU, Hartl R. Pedicle screw navigation: a systematic review and meta-analysis of perforation risk for computer-navigated versus freehand insertion. *J Neurosurg Spine.* 2012;17(2):113–122.
41. Tian NF, Xu HZ. Image-guided pedicle screw insertion accuracy: a meta-analysis. *Int Orthop.* 2009;33(4):895–903.
42. Kosmopoulos V, Schizas C. Pedicle screw placement accuracy: a meta-analysis. *Spine.* 2007;32(3):111.
43. Wood M, Mannion R. A comparison of CT-based navigation techniques for minimally invasive lumbar pedicle screw placement. *J Spinal Disord Tech.* 2011;24(1):1.

55

Postoperative Spinal Deformities: Kyphosis, Nonunion, and Loss of Motion Segment

AVERY L. BUCHHOLZ, JOHN C. QUINN, CHRISTOPHER I. SHAFFREY

HIGHLIGHTS

- Proximal junctional kyphosis and proximal junctional failure are separate entities and must be recognized and cared for appropriately.
- The best treatment for pseudarthrosis is to prevent it from happening in the first place with meticulous placement of instrumentation and bone preparation.
- Maintaining and restoring lumbar lordosis in association with pelvic parameters can help prevent adjacent segment disease.

RED FLAGS

- Smoking
- Osteoporosis
- Advanced age

Background

Lumbar spine instrumentation and fusion is a commonly indicated treatment for infection, tumors, trauma, deformity, and degenerative disease. With broad indications and continued improvement in surgical techniques and technology, there has been a tremendous increase in the number of lumbar spine fusions performed in the last decade.[1] Unfortunately, these surgeries can result in unplanned complications such as proximal disease, failure of fusion, and loss of motion with associated adjacent level disease, all of which can be problematic for patients and the treating physician. The purpose of this chapter is to discuss each of these fusion-related complications and provide some insight into how to properly manage them.

Proximal Junctional Kyphosis

With the advent of modern instrumentation and selective fusions, junctional kyphosis at the transition from fused to mobile segments may be a common radiographic finding. After long-segment spinal instrumentation, proximal junctional kyphosis (PJK) can be seen as a postoperative complication (Fig. 55.2). In adult spinal deformity surgery, the reported incidence ranges from 11.0% to 52.9%; however, the description and criteria for defining PJK and its clinical impact vary in the literature.[2–8] PJK has traditionally been defined by a 10 degree or greater increase in kyphosis at the proximal junction as measured on a sagittal radiograph with a Cobb angle from the caudal end plate of the uppermost instrumented vertebrae (UIV) to the cephalad end plate of the vertebrae two segments cranial to the UIV. This measurement was reported by Glattes et al. and has been validated in several subsequent studies.[2,9] Although PJK, as defined above, may have a high postoperative occurrence rate, the significance of PJK remains debatable. Some reports indicate that PJK is only a radiographic phenomenon with little clinical significance, whereas others indicate that PJK is associated with significant pain, neurologic deficit, and need for revision surgery.[4,10,11] A recent review of causes for hospital readmission after adult deformity surgery reported that PJK was the most common postoperative complication requiring surgical treatment in a cohort of 836 patients.[12]

Despite some benign reports of PJK, investigators have recognized a subset of patients with a more severe version of PJK and an increased need for revision surgery. In addition to increased deformity and pain, these patients are at an increased neurologic risk. The term proximal junctional failure (PJF) is used to define this group and to distinguish it from PJK. PJF is associated not only with an increase in kyphosis but also with structural failure. The structural failure occurs at either the UIV or the vertebrae immediately proximal to the fusion construct (UIV +1).[13] Structural failure is considered a vertebral body fracture, disruption of the posterior osseoligamentous complex, or both. Unlike traditional PJK, PJF has a clear association with increased pain, spinal instability, risk of neurologic injury, and need for revision surgery.[13,14]

Risk factors for developing PJK/PJF have been identified and include advanced patient age, poor bone quality, posterior spinal ligamentous disruption, instrumentation rigidity, fusion to the sacrum, and postoperative spinal alignment.[2] With respect to adult patients, Kim et al. found age over 55 to be a significant risk factor for the development of PJK. They also found combined anterior/posterior fusions to have higher PJK rates than posterior-alone procedures.[4] Yagi et al. found higher rates of PJK in patients with fusion to the sacrum.[11] Some cases of PJK may develop from structural damage. Studies on adolescent patients have shown an increased incidence of PJK with posterior instrumentation compared with an anterior approach.[15] The conclusion was that disruption of the posterior tension band from surgery and deformity correction forces applied during surgery results in an increased incidence of PJK. Ligamentum flavum damage has also been attributable to PJK progression. Vertebral body fractures have been associated with the mechanical stress generated by pedicle screw instrumentation at the proximal junction. This has been shown to be higher with inclusion of the sacrum.[16] Yagi et al. also associated fusion of the sacrum with higher PJK rates.[11] Both of these reports support the idea that correction forces, and possibly surgical dissection, contribute to PJK and PJF.[11,16]

The occurrence of PJK is most prevalent in the early postoperative period. Kim et al. reported PJK to be most common in the first 8 weeks after surgery with 59% of patients progressing in this time.[4] In a review of adolescent idiopathic scoliosis patients, Kim et al. found a lower prevalence of PJK (26%) with no significant progression from 2 years on.[10] It appears that the most dramatic progression of PJK occurs in the first 3 to 6 months.

Patients who undergo greater sagittal realignment are also at higher risk of PJK/PJF. In a study by Hart et al., patients who experienced PJF had a greater number of pedicle subtraction osteotomies, an increase in lumbar lordosis, pelvic-incidence and lumbar lordosis mismatch reduction, and sagittal vertical axis (SVA) correction.[14] More importantly, from a clinical perspective there is evidence that patients with PJF do worse clinically than patients without this complication. Hostin et al. reported on their experience with 1218 adult deformity surgeries. There were 68 cases of PJF (5.6%) with 28 of those patients undergoing revision surgery within 6 months of the operation. Patients undergoing revision surgery were identified with PJF on average 9 weeks after the initial surgery compared with 13 weeks for patients who did not have revision surgery.[13] This again demonstrates the impact of mechanical failure as opposed to recurrent deformity. There is a clear clinical significance with the occurrence of PJF given the frequent need for extension of instrumentation.

Several strategies have been proposed to mitigate the occurrence of PJK/PJF, including preservation of the posterior ligament complex and adjacent facet joints, use of vertebral augmentation with polymethyl methacrylate (PMMA) to prevent vertebral compression fractures, and use of less rigid fixation at the proximal terminal junction of the construct with transitional rods, transverse process hooks, and dynamic stabilization techniques. Cadaveric models have shown a reduced incidence of junctional fractures with vertebroplasty. Kebaish et al. demonstrated this with 18 cadaveric spine specimens in an axial loading model showing 5 out of 6 fractures in the control group, 6/6 with cement at UIV, and only one fracture in the UIV +1 cement group.[17] This has also been demonstrated in clinical practice with a report of 8% PJK rates and 5% PJF rates in 41 patients treated with prophylactic UIV +1 vertebroplasty.[18] Additional data is needed, but this treatment may prove to be advantageous in reducing PJK rates. There has been no good data to support transitional rods or the use of hooks over pedicle screws at the upper levels of instrumentation. Percutaneous instrumentation has also not produced a decrease in PJK over open screw placement.

One technique that does seem to offer the potential to reduce the occurrence of PJK/PJF is the use of junctional tethers. Using a polyester tether such as woven polyethylene Mersilene tape (Ethicon, Somerville, NJ), the spinous processes are interwoven in an attempt to dissipate forces at the proximal junction. Although their clinical effectiveness remains under investigation, Bess et al. recently provided a finite element analysis that demonstrated that posterior tethers created a more gradual transition in range-of-motion and adjacent-segment stress from the instrumented to noninstrumented spine.[19] There are numerous techniques for the application of these tethers. Most simply, the spinous processes of the UIV +1 and UIV −1 are tethered together by passing the Mersilene tape through each and tying it together. Recently at our institution, we have begun tying the Mersilene tape from the UIV +1 to a crosslink and creating distraction to increase tension on the Mersilene tape (Fig. 55.1). In a retrospective review, our data shows a 40.8% PJK rate with no tether, 34.3% with standard tether technique, and 19% with use of a crosslink. This is pending publication.

Current management for PJK involves both conservative and surgical interventions. When diagnosed radiographically, PJK may be followed with routine imaging and close observation. Some patients will remain asymptomatic. Other patients may be managed by pain medications, physical therapy to strengthen the back, or epidural injections. We have found aquatics-based physical therapy programs to be most effective because they unload the spine and allow patients to increase their activity level with reduced pain. Surgical management when needed involves extension of the fusion superiorly to correct the deformity. Regardless of where the fusion ends, PJK will remain a risk factor.

Nonunion

Pseudarthrosis is a well-reported complication of lumbar spine surgery. Its diagnosis is based on appropriate clinical history and imaging findings or implant failure, loss of fixation, deformity, or radiolucencies. However, the presentation is unpredictable, and it can occur up to a decade postoperatively despite the presence of solid bone formation at earlier time points. Surgery for spinal deformity correction relies heavily on arthrodesis across several

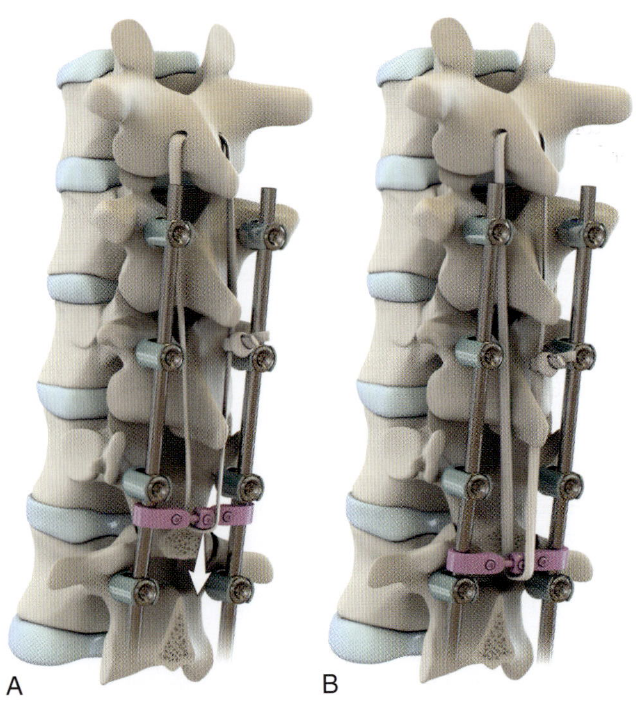

• **Fig. 55.1** (A) Illustration of Mersilene tether tied from the UIV +1 spinous process to a crosslink device. The tape is tied tight with the crosslink in a cephalad position. (B) With the Mersilene tied tightly, the crosslink is distracted, putting increased tension on the tether and adding support to the transition from instrumented to noninstrumented segments.

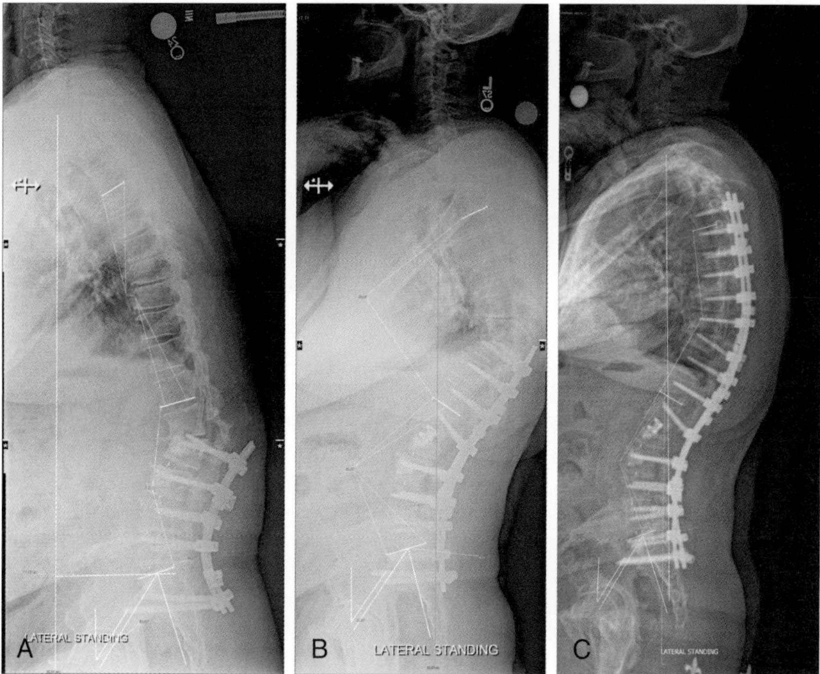

• **Fig. 55.2** (A) Preoperative standing lateral radiograph showing loss of sagittal balance, lordosis, and proximal junctional kyphosis (PJK) with a pelvic incidence (PI) 49 degrees, pelvic tilt (PT) 33 degrees, lumbar lordosis (LL) 2 degrees, and thoracic kyphosis (TK) 15 degrees and an 11-cm SVA. (B) T10 to iliac with L2 PSO postoperative standing lateral radiograph showing PJK. Measurements include PI 49 degrees, PT 35 degrees, LL 50 degrees, and TK 59 degrees and a −1-cm SVA. Kyphosis is 50 degrees across the PJK segment. (C) T4 to iliac extension postoperative standing lateral radiograph. Measurements include PI 49 degrees, PT 30 degrees, LL 49 degrees, and TK 46 degrees and a −1-cm SVA. Restored sagittal alignment.

levels of the spinal column. To achieve a solid fusion, locally harvested autologous bone graft is used along with supplemented allograft. Occasionally osteoinductive and osteoconductive agents are used as well. Fusion in children and adolescents is rarely a concern due to high bone quality. In adult patients nonunion is a real concern and must be monitored closely. Rates of pseudarthrosis after lumbar spine fusion have ranged from 5% to 35% with a higher incidence in surgeries spanning three or more levels.[1] Pseudarthrosis should be suspected when a patient presents with recurrent pain and/or neurologic symptoms during long-term follow-up from fusion or in the presence of instrumentation failure. A mechanical exacerbation of symptoms may suggest instability at the surgical site. Diagnosis can be difficult because symptoms are not specific to pseudarthrosis but may be attributable to other causes, such as infection or adjacent segment disease (ASD). A pain-free interval in the postoperative period is a useful clue into the history. Patients with no symptom relief postoperatively should be studied further to rule out additional causes.

It is often difficult to predict when or whether a pseudarthrosis will become symptomatic for patients. DePalma and Rothman retrospectively reviewed outcomes in patients with radiographic evidence of pseudarthrosis compared with those in matched controls with a successful lumbar fusion and found no significant difference between the two groups in terms of subjective satisfaction, symptom relief, or return to activity.[20] More recent studies, however, suggest that a solid fusion correlates with improved long-term outcomes and decreased symptom severity. Kornblum et al. reported on patients with symptomatic spinal stenosis and spondylolisthesis treated with posterolateral arthrodesis. Eighty-six percent of patients with a solid fusion had "excellent" or "good" long-term outcomes compared with only 56% of patients with a pseudarthrosis.[21] It remains unclear why some patients can tolerate a nonunion with good long-term clinical outcomes, whereas others require surgical treatment. Local factors that can lead to nonunions include poor preparation or decortication of the fusion surface, insufficient viable graft material, vascular insufficiency, smoking, poor nutrition, or metabolic problems. Meticulous surgical preparation and adequate-quality bone graft will minimize the risk for fusion failure. Global parameters may also contribute to pseudarthrosis. Malalignment of the spine with poor sagittal balance, insufficient compression forces, and inadequate stability at the fusion site all contribute. These mechanical concerns become increasingly significant when fusions extend across transition zones such as the lumbosacral junction. In the adult population, a correlation between poor postoperative sagittal alignment and pseudarthrosis has been noted.[5]

The assessment of fusion can be difficult. Plain radiographs are often the initial assessment for pseudarthrosis and other diagnoses given their availability and relatively low cost, but the radiographic presentation of nonunions can vary. In a study using plain radiographs, Kim et al. found an average of 3.5 years (range: 12–131 months) before fusion failure could be detected.[22] In a similar study, Dickson et al. showed that out of 18 patients with known pseudarthrosis, only 13 (72%) were detected by radiographs 2 years postoperatively.[23] This data along with other findings suggests that annual radiographic follow-up should be implemented for multilevel fusions even if bony union is apparent at early time points. Computed tomography (CT) imaging has the strongest correlation of fusion assessment and should be obtained if a nonunion is in question. Although there are no universally accepted criteria for pseudarthrosis with an interbody fusion, most studies use the following to identify a nonunion: motion on dynamic films, absence of continuous trabecular bone between adjacent vertebrae, gas in the disc space, and periimplant radiolucency. Current radiographic guidelines for successful lumbar fusion include less than 3 mm of translation motion and less than 5 degrees of angular motion on flexion and extension radiographs.[24] As CT technology advances, so does our ability to detect pseudarthrosis. Shah et al. reported bridging trabecular bone to be appreciated on 95% of thin-section CT scans compared with 4% of plain films 6 months postoperatively. These authors suggest that thin-section CT should be the modality of choice for the detection of pseudarthrosis.[25]

Additional methods used to detect pseudarthrosis include bone scintigraphy and positron emission tomography (PET) scans. Bone scintigraphy uses radiographic tracer to localize tissue with high metabolic activity (indicating active tissue changes or repair). This is more commonly used to detect infections, neoplasm, and occult fractures. It currently remains a poor choice for the detection of pseudarthrosis due to poor sensitivity. Similarly, PET scans detect gamma ray emission from positron-emitting radioactive tracers, which have an affinity for metabolically active cells. It has recently been suggested that tracers, which are used more commonly for detection of infections and neoplasm, can also measure bone graft healing by correlating increased uptake at the fusion site. Although studies have shown this to be a modality for monitoring active bone formation, little data exists on clinical applications and correlation with rates of nonunion.

The treatment of pseudarthrosis varies but is almost always surgical.[24] In cases of asymptomatic patients, they may be observed and followed closely with radiographs and routine evaluation. When symptomatic, patients will often experience pain in the axial spine with occasional radicular symptoms. A delayed fusion with no evidence of instrumentation loosening may be treated with bracing, activity limitation, and observation. Primary principles of surgery include stabilization of the existing posterior fixation and regrafting. Treatments may require a circumferential fusion with anterior lumbar interbody fusion (ALIF) or lateral lumbar or posterior lumbar interbody fusion. Interbody devices allow for increased surface area under compressive forces, creating an ideal environment for fusion. Advances in biologics, allograft materials, and growth factor augmentation have all improved arthrodesis. The ideal material demonstrates osteoinductive, osteoconductive, and/or osteogenic properties. Iliac crest bone graft has been the gold standard autograft bone material; however, complications with harvest and limitations in supply have led to the development of additional agents. A review of posterolateral lumbar fusion rates reported iliac crest fusion rate of 79%, allograft bone 52%, ceramics 87%, demineralized bone matrices 89%, autologous bone marrow 74%, and bone morphogenetic properties 94%.[26] Implants must be solidly anchored and screws increased in size as needed. Osteoporotic bone requires segmental fixation, and when a fusion extends to the sacrum, supplemental instrumentation with iliac screws is often required.

The best treatment for pseudarthrosis is to prevent it from occurring at the initial operation. Improvements in bone graft materials, instrumentation, and techniques have all led to decreased rates of nonunion. Treatment of pseudarthrosis has also benefited from these advancements. Another critical aspect of pseudarthrosis prevention is the assessment of the patient's preoperative condition. Risk factors such as alcoholism, osteoporosis, advanced age, malnutrition, and tobacco use have all been attributed to decreased fusion rates. During surgery for pseudarthrosis, emphasis must be placed on bone preparation and arthrodesis. This involves aggressive removal of fibrous tissue, renewed grafting with autologous bone, and revision instrumentation when necessary. Poor alignment must be addressed with evaluation of sagittal parameters. This may involve osteotomies or corrective maneuvers. The importance of proper alignment is increased with the length of fusion and extension across junctional zones.

Loss of Motion Segment and Adjacent Segment Disease

ASD is a clinical deterioration of adjacent vertebral levels after a spine fusion and is a recognized outcome with a mean annual incidence of 2.9% in the cervical spine and 3.9% in the lumbar spine.[27,28] ASD occurs as a result of increased degeneration of spine levels neighboring a fused segment, theoretically from increased biomechanical stress and physiologic loading. Pathology can be difficult to differentiate from the natural history of normal spinal degeneration, but breakdown of these adjacent levels has been identified as a cause of postoperative pain and disability.

Many studies have looked at the prevalence of clinical symptoms associated with ASD. In a study of patients with one- or two-level lumbar fusion, Cheh et al. showed that 43% and 24% of patients develop radiographic and clinically symptomatic ASD, respectively.[29] Ghiselli et al. reported a retrospective review of 215 patients after posterior lumbar fusion. These patients had a reoperation rate associated with ASD of 16.5% in the first 5 years and 36.1% at 10 years.[28] A similar study by Gillet found a reoperation rate of 20% over a 2- to 15-year follow-up period.[30] Penta et al. looked at magnetic resonance images 10 years after lumbar fusion and found radiographically diagnosed ASD in 32% of patients.[31] Part of the difficulty in diagnosing ASD stems from the discrepancies in its definition. Some studies use radiographic deterioration as evidence for ASD, whereas others rely on the need for reoperation. As a way to better inform the patient and the surgeon, we favor using a discrete end point of surgery as a way to predict and determine ASD.

The risk factors that lead to ASD have been studied, with age being the most influential factor and those over age 60 being at highest risk.[29] Higher ASD rates have also been seen in postmenopausal women. Other risk factors, including positive smoking history and increased fusion length, have been studied with conflicting reports. One risk factor that does seem to have a strong association with ASD is the preoperative anatomic alignment of the spine. In some reports, a diagnosis of degenerative scoliosis alone increases the risk of ASD.[32] A retrospective study by Kumar et al. showed that patients with a normal C7 plumb line and sacral inclination had the lowest rates of ASD.[33] Sacral slope ≤35 degrees was associated with increased ASD and can be interpreted as a failure to restore sagittal alignment with compensation by pelvic retroversion. Failure to maintain proper spinal alignment during a fusion can result in accelerated adjacent degeneration.[34–36]

Not restoring adequate lumbar lordosis during lumbar fusion may result in mechanical low back pain, sagittal malalignment, and increased risk of adjacent segment degeneration. Umehara et al. described the biomechanical effect of postoperative hypolordosis in lumbar fusion on instrumented and adjacent spinal segments. They described accelerated adjacent segment deterioration by loading motion segments in a nonphysiologic way. Hypolordosis also increased stress on the interbody implant with increased loading on the posterior implants from repetitive extension in the lumbar spine.[37] In 2001, Izumi and Kumano assessed lumbar alignment before and after fusion operations and found that cases of degenerative changes in adjacent segments were increased in patients with postoperative loss of lordosis of 10 degrees.[38] Rothenfluh et al. found a higher incidence of ASD with larger pelvic incidence (PI)-lumbar lordosis (LL) mismatch. The authors also found that patients with postoperative PI-LL mismatch underwent revision surgery with tenfold greater frequency than patients with appropriate postoperative sagittal alignment.[39]

Treatment for ASD is complicated by the risk associated with revision surgery and the potential for further degenerative disease. Priorities should be dictated by the patient's age and degree of symptoms, with conservative measures being appropriate in most cases. When surgical management is indicated, restoring and maintaining spinal alignment is a proven way to improve patient outcomes and reduce the incidence of future ASD.

SURGICAL REWIND

My Worst Case

- A 71-year-old-male with 6 prior lumbar surgeries over a 5-year period. Patient has developed a progressive and severe kyphotic deformity above his L2 through iliac instrumentation and now has severe sagittal imbalance.
- Patient underwent an extended L2 pedicle subtraction osteotomy with extension of instrumentation and fusion from iliac to T10. A Mersilene tape tether was placed from T9 to T11.
- At the 6-month postoperative visit, patient was noted to have significant PJK measuring 50 degrees. Patient had localized pain and failed conservative management on close follow-up. Patient elected for surgical management with extension of instrumentation and fusion to T4 with reduction of kyphosis.

NEUROSURGICAL SELFIE

- In all phases of spine care, proper attention must be paid to pelvic parameters and sagittal balance. Any surgical intervention must prioritize restoration and maintenance of lumbar lordosis with attention to spinal alignment.
- Although some risk factors are unavoidable (advanced age, scoliosis), others such as quality of bone, smoking cessation, and nutrition should be maximized before surgery. We routinely consult endocrine for help in managing osteopenia and osteoporosis.
- Meticulous attention to proper fusion at the initial surgery is the best prevention for pseudarthrosis. When a nonunion does occur, extra effort must be made to remove fibrous tissue from bone surfaces and prepare a new arthrodesis surface. Biologics are helpful in both initial and subsequent surgeries.

References

1. Deyo RA, Mirza SK, Martin BI, Kreuter W, Goodman DC, Jarvik JG. Trends, major medical complications, and charges associated with surgery for lumbar spinal stenosis in older adults. *JAMA.* 2010;303(13):1259–1265.
2. Glattes RC, Bridwell KH, Lenke LG, Kim YJ, Rinella A, Edwards C 2nd. Proximal junctional kyphosis in adult spinal deformity following long instrumented posterior spinal fusion: incidence, outcomes, and risk factor analysis. *Spine.* 2005;30(14):1643–1649.
3. Ha Y, Maruo K, Racine L, et al. Proximal junctional kyphosis and clinical outcomes in adult spinal deformity surgery with fusion from the thoracic spine to the sacrum: a comparison of proximal and distal upper instrumented vertebrae. *J Neurosurg Spine.* 2013;19(3):360–369.
4. Kim YJ, Bridwell KH, Lenke LG, Glattes CR, Rhim S, Cheh G. Proximal junctional kyphosis in adult spinal deformity after segmental posterior spinal instrumentation and fusion: minimum five-year follow-up. *Spine.* 2008;33(20):2179–2184.
5. Park SJ, Lee CS, Chung SS, Lee JY, Kang SS, Park SH. Different risk factors of proximal junctional kyphosis and proximal junctional failure following long instrumented fusion to the sacrum for adult spinal deformity: survivorship analysis of 160 patients. *Neurosurgery.* 2017;80(2):279–286.
6. Reames DL, Kasliwal MK, Smith JS, Hamilton DK, Arlet V, Shaffrey CI. Time to development, clinical and radiographic characteristics, and management of proximal junctional kyphosis following adult thoracolumbar instrumented fusion for spinal deformity. *J Spinal Disord Tech.* 2015;28(2):E106–E114.
7. Smith JS, Klineberg E, Lafage V, et al. Prospective multicenter assessment of perioperative and minimum 2-year postoperative complication rates associated with adult spinal deformity surgery. *J Neurosurg Spine.* 2016;25(1):1–14.
8. Yan C, Li Y, Yu Z. Prevalence and consequences of the proximal junctional kyphosis after spinal deformity surgery: a meta-analysis. *Medicine (Baltimore).* 2016;95(20):e3471.
9. Sacramento-Dominguez C, Vayas-Diez R, Coll-Mesa L, et al. Reproducibility measuring the angle of proximal junctional kyphosis using the first or the second vertebra above the upper instrumented vertebrae in patients surgically treated for scoliosis. *Spine.* 2009; 34(25):2787–2791.
10. Kim YJ, Lenke LG, Bridwell KH, et al. Proximal junctional kyphosis in adolescent idiopathic scoliosis after 3 different types of posterior segmental spinal instrumentation and fusions: incidence and risk factor analysis of 410 cases. *Spine.* 2007;32(24):2731–2738.
11. Yagi M, Akilah KB, Boachie-Adjei O. Incidence, risk factors and classification of proximal junctional kyphosis: surgical outcomes review of adult idiopathic scoliosis. *Spine.* 2011;36(1):E60–E68.
12. Schairer WW, Carrer A, Deviren V, et al. Hospital readmission after spine fusion for adult spinal deformity. *Spine.* 2013;38(19):1681–1689.
13. Hostin R, McCarthy I, O'Brien M, et al. Incidence, mode, and location of acute proximal junctional failures after surgical treatment of adult spinal deformity. *Spine.* 2013;38(12):1008–1015.
14. Hart R, McCarthy I, O'Brien M, et al. Identification of decision criteria for revision surgery among patients with proximal junctional failure after surgical treatment of spinal deformity. *Spine.* 2013;38(19):E1223–E1227.
15. Rhee JM, Bridwell KH, Won DS, Lenke LG, Chotigavanichaya C, Hanson DS. Sagittal plane analysis of adolescent idiopathic scoliosis: the effect of anterior versus posterior instrumentation. *Spine.* 2002;27(21):2350–2356.
16. Watanabe K, Lenke LG, Bridwell KH, Kim YJ, Koester L, Hensley M. Proximal junctional vertebral fracture in adults after spinal deformity surgery using pedicle screw constructs: analysis of morphological features. *Spine.* 2010;35(2):138–145.
17. Kebaish KM, Martin CT, O'Brien JR, LaMotta IE, Voros GD, Belkoff SM. Use of vertebroplasty to prevent proximal junctional fractures in adult deformity surgery: a biomechanical cadaveric study. *Spine J.* 2013;13(12):1897–1903.
18. Martin CT, Skolasky RL, Mohamed AS, Kebaish KM. Preliminary results of the effect of prophylactic vertebroplasty on the incidence of proximal junctional complications after posterior spinal fusion to the low thoracic spine. *Spine Deform.* 2013;1(2):132–138.
19. Bess S, Harris JE, Turner AW, et al. The effect of posterior polyester tethers on the biomechanics of proximal junctional kyphosis: a finite element analysis. *J Neurosurg Spine.* 2017;26(1):125–133.
20. DePalma AF, Rothman RH. The nature of pseudarthrosis. *Clin Orthop Relat Res.* 1968;59:113–118.
21. Kornblum MB, Fischgrund JS, Herkowitz HN, Abraham DA, Berkower DL, Ditkoff JS. Degenerative lumbar spondylolisthesis with spinal stenosis: a prospective long-term study comparing

fusion and pseudarthrosis. *Spine*. 2004;29(7):726–733, discussion 733–734.
22. Kim YJ, Bridwell KH, Lenke LG, Cho KJ, Edwards CC 2nd, Rinella AS. Pseudarthrosis in adult spinal deformity following multisegmental instrumentation and arthrodesis. *J Bone Joint Surg Am*. 2006;88(4):721–728.
23. Dickson DD, Lenke LG, Bridwell KH, Koester LA. Risk factors for and assessment of symptomatic pseudarthrosis after lumbar pedicle subtraction osteotomy in adult spinal deformity. *Spine*. 2014;39(15):1190–1195.
24. Chun DS, Baker KC, Hsu WK. Lumbar pseudarthrosis: a review of current diagnosis and treatment. *Neurosurg Focus*. 2015;39(4):E10.
25. Shah RR, Mohammed S, Saifuddin A, Taylor BA. Comparison of plain radiographs with CT scan to evaluate interbody fusion following the use of titanium interbody cages and transpedicular instrumentation. *Eur Spine J*. 2003;12(4):378–385.
26. Hsu WK, Nickoli MS, Wang JC, et al. Improving the clinical evidence of bone graft substitute technology in lumbar spine surgery. *Global Spine J*. 2012;2(4):239–248.
27. Hilibrand AS, Carlson GD, Palumbo MA, Jones PK, Bohlman HH. Radiculopathy and myelopathy at segments adjacent to the site of a previous anterior cervical arthrodesis. *J Bone Joint Surg Am*. 1999;81(4):519–528.
28. Ghiselli G, Wang JC, Bhatia NN, Hsu WK, Dawson EG. Adjacent segment degeneration in the lumbar spine. *J Bone Joint Surg Am*. 2004;86-A(7):1497–1503.
29. Cheh G, Bridwell KH, Lenke LG, et al. Adjacent segment disease following lumbar/thoracolumbar fusion with pedicle screw instrumentation: a minimum 5-year follow-up. *Spine*. 2007;32(20): 2253–2257.
30. Gillet P. The fate of the adjacent motion segments after lumbar fusion. *J Spinal Disord Tech*. 2003;16(4):338–345.
31. Penta M, Sandhu A, Fraser RD. Magnetic resonance imaging assessment of disc degeneration 10 years after anterior lumbar interbody fusion. *Spine*. 1995;20(6):743–747.
32. Alentado VJ, Lubelski D, Healy AT, et al. Predisposing characteristics of adjacent segment disease after lumbar fusion. *Spine*. 2016;41(14):1167–1172.
33. Kumar MN, Baklanov A, Chopin D. Correlation between sagittal plane changes and adjacent segment degeneration following lumbar spine fusion. *Eur Spine J*. 2001;10(4):314–319.
34. Axelsson P, Johnsson R, Stromqvist B. The spondylolytic vertebra and its adjacent segment. Mobility measured before and after posterolateral fusion. *Spine*. 1997;22(4):414–417.
35. Hayes MA, Tompkins SF, Herndon WA, Gruel CR, Kopta JA, Howard TC. Clinical and radiological evaluation of lumbosacral motion below fusion levels in idiopathic scoliosis. *Spine*. 1988;13(10): 1161–1167.
36. Jackson RP, McManus AC. Radiographic analysis of sagittal plane alignment and balance in standing volunteers and patients with low back pain matched for age, sex, and size. A prospective controlled clinical study. *Spine*. 1994;19(14):1611–1618.
37. Umehara S, Zindrick MR, Patwardhan AG, et al. The biomechanical effect of postoperative hypolordosis in instrumented lumbar fusion on instrumented and adjacent spinal segments. *Spine*. 2000;25(13):1617–1624.
38. Izumi Y, Kumano K. Analysis of sagittal lumbar alignment before and after posterior instrumentation: Risk factor for adjacent unfused segment. *Eur J Orthop Surg Traumatol*. 2001;11(1):9–13.
39. Rothenfluh DA, Mueller DA, Rothenfluh E, Min K. Pelvic incidence-lumbar lordosis mismatch predisposes to adjacent segment disease after lumbar spinal fusion. *Eur Spine J*. 2015;24(6):1251–1258.

56

Complications of Minimally Invasive Spinal Surgery

GEORGE M. GHOBRIAL, HSUAN-KAN CHANG, MICHAEL Y. WANG

HIGHLIGHTS

- Complication avoidance in minimally invasive spinal surgery begins with careful preoperative selection of all candidates in the clinic.
- Competency in minimally invasive spinal surgery requires an understanding of specific anatomic corridors utilized in minimally invasive spinal approaches. At the least, a full understanding of the relevant anatomy can avert major neurovascular injury.
- Uncomplicated access of the lateral disc space can still be complicated by subsidence in the long run. Iatrogenic end plate injury due to aggressive disc space preparation can be viewed as a procedural complication because subsidence reverses indirect decompression.
- Tubular approaches have a higher learning curve and carry an increased risk for durotomy and nerve root injury. Careful preoperative consideration should go into the selection of these patients because severely spondylotic or morbidly obese patients can lead to increased operative durations, time spent in the prone position, increased anesthesia, airway edema, and all other associated morbidity.
- The minimally invasive spinal posterior cervical foraminotomy minimizes muscular detachment of paraspinal neck musculature that is key in preserving normal cervical alignment. Utilization of decompression-only procedures, even muscle splitting approaches in patients with preoperative cervical kyphosis, should be done with careful consideration because there is still an elevated risk for worsening cervical deformity by loss of cervical lordosis and increased cervical sagittal malalignment.

Background

One of the fundamental tenets of minimally invasive spinal (MIS) surgery is the improvement of short-term outcomes through the limitation of approach-related morbidity.[1,2] Tubular access for posterior cervical and lumbar pathology, lateral lumbar transpsoas surgery, minimally invasive lumbar interbody fusion, and percutaneous instrumentation have all grown in popularity with the common goal of lowering surgical morbidity, cost, and maximizing outcomes. In this chapter, the authors discuss select versatile MIS approaches such as the lateral lumbar interbody fusion (LLIF) and posterior paraspinal approaches to the lumbar and cervical spine. An emphasis on complication avoidance as well as intraoperative and postoperative complication management is made.

Anatomic Insights

Posterior Cervical Approach

The posterior approach to the cervical spine in an MIS fashion entails an understanding of the posterior cervical musculature. Normal cervical lordosis (CL) is a relatively modern research focus, consisting of studies of asymptomatic adults.[3,4] In general, due to the lack of consensus on normal cervical alignment, there is a debate over the concept of cervical deformity.[3] Yukawa et al. evaluated 1200 asymptomatic adults, finding the mean CL to be 13.9 ± 12.3 degrees and a range of motion of 55 degrees.[4] Generally, a trend in the literature shows common cervical deformity criteria to include either CL less than 10 degrees, CL less than 0 degrees (kyphosis), or greater than 4 cm of cervical positive sagittal malalignment (CPSM), which is the difference in plumb lines between the centra of C2 and C7.[5,6] Cervical deformity should not be an afterthought when planning even MIS posterior cervical surgery because the CL of the neck is maintained by the extensor musculature.[7] Reduction in this tension band will result in gradual loss of lordosis. Detachment of the posterior muscular attachments from the spinous processes in the midline posterior cervical approach for laminectomy is widely performed with an instrumented fusion. The deep muscular attachments consist of the semispinalis cervices and multifidus muscles, and are avoidable in decompression surgery from a paramedian muscle-splitting approach. Even a single-level posterior foraminotomy, which entails the subperiosteal release of the muscle fibers from the lamina and drilling of less than 50% of a unilateral facet, is still observed to result in a loss of CL <10 degrees, an occurrence more common in patients with preoperative cervical deformity.[8] This can be done with a tubular retractor. Shiraishi et al. describe their experience with 79 patients utilizing a curvilinear paramedian fascial incision to allow for access to the laminar facet junction by splitting the semispinalis cervices and interspinales muscles.[7] This technique was not observed to result in cervical kyphosis; however, their follow-up was limited.

Lateral Lumbar Transpsoas Approach

Nerve Injury

Ozgur et al.[9] first published results with the LLIF in 2006, describing an MIS surgical corridor to the lumbar disc and vertebral body. This lateral transpsoas, retroperitoneal approach has demonstrated in approximately 10 years to be versatile in addressing a variety of posterior degenerative indications with a low complication rate[10]:

degenerative scoliosis[11] and global sagittal imbalance,[12] neoplasms,[13,14] osteodiscitis,[15] and thoracolumbar trauma.[1] The attempt to expand this approach illustrates the desire of surgeons and patients to overcome the morbidity attributed to dissection of the posterior musculature. Meticulous technique and surgeon awareness of critical neurovascular and retroperitoneal structures are key in avoidance of devastating injury.

The LLIF is unique in that every surgical step requires a broad anatomic knowledge to avoid injury. The muscular anatomy of the abdominal wall consists of three layers: the external oblique, internal oblique, and transversalis muscles, from superficial to deep. Injury to the subcostal nerve, arising from the T12 nerve root, can occur as the nerve runs between the transversus abdominus and internal oblique muscles and results in pseudohernia.[16,17] The iliohypogastric (L1 supplied) runs anterior to the quadratus lumborum muscle, with an anterior branch running between the transversus abdominis and internal oblique layers susceptible to injury through approach or by heat transfer by monopolar cautery. The ilioinguinal nerve courses more posteriorly, but can travel ventral and inferior before piercing the transversus abdominis muscle to enter the inguinal canal. Injury to these sensory nerves can result in numbness or a painful neuroma. Deep to the muscular layer lies the peritoneal fascia and retroperitoneum. The abdominal fat and bowel are swept anteriorly with the psoas being the next anatomic structure of intended entry. The femoral nerve takes a more posterior to anterior position within the psoas muscle as one descends from cranial to caudal, with the greatest risk for injury at the L4–L5 disc space.[18] Lastly, thc gcnitofemoral arises from L1 and L2, traveling obliquely from a posterior to anterior direction on its eventual course to the abdominal wall.[1]

Vascular Injury

The most feared complication of lateral surgery is catastrophic venous injury or arterial injury. A systematic approach to reviewing each individual patient's anatomy is key to avoiding injury. Hu et al. demonstrated in an magnetic resonance imaging (MRI) study of the relevant vascular anatomy for the LLIF that the vena cava migrates laterally from L1 to L5 in most patients (up to 70%), and therefore an increased risk of venous injury on a right-sided approach is noted at the L4–L5 disc space.[19,20] The importance to understanding where the vessels lie on each patient's MRI is due to variations in individual anatomy. Another finding in the transitional lumbosacral zone is a lower sacral slope and a more triangular shape of the vertebral bodies, giving L5 more of an appearance seen in S1.[21] Great care must be taken not to deviate medially and anteriorly along the side of the triangular vertebral body, but even more so here as the iliac vein has a more lateral course and runs at the greatest risk for injury.

Adult Degenerative Scoliosis

Adult degenerative scoliosis and adult spinal deformity (ASD) represent challenges in identifying safe working corridors and pose increased risk for vascular injury, bowel injury, or retroperitoneal injury. Blizzard et al. reported an arterial avulsion from an unidentified source injury retractor placement on the convexity of a multilevel degenerative scoliosis correction.[22] After retractor expansion, episodic arterial bleeding was encountered; however, it was quickly controlled after immediate placement of vascular clips on what was thought to be a segmental artery. Because no further blood loss was encountered, the surgical course continued, and the scheduled T12 to L5 LLIF proceeded. The patient presented with delayed back pain symptoms several days later, with a computed tomography (CT) of the abdomen demonstrating a delayed renal infarction, indicating a left renal artery occlusion by the vascular clips.[22] The renal pole will often appear within the trajectory or dorsal to the approach in thoracolumbar junction treatment of a degenerative scoliosis curve. In adult idiopathic scoliosis, or adolescent idiopathic scoliosis in the adult, significant rotation can occur in tandem with the typical lumbar degenerative curve. Careful review of the preoperative anatomy can mean life and death because the prevertebral vessels may be in a different location adjacent to the vertebral body. Another case report of vascular injury resulted from lumbar two-segmental artery injury and coagulation, which presented with hemodynamic compromise 48 hours after the uneventful L2–3 LLIF. This pseudoaneurysm was successfully managed with endovascular coil and glue embolization.[23]

Posterior Paraspinal Lumbar Approach

The posterior lumbar paraspinal muscle-splitting approach is similar to the cervical paraspinal muscular approach in terms of surgical goals, which are to decrease postoperative axial pain, facilitate faster recovery, and to limit deformity due to surgical destabilization of the posterior spinal attachments. Watkins described a paraspinal muscular approach between the sacrospinalis muscles medially and the quadratus lumborum laterally.[24,25] All paraspinal muscular approaches are commonly mistaken for and often referred to as the Wiltse approach. The Wiltse approach is more medial and describes an intermuscular approach between the multifidus and longissimus muscles.[26] Due to the lack of clearly identifiable landmarks, this approach can be difficult. The use of an MIS retractor will obviate the direct visualization that is afforded by a large incision. Vialle et al. evaluated 50 cadavers in an attempt to clarify the approach.[25] They found the appropriate distance from midline to be a mean of 4.04 cm at which the surgeon would most easily encounter the natural cleavage plane between the multifidus and longissimus muscles.[25,27] Most techniques utilizing MIS tubular retractors in the posterior lumbar spine use fluoroscopy for guidance and therefore relegate the nuances of intraoperative anatomic identification of paraspinal muscles to an academic exercise. Instead, the safe use of tubular retractors with paraspinal approaches is through safe technique with K-wire and dilator placement under fluoroscopic guidance.

Prevention

Lateral Retroperitoneal Transpsoas Approach (LLIF)

Complication avoidance starts with patient selection. Although the indications for management with a lateral approach are expanding, there are numerous pathologies that are relatively contraindicated, or are only recommended after considerable experience with the LLIF is gained. For example, the use of the LLIF for anterior column release and placement of a hyperlordotic cage for the restoration of lumbar lordosis in flatback deformity may be a less invasive alternative than a PSO in an elderly patient with progressive decline in function; this is not a typical procedure for a surgeon with limited experience.[12]

Neurologic Injury

The dissection of the psoas muscle should not continue without an understanding of the relationship of the dilator position in the psoas muscle with respect to the femoral nerve. There are numerous reports regarding the location of the nerve within the psoas muscle. In one anatomic study, Uribe et al. divide the discs into four equal zones, numbered anterior to posterior, as a way to create a helpful understanding of the position of the lumbosacral plexus and femoral nerve in relation to anteroposterior position along the disc space.[28] For example, in their study, at L2–3, all of the nerves were in the posterior zone (IV), except with the genitofemoral nerve crossing fairly reliably in the midpoint of the L2–3 disc (between zones 2 and 3)(II). The genitofemoral nerve is a sensory nerve, and its location cannot be determined by stimulus-evoked electromyography (EMG). Injury could result in perineal numbness, or a neuroma can potentially result from transection. Thigh flexion weakness can occur, and most often, this weakness improves. One additional consideration is the use of neuromuscular blockade during intubation, which in a team with inconsistent anesthesia providers, this administration could occur without communication to the team. The rationale for neuromuscular blockade with posterior surgery is that the half-life is short enough to allow stimulus-evoked or continuous EMG, or motor-evoked potential use by the appropriate needed time point. However, with a lateral approach, the time to access and stimulate the psoas muscle occurs much earlier, most often before the neuromuscular blockade would wear off.

Vascular Injury

The most feared complication of lateral surgery is catastrophic venous injury or arterial injury. This cannot be overstressed, that successful implementation of MIS spinal surgery requires the proper selection of patients. Therefore always review the preoperative vascular anatomy on the axial MRI imaging, noting in particular the course of the iliac bifurcation and level. Always evaluate the position of the nerves within the psoas, which is posteriorly located, and any anterior vasculature. This gives you an estimation of your working corridor.

Anatomic radiographic studies have shown a consistent relationship with a high iliac bifurcation, resulting in a frequent lateral course of the iliac vein across the L4–5 disc space.[21] As mentioned above, a lumbosacral transitional vertebra can occur, and the patient can have six lumbar vertebrae, such that the iliac bifurcation occurs a level higher than in most patients. Vascular or neurologic injury is a possibility (Fig. 56.2). In a retrospective review of 351 patients that underwent LLIF at L4–5, 2.8% (n = 6) patients were noted to have a lumbarized sacrum, meaning that they had six lumbar vertebrae and a mobile L6–S1 disc space.[29] Sharp injury to retroperitoneal viscera and vascular structures is a life-threatening procedural complication, as illustrated in a case report where anterior migration of a retractor blade resulted in catastrophic common iliac vein injury and subsequent death.[30] Understanding the relevant vascular anatomy is key to preventing life-threatening complication. The vena cava has been shown to migrate laterally from L1 to L5 and in 70% of patients is at considerable risk for injury from a right-sided approach at the L4–L5 level.[19,20] Another iliac vein injury has been reported at the L4–5 level from a right-sided approach due to an early iliac vein bifurcation, and a relatively narrow working corridor on preoperative MRI.[31] Adult degenerative scoliosis represents another challenge in identifying safe working corridors and poses a risk for vascular injury. One example of this was reported by Blizzard et al., who reported an arterial injury during adult scoliosis correction.[22] During retractor expansion, episodic arterial bleeding was identified, requiring intraoperative vascular surgery assistance. The bleeding was promptly controlled with vascular clip application, allowing the T12 to L5 LLIF to proceed due to low blood loss. However, delayed renal infarction resulted, due to injury to the left renal artery.[22] In another patient, a delayed left L2 lumbar artery pseudoaneurysm was diagnosed after hemodynamic compromise, which occurred 48 hours after an uneventful L2–3 LLIF. This was successfully managed with endovascular coil and glue embolization.[23]

In most instances, brisk bleeding should be tamponaded immediately with pressure held for several minutes. Most injuries along this approach are venous and will be controlled when substantial pressure is held. Use of immediate cautery at the location of a small injury to the lumen of a large vein will convert this injury to a large tear, and a less controllable source of bleeding. In the event of uncontrolled bleeding, an immediate decision should be to call for blood, notify the anesthesiologist, call for the assistance of a general surgeon, and extend the incision to allow for a wider exposure and superior vessel control.

Subsidence

Subsidence is a serious complication of LLIF or any procedure that relies on indirect decompression of the pathology, which is often from foraminal stenosis, subarticular recess stenosis, or ligamentous hypertrophy and central canal stenosis. Many intraoperative decisions can impact the development of subsidence, which varies in the literature from 0.3% to 22%.[32–34] Multiple patient-specific risk factors for subsidence can include an elderly patient,[35] T score less than −2.5 on femoral neck bone densitometry,[36,37] recombinant human bone morphogenetic protein-2 use (rhBMP-2),[35] and increased surgical complexity.[11,38] As a percentage of troublesome levels, the L4–5 level is also at a relatively elevated risk for subsidence due to a high iliac crest, which can force the angle of entry from orthogonal to tangential, resulting in elevated forces directed into end plates. Moreover, as with any MIS procedure, poor fluoroscopy visualization commonly facilitated by patient body-habitus resulting in poor penetration of x-rays can affect the clarity of end plate margins and increase the change of a nonorthogonal trajectory. Overall, subsidence rates have been estimated to range from 0.3% to 22%, largely the work of retrospective radiographic case-control studies.[32–34] Several studies have implicated surgeon decision-making as a risk factor for subsidence, namely by overly aggressive graft height in a collapsed disc space. Tohmeh et al. found that increased cage height and decreased length and width correlate with increased subsidence at the 1-year mark.[39] Le et al. found in an analysis of subsidence risk factors that overdistraction of the end plates by improperly large grafts may be the most important of the three-dimensional parameters in terms of subsidence risk. In their study, they found the majority of subsidence cases to occur at 12 mm or greater, ultimately recommending a 10-mm cage maximum in either parallel or lordotic geometries.[32] Satake et al. noted similar findings, with the incidence in end plate injury ranging from 8.3% to 21.4% when increasing from 10 to 12 mm in craniocaudal graft height (+13.1%), respectively.[40]

This was followed by overly narrow cage widths as the second most common predictor of subsidence in the postoperative period.[32] However, the risk of neurovascular injury by exceeding the anteroposterior diameter of the working channel between the nerve and vascular structures outweighs the risk of subsidence. Graft length is also important, but the issue of undersized grafts and lack of appropriate contact with the denser cortical apophyseal ring is relatively less common than oversizing a graft. An undersized graft has been biomechanically shown to have a greater peak load to failure. One additional caveat to the appropriate graft length is that in rotational deformities and an oversized graft, exceeding the depth of the contralateral annular ring with any instrument could result in injury to the vena cava, aorta, or bowel. It is recommended to note the depth of each instrument with fluoroscopy and to have the surgeon use his or her nondominant hand to maintain this position along the instrument; the hand becomes a positive stop on the patient's body, preventing bottoming out. There are many systems for preventing this sort of complication because this complication can occur with any form of lumbar interbody access. One last topic is the use of rhBMP-2 in LLIF, which is quite commonplace. High dosages of rhBMP-2 (>2 mg) have not been shown to raise the fusion rates beyond lower doses, such as 1 to 2 mg.[32] RhBMP-2 is thought to accelerate the cortical uptake of graft and in turn to result in an earlier risk of developing subsidence. This earlier subsidence, when studied, did not carry out significantly. Subsidence is an area that warrants further study with an attention to standardized definitions of the term, or a focus on linear representations of subsidence measurements.[32]

Durotomy

A dural tear is one of the most common complications of spinal surgery, particularly in revision surgery, deformity, and MIS spinal surgery. In most cases, the dura can be repaired primarily and made watertight. Adjuncts include fibrin sealant, a dural patch, flat bed rest, and lumbar cerebrospinal fluid (CSF) diversion. It is rarely encountered where the wound needs to be extended to allow for a definitive closure.

Lateral extracavity, retropleural approaches have been popularized for the treatment of mid- to low-thoracic central and paracentral disc herniations, with and without calcifications. In many instances these approaches can remain extrapleural, and a plane of dissection along the excised rib provides a clear working channel to resect the calcified disc herniation. In the even of a frank CSF leak, seen in trauma or with a calcified, adherent disc herniation, the CSF leak may or may not be in the field of view. If the repair is not visualized, an alloderm patch can be sutured over the potential area followed by fibrin glue. This should be followed by intraoperative lumbar drain placement and CSF diversion, possibly with a chest tube, as well by monitoring fluid collection at the wound bed and in the pleural cavity. The concern is that a large CSF collection can develop within the thoracic cavity due to the large cavity and due to the negative pleural pressure. Flat bed rest and steady CSF drainage at 10 cc/h for a minimum of 2 days will help facilitate closure; in addition, there should be careful observation for the development of severe headaches. It is important to be aware of the development of hygromas or subdural hemorrhage, which is a potential risk from CSF fistula formation.

SURGICAL REWIND

My Worst Cases

Case 1

A 77-year-old male underwent a stand-alone MIS LLIF for rostral adjacent-segment degeneration at L3–4. The operation was uneventful, and the intraoperative fluoroscopic image showed proper position of the cage at the center (Fig. 56.1A). Increasing low back pain gradually developed postoperatively. Follow-up radiographic imaging demonstrated lateral cage

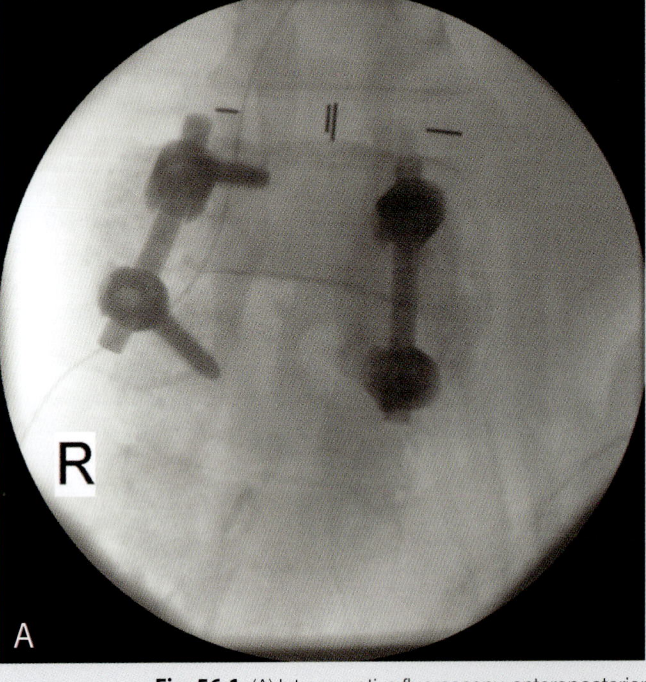

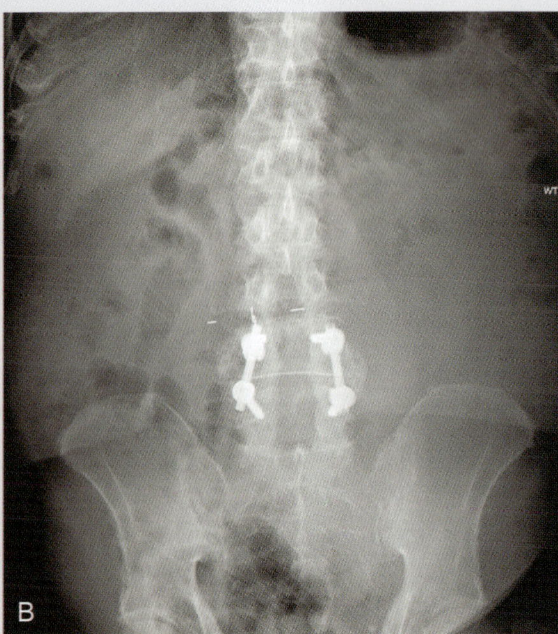

• **Fig. 56.1** (A) Intraoperative fluoroscopy, anteroposterior view demonstrating final poly ether ether ketone (PEEK) cage placement at the L3–4 disc space using the lateral lumbar transpsoas interbody approach. (B) Lateral radiograph, demonstrating interbody graft migration.

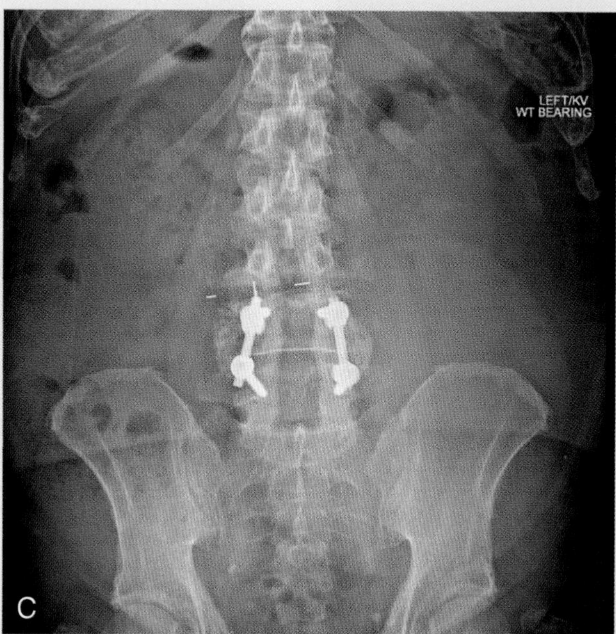

• **Fig. 56.1, cont'd** (C) Lateral radiograph, demonstrating stable interbody positioning.

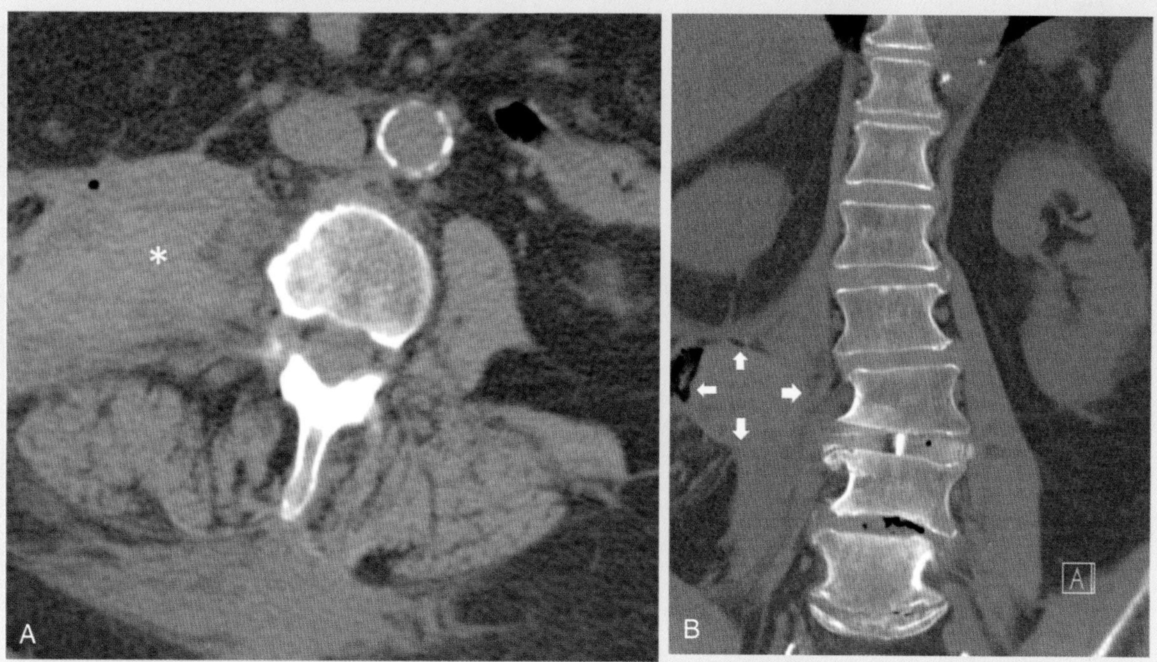

• **Fig. 56.2** (A) Computed tomography (CT) of the abdomen, axial view. A right-sided psoas hematoma is shown (asterisk). (B) CT of the abdomen, sagittal view. Demonstrating the craniocaudal extent of the right-sided psoas hematoma with presumed displacement of the lumbosacral plexus (not shown).

migration 2 months postoperatively (Fig. 56.1B). Strict bracing and activity limitation were instructed to the patient. Further follow-up images demonstrated stable status in cage migration at 4 and 6 months after surgery (Fig. 56.1C). The patient stated his back pain also improved during further clinic visit.

Case 2

A 70-year-old female underwent a stand-alone right-sided MIS LLIF for degenerative disc disease at L3–4. After surgery, on postoperative day 1, she started to develop progressive right thigh weakness over 3 days. A CT scan revealed that there was an accumulation of right psoas muscle hematoma on postoperative day 3. The patient underwent hematoma evacuation with subsequent drain placement under continuous aspiration. Further follow-up CT scan showed resolution of hematoma on postoperative day 7. The patient's thigh weakness improved with physical therapy over the following 3-month interim.

NEUROSURGICAL SELFIE MOMENT

The MIS spine surgery has a steep learning curve with technical challenges to the surgeon. The MIS surgery is not without complications. The complication rate may be higher than with open procedures during the learning curve period. The advantages of MIS surgery include reduced blood loss, superior cosmesis, decreased pain, less tissue dissection, and quicker recovery. These must be balanced against potentially serious complications of MIS surgery like vascular injury and nerve root avulsion. Careful preoperative selection of candidates and a thorough understanding of the surgical corridor are essential for a successful surgery.

References

1. Lehmen JA, Gerber EJ. MIS lateral spine surgery: a systematic literature review of complications, outcomes, and economics. *Eur Spine J.* 2015;24(suppl 3):287–313.
2. Wang MY, Lerner J, Lesko J, McGirt MJ. Acute hospital costs after minimally invasive versus open lumbar interbody fusion: data from a US national database with 6106 patients. *J Spinal Disord Tech.* 2012;25(6):324–328.
3. Scheer JK, Tang JA, Smith JS, et al. Cervical spine alignment, sagittal deformity, and clinical implications: a review. *J Neurosurg Spine.* 2013;19(2):141–159.
4. Yukawa Y, Kato F, Suda K, Yamagata M, Ueta T. Age-related changes in osseous anatomy, alignment, and range of motion of the cervical spine. Part I: radiographic data from over 1,200 asymptomatic subjects. *Eur Spine J.* 2012;21(8):1492–1498.
5. Passias PG, Oh C, Jalai CM, et al. Predictive model for cervical alignment and malalignment following surgical correction of adult spinal deformity. *Spine.* 2016;41(18):E1096–E1103.
6. Smith JS, Ramchandran S, Lafage V, et al. Prospective multi-center assessment of early complication rates associated with adult cervical deformity surgery in 78 patients. *Neurosurgery.* 2016;79(3): 378–388.
7. Shiraishi T, Kato M, Yato Y, et al. New techniques for exposure of posterior cervical spine through intermuscular planes and their surgical application. *Spine.* 2012;37(5):E286–E296.
8. Jagannathan J, Sherman JH, Szabo T, Shaffrey CI, Jane JA. The posterior cervical foraminotomy in the treatment of cervical disc/ osteophyte disease: a single-surgeon experience with a minimum of 5 years' clinical and radiographic follow-up. *J Neurosurg Spine.* 2009;10(4):347–356.
9. Ozgur BM, Aryan HE, Pimenta L, Taylor WR. Extreme Lateral Interbody Fusion (XLIF): a novel surgical technique for anterior lumbar interbody fusion. *Spine J.* 2006;6(4):435–443.
10. Rodgers WB, Gerber EJ, Patterson J. Intraoperative and early postoperative complications in extreme lateral interbody fusion: an analysis of 600 cases. *Spine.* 2011;36(1):26–32.
11. Isaacs RE, Hyde J, Goodrich JA, Rodgers WB, Phillips FM. A prospective, nonrandomized, multicenter evaluation of extreme lateral interbody fusion for the treatment of adult degenerative scoliosis: perioperative outcomes and complications. *Spine.* 2010;35(26 supp l):S322–S330.
12. Saigal R, Mundis GM Jr, Eastlack R, Uribe JS, Phillips FM, Akbarnia BA. Anterior column realignment (ACR) in adult sagittal deformity correction: technique and review of the literature. *Spine.* 2016;41(suppl 8):S66–S73.
13. Boah AO, Perin NI. Lateral access to paravertebral tumors. *J Neurosurg Spine.* 2016;24(5):824–828.
14. Serak J, Vanni S, Levi AD. The extreme lateral approach for treatment of thoracic and lumbar vertebral body metastases. *J Neurosurg Sci.* 2015;9. [Epub ahead of print].
15. Blizzard DJ, Hills CP, Isaacs RE, Brown CR. Extreme lateral interbody fusion with posterior instrumentation for spondylodiscitis. *J Clin Neurosci.* 2015;22(11):1758–1761.
16. Dakwar E, Le TV, Baaj AA, et al. Abdominal wall paresis as a complication of minimally invasive lateral transpsoas interbody fusion. *Neurosurg Focus.* 2011;31(4):E18.
17. Plata-Bello J, Roldan H, Brage L, Rahy A, Garcia-Marin V. Delayed abdominal pseudohernia in young patient after lateral lumbar interbody fusion procedure: case report. *World Neurosurg.* 2016;91:671.e13–671.e16.
18. Benglis DM, Vanni S, Levi AD. An anatomical study of the lumbosacral plexus as related to the minimally invasive transpsoas approach to the lumbar spine. *J Neurosurg Spine.* 2009;10(2):139–144.
19. Hu WK, He SS, Zhang SC, et al. An MRI study of psoas major and abdominal large vessels with respect to the X/DLIF approach. *Eur Spine J.* 2011;20(4):557–562.
20. Moro T, Kikuchi S, Konno S, Yaginuma H. An anatomic study of the lumbar plexus with respect to retroperitoneal endoscopic surgery. *Spine.* 2003;28(5):423–428, discussion 427–428.
21. Josiah DT, Boo S, Tarabishy A, Bhatia S. Anatomical differences in patients with lumbosacral transitional vertebrae and implications for minimally invasive spine surgery. *J Neurosurg Spine.* 2017;26(2):137–143.
22. Blizzard DJ, Gallizzi MA, Isaacs RE, Brown CR. Renal artery injury during lateral transpsoas interbody fusion: case report. *J Neurosurg Spine.* 2016;25(4):464–466.
23. Santillan A, Patsalides A, Gobin YP. Endovascular embolization of iatrogenic lumbar artery pseudoaneurysm following extreme lateral interbody fusion (XLIF). *Vasc Endovascular Surg.* 2010;44(7): 601–603.
24. Watkins MB. Posterolateral bonegrafting for fusion of the lumbar and lumbosacral spine. *J Bone Joint Surg Am.* 1959;41-A(3):388–396.
25. Vialle R, Wicart P, Drain O, Dubousset J, Court C. The Wiltse paraspinal approach to the lumbar spine revisited: an anatomic study. *Clin Orthop Relat Res.* 2006;445:175–180.
26. Wiltse LL. The paraspinal sacrospinalis-splitting approach to the lumbar spine. *Clin Orthop Relat Res.* 1973;91:48–57.
27. Vialle R, Court C, Khouri N, et al. Anatomical study of the paraspinal approach to the lumbar spine. *Eur Spine J.* 2005;14(4):366–371.
28. Uribe JS, Arredondo N, Dakwar E, Vale FL. Defining the safe working zones using the minimally invasive lateral retroperitoneal transpsoas approach: an anatomical study. *J Neurosurg Spine.* 2010;13(2): 260–266.
29. Smith WD, Youssef JA, Christian G, Serrano S, Hyde JA. Lumbarized sacrum as a relative contraindication for lateral transpsoas interbody fusion at L5-6. *J Spinal Disord Tech.* 2012;25(5):285–291.
30. Assina R, Majmundar NJ, Herschman Y, Heary RF. First report of major vascular injury due to lateral transpsoas approach leading to fatality. *J Neurosurg Spine.* 2014;21(5):794–798.
31. Buric J, Bombardieri D. Direct lesion and repair of a common iliac vein during XLIF approach. *Eur Spine J.* 2016;25(suppl 1):89–93.
32. Le TV, Baaj AA, Dakwar E, et al. Subsidence of polyetheretherketone intervertebral cages in minimally invasive lateral retroperitoneal transpsoas lumbar interbody fusion. *Spine.* 2012;37(14):1268–1273.
33. Malham GM, Ellis NJ, Parker RM, et al. Maintenance of segmental lordosis and disc height in standalone and instrumented Extreme Lateral Interbody Fusion (XLIF). *Clin Spine Surg.* 2017;30(2): E90–E98.
34. Marchi L, Abdala N, Oliveira L, Amaral R, Coutinho E, Pimenta L. Radiographic and clinical evaluation of cage subsidence after stand-alone lateral interbody fusion. *J Neurosurg Spine.* 2013;19(1): 110–118.
35. Vaidya R, Sethi A, Bartol S, Jacobson M, Coe C, Craig JG. Complications in the use of rhBMP-2 in PEEK cages for interbody spinal fusions. *J Spinal Disord Tech.* 2008;21(8):557–562.
36. Belkoff SM, Maroney M, Fenton DC, Mathis JM. An in vitro biomechanical evaluation of bone cements used in percutaneous vertebroplasty. *Bone.* 1999;25(2 suppl):23S–26S.

37. Hou Y, Luo Z. A study on the structural properties of the lumbar endplate: histological structure, the effect of bone density, and spinal level. *Spine*. 2009;34(12):E427–E433.
38. Park SH, Park WM, Park CW, Kang KS, Lee YK, Lim SR. Minimally invasive anterior lumbar interbody fusion followed by percutaneous translaminar facet screw fixation in elderly patients. *J Neurosurg Spine*. 2009;10(6):610–616.
39. Tohmeh AG, Khorsand D, Watson B, Zielinski X. Radiographical and clinical evaluation of extreme lateral interbody fusion: effects of cage size and instrumentation type with a minimum of 1-year follow-up. *Spine*. 2014;39(26):E1582–E1591.
40. Satake K, Kanemura T, Yamaguchi H, Segi N, Ouchida J. Predisposing factors for intraoperative endplate injury of extreme lateral interbody fusion. *Asian Spine J*. 2016;10(5):907–914.

57 Complications of Surgery for Intrinsic Spinal Cord Tumors

VINAYAK NARAYAN, AQUEEL PABANEY, ANIL NANDA

HIGHLIGHTS

- Intramedullary spinal cord tumors are rare and challenging entities, comprising 16% to 58% of all primary spinal cord and 2% to 8.5% of all primary central nervous system tumors in the adult and pediatric populations.
- Common complications encountered with spinal cord tumor surgery include intraoperative damage to spinal cord tracts leading to motor and sensory deficits, and cerebrospinal fluid leak.
- When approaching the lower thoracic spinal cord levels, the surgeon should investigate the location of the artery of Adamkiewicz.
- Complications can be avoided by use of intraoperative monitoring, neuronavigation, and careful examination of patient imaging.

Introduction

Intramedullary spinal cord (IMSC) tumors are rare and challenging entities, comprising 16% to 58% of all primary spinal cord and 2% to 8.5% of all primary central nervous system tumors in the adult and pediatric population.[1,2] The ependymoma, astrocytoma, and hemangioblastoma correspond to more than 90% of all IMSC tumors.[3] Other IMSC tumors such as glioma, cavernoma, hamartoma, metastases, inclusion tumor, cyst, neurocytoma, melanocytoma, and lipoma are rarely encountered. Several genetic factors have been associated with IMSC tumors. Neurofibromatosis type 1 (NF1), neurofibromatosis type 2 (NF2), and von Hippel-Lindau disease (VHL) are the most common genetic diseases that are prone to cause the development of astrocytoma, ependymoma, and hemangioblastoma, respectively. Approximately 20% of patients affected by NF1 and NF2 will develop an IMSC tumor. 15% to 25% of hemangioblastomas are associated with VHL syndrome, an autosomal dominant condition with incomplete penetrance and incomplete expression.[4]

IMSC tumors are particularly related to syringomyelia (25%–58%), especially those tumors located in the lower cervical and upper thoracic spine.[5] The occurrence of a syrinx is seen as a sign of a favorable outcome after resection because it denotes a noninfiltrative tumor and a rapid postoperative recovery after the resolution of the fluid-filled cavity. Half of the syringes occur above the tumor, whereas 40% are above and below, and only 10% are primarily below the tumor.

Anatomic Insights

The spinal cord (SC) has a cylindrical shape that is slightly flattened in the anteroposterior axis. It follows the curvature of the vertebral column and shows two characteristic enlargements, namely the cervical and lumbar ones, where motor neurons related to the upper and lower limbs concentrate. The conus medullaris is aligned to the first lumbar vertebra and gives rise to more than 50 rootlets over a length of <3 cm. The SC is covered by the flexible vertebral column and the meninges. At the spinal level, the dura is arranged in three layers, contrary to the two-layer intracranial dura. The internal layer is in continuity with the inner dural layer of the head, the middle layer is connected to the external dural layer of the head, and the external layer continues as the periosteum of the skull. Under and loosely attached to the dura is the arachnoid layer, which contains the subarachnoid space filled with cerebrospinal fluid (CSF). It also extends to the dural sac. The arachnoid covers the spinal nerves toward the root sleeves, where it fuses with the dura. Within the subarachnoid space, several septations have been described, especially in the posterior space, where there is a longitudinal dorsal or dorsolateral septum from the arachnoid to the spinal pial surface dividing the subarachnoid space into left and right halves. The pia mater is the innermost meningeal layer and encases the spinal cord. It provides a barrier between the subarachnoid space and the perivascular spaces. The pia is firmly attached to the dura by 21 pairs of extensions, called the denticulate ligaments. They run alongside the spinal cord to the level of the conus medullaris, where they end between the last thoracic and the first lumbar nerves. In the center of the SC lies the central canal. It consists of the remnants of the neural tube central cavity lined by ependymal cells and filled with CSF. The anterior and posterior commissures enclose the central canal. The gray matter horns are somatotopically organized and contain different classes of functional neurons. As a result, motor neurons that innervate axial muscles are medially located in the ventral horn, whereas motor neurons that control distal limb movements are located more laterally. Finally, motor neurons responsible for controlling proximal limb muscles lie in between. The posterior horn has a layered neuronal organization that is based on synaptic inputs and outputs. The superficial layers receive exteroceptive sensory information about pain, temperature, and light touch, and generate the contralateral spinothalamic tracts.

The deep layers are involved with proprioceptive information and contribute to the ipsilateral spinocerebellar tracts. The posterior cervical horn also includes the spinal nucleus of the trigeminal nerve. The white matter is organized in tracts associated with major motor or sensory functions. The posterior column enlarges, as the SC ascends, to include more axons carrying fine-touch, vibration, and proprioceptive information from the lower limbs medially (fasciculus gracilis) and the upper limbs laterally (fasciculus cuneatus). The lateral column contains the two most prominent ascending tracts, namely the lateral spinothalamic and the spinocerebellar ones, and one descending tract, the lateral corticospinal tract. Finally, the anterior spinothalamic and corticospinal tracts are found in the anterior column. The spinal vascular anatomy starts in the segmental extraspinal arteries, which correspond to the pathways of blood from the aorta and provide the arterial supply to not only the cord, but also to the nerve roots, dura, and paraspinal musculature. Each segmental artery has a ventral and a dorsal branch. The dorsal division gives off a spinal branch, which splits into the retrocorporeal (anterior spinal canal), prelaminar (posterior spinal canal), and radicular arteries. The radicular artery is termed the radiculomeningeal artery when it feeds the nerve roots and dura at every level. On the other hand, if these arteries take part in the cord vascular network, they are better termed radiculomedullary arteries if they supply the anterior spinal artery (ASA), and radiculopial or posterior radiculomedullary arteries if they supply the posterior spinal arteries (PSAs) and surface vasocorona of the SC. The artery of Adamkiewicz is also known as the great radicular artery or even as arteria radiculomedullaris magna and has a left-sided predominance. As the artery pierces the dura, a slight caudal turn may occasionally be seen. The artery then joins the ventral root on its way to the ventral surface of the SC, where the artery anastomoses with the ASA at or just before its typical and characteristic hairpin turn. The PSAs receive approximately 10 to 28 feeders, which can also demonstrate a hairpin configuration in the paramedian locations.

RED FLAGS

- Variability in vascular supply of spinal cord.
- Imaging including magnetic resonance imaging (MRI) and angiogram should be carefully reviewed to differentiate between neoplastic and vascular pathologies.
- Previous surgery or radiation therapy.

Prevention

Several maneuvers can be undertaken to avoid major complications during intrinsic spinal cord tumor surgery. A careful examination of imaging studies should be undertaken. Attention should be paid to the location of the tumor (intramedullary vs extramedullary), vascular congestion, presence of syrinx, and concurrent tumors. A detailed neurologic examination should be carried out to document preoperative deficits. In selected cases, it might be prudent to obtain a spinal angiogram to identify the artery of Adamkiewicz. Intraoperatively, neuromonitoring must be employed to provide real-time feedback during tumor resection.[6] The use of tools such as a microscope, microinstruments, and devices like ultrasonic aspirators is indispensable for safe resection of these tumors.

Vascular Injury

Every attempt should be made to preserve all arteries and veins to prevent the development of arterial or venous infarctions. If a vascular sacrifice is inevitable, a temporary occlusion should be performed and any changes in neuromonitoring should be noted. If no worsening of neuromonitoring occurs, then that vessel can be sacrificed.

Parenchymal Injury

Spinal cord tissue should be very delicately handled using microinstruments and by employing microsurgical techniques. Direct handling of the spinal cord should be avoided, and the surgeon should make use of dentate ligaments, arachnoid, and pia mater to mobilize the spinal cord. Bipolar coagulation should be sparingly used to avoid thermal injury to the spinal cord. A combination of sharp and blunt dissection should be carried out, and generous use of hemostatic agents such as Gelfoam, Floseal, or Oxycel should be used to control minor bleeders. In addition, when making a myelotomy, the surgeon should ensure midline position to cause minimal damage to the posterior columns.[7] Arachnoid knife or a sharp blade should be used for myelotomy, and the cavity should be enlarged using spreading motions of the bipolar and cotton balls; use of fixed retractors is highly discouraged.

CSF Leak

Although not a direct consequence of spinal cord surgery, CSF leak can ruin a good day's work. It is imperative that the surgeon pay utmost attention to a meticulous, watertight closure at the end of the case. Dural stitches should be placed not more than 1 mm apart and tension exerted when running the suture. Dural sealants can be used to supplement the closure as well.

In addition to these, several other complications such as operative site hematoma, arachnoiditis, sepsis, meningocele, pulmonary embolism, and cervical kyphosis may also be encountered in IMSC tumor surgery.

SURGICAL REWIND

My Worst Case

A 31-year-old female patient presented with difficulty in walking and numbness in both feet. Her weakness worsened progressively. MRI of dorsal spine showed a D7 to D9 intramedullary lesion that was enhancing on contrast injection. (Fig. 57.1A–C) A detailed discussion was held with the patient and her family regarding the prognosis and possible complications like neurologic deterioration. A detailed informed consent in this regard was taken. She underwent D7 to D9 laminectomy. The spinal cord appeared widened and full at the level of lesion. The tumor was decompressed. Postoperatively her neurologic status further worsened and became paraplegic with sphincter involvement. Postoperative MRI revealed complete excision of tumor (Fig. 57.1D and E), and the pathology showed cellular ependymoma. She was sent for rehabilitation and gradually regained power in her lower limbs. She is now able to ambulate with the aid of a walker. Her recent MRI showed no tumor recurrence (Fig. 57.1F and G). Intramedullary tumors at critical locations like the cervical and thoracic spinal cord are well known to cause neurologic deterioration, and detailed discussion with the patient and the family before the surgery is essential in this regard.

Continued

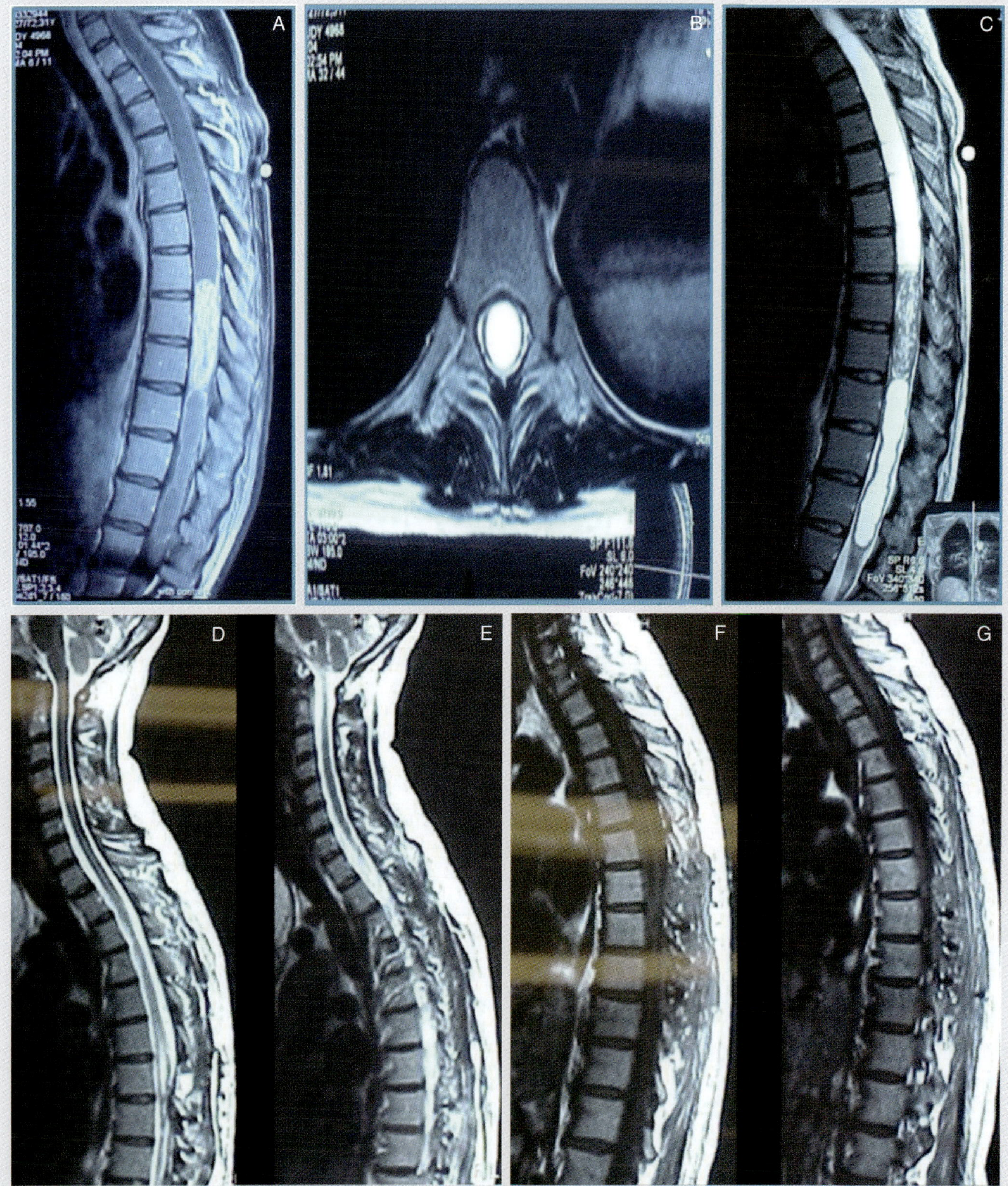

• **Fig. 57.1** (A–C) Preoperative magnetic resonance imaging (MRI) showing the tumor; (D and E) postoperative MRI showing complete excision of tumor; (F and G) follow-up MRI showing no tumor recurrence.

NEUROSURGICAL SELFIE MOMENT

Complications in spinal cord tumor surgery are not uncommon. A careful balance between tumor decompression and spinal cord protection with neuromonitoring is required. Ischemic injury to the compressed cord should be kept in mind during the tumor dissection and manipulation. A detailed informed consent is important in dealing with high-risk cases.

References

1. Malis LI. Intramedullary spinal cord tumors. *Clin Neurosurg.* 1978;25:512–539.
2. Stein BM, McCormick PC. Intramedullary neoplasms and vascular malformations. *Clin Neurosurg.* 1992;39:361–387.
3. Brotchi J. Intrinsic spinal cord tumor resection. *Neurosurgery.* 2002; 50(5):1059–1063.
4. Neumann HPH, Eggert HR, Weigel K, Friedburg H, Wiestler OD, Schollmeyer P. Hemangioblastomas of the central nervous system. *J Neurosurg.* 1989;70(1):24–30.
5. Samii M, Klekamp J. Surgical results of 100 intramedullary tumors in relation to accompanying syringomyelia. *Neurosurgery.* 1994;35(5): 865–873.
6. Ng Z, Ng S, Nga V, et al. Intradural spinal tumors—review of postoperative outcomes comparing intramedullary and extramedullary tumors from a single institution's experience. *World Neurosurg.* 2018;109: 229–232.
7. Brotchi J, Fischer G. Spinal cord ependymomas. *Neurosurg Focus.* 1998;4(5):e2.

58

Complications of Surgery for Vertebral Body Tumors

MICHAEL A. GALGANO, HESHAM SOLIMAN, JARED FRIDLEY, ZIYA L. GOKASLAN

Introduction

Vertebral column neoplasms can be categorized as primary or malignant in origin, based on whether they arise directly from spinal osseous structures or extraspinal locations, respectively. The management of such tumors varies greatly from one patient to the next. Many primary spinal tumors are relatively resistant to chemotherapy and radiation, thus often necessitating extensive multidisciplinary operations to achieve maximal cytoreduction in such a way that negative margins are achieved. Unlike the treatment of primary tumors, the treatment of metastatic spine tumors remains palliative in nature. With new adjuvant therapies for these tumors, whether primary or metastatic, there is a myriad of options available to devise a tailored treatment plan on a case-by-case basis. In this chapter, we will be discussing potential complications that can be encountered during resection of vertebral column neoplasms.

The management goal with primary vertebral column neoplasms is to provide long-term disease-free intervals and ultimately to eradicate the neoplastic process. En bloc tumor resection for most primary spinal tumors gives patients the best chance at achieving this goal. Primary tumors can be subdivided into benign, locally malignant, and malignant. Benign primary vertebral tumors include aneurysmal bone cysts, chondromas and enchondromas, hemangiomas, osteoid osteomas, and osteoblastomas. The most common locally malignant and malignant primary vertebral tumors are chordomas and sarcomas, respectively.[1] Giant cell tumors, chordoma, and chondrosarcoma have shown better local control rates with en bloc resection versus intralesional resection: 92.3%,78%, 82% versus 72.2%, 22%, 0%.[2] This advantage may be negated in patients who have had a prior biopsy with contamination of the biopsy tract followed by tumor resection.[2,3]

Unlike primary spinal tumors, surgical treatment of metastatic vertebral column tumors is palliative with the goals primarily being preservation or improvement of neurologic function, and restoration or maintenance of spinal stability.[4] The neurologic, oncologic, mechanical, and systemic (NOMS) criteria are a widely accepted working algorithm for decision-making in regard to metastatic spinal tumors.[5] This framework guides the spinal surgeon through a process evaluating the patient's neurologic condition, oncologic status, mechanical stability, and overall systemic disease burden. Radiation, whether stereotactic body radiotherapy (SBRT) or conventional external beam radiation therapy (EBRT), is the mainstay of treatment after surgery and, along with appropriate chemotherapy, may improve local disease control. One of the potential complications of SBRT is the increased rate of vertebral body fractures, which needs to be taken into account when planning surgical intervention.[6]

Consideration of the appropriate management plan for the patient harboring a vertebral column tumor depends on several factors, such as the lesion location and goals of surgery as well as the patient's general condition, lung capacity, prior surgery, or radiation. Spinal instrumentation and arthrodesis are generally performed for stabilization purposes and deformity correction. The longer the expected survival of the patient, the more important achieving an osseous fusion becomes. Other interventions such as vertebroplasty/kyphoplasty (VP/KP), radiofrequency ablation (RFA), and laser interstitial thermal ablation (LITT) are becoming more widely accepted adjuncts to the overall management of patients harboring spinal neoplasms. These adjuvant procedures may be incorporated into the surgical plan or performed as outpatient procedures before or after surgery by an interventionalist. Preoperative embolization may also be appropriate for hypervascular tumors before surgery.

Complications during the resection of vertebral column neoplasms can be categorized into approach-related morbidities, challenges achieving stabilization and fusion, wound healing problems, length-of-surgery related problems, and intraoperative hemorrhage. Understanding these types of complications will hopefully help minimize patient morbidity by helping the surgical practitioner prevent the problem from happening and dealing with it effectively if it does occur.

Approach-Related Morbidity

Spinal tumor resection can be separated into three separate parts: (1) maximum safe tumor resection, (2) neural element decompression, and (3) spinal stabilization. These different facets of surgery are influenced by tumor location and size as well as by involvement of vertebral bone, neural elements, and extraspinal tissue. Although it may be possible to accomplish all three surgical goals from one approach, in many cases multiple approaches may be needed to safely resect tumor and reconstruct the spine. It is of utmost importance that the spinal surgeon has a solid understanding not just of the involved segmental spinal anatomy, but also of the surrounding visceral and soft tissue structures that can be encountered en route.

Resection of tumors in the ventral cervical spine will almost always be through a standard anterior neck dissection. Anticipated complications of dissection include injury to the pharynx, esophagus, trachea, larynx, and nearby neurovascular structures of the neck. It is reasonable to obtain a preoperative assessment of the vocal cords by an ENT surgeon in revision surgeries for this approach. Having this knowledge may influence the side of the approach taken for the subsequent surgery. It may be difficult at times to discern typically reliable anatomic landmarks such as the uncinate process with extensive tumor infiltration. The surgeon's sense for the midline may thus be compromised. One may consider obtaining an AP x-ray with a bent spinal needle placed inside the disc space to have a better understanding of the midline. The cervical spine is a unique anatomic segment in that the vertebral arteries course within the osseous structures (transverse foramina) from C6 to the atlas. Because of this intimate relationship between vascular and osseous structures, the vertebral arteries are at risk of injury while attempting to resect certain cervical spine tumors. This becomes relevant in the resection of tumors encasing the vertebral arteries. Resection of primary tumors encasing one vertebral artery often requires preoperative embolization in an effort to achieve an en bloc excision. Preoperative balloon occlusion testing is necessitated before permanently embolizing the vertebral artery. Unintended vertebral artery injury during resection of metastatic tumors adjacent to the vertebral artery can have disastrous consequences from hemorrhage and potentially posterior fossa infarcts. In the event of a vertebral artery injury, it is the senior author's recommendation to pack it with hemostatic material and complete the procedure, followed by angiography, rather than aborting the procedure.

When a primary cervical spine tumor encompasses a nearby vertebral artery, sacrifice of that vessel should be considered in an effort to achieve negative margins during an en bloc resection (Fig. 58.1). A preoperative diagnostic angiogram of both carotid arteries and vertebral arteries is essential to ascertain the collateral blood flow to the posterior circulation. A balloon occlusion test of the vertebral artery of interest must be performed to ensure that the patient has adequate posterior fossa perfusion from the contralateral vertebral artery or from the anterior circulation via the posterior communicating arteries. It is preferred to perform endovascular embolization before open surgical ligation of a vertebral artery.[7] This allows occlusion of the vertebral artery in a controlled setting. The alternative would require dissecting the vertebral artery out of the tumor, which harbors significant risks. Unilateral vertebral artery ligation has been shown to be relatively safe in a small case series,[8] although distal embolization of occlusion material may occur, leading to posterior fossa infarcts. Instrumenting the cervical spine also poses a significant risk to the vertebral arteries, particularly at C1 and C2, due to the complex course of the vertebral artery and the unique bony anatomy of the craniocervical junction. Performing tumor resection in separate stages may be a useful strategy if intraoperative ligation of the vertebral artery is performed to ascertain the patient's neurologic function before placement of instrumentation that could injure the remaining patent vertebral artery.

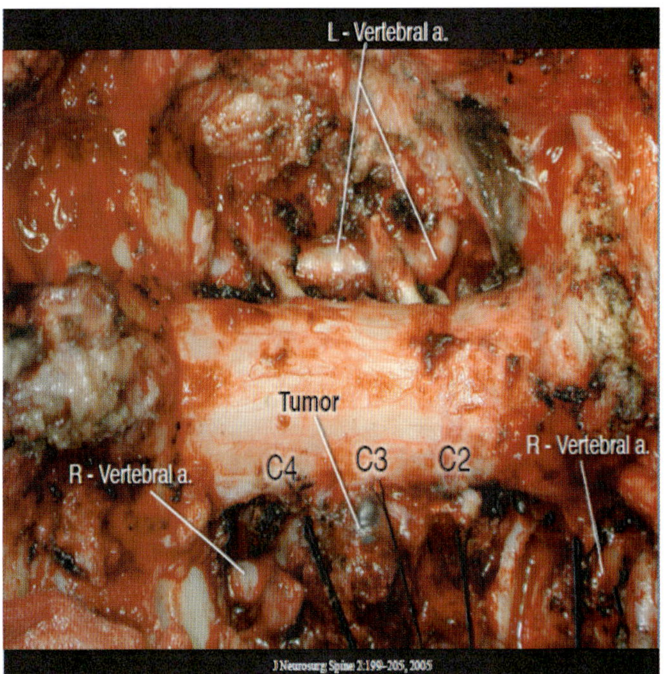

• **Fig. 58.1** Right-sided cervical nerve root and vertebral artery ligation. (Permission of use granted by Rhines LD, Fourney DR, Siadati A, Suk I, Gokaslan ZL. En bloc resection of multilevel cervical chordoma with C-2 involvement. Case report and description of operative technique. *J Neurosurg Spine*. 2005;2(2):199–205.)

In an effort to achieve an en bloc excision of a primary cervical spinal tumor, nerve roots may also need to be sacrificed. Having a candid conversation with the patient before this undertaking is extremely important in an effort to manage postoperative expectations of neurologic function. Ligation of the C2 and C3 nerve roots carries little morbidity, aside from the potential for occipital neuralgia, due to lack of motor innervation, whereas C3–5 nerve root ligation can cause unilateral diaphragm paralysis. Lower cervical nerve root sacrifice has a more clinically relevant effect on the patient's motor and sensory function. C5 and C6 nerve root sacrifice can cause deltoid and biceps weakness, respectively. C7 nerve root ligation can cause triceps weakness, although typically without significant clinical impact, and C8 and T1 nerve root ligation can cause significant functional impairment with fine motor tasks of the hand. A neurovascular-sparing en bloc resection has been described for specific cervical primary tumors, which spares the nerve roots and vertebral arteries with utilization of multiple osteotomies, paying special attention to removal of the lateral transverse foramen.[9]

Complex retropharyngeal approaches may be utilized on rare occasions to fully access a primary tumor of the upper cervical spine (Fig. 58.2). This oftentimes necessitates preoperative tracheostomy and gastrostomy tube placement. Cerebrospinal fluid (CSF) leaks during such approaches may also be very challenging to manage. High cervical neoplasms are associated with significant surgical morbidities.

Thoracic vertebral column tumors may involve adjacent vasculature and mediastinal structures. Extensive vascular reconstruction may be required after an en bloc spondylectomy if the aorta is intimately involved, with a primary thoracic spine tumor necessitating excision of part of the aorta in an effort to obtain negative margins.[10] Such lesions often require a combined anterior-posterior approach, necessitating the utilization of operative corridors through the thoracic cavity. Nerve root ligation is often necessary to gain access to the ventral compartment of the spine from a posterior approach. This may be the case if there is significant ventral epidural disease and a transpedicular, costotransversectomy, or extracavitary approach is being undertaken to achieve access. Aside from T1 innervation of hand intrinsics, thoracic nerve root ligation is well tolerated.[11] When performing complex thoracolumbar approaches, the artery of Adamkiewicz must be avoided. This artery usually

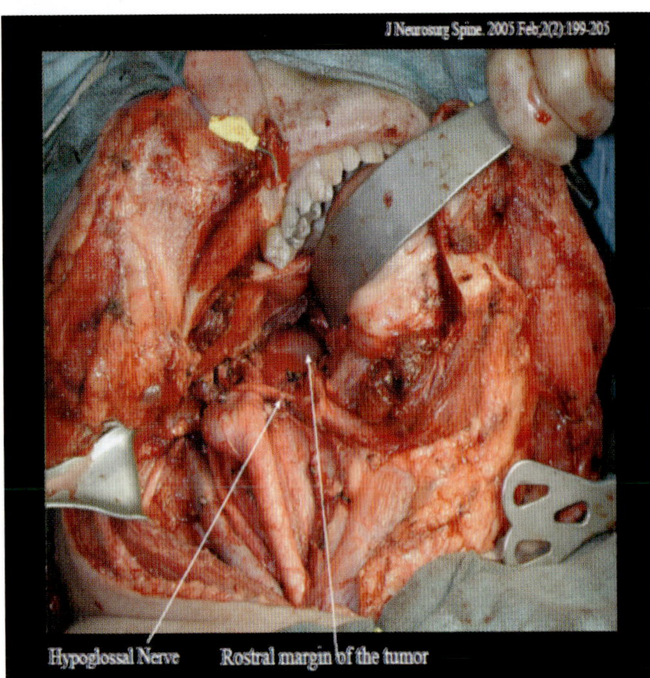

• **Fig. 58.2** Complex retropharyngeal approach for resection of a cervical chordoma. (Permission of use granted by Rhines LD, Fourney DR, Siadati A, Suk I, Gokaslan ZL. En bloc resection of multilevel cervical chordoma with C-2 involvement. Case report and description of operative technique. *J Neurosurg Spine*. 2005;2(2):199–205.)

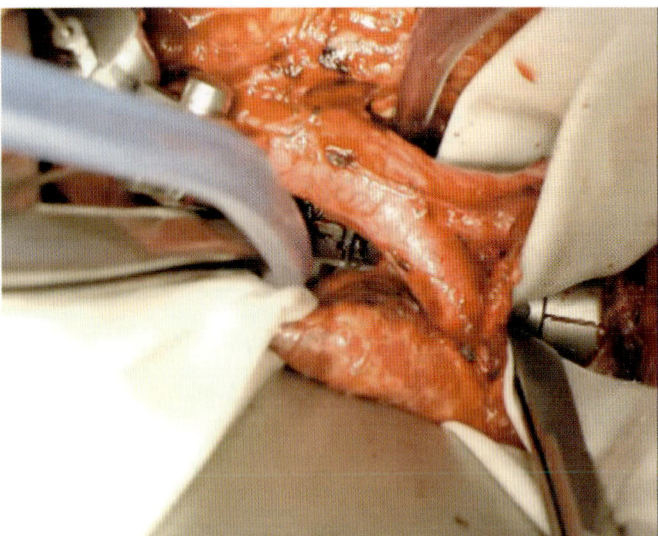

• **Fig. 58.3** Retraction of the inferior vena cava and visualization of the aortic bifurcation en route to the anterior lumbar spine. (Permission of use granted by Clarke MJ, Hsu W, Suk I, et al. Three-level en bloc spondylectomy for chordoma. *Neurosurgery*. 2011;68(2 Suppl Operative):325–33.)

arises between T9 and T12. It is a major blood source to the spinal cord. Identification of the artery of Adamkiewicz on preoperative angiography is helpful when contemplating ligation of multiple segmental vessels. Injury can lead to spinal cord hypoperfusion and ischemia, causing significant neurologic dysfunction. In an anterior vertebrectomy through a transthoracic or lateral extracavitary approach, there is a risk of injury to the thoracic duct, which can lead to chylothorax in addition to the anticipated pneumothorax/hemothorax.[12] Chylothorax is a challenging condition to treat because it often requires significant dietary modification and potentially decompression of the pleural space with tube thoracostomy or repeated thoracentesis. The posterior thoracic spine approach was found to have a higher incidence of wound infection compared with anterior approaches (26.7% vs 4.5%), in addition to a higher rate of deep vein thrombosis (DVT; 15.6% vs 0%).[13] In patients where the pleura is violated for tumor access, the duration of chest tube use was greater in the combined anterior/posterior approach group compared with the anterior-only group.[13] The overall rate of complications was higher in patients who underwent a combined simultaneous anterior and posterior approach than in patients who were treated using a single posterior approach (53.24% vs 32.1%).[2]

Lumbar spine tumors with significant ventral disease can be particularly challenging to surgically resect from a posterior-only approach due to the significant neurologic morbidity that can occur with lumbar nerve root injury. In some patients with primarily upper lumbar spine tumors, L1 and L2 nerve root ligation can be well tolerated, so a posterior-only approach can be considered. A combined anterior-posterior approach must be undertaken for primary tumors involving L3 and below.[14] Ligating nerve roots anywhere from L3 to L5 can cause significant motor and sensory impairment. An anterior approach to the lumbar spine would potentially necessitate mobilization of the inferior vena cava (IVC), aorta, or their branches, thus placing these vessels at risk of injury during surgery.

The iliac vessels and rectum are in close proximity when operating on sacral tumors (Fig. 58.3). During a sacrectomy for a primary bone tumor, sacrifice of the sacral nerve roots may be warranted to obtain an en bloc resection. Vascular reconstruction may also be needed if the iliac vessels are intimately involved with the tumor. Inevitably, bowel, bladder, and sexual function are significantly altered with sacrectomies, depending on how rostral the sacral amputation is. The higher the sacral amputation, the more likely it is that bowel/bladder will be adversely affected. It has also been shown that preoperative functional status in the context of bowel/bladder function is predictive of long-term function.[15] Historically, surgery for high sacral primary neoplasms was performed via an anterior/posterior approach. The anterior approach gives the surgeon direct access and visualization of the rectum and vasculature ventral to the sacrum. This technique does carry the inherent risks of an open laparotomy, including bowel injury. In addition, there is less control of the thecal sac and its neural elements distal to S1 utilizing an anterior-only approach, and hence it is often combined with a posterior approach.[16] Posterior-only approaches to sacral neoplasms have been described, which can avoid some of the described approach-related morbidities.[17] The posterior approach gives the surgeon direct access to the sacral nerve roots should it be necessary to ligate them distal to S1. A posterior-only approach may be feasible when there is no rectal invasion by the tumor, the tumor is above L5/S1, and there is no iliac vessel involvement.[16]

Approaches to any vertebral column tumor carry an inherent risk of injury to the spinal cord or nerve roots. Intraoperative neuromonitoring can alert the surgeon to potential damage, often before permanent injury has occurred. Routine use of somatosensory evoked potentials, motor evoked potentials, and electromyography is a valuable asset to avoid permanent neurologic injury. Damage to the dura and resultant CSF leaks are also concerns. Avoidance is crucial, but primary repair is similarly important if a dural tear is encountered during surgery. If the dural tear is not easily repairable due to its inherent morphology or ventral location, a strong

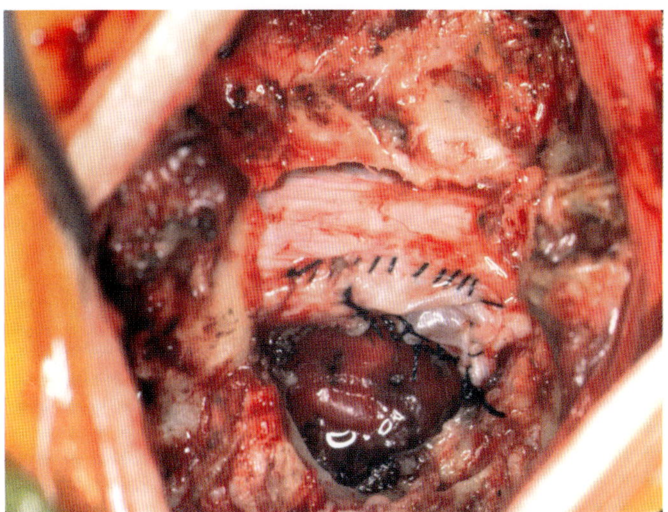

• **Fig. 58.4** Ventral-lateral dural repair utilizing a dural substitute.

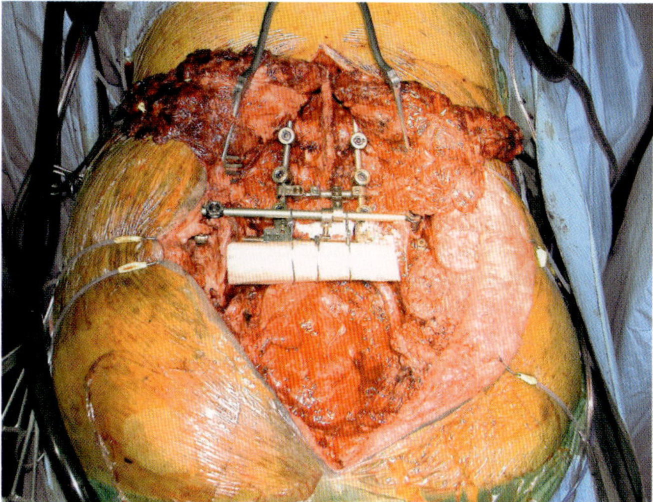

• **Fig. 58.5** Lumbopelvic reconstruction after sacrectomy for a chordoma. (Permission of use granted by Rhines LD, Fourney DR, Siadati A, Suk I, Gokaslan ZL. En bloc resection of multilevel cervical chordoma with C-2 involvement. Case report and description of operative technique. *J Neurosurg Spine*. 2005;2(2):199–205.)

myofascial closure is strongly recommended. Additional musculocutaneous flaps can augment closure and prevent subarachnoid-cutaneous fistulas postoperatively. A transpedicular approach to the ventral thecal sac has been described, whereby a Gore-Tex sling is utilized and sutured around the thecal sac as a means of closing a challenging ventral dural tear (Fig. 58.4). This technique was first utilized for ventral thoracic spinal cord herniation.[18]

Challenges Maintaining Stabilization and Achieving Fusion

The main goal of en bloc resection of primary vertebral column tumors is long-term disease-free survival. Unlike most patients with metastatic spine disease, patients with primary tumors may live for many years. This necessitates making an osseous fusion a high priority in these patients to reduce the risk of pseudarthrosis and hardware failure. En bloc tumor resections are biomechanically destabilizing surgeries because the integrity of the anterior, middle, and posterior column is often disrupted, necessitating circumferential multisegment instrumentation for stabilization. Pseudarthrosis and delayed instrumentation failure are potential challenges with long, complex constructs after tumor resection. Spinal instrumentation has a high risk of failure in these patients if osseous fusion does not occur. Screw-rod techniques are utilized for posterior and middle column support, whereas titanium or polyetheretherketone (PEEK) cages packed with allograft are often placed for anterior column support.[19] Novel techniques to create customized spinal implants that achieve optimal biomechanical stability are currently being investigated. The implantation of a 3D-printed, patient-specific artificial vertebral body has been described in a patient who underwent a high cervical spondylectomy for Ewing's sarcoma.[20] Resection of cranio-cervical tumors requiring complex occipital-cervical instrumentation may predispose to pseudarthrosis, and postoperative halo-vest immobilization can be used to maximize osseous fusion.

Lumbopelvic primary tumors present an especially unique and challenging situation when the lumbar pedicles are removed to maintain negative margins, making lumbar fixation difficult. However, bicortical transvertebral body screws can act as a surrogate for the missing pedicles. This novel instrumentation technique is known as creating "false pedicles." In such extensive lumbopelvic reconstructive surgeries, it is important to rebuild the pelvis in an effort to support the standing axial load (Fig. 58.5).[21] In addition to the biomechanical strains placed on the spine after such an extensive destabilizing surgery, postoperative radiation in this patient population predisposes them to nonunion. Lumbopelvic reconstructions generally include a complex screw-rod construct, and a vascularized fibular graft can be the primary strut between the lumbar spine and pelvis. Vascularized osseous grafting is often done by plastic surgeons. Cadaveric allograft struts can also be utilized for this as well. Dead space between the graft and host bone makes obtaining a solid fusion more difficult, and synthetic grafts, which are frequently utilized, can cause immunologic rejection. Resected extracorporeal-irradiated tumor-bearing sacral bone has also been used as an alternative for bone graft after sacrectomy.[22] Long-term bone fusion is an absolute priority after wide en bloc excision of primary vertebral column neoplasms, due to the potential for long-term survival.

Wound Complications

Problems with wound healing are unfortunately a common postoperative hurdle that patients harboring spinal column tumors must deal with. Individuals afflicted with metastatic disease to the spine often receive adjuvant chemotherapy and radiation. Many chemotherapeutic agents place patients into an immunocompromised state, rendering the patient unable to optimally fight off infections. Radiation to a recently operated surgical site is notorious for inhibiting optimal wound healing.

Patients with primary spinal tumors also very frequently encounter wound complications, due in part to large soft tissue defects created in an effort to obtain negative margins around the primary site of the tumor. Larger defects are created if there is soft tissue tumor invasion. In a study among patients treated with en bloc resection, one-third required reoperation as a result of wound dehiscence within 30 days of surgery.[23] Additionally, patients with multiple comorbidities such as diabetes may have decreased wound healing capacity.[6,24] Medical optimization measures such as smoking cessation, diabetes control, and staying in a good nutritional state before surgery are invaluable prophylactic approaches that can be taken.

A prophylactic measure that can be undertaken in surgeries that necessitate complex soft tissue reconstructive challenges is the use of well-vascularized musculocutaneous flaps. A systematic review of the literature found that among patients with spinal neoplasms, 28% of these patients received prophylactic muscular flaps at the initial surgery. The primary indications were instrumentation, previous irradiation, and previous surgery.[24,25] A separate study found a statistically significant difference in the incidence of complications in patients who underwent prophylactic soft tissue reconstruction (20%) as opposed to those who did not (45%).[6]

Musculocutaneous flaps are able to inhibit bacterial growth, thus helping to prevent surgical site infection.[24] These flaps also tend to enhance blood flow, thereby improving the oxygen-rich environment, which increases bacterial elimination.[26] Patients with cervical and lumbosacral neoplasms requiring soft tissue reconstruction tend to have a higher rate of wound complications, as opposed to their thoracic counterparts.[6] This is predominantly due to the lack of anatomically available soft tissue in the cervical and lumbosacral spine that can be utilized as flaps. The thoracic spine regional anatomy harbors an easily accessible multitude of muscles that can be utilized.

Length of Surgery-Related Complications

DVT and pulmonary embolism (PE) are responsible for significant morbidity and mortality in spine tumor surgery. The prevalence of DVT after spine surgery is estimated to be between 0.3% and 15.5%.[27] Utilization of prophylactic subcutaneous unfractionated heparin is essential in this patient population. The risk of DVT/PE is known to be higher in patients harboring a neoplastic process. Prophylactic placement of an IVC filter in this patient population has been advocated by some,[28,29] although the risk of a DVT/PE is not mitigated by its placement.

Postoperative visual loss (POVL) is a rare complication often related to length of surgery and can have devastating effects with permanent visual loss being the most feared outcome. POVL has an incidence of 0.0008% to 0.002% in the general surgical population, but a 0.09% to 0.20% incidence after spinal surgery.[30] POVL diagnoses included anterior (AION) and posterior (PION) ischemic optic neuropathy, central retinal artery occlusion (CRAO), and cortical blindness (CB). Usually irreversible, PION is the most common entity and is specifically associated with prone positioning, prolonged procedures, hemodilution, facial edema, significant blood loss, hypotension, and comorbidities such as diabetes, hypertension, atherosclerosis, and smoking.[30] Although rare, this devastating complication should be included in the preoperative discussion and surgical consent. Precautionary measures that minimize the risk of PION include caution during positioning, avoiding direct pressure on the orbits, staging high-risk procedures, maximizing hemostasis, avoiding large crystalloid infusions, and keeping the head at or above the heart.[30]

Intraoperative Hemorrhage

Intraoperative blood loss is a common cause of morbidity during resection of spinal tumors. Rates of massive blood loss (>5000 mL) have been known to occur in 43% of cases of en bloc resections.[31] Many primary malignant bone tumors demonstrate increased vascularity on angiography, although this can be variable with chordomas.[32] Metastatic tumors originating from vascular visceral structures tend to be problematic in the operating room because intralesional resections are generally undertaken for nonprimary bone tumors. Preoperative thoracolumbar angiography can sometimes identify the dominant radicular artery that supplies the spinal cord, although this does not typically alter the side of approach or preclude resection. Preoperative embolization of distal tumor vasculature has been widely recommended to decrease intraoperative hemorrhage, especially in more vascular pathologies, such as renal cell carcinoma.[33] Avoiding embolization of large arterial feeders minimizes unwanted collateral vessel occlusion, tissue ischemia, and infarction.[32] Preoperative embolization should occur about 1 to 2 days before the planned surgery to minimize blood supply and maximize benefit.[32]

With regard to the cervical region, the anatomy and physiology of the vertebral artery needs to be carefully assessed because damage to this structure can cause catastrophic bleeding and devastating posterior circulation infarcts (Fig. 58.6). Even when the vertebral

SURGICAL REWIND

My Worst Case

A 40-year-old female presents to the neurosurgery clinic with a past medical history of neurofibromatosis type 1 NF-1. Five years previously, she underwent a posterior thoracic approach for T6 corpectomy and multilevel stabilization for a circumferential plexiform neurofibroma. Subsequent imaging revealed rapid growth of the tumor over a short period of time from the last follow-up (Figs 58.7 and 58.8). A computed tomography–guided biopsy revealed malignant transformation of the neurofibroma. The patient subsequently underwent a two-stage surgical procedure. The first stage was a posterior approach to the thoracic spine T2 through T10 fixation and fusion with resection of T5, T6, and T7 vertebral bodies, cage reconstruction, and mobilization of the tumor. In the second stage, a left-sided thoracotomy and complete removal of the tumor with decompression of the spinal cord were undertaken. The patient's postoperative course was complicated with a persistent CSF–pleural fistula, leading to a left-sided pleural effusion with respiratory compromise (Fig. 58.9). The patient was taken back to the operating room, where the CSF leak from the dura was repaired and a complex plastic closure of the incision was performed. A lumbar drain was left in place for several days. This was unfortunately complicated by intracranial hypotension with subsequent subdural hygromas. The patient was eventually weaned off the lumbar drain. The patient postoperatively did well eventually and was discharged from the hospital with no further evidence of CSF leak (Fig. 58.10).

CSF–pleural fistulas are unfortunate complications that are not uncommon for such procedures as described above. In an effort to give the patient a maximum survival benefit and disease-free interval, en bloc excision is the surgical goal. These types of surgeries carry a very high complication profile, given the complexity and extraspinal anatomy that must be traversed to resect these tumors. CSF–pleural fistulas should be dealt with on an urgent basis, before severe respiratory compromise. First-line treatment entails pleural fluid drainage and direct repair of the dural defect. CSF diversion can be considered as an adjunctive measure.

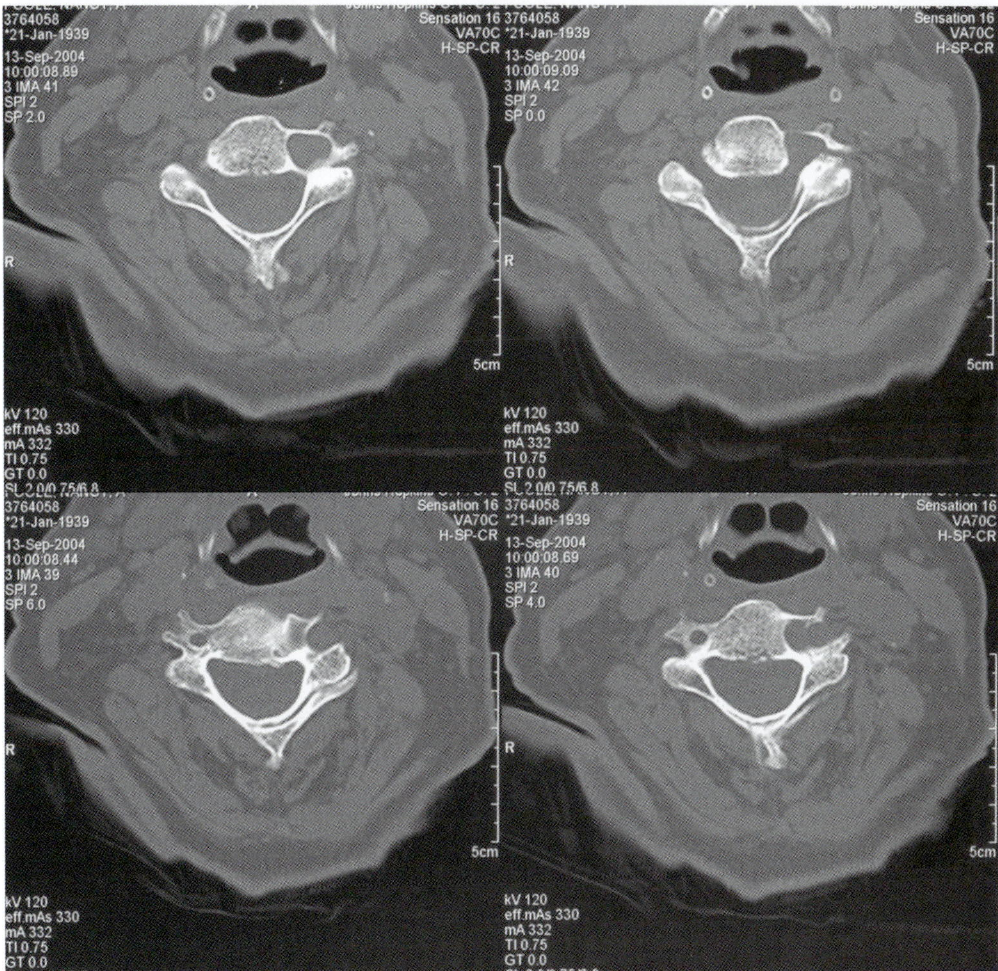

• **Fig. 58.6** Axial cervical spine computed tomography scan displaying a medially situated left-sided vertebral artery.

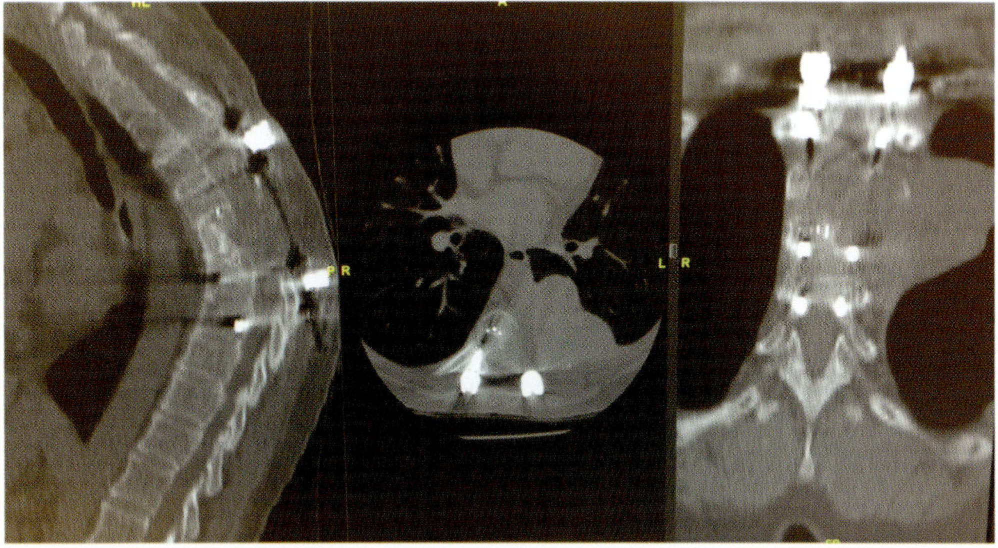

• **Fig. 58.7** Sagittal, axial, and coronal computed tomography scan depicting a previously reconstructed mid-thoracic spine, with recurrence of a large paraspinal malignant nerve sheath neurofibroma.

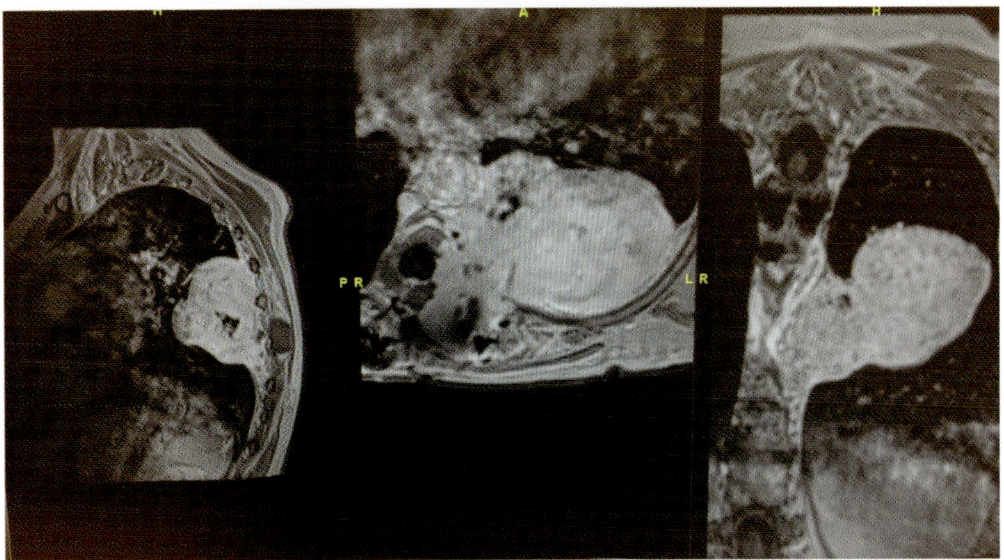

• **Fig. 58.8** Sagittal, axial, and coronal postcontrast T1 magnetic resonance imaging scan depicting an avidly enhancing recurrent mid-thoracic paraspinal malignant nerve sheath with encroachment upon the spinal cord.

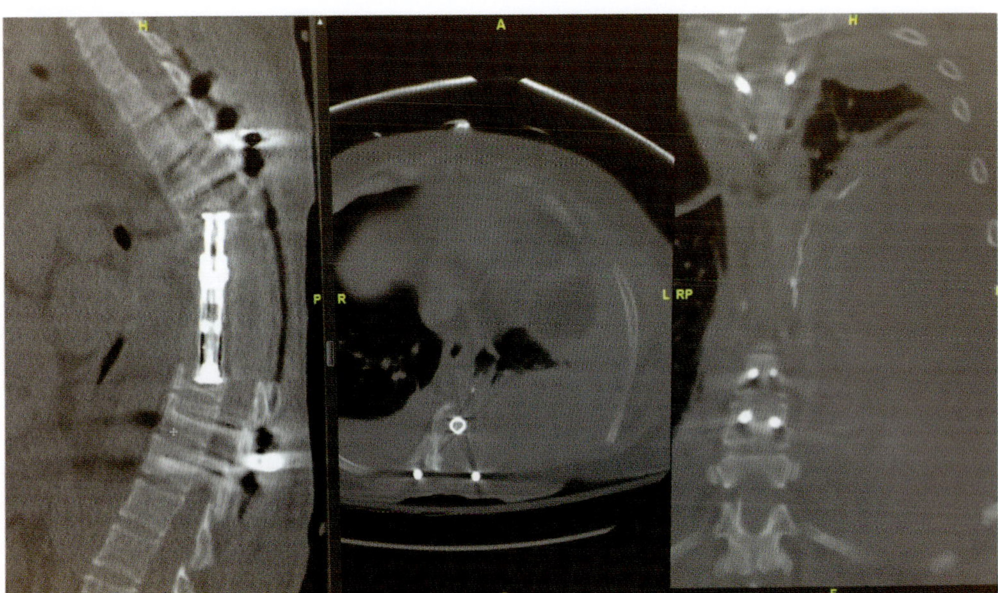

• **Fig. 58.9** Postoperative computed tomography scan depicting a large left-sided cerebrospinal fluid pleural effusion after en bloc.

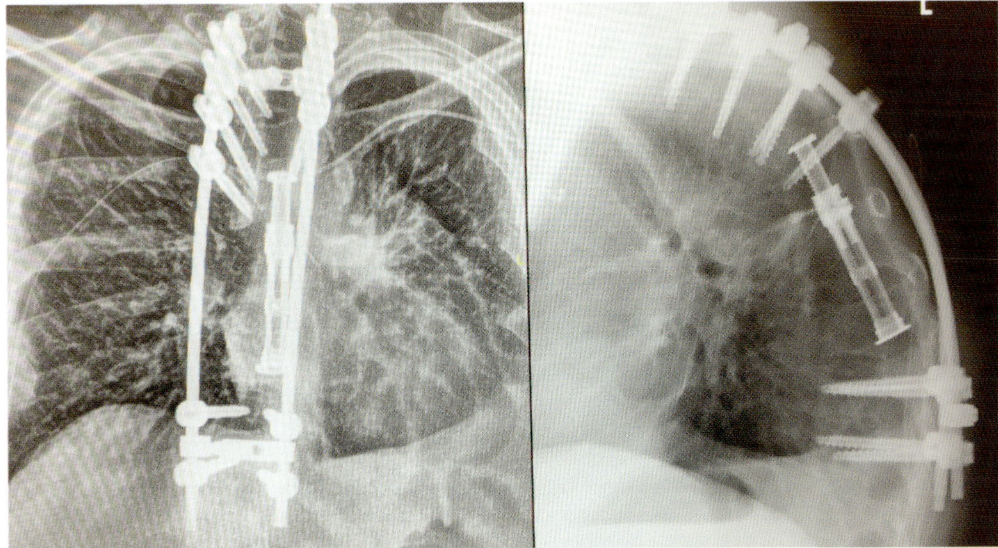

• **Fig. 58.10** Thoracic x-rays revealing instrumentation from T2 to T10, anterior column reconstruction with an expandable cage, and resolution of the left-sided cerebrospinal fluid pleural effusion.

artery is not directly involved by the tumor, it is frequently very challenging to achieve complete en bloc resection while preserving both vertebral arteries. As stated earlier in the chapter, a balloon occlusion test is recommended to assess the safety of sacrificing one vertebral artery.[8] Endovascular occlusion is preferred over open surgical ligation to avoid intraoperative hemorrhage associated with the abundant venous plexus of the transverse foramina.[34] The spinal level of the most proximal level of embolization should be known before surgery because it is still possible to lacerate the vertebral arterial stump, which can potentially lead to significant blood loss.

Conclusion

Although the surgical management of spinal tumors is often technically rewarding, significant complications along with serious expected morbidities often occur. Vertebral column neoplasms do not often respect anatomic boundaries, thereby leading to invasion of soft tissue and visceral structures, complicating their resection. Surrounding each spinal segment is a unique 360-degree network of visceral organs and neurovascular structures that must be taken into account when planning a vertebral column tumor resection. The mainstay of diminishing complications relating to surgery lies in exceptional preparation, from understanding the relational anatomy to ensuring that the patient is medically optimized before surgery. It should be understood that spine tumor surgery necessitates a multidisciplinary approach to optimize outcomes and decrease the rate of complications.

References

1. Quintan LM. Primary vertebral tumors—and Enneking was right. *World Neurosurg*. 2017;775–776.
2. Boriani S, Gasbarrini A, Bandiera S, Ghermandi R, Lador R. Predictors for surgical complications of en bloc resections in the spine: review of 220 cases treated by the same team. *Eur Spine J*. 2016;25:3932–3941.
3. Luksanapruksa P, Buchowski JM, Singhatanadgige W, Bumpass DB. Systematic review and meta-analysis of en bloc vertebrectomy compared with intralesional resection for giant cell tumors of the mobile spine. *Global Spine J*. 2016;6:798–803.
4. Goel A. Surgery for malignant spinal tumors: beyond the lure of the "technically sweet". *World Neurosurg*. 2017;777–778.
5. Laufer I, Rubin DG, Lis E, et al. The NOMS framework: approach to the treatment of spinal metastatic tumors. *Oncologist*. 2013;18:744–751.
6. Chang DW, Friel MT, Youssef AA. Reconstructive strategies in soft tissue reconstruction after resection of spinal neoplasms. *Spine*. 2007;32:1101–1106.
7. Mattei TA, Mendel E. En bloc resection of primary malignant bone tumors of the cervical spine. *Acta Neurochir (Wien)*. 2014;156:2159–2164.
8. Hoshino Y, Kurokawa T, Nakamura K, et al. A report on the safety of unilateral vertebral artery ligation during cervical spine surgery. *Spine*. 1996;21:1454–1457.
9. Stulik J, Barna M, Vyskocil T, Nesnidal P, Kryl J, Klezl Z. Total en bloc spondylectomy of C3: a new surgical technique and literature review. *Acta Chir Orthop Traumatol Cech*. 2015;82:261–267.
10. Gosling T, Pichlmaier MA, Langer F, Krettek C, Hufner T. Two-stage multilevel en bloc spondylectomy with resection and replacement of the aorta. *Eur Spine J*. 2013;22(suppl 3):S363–S368.
11. Yokogawa N, Murakami H, Demura S, et al. Motor function of the upper-extremity after transection of the second thoracic nerve root during total en bloc spondylectomy. *PLoS ONE*. 2014;9:e109838.
12. Sugimoto S, Tanaka M, Suzawa K, et al. Pneumocephalus and chylothorax complicating vertebrectomy for lung cancer. *Ann Thorac Surg*. 2015;99:1425–1428.
13. Xu R, Garces-Ambrossi GL, McGirt MJ, et al. Thoracic vertebrectomy and spinal reconstruction via anterior, posterior, or combined approaches: clinical outcomes in 91 consecutive patients with metastatic spinal tumors. *J Neurosurg Spine*. 2009;11:272–284.
14. Kawahara N, Tomita K, Murakami H, Demura S. Total en bloc spondylectomy for spinal tumors: surgical techniques and related basic background. *Orthop Clin North Am*. 2009;40:47–63, vi.
15. Moran D, Zadnik PL, Taylor T, et al. Maintenance of bowel, bladder, and motor functions after sacrectomy. *Spine J*. 2015;15:222–229.
16. Clarke MJ, Dasenbrock H, Bydon A, et al. Posterior-only approach for en bloc sacrectomy: clinical outcomes in 36 consecutive patients. *Neurosurgery*. 2012;71:357–364, discussion 364.
17. Zang J, Guo W, Yang R, Tang X, Li D. Is total en bloc sacrectomy using a posterior-only approach feasible and safe for patients with malignant sacral tumors? *J Neurosurg Spine*. 2015;22:563–570.
18. Chaichana KL, Sciubba DM, Li KW, Gokaslan ZL. Surgical management of thoracic spinal cord herniation: technical consideration. *J Spinal Disord Tech*. 2009;22:67–72.
19. Lewandrowski KU, Hecht AC, DeLaney TF, Chapman PA, Hornicek FJ, Pedlow FX. Anterior spinal arthrodesis with structural cortical allografts and instrumentation for spine tumor surgery. *Spine*. 2004;29:1150–1158, discussion 1159.
20. Xu N, Wei F, Liu X, et al. Reconstruction of the upper cervical spine using a personalized 3d-printed vertebral body in an adolescent with Ewing sarcoma. *Spine*. 2016;41:E50–E54.
21. Mendel E, Mayerson JL, Nathoo N, Edgar RL, Schmidt C, Miller MJ. Reconstruction of the pelvis and lumbar-pelvic junction using 2 vascularized autologous bone grafts after en bloc resection for an iliosacral chondrosarcoma. *J Neurosurg Spine*. 2011;15:168–173.
22. Nishizawa K, Mori K, Saruhashi Y, Takahashi S, Matsusue Y. Long-term clinical outcome of sacral chondrosarcoma treated by total en bloc sacrectomy and reconstruction of lumbosacral and pelvic ring using intraoperative extracorporeal irradiated autologous tumor-bearing sacrum: a case report with 10 years follow-up. *Spine J*. 2014;14:e1–e8.
23. Groves ML, Zadnik PL, Kaloostian P, et al. Epidemiologic, functional, and oncologic outcome analysis of spinal sarcomas treated surgically at a single institution over 10 years. *Spine J*. 2015;15:110–114.
24. Chieng LO, Hubbard Z, Salgado CJ, Levi AD, Chim H. Reconstruction of open wounds as a complication of spinal surgery with flaps: a systematic review. *Neurosurg Focus*. 2015;39:E17.
25. Garvey PB, Rhines LD, Dong W, Chang DW. Immediate soft-tissue reconstruction for complex defects of the spine following surgery for spinal neoplasms. *Plast Reconstr Surg*. 2010;125:1460–1466.
26. Eshima I, Mathes SJ, Paty P. Comparison of the intracellular bacterial killing activity of leukocytes in musculocutaneous and random-pattern flaps. *Plast Reconstr Surg*. 1990;86:541–547.
27. Yoshioka K, Kitajima I, Kabata T, et al. Venous thromboembolism after spine surgery: changes of the fibrin monomer complex and D-dimer level during the perioperative period. *J Neurosurg Spine*. 2010;13:594–599.
28. Leon L, Rodriguez H, Tawk RG, Ondra SL, Labropoulos N, Morasch MD. The prophylactic use of inferior vena cava filters in patients undergoing high-risk spinal surgery. *Ann Vasc Surg*. 2005;19:442–447.
29. Rosner MK, Kuklo TR, Tawk R, Moquin R, Ondra SL. Prophylactic placement of an inferior vena cava filter in high-risk patients undergoing spinal reconstruction. *Neurosurg Focus*. 2004;17:E6.

30. Li A, Swinney C, Veeravagu A, Bhatti I, Ratliff J. Postoperative visual loss following lumbar spine surgery: a review of risk factors by diagnosis. *World Neurosurg*. 2015;84:2010–2021.
31. Fisher CG, Keynan O, Boyd MC, Dvorak MF. The surgical management of primary tumors of the spine: initial results of an ongoing prospective cohort study. *Spine*. 2005;30:1899–1908.
32. Gottfried ON, Schmidt MH, Stevens EA. Embolization of sacral tumors. *Neurosurg Focus*. 2003;15:E4.
33. Berkefeld J, Scale D, Kirchner J, Heinrich T, Kollath J. Hypervascular spinal tumors: influence of the embolization technique on perioperative hemorrhage. *AJNR Am J Neuroradiol*. 1999;20:757–763.
34. Mattei TA, Mendel E. En bloc resection of primary malignant bone tumors of the cervical spine. *Acta Neurochir (Wien)*. 2014;156: 2159–2164.

59

Complications of Surgery for Spinal Vascular Malformations

RAMI O. ALMEFTY, ROBERT F. SPETZLER

HIGHLIGHTS

- Spinal vascular malformations are complex lesions with potentially devastating consequences in the event of spinal cord injury.
- A thorough knowledge of the anatomy and pathophysiology is critical to safely treat patients with these lesions.
- The pial resection technique makes resection of intradural intramedullary spinal arteriovenous malformations safe and effective, with excellent neurologic and angiographic results.

Background

Spinal vascular malformations are complex lesions that represent a clinically significant management challenge. Our understanding of their pathophysiology and our ability to treat these lesions have grown substantially with improvements in microsurgery, endovascular techniques, and neuroimaging.[1,2] We have developed a modified classification system of these lesions based on their anatomy and pathophysiology.[3] Classification helps organize our understanding and guide the management of spinal vascular malformations, particularly arteriovenous malformations (AVMs). This chapter focuses on the surgical treatment of intradural intramedullary AVMs because dorsal intradural arteriovenous fistulae are less complex and thus less technically challenging, and other spinal vascular malformations are less commonly treated surgically. Intradural intramedullary AVMs, also known as type II or glomus AVMs, are located, at least partially, in the spinal cord parenchyma but frequently bridge the pial surface. We have pioneered the use of the pial resection technique for their removal, which we have applied with excellent results. The pial resection technique is often used in conjunction with preoperative embolization (Fig. 59.1).[4]

Anatomic Insights

Arterial

Longitudinal arteries: The spinal cord vasculature can be conceptualized as a grid with longitudinally oriented vessels fed by transversely oriented vessels. The longitudinal vessels are the single anterior spinal artery and the paired posterior spinal arteries. The anterior spinal artery arises from the bilateral vertebral arteries and runs continuously in the anterior median fissure in the anterior midline. It supplies approximately two-thirds of the spinal cord, including most of the gray matter via both small penetrating and circumferential arteries around the pial surface. The posterior spinal arteries are paired discontinuous arteries that arise from the vertebral arteries and run medial to the dorsal root entry zone. They supply the posterior spinal cord, which comprises approximately one-third of the spinal cord, including the dorsal columns and a small contribution to the central gray matter via small circumferential pial branches.

Segmental arteries: As the longitudinal arteries descend the spinal cord, they are fed by transversally oriented arteries known as *segmental arteries*. The segmental arteries vary in their origin and their termination. In the cervical spine, they typically arise from the vertebral arteries and the thyrocervical trunk. In the lumbar and thoracic spine, they typically originate from the aorta and iliac arteries. The segmental arteries have numerous and variable transverse and longitudinal anastomoses. Each segmental artery sends a branch to the vertebral bodies before continuing to its final branch point in front of the transverse process. It then divides into an intercostal branch and a dorsal branch. The intercostal branch supplies the ribs and musculature. Along its route, the dorsal branch supplies the posterior elements of the spine and the dural and epidural elements. The continuation of the dorsal branch has one of three possibilities and has been referred to by different nomenclature. The number and location of each branch type are highly variable. At some levels, the artery does not contribute to the spinal cord and supplies only the dura and nerve root; this variation is best termed a *radicular artery*. Alternatively, the segmental artery may connect with the posterior spinal artery and supply the nerve root and posterior spinal cord, at which point it is best referred to as a *posterior radiculopial artery*. Finally, it can connect to the anterior spinal artery and supply the nerve root, pia, and intramedullary spinal cord, where it is known as an *anterior radiculomedullary artery*. The large anterior radiculomedullary artery in the thoracolumbar spine is known by the eponymous term the *artery of Adamkiewicz*.[5]

Venous

The venous anatomy of the spinal cord is similarly organized and plays a critical role in the pathophysiology of AVM lesions.

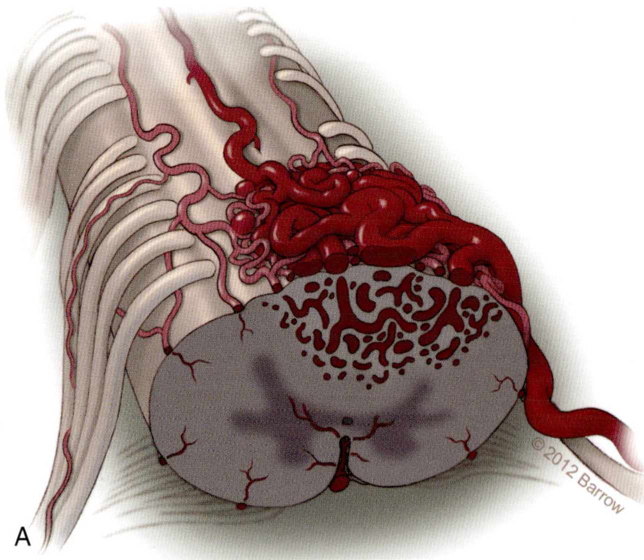

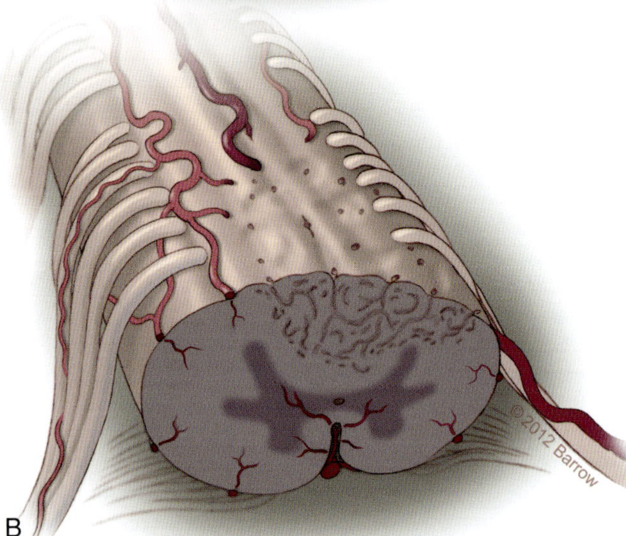

• **Fig. 59.1** (A) Illustration of a glomus spinal arteriovenous malformation (AVM) affecting the posterior spinal cord. The AVM nidus extends through the spinal parenchyma into the extrapial space. Associated feeding arteries arising from the posterior arteries, intranidal aneurysms, and arterialized draining veins are present. (B) The extrapial portion of the AVM nidus has been resected, leaving the parenchymal portion of the nidus. Despite subtotal nidal resection, the glomus spinal AVM has been essentially devascularized and obliterated. (Used with permission from Barrow Neurological Institute, Phoenix, Arizona.)

A network of intramedullary veins drains into the longitudinally oriented intradural extramedullary network, which is connected to the longitudinal epidural plexus through the dura by radicular veins.[6]

RED FLAGS

- Complex, diffuse AVMs with multiple arterial feeders
- Arterial supply from radiculomedullary arteries
- Ventral location
- Location primarily deep within the spinal cord parenchyma with little pial presentation

Prevention

The single best method for avoiding complications from spinal vascular malformations is a thorough understanding of the pathophysiology of spinal AVMs and of both normal and pathologic anatomy. The next critical factor is to proceed with embolization and resection with the understanding that leaving residual AVM is far better than causing a devastating neurologic injury.

AVM Management

During AVM resection, the best way to avoid ischemic damage or direct injury to the spinal cord is to avoid extensive dissection within the spinal cord itself and to use embolization judiciously. In the event of either of these complications, treatment may include corticosteroids, avoidance of hypotension and hypoperfusion, and supportive care. Immediate postoperative decline is not unusual, but patients frequently recover over time with rehabilitative therapy.[7]

Patients must also be monitored for late sequelae, such as tethering, recurrence, or deformity development. New or worsening symptoms should prompt investigation. Tethering is not uncommon, and patients respond well to detethering.[4] We prefer to perform a laminoplasty rather than a laminectomy to facilitate reoperation and to help avoid the development of a deformity.

SURGICAL REWIND

My Worst Cases

Case 1

We have emphasized the importance of the pial resection technique, which allows the safe and effective resection of difficult spinal AVMs that would not have been resectable previously. The following case demonstrates an example of a dissection that was extended subpially. A young girl previously presented with a headache and cranial subarachnoid hemorrhage. Angiography showed a cervical AVM. The patient was neurologically intact. The patient underwent cervical laminoplasty for resection. During the procedure, the dissection suboptimally extended subpially. Postoperative angiography confirmed complete obliteration of the AVM. Postoperatively, the patient remained with full strength but developed right leg numbness and proprioceptive loss (Fig. 59.2).

Case 2

Embolization is an important adjunct to surgical resection and can facilitate surgery. However, because of the tenuous vascular supply to the spinal cord, embolization must be used judiciously. In this case, we describe a young girl who experienced a previous hemorrhage related to a conus medullaris AVM. The patient underwent evacuation of the hematoma and decompression at an external hospital and had an excellent recovery. She later presented to our institution for definitive treatment. She underwent preoperative embolization followed by surgical resection. After surgery, there was persistent AVM filling through a single arterial feeder, which could likely be cured with embolization. The single arterial feeder was embolized with glue, which obliterated the AVM. After the final embolization, the patient became severely paraparetic, with sensory loss, and loss of bowel and bladder control. The patient's symptoms were managed with blood pressure augmentation, the avoidance of hypotension, and corticosteroids. Because propagation of a thrombus was potentially involved, the patient also received aspirin and heparin. The patient had only short-term follow-up but began to show improvement (Fig. 59.3).

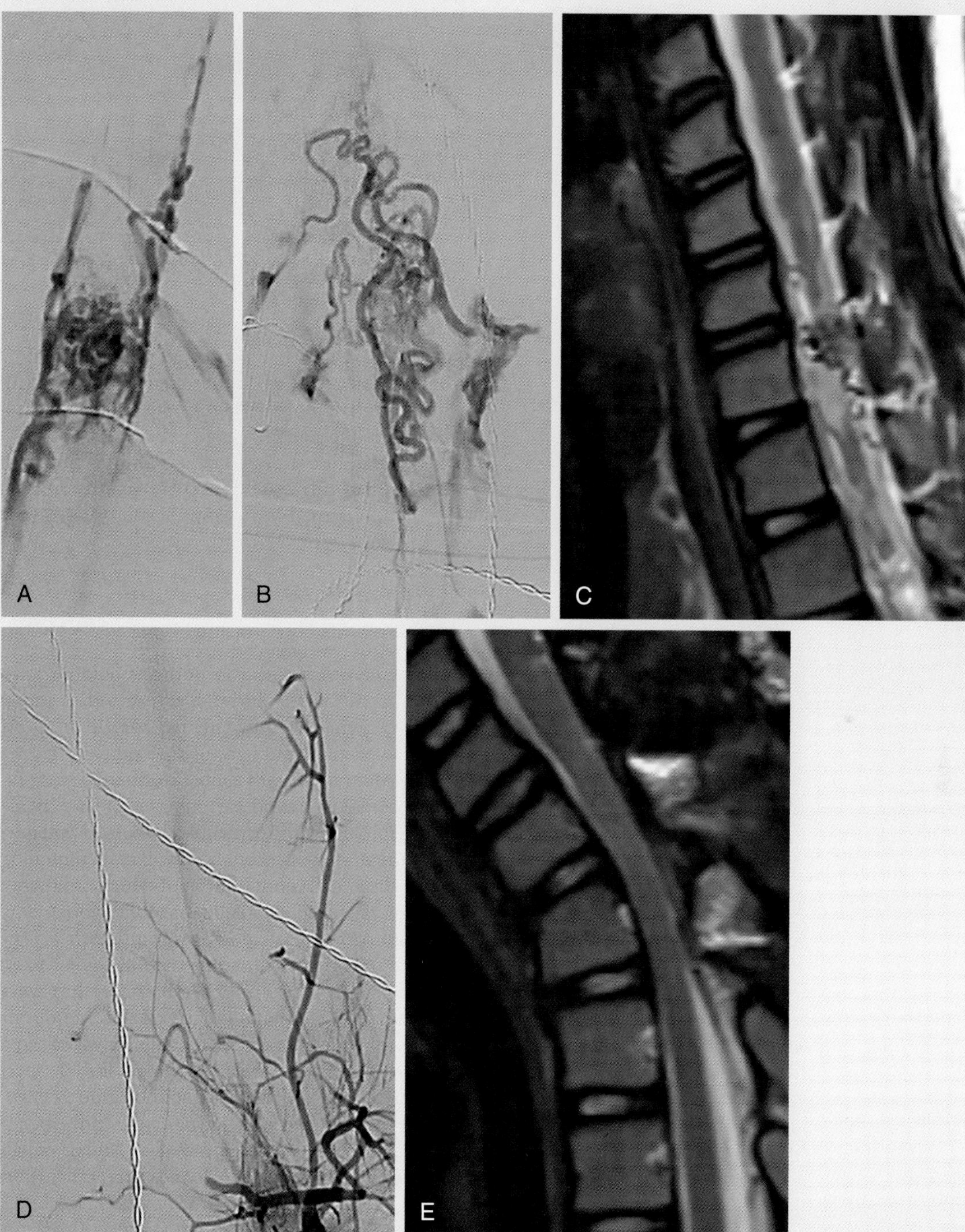

• **Fig. 59.2** Preoperative (A) lateral and (B) anteroposterior (AP) digital subtraction angiograms of left costocervical trunk and (C) sagittal T2-weighted magnetic resonance image (MRI) showing the intramedullary arteriovenous malformation. (D) Postoperative AP digital subtraction angiogram of left costocervical trunk. (E) Sagittal T2-weighted MRI demonstrating the complete resection. (Used with permission from Barrow Neurological Institute, Phoenix, Arizona.)

Continued

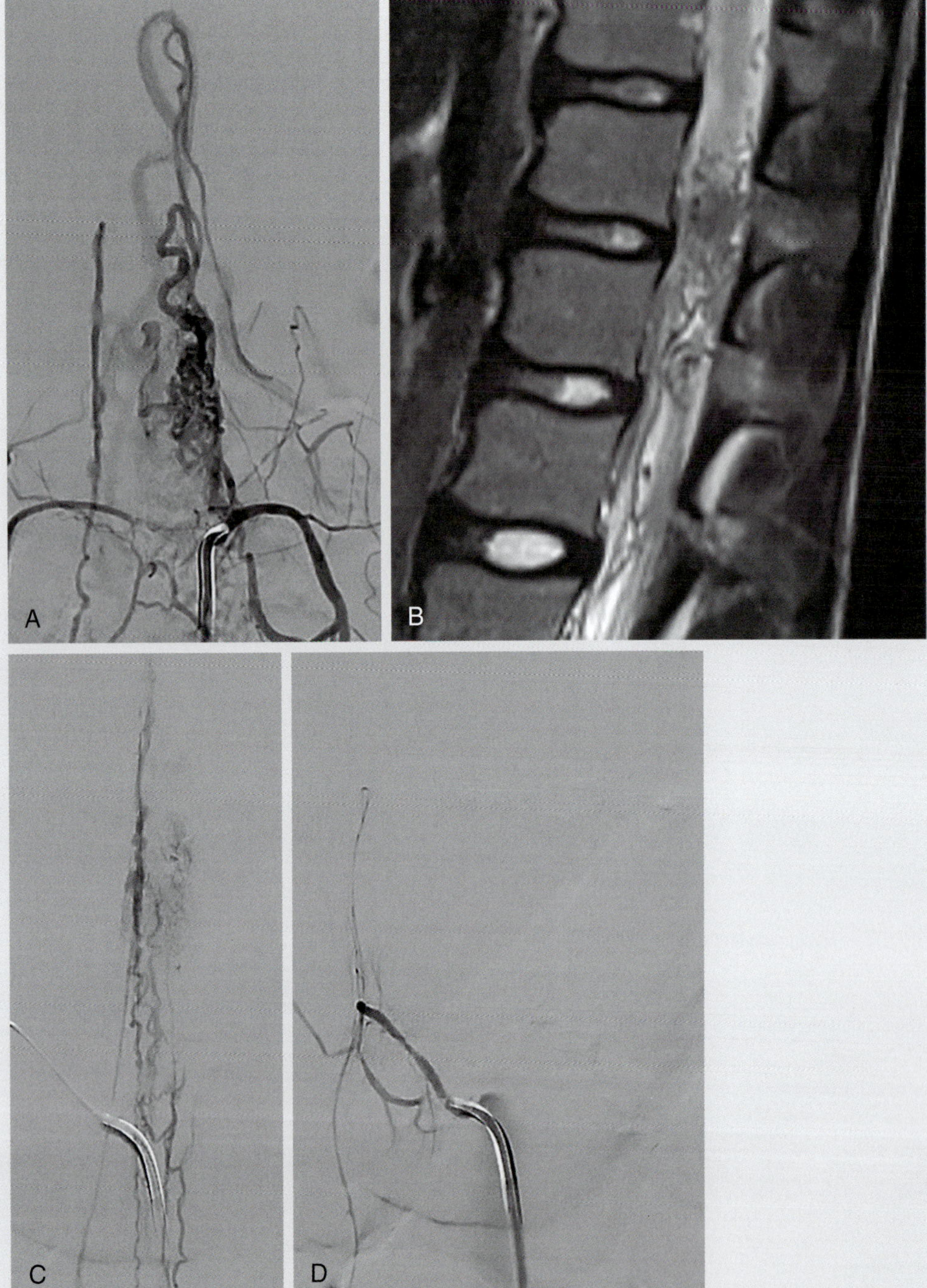

• **Fig. 59.3** Preoperative (A) anteroposterior digital subtraction angiogram and (B) sagittal T2-weighted magnetic resonance image demonstrating the intramedullary arteriovenous malformation (AVM). Anteroposterior digital subtraction angiograms of (C) right L1 injection postsurgical resection showing residual AVM through a single remaining feeder and (D) postembolization injection showing no residual filling. (Used with permission from Barrow Neurological Institute, Phoenix, Arizona.)

NEUROSURGICAL SELFIE MOMENT

Spinal vascular malformations represent a considerable management challenge because of their complexity and the often irremediable nature of spinal cord damage. The management of complications is aimed at prevention, which is best achieved by developing comprehensive knowledge of the normal and pathologic anatomy, implementing the strategic use of embolization, and developing expertise in microsurgical techniques. The pial resection technique facilitates the safe resection of spinal AVMs, and the temptation to follow the AVM nidus into the spinal cord parenchyma must be resisted. Supportive care, corticosteroids, and blood pressure augmentation can help reduce neurologic complications, such as edema, and can help optimize perfusion.

References

1. Rangel-Castilla L, Russin JJ, Zaidi HA, et al. Contemporary management of spinal AVFs and AVMs: lessons learned from 110 cases. *Neurosurg Focus*. 2014;37(3):E14.
2. Flores BC, Klinger DR, White JA, Batjer HH. Spinal vascular malformations: treatment strategies and outcome. *Neurosurg Rev*. 2017;40(1): 15–28.
3. Kim LJ, Spetzler RF. Classification and surgical management of spinal arteriovenous lesions: arteriovenous fistulae and arteriovenous malformations. *Neurosurgery*. 2006;59(5 suppl 3):S195–S201, discussion S3–S13.
4. Velat GJ, Chang SW, Abla AA, Albuquerque FC, McDougall CG, Spetzler RF. Microsurgical management of glomus spinal arteriovenous malformations: pial resection technique: clinical article. *J Neurosurg Spine*. 2012;16(6):523–531.
5. Bolton B. The blood supply of the human spinal cord. *J Neurol Psychiatry*. 1939;2(2):137–148.
6. Gillilan LA. Veins of the spinal cord: anatomic details; suggested clinical applications. *Neurology*. 1970;20(9):860–868.
7. Wilson DA, Abla AA, Uschold TD, McDougall CG, Albuquerque FC, Spetzler RF. Multimodality treatment of conus medullaris arteriovenous malformations: 2 decades of experience with combined endovascular and microsurgical treatments. *Neurosurgery*. 2012;71(1): 100–108.

60

Complications of Surgery and Radiosurgery in Spinal Metastasis

IBRAHIM HUSSAIN, ILYA LAUFER, MARK BILSKY

HIGHLIGHTS

- Hemorrhage, wound dehiscence/infection, and hardware failure are the most common complications during and after spinal tumor surgery.
- Esophagitis, myelopathy, and development of vertebral body compression fractures are the most common significant complications after spinal tumor radiosurgery.
- Many of these complications can be mitigated by appropriate preoperative management; however, subsequent interventions still may be required with the goal of preventing systemic deterioration and preserving quality of life.

Background

Technologic and medical breakthroughs in the diagnosis and treatment of metastatic disease have markedly increased life expectancy in patients with cancer. While effective chemotherapy, biologics, and immunotherapy have had profound impact with specific tumors, advances in radiation therapy and a better understanding of optimal surgical strategies have concordantly played a vital role in the multidisciplinary management of these patients. The spine represents the most common skeletal site for metastatic disease, affecting up to 30% of patients with solid organ malignancies.[1,2] Radiation and surgery are the principal modalities used to achieve local tumor control in the setting of spine metastases. The NOMS decision framework takes into account four sentinel decision points: Neurologic, Oncologic, Mechanical Stability, and Systemic Disease.[3-7] This framework can integrate evidence-based guidelines to determine the optimal treatment strategy. Stereotactic radiosurgery (SRS) represents a significant advance over conventional external beam radiation (cEBRT) because responses to SRS are both histology- and volume-independent when used in the upfront setting or as a postoperative adjuvant treatment.[8] From an oncologic perspective, tumoral responses are no longer dictated by the radioresistance seen with cEBRT for most solid tumor malignancies. Despite exponentially better tumor control achieved with SRS, surgery continues to play a critical role in the treatment of patients with neurologic indications, including high-grade epidural spinal cord compression (ESCC) with or without myelopathy, and the treatment of radioresistant tumors and mechanical instability. Superior outcomes have been demonstrated in patients with symptomatic solid tumor ESCC treated with surgical decompression and stabilization compared with radiotherapy alone.[9,10]

Despite significant advances in surgery and radiation, treatment-related complications need to be weighed carefully in decision-making. Operative techniques and instrumentation have improved, but oncologic and medical comorbidities can significantly impact surgical outcomes. Additionally, the last decade has witnessed tremendous advances in the technology used to deliver SRS, and significant effort from multiple institutions has centered on defining optimal tumoricidal doses while minimizing toxicity to organs at risk. Tight dose constraints have been established to prevent injuries to structures such as the spinal cord, esophagus, and vertebral body. These complications can significantly diminish quality of life, but improved outcomes can be achieved by identifying and treating risk factors and aggressively managing complications.

RED FLAGS

- Thrombocytopenia that does not respond to transfusion is an absolute contraindication to proceeding with surgery.
- Reoperations, previously irradiated tissue, neutropenia, and vascular endothelial growth factor (VEGF) inhibitor therapy (e.g., bevacizumab) represent risk factors for wound complications.
- Known risk factors for hardware failure requiring possible revision surgery include the following: extensive tumor involvement of the pedicle and vertebral body, previously irradiated bone, osteoporosis, extensive chest wall resection, and constructs greater than six contiguous spinal levels.
- Radiosurgery of spinal metastases can cause radiation-induced complications of the esophagus, brachial plexus, and spinal cord and can predispose treated vertebrae to compression fractures.

Prevention

Tumor Hemorrhage

Hypervascular tumors should be considered for preoperative digital subtraction angiography (DSA) to identify the vascular anatomy supplying spinal metastases and to assess the potential to embolize large arterial feeders to the tumor.[11,12] A laundry list of tumors that often benefit from preoperative embolization is provided in Table 60.1. In general, tumors originating from vascular organs, such as the kidney and thyroid gland, frequently exhibit hypervascularity, as do tumors with "angio" or "hemangio" in their name. The most significant misnomer is solitary fibrous tumor, which was previously called hemangiopericytoma and was found

TABLE 60.1 Hypervascular Solid Organ Spinal Metastases
Renal cell carcinoma
Hemangiopericytoma (solitary fibrous tumor)
Follicular/papillary thyroid carcinoma
Neuroendocrine tumors
Paraganglioma
Hepatocellular carcinoma
Cholangiocarcinoma
Angiosarcoma

consistently to be the most hypervascular tumor on the list. A tumor blush is often visible on angiographic injection of the segmental arteries feeding the tumor, with the intensity of the blush indicative of the vascularity of the tumor. Infusion of polyvinyl alcohol particles and liquid embolics (e.g., *N*-butyl cyanoacrylate [NBCA]) and deployment of detachable platinum coils have been described as effective embolization methods. When tumors are not supplied by a radiculomedullary artery, such as the artery of Adamkiewicz, selective embolization can be performed with extremely low complication rates or significant long-term morbidity.[11] Reduction in intraoperative blood loss by up to 50% can be seen, ultimately resulting in fewer blood transfusions and hypotensive episodes.[13,14] The timing between embolization and surgery remains unclear, although most centers will operate within 72 hours of embolization to obviate revascularization of the tumor.[15]

Other significant considerations for tumor hemorrhage are related to systemic issues preventing normal clotting. Coagulopathy and thrombocytopenia including those related to liver dysfunction (especially in the setting of hepatocellular carcinoma), factor deficiencies, or marrow suppression related to chemotherapy or wide-field radiation are primary factors. Appropriate transfusion of fresh frozen plasma (FFP) and/or platelets as well as vitamin K replacement are critical to reducing blood loss. Understanding of the timing of nadir counts related to chemotherapy can often be used to anticipate recovery. Discontinuing medications that impact platelet function (e.g., nonsteroidal antiinflammatories) or cause low platelets (e.g., heparin-induced thrombocytopenia) may often allow clotting abnormalities to correct. One contraindication to surgery is thrombocytopenia secondary to marrow suppression from wide-field irradiation or advanced disease. Chronic thrombocytopenia cannot be managed effectively because these patients often sustain uncontrolled intraoperative or postoperative hemorrhage with the need for massive platelet transfusions, often resulting in compressive clot at the laminectomy site. Early hematology consultation and bone marrow biopsy are often helpful in establishing the etiology and expected time to recovery of clotting disorders.

Wound Complications

Wound breakdown, dehiscence, and infection are the most common complications after instrumented spine procedures for metastatic disease. Major factors impacting wound healing include systemic therapy (e.g., glucocorticoids, biologics, or chemotherapy), poorly controlled diabetes mellitus, and hypoalbunemia from poor nutrition. Surgical risk factors include significant blood loss and increased length of surgery. Neutropenia with an absolute neutrophil count (ANC) less than 1000 cells per microliter also signifies poor immunologic function and conveys a higher chance of infection. Treatment with granulocyte colony- stimulating factor (G-CSF), such as Neupogen (Amgen, Thousand Oaks, CA), will often correct the neutropenia within 24 hours of infusion, reducing operative risks. Previously irradiated tissue, particularly preoperative cEBRT within 6 weeks of surgery, results in a very high risk of infection.[16] With the integration of neoadjuvant radiation into spine treatment paradigms, it is important to note that SRS reduces the rate of wound problems compared with cEBRT.[16]

Management

Tumor Hemorrhage

Intraoperative control of tumor hemorrhage can be addressed by a number of strategies. Direct cauterization with monopolar and bipolar cautery can be used; however, monopolar cautery should be avoided when near the thecal sac, spinal cord, or nerve roots to prevent thermal injury. Radiofrequency energy bipolar sealers with built-in saline irrigation, such as the Aquamantys (Medtronic, Fridley, MN), are also excellent tools for controlling bleeding without char or smoke. Hemostatic matrix agents, thrombin, and direct pressure with cottonoids can also be used as needed. Compression with rolled strips of thrombin-soaked Avitene (Bard, New Providence, NJ) balls packed into the vertebrectomy defect is superb for controlling bleeding. Intermittent irrigation with 3% hydrogen peroxide can serve as both hemostatic control agent and bactericide. Even in cases where intraoperative hemostasis is adequately achieved, postoperative hemorrhage can result in rapid neurologic deterioration. Early identification and correction of coagulopathy should be addressed, especially in high-risk patients with hepatocellular carcinoma, multiple myeloma, and lymphoma.[17] Hypothermia can induce coagulopathy that can contribute to intraoperative tumoral hemorrhage. In vitro, animal, and clinical studies have demonstrated that temperatures below 35°C can induce platelet dysfunction, decreased platelet count, and diminished synthesis of clotting enzymes and plasminogen activator inhibitors.[18] Furthermore, a progressive decrease in body temperature correlates with delays in the initiation of thrombus formation.[18] Appropriate intraoperative management can help reduce the occurrence of these phenomena with the use of body warmers and infusion of warmed intravenous fluids.

Coagulopathy can often be recognized intraoperatively as previously clotted blood begins to lyse or be predicted based on excessive blood loss of greater than 2 liters or transfusion of greater than 5 units of packed red blood cells (pRBCs). If possible, FFP and platelets should be given intraoperatively rather than in the postoperative period. Postoperative transfusion may result in tenacious local clot that cannot be evacuated even with epidural drains. Should evidence of an epidural hematoma develop with an acutely worsening neurologic examination or spinal cord compression as determined by imaging, expeditious return to the operating room for exploration and hematoma evacuation can salvage a good neurologic outcome. Subfascial/epidural drains are often used postoperatively to prevent subacute hematoma complications; however, their utility in mitigating emergent epidural hematomas is less clear.[19]

Wound Infection and Dehiscence

Surgical site infections, osteomyelitis, and paraspinal abscesses after spine tumor surgeries range from 9% to 14%, with *Staphylococcus aureus* being the most common organism.[20] Perioperative antibiotics should be given within one hour of skin incision and continued for 24 hours postoperatively in all cases. Vancomycin powder placed in the wound before wound closure is associated with a lower rate of deep spinal wound infection with minimal side effects.[21] In nonseptic patients who develop small postoperative collections concerning for infection, image-guided biopsy of the lesion should be attempted to isolate an organism. Systemic antibiotic treatment should then be tailored for the organism and its sensitivities. For large abscesses with thick capsules that are unlikely to be resolved by systemic treatment alone, wound exploration, washout, and debridement may be required. Assistance from infectious disease specialists in most cases is advised.

For patients requiring wound revision surgeries due to wound infection, dehiscence, or symptomatic pseudomeningocele, complex closures performed with the assistance of plastic surgeons have resulted in better outcomes and decreased occurrence of developing further complications.[22-24] The use of local rotational or transpositional flaps (e.g., trapezius or latissimus turnover flaps) provides vascularized tissue to the defective area that accelerates healing and can aid in bacterial clearance.[25] These flaps are critically important in the setting of previously irradiated tissue.

Another major consideration for preventing wound infections and dehiscence is the timing and order of radiotherapy and surgery. Complications are significantly reduced when surgery is followed by radiotherapy as opposed to radiotherapy followed by surgery.[26] Advances in intensity modulated image-guided radiotherapy (IMRT) allow radiation oncologists to target spinal tumors using multiple beam trajectories and in the postoperative setting; generally results in a significantly lower dose to the region of the healing skin incision compared with cEBRT, which delivers a significant dose to the operative corridor.

Cerebrospinal Fluid (CSF) Leak

The majority of spine tumor surgeries are for epidural lesions; therefore incidental durotomies can become a major source of morbidity. Durotomies are typically managed based on the size of the defect. A primary closure should always be attempted. Muscle patches and dural/fibrin sealants are commonly used. For large defects, dural patch grafts such as Dura-Guard (Baxter, Deerfield, IL) can effectively create a watertight repair. A Valsalva maneuver intraoperatively should confirm a watertight closure. In cases where this cannot be achieved or patients are otherwise at high risk for pseudomeningocele formation, a lumbar drain can be placed. Drainage of 10 mL per hour is often used with the goal to taper down drainage until the leak is confirmed as sealed; however, the hourly drainage volume can be increased, if needed, as long as the patient does not develop a low-pressure headache or subdural collections on imaging. Patient positioning is also important because lower thoracic and lumbar CSF leaks are best managed by keeping patients flat for at least 24 hours postoperatively; in comparison, the head of the bed is kept up for patients with cervical and upper thoracic leaks. Postoperative signs and symptoms of intracranial hypotension should be assessed, including positional headaches improved with recumbency, altered mental status, and fluid drainage directly from the wound. Vacuum-assisted subfascial drains should be used with extreme caution because the negative pressure generated can exacerbate small dural defects and prevent proper healing.[27] Likewise, lateral and anterior approach surgeries requiring chest tube insertion are at high risk for the same issue if kept on suction. High-volume thin output from subfascial drains or chest tubes should raise concern that a CSF leak persists. In cases refractory to conservative management, re-exploration to identify and primarily repair the defect may be required. For many of these situations, plastic surgery assistance is recommended with complex closures utilizing local rotational flaps; in severe cases, omental rotational or free flaps may be required.[28]

Hardware Failure

Hardware failure is characterized by screw pullout, rod fracture, or interbody device migration. Risk factors include previous irradiation, extensive pedicle/vertebral body tumor involvement, postmenopausal or androgen blockade–induced osteoporosis, junctional spine instrumentation (cervicothoracic or thoracolumbar), and chest wall resection.[22,29] Strategies to prevent screw pullout include cement augmentation of pedicle screws with polymethyl methacrylate (PMMA) in the thoracic and lumbar spine, which improves pullout strength and biomechanical stability of implanted instrumentation.[30-32] The recent US Food and Drug Administration approval of fenestrated screws allows the injection of cement material directly into the screw to support fixation. Construct length is also an important factor for hardware failure. Extending constructs one to two levels when there is extensive multilevel tumor involvement can decrease stress on the entire construct by distributing shearing forces.

Radiation Toxicity

Understanding radiation dose and fractionation when treating spinal metastases can help reduce the incidence of radiation toxicity. Collateral effects to the skin, esophagus, peripheral nerves, and spinal cord have been reported, manifested as symptoms such as dysphagia, odynophagia, radiculopathy, myelopathy, or other focal sensorimotor deficit.[33,34] Strict dose constraints for all organs at risk have been established to minimize toxicity. In certain cases, organ displacement via saline infusion into the retroperitoneum can be used to displace also the kidney or bowel several centimeters, creating a more favorable target for SRS of thoracolumbar spine metastases.

Radiation-induced myelopathy is a rare complication but can also cause neurologic deficits based on the dose received by the spinal cord. Occurring infrequently in about 0.4% of treated patients, it has a typical time frame of 6 months for development of symptoms.[8,35] A maximal spinal cord dose constraint of 14 or 10 Gy to 10% of the spinal cord minimizes the occurrence of myelopathy.[8] Although studies have failed to show reliable treatment strategies for this complication, steroid administration has been reported with varying degrees of success.

Non-neurologic Injury

Radiation-induced esophagitis is the most common side effect of radiosurgery to the cervical and thoracic spine.[34] Patients typically present with dysphagia and odynophagia, and although most cases are self-limited, more serious complications can occur. Mild cases can be treated by slow transition to a mechanical soft diet and application of topical anesthetics (e.g., 2% viscous xylocaine) to help reduce symptoms until inflammation subsides.[36] Radiation-induced strictures can develop, but multiple repeat dilations place patients at risk of esophageal perforation. High dose, single-fraction paraspinal SRS has demonstrated a low rate (~7%) of grade 3 or higher acute or late esophageal toxicity,[37] and more recent dose constraints have decreased this risk further.

Radiation recall is the phenomenon of local inflammatory reaction that occurs in an area of irradiation after the administration of certain chemotherapeutic agents. This is a poorly understood complication of cancer treatment; however, it can result in profound complications, especially to tissues in the vicinity of previous surgery. The most common agents that have been shown to induce radiation recall include the anthracyclines, taxanes, antimetabolites, and epidermal growth factor receptor (EGFR) inhibitors.[38] The severity of radiation recall varies widely; however, severe cases can result in esophageal perforation and skin necrosis and ulceration. When it occurs in the paraspinal region after surgical intervention, the risk of wound dehiscence significantly increases. Although the prediction is unclear as to which patients will be affected and in what time frame, appropriate management, including immediate cessation of the offending agent, should be underscored.

De novo and progressive vertebral compression fractures (VCFs) after spinal radiosurgery range from 3% to 40%,[39,40] with a median time to fracture of 3 to 11 months. However, the SRS-associated symptomatic fracture risk requiring surgical intervention is quite low at approximately 7%, and independent of administered dose. For patients with pain refractory to conservative measures, percutaneous cement augmentation, pedicle screws, or open surgery should be considered. Excellent pain outcomes after these interventions are reported in the 80% to 90% range.[39]

SURGICAL REWIND

My Worst Case

A 51-year-old man presented with right-sided subscapular pain and was diagnosed with a Pancoast tumor (Fig. 60.1A). He underwent neoadjuvant chemoradiation consisting of cisplatin/etoposide and 5760 cGy in 32 fractions. He underwent a right thoracotomy for upper lobectomy with chest wall resection and right-sided T1–T4 facetectomy, T2 and T3 pedicle excision, and C7–T6 posterior instrumented stabilization and fusion (Fig. 60.1B). Four weeks later, he presented with exposed hardware due to a wound dehiscence (Fig. 60.1C). The wound was debrided, and plastic surgery service performed myocutaneous flap reconstruction using the left trapezius muscle. Two months later he presented with a new incisional dehiscence and underwent additional debridement and flap revision (Fig. 60.1D). Three years after the initial surgery, the patient developed a chin-on-chest deformity (Fig. 60.1E) that required C2–T10 posterior instrumented fusion with C7–T1 Smith-Petersen osteotomy (Fig. 60.1F).

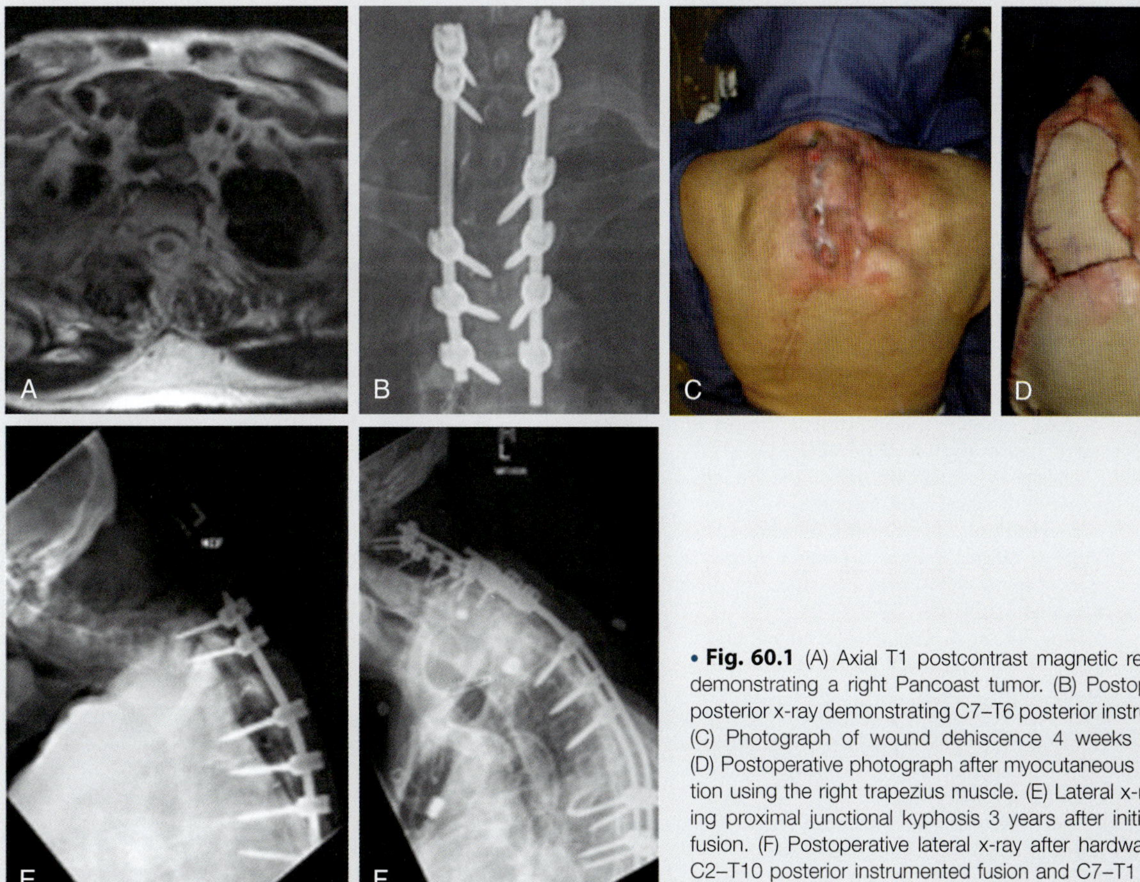

• **Fig. 60.1** (A) Axial T1 postcontrast magnetic resonance image demonstrating a right Pancoast tumor. (B) Postoperative anteroposterior x-ray demonstrating C7–T6 posterior instrumented fusion. (C) Photograph of wound dehiscence 4 weeks postoperatively. (D) Postoperative photograph after myocutaneous flap reconstruction using the right trapezius muscle. (E) Lateral x-ray demonstrating proximal junctional kyphosis 3 years after initial instrumented fusion. (F) Postoperative lateral x-ray after hardware revision with C2–T10 posterior instrumented fusion and C7–T1 Smith-Petersen osteotomy.

NEUROSURGICAL SELFIE MOMENT

The overall oncologic management of patients with metastatic disease is fraught with many challenges. With patients living longer due to advances in care, optimal surgical and radiation options for treating spinal metastases are paramount to preserving quality of life in these individuals. A multidisciplinary approach to managing these patients, involving interventional radiologists, radiation oncologists, and plastic surgeons, among others, has demonstrated enormous benefits in preventing and managing complications. Preoperative attention to vascular blood supply, dosing constraints, and systemic risk factors for hemorrhage and infection can help reduce the occurrence of complications. Similarly, intraoperative adjuncts such as cement augmentation, body warmers, radiofrequency cauterization devices, and intraoperative neurophysiologic monitoring can also mitigate surgical and hardware-related complications. Each patient should ultimately be evaluated on a case-by-case basis for the ideal treatment strategy.

References

1. Kakhki VR, Anvari K, Sadeghi R, et al. Pattern and distribution of bone metastases in common malignant tumors. *Nucl Med Rev Cent East Eur.* 2013;16(2):66–69.
2. Ortiz. Gomez JA. The incidence of vertebral body metastases. *Int Orthop.* 1995;19(5):309–311.
3. Laufer I, Rubin DG, Lis E, et al. The NOMS framework: approach to the treatment of spinal metastatic tumors. *Oncologist.* 2013;18(6):744–751.
4. Bilsky MH, Laufer I, Fourney DR, et al. Reliability analysis of the epidural spinal cord compression scale. *J Neurosurg Spine.* 2010;13(3):324–328.
5. Fisher CG, DiPaola CP, Ryken TC, et al. A novel classification system for spinal instability in neoplastic disease: an evidence-based approach and expert consensus from the Spine Oncology Study Group. *Spine.* 2010;35(22):E1221–E1229.
6. Fisher CG, Schouten R, Versteeg AL, et al. Reliability of the Spinal Instability Neoplastic Score (SINS) among radiation oncologists: an assessment of instability secondary to spinal metastases. *Radiat Oncol.* 2014;9:69.
7. Fisher CG, Versteeg AL, Schouten R, et al. Reliability of the spinal instability neoplastic scale among radiologists: an assessment of instability secondary to spinal metastases. *AJR Am J Roentgenol.* 2014;203(4):869–874.
8. Yamada Y, Katsoulakis E, Laufer I, et al. The impact of histology and delivered dose on local control of spinal metastases treated with stereotactic radiosurgery. *Neurosurg Focus.* 2017;42(1):E6.
9. Patchell RA, Tibbs PA, Regine WF, et al. Direct decompressive surgical resection in the treatment of spinal cord compression caused by metastatic cancer: a randomised trial. *Lancet.* 2005;366(9486):643–648.
10. Moussazadeh N, Laufer I, Yamada Y, et al. Separation surgery for spinal metastases: effect of spinal radiosurgery on surgical treatment goals. *Cancer Control.* 2014;21(2):168–174.
11. Nair S, Gobin YP, Leng LZ, et al. Preoperative embolization of hypervascular thoracic, lumbar, and sacral spinal column tumors: technique and outcomes from a single center. *Interv Neuroradiol.* 2013;19(3):377–385.
12. Robial N, Charles YP, Bogorin I, et al. Is preoperative embolization a prerequisite for spinal metastases surgical management? *Orthop Traumatol Surg Res.* 2012;98(5):536–542.
13. Prince EA, Ahn SH. Interventional management of vertebral body metastases. *Semin Intervent Radiol.* 2013;30(3):278–281.
14. Wilson MA, Cooke DL, Ghodke B, et al. Retrospective analysis of preoperative embolization of spinal tumors. *AJNR Am J Neuroradiol.* 2010;31(4):656–660.
15. Hong CG, Cho JH, Suh DC, et al. Preoperative embolization in patients with metastatic spinal cord compression: mandatory or optional? *World J Surg Oncol.* 2017;15(1):45.
16. Keam J, Bilsky MH, Laufer I, et al. No association between excessive wound complications and preoperative high-dose, hypofractionated, image-guided radiation therapy for spine metastasis. *J Neurosurg Spine.* 2014;20(4):411–420.
17. Kumar N, Zaw AS, Khine HE, et al. Blood loss and transfusion requirements in metastatic spinal tumor surgery: evaluation of influencing factors. *Ann Surg Oncol.* 2016;23(6):2079–2086.
18. Polderman KH. Mechanisms of action, physiological effects, and complications of hypothermia. *Crit Care Med.* 2009;37(suppl 7): S186–S202.
19. Ahn DK, Kim JH, Chang BK, et al. Can we prevent a postoperative spinal epidural hematoma by using larger diameter suction drains? *Clin Orthop Surg.* 2016;8(1):78–83.
20. Omeis IA, Dhir M, Sciubba DM, et al. Postoperative surgical site infections in patients undergoing spinal tumor surgery: incidence and risk factors. *Spine.* 2011;36(17):1410–1419.
21. Okafor R, Molinari W, Molinari R, et al. Intrawound vancomycin powder for spine tumor surgery. *Global Spine J.* 2016;6(3):207–211.
22. Mesfin A, Sciubba DM, Dea N, et al. Changing the adverse event profile in metastatic spine surgery: an evidence-based approach to target wound complications and instrumentation failure. *Spine.* 2016;41(suppl 20):S262–S270.
23. Sciubba DM, Goodwin CR, Yurter A, et al. A systematic review of clinical outcomes and prognostic factors for patients undergoing surgery for spinal metastases secondary to breast cancer. *Global Spine J.* 2016;6(5):482–496.
24. Chang DW, Friel MT, Youssef AA. Reconstructive strategies in soft tissue reconstruction after resection of spinal neoplasms. *Spine.* 2007;32(10):1101–1106.
25. Vitaz TW, Oishi M, Welch WC, et al. Rotational and transpositional flaps for the treatment of spinal wound dehiscence and infections in patient populations with degenerative and oncological disease. *J Neurosurg.* 2004;100(suppl 1 Spine):46–51.
26. Ghogawala Z, Mansfield FL, Borges LF. Spinal radiation before surgical decompression adversely affects outcomes of surgery for symptomatic metastatic spinal cord compression. *Spine.* 2001;26(7): 818–824.
27. Niu T, Lu DS, Yew A, et al. Postoperative cerebrospinal fluid leak rates with subfascial epidural drain placement after intentional durotomy in spine surgery. *Global Spine J.* 2016;6(8):780–785.
28. Epstein NE. When does a spinal surgeon need a plastic surgeon? *Surg Neurol Int.* 2013;4(suppl 5):S299–S300.
29. Amankulor NM, Xu R, Iorgulescu JB, et al. The incidence and patterns of hardware failure after separation surgery in patients with spinal metastatic tumors. *Spine J.* 2014;14(9):1850–1859.
30. Jang JS, Lee SH, Rhee CH, et al. Polymethylmethacrylate-augmented screw fixation for stabilization in metastatic spinal tumors. Technical note. *J Neurosurg.* 2002;96(suppl 1):131–134.
31. Frankel BM, Jones T, Wang C. Segmental polymethylmethacrylate-augmented pedicle screw fixation in patients with bone softening caused by osteoporosis and metastatic tumor involvement: a clinical evaluation. *Neurosurgery.* 2007;61(3):531–537, discussion 537–538.
32. Amendola L, Gasbarrini A, Fosco M, et al. Fenestrated pedicle screws for cement-augmented purchase in patients with bone softening: a review of 21 cases. *J Orthop Traumatol.* 2011;12(4): 193–199.
33. Sahgal A, Weinberg V, Ma L, et al. Probabilities of radiation myelopathy specific to stereotactic body radiation therapy to guide safe practice. *Int J Radiat Oncol Biol Phys.* 2013;85(2):341–347.
34. Sharma M, Bennett EE, Rahmathulla G, et al. Impact of cervicothoracic region stereotactic spine radiosurgery on adjacent organs at risk. *Neurosurg Focus.* 2017;42(1):E14.
35. Gibbs IC, Patil C, Gerszten PC, et al. Delayed radiation-induced myelopathy after spinal radiosurgery. *Neurosurgery.* 2009;64(suppl 2):A67–A72.

36. Iyer R, Jhingran A. Radiation injury: imaging findings in the chest, abdomen and pelvis after therapeutic radiation. *Cancer Imaging*. 2006;6:S131–S139.
37. Cox BW, Jackson A, Hunt M, et al. Esophageal toxicity from high-dose, single-fraction paraspinal stereotactic radiosurgery. *Int J Radiat Oncol Biol Phys*. 2012;83(5):e661–e667.
38. Burris HA 3rd, Hurtig J. Radiation recall with anticancer agents. *Oncologist*. 2010;15(11):1227–1237.
39. Boehling NS, Grosshans DR, Allen PK, et al. Vertebral compression fracture risk after stereotactic body radiotherapy for spinal metastases. *J Neurosurg Spine*. 2012;16(4):379–386.
40. Chang JH, Shin JH, Yamada YJ, et al. Stereotactic body radiotherapy for spinal metastases: what are the risks and how do we minimize them? *Spine*. 2016;41(suppl 20):S238–S245.

61 Spinal Fracture Complications

ROBERT F. HEARY, M. OMAR IQBAL

HIGHLIGHTS

- Traumatic spinal fractures are a leading cause of morbidity in the trauma patient.
- Spinal stability is defined as the ability of the spine to resist displacement of structures under physiologic loads so as to prevent injury or irritation to neural elements.
- The spine is divided into three regions with specific anatomic properties that must be considered in traumatic spinal fracture repair.
- The traumatic spine must be assessed and managed differently than degenerative pathology.
- The complications or sequelae of traumatic spinal fractures can be mitigated with appropriate preoperative and perioperative considerations for the trauma patient.
- The goal in the management of spinal fractures is the restoration of alignment, the preservation of neurologic function, and the mitigation of posttraumatic pain.

Background

Traumatic spinal fractures represent a minority of injuries seen in the trauma population, but they account for a substantial cost to the health care system and represent a burden on society.[1–3] Depending on the population studied, variation in the literature exists regarding the order of the common mechanisms of injury.[4,5] The most common mechanisms include motor vehicle accident and high-energy fall from a height. Injuries caused by violent assaults vary depending on the region of the United States that is studied. The character and location of injury to the spine correlate with the mechanism of injury. The thoracolumbar junction is the most common site of injury, comprising over 80% of all spinal traumas.[6] The highest number of complete motor and sensory neurologic deficits are found in cervical spine injuries. Prehospital immobilization and the early recognition and management of acute spinal fractures are critical to reduce the morbidity of this traumatic injury. Preoperative complications often result from failure to identify spinal fractures and/or ligamentous injuries, whereas postoperative complications often result in delayed instability after either conservative or operative treatment of spinal injuries resulting in posttraumatic kyphosis or delayed painful angulation of the posttraumatic spine.[7,8] Neurologic deficits can also occur and/or be detected in the postoperative period. As such, vigilance in the postoperative follow-up is necessary regardless of whether operative or nonoperative treatment was chosen.

Anatomic Insights

The spine is a complex structure that exists as a combination of three subsystems: (1) the vertebrae providing an osseous structural frame; (2) intervertebral discs, apophyseal joints, and ligaments providing dynamic support; and (3) the coordination of muscle response through neural control. Instability occurs with anatomic disruption by trauma or disease of any one or combination of these systems. Panjabi and White elegantly defined spinal stability as "the ability of the spine to resist displacement of vertebral structures under physiologic loads such that neither damage nor irritation to neural elements can occur, while also preventing the development of deformity or pain due to structural change" (Fig. 61.1).[9]

The spine is composed of 25 vertebrae further divided into three distinct regions, each with its own common size, orientation, and relationship to surrounding structures that contribute to the functionality of the axial skeleton: (1) cervical, (2) thoracic, and (3) lumbosacral segments.

The vertebrae are composed of an inner highly porous, cancellous bone and a dense outer cortical shell. The vertebral end plates provide an even distribution of mechanical loads, and prevent disc extrusion into the vertebral bodies. The posterior elements of the vertebrae include a neural arch and transverse, spinous, and articular processes (inferior and superior facets). The neural arch is a ringed structure with its anterior portion attached to the vertebral body (pedicles) and the posterior half (laminae). The superior articular process of the vertebra below and inferior articular process of the vertebra above comprise the facet joint of each motion segment and limit the extent of torsion and shear. The orientation of these facet joints changes, depending on the spinal region, thereby modulating their respective functions. Most of the axial load sharing occurs in the vertebral body and intervertebral discs, or anterior column, with 10% to 20% distributed posteriorly to the facet. This value can go to as high as 70% during hyperextension.[10] The transverse and spinous processes provide attachment points to ligaments and skeletal muscles that are responsible for spinal motion.

The intervertebral disc is composed of two parts: an inner gelatinous nucleus pulposus and an outer annulus fibrosis. The compressive loads are distributed across the gelatinous structure in between the vertebral bodies. Flexion and lateral bending result

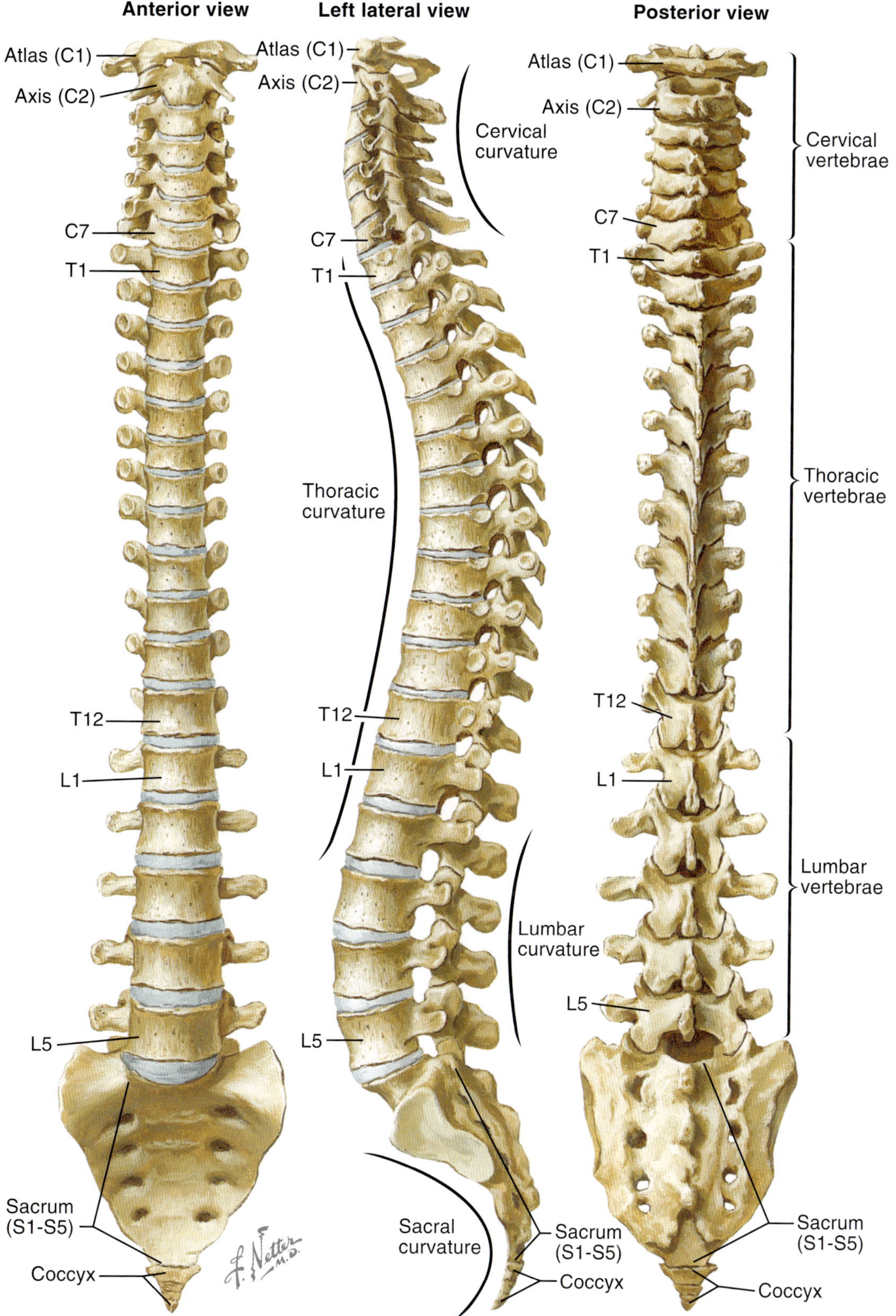

• **Fig. 61.1** Spinal anatomy. (H.R. Winn. *Youmans and Winn Neurological Surgery*. 7th ed. Philadelphia, PA: Elsevier; 2017. Fig. 273.1, p. 2260.)

in loading conditions that cause as much as a 50% increase in annulus deformation and that cause increases in nuclear pressure such that traumatic annulus tearing and subsequent herniation of the disc material can occur.[11]

Spinal ligaments provide low resistance to motion under physiologic loads, while distributing uniaxial tensile loads from one bone to another during loads beyond this range. These tasks are performed by seven subaxial spinal ligaments, which can be divided into intrasegmental systems that hold the functional spinal unit together and intersegmental systems that hold multiple vertebrae together. The posterior ligamentous complex (PLC) and paraspinal muscles form the posterior tension band of the spinal column that counterbalances the compressive force on the anterior column.

Cervical Spine

The occiput–C1 articulation is the most important segment involved in flexion-extension of the cervical spine (Fig. 61.2).[12] The occipital condyles articulate with the lateral masses of C1 to permit flexion and extension with limited rotation and lateral bending. There are several critical ligamentous structures at this segment that hold the occiput and cervical spine together; they are beyond the scope of this chapter. The hypoglossal nerve traverses the medial-superior aspect of each occipital condyle through the hypoglossal canal. As many as 40% of patients with occipital condyle fractures have lower cranial nerve injuries, primarily CN XII, some of which can develop in a delayed fashion.[13] Osseous and/or ligamentous fractures at this segment can lead to atlanto-occipital dissociation, which is frequently a fatal injury.

The atlas, or C1 vertebra, is the first of the cervical vertebrae and exists as a bony ring surrounding the spinal cord. The anterior and posterior arches are located anterior and posterior, respectively, to the lateral masses that articulate with the occiput. The vertebral arteries course laterally to the bony ring through the transverse foramina. A burst fracture that includes a fracture through both arches is known as a Jefferson fracture. Most of these fractures can be managed conservatively. The extent of ligamentous injury can be extrapolated by the overhang of the C1 lateral mass on C2. Although this threshold has recently come into question, a bilateral combined value of greater than 7 mm indicates a significant ligamentous disruption that implies instability requiring fixation at this level. This radiographic finding is known as the rule of Spence.[14]

C2 is composed of a vertebral body, the odontoid process or dens, and the foramen transversarium. The odontoid process is tightly held to the ventral portion of the C1 ring by the transverse atlantal ligament. The C1–C2 complex allows more rotation than any other spinal segment. This region accounts for approximately 50% of all rotation of the cervical spine. C2 fractures are classified as odontoid fractures (Types I–III), hangman's fractures (bilateral traumatic spondylolisthesis through the pars interarticularis), facet fractures, or injuries to the foramen transversarium. Between 50% and 70% of fractures at this level are odontoid fractures and are associated with other spine injuries in 34% of patients.[15] Anderson and D'Alonzo classified these fractures into three types.[16] Type I is a fracture through the upper part of the odontoid process, which likely results from an avulsion of one of the alar ligaments and is considered stable. Type II fractures represent nearly 70% of all odontoid fractures and occur at the junction between the odontoid process and the vertebral body.[15] These were later subclassified to account for treatment consequences of the subtle differences in fracture pattern.[17] These fractures are generally considered unstable; however, treatment remains controversial because many authors have reported significant healing with conservative measures. Type III odontoid fractures extend into the body of the axis and are often managed conservatively unless significant comminution and/or displacement occurs. Hangman's fractures, or bilateral traumatic spondylolisthesis through the pars interarticularis, are the second most common type of axis fractures. These fractures result from either axial loading from the skull—through the occipital condyles and the C1–C2 lateral masses, where they converge at the base of C2, passing through the weak pars interarticularis[18]—or from hyperextension and distraction (execution by hanging).[19]

The subaxial cervical spine spans from C3 to C7. The lordosis of the cervical spine affords greater mobility in this segment. The facet joint complex is coronally oriented and provides stability to the subaxial spine, and injury to the facet capsule or fracture can result in decreased biomechanical stability.[20] The PLC provides support during flexion-extension, whereas the facets support axial rotation as well as flexion and extension. Superior articulating facets transition from a posteromedial orientation at C3 to a posterolateral orientation at C7.[21] Facet fractures range from minor nondisplaced fractures to varying degrees of subluxations and dislocations. A variety of classification systems have been developed to describe subaxial cervical injuries with little consensus. The following subtypes of injury are based on the AOSpine system (Subaxial Cervical Spine Injury Classification System).[22] Compression injuries result in compression fractures, with or without retropulsion (burst) of the vertebral body and/or the spinous processes and laminae. Tension band injuries involve either the anterior or posterior tension band of the cervical spine. These injuries can include osseous and/or ligamentous structures. They involve fractures or disruptions through the vertebral body or disc with an intact posterior hinge that prevents displacement. Translational injuries result from displacement of one vertebral body over another in any direction, often resulting in vertebral body and/or posterior element fractures. The vertebral arteries are encased by the transverse foramina from C6 to C1. As such, fractures through the transverse foramina or hyperextension of the cervical spine can lead to blunt vascular injury.

Thoracic Spine

The thoracic spine is aligned in kyphosis and structurally rendered more rigid by the rib cage that articulates with it (Fig. 61.3). The mobility of the lordotic cervical spine meets the rigidity of the thoracic spine at the C7–T1 disc space, creating unique biomechanical properties of the cervico-thoracic junction that predispose this region to high-velocity injuries. The facets transition from a coronal orientation in the upper thoracic spine to a sagittal orientation in the lumbar spine. The apex of the thoracic kyphosis is at approximately the T8 vertebral level, which also corresponds to the narrowest cross-sectional area of the spinal canal.[23] The thoracolumbar junction (T10–L2) is another biomechanical transition zone from a stiff rostral kyphotic thoracic spine to a more flexible caudal lordotic lumbar spine, which predisposes this region to high-velocity injuries.

The Subaxial Cervical Spine Injury Classification (SLIC) system describes the morphology of upper thoracic spine fractures as well as those of the cervical spine; included are categories for compression, burst, distraction, and rotational-translational injuries. Compression injuries are due to axial loading and result in loss of height of the anterior column (a flexion teardrop fracture). High axial loading forces will disrupt the posterior wall of the vertebral bodies and result in burst fractures with retropulsion of bone

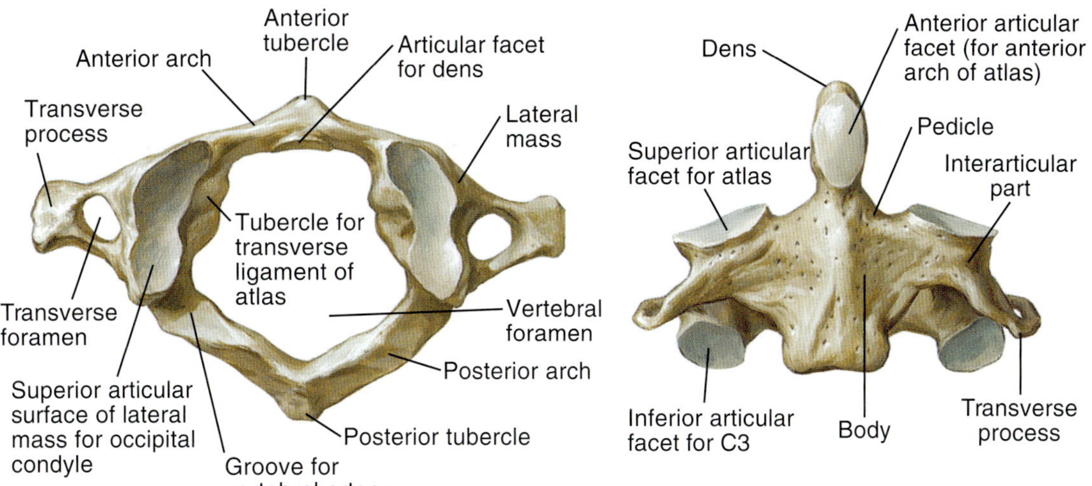
Anterior arch
Anterior tubercle
Articular facet for dens
Transverse process
Lateral mass
Tubercle for transverse ligament of atlas
Transverse foramen
Vertebral foramen
Posterior arch
Superior articular surface of lateral mass for occipital condyle
Posterior tubercle
Groove for vertebral artery
Atlas (C1): superior view
Dens
Anterior articular facet (for anterior arch of atlas)
Pedicle
Superior articular facet for atlas
Interarticular part
Inferior articular facet for C3
Body
Transverse process
Axis (C2): anterior view

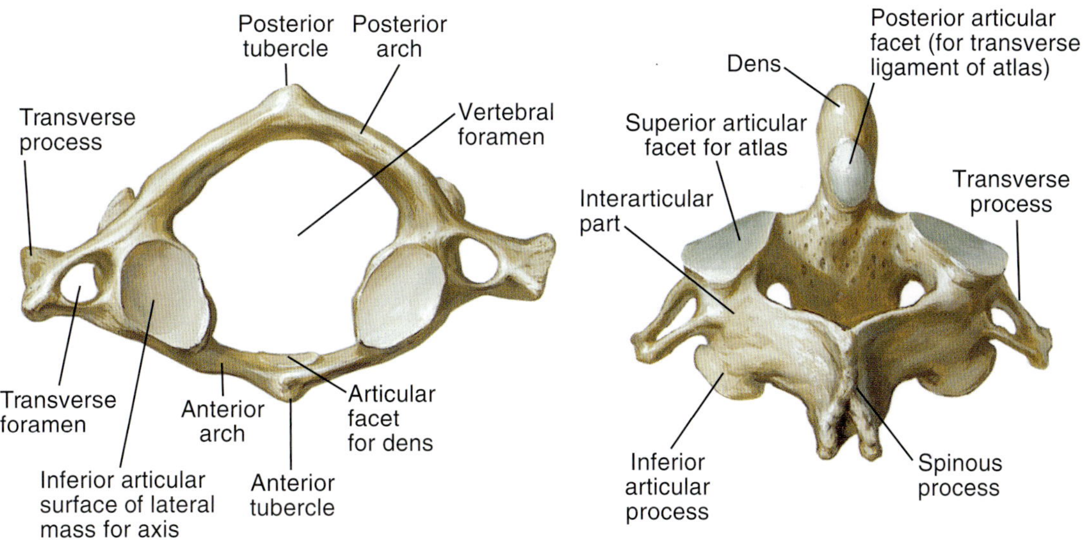
Posterior tubercle
Posterior arch
Transverse process
Vertebral foramen
Transverse foramen
Anterior arch
Articular facet for dens
Inferior articular surface of lateral mass for axis
Anterior tubercle
Atlas (C1): inferior view
Dens
Posterior articular facet (for transverse ligament of atlas)
Superior articular facet for atlas
Transverse process
Interarticular part
Inferior articular process
Spinous process
Axis (C2): posterosuperior view

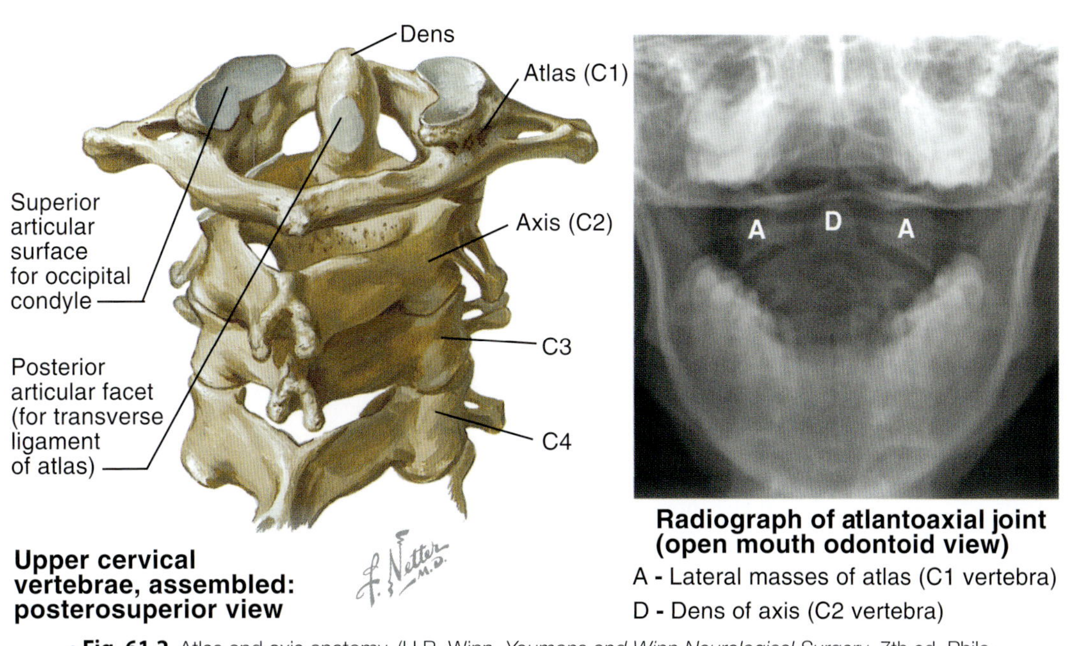
Dens
Atlas (C1)
Superior articular surface for occipital condyle
Axis (C2)
C3
Posterior articular facet (for transverse ligament of atlas)
C4
Upper cervical vertebrae, assembled: posterosuperior view
A
D
A
Radiograph of atlantoaxial joint (open mouth odontoid view)
A - Lateral masses of atlas (C1 vertebra)
D - Dens of axis (C2 vertebra)

• **Fig. 61.2** Atlas and axis anatomy. (H.R. Winn. *Youmans and Winn Neurological Surgery*. 7th ed. Philadelphia, PA: Elsevier; 2017. Fig. 273.2, p. 2261.)

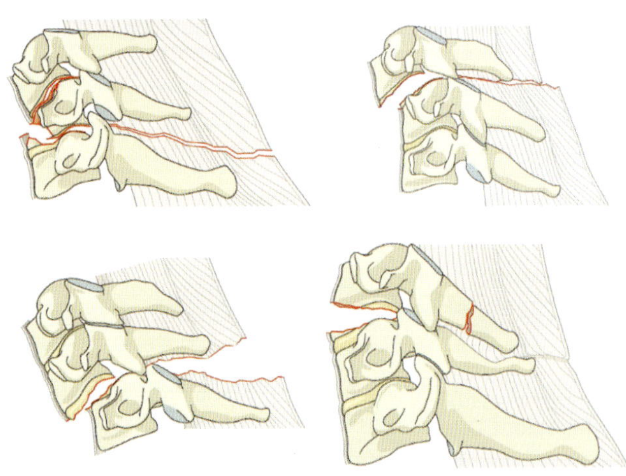

• **Fig. 61.3** Subluxation of cervical facet. (H.R. Winn. *Youmans and Winn Neurological Surgery*. 7th ed. Philadelphia, PA: Elsevier; 2017. Fig. 306.15, p. 2524.)

from the posterior aspect of the vertebral body into the spinal canal, which may cause significant neurologic injuries. Distraction injuries result from hyperextension of the thoracic spine, which may cause anterior ligamentous structures, including the anterior longitudinal ligament (ALL), to avulse the anterior inferior corner of the vertebral body, resulting in an extension teardrop fracture and a wider intervertebral space seen on imaging. Rotational-translational injuries are characterized by one vertebral body being rotated or translated beyond physiologic thresholds with respect to another. Unilateral and bilateral facet dislocations, floating lateral masses, and bilateral pedicle fractures are representative of this type of injury.

Lumbar Spine

The lumbar spine is distinguished by the largest vertebral bodies in the spine, which subserve the largest axial loads. The pedicles are robust and increase in angulation from 0 degrees at L1 to 30 degrees at L5. The transverse processes originate increasingly anteriorly at more caudal segments and are attached to ligaments in the rigid pelvis at the more caudal segments. High-velocity injuries including falls from a height make the transverse processes prone to fracture. The facets are sagittally oriented to facilitate flexion and extension along this highly mobile lordotic segment.

A variety of classification systems have been developed over time to describe different injury patterns in the lumbar spine.[24–26] The Thoracolumbar Injury Classification and Severity Score (TLICS) classifies injuries of the thoracolumbar junction and, by extension, the lumbar spine according to morphology, neurologic status, and integrity of the PLC to guide treatment decisions.[24,27] The morphology of fractures includes compression, burst, translation, and rotation. Compression fractures of the vertebral body are visualized as a loss of height on radiographic imaging. The presence of short tau inversion recovery (STIR) signal on magnetic resonance imaging (MRI) distinguishes acute from chronic fractures in the anterior column. Burst fractures are compression fractures with retropulsion of the vertebral bone dorsally into the spinal canal. Translation/rotation injuries are sustained by rotational forces applied simultaneously with a flexion movement at the thoracolumbar spine, leading to complete disruption of the PLC and extension through the anterior disc and vertebral body. These are often associated with facet fractures and are usually unstable. Fracture dislocations are defined by the translation of the cephalad vertebrae compared with the adjacent caudal vertebrae. The facets are often disarticulated or fractured, and displacement of the vertebral body can range from 10% to complete spondyloptosis. Another fracture pattern similar to flexion-distraction injuries is the eponymous Chance fracture. In this injury, the fracture line extends from the posterior spinous process through the pedicles, vertebral body, and the PLC. The injury primarily involves bone, but can occur through the soft tissues as a so-called "ligamentous Chance fracture" (Figs 61.4 and 61.5).

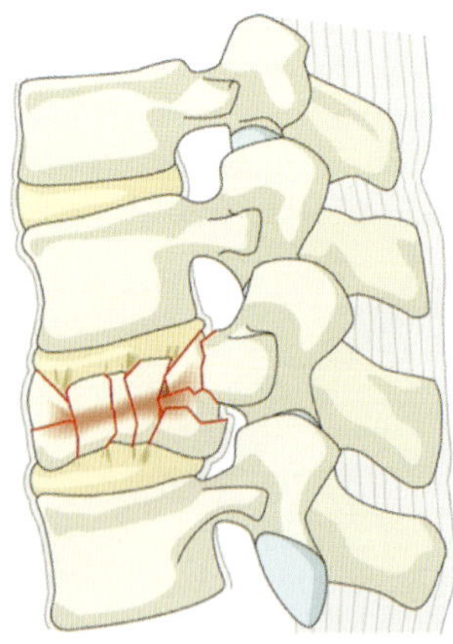

• **Fig. 61.4** Burst fracture. (H.R. Winn. *Youmans and Winn Neurological Surgery*. 7th ed. Philadelphia, PA: Elsevier; 2017. Table 309.3, 2542.)

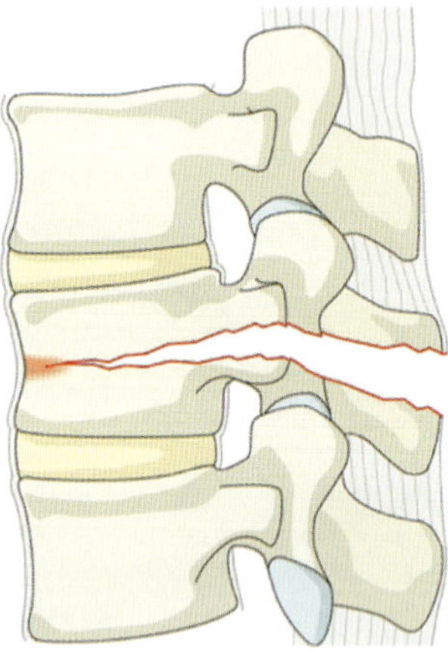

• **Fig. 61.5** Chance fracture. (H.R. Winn. *Youmans and Winn Neurological Surgery*. 7th ed. Philadelphia, PA: Elsevier; 2017. Table 309.3, p. 2542.)

The conus medullaris ends between T11 and L3, most often at the middle third of the L1 vertebra.[28] Distally, the conus gives rise to the cauda equina exiting as nerve roots at their respective neural foramen. The large number of nerve roots exiting at the level of the conus medullaris explains the mixed upper and lower motor neuron injuries that occur frequently in thoracolumbar trauma.

RED FLAGS

- Condylar-cervical interval greater than 4 mm—Atlanto-occipital dislocation (AOD)
- Greater than 7-mm displacement laterally of C1 on C2—Transverse ligament disruption

- Fracture through transverse foramen of cervical spine—Vertebral artery injury
- C7 spinous process fracture (clay shoveler's)—Facet fracture or unilateral jumped facet
- High-velocity bony injury in thoracolumbar junction carries 25% risk for spinal cord injury and 30% risk for intraabdominal injury.[42]
- High-velocity bony injuries of thoracolumbar junction have an associated 50% risk of neurologic injury.[43]
- Smoking, diabetes mellitus, steroid use—Risk of nonunion
- Spondyloarthropathies including diffuse idiopathic skeletal hyperostosis (DISH) and ankylosing spondylitis
- Age >60, neurologic deficit, polytrauma, and spondylosis are all associated with having additional clinically relevant MRI findings.[40,41]
- Incompetence of PLC is inferred through splaying or avulsion fractures of spinous processes, widening of facet joints, disruption in ligamentum flavum or posterior longitudinal ligament on MRI, and interspinous edema.
- Risk of orthosis noncompliance in young males with risk-taking behavior
- Four main causes of incorrect primary therapy: nonobservance of anatomy and function of the spine, incorrect appraisal of injury, inadequate primary therapy, and mistakes in surgical technique or tactics.[39]

Prevention of Complications

A. *Preoperative Prevention*

The prevention of complications from spinal fractures begins at the prehospital level with emergency medical services (EMS). Clinical evidence reveals that EMS technicians can be trained to identify spinal injuries and to immobilize to a level similar to that of emergency medicine physicians. Current recommendations include the use of a cervical collar, head immobilization, and a spinal board in appropriately triaged patients to prevent secondary neurologic injuries from spinal trauma.[29] Once the patient arrives in the trauma bay, it is critical to achieve and maintain stable hemodynamic parameters to optimize spinal cord perfusion. All patients with suspected spinal cord injury must get appropriate imaging, which in 2017 includes computed tomography (CT) scanning of the cervical, thoracic, and lumbar spines with coronal and sagittal reformatted images.[30,31] After a thorough physical examination and review of imaging, the injury must be classified according to SLIC for subaxial cervical spine or the TLICS system for thoracolumbar fractures. If a cervical facet subluxation is found, reduction should be attempted as soon as possible with preoperative traction in the trauma bay or radiology suite. If unsuccessful, intraoperative traction during definitive fixation will be necessary.

B. *Perioperative Prevention*

Perioperative prevention includes appropriate decision-making regarding the surgical plan. Absolute indications for surgery include progressive neurologic compromise and catastrophic instability. Failure to appropriately address the instability will result in a pseudarthrosis, or bony nonunion, or instrumentation failure. An instrumented construct that is not long enough, for example, may result in postoperative kyphosis.[32] Certain operative approaches are favored for specific pathology. For example, for retropulsed fragments in the canal, some authors argue an anterior, retroperitoneal approach is the most effective at achieving neural decompression.[33–35] Others have studied anteroposterior versus posterolateral decompression and instrumented fusion and found no statistical difference in radiologic and functional outcomes in the treatment of thoracolumbar burst fractures.[36] The essential point is that, regardless of the orientation for the approach, the spinal canal must be adequately decompressed to place the neural elements in an ideal environment for recovery while preserving the long-term stability of the spine in the process. Appropriate positioning while maintaining inline stability of the spine is critical when flipping a patient prone for posterior approaches.

The assessment and management of traumatic spinal fractures is very different from that of degenerative pathology. The traumatic spine is often misaligned, whereas the degenerative spine often maintains normal alignment. This is an important distinction to make because this will help determine which approach one should take in restoring normal alignment. An advantage of correcting traumatic injuries is the greater likelihood of young males, who typically have strong bones, being involved, which provides some benefits for both fixation and deformity correction. Traumatic spinal fractures often result in subluxation, rotation, and/or translational injuries that must be identified and addressed. The length of construct will have to be appropriate to achieve and maintain sagittal alignment. When operating on the traumatized spine, one should also expect to encounter distorted anatomy during surgery. A thorough review of the preoperative imaging, followed by formulation and then execution of a surgical plan with alternative options if further instability or comminution is encountered during surgery, is paramount to a successful operation.

A successful and timely fusion is also critical to the successful treatment of traumatic spinal fractures. We strongly advocate the use of autologous iliac crest bone graft in the treatment of patients with trauma and polytrauma. The excellent fusion rate and time to fusion conferred by autologous iliac crest bone graft afford patients with traumatic instability a favorable chance at fusion, with earlier return to work and sooner removal of any external orthoses. The morbidity of donor site pain is well reported in the literature, with 3% of patients reporting unacceptable long-term pain.[37]

After surgery, we do advocate use of an orthosis in the traumatic spine fracture patient. Instrumentation will reduce micro-motion, whereas a spinal orthosis will reduce macro-motion of the healing construct and provide an optimal chance for fusion. The orthosis will also have a psychological impact on the patients, their families, and their caretakers, by reminding the patient that he or she has had surgery on the spine, thereby reducing aggressive or excessive activity.

Sequelae of Spinal Fractures

- Spinal infection
- Progressive neurologic deficit or other spinal cord injury
- Spinal deformity resulting in abnormal gait or posture
- Malplaced instrumentation and/or pseudarthrosis
- Persistent or worsening axial pain

The most common complication after conservative or operative management of spinal injury is posttraumatic kyphosis or delayed painful angulation of the posttraumatic spine.[7,8] Posttraumatic kyphosis often results from flexion-compression injuries to the anterior column and can occur at any level, although most commonly at the thoracolumbar junction. Altered sagittal alignment results in stress on facets and intervertebral shear, and it potentiates instability, thereby accelerating degenerative processes. Severe spinal cord injury can result in neuropathic spinal arthropathy (Charcot spine), producing pain and instability. Persistent pain will occur in as many as 94% of patients with delayed posttraumatic kyphotic deformity.[38] A localized kyphotic deformity of greater than 30 degrees is associated with chronic continued pain in the area of kyphosis.[8] Progressive neurologic deficit can occur in as many as 27% of patients with posttraumatic deformity; these deficits include bowel and bladder dysfunction, progressive extremity weakness, and sensory dysesthesias. Traumatic spinal fracture leading to complete spinal cord injury is, of course, the worst complication on the spectrum of injury.

Unfortunately, postoperative infections are not uncommon in the setting of polytrauma. Patients with polytrauma may have other sources of infection; for example, as a result of abdominal viscera penetration, or as a result of a foreign body having contact with the instrumented construct. Furthermore, the increased cortisol levels secondary to the stress response diminish the immune system and the ability to fight infection. In our own experience at a Level 1 trauma center, the postoperative infection rates have been substantially higher on polytrauma patients than in routine elective cases for degenerative disease.

Malpositioned instrumentation in corrective surgery for traumatic deformity is a potential complication after treatment for traumatic spinal fractures. As mentioned earlier, the alignment may be compromised with multilevel spinal injury, and failure to address the malalignment may result in malpositioned instrumentation if the deformity is not reduced appropriately. In addition, comminuted fractures may distort normal anatomy and lead to poorly placed spinal instrumentation such as pedicle screws.

Management

Assessment of delayed posttraumatic instability includes imaging modalities not otherwise employed in the acute setting of initial injury. When a patient presents for evaluation of a delayed posttraumatic complication from surgery or conservative management, it is imperative that a new set of imaging is obtained at the time of presentation to the office to establish a reference point from which the problem can then be assessed and managed. We have routinely obtained postoperative CT scans in the immediate postoperative period for the past 2+ decades. This allows us to compare any changes in alignment, at a delayed time point, with the appearance in the immediate postoperative period. Standing 36-in.-long cassette radiographs can be utilized to assess for global and regional alignment. Flexion/extension radiographs are used to assess for fixed or dynamic instability. Fine-cut (<3 mm) CT slices or, alternatively, CT-myelography in the setting of prior instrumentation can be used to determine central and foraminal neural compression, pseudarthrosis, and other instrumentation failure. MRI aids in assessing soft tissue structures including facet capsules, PLC, and the spinal cord, and aids in assessing the adjacent levels above and below the fixated segments. It is essential to preoperatively determine tethering, neural compression, or syrinx formation to avoid iatrogenic injuries.[39] Electrophysiology may be used as an adjunct to confirm radicular pathology when imaging is equivocal. After sufficient characterization of the posttraumatic injury, an appropriate operative plan can be determined with the goals of alleviating pain, preventing further neurologic injury, and restoring anatomic alignment. An important tenet to consider when performing revision surgery is to change the approach from the index operation. One should not assume that the failure of the first operation is from the technique of the initial surgeon. Instead, doing something different the second time around after rethinking the problem is often the better thing to do.

SURGICAL REWIND

My Worst Case

A 32-year-old male presented with intractable back pain. He had a fall from a height in Central America at the age of 16 years and was treated "conservatively" for an L2 burst fracture. He was unemployable due to severe pain resulting from a kyphotic deformity. At the time of his initial evaluation, he was found to have a chronic L2 burst fracture with kyphosis measuring 47 degrees from the top of L1 to the bottom of L3 (Fig. 61.6).

He underwent a pedicle subtraction osteotomy (PSO) with stabilization from T12 to L4 using a bilateral pedicle screw construct with correction of the kyphotic deformity. He recovered very well from the surgery until postoperative day 3, when he got out of bed in a thoraco-lumbo-sacral orthosis (TLSO) brace and lost sensation and motor power from the waist downward.

A STAT CT-myelogram was performed that demonstrated a complete block of the myelographic dye at the L3 pedicle level. His alignment on the post-myelographic CT scan showed an 18-degree lordosis from L1 to L3 (a 65-degree correction of sagittal alignment compared with his preoperative imaging).

He was immediately returned to the operating room, where laminectomies of L1 and L3 were performed (Fig. 61.7). At the index surgery, a laminectomy of L2 had been performed with modest laminotomies of the inferior aspect of the L1 lamina and the superior aspect of the L3 lamina.

During the revision surgery, all nerves were noted to be freed of any compression, and the dura was "unkinked." The instrumentation construct was not modified.

On emerging from anesthesia, he demonstrated movement and sensation in both lower extremities. Neurologic improvement was rapid over the next 3 days back to his baseline preoperative levels.

At 2 years postoperatively, he was neurologically intact and pain free. Plain film radiographs showed solid fusions from T12 to L4 with no lucencies or instrumentation issues noted (Figs 61.8 and 61.9).

Ten years after surgery, at age 42, he remains pain free and neurologically intact. He had become employed, for the first time in his life, at age 35 years (3 years postoperatively) in a housekeeping job that he was continuing to work at 10 years after surgery.

Teaching point: If a PSO is performed, a correction of approximately 35 degrees can be expected for a single level. In the case presented, the laminae of L1 and L3 apposed each other and blocked visualization of the spinal dura. At the time of the emergency revision surgery, clear kinking of the dura was identified and able to be released. In the future, if greater than 40 degrees of correction is obtained during a PSO procedure, performing an additional level of posterior decompression above and below the index level should be strongly considered.

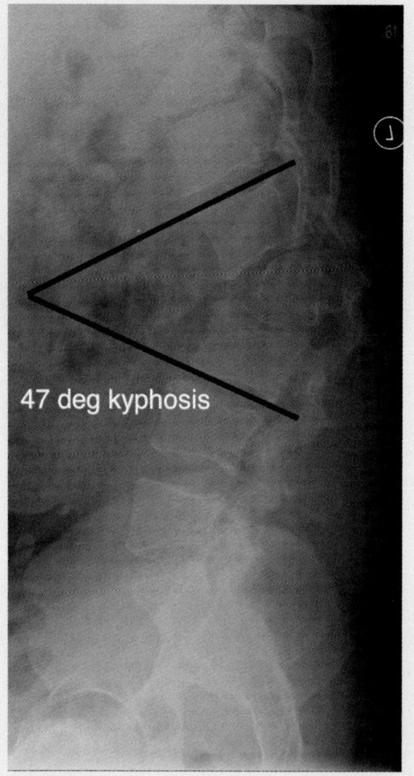

• **Fig. 61.6** Preoperative lateral lumbar x-ray.

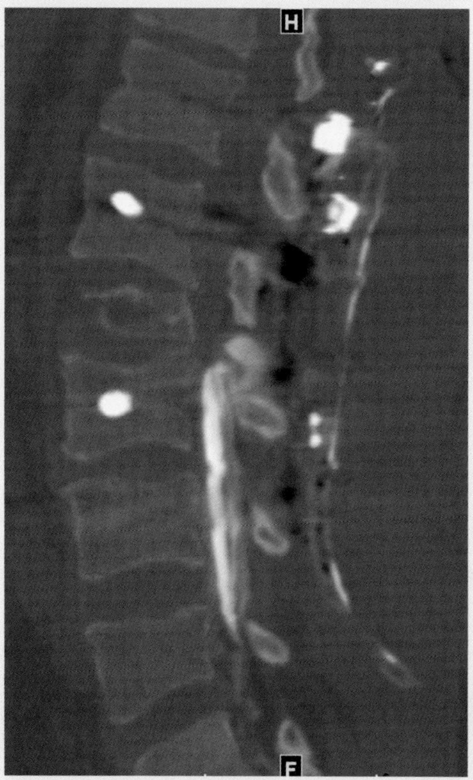

• **Fig. 61.7** Sagittal computed tomography myelogram.

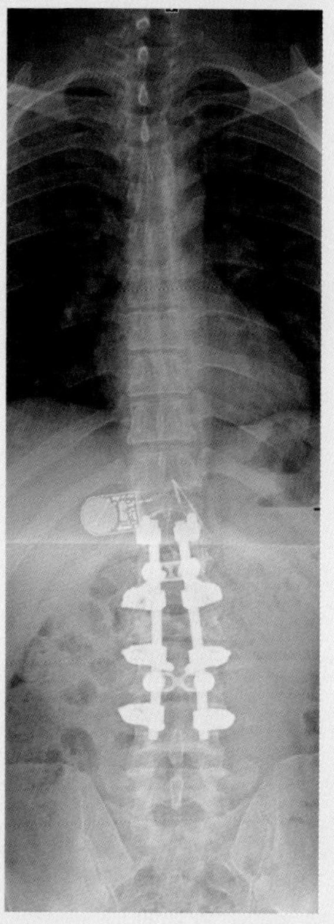

• **Fig. 61.8** Postoperative AP scoliosis series x-ray.

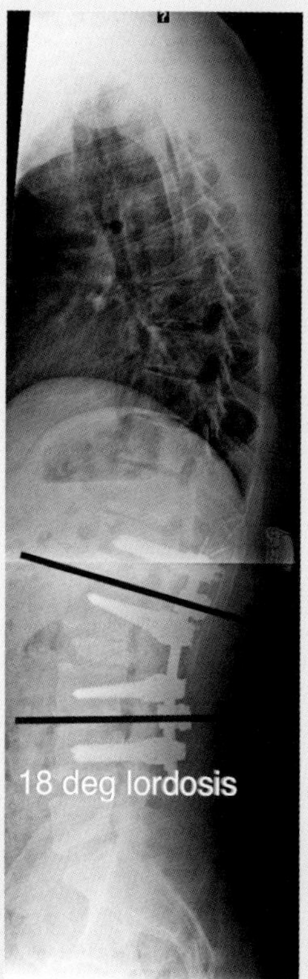

• **Fig. 61.9** Postoperative lateral scoliosis series x-ray.

NEUROSURGICAL SELFIE MOMENT

Traumatic spinal fractures must be assessed and managed differently from other spinal pathology, including degenerative, neoplastic, or infectious. Establishing stability, restoring alignment, and decompressing neural elements are critical to the successful repair of spinal fractures. Patients with polytrauma should receive special consideration in terms of infection prophylaxis, instrumentation positioning, and fusion techniques. Management of posttraumatic spinal fracture complications begins with fresh imaging, comparison with the immediate postoperative images, and characterization of the problem followed by a new approach at an operative solution when feasible.

References

1. Rivara FP, Grossman DC, Cummings P. Injury prevention. *NEJM*. 1997;337(8):543–548.
2. Sekhon LH, Fehlings MG. Epidemiology, demographics, and pathophysiology of acute spinal cord injury. *Spine*. 2001;26(24 suppl):S2–S12.
3. Vaccaro AR, Lin S, Balderston RA, Cotier JM, An HS, Sun S. Noncontiguous injuries of the spine. *J Spinal Disord*. 1992;5(3): 320–329.
4. El-Faramawy A, El-Menyar A, Zarour A, et al. Presentation and outcome of traumatic spinal fractures. *J Emerg Trauma Shock*. 2012;5(4):316–320.
5. Wang H, Zhang Y, Xiang Q, et al. Epidemiology of traumatic spinal fractures: experience from medical university–affiliated hospitals in Chongqing, China, 2001–2010. *J Neurosurg Spine*. 2012;17(5): 459–468.
6. Wang H, Liu X, Zhao Y, et al. Incidence and pattern of traumatic spinal fractures and associated spinal cord injury resulting from motor vehicle collisions in China over 11 years: An observational study. *Medicine (Baltimore)*. 2016;95(43):e5220.
7. Khoueir P, Oh BC, Wang MY. Delayed posttraumatic thoracolumbar spinal deformities: diagnosis and management. *Neurosurgery*. 2008;63(3 suppl):117–124.
8. Schoenfeld AJ, Wood KB, Fisher CF, et al. Posttraumatic kyphosis: current state of diagnosis and treatment: results of a multinational survey of spine trauma surgeons. *J Spinal Disord Tech*. 2010;23(7):e1–e8.
9. Panjabi MM, White AA 3rd. Basic biomechanics of the spine. *Neurosurgery*. 1980;7(1):76–93.
10. Lorenz M, Patwardhan A, Vanderby R Jr. Load-bearing characteristics of lumbar facets in normal and surgically altered spinal segments. *Spine*. 1983;8(2):122–130.
11. Adams MA, Dolan P. Recent advances in lumbar spinal mechanics and their clinical significance. *Clin Biomech (Bristol, Avon)*. 1995;10(1):3–19.
12. Goel ACF. *The craniovertebral junction: diagnosis, pathology, surgical techniques*. Stuttgart: Theime; 2011.
13. Anderson PA, Montesano PX. Morphology and treatment of occipital condyle fractures. *Spine*. 1988;13(7):731–736.
14. Spence KF Jr, Decker S, Sell KW. Bursting atlantal fracture associated with rupture of the transverse ligament. *J Bone Joint Surg Am*. 1970;52(3):543–549.
15. Greene KA, Dickman CA, Marciano FF, Drabier JB, Hadley MN, Sonntag VK. Acute axis fractures. Analysis of management and outcome in 340 consecutive cases. *Spine*. 1997;22(16):1843–1852.
16. Anderson LD, D'Alonzo RT. Fractures of the odontoid process of the axis. *J Bone Joint Surg Am*. 1974;56(8):1663–1674.
17. Grauer JN, Shafi B, Hilibrand AS, et al. Proposal of a modified, treatment-oriented classification of odontoid fractures. *Spine J*. 2005;5(2):123–129.
18. Schneider RC, Livingston KE, Cave AJ, Hamilton G. "Hangman's fracture" of the cervical spine. *J Neurosurg*. 1965;22:141–154.
19. Wood-Jones F. The ideal lesion produced by judicial hanging. *Lancet*. 1913;181(4662):53.
20. Nadeau M, McLachlin SD, Bailey SI, Gurr KR, Dunning CE, Bailey CS. A biomechanical assessment of soft-tissue damage in the cervical spine following a unilateral facet injury. *J Bone Joint Surg Am*. 2012;94(21):e156.
21. Panjabi MM, Oxland T, Takata K, Goel V, Duranceau J, Krag M. Articular facets of the human spine. Quantitative three-dimensional anatomy. *Spine*. 1993;18(10):1298–1310.
22. Vaccaro AR, Koerner JD, Radcliff KE, et al. AOSpine subaxial cervical spine injury classification system. *Eur Spine J*. 2016;25(7):2173–2184.
23. Ko HY, Park JH, Shin YB, Baek SY. Gross quantitative measurements of spinal cord segments in human. *Spinal Cord*. 2004;42(1): 35–40.
24. Bono CM, Vaccaro AR, Hurlbert RJ, et al. Validating a newly proposed classification system for thoracolumbar spine trauma: looking to the future of the thoracolumbar injury classification and severity score. *J Orthop Trauma*. 2006;20(8):567–572.
25. Dai LY, Jin WJ. Interobserver and intraobserver reliability in the load sharing classification of the assessment of thoracolumbar burst fractures. *Spine*. 2005;30(3):354–358.
26. McCormack T, Karaikovic E, Gaines RW. The load sharing classification of spine fractures. *Spine*. 1994;19(15):1741–1744.
27. Patel AA, Vaccaro AR, Albert TJ, et al. The adoption of a new classification system: time-dependent variation in interobserver reliability of the thoracolumbar injury severity score classification system. *Spine*. 2007;32(3):E105–E110.
28. Soleiman J, Demaerel P, Rocher S, Maes F, Marchal G. Magnetic resonance imaging study of the level of termination of the conus medullaris and the thecal sac: influence of age and gender. *Spine*. 2005;30(16):1875–1880.
29. Ahn H, Singh J, Nathens A, et al. Pre-hospital care management of a potential spinal cord injured patient: a systematic review of the literature and evidence-based guidelines. *J Neurotrauma*. 2010;28(8): 1341–1361.
30. Como JJ, Diaz JJ, Dunham CM, et al. Practice management guidelines for identification of cervical spine injuries following trauma: update from the eastern association for the surgery of trauma practice management guidelines committee. *J Trauma*. 2009;67(3): 651–659.
31. Sixta S, Moore FO, Ditillo MF, et al. Screening for thoracolumbar spinal injuries in blunt trauma: an Eastern Association for the Surgery of Trauma practice management guideline. *J Trauma Acute Care Surg*. 2012;73(5 suppl 4):S326–S332.
32. Keene JS, Lash EG, Kling TF Jr. Undetected posttraumatic instability of "stable" thoracolumbar fractures. *J Orthop Trauma*. 1988;2(3):202–211.
33. McAfee PC, Bohlman HH, Yuan HA. Anterior decompression of traumatic thoracolumbar fractures with incomplete neurological deficit using a retroperitoneal approach. *J Bone Joint Surg Am*. 1985;67(1):89–104.
34. McDonough PW, Davis R, Tribus C, Zdeblick TA. The management of acute thoracolumbar burst fractures with anterior corpectomy and Z-plate fixation. *Spine*. 2004;29(17):1901–1908, discussion 1909.
35. Schnee CL, Ansell LV. Selection criteria and outcome of operative approaches for thoracolumbar burst fractures with and without neurological deficit. *J Neurosurg*. 1997;86(1):48–55.
36. Lin B, Chen ZW, Guo ZM, Liu H, Yi ZK. Anterior approach versus posterior approach with subtotal corpectomy, decompression, and reconstruction of spine in the treatment of thoracolumbar burst fractures: a prospective randomized controlled study. *J Spinal Disord Tech*. 2011.
37. Heary RF, Schlenk RP, Sacchieri TA, Barone D, Brotea C. Persistent iliac crest donor site pain: independent outcome assessment. *Neurosurgery*. 2002;50(3):510–516, discussion 516–517.
38. Malcolm BW, Bradford DS, Winter RB, Chou SN. Post-traumatic kyphosis. A review of forty-eight surgically treated patients. *J Bone Joint Surg Am*. 1981;63(6):891–899.

39. Harms J, Stoltze D. The indications and principles of correction of post-traumatic deformities. *Eur Spine J*. 1992;1(3):142–151.
40. Pourtaheri S, Emami A, Sinha K, et al. The role of magnetic resonance imaging in acute cervical spine fractures. *Spine J*. 2014;14(11):2546–2553.
41. Vaccaro AR, Hulbert RJ, Patel AA, et al. The subaxial cervical spine injury classification system: a novel approach to recognize the importance of morphology, neurology, and integrity of the disco-ligamentous complex. *Spine*. 2007;32(21):2365–2374.
42. Chapman JR, Agel J, Jurkovich GJ, Bellabarba C. Thoracolumbar flexion-distraction injuries: associated morbidity and neurological outcomes. *Spine*. 2008;33(6):648–657.
43. Saboe LA, Reid DC, Davis LA, Warren SA, Grace MG. Spine trauma and associated injuries. *J Trauma*. 1991;31(1):43–48.

62

Posttraumatic Syringomyelia

RASHAD JABARKHEEL, SIRAJ GIBANI, YI-REN CHEN, JOHN K. RATLIFF

HIGHLIGHTS

- Posttraumatic syringomyelia is a syrinx that forms within the spinal cord in a delayed fashion after spinal cord injury due to impaired cerebrospinal fluid flow.
- Posttraumatic syringomyelia is an underappreciated complication after spinal cord injury. Among spinal cord injury patients, 1% to 9% report symptomatic syringomyelia, and another 21% to 28% have a syrinx on magnetic resonance imaging.
- The degree of spinal stenosis after initial spinal cord injury is associated with increased risk of developing posttraumatic syringomyelia.
- Prevention of posttraumatic syringomyelia in spinal cord injury patients depends on successful decompression and restoration of cerebrospinal fluid flow after initial injury. Avoidance of activities that increase venous pressure may be helpful.
- Magnetic resonance imaging is the imaging modality of choice for detecting syringomyelia.
- Surgical treatment of posttraumatic syringomyelia is indicated for patients with new symptoms of progressive neurologic deterioration.
- Initial surgical management of posttraumatic syringomyelia is arachnoidolysis. Characteristics of the syrinx determined either preoperatively or intraoperatively may indicate the need for shunting.
- Intraoperative ultrasonography is useful in detecting subarachnoid adhesions.
- The rate of reoperation for posttraumatic syringomyelia is high. Spinal cord traction and bleeding during surgery may lead to recurrent arachnoid adhesions.

Background

Syringomyelia is a broad term that is used to describe a condition in which a syrinx forms within the spinal cord resulting from disruption to normal cerebrospinal fluid (CSF) flow. This may lead to progressive myelopathy. As described by Milhorat, there are many different types of syringomyelia depending on the location of the syrinx within the spinal cord and the underlying etiology.[1] In the case of the most common type of syringomyelia, associated with Chiari I malformations, CSF flow is disrupted by the protrusion of the cerebellar tonsils through the foramen magnum. The protrusion of the cerebellar tonsils occludes the subarachnoid space at the level of the foramen magnum and leads to increased cervical CSF pulse pressure waves. Over time this leads to the formation of a syrinx within the central canal as the walls of the central canal struggle to tolerate the higher than normal CSF pressures.[2] Approximately 12% to 22.9% of patients with a Chiari I malformation develop a syrinx on magnetic resonance imaging (MRI).[3] The syrinxes seen with Chiari I malformations are described as noncommunicating central canal syrinxes, meaning that they are cystic dilations of the central canal in which the syrinx does not communicate with the fourth ventricle.

Posttraumatic syringomyelia describes a condition in which a syrinx forms within the spinal cord after spinal cord injury. Syrinx formation often results in progressive myelopathy. In contrast to syringomyelia due to Chiari malformations, posttraumatic syringomyelia generally consists of noncommunicating extracanalicular syrinxes, with cystic dilations of the spinal cord that are outside of the central canal.[1] In posttraumatic syringomyelia the cause of obstruction to CSF flow is not at the level of the foramen magnum, in contrast to the more common Chiari malformation, but instead at the site of the initial spinal cord injury. Specifically, in posttraumatic syringomyelia there is obstruction of CSF flow at the site of initial trauma due to increased subarachnoid adhesions and narrowing of the subarachnoid space due to scarring from the initial trauma. This obstruction to CSF flow at the level of the initial trauma results in increased CSF pulse pressure in the subarachnoid space.

According to the intramedullary pulse pressure theory, the increased CSF pulse pressure leads to the formation of a syrinx as the CSF flow is diverted by (1) traveling through Rudolf-Virchow spaces into the parenchyma of the spinal cord and (2) passing through the narrowing of the subarachnoid space with an increased velocity and decreased pressure due to Bernoulli's equation. The CSF flow into the spinal cord contributes to the formation of a syrinx by directly increasing the extracellular fluid within the cord. The CSF that flows along the outside of the cord past the narrowing contributes to the formation of a syrinx by decreasing the pressure on the outside of the cord and thus allowing it to balloon from within (Fig. 62.1).[4]

Posttraumatic syringomyelia typically presents in a delayed fashion from months to decades after spinal cord injury.[5] The symptoms of posttraumatic syringomyelia typically progress gradually. Rarely, sudden deterioration has also been reported.[6] The most common presenting symptoms are pain and sensory loss followed by motor weakness. Pain is typically intermittent at or above the level of the initial injury and may be described as burning, dull, or aching. Coughing, sneezing, and straining often exacerbate the pain due to increased venous pressure.[7–9] Sensory loss is also typically at or above the level of the initial injury and can come in a variety of forms, from a combination of loss of pain and temperature sensation, to a combination of loss of pain and proprioception.[5] Motor weakness typically begins after symptoms of sensory loss and presents as new loss of motor function above the level of previous injury.[6] New loss of deep tendon reflexes may be an early sign of posttraumatic syringomyelia.[5]

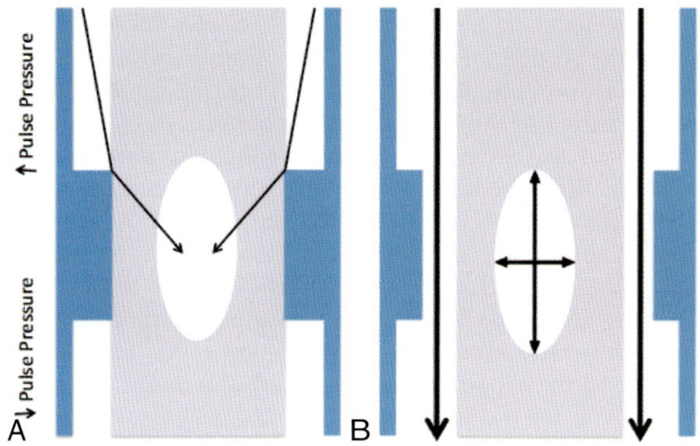

• **Fig. 62.1** *Intramedullary Pulse Pressure Theory*. Narrowing of the subarachnoid space causes an increase in the cerebrospinal fluid (CSF) pulse pressure superiorly. CSF flow is diverted near this area of narrowing either by traveling through Rudolf-Virchow spaces into the parenchyma of the spinal cord as seen in (A), or by passing through the narrowing with an increased velocity due to Bernoulli's equation as seen in (B). The CSF flow into the spinal cord contributes to the formation of a syrinx by directly increasing the extracellular fluid within the cord. The CSF that flows along the outside of the cord past the narrowing contributes to the formation of a syrinx by decreasing the pressure on the outside of the cord and thus allowing the cord to balloon from within. (Figure adapted from Greitz D. Unraveling the riddle of syringomyelia. *Neurosurgical review.* 2006;29(4):251-263; discussion 64.)

Posttraumatic syringomyelia is underappreciated as a source of morbidity after spinal cord injury. According to the National Spinal Cord Injury Database, between 183,000 and 230,000 individuals in the United States live with spinal cord injury. In this population, between 1% and 9% report symptomatic syringomyelia. Between 1 and 30 years after injury, 21% to 28% will be found to have a syrinx, and another 30% to 50% will have some degree of spinal cystic change.[6]

Anatomic Insight

Syrinxes associated with posttraumatic syringomyelia are often irregular in shape and can occur anywhere along the spinal cord depending on the location and extent of the initial spinal cord injury. Most syrinxes are located near the initial trauma site with approximately 4% extending caudally, 81% rostrally, and 15% in both directions.[5] Notably, posttraumatic syrinxes can communicate directly with the CSF in the subarachnoid space if found near the ventromedian fissure or a dorsal nerve root entry zone.[10] Most posttraumatic syrinxes are found in the central and dorsolateral gray matter, whereas approximately 9% are found solely in the dorsal columns.[6] In terms of size, the average syrinx length is between 6.5 and 7.8 spinal segments long.[9,11]

RED FLAGS

- Patients may have a progressing syrinx but no symptoms if they have already lost neurologic function in that area from their initial injury.
- Asymptomatic syringomyelia must be monitored to avoid progression into the brainstem and, consequently, syringobulbia.
- Excess spinal cord traction and bleeding during surgery for initial spinal cord injury may lead to arachnoid adhesions and, consequently, posttraumatic syringomyelia.

Risk Factors

Perrouin-Verbe et al. found a strong correlation between the degree of spinal canal stenosis after injury and the risk of developing posttraumatic syringomyelia.[9] Schurch et al. and Abel et al. similarly found that the degree of cord compression and kyphosis at the site of injury was associated with an increased risk of developing posttraumatic syringomyelia.[12,13] Another positive risk factor for posttraumatic syringomyelia is the severity of the initial injury. In a retrospective analysis of 600 patients with posttraumatic syringomyelia, Edgar and Quail found that 82% of their patients had a complete spinal cord injury, much higher than the approximately 47% found in the overall spinal cord injury population.[14] Similarly, el Masry and Biyani found the incidence of posttraumatic syringomyelia to be twice as high in patients with complete spinal cord injury as compared with patients with incomplete injury.[15,16]

In terms of risk factors associated with the rate of progression to syringomyelia after an injury, it has been found that increasing age and spinal instrumentation without decompression lead to earlier onset of posttraumatic syringomyelia. It is unclear whether the severity of initial injury or the level at which injury takes place is associated with an earlier onset of posttraumatic syringomyelia.[17,18]

Prevention

Given the risk factors mentioned above for the development of posttraumatic syringomyelia, its prevention is contingent on alleviating anatomic factors such as spinal stenosis and spinal misalignment, each of which may lead to obstruction of CSF flow after initial injury. Prevention of posttraumatic syringomyelia in spinal cord injury patients is predicated on the restoration and maintenance of normal CSF flow. With that said, the measures a neurosurgeon should take to ensure a restoration of normal CSF flow with the hopes of preventing posttraumatic syringomyelia after initial spinal cord injury remain unclear. No comprehensive studies thus far have looked at the incidence of posttraumatic syringomyelia in spinal cord injury patients who received either stabilization alone or stabilization combined with decompression. Based on the limited available evidence, some groups recommend spinal stabilization and realignment, but not additional direct surgical decompression for the purposes of reducing the risk of posttraumatic syringomyelia in cases of complete spinal cord injury.[16]

Management

Management of posttraumatic syringomyelia is controversial. A review of the literature reveals an array of reports that conclude with discrepant recommendations regarding timing of surgical treatment as well as choice of operative approach. The indications for surgical treatment of posttraumatic syringomyelia vary in large part because collectively the outcomes of treatment are unpredictable and typically short lasting. For example, in a series of 53 patients treated with both arachnoidolysis and duraplasty, or shunting, Lee et al. found improvement rates ranging from 20% to 76% depending on the specific symptom in question.[19] Some authors recommend surgical treatment for patients who have motor symptoms resulting from posttraumatic syringomyelia; surgical treatment more often results in positive outcomes for motor symptoms than it does for sensory or pain symptoms.[16] Other authors, however, recommend surgical treatment for all patients with new symptoms of progressive neurologic deterioration resulting from a syrinx.[6,20,21]

The goal of surgical treatment for posttraumatic syringomyelia is to correct the anatomic deformity that led to the obstruction of CSF flow and thus produced the formation of the syrinx. Most authors currently recommend arachnoidolysis and duraplasty as first-line treatment for posttraumatic syringomyelia, with shunting procedures reserved for cases that (1) are refractory to arachnoidolysis, (2) have extensive arachnoid adhesions, or (3) are without cord tethering on ultrasound.[6,19,20] MRI is the imaging modality of choice for detecting and monitoring the progression of a posttraumatic syrinx.[22]

Arachnoidolysis and Duraplasty

Arachnoidolysis and duraplasty are recommended as first-line treatment for posttraumatic syringomyelia. The goal of this surgery is correcting the mechanism (Fig. 62.1A and B) by which the syrinx forms, according to the intramedullary pulse pressure theory. By clearing the arachnoid scarring, CSF flow is restored, with the goal that the syrinx collapses or ceases to expand.

In performing arachnoidolysis and duraplasty for posttraumatic syringomyelia, there are a couple of key concepts to keep in mind to minimize postoperative complications. Throughout the operation it is critical to minimize bleeding and, in particular, to minimize bleeding before opening the dura. Contamination of blood into the subdural space may increase the likelihood of new arachnoid adhesions. After the laminectomy is performed and the dura is exposed, ultrasound is useful to detect the extent of the arachnoid adhesions and consequently the optimal location for dura opening. Once durotomy is achieved, arachnoidolysis should be performed with sharp dissection under the microscope. Sharp dissection is important because excess traction during dissection may result in an increased likelihood of new arachnoid adhesions.[6]

Shunting

Various shunting procedures may be performed to treat posttraumatic syringomyelia. Options for shunting procedures include syringosubarachnoid, syringopleural, and syringoperitoneal

SURGICAL REWIND

My Worst Case

A 46-year-old male presents status post a motorcycle motor vehicle accident (MVA) with a T3 ASIA A spinal cord injury. He was initially treated with external immobilization for the fracture; he did not undergo operative decompression or stabilization. Immediate postinjury films showed cord compression and cord contusion (Fig. 62.3A and B).

Within approximately 2 years of his initial presentation, he developed new left upper extremity burning pain, scapular pain, and difficulty with left hand grip. He reported inability to complete fine motor tasks with his left hand and disturbing numbness and tinging (N/T) over his left hand. He had difficulty with using a wheelchair and developed difficulty with transfers.

New imaging showed a large thoracic and cervical syrinx, tracking to the C2 level (Fig. 62.2A and B).

The patient was operatively treated with a thoracic laminectomy, an exploration with lysis of dense intradural adhesions, and a stabilization of his fracture.

Postoperatively, the patient noted stabilization of his clinical complaints but no improvement of his posttraumatic syrinx. Radiographically, the syrinx remained stable.

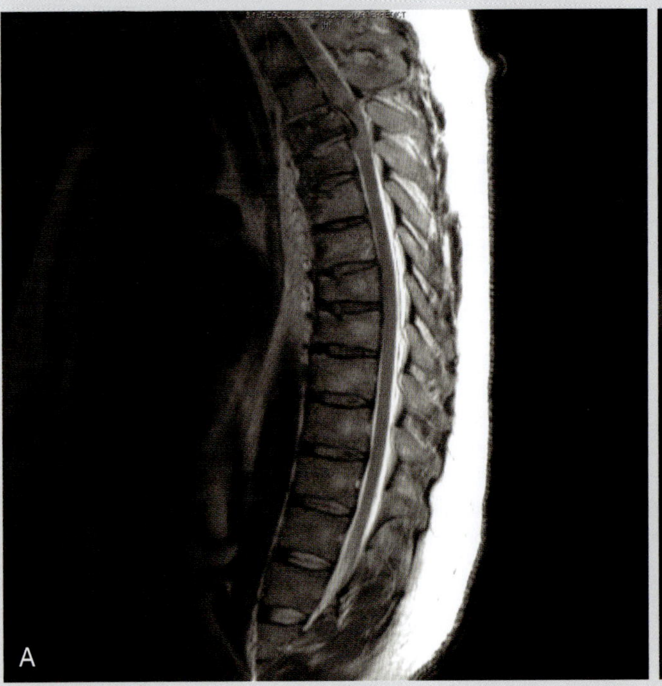

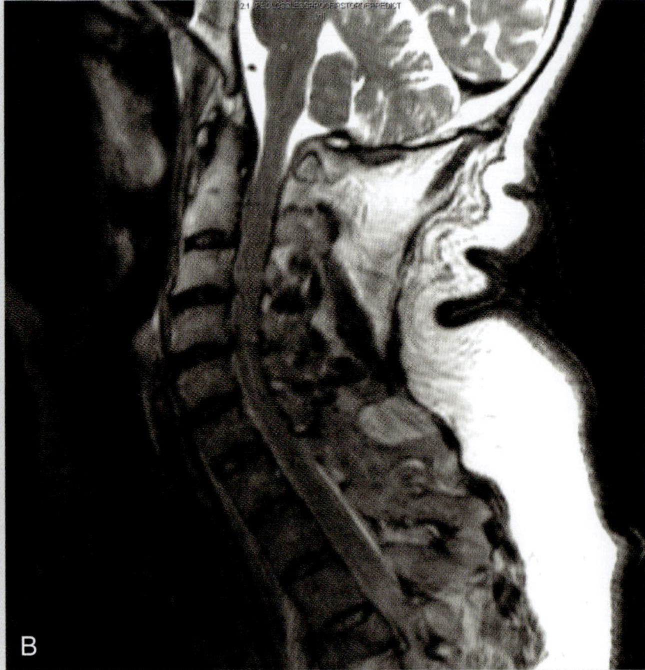

• **Fig. 62.2** Large thoracic (A) and cervical (B) syrinx, tracking to the C2 level.

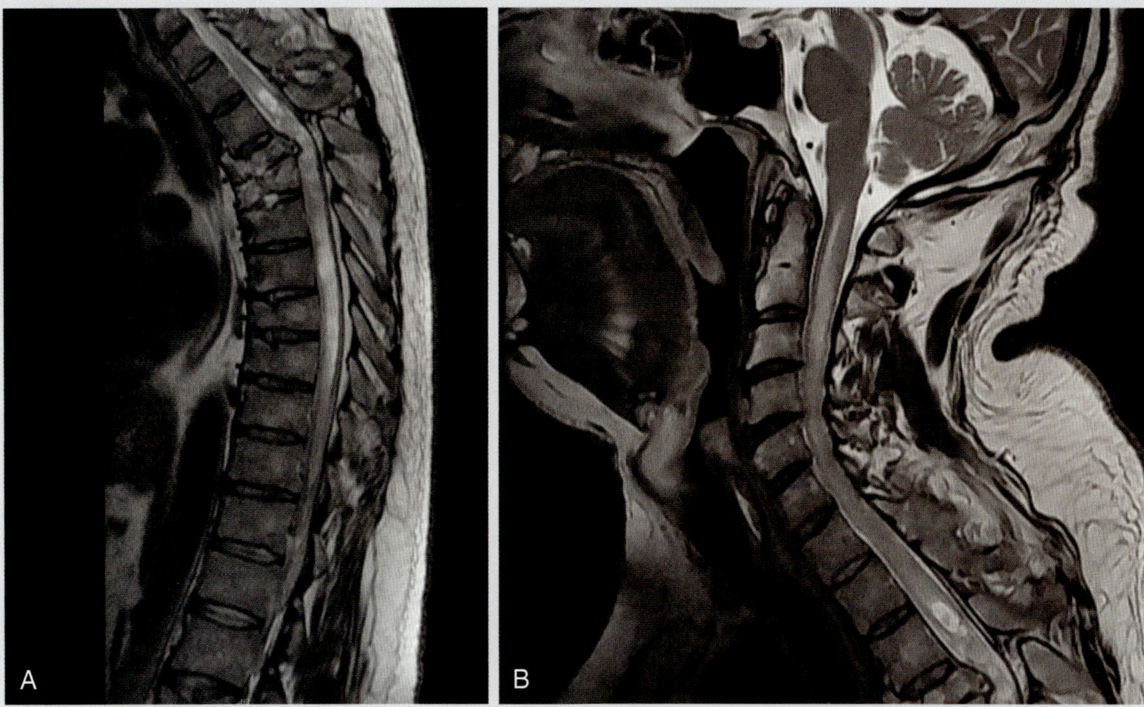

• **Fig. 62.3** Immediate postinjury MRI shows cord compression and cord contusion. (A) MRI thoracic. (B) MRI cervical.

diversion. There is inconclusive evidence as to which procedure leads to better patient outcomes.[6] All of the shunting procedures are similar in that they offer a direct way to drain a syrinx when restoration of CSF flow through arachnoidolysis or other methods is ineffective or not feasible. Many of the techniques used to minimize postoperative complications in arachnoidolysis are also applicable in the context of shunting procedures. Surgical approach should minimize factors that are associated with increased risk of new arachnoid adhesions, such as excess bleeding into the subdural space and excess spinal cord traction. Intraoperative ultrasound is again useful here for determining the optimal location for dural opening and shunt placement. Choice of site for myelotomy should be based on patient neurologic deficit, syrinx morphology, and plan for diversion. Usually anatomic considerations guide the site for shunt insertion.

Challenges unique to shunting for treatment of posttraumatic syringomyelia include high rates of shunt failure. In one study, Sgouros and Williams reported shunt failure rates of 49% within 6 years of surgery.[23] Insertion of additional side holes into the shunt may decrease the incidence of shunt failure.[6]

References

1. Milhorat TH. Classification of syringomyelia. *Neurosurg Focus.* 2000;8(3):E1.
2. Heiss JD, Patronas N, DeVroom HL, et al. Elucidating the pathophysiology of syringomyelia. *J Neurosurg.* 1999;91(4):553–562.
3. Kahn EN, Muraszko KM, Maher CO. Prevalence of Chiari I malformation and syringomyelia. *Neurosurg Clin N Am.* 2015;26(4):501–507.
4. Greitz D. Unraveling the riddle of syringomyelia. *Neurosurg Rev.* 2006;29(4):251–263, discussion 64.
5. Biyani A, el Masry WS. Post-traumatic syringomyelia: a review of the literature. *Paraplegia.* 1994;32(11):723–731.
6. Brodbelt AR, Stoodley MA. Post-traumatic syringomyelia: a review. *J Clin Neurosci.* 2003;10(4):401–408.
7. Balmaseda MT Jr, Wunder JA, Gordon C, Cannell CD. Posttraumatic syringomyelia associated with heavy weightlifting exercises: case report. *Arch Phys Med Rehabil.* 1988;69(11):970–972.
8. Vernon JD, Silver JR, Ohry A. Post-traumatic syringomyelia. *Paraplegia.* 1982;20(6):339–364.
9. Perrouin-Verbe B, Lenne-Aurier K, Robert R, et al. Post-traumatic syringomyelia and post-traumatic spinal canal stenosis: a direct relationship: review of 75 patients with a spinal cord injury. *Spinal Cord.* 1998;36(2):137–143.
10. Milhorat TH, Capocelli AL Jr, Anzil AP, Kotzen RM, Milhorat RH. Pathological basis of spinal cord cavitation in syringomyelia: analysis of 105 autopsy cases. *J Neurosurg.* 1995;82(5):802–812.
11. Kim HG, Oh HS, Kim TW, Park KH. Clinical features of post-traumatic syringomyelia. *Korean J Neurotrauma.* 2014;10(2):66–69.
12. Schurch B, Wichmann W, Rossier AB. Post-traumatic syringomyelia (cystic myelopathy): a prospective study of 449 patients with spinal cord injury. *J Neurol Neurosurg Psychiatry.* 1996;60(1):61–67.
13. Abel R, Gerner HJ, Smit C, Meiners T. Residual deformity of the spinal canal in patients with traumatic paraplegia and secondary changes of the spinal cord. *Spinal Cord.* 1999;37(1):14–19.
14. Edgar R, Quail P. Progressive post-traumatic cystic and non-cystic myelopathy. *Br J Neurosurg.* 1994;8(1):7–22.
15. el Masry WS, Biyani A. Incidence, management, and outcome of post-traumatic syringomyelia. In memory of Mr Bernard Williams. *J Neurol Neurosurg Psychiatry.* 1996;60(2):141–146.

16. Bonfield CM, Levi AD, Arnold PM, Okonkwo DO. Surgical management of post-traumatic syringomyelia. *Spine*. 2010;35(21 suppl):S245–S258.
17. Ko HY, Kim W, Kim SY, et al. Factors associated with early onset post-traumatic syringomyelia. *Spinal Cord*. 2012;50(9):695–698.
18. Vannemreddy SS, Rowed DW, Bharatwal N. Posttraumatic syringomyelia: predisposing factors. *Br J Neurosurg*. 2002;16(3):276–283.
19. Lee TT, Alameda GJ, Camilo E, Green BA. Surgical treatment of post-traumatic myelopathy associated with syringomyelia. *Spine*. 2001;26(24 suppl):S119–S127.
20. Klekamp J. Treatment of posttraumatic syringomyelia. *J Neurosurg Spine*. 2012;17(3):199–211.
21. Falci SP, Indeck C, Lammertse DP. Posttraumatic spinal cord tethering and syringomyelia: surgical treatment and long-term outcome. *J Neurosurg Spine*. 2009;11(4):445–460.
22. Sett P, Crockard HA. The value of magnetic resonance imaging (MRI) in the follow-up management of spinal injury. *Paraplegia*. 1991;29(6):396–410.
23. Sgouros S, Williams B. Management and outcome of posttraumatic syringomyelia. *J Neurosurg*. 1996;85(2):197–205.

63

Complications of Surgery for Peripheral Nerve Injuries and Tumors

THOMAS J. WILSON, ROBERT J. SPINNER

HIGHLIGHTS

- Prevention of reconstruction failure depends on choosing the appropriate reconstructive strategy for the right time frame and optimizing the surgical technique.
- For upper trunk injuries with failure of primary nerve reconstruction, additional options exist including free-functioning muscle transfer, tendon transfers, and shoulder fusion.
- For nerve sheath tumors, rapid growth, neurologic deficits, being fixed rather than mobile on palpation, and significant spontaneous pain warrant further evaluation for malignancy.
- When a nerve sheath tumor is unexpectedly diagnosed as a malignant nerve sheath tumor or other malignant tumor, a multidisciplinary sarcoma team should be employed to evaluate for metastatic disease and plan for definitive resection with or without chemotherapy and radiation.

Background—Nerve Injuries

Injury to the brachial plexus can occur secondary to penetrating trauma or trauma that induces stretch in the nerves comprising the brachial plexus. Brachial plexus injuries are reported to occur in approximately 1% of polytrauma patients, with motor vehicle accidents being the most common mechanism of injury.[1] Among motor vehicle accidents, motorcycle and snowmobile accidents carry a substantially higher risk than automobile accidents. Supraclavicular brachial plexus injuries are significantly more common than infraclavicular brachial plexus injuries in the polytrauma setting.[1]

Seddon classified nerve injuries into three groups: (1) neurapraxic, (2) axonotmetic, and (3) neurotmetic. Neurapraxic injury is the mildest form; the axon remains intact, as well as the epineurium, perineurium, and endoneurium. Wallerian degeneration does not occur. There is a focal physiologic conduction block with intact conduction distal to the site of injury and proximal to the site of injury but not across the injured segment. Spontaneous recovery is the norm and usually occurs within days or weeks. Axonotmetic injuries are characterized by partial or complete axon disruption with preservation of the epineurium and perineurium. Wallerian degeneration occurs distal to the injury, and after Wallerian degeneration occurs, conduction distal to the injury is lost. Spontaneous recovery can occur. Finally, neurotmetic injuries, the most severe form, are characterized by disruption of the axon and surrounding connective tissue, including the perineurium and epineurium. Wallerian degeneration occurs distal to the site of injury. Spontaneous recovery is not possible.[2]

A common mechanism of injury involves a sudden increase in the angle between the neck and the shoulder, stretching the brachial plexus, particularly the upper brachial plexus. Options for management depend on the segment(s) of the brachial plexus that are injured, the severity of the injury, and the timing of presentation. Potential management options include conservative management allowing for spontaneous recovery; neurolysis, nerve graft repair, and nerve transfer (primary nerve surgery); and other soft tissue or bony reconstruction strategies, including tendon transfer, free muscle transfer, and joint fusion (secondary surgery).

Anatomic Insights

The brachial plexus is comprised of the C5–T1 spinal nerves. The C5 and C6 nerves join to form the upper trunk of the brachial plexus. With injury to the upper brachial plexus, there is loss of shoulder abduction (deltoid and supraspinatus), shoulder external rotation (infraspinatus), forearm supination (biceps), and elbow flexion (biceps, brachialis, and brachioradialis). Reconstructive strategies target restoration of these movements. Other nerves related to the upper brachial plexus include the phrenic, dorsal scapular, and long thoracic nerves. The phrenic nerve receives contributions from C3, C4, and C5 and innervates the diaphragm. The dorsal scapular nerve arises from the proximal aspect of the C5 nerve root to innervate the levator scapulae and rhomboids. The long thoracic nerve receives contributions from C5, C6, and C7, with the contributions arising proximally, ultimately innervating the serratus anterior.

Although the Seddon classification of nerve injuries is important in determining the likelihood of spontaneous recovery, an additional classification system is important for determining both the possibility of spontaneous recovery and the options for nerve reconstruction when necessary. This system dichotomizes nerve injuries based on the anatomic position of the injury relative to the dorsal root ganglion into preganglionic versus postganglionic injuries. Preganglionic injuries generally do not have a chance for spontaneous recovery, and in cases of nerve reconstruction, nerve graft repair is not an option because a viable nerve stump will not be present to graft into. Postganglionic injuries may or may not have a chance of spontaneous recovery, depending on the extent of the injury, but in cases of nerve reconstruction, a viable nerve stump will generally be present, allowing for nerve graft repair as an option.

In the setting of upper brachial plexus injuries, clinical, electrodiagnostic, and imaging features can be clues to pre- versus postganglionic status. Clinically, examination of the rhomboids and serratus anterior is important, since the takeoffs of the nerves or contributions to the nerves that innervate these muscles occur so proximally on C5 and C6. Loss of innervation to the rhomboids and/or serratus anterior suggests a very proximal injury. Although it does not confirm a preganglionic injury, it makes it more likely. Similarly, electromyography (EMG) can be used to determine whether the rhomboids and serratus anterior have been affected by the injury (i.e., presence of fibrillation potentials). An additional clue comes with sensory nerve action potential (SNAP) testing. In cases of postganglionic injury, both motor nerve action potentials and SNAPs are lost, whereas in cases of preganglionic injury, the motor nerve action potential is lost, but the SNAP is preserved. Similarly, an elevated hemidiaphragm on imaging (e.g., inspiration/expiration chest films, ultrasound, computed tomography [CT] scan) suggests involvement of the phrenic nerve. Although not diagnostic of a preganglionic injury, involvement of the phrenic nerve suggests a proximal and severe injury. Cervical radiographs showing spinal fractures are also associated with preganglionic injuries. Both CT and magnetic resonance (MR) myelography can also be used to look for signs of nerve root avulsion (preganglionic injury). The most common signs are the presence of a pseudomeningocele or pseudomeningocele with absent rootlets.

In cases of preganglionic injuries, nerve transfer is the procedure of choice. Because of the improved results with newer types of nerve transfers, nerve transfers are being increasingly used by many surgeons, in lieu of nerve grafting, in select cases of postganglionic injury or in cases where patients present late (i.e., after the typical window for nerve surgery). When performing nerve transfers, surgeons must understand the anatomy of the potential donor nerves to maximize outcomes and minimize donor morbidity. Probably the most common nerve transfers employed for upper brachial plexus injuries include spinal accessory nerve to suprascapular nerve and/or radial nerve triceps branch to axillary nerve for shoulder (C5) targets; and ulnar nerve fascicle to musculocutaneous nerve biceps branch (Oberlin transfer) with or without median nerve fascicle to musculocutaneous nerve brachialis branch for elbow flexion (C6) targets. In this situation, an ideal donor nerve is purely motor with a large number of motor axons, has sufficient length to allow coaptation to the target nerve in a tension-free manner without an intervening graft, has a redundant or expendable function, and has an action that is synergistic to the action of the target nerve.[3]

The spinal accessory nerve comprises approximately 1500 motor axons, innervating both the sternocleidomastoid and trapezius muscles.[4] The spinal accessory nerve emerges from beneath the sternocleidomastoid to run on the anterior surface of the trapezius, innervating the trapezius along its course. Transection of the spinal accessory nerve for use as a donor should occur distal to the first motor branch to the trapezius to allow continued partial innervation of the trapezius and to avoid the morbidity associated with complete denervation of the trapezius. Sufficient length of the spinal accessory nerve can typically be isolated to allow coaptation to the suprascapular nerve in a tension-free manner without an intervening graft. Debate exists as to whether the spinal accessory nerve should be used as a donor in this way or whether the trapezius muscle should be preserved and used instead for tendon transfer.

The radial nerve innervates all three heads of the triceps muscle. The redundant function of the heads of the triceps makes individual nerve branches to the triceps good candidates to be used as donor nerves. Furthermore, the synergistic function of the triceps and the deltoid muscles makes the triceps nerve branches good candidates for nerve transfer, specifically to the axillary nerve. Each of the branches to the three heads has theoretical advantages. The long head of the triceps is mechanically the least important for elbow extension, making use of the nerve branch to the long head theoretically the branch associated with the lowest donor morbidity. The branch to the long head also is the largest and contains the highest number of motor axons. The significant downside is that the length of the branch to the long head is typically short, making obtaining enough length for tension-free coaptation to the axillary nerve difficult.[5–8] The branch to the medial head of the triceps is longer, making it significantly easier to achieve sufficient length.[7] Care must be taken when isolating the specific triceps branch intended for nerve transfer to avoid damage to the main trunk of the radial nerve and weakening of wrist/finger extension.

A single fascicle of the ulnar nerve can be transferred to the biceps branch of the musculocutaneous nerve (Fig. 63.1). The close proximity of the ulnar nerve to the biceps branch in the upper arm means that only a short length is needed for a tension-free coaptation. The ideal donor nerve fascicle supplies only, or at least predominantly, the flexor carpi ulnaris. By utilizing a fascicle innervating the flexor carpi ulnaris, which is redundantly innervated by multiple fascicles, donor morbidity is minimized (also, other median nerve innervated wrist flexors exist, minimizing donor morbidity). The fascicle innervating predominantly the flexor carpi ulnaris is typically located in the anterior-medial portion of the nerve.[9]

Elbow flexion can be supplemented by reinnervating the brachialis via median nerve fascicle transfer to the brachialis branch of the musculocutaneous nerve. Similar to the ulnar fascicle transfer, the close proximity of the median nerve to the brachialis branch means that only a short length is needed for a direct tension-free repair and that the coaptation sits close to the motor end plate of the brachialis muscle, requiring only a short distance of nerve regeneration. The ideal fascicles for transfer innervate predominantly the flexor digitorum superficialis and flexor carpi radialis. Such a fascicle typically is located in the anterior-medial portion of the nerve. The fascicles ultimately giving rise to the anterior interosseous nerve are to be avoided as donors. These fascicles typically are located in the posterior-medial nerve.[10] Understanding the fascicular topography and performing careful interfascicular dissection are critical to avoiding undue injury to the median nerve.

Although these are likely the most commonly employed nerve transfer strategies with upper brachial plexus injuries, a variety of other donor nerves and nerve transfer strategies have also been described and are available in the surgical armamentarium. Add to these nerve graft repair and secondary reconstructive strategies and there is a wide array of choices. Potential complications include injury to surrounding nerves or donor nerves, vascular injury because the brachial plexus lies in close proximity to major vascular structures, pneumothorax (the brachial plexus lies in close proximity to the apex of the lung, or during intercostal nerve isolation for transfer, if that strategy is employed), chyle leak or chylothorax (particularly on the left side due to the proximity of the thoracic duct), phrenic nerve injury with paralysis of a hemidiaphragm, and failure of the reconstruction. Failure of the reconstruction to achieve satisfactory restoration of function is the most common complication among the list. This complication will be our focus.

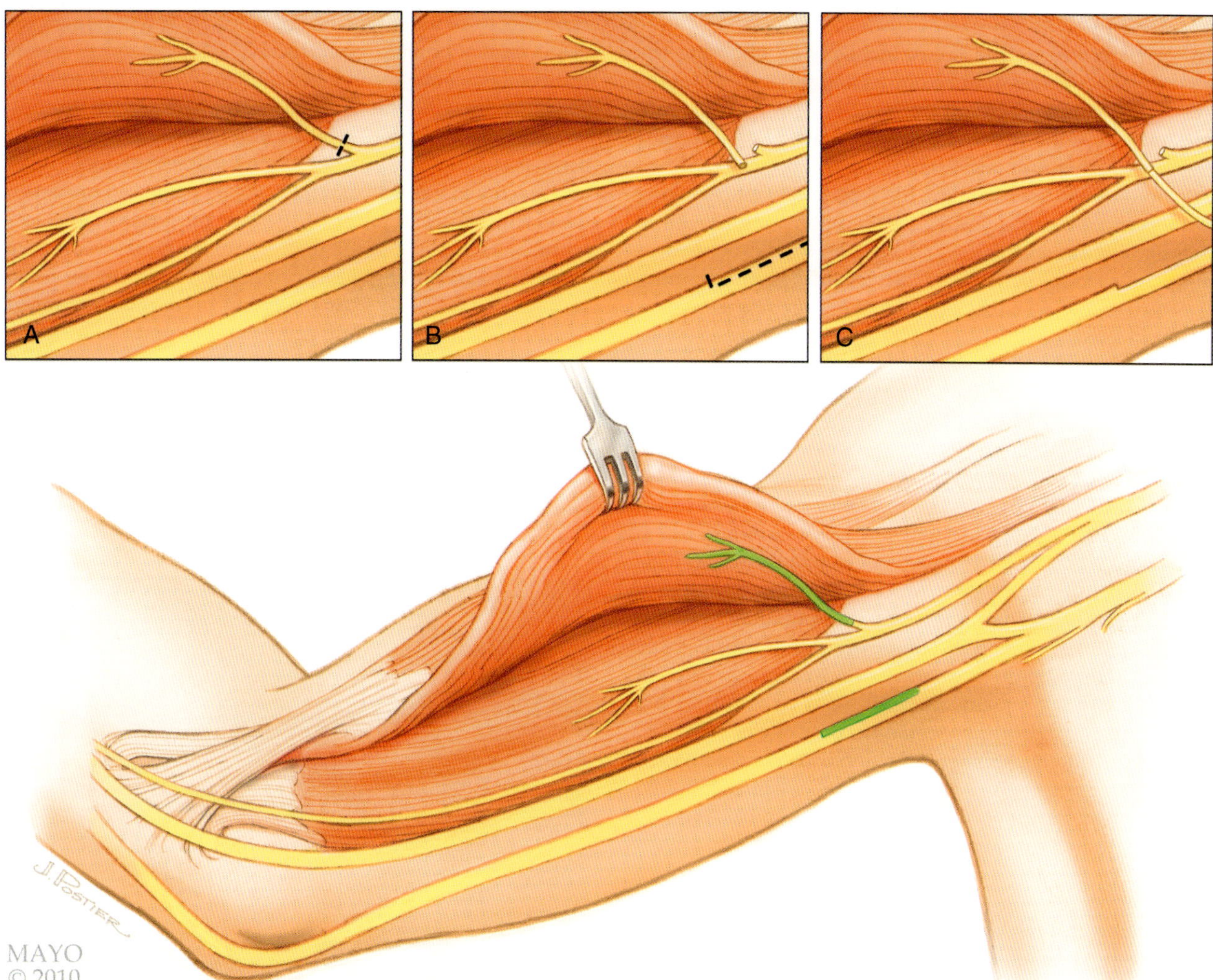

• **Fig. 63.1** Diagram of the Oberlin transfer: ulnar nerve fascicle to biceps branch of the musculocutaneous nerve. (A) The biceps branch of the musculocutaneous nerve is isolated and transected proximally. (B) Interfascicular dissection of the ulnar nerve is performed to isolate a fascicle that supplies the flexor carpi ulnaris solely or at least predominantly. The fascicle is then transected distally to be used as a donor. (C) A direct tension-free coaptation is performed between the ulnar fascicle and the biceps branch. (Used with permission of Mayo Foundation for Medical Education and Research. All rights reserved.)

RED FLAGS

Debate continues regarding nerve graft repair versus nerve transfer as the optimal reconstructive strategy when both are options. To employ a nerve graft repair strategy requires a viable nerve stump to graft into. An injured, unhealthy nerve stump is a risk factor for failure. There is no way to completely reliably determine the health of the nerve stump. A combination of visual inspection, intraoperative electrophysiologic testing and, in some cases, intraoperative histologic analysis is used to determine whether a nerve stump is viable. To adequately prepare the nerve stump for grafting, the nerve must be resected back to healthy tissue with a normal fascicular pattern. Grafting into a damaged, unhealthy nerve is a risk factor for failure.

The length of nerve graft has also been associated with outcomes, with longer nerve graft length being associated with poorer outcome.[11,12] The data, however, are mixed in this regard, with some studies showing no correlation between nerve graft length and outcome.[13] Longer graft lengths may be a red flag, but this remains to be proven conclusively.

From the time of injury, it is a race against time to restore innervation before the muscle and neuromuscular junction are irreparably damaged.[14] Prolonged delay from injury to reconstruction is a red flag for failure. Nerve transfers can be performed in a more delayed fashion than nerve graft repair due to the shorter distance of nerve regeneration required to reach the motor end plate, but prolonged delay, whether nerve graft or transfer is employed, is a risk factor for poor outcome. Although not a hard-and-fast rule, nerve graft repair beyond approximately 6 months after injury and nerve transfer beyond approximately 9 months after injury have progressively more risk of failure the further beyond these time points one gets.

Nerve transfers borrow function from another nerve. The success of this strategy depends on the integrity and health of the donor nerve. For example, the Oberlin nerve transfer borrows a nerve fascicle innervating the flexor carpi ulnaris from the ulnar nerve to reinnervate the biceps branch of the musculocutaneous nerve. If the flexor carpi ulnaris is weak on examination, is this still a viable option? How weak is too weak for the nerve still to be considered a viable donor? These questions remain to be answered. It is clear, however, that injury to the donor nerve is a risk factor for reconstruction failure.

Prevention

Prevention of reconstruction failure depends on choosing the appropriate reconstructive strategy, optimizing surgical technique, and appropriately timing surgical intervention. Time from injury to surgery should be minimized while still allowing sufficient time to determine whether spontaneous recovery will occur. For closed injuries, the optimal time window for surgical decision-making is between 3 and 6 months postinjury. A combination of clinical examination, electrodiagnostics, and imaging should be used to determine the need for surgery. In cases of delayed presentation, nerve transfer strategies, rather than nerve graft repair, should be strongly considered.

The reconstructive strategy should be optimized to lessen the risk of failure. Data suggest that in upper brachial plexus injury, the Oberlin transfer (ulnar fascicle to biceps branch) has better outcomes than any other nerve transfer strategy and also better outcomes compared with nerve graft repair.[13,15,16] Double fascicular transfer utilizing a fascicle from the median nerve transferred to the brachialis branch plus the Oberlin nerve transfer, which intuitively would have improved outcomes compared with a single fascicular transfer, has been shown to have outcomes similar to those with single transfer using the Oberlin technique.[17,18] If the ulnar nerve is partially injured and the flexor carpi ulnaris is weak, consideration should be given to an alternative strategy (though how weak is too weak remains unclear), so as to avoid further injury to the ulnar nerve or suboptimal recovery of elbow flexion.

For reconstruction of shoulder abduction and external rotation when nerve graft repair is possible, a number of potential permutations exist with combinations of nerve graft repair, spinal accessory nerve to suprascapular nerve transfer, radial nerve triceps branch to axillary nerve transfer, and trapezius tendon transfer (which requires not utilizing the spinal accessory nerve as a donor). Two recent systematic analyses suggest that dual nerve transfer yields improved results for shoulder abduction compared with single nerve transfer, nerve graft, or combined nerve transfer and nerve graft.[13,16] The role of trapezius tendon transfer relative to spinal accessory nerve transfer remains unclear.

When nerve graft repair is utilized, surgical technique is important in preventing or minimizing the risk of failure. Intraoperative electrophysiologic testing with somatosensory motor evoked potentials and motor evoked potentials can be used to confirm that the nerve stump is in continuity with the spinal cord and is viable. Nerve action potentials also can be used to determine a preganglionic versus postganglionic injury and to document regeneration across a postganglionic injury (i.e., a neuroma-in-continuity). The nerve stump must be prepared adequately to receive a graft. The damaged end should be resected back to bleeding, healthy-appearing nerve with normal fascicular architecture. We confirm this visually, though confirmation with histologic analysis is performed at some centers.[19] The nerve graft should be cabled to create a size match between the nerve stump and cabled graft. Each coaptation should be secured with several fine microsutures, often supplemented with fibrin glue. We also wrap the coaptation site with a collagen nerve wrap because there are some data in animal models indicating that this improves outcomes.[20] Finally, the graft length should be minimized while still allowing for a tension-free repair.

Management

In cases of upper brachial plexus injury, the primary goal of reconstruction is restoration of elbow flexion. When the feared complication of reconstruction failure occurs, the primary focus continues to be restoration of elbow flexion. It is important to know that in cases of primary reconstruction failure, secondary options exist and good outcomes can still be achieved. When other techniques to augment elbow flexion with tendon transfers (i.e., latissimus dorsi or pectoralis major) or Steindler flexorplasty (advancement of the flexor-pronator origin) are not possible (because of donor weakness), free-functioning muscle transfer is a good option. In our experience, the gracilis muscle is preferred. Because the gracilis muscle remains normally innervated in the thigh, there are no time constraints on when free-functioning gracilis muscle transfer can be performed (as there are for nerve graft repair and nerve transfer strategies).

Although the technical details are beyond the scope of this chapter, the gracilis muscle can be harvested from the lower limb and transferred to the arm to restore elbow flexion (Fig. 63.2). Arterial supply to the donor muscle is typically from the thoracoacromial trunk, and venous outflow is typically via the cephalic vein. The gracilis is transferred with a skin paddle to allow postoperative monitoring of the viability of the muscle. Innervation is provided

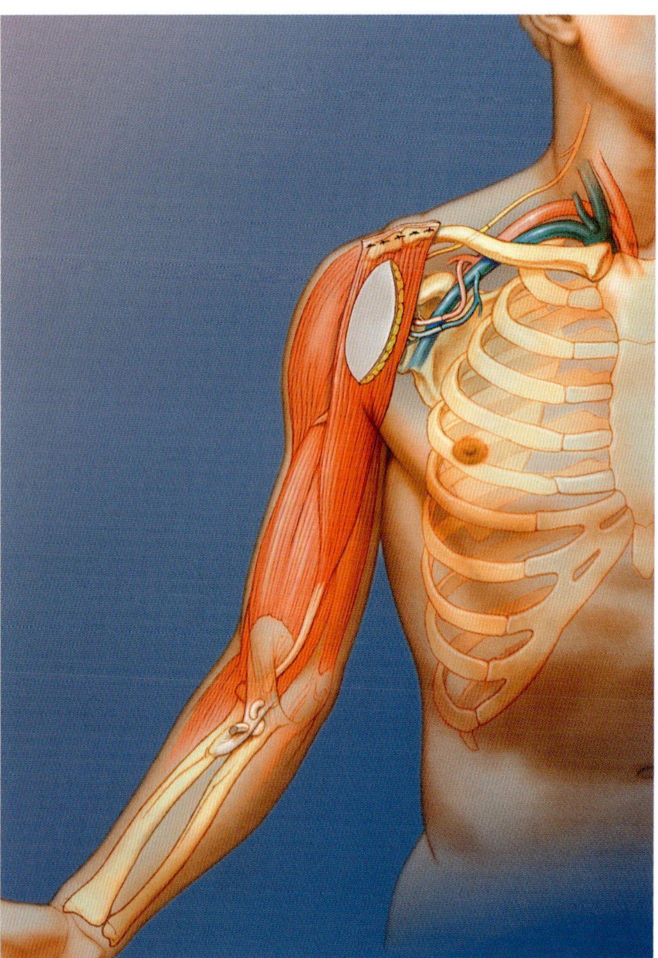

• **Fig. 63.2** Diagram of a gracilis free-functioning muscle transfer for elbow flexion. Proximally, the gracilis is attached to the acromion process and lateral clavicle. Distally, the gracilis tendon is woven into the biceps tendon. The thoracoacromial trunk artery and cephalic vein are used for vascular inflow and outflow. The spinal accessory nerve was transferred to the obturator nerve branch to the gracilis for innervation. Alternatively, intercostal nerves are commonly used as donor nerves. (Used with permission of Mayo Foundation for Medical Education and Research. All rights reserved.)

by intercostal nerve transfer using two to three intercostal nerves. The proximal muscle is secured to the acromion and lateral clavicle. The distal tendon of the gracilis muscle is typically attached to the biceps tendon in cases of isolated upper brachial plexus injury but may be attached more distally to the radius. In addition to elbow flexion, transfer of the gracilis muscle aids in shoulder stability. Approximately 70% of free-functioning gracilis muscle transfer patients in whom intercostal nerve transfer was used to innervate the gracilis achieve Medical Research Council grade 3 or better elbow flexion strength.[21]

In cases of failure to achieve shoulder stability, shoulder abduction, or external rotation, options include trapezius tendon transfer and glenohumeral joint fusion. Trapezius tendon transfer is designed mainly to achieve shoulder external rotation. Glenohumeral joint fusion can stabilize the shoulder, improve pain and, counterintuitively, improve motion.[22,23]

Background—Peripheral Nerve Tumors

Schwannomas and neurofibromas account for the vast majority of peripheral nerve sheath tumors (PNSTs). These tumors can occur sporadically or can be associated with genetic disorders such as neurofibromatosis 1 (NF1) and 2 (NF2) and schwannomatosis. The incidence is approximately 2:100,000 sporadically.[24] Malignant transformation is exceedingly rare in sporadic tumors, with an incidence of approximately 0.001%. In comparison, patients with NF1 have a 10% lifetime risk of malignant transformation of a neurofibroma.[25] Neurofibromas have a significantly higher risk of malignant degeneration in comparison with schwannomas, and malignant degeneration is most closely associated with NF1 compared with schwannomatosis. When a patient presents with a PNST, it is important for the clinician to discern the likelihood that the tumor is sporadic versus genetic disorder–associated and the likelihood that the mass is benign versus malignant.

Malignant peripheral nerve sheath tumors (MPNSTs) account for approximately 5% to 10% of soft tissue sarcomas. They arise sporadically (~50%), associated with NF1 (~20%–50%), and associated with radiation (~10%, on average 15 years after radiation).[26–29] Internal plexiform neurofibromas appear to have the highest risk of malignant degeneration at approximately 10%.[30]

NF1 is an autosomal dominant disorder that occurs in approximately 1:3500 live births. Approximately 50% of cases occur as the result of a spontaneous mutation. Diagnosis of NF1 requires two or more of the following criteria:

1. Six or more café-au-lait spots of sufficient size depending on age
2. Axillary or inguinal freckling (>2 freckles)
3. Two or more neurofibromas or one plexiform neurofibroma
4. Optic nerve glioma
5. Two or more Lisch nodules
6. Typical osseous abnormality
7. First-degree relative with NF1[31]

NF2 is an autosomal dominant disorder. Approximately 50% of cases occur as the result of a spontaneous mutation.[32] The most common, though not universal, feature of the disorder is the presence of bilateral vestibular schwannomas. Multiple sets of diagnostic criteria have been proposed, but according to the National Neurofibromatosis Foundation, diagnosis of definite NF2 requires:

1. Bilateral vestibular schwannomas

Or

2. First-degree relative with NF2 AND a unilateral vestibular schwannoma <30 years of age *or* at least two of the following:

SURGICAL REWIND

My Worst Case

A 23-year-old man was involved in a snowmobile accident and suffered a fracture of both the radius and ulna requiring operative repair as well as a brachial plexus injury. Physical examination and electrodiagnostics suggested injury to C5, C6, and C7. Physical examination findings included supraspinatus/deltoid 0/5, biceps/brachialis/brachioradialis 0/5, infraspinatus 0/5, pectoralis major 2/5, latissimus dorsi 1/5, triceps 4/5, and wrist extension (both extensor carpi radialis and ulnaris) 4–/5. Imaging did not reveal any evidence of pseudomeningoceles to suggest avulsions, and SNAPs were absent on electrodiagnostic testing, also supporting postganglionic injuries. At 6 months postinjury there was no recovery of shoulder abduction, shoulder external rotation, or elbow flexion.

A supraclavicular brachial plexus exploration was performed. Exploration revealed a viable C5 nerve stump, with no available C6 nerve stump. Nerve graft repair was done using sural nerve grafting from C5 to the suprascapular nerve and posterior division of the upper trunk. An Oberlin transfer (ulnar nerve fascicle to biceps branch of the musculocutaneous) was then performed to reconstruct elbow flexion. The operation was completed uneventfully.

At 15 months after the reconstruction, he had no recovery of supraspinatus, infraspinatus, deltoid, or biceps function. EMG also showed no signs of reinnervation of these muscles, with no motor units. The lack of recovery, particularly the lack of biceps recovery, is a devastating complication. Over 90% of patients achieve grade 4 or better elbow flexion with the Oberlin transfer.[15] Patients expect recovery. This is a particularly devastating complication in the setting of a normally functioning hand. With no recovery, he was offered a gracilis free-functioning muscle transfer targeting elbow flexion and elected to proceed with this reconstruction.

He was taken to the operating room, where the gracilis muscle was harvested. The spinal accessory nerve was transferred to the obturator motor branch to the gracilis to innervate the muscle. The thoracoacromial trunk artery and cephalic vein were used for vascular inflow and outflow of the muscle. The proximal gracilis muscle was sewn into the clavicle while the distal tendon of the gracilis was woven into the biceps tendon. The operation was completed uneventfully, and the patient recovered well postoperatively.

Elbow flexion progressively recovered postoperatively. By 3 years after the free- functioning muscle transfer, he had grade 4–/5 elbow flexion. Paralysis of his shoulder, however, persisted. Five years after his initial injury, he underwent secondary tendon transfers for shoulder reconstruction. He underwent upper trapezius to infraspinatus insertion tendon transfer and levator scapulae augmented with posterior tibialis autograft to supraspinatus insertion tendon transfer. Eighteen months later, he had recovered a stable shoulder with 10 degrees of external rotation and 30 degrees of abduction.

NEUROSURGICAL SELFIE MOMENT

Failure to achieve satisfactory restoration of movement after upper brachial plexus injury and brachial plexus reconstruction is a feared but not uncommon complication. The risk of reconstruction failure is minimized by selecting the optimal reconstructive strategy, minimizing the delay between injury and reconstruction, and through optimizing the technical nuances of the reconstruction. When failure occurs, it is important to know and to remember that additional options exist. These options include free-functioning gracilis muscle transfer with intercostal nerve transfer for innervation targeting restoration of elbow flexion, along with trapezius tendon transfer or glenohumeral joint fusion to improve stability and movement of the shoulder. Good outcomes can still be achieved for patients with upper brachial plexus injuries, despite initial failure.

meningioma, glioma, neurofibroma, schwannoma, or posterior subcapsular lenticular opacity[33]

Malignant degeneration is not typically associated with schwannomatosis, though multiple nerve sheath tumors are a consistent feature of the disorder. The majority of cases of schwannomatosis are sporadic, with only an estimated 15% to 25% of cases being inherited.[34] The annual incidence of schwannomatosis is thought to be approximately 1–2 : 1,000,000.[35] The diagnostic criteria for definite schwannomatosis are:

1. Age >30 *and* at least two nonvestibular schwannomas (one with pathologic confirmation) *and* no evidence of vestibular schwannoma on magnetic resonance imaging (MRI) *and* no NF2 mutation

Or

2. At least one nonvestibular schwannoma (pathologically confirmed) *and* first-degree relative who meets criteria in #1[36]

Evaluation of a patient presenting with a nerve sheath tumor (or what appears to be a nerve sheath tumor) begins with a careful history and physical examination. Depending on the findings, additional testing may be warranted and helpful, including electrodiagnostic studies, ultrasound, and/or MRI. In cases where atypical features are present, a positron emission tomography (PET) scan may be helpful. Options for management include percutaneous biopsy, open biopsy, resection, and conservative management with serial MRIs. Each of these options has its role in the management of such lesions. Appropriate evaluation is vital to avoiding the complication to be discussed here, misdiagnosing a malignant nerve sheath tumor as benign or, in some cases, mistaking another malignancy (not a nerve sheath tumor at all) for a benign nerve sheath tumor and undertaking a management strategy for a benign lesion inappropriately.

Anatomic Insights

Schwannomas and neurofibromas both can arise in any peripheral nerve. Although these tumors arise within the epineurium of the nerve, the relationship of the mass to the fascicular architecture of the nerve differs between the two pathologic entities. Schwannomas typically arise from and involve only a single fascicle, whereas neurofibromas typically involve more than one nerve fascicle.

Schwannomas and neurofibromas cannot be reliably distinguished on imaging. Benign PNSTs have some characteristic features on MRI. Benign PNSTs typically have distinct borders and are usually round or fusiform in shape. On T1-weighted sequences, these masses are usually iso- or slightly hypointense to skeletal muscle but on postcontrast sequences show avid contrast enhancement. On T2-weighted sequences, the masses are typically hyperintense to skeletal muscle. The target sign and split fat sign are both associated with benign PNSTs, though they are not uniformly present. The target sign gets its name from the targetlike appearance created by a rim of T2-hyperintensity surrounding central T2-hypointensity. The split fat sign is typically seen on T1-weighted sequences without fat suppression. A thin rim of fat can be seen around the mass.

RED FLAGS

A thorough history and physical examination can reveal a number of red flags that should raise suspicion of a malignant rather than benign nerve sheath tumor. Benign nerve sheath tumors typically are slow-growing, mobile, and present with pain on palpation but with little spontaneous pain. Rapid growth, being fixed rather than mobile on palpation, and the presence of considerable spontaneous pain warrant further evaluation for malignancy. A neurologic deficit as the presenting symptom is rare for benign nerve sheath tumors (~2%–5%).[37] Thus, presentation with a neurologic deficit should also raise suspicion of malignancy. Tinel's test can yield pain or tingling in the distribution of the affected nerve with either benign or malignant tumors and should not necessarily be considered a red flag for malignancy.

Imaging should also be thoroughly reviewed to identify red flags suggestive of malignancy. MRI features cannot reliably distinguish between benign and malignant, but several features should prompt consideration of further evaluation for malignancy. These features include size >5 cm, peripheral enhancement, perilesional edema, and intratumoral cystic change.[38] Furthermore, rapid growth on serial MRIs should also raise suspicion.

Abnormal PET scan findings should also be considered a red flag for malignancy. Standard uptake value (SUV) maximum thresholds have been proposed, as have thresholds for the SUV tumor-to-liver ratio to distinguish benign from malignant. An SUVmax >6.1 is considered suggestive of a malignant nerve sheath tumor, as is a tumor-to-liver ratio >1.5. However, these thresholds are not perfectly predictive. There is considerable overlap in SUVmax values of MPNSTs and benign PNSTs, particularly schwannomas, which often demonstrate higher SUVmax than neurofibromas.[39–42]

Prevention

The keys to preventing misdiagnosis of a malignant nerve sheath tumor (or other malignancy) as benign are taking a thorough history, performing a detailed physical/neurologic examination, and utilizing appropriate imaging studies to recognize red flags. When red flags are recognized, more advanced imaging techniques and biopsy of the lesion should be considered before endeavoring upon resection. Biopsy should be used judiciously, as percutaneous biopsy carries its own set of risks, including nerve injury and scarring, that will make later resection of benign lesions more difficult, exposing the patient to additional risk of neurologic injury. Accordingly, biopsy should be reserved for those cases in which red flags are present.

Management

In cases where a nerve sheath tumor is thought to be benign and is resected, only later to be diagnosed as a malignancy, it is important to change the management paradigm to one appropriate for a sarcoma. Resection of benign nerve sheath tumors is performed in a function-sparing manner, where preservation of function, rather than complete resection, is the priority. In contrast, MPNSTs and other malignancies are managed with aggressive surgical removal of the tumor with wide, histologically negative margins, even at the expense of function. Once the diagnosis of a malignant nerve sheath tumor or other malignancy has been made, it is important to take a multidisciplinary approach to management to develop a consensus regarding further surgery, radiation therapy, and chemotherapy.

Approximately 10% to 16% of patients have metastatic disease at the time of diagnosis of an MPNST.[43] As a result, performing a metastatic workup (e.g., CT chest, abdomen, pelvis) is an important part of determining optimal management. Local control is an important factor in determining the risk of both metastasis and mortality. In the absence of metastatic disease, management of a misdiagnosed MPNST or other malignancy will typically include a second stage of surgery to achieve local control with aggressive resection and negative margins. Although it has only a modest positive effect on survival, the Oncology Consensus Group recommends adjuvant radiation therapy, whether or not negative surgical margins are achieved. The typical radiation treatment regimen consists of 6000 to 7000 cGy to the operative field and a 5-cm field margin.[44] Chemotherapy is typically reserved for metastatic MPNSTs or some high-risk tumors. In general, MPNSTs are relatively chemoresistant.

SURGICAL REWIND

My Worst Case

A 50-year-old woman presented with pain in the lateral leg for at least 10 years. Over that time, she had two imaging studies reportedly read as normal. The pain worsened over the 2 years before presentation. The pain was particularly exacerbated by contact or bumping the proximal lateral leg. She complained of night pain and difficulty sleeping. She denied weakness. She denied constitutional symptoms. On physical examination, she had a slight prominence of the midportion of the lateral leg, with pain on palpation that was nonradiating. Her sensory and motor examinations were normal.

An MR imaging study revealed a T2-hyperintense, contrast-enhancing mass posteromedial to the peroneus muscles abutting the fibular shaft (Fig. 63.3). The mass appeared well-circumscribed, without muscular or osseous invasion. There was a small amount of edema in the surrounding musculature apparent on the T2-weighted sequences. This was thought to be most consistent with a benign PNST, most likely an intramuscular schwannoma.

She was taken to the operating room for resection of the mass. Intraoperatively, a well-circumscribed, slightly irregular mass was encountered within the peroneus musculature (Fig. 63.4). The mass was mobilized circumferentially and resected without violation of the capsule. What appeared to be a small nerve twig was encountered on the distal aspect of the mass, and this was cut and sent with the specimen. Frozen section pathology was read as a spindle cell neoplasm, consistent with a cellular schwannoma.

Final pathology later returned as a monophasic synovial sarcoma. The complication of misdiagnosis is significant due to the likelihood of positive margins remaining after the initial operation and contamination and seeding of the surgical field with malignant cells, making the risk of local recurrence higher and the definitive operation more difficult. In retrospect, several features should have raised suspicion and prompted consideration of a biopsy. First, the pain was somewhat atypical for a benign nerve sheath tumor in that it included night pain. Next, several imaging features were atypical for a benign nerve sheath tumor, including the homogeneous T2-hyperintensity without a target sign or areas of T2-hypointensity, somewhat irregular borders, slight perilesional edema within the surrounding muscle, and the intimate association of the tumor with the bone, which is unusual for a benign nerve sheath tumor but typical of a synovial sarcoma.

Due to the diagnosis of a synovial sarcoma, she was then referred for management by a multidisciplinary sarcoma team. Metastatic workup did not reveal any evidence of metastatic disease. A follow-up MRI did not show any evidence of persistent/residual tumor. Her treatment plan consisted of radiation therapy followed by definitive surgery with wide excision. She received external beam radiation therapy for a total of 50 Gy over 28 fractions. Definitive surgery was then performed with wide excision of the tumor bed, including the lateral compartment muscles and the fibula (Fig. 63.5).

Postoperatively, she recovered well. She is now approximately 11 years out from her initial resection. She has not had any evidence of local

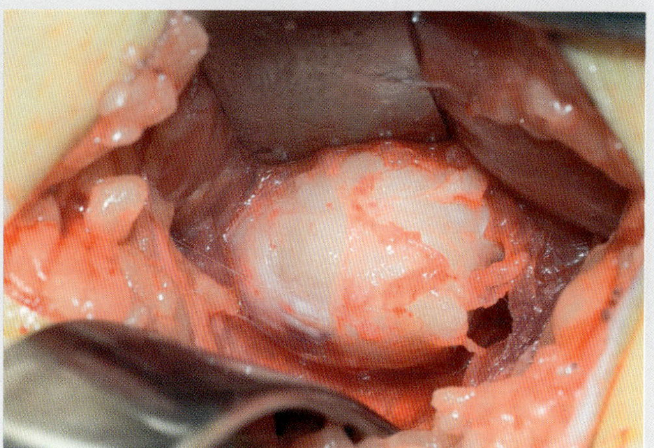

• **Fig. 63.4** Intraoperative photograph of a well-circumscribed, slightly irregular mass within the peroneus musculature.

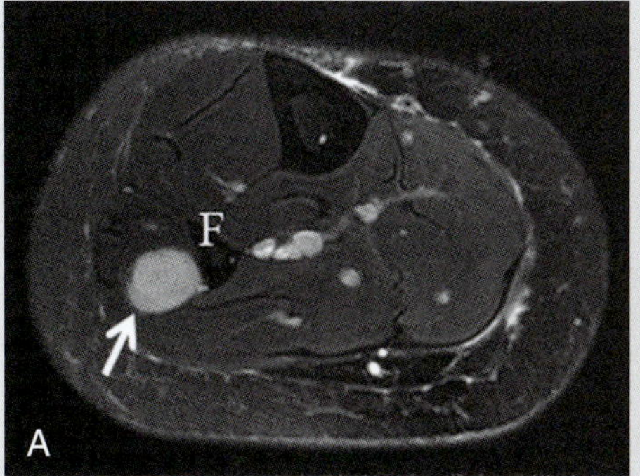

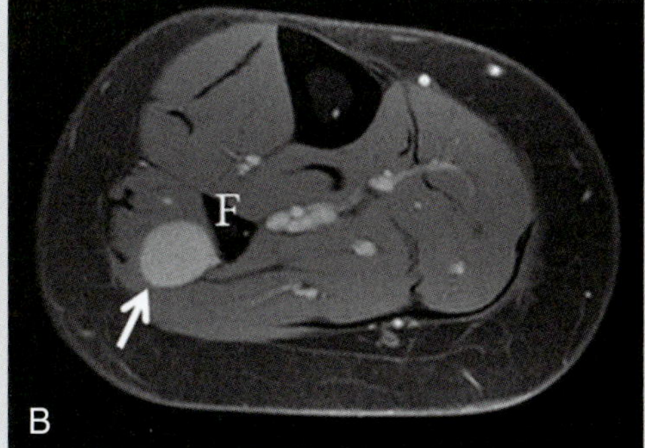

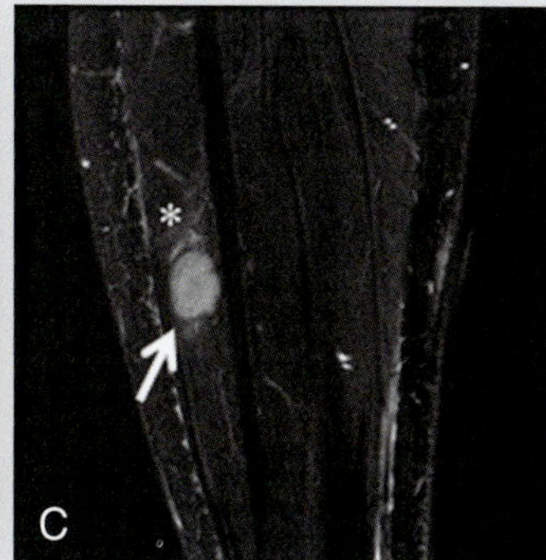

• **Fig. 63.3** Preoperative magnetic resonance study. (A) Axial, T2-weighted; (B) axial spoiled-gradient postgadolinium; and (C) coronal oblique, T2-weighted images showing a well-circumscribed, T2-hyperintense, contrast-enhancing mass *(white arrows)* within the lateral compartment of the leg, abutting the fibula (F). There is mild associated edema *(asterisk)* within the peroneus musculature.

Continued

recurrence or metastatic disease but continues to be followed. Fortunately, resection of the lateral compartment musculature and partial resection of the fibula are tolerated well, with little morbidity. In other circumstances, such as tumors in the anterior or posterior compartment, the second-stage operation could potentially have significantly more morbidity associated with it, adding impact to the initial complication of misdiagnosis.

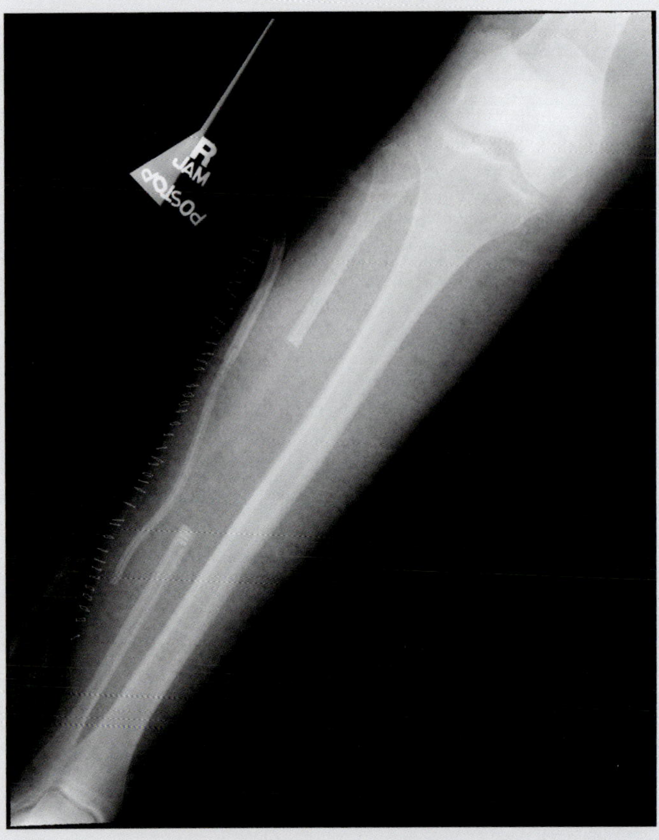

• **Fig. 63.5** An x-ray demonstrating the fibular resection performed as part of the definitive surgery for a synovial sarcoma.

NEUROSURGICAL SELFIE MOMENT

There is no perfect way to decipher benign from MPNSTs. As a result, if a surgeon encounters enough patients with nerve sheath tumors, the complication of misdiagnosis of an MPNST as benign will occur. It is important to minimize the risk of this occurring by recognizing the red flags for malignancy in the history and physical examination and on the imaging studies. Biopsy should be used judiciously but should be used in cases where red flags are present. We try to review the imaging of every case of a peripheral nerve tumor with an experienced musculoskeletal radiologist. We recognize that the complication of misdiagnosis does occur despite our best attempts to avoid it. When it does occur, a multidisciplinary approach needs to be employed. Metastatic workup should be performed, and consideration should be given to a second stage, aggressive resection, radiation therapy, and/or chemotherapy.

References

1. Midha R. Epidemiology of brachial plexus injuries in a multitrauma population. *Neurosurgery*. 1997;40(6):1182–1188; discussion 1188–1189.
2. Seddon HJ. A classification of nerve injuries. *Br Med J*. 1942; 2(4260):237–239.
3. Ray WZ, Chang J, Hawasli A, Wilson TJ, Yang L. Motor nerve transfers: a comprehensive review. *Neurosurgery*. 2016;78(1):1–26.
4. Vathana T, Larsen M, de Ruiter GC, Bishop AT, Spinner RJ, Shin AY. An anatomic study of the spinal accessory nerve: extended harvest permits direct nerve transfer to distal plexus targets. *Clin Anat*. 2007;20(8):899–904.
5. Travill AA. Electromyographic study of the extensor apparatus of the forearm. *Anat Rec*. 1962;144:373–376.
6. Lee JY, Kircher MF, Spinner RJ, Bishop AT, Shin AY. Factors affecting outcome of triceps motor branch transfer for isolated axillary nerve injury. *J Hand Surg Am*. 2012;37(11):2350–2356.
7. Bertelli JA, Santos MA, Kechele PR, Ghizoni MF, Duarte H. Triceps motor nerve branches as a donor or receiver in nerve transfers. *Neurosurgery*. 2007;61(5 suppl 2):333–338; discussion 338–339.
8. Kostas-Agnantis I, Korompilias A, Vekris M, et al. Shoulder abduction and external rotation restoration with nerve transfer. *Injury*. 2013;44(3): 299–304.
9. Oberlin C, Ameur NE, Teboul F, Beaulieu JY, Vacher C. Restoration of elbow flexion in brachial plexus injury by transfer of ulnar nerve fascicles to the nerve to the biceps muscle. *Tech Hand Up Extrem Surg*. 2002;6(2):86–90.
10. Ray WZ, Pet MA, Yee A, Mackinnon SE. Double fascicular nerve transfer to the biceps and brachialis muscles after brachial plexus injury: clinical outcomes in a series of 29 cases. *J Neurosurg*. 2011; 114(6):1520–1528.

11. Samii A, Carvalho GA, Samii M. Brachial plexus injury: factors affecting functional outcome in spinal accessory nerve transfer for the restoration of elbow flexion. *J Neurosurg*. 2003;98(2):307–312.
12. Ricardo M. Surgical treatment of brachial plexus injuries in adults. *Int Orthop*. 2005;29(6):351–354.
13. Ali ZS, Heuer GG, Faught RW, et al. Upper brachial plexus injury in adults: comparative effectiveness of different repair techniques. *J Neurosurg*. 2015;122(1):195–201.
14. Carlsen BT, Bishop AT, Shin AY. Late reconstruction for brachial plexus injury. *Neurosurg Clin N Am*. 2009;20(1):51–64; vi.
15. Leechavengvongs S, Witoonchart K, Uerpairojkit C. Thuvasethakul P, Ketmalasiri W. Nerve transfer to biceps muscle using a part of the ulnar nerve in brachial plexus injury (upper arm type): a report of 32 cases. *J Hand Surg Am*. 1998;23(4):711–716.
16. Garg R, Merrell GA, Hillstrom HJ, Wolfe SW. Comparison of nerve transfers and nerve grafting for traumatic upper plexus palsy: a systematic review and analysis. *J Bone Joint Surg Am*. 2011;93(9):819–829.
17. Martins RS, Siqueira MG, Heise CO, Foroni L, Teixeira MJ. A prospective study comparing single and double fascicular transfer to restore elbow flexion after brachial plexus injury. *Neurosurgery*. 2013;72(5):709–714; discussion 714–715; quiz 715.
18. Carlsen BT, Kircher MF, Spinner RJ, Bishop AT, Shin AY. Comparison of single versus double nerve transfers for elbow flexion after brachial plexus injury. *Plast Reconstr Surg*. 2011;127(1):269–276.
19. Malessy MJ, van Duinen SG, Feirabend HK, Thomeer RT. Correlation between histopathological findings in C-5 and C-6 nerve stumps and motor recovery following nerve grafting for repair of brachial plexus injury. *J Neurosurg*. 1999;91(4):636–644.
20. Lee JY, Parisi TJ, Friedrich PF, Bishop AT, Shin AY. Does the addition of a nerve wrap to a motor nerve repair affect motor outcomes? *Microsurgery*. 2014;34(7):562–567.
21. Maldonado AA, Kircher MF, Spinner RJ, Bishop AT, Shin AY. Free functioning gracilis muscle transfer versus intercostal nerve transfer to musculocutaneous nerve for restoration of elbow flexion after traumatic adult brachial pan-plexus injury. *Plast Reconstr Surg*. 2016;138(3):483e–488e.
22. Chammas M, Goubier JN, Coulet B, Reckendorf GM, Picot MC, Allieu Y. Glenohumeral arthrodesis in upper and total brachial plexus palsy. A comparison of functional results. *J Bone Joint Surg Br*. 2004;86(5):692–695.
23. Atlan F, Durand S, Fox M, Levy P, Belkheyar Z, Oberlin C. Functional outcome of glenohumeral fusion in brachial plexus palsy: a report of 54 cases. *J Hand Surg Am*. 2012;37(4):683–688.
24. Sandberg AA, Stone JF. *The genetics and molecular biology of neural tumors*. 1st ed. New York, NY: Humana Press; 2008.
25. Baehring JM, Betensky RA, Batchelor TT. Malignant peripheral nerve sheath tumor: the clinical spectrum and outcome of treatment. *Neurology*. 2003;61(5):696–698.
26. Ducatman BS, Scheithauer BW. Postirradiation neurofibrosarcoma. *Cancer*. 1983;51(6):1028–1033.
27. Ducatman BS, Scheithauer BW, Piepgras DG, Reiman HM, Ilstrup DM. Malignant peripheral nerve sheath tumors. A clinicopathologic study of 120 cases. *Cancer*. 1986;57(10):2006–2021.
28. Fuchs B, Spinner RJ, Rock MG. Malignant peripheral nerve sheath tumors: an update. *J Surg Orthop Adv*. 2005;14(4):168–174.
29. James AW, Shurell E, Singh A, Dry SM, Eilber FC. Malignant peripheral nerve sheath tumor. *Surg Oncol Clin N Am*. 2016;25(4):789–802.
30. McGaughran JM, Harris DI, Donnai D, et al. A clinical study of type 1 neurofibromatosis in northwest England. *J Med Genet*. 1999; 36(3):197–203.
31. Tonsgard JH. Clinical manifestations and management of neurofibromatosis type 1. *Semin Pediatr Neurol*. 2006;13(1):2–7.
32. Evans DG, Huson SM, Donnai D, et al. A genetic study of type 2 neurofibromatosis in the United Kingdom. I. Prevalence, mutation rate, fitness, and confirmation of maternal transmission effect on severity. *J Med Genet*. 1992;29(12):841–846.
33. Gutmann DH, Aylsworth A, Carey JC, et al. The diagnostic evaluation and multidisciplinary management of neurofibromatosis 1 and neurofibromatosis 2. *JAMA*. 1997;278(1):51–57.
34. Plotkin SR, Blakeley JO, Evans DG, et al. Update from the 2011 International Schwannomatosis Workshop: from genetics to diagnostic criteria. *Am J Med Genet A*. 2013;161A(3):405–416.
35. Antinheimo J, Sankila R, Carpen O, Pukkala E, Sainio M, Jaaskelainen J. Population-based analysis of sporadic and type 2 neurofibromatosis-associated meningiomas and schwannomas. *Neurology*. 2000;54(1):71–76.
36. MacCollin M, Chiocca EA, Evans DG, et al. Diagnostic criteria for schwannomatosis. *Neurology*. 2005;64(11):1838–1845.
37. Donner TR, Voorhies RM, Kline DG. Neural sheath tumors of major nerves. *J Neurosurg*. 1994;81(3):362–373.
38. Wasa J, Nishida Y, Tsukushi S, et al. MRI features in the differentiation of malignant peripheral nerve sheath tumors and neurofibromas. *AJR Am J Roentgenol*. 2010;194(6):1568–1574.
39. Salamon J, Papp L, Toth Z, et al. Nerve sheath tumors in neurofibromatosis type 1: assessment of whole-body metabolic tumor burden using F-18-FDG PET/CT. *PLoS ONE*. 2015;10(12):e0143305.
40. Benz MR, Czernin J, Dry SM, et al. Quantitative F18-fluorodeoxyglucose positron emission tomography accurately characterizes peripheral nerve sheath tumors as malignant or benign. *Cancer*. 2010;116(2):451–458.
41. Brahmi M, Thiesse P, Ranchere D, et al. Diagnostic accuracy of pet/ct-guided percutaneous biopsies for malignant peripheral nerve sheath tumors in neurofibromatosis type 1 patients. *PLoS ONE*. 2015; 10(10):e0138386.
42. Combemale P, Valeyrie-Allanore L, Giammarile F, et al. Utility of 18F-FDG PET with a semi-quantitative index in the detection of sarcomatous transformation in patients with neurofibromatosis type 1. *PLoS ONE*. 2014;9(2):e85954.
43. Anghileri M, Miceli R, Fiore M, et al. Malignant peripheral nerve sheath tumors: prognostic factors and survival in a series of patients treated at a single institution. *Cancer*. 2006;107(5):1065–1074.
44. Ferner RE, Gutmann DH. International consensus statement on malignant peripheral nerve sheath tumors in neurofibromatosis. *Cancer Res*. 2002;62(5):1573–1577.

Index

Page numbers followed by "*f*" indicate figures, "*t*" indicate tables, and "*b*" indicate boxes.

B

C

D